MASTERY OF SURGERY

Mastery of Plastic and Reconstructive Surgery

Volume I

Edited by

Mimis Cohen, M.D.

Professor, Departments of Surgery and Pediatrics, University of Illinois
College of Medicine; Chief, Divisions of Plastic Surgery, University of
Illinois Hospital and Cook County Hospital, Chicago

Foreword by

Robert M. Goldwyn, M.D.

Clinical Professor of Surgery, Harvard Medical School;
Head, Division of Plastic Surgery, Beth Israel Hospital, Boston

In conjunction with

Catherine Judge Allen, M.A.
Publications Editor, University of Illinois College of Medicine, Chicago

Little, Brown and Company
Boston/New York/Toronto/London

Library of Congress Cataloging-in-Publication Data

Mastery of plastic and reconstructive surgery / edited by Mimis Cohen.
    p.   cm.
  Includes bibliographical references and index.
  ISBN 0-316-15003-7
  1. Surgery, Plastic. I. Cohen, Mimis.
  [DNLM: 1. Surgery, Plastic—methods.   WO 600 M423 1994]
RD118.M386 1994
617.9'5—dc20
DNLM/DLC
for Library of Congress   93-33838
                                                    CIP

Volume I ISBN: 0-316-14998-5

Printed in the United States of America
MV-NY

Editorial: Nancy E. Chorpenning, Robert Stuart
Production Editor: Kellie Cardone
Copyeditors: Catherine Judge Allen, Sylvia Hines
Indexer: Alexandra Nickerson
Production Supervisor: Cate Rickard
Cover Designer: Cate Rickard

To my father and first teacher of the art and craft of surgery
Dr. Nissim Cohen

To my mother
Nina Cohen

To my wife
Andrea Biel-Cohen

And to my daughter
Saranna

Contents

Foreword by Robert M. Goldwyn   xvii
Series Introduction by Lloyd M. Nyhus and Robert J. Baker   xix
Preface   xxi
Contributing Authors   xxiii

Volume I

I. GENERAL PRINCIPLES AND TECHNIQUES

1. Wound Healing   3
    Beatriz H. Porras-Reyes and Thomas A. Mustoe

2. Basic Principles and Techniques in Plastic Surgery   14
    Norman Weinzweig and Jeffrey Weinzweig

3. Scar Revision   34
    Maher Anous, David T. Netscher, and Samuel Stal

Tissue Transfer
4. Skin Grafts   45
    Henry C. Vasconez

5. Flaps: Physiology, Principles of Design, and Pitfalls   56
    B. George H. Lamberty and Ciaran Healy

6. Skin Flaps, Fasciocutaneous Flaps, and Musculocutaneous Flaps   71
    Luis O. Vasconez, Mabel Gamboa-Bobadilla, and Michael P. Bentley

7. Tissue Transfer: Fat, Dermal, Muscle, Cartilage, and Fascial Grafts   88
    W. Thomas Lawrence and Mark S. Potenza

8. The Omentum in Reconstructive Surgery   95
    Michael A. Marschall, Elias G. Gikas, and Mimis Cohen

9. Bone Grafts   102
    John W. Polley

10. Bone Substitutes   113
Harvey M. Rosen

11. Flexor Tendon Grafting   120
Hani S. Matloub, Christopher D. Prevel, N. John Yousif, and James R. Sanger

12. Nerve Grafting   127
Warren C. Breidenbach and Waqar Aziz

Special Techniques

13. Principles of Craniomaxillofacial Surgery   135
Ian T. Jackson

14. Principles of Rigid Bony Fixation of the Craniofacial Skeleton   169
Hans-G. Luhr

15. Reconstruction Using Soft Tissue Expansion   201
Ernest K. Manders

16. Blunt Suction-Assisted Lipectomy   216
Gregory P. Hetter

17. Lasers in Plastic Surgery   252
Lovic W. Hobby

18. Three-Dimensional Imaging: An Adjunct to Craniomaxillofacial Reconstruction   271
Bryant A. Toth and Bryan G. Forley

II. SKIN AND ADNEXA

19. Benign Skin Tumors   295
Brian Cook, Susan D. Gass, Michael D. Lichter, Stephanie F. Marschall, and Lawrence M. Solomon

20. Premalignant Skin Tumors, Basal Cell Carcinoma, and Squamous Cell Carcinoma   309
David T. Netscher, Maher Anous, and Melvin Spira

21. Principles of Mohs Micrographic Surgery   333
June K. Robinson

22. Malignant Melanoma   341
Steven D. Macht and Joseph G. DeSantis

23. Vascular Malformations   352
Hugh G. Thomson and Patricia E. Burrows

24. Lymphedema   374
Bernard McC. O'Brien and P. A. Vinod Kumar

25. Hidradenitis Suppurativa   384
Norman Weinzweig

26. Thermal Burns: Resuscitation and Initial Management   396
John O. Kucan

27. Burn Wounds: Excision and Grafting   407
Jeremy J. Burdge and Robert L. Ruberg

28. Reconstruction of Burn Deformities of the Head and Neck   416
Bruce M. Achauer

29. Reconstruction of Burn Deformities of the Extremities and Trunk   429
Warren L. Garner and David J. Smith, Jr.

30. Electrical and Chemical Injuries   441
     Martin C. Robson and Peter G. Hayward

31. Radiation Injuries   452
     Ross Rudolph

III. HEAD AND NECK

Congenital Anomalies

32. Craniofacial Embryology   459
     Robert M. Greene and Wayde M. Weston

33. The Cleft Palate–Craniofacial Team   471
     Howard Aduss

34. The Clinical Use of Cephalometrics   475
     R. Bruce Ross

35. The Classification and Management of Facial Clefts   486
     J. C. van der Meulen

36. Craniosynostosis and Craniofacial Dysostosis   499
     Daniel Marchac and Dominique Renier

37. Frontoethmoidal Meningoencephalocele   516
     David J. David and Richard H. C. Harries

38. Mandibulofacial Dysostosis   527
     H. F. Sailer, Klaus W. Grätz, and Michael C. Locher

39. Hemifacial Microsomia   536
     Douglas K. Ousterhout and Karin Vargervik

40. Unilateral Cleft Lip   548
     Janusz Bardach

41. Bilateral Cleft Lip   566
     M. Samuel Noordhoff

42. Primary Correction of the Nasal Deformity Associated with Cleft
     Lip   581
     Kenneth E. Salyer

43. Cleft Palate   595
     Don LaRossa

44. Secondary Soft Tissue Procedures for Cleft Lip and Palate   605
     Michael B. Lewis

45. Velopharyngeal Insufficiency   619
     Bonnie E. Smith and Thomas W. Guyette

46. Pharyngeal Flaps for the Correction of Velopharyngeal
     Insufficiency   632
     William C. Trier

47. Sphincter Pharyngoplasty   643
     Roger C. Mixter and Stanley J. Ewanowski

48. Orthodontic Management for Patients with Cleft Lip and Palate   648
     Alvaro A. Figueroa and Howard Aduss

49. Secondary Bone Grafting of Residual Alveolar Clefts   669
     Mimis Cohen

50. The Correction of Secondary Skeletal Deformities in Adolescent Patients
     with Cleft Lip and Palate   682
     Jeffrey C. Posnick

51. Secondary Correction of the Nasal Deformity Associated with Cleft Lip   702
Mimis Cohen

52. Maxillary Deformities: Orthognathic Surgery   720
James A. Lehman, Jr.

53. Mandibular Deformities: Orthognathic Surgery   742
H. P. M. Freihofer

54. Prosthetic Management for Patients with Cleft Lip and Palate   759
David J. Reisberg

55. Congenital Deformities of the External Ear   776
Kunihiro Kurihara

56. Congenital Ptosis of the Eyelid   800
Allen M. Putterman

57. Congenital Masses and Sinuses of the Head and Neck   809
Diane V. Dado

58. Facial Reanimation: Cross-Face Nerve Grafting and Muscle Transplantation   822
Ronald M. Zuker

Index [1]

Volume II

Tumors

59. Reconstruction of Defects of the Scalp and Skull   830
Kenneth C. Shestak and Sai S. Ramasastry

60. Principles of Facial Reconstruction   842
Frederick J. Menick

61. Reconstruction of the Eyelids   864
Glenn W. Jelks and Elizabeth B. Jelks

62. Reconstruction of the Nose   883
Frederick J. Menick and Gary C. Burget

63. Reconstruction of the Lips   906
Miroslaw F. Stranc

64. Carcinoma of the Oropharynx   921
Henry C. Vasconez and Edward A. Luce

65. Principles of Composite Resection and Neck Dissection for Carcinoma of the Oropharynx   931
David L. Larson

66. Principles of Chemotherapy for Oropharyngeal Cancer   939
Kirk Heyne and Waun Ki Hong

67. Principles of Radiation Therapy for Oropharyngeal Cancer   945
Nora A. Janjan

68. Oral and Pharyngeal Reconstruction with Transposition Flaps   956
Stephen J. Mathes and Joseph L. Kiener

69. Oral and Pharyngeal Reconstruction with Free Tissue Transfer   966
Michael J. Miller and William M. Swartz

70. Reconstruction of the Mandible and the Floor of the Mouth   982
James R. Sanger, N. John Yousif, and Hani S. Matloub

71. Carcinoma of the Base of the Skull: Paranasal Sinuses and Orbits   1000
Ivo P. Janecka

72. Cancer of the Larynx   1008
William W. Dzwierzynski and Riley S. Rees

73. Prosthetic Rehabilitation After Operations for Cancer of the Head and Neck   1018
David J. Reisberg

74. Tumors of the Salivary Glands   1034
Mark S. Granick and Mark P. Solomon

75. Facial Reanimation   1045
Alfonso Oliva, Harry J. Buncke, Gregory M. Buncke, and William C. Lineaweaver

Maxillofacial Trauma

76. The Initial Management of Patients with Facial Trauma   1060
Craig D. Hall, Sidney B. Eisig, and Charles D. Hanf

77. Radiologic Evaluation of Maxillofacial Trauma   1069
Bradley G. Langer and D. G. Spigos

78. Primary Repair and Secondary Reconstruction of Facial Soft Tissue Injuries   1083
Rod J. Rohrich and Denton Watumull

79. Correction of Traumatic Ptosis of the Eyelid and Reconstruction of the Lacrimal System   1101
Frank A. Nesi, John D. Siddens, and Kevin L. Waltz

80. Fractures of the Frontal Sinus   1109
M. Haskell Newman

81. Fractures of the Zygoma   1119
Walter G. Sullivan and Richard J. L. Phillips

82. Fractures of the Nose   1126
Rudolph F. Dolezal

83. Fractures of the Orbit and Nasoethmoidal Bones   1136
Paul N. Manson and Bernard L. Markowitz

84. Fractures of the Maxilla   1156
Michael J. Yaremchuk

85. Fractures of the Mandible   1165
Karsten K. H. Gundlach

86. Complex Facial Fractures: Gunshot Wounds to the Face   1181
J. S. Gruss

87. Facial Fractures in Children and Adolescents   1188
Richard C. Schultz

88. Secondary Reconstruction of Soft Tissue Deformity Associated with Orbital Trauma   1199
S. Anthony Wolfe

89. Traumatic Deformities and Reconstruction of the Temporomandibular Joint   1220
David Mendes and Jonathan S. Jacobs

IV. THE TRUNK

90. Congenital Anomalies of the Chest Wall   1233
Alan E. Seyfer

91. Meningomyelocele   1240
Dennis E. McDonnell and Alan E. Seyfer

92. Reconstruction of the Chest Wall   1248
Mimis Cohen

93. Intrathoracic Transposition of Soft Tissue   1268
N. Bradly Meland and Phillip G. Arnold

94. Prophylactic Subcutaneous Mastectomy and Reconstruction   1276
John R. Jarrett

95. Immediate Reconstruction of the Breast After Mastectomy   1283
R. Barrett Noone

96. Immediate and Delayed Breast Reconstruction with Tissue Expanders   1295
Jack Fisher and Dennis C. Hammond

97. Delayed Breast Reconstruction with Autogenous Tissue   1309
G. Patrick Maxwell, John W. Polley, and Gustavo E. Galante

98. Breast Reconstruction with Free Tissue Transfer   1324
James C. Grotting

99. Nipple-Areolar Reconstruction   1342
John W. Little

100. Reconstruction of the Abdominal Wall and Groin   1349
Dennis J. Hurwitz and Ronald R. Hollins

101. Reconstruction of Hip and Pelvic Defects   1360
N. Bradly Meland

102. Pressure Sores   1371
Michael A. Marschall and Mimis Cohen

103. Developmental Anomalies of the Male and Female Genitalia   1387
Charles E. Horton, Charles E. Horton, Jr., and John A. Dean

104. Reconstruction and Construction of the Penis   1400
Lawrence J. Gottlieb and Laurence A. Levine

Index [1]

Volume III

V. THE UPPER EXTREMITY

105. Hand-Skin Incisions   1415
James Thomas Nolan, Jerry E. Nye, and Mark Nissenbaum

106. Congenital Anomalies of the Hand   1424
Joseph Upton and Charles Hergrueter

107. Tumors of the Hand   1454
J. L. Posch

108. Hand Infections   1467
William C. Lineaweaver

109. Initial Evaluation and Management of Hand Injuries   1480
James D. Schlenker and Christ P. Koulis

110. Fingernail and Fingertip Injuries   1493
Carl N. Williams, Jr. and Robert R. Schenck

111. Hand and Wrist Fractures   1508
Alan E. Freeland and Michael E. Jabaley

112. Injuries to the Joints and Ligaments of the Upper Extremity   1531
Richard E. Brown and Robert L. Walton

113. Acute Flexor Tendon Injuries   1550
John S. Taras and James M. Hunter

114. Late Flexor Tendon Reconstruction and Tendon Grafting   1557
James W. Strickland

115. Extensor Tendon Injuries   1572
Elvin G. Zook and Richard E. Brown

116. Tendon Transfers   1579
Neil Ford Jones

117. Nerve Injuries: Primary Repair and Reconstruction   1598
Susan E. Mackinnon

118. Amputations: Revascularization and Replantation   1625
Robert C. Russell, Beth Bergman, and Brent Graham

119. Soft Tissue Coverage of the Hand and Upper Extremity   1645
Benjamin E. Cohen and Gary S. Branfman

120. Salvage of a Mutilated Hand   1658
Luis R. Scheker

121. Thumb Reconstruction and Pollicization by Conventional Techniques   1682
Vincent R. Hentz

122. Toe-to-Hand Transplantation   1699
Gregory M. Buncke, Harry J. Buncke, Alfonso Oliva, and William C. Lineaweaver

123. Rheumatoid Disease of the Hand and Wrist   1710
Robert Lee Wilson and Hugh Allen Frederick

124. Dupuytren Contracture   1720
Lynn D. Ketchum

125. Wrist Pain   1728
V. Leroy Young and Jeffrey P. Groner

126. Rehabilitation of Hand Injuries   1745
Shirley W. Chan, Joanne M. Jaglowski, and Rhonda Kaplan

VI. THE LOWER EXTREMITY

127. Lower Extremity Trauma: Principles of Evaluation and Early Management   1767
Dennis Mess

128. Lower Extremity Reconstruction: Management of Soft Tissue Defects   1773
Foad Nahai and Tim R. Love

129. Lower Extremity Reconstruction: Management of Bony Defects   1800
Clayton R. Perry

130.   Chronic Osteomyelitis   1809
       Thomas R. Stevenson

131.   Reconstruction and Rehabilitation of the Mutilated Foot   1820
       Hans U. Steinau, R. Büttemeyer, and B. Claudi

132.   Leg Ulcers   1828
       Stan J. Monstrey, Sai S. Ramasastry, Prakash C. Mullick, and Kenneth C.
       Shestak

133.   The Diabetic Foot   1839
       Lawrence B. Colen

VII. AESTHETIC SURGERY

134.   Contouring of the Facial Skeleton   1863
       Linton A. Whitaker

135.   Facial Rejuvenation: Facelift   1873
       Bruce F. Connell and Timothy J. Marten

136.   Facial Rejuvenation in Men   1903
       John Q. Owsley and Bernard S. Alpert

137.   Facial Rejuvenation: Subperiosteal Facelift   1910
       Oscar M. Ramirez

138.   Blepharoplasty   1920
       Stanley A. Klatsky

139.   Transconjunctival Blepharoplasty   1941
       Bruno Ristow

140.   Forehead-Lifts   1948
       Bruno Ristow

141.   Brow-Lift   1958
       Stanley A. Klatsky

142.   Oculoplastic Surgery   1968
       Michael Paul Vincent

143.   Ancillary Procedures for Facial Rejuvenation   1979
       Jack A. Friedland and Daniel C. Mills II

144.   Perioral Rejuvenation   1990
       Harvey W. Austin

145.   Primary Rhinoplasty: Basic Techniques   1999
       Mark B. Constantian

146.   Correction of Difficult Nasal Deformities   2021
       Peter McKinney and William J. Koenig

147.   Secondary Rhinoplasty   2033
       Rodolphe Meyer

148.   Aesthetic Facial Surgery in African-Americans   2050
       W. Earle Matory, Jr.

149.   Aesthetic Facial Surgery in Orientals   2059
       Khoo Boo-Chai

150.   Hair Restoration in Male Pattern Baldness   2088
       Paul S. Howard

151. Augmentation Mammaplasty   2099
Scott L. Spear and Konrad L. Dawson

152. Inferior Pedicle Breast Reduction   2114
Robert W. Bernard and Daniel C. Morello

153. The Parenchymal Pedicle Technique for Reduction
Mammaplasty   2126
Robert L. Walton and Federico Gonzalez

154. Reduction of Large Breasts by a Combination of Liposuction and
Vertical Mammaplasty   2143
Madeleine Lejour

155. Correction of Breast Ptosis by Vertical Mammaplasty   2157
Madeleine Lejour

156. Abdominal Contour Operations   2165
Alan Matarasso

157. Body Contouring with Suction-Assisted Lipectomy   2186
Bahman Teimourian and Saeed Marefat

158. Body Contouring: Trunk- and Thigh-Lifts   2201
Ted E. Lockwood

159. Brachioplasty and Brachial Suction-Assisted Lipoplasty   2219
Peter A. Vogt and Ricardo Baroudi

160. Aesthetic Procedures for the Lower Extremity   2237
Adrien Aiache

Index [1]

Foreword

When Mimis Cohen discussed this herculean undertaking with me, I was skeptical about its necessity and value. Unlike a generation ago, today our specialty does not lack literary documentation. In addition to plastic surgery journals—and there are more than a dozen worldwide—hundreds of books on a seemingly infinite variety of subjects are available. Annually and unremittingly books appear, many on the same topic. My skepticism continued until I saw the copyedited version. In fact, I was reluctant to write a foreword until the product was in hand so that I could be certain that this three-volume set was worthwhile and needed. It is. Why? Because it gives the reader useful information from those of acknowledged experience on the highways and byways of plastic surgery. The authors have honored their instructions to avoid the usual and often tedious textbook approach to a specific condition, its history, diagnosis,

and treatment. Rather they have described succinctly and clearly their analysis of a problem and their treatment. The illustrations reinforce the text, enabling the reader to get what he or she wants without having to meander through a maze. This book is mercifully free of rococco. Yet, the pages do not read like telegrams strung together. It is not only readable but it is memorable—in the sense that it fosters retention. To write something that is read and to read something that is remembered satisfy the objectives of both author and reader.

One can go through this book, volume by volume, without a specific order, just to pick up a new fact, good advice, or a different perspective. As is more likely to happen, however, this book will be an instant resource for the hard-pressed surgeon planning a pending procedure or puzzling over a patient seen that day.

It would be sensible for me to stop at this point, having praised, and honestly so, what Dr. Cohen has put together. Yet I cannot resist adding a thought that perhaps as a guest in somebody else's book, I should keep to myself. And that concerns the title. Perhaps it is my cynicism or my dissatisfaction with my own results or my "I'm from Missouri" attitude about the results of others, but I wish that this book had added to its title *"Toward" Mastery of Plastic and Reconstructive Surgery*. Who among us has really mastered any condition or procedure, except perhaps the drainage of an abscess? Furthermore, the perfect execution of an operation is not always synonymous with the optimal treatment of the illness (e.g., radical mastectomy for breast cancer). This philosophic quibbling aside, this *is* a project worth the effort, and its culmination—this impressive book—does credit to its editor, its authors, and its publisher.

Robert M. Goldwyn, M.D.

Series Introduction

We are genuinely pleased that *Mastery of Plastic and Reconstructive Surgery* is part of the Mastery of Surgery series. Although we knew when this project was initiated that Dr. Cohen would expend much effort to produce an excellent text–atlas, he and his colleagues have far exceeded our expectations.

This three-volume opus is exhaustive in scope, and the information is of the highest quality. Leaders in plastic and reconstructive surgery and allied disciplines have generously shared their talents and skills through their contributions. Twelve nations are represented in the list of contributors, lending an international scope to the work.

We congratulate Mimis Cohen for a monumental task well done. He is responsible for the overall quality of the final product, and Little, Brown and Company is responsible for excellent editorial supervision and another quality production.

Lloyd M. Nyhus, M.D.
Robert J. Baker, M.D.

Preface

When invited to edit these volumes of *Mastery of Plastic and Reconstructive Surgery,* I accepted the challenge without reservation, even though several surgical textbooks available covered the entire scope of the field of plastic surgery. I was familiar with *Mastery of Surgery,* first published in 1984 and revised in 1992, and was well aware of the unique format that made the book so successful. As mentioned in the preface to the first edition, "it was decided to take the format of this work beyond that of an atlas that would simply show the steps in an operation. Instead, the format is directed toward showing the reader how to improve performance of the procedures described by emphasizing the refinements of technique developed by the respective authors and which they, through personal experience, have found to work well."

Mastery of Plastic and Reconstructive Surgery was designed with the same philosophy in an effort to assist the reader in mastering the various techniques and procedures of the specialty. Although each chapter includes some historical information, the emphasis is placed on the surgical anatomy of an area and on each author's specific approach to the evaluation and management of a particular problem. The authors were asked to focus on describing their preferred surgical techniques in detail. They were also asked to emphasize ways to improve surgical results and ways to prevent and manage complications. I encouraged them to include as many drawings or photographs as necessary to illustrate their points. Because of this personal approach, several well-accepted techniques are only briefly described.

The authors were selected from among the world's authorities. They are well known for their many publications and contributions to the field as well as for their teaching credentials. I thank them for the time and effort they contributed to this project.

I express my deep appreciation to Ms. Catherine Judge Allen for her painstaking review of all the chapters. Her contribution to the final organization and continuity of the text is invaluable. My secretaries, Christine Saliga-Sullivan and Amy Onstott, worked hard typing and retyping manuscripts and spent many hours on the telephone communicating with the authors and their secretaries.

The team at Little, Brown—Nancy Chorpenning, Rob Stuart, and Kellie Cardone—also outdid themselves in encouraging me and helping me with every detail.

I hope that the readers will, as Drs. Nyhus and Baker hoped in their preface to the first edition of *Mastery of Surgery,* derive as much pleasure and benefit from reading this book as I did from compiling and editing it.

M. C.

Contributing Authors

Bruce M. Achauer, M.D.

Associate Adjunct Professor of Surgery, University of California, Irvine, College of Medicine, Irvine; Chief of Plastic Surgery, Children's Hospital of Orange County, Orange, California
Chapter 28. *Reconstruction of Burn Deformities of the Head and Neck*

Howard Aduss, D.D.S.

Professor of Orthodontics, Department of Pediatrics, Craniofacial Center, University of Illinois College of Medicine, Chicago
Chapter 33. *The Cleft Palate–Craniofacial Team*
Chapter 48. *Orthodontic Management for Patients with Cleft Lip and Palate*

Adrien Aiache, M.D.

Attending Physician, Department of Surgery, Beverly Hills Medical Center, Los Angeles
Chapter 160. *Aesthetic Procedures for the Lower Extremity*

Bernard S. Alpert, M.D.

Associate Clinical Professor, Division of Plastic and Reconstructive Surgery, University of California, San Francisco, School of Medicine; Chief, Department of Plastic Surgery, Davies Medical Center, San Francisco
Chapter 136. *Facial Rejuvenation in Men*

Maher Anous, M.D.

Assistant Professor, Division of Plastic Surgery, Baylor College of Medicine; Attending Physician, The Methodist Hospital, Houston
Chapter 3. *Scar Revision*
Chapter 20. *Premalignant Skin Tumors, Basal Cell Carcinoma, and Squamous Cell Carcinoma*

Phillip G. Arnold, M.D.

Professor and Chairman, Division of Plastic Surgery, Mayo Medical School; Plastic Surgery Consultant, Mayo Clinic, Rochester, Minnesota
Chapter 93. *Intrathoracic Transposition of Soft Tissue*

Harvey W. Austin, M.D.

Attending Surgeon, Reston Hospital Center, Reston, Virginia
Chapter 144. *Perioral Rejuvenation*

Waqar Aziz, M.D.

Senior Fellow, Christine M. Kleinert Institute, Louisville, Kentucky
Chapter 12.   Nerve Grafting

Janusz Bardach, M.D.

Professor Emeritus of Plastic Surgery, University of Iowa College of Medicine, Iowa City, Iowa
Chapter 40.   Unilateral Cleft Lip

Ricardo Baroudi, M.D.

Attending Plastic Surgeon, Hospital Samaritano, Campinas City, Brazil
Chapter 159.   Brachioplasty and Brachial Suction-Assisted Lipoplasty

Michael P. Bentley, M.D.

Staff Plastic Surgeon, Jackson Hospital, Montgomery, Alabama
Chapter 6.   Skin Flaps, Fasciocutaneous Flaps, and Musculocutaneous Flaps

Beth Bergman, M.D.

Former Microsurgery Research Fellow, Division of Plastic Surgery, Southern Illinois University School of Medicine, Springfield, Illinois
Chapter 118.   Amputations: Revascularization and Replantation

Robert W. Bernard, M.D.

Chief, Emeritus, Department of Plastic Surgery, White Plains Hospital; Chief, Department of Plastic Surgery, United Hospital, Port Chester, New York
Chapter 152.   Inferior Pedicle Breast Reduction

Khoo Boo-Chai, M.D.

Professor, Department of Plastic Surgery, Third Teaching Hospital, Beijing Medical University, Beijing
Chapter 149.   Aesthetic Facial Surgery in Orientals

Gary S. Branfman, M.D.

Director, Victoria Plastic Surgery Center, Victoria, Texas
Chapter 119.   Soft Tissue Coverage of the Hand and Upper Extremity

Warren C. Breidenbach, M.D.

Clinical Assistant Professor, Division of Plastic and Reconstructive Surgery, University of Louisville School of Medicine; Staff Physician, Louisville Hand Surgery, Louisville, Kentucky
Chapter 12.   Nerve Grafting

Richard E. Brown, M.D.

Assistant Professor, Department of Surgery, Southern Illinois University School of Medicine, Springfield, Illinois
Chapter 112.   Injuries to the Joints and Ligaments of the Upper Extremity
Chapter 115.   Extensor Tendon Injuries

Gregory M. Buncke, M.D.

Assistant Clinical Professor, Department of Surgery, University of California, San Francisco, School of Medicine, San Francisco; Attending Surgeon, Microsurgical Replantation Transplantation Department, University of California, Davis, Medical Center, Sacramento, California
Chapter 75.   Facial Reanimation
Chapter 122.   Toe-to-Hand Transplantation

Harry J. Buncke, M.D.

Clinical Professor, Department of Surgery, University of California, San Francisco, School of Medicine, San Francisco; Director, Microsurgical Replantation Transplantation Department, University of California, Davis, Medical Center, Sacramento, California
Chapter 75.   Facial Reanimation
Chapter 122.   Toe-to-Hand Transplantation

Jeremy J. Burdge, M.D.

Clinical Assistant Professor, Division of Plastic Surgery, Ohio State University College of Medicine, Columbus, Ohio
Chapter 27.   Burn Wounds: Excision and Grafting

Gary C. Burget, M.D.

Clinical Assistant Professor, Division of Plastic and Reconstructive Surgery, University of Chicago Pritzker School of Medicine, Chicago
Chapter 62.   Reconstruction of the Nose

Patricia E. Burrows, M.D.

Associate Professor of Radiology, University of Toronto Faculty of Medicine; Staff Radiologist, Department of Diagnostic Imaging, Hospital for Sick Children, Toronto
Chapter 23. Vascular Malformations

R. Büttemeyer, M.D.

Professor, Department of Plastic Surgery and Burn Unit, University Hospital, Bochum, Germany
Chapter 131. Reconstruction and Rehabilitation of the Mutilated Foot

Shirley W. Chan, O.T.R., C.V.E., C.H.T.

Hand Therapy Supervisor, Occupational Therapy Department, Davies Medical Center, San Francisco
Chapter 126. Rehabilitation of Hand Injuries

B. Claudi, M.D.

Professor and Chief, Trauma Service, Technical University and R. D. Tsar Hospital, München, Germany
Chapter 131. Reconstruction and Rehabilitation of the Mutilated Foot

Benjamin E. Cohen, M.D.

Academic Chief and Director, Plastic Surgery Residency Program, and Director, Microsurgical Research and Training Laboratory, St. Joseph's Hospital, Houston
Chapter 119. Soft Tissue Coverage of the Hand and Upper Extremity

Mimis Cohen, M.D.

Professor, Departments of Surgery and Pediatrics, University of Illinois College of Medicine; Chief, Divisions of Plastic Surgery, University of Illinois Hospital and Cook County Hospital, Chicago
Chapter 8. The Omentum in Reconstructive Surgery
Chapter 49. Secondary Bone Grafting of Residual Alveolar Clefts
Chapter 51. Secondary Correction of the Nasal Deformity Associated with Cleft Lip
Chapter 92. Reconstruction of the Chest Wall
Chapter 102. Pressure Sores

Lawrence B. Colen, M.D.

Associate Professor, Department of Plastic and Reconstructive Surgery, Eastern Virginia Medical School of the Medical College of Hampton Roads, Norfolk, Virginia
Chapter 133. The Diabetic Foot

Bruce F. Connell, M.D.

Clinical Professor of Plastic Surgery, University of California, Irvine, College of Medicine, Irvine, California
Chapter 135. Facial Rejuvenation: Facelift

Mark B. Constantian, M.D.

Clinical Instructor in Surgery, Harvard Medical School, Boston; Active Staff, Department of Plastic Surgery, Nashua Memorial Hospital, Nashua, New Hampshire
Chapter 145. Primary Rhinoplasty: Basic Techniques

Brian Cook, M.D.

Assistant Professor, Department of Dermatology, University of Illinois College of Medicine; Director of Mohs and Dermatologic Surgery, University of Illinois Hospital, Chicago
Chapter 19. Benign Skin Tumors

Diane V. Dado, M.D.

Associate Professor, Departments of Surgery and Pediatrics, Loyola University of Chicago Stritch School of Medicine; Attending Physician, Department of Surgery, Foster G. McGaw Hospital of Loyola University, Maywood, Illinois
Chapter 57. Congenital Masses and Sinuses of the Head and Neck

David J. David, A.C., M.B., F.R.C.S., F.R.A.C.S.

Head, Australian Craniofacial Unit, Adelaide Medical Centre for Women and Children, North Adelaide, South Australia
Chapter 37. Frontoethmoidal Meningoencephalocele

Konrad L. Dawson, M.D.

Instructor, Division of Plastic Surgery, Georgetown University Medical Center, Washington
Chapter 151. Augmentation Mammaplasty

John A. Dean, M.D.	Chief Resident, Department of Plastic Surgery, Eastern Virginia Medical School of the Medical College of Hampton Roads, Norfolk, Virginia *Chapter 103. Developmental Anomalies of the Male and Female Genitalia*
Joseph G. DeSantis, M.D.	Assistant Clinical Professor, Division of Plastic and Reconstructive Surgery, George Washington University School of Medicine and Health Sciences, Washington *Chapter 22. Malignant Melanoma*
Rudolph F. Dolezal, M.D.	Clinical Associate Professor, Department of Surgery, University of Illinois College of Medicine, Chicago; Attending Physician, University of Illinois Hospital and Lutheran General Hospital, Park Ridge, Illinois *Chapter 82. Fractures of the Nose*
William W. Dzwierzynski, M.D.	Assistant Professor, Department of Surgery, Medical College of Wisconsin; Attending Surgeon, MCW Clinic Froedtert Memorial Lutheran Hospital, Milwaukee *Chapter 72. Cancer of the Larynx*
Sidney B. Eisig, D.D.S.	Assistant Professor, Department of Dentistry/Oral and Maxillofacial Surgery, Albert Einstein College of Medicine of Yeshiva University, and Montefiore Medical Center, Bronx, New York *Chapter 76. The Initial Management of Patients with Facial Trauma*
Stanley J. Ewanowski, Ph.D.	Emeritus Professor, Department of Rehabilitation Medicine and Communicative Disorders, University of Wisconsin Medical School, Madison, Wisconsin *Chapter 47. Sphincter Pharyngoplasty*
Alvaro A. Figueroa, D.D.S.	Associate Professor, Departments of Surgery and Pediatrics, University of Illinois College of Medicine, and Department of Orthodontics, University of Illinois College of Dentistry; Attending, Craniofacial Center, University of Illinois College of Medicine, and Consultant, Cleft Palate Team, Cook County Hospital, Chicago *Chapter 48. Orthodontic Management for Patients with Cleft Lip and Palate*
Jack Fisher, M.D.	Assistant Clinical Professor, Division of Plastic Surgery, Vanderbilt University School of Medicine; Attending Physician, Institute of Aesthetic and Reconstructive Surgery, Mid-State Baptist Hospital, Nashville, Tennessee *Chapter 96. Immediate and Delayed Breast Reconstruction with Tissue Expanders*
Bryan G. Forley, M.D.	Attending Physician, Department of Plastic and Reconstructive Surgery, St. Francis Memorial Hospital, San Francisco *Chapter 18. Three-Dimensional Imaging: An Adjunct to Craniomaxillofacial Reconstruction*
Hugh Allen Frederick, M.D.	Hand Surgery Fellow, Good Samaritan Hospital, Phoenix *Chapter 123. Rheumatoid Disease of the Hand and Wrist*
Alan E. Freeland, M.D.	Professor, Department of Orthopedic Surgery, University of Mississippi School of Medicine; Attending Physician, Department of Orthopedic Surgery, University of Mississippi Hospital, Jackson, Mississippi *Chapter 111. Hand and Wrist Fractures*
H.P.M. Freihofer, M.D., D.M.D., Ph.D.	Chairholder and Head, Department of Oral and Maxillofacial Surgery, University Hospital, Nijmegen, The Netherlands *Chapter 53. Mandibular Deformities: Orthognathic Surgery*
Jack A. Friedland, M.D.	Chief, Plastic Surgery Service of Children's Rehabilitative Services for the State of Arizona; Attending Physician, St. Joseph's Hospital, Phoenix *Chapter 143. Ancillary Procedures for Facial Rejuvenation*
Gustavo E. Galante, M.D.	Former Fellow, Institute of Aesthetic and Reconstructive Surgery, Mid-State Baptist Hospital, Nashville, Tennessee *Chapter 97. Delayed Breast Reconstruction with Autogenous Tissue*

Mabel Gamboa-Bobadilla, M.D.	Research Assistant Professor, Division of Plastic Surgery, University of Alabama School of Medicine, Birmingham, Alabama *Chapter 6. Skin Flaps, Fasciocutaneous Flaps, and Musculocutaneous Flaps*
Warren L. Garner, M.D.	Assistant Professor, Department of Surgery, University of Michigan Medical School; Attending Physician, Department of Plastic Surgery, University of Michigan Medical Center, Ann Arbor, Michigan *Chapter 29. Reconstruction of Burn Deformities of the Extremities and Trunk*
Susan D. Gass, M.D.	Resident, University of Illinois College of Medicine; Resident, Department of Dermatology, University of Illinois Hospital, Chicago *Chapter 19. Benign Skin Tumors*
Elias G. Gikas, M.D.	Attending Surgeon, Department of Plastic Surgery, Swedish Covenant Hospital, Chicago *Chapter 8. The Omentum in Reconstructive Surgery*
Federico Gonzalez, M.D.	Associate Professor, Department of Surgery, University of Missouri—Kansas City School of Medicine; Chief of Plastic and Reconstructive Surgery and Program Director, Truman Medical Center, Kansas City, Missouri *Chapter 153. The Parenchymal Pedicle Technique for Reduction Mammaplasty*
Lawrence J. Gottlieb, M.D.	Associate Professor of Clinical Surgery, University of Chicago Pritzker School of Medicine; Co-Director of Genitourinary Reconstructive Program, Department of Surgery, University of Chicago Medical Center, Chicago *Chapter 104. Reconstruction and Construction of the Penis*
Brent Graham, M.D.	Microsurgery Research Fellow, Division of Plastic Surgery, Southern Illinois University School of Medicine, Springfield, Illinois *Chapter 118. Amputations: Revascularization and Replantation*
Mark S. Granick, M.D.	Professor, Department of Surgery, Medical College of Pennsylvania; Co-Chief, Department of Plastic Surgery, Medical College Hospitals, Philadelphia *Chapter 74. Tumors of the Salivary Glands*
Klaus W. Grätz, M.D., D.D.S.	Senior Physician, Department of Craniomaxillofacial Surgery, University of Zurich, and University Hospital, Zurich, Switzerland *Chapter 38. Mandibulofacial Dysostosis*
Robert M. Greene, Ph.D.	Professor, Department of Anatomy, Jefferson Medical College of Thomas Jefferson University, Philadelphia *Chapter 32. Craniofacial Embryology*
Jeffrey P. Groner, M.D.	Assistant Professor, Division of Plastic and Reconstructive Surgery, Washington University School of Medicine; Attending Physician, Barnes Hospital, St. Louis *Chapter 125. Wrist Pain*
James C. Grotting, M.D.	Associate Professor, Department of Surgery, University of Alabama School of Medicine; Attending Physician, Division of Plastic Surgery, University of Alabama Hospitals, Birmingham, Alabama *Chapter 98. Breast Reconstruction with Free Tissue Transfer*
J. S. Gruss, M.B., F.R.C.S. (C)	Professor, Department of Surgery, University of Washington Medical School; Attending Staff, Department of Plastic Surgery, Children's Hospital and Medical Center, Seattle *Chapter 86. Complex Facial Fractures: Gunshot Wounds to the Face*
Karsten K. H. Gundlach, M.D., D.M.D., M.S.D.	Professor and Chairman, Department of Maxillofacial Surgery, Rostock University, Rostock, Germany *Chapter 85. Fractures of the Mandible*

Thomas W. Guyette, Ph.D.

Assistant Professor, Department of Pediatrics, Craniofacial Center, University of Illinois College of Medicine, Chicago
Chapter 45. *Velopharyngeal Insufficiency*

Craig D. Hall, M.D.

Associate Professor, Department of Surgery, University of Medicine and Dentistry of New Jersey, Robert Wood Johnson Medical School, Piscataway; Craniofacial Surgeon, Hackensack Medical Center, Hackensack, New Jersey
Chapter 76. *The Initial Management of Patients with Facial Trauma*

Dennis C. Hammond, M.D.

Attending Surgeon, Department of Plastic and Reconstructive Surgery, Grand Rapids Area Medical Education Center, Grand Rapids, Michigan
Chapter 96. *Immediate and Delayed Breast Reconstruction with Tissue Expanders*

Charles D. Hanf, M.D.

Assistant Professor, Departments of Surgery and Anesthesiology, Albert Einstein College of Medicine of Yeshiva University; Assistant Attending Surgeon, Departments of Surgery and Anesthesia, Montefiore Medical Center, Bronx, New York
Chapter 76. *The Initial Management of Patients with Facial Trauma*

Richard H. C. Harries, B.M., B.S., B.Sc.

Craniofacial Registrar, Australian Craniofacial Unit, Adelaide Medical Centre for Women and Children, North Adelaide, South Australia
Chapter 37. *Frontoethmoidal Meningoencephalocele*

Peter G. Hayward, M.B.B.S., F.R.A.C.S.

Senior Research Fellow, Department of Surgery, University of Melbourne; Consultant and Plastic Surgeon, St. Vincent's Hospital, Melbourne, Australia
Chapter 30. *Electrical and Chemical Injuries*

Ciaran Healy, F.R.C.S.

Supervisor in Anatomy and Registrar, Department of Plastic Surgery, Addenbrooke's Hospital, Cambridge, England
Chapter 5. *Flaps: Physiology, Principles of Design, and Pitfalls*

Vincent R. Hentz, M.D.

Associate Professor, Department of Surgery, Stanford University School of Medicine; Chief, Division of Hand Surgery, Stanford University Hospital, Stanford, California
Chapter 121. *Thumb Reconstruction and Pollicization by Conventional Techniques*

Charles Hergrueter, M.D.

Instructor in Surgery, Harvard Medical School; Attending Physician, Brigham and Women's Hospital, Boston
Chapter 106. *Congenital Anomalies of the Hand*

Gregory P. Hetter, M.D.

Assistant Clinical Professor, Department of Surgery, University of Nevada School of Medicine, Reno; Assistant Chief, Department of Plastic Surgery, Sunrise Hospital, Las Vegas
Chapter 16. *Blunt Suction-Assisted Lipectomy*

Kirk Heyne, M.D.

Assistant Internist, University of Texas Medical School at Houston; Clinical Instructor, Head, Neck, and Thoracic Medical Oncology, The University of Texas M. D. Anderson Cancer Center, Houston
Chapter 66. *Principles of Chemotherapy for Oropharyngeal Cancer*

Lovic W. Hobby, M.D.

Chief, Plastic Surgery Service, Piedmont Hospital, Atlanta
Chapter 17. *Lasers in Plastic Surgery*

Ronald R. Hollins, D.M.D., M.D.

Assistant Professor and Chief, Division of Plastic and Reconstructive Surgery, University of Nebraska College of Medicine, Omaha, Nebraska
Chapter 100. *Reconstruction of the Abdominal Wall and Groin*

Waun Ki Hong, M.D.

Professor of Medicine and Chief, Section of Head, Neck, and Thoracic Medical Oncology, The University of Texas M. D. Anderson Cancer Center, Houston
Chapter 66. *Principles of Chemotherapy for Oropharyngeal Cancer*

Charles E. Horton, M.D.

Professor, Department of Plastic Surgery, Eastern Virginia Medical School of the Medical College of Hampton Roads, Norfolk, Virginia
Chapter 103. *Developmental Anomalies of the Male and Female Genitalia*

Charles E. Horton, Jr., M.D.

Assistant Professor, Department of Urology, Eastern Virginia Medical School of the Medical College of Hampton Roads; Attending Physician, Norfolk General Hospital, Norfolk, Virginia
Chapter 103. *Developmental Anomalies of the Male and Female Genitalia*

Paul S. Howard, M.D.

Assistant Professor, Department of Surgery, University of Alabama School of Medicine; Attending Surgeon, University of Alabama Hospitals, Birmingham, Alabama
Chapter 150. *Hair Restoration in Male Pattern Baldness*

James M. Hunter, M.D.

Distinguished Professor, Department of Orthopaedic Surgery, Jefferson Medical College of Thomas Jefferson University; Attending Staff, Thomas Jefferson University Hospital, Philadelphia
Chapter 113. *Acute Flexor Tendon Injuries*

Dennis J. Hurwitz, M.D.

Clinical Associate Professor, University of Pittsburgh School of Medicine; Attending Staff, Magee-Women's Hospital, Pittsburgh, Pennsylvania
Chapter 100. *Reconstruction of the Abdominal Wall and Groin*

Michael E. Jabaley, M.D.

Clinical Professor, Departments of Plastic and Orthopedic Surgery, University of Mississippi School of Medicine, Jackson, Mississippi
Chapter 111. *Hand and Wrist Fractures*

Ian T. Jackson, M.D.

Director, Institute of Craniofacial and Reconstructive Surgery, Chief, Department of Plastic Surgery, and Director of Training Program, Providence Hospital, Southfield, Michigan
Chapter 13. *Principles of Craniomaxillofacial Surgery*

Jonathan S. Jacobs, D.M.D., M.D.

Associate Professor, Department of Plastic Surgery, Eastern Virginia Medical School of the Medical College of Hampton Roads, Norfolk, Virginia
Chapter 89. *Traumatic Deformities and Reconstruction of the Temporomandibular Joint*

Joanne M. Jaglowski, M.A., O.T.R., C.H.T.

Senior Hand Therapist, Davies Medical Center, San Francisco
Chapter 126. *Rehabilitation of Hand Injuries*

Ivo P. Janecka, M.D.

Professor, Department of Otolaryngology and Neurological Surgery, University of Pittsburgh School of Medicine; Director, Center for Cranial Base Surgery, Pittsburgh, Pennsylvania
Chapter 71. *Carcinoma of the Base of the Skull: Paranasal Sinuses and Orbits*

Nora A. Janjan, M.D.

Associate Professor of Radiotherapy and Attending Physician, The University of Texas M. D. Anderson Cancer Center, Houston
Chapter 67. *Principles of Radiation Therapy for Oropharyngeal Cancer*

John R. Jarrett, M.D.

Attending Surgeon, Sacred Heart Medical Center, Eugene, Oregon
Chapter 94. *Prophylactic Subcutaneous Mastectomy and Reconstruction*

Elizabeth B. Jelks, M.D.

Clinical Instructor, Department of Ophthalmology, New York University School of Medicine, New York
Chapter 61. *Reconstruction of the Eyelids*

Glenn W. Jelks, M.D.

Associate Professor, Department of Surgery, New York University School of Medicine, New York
Chapter 61. *Reconstruction of the Eyelids*

Neil Ford Jones, M.D.

Professor and Chief of Hand Surgery, Division of Plastic and Reconstructive Surgery, University of California, Los Angeles, UCLA School of Medicine, Los Angeles
Chapter 116. Tendon Transfers

Rhonda Kaplan, M.S., O.T.R., C.H.T.

Senior Hand Therapist, Davies Medical Center, San Francisco
Chapter 126. Rehabilitation of Hand Injuries

Lynn D. Ketchum, M.D.

Clinical Professor, Department of Surgery, University of Kansas School of Medicine, Kansas City; Attending Surgeon, Department of Plastic and Hand Surgery, Humana Medical Center, Overland Park, Kansas
Chapter 124. Dupuytren Contracture

Joseph L. Kiener, M.D.

Clinical Assistant Professor, Department of Surgery, University of Nevada School of Medicine, Reno, Nevada
Chapter 68. Oral and Pharyngeal Reconstruction with Transposition Flaps

Stanley A. Klatsky, M.D.

Assistant Professor, Division of Plastic Surgery, Johns Hopkins University School of Medicine, Baltimore; President, Medical Staff, and Chief, Division of Plastic and Reconstructive Surgery, Baltimore County General Hospital, Randallstown, Maryland
Chapter 138. Blepharoplasty
Chapter 141. Brow-Lift

William J. Koenig, M.D.

Instructor of Clinical Surgery, Northwestern University Medical School, Chicago
Chapter 146. Correction of Difficult Nasal Deformities

Christ P. Koulis, D.M.D.

Resident, General Surgery, University of Illinois College of Medicine, Chicago
Chapter 109. Initial Evaluation and Management of Hand Injuries

John O. Kucan, M.D.

Professor of Surgery, Southern Illinois University School of Medicine; Director, Memorial Burn Center, Memorial Medical Center, Springfield, Illinois
Chapter 26. Thermal Burns: Resuscitation and Initial Management

P. A. Vinod Kumar, M.B.B.S., M.S., M.Ch., M.N.A.M.S.

Senior Research Fellow, Microsurgery Research Centre, St. Vincent's Hospital, Victoria, Australia
Chapter 24. Lymphedema

Kunihiro Kurihara, M.D.

Associate Professor, Department of Plastic Surgery, Jikei University School of Medicine; Chief and Director, Department of Plastic and Reconstructive Surgery, Jikei University Kashiwa Hospital, Tokyo
Chapter 55. Congenital Deformities of the External Ear

B. George H. Lamberty, M.A., M.B., B.Ch., F.R.C.S.

Associate Lecturer, Clinical School, University of Cambridge; Consultant, Plastic and Reconstructive Surgeon, Department of Plastic Surgery, Addenbrooke's Hospital, Cambridge, England
Chapter 5. Flaps: Physiology, Principles of Design, and Pitfalls

Bradley G. Langer, M.D.

Assistant Professor, Department of Radiology, University of Illinois College of Medicine; Chairman and Program Director, Department of Radiology, Cook County Hospital, Chicago
Chapter 77. Radiologic Evaluation of Maxillofacial Trauma

Don LaRossa, M.D.

Associate Professor, Division of Plastic Surgery, University of Pennsylvania School of Medicine; Attending Physician, Children's Hospital of Philadelphia and Hospital of the University of Pennsylvania, Philadelphia
Chapter 43. Cleft Palate

David L. Larson, M.D.

Professor and Chairman, Division of Plastic and Reconstructive Surgery, Medical College of Wisconsin, Milwaukee
Chapter 65.   *Principles of Composite Resection and Neck Dissection for Carcinoma of the Oropharynx*

W. Thomas Lawrence, M.D.

Professor, Department of Surgery, Chief, Division of Plastic and Reconstructive Surgery and Surgery of the Hand, University of North Carolina at Chapel Hill School of Medicine, Chapel Hill, North Carolina
Chapter 7.   *Tissue Transfer: Fat, Dermal, Muscle, Cartilage, and Fascial Grafts*

James A. Lehman, Jr., M.D.

Professor, Division of Plastic Surgery, Northeastern Ohio Universities College of Medicine, Rootstown; Fellowship Director, Division of Plastic Surgery, Children's Hospital Medical Center of Akron, Akron, Ohio
Chapter 52.   *Maxillary Deformities: Orthognathic Surgery*

Madeleine Lejour, M.D.

Professor, Department of Plastic Surgery, Free University of Brussels; Head, Department of Plastic Surgery, University Hospital Brugman, Brussels, Belgium
Chapter 154.   *Reduction of Large Breasts by a Combination of Liposuction and Vertical Mammaplasty*
Chapter 155.   *Correction of Breast Ptosis by Vertical Mammaplasty*

Laurence A. Levine, M.D.

Assistant Professor of Surgery, University of Chicago Pritzker School of Medicine; Co-Director of the Genitourinary Reconstructive Program, Department of Surgery, University of Chicago Medical Center, Chicago
Chapter 104.   *Reconstruction and Construction of the Penis*

Michael B. Lewis, M.D.

Associate Professor, Department of Surgery, Tufts University School of Medicine; Chief, Division of Plastic Surgery, New England Medical Center Hospitals, Boston
Chapter 44.   *Secondary Soft Tissue Procedures for Cleft Lip and Palate*

Michael D. Lichter, M.D.

Clinical Assistant Professor, Department of Dermatology, University of Illinois College of Medicine, Chicago
Chapter 19.   *Benign Skin Tumors*

William C. Lineaweaver, M.D.

Associate Professor, Division of Plastic Surgery and Division of Hand Surgery, Stanford University Medical Center, Stanford, California
Chapter 75.   *Facial Reanimation*
Chapter 108.   *Hand Infections*
Chapter 122.   *Toe-to-Hand Transplantation*

John W. Little, M.D.

Professor, Division of Plastic Surgery, Georgetown University Medical Center, Washington
Chapter 99.   *Nipple-Areolar Reconstruction*

Michael C. Locher, M.D., D.D.S.

Senior Physician, Department of Craniomaxillofacial Surgery, University of Zurich, Zurich, Switzerland
Chapter 38.   *Mandibulofacial Dysostosis*

Ted E. Lockwood, M.D.

Assistant Clinical Professor, Division of Plastic Surgery, University of Missouri—Kansas City School of Medicine, Kansas City, Missouri; Attending Plastic Surgeon, Humana Hospital of Overland Park, Overland Park, Kansas
Chapter 158.   *Body Contouring: Trunk- and Thigh-Lifts*

Tim R. Love, M.D.

Attending Physician, The Center for Plastic and Reconstructive Surgery, Orlando, Florida
Chapter 128.   *Lower Extremity Reconstruction: Management of Soft Tissue Defects*

Edward A. Luce, M.D.

Professor and Chief, Division of Plastic Surgery, University of Kentucky College of Medicine, Lexington, Kentucky
Chapter 64. Carcinoma of the Oropharynx

Hans-G. Luhr, M.D., D.M.D.

Professor and Chairman, Department of Maxillofacial Surgery, University of Goettingen, Goettingen, Germany
Chapter 14. Principles of Rigid Bony Fixation of the Craniofacial Skeleton

Steven D. Macht, M.D.

Clinical Professor, Department of Plastic Surgery, George Washington University School of Medicine and Health Sciences, Washington
Chapter 22. Malignant Melanoma

Susan E. Mackinnon, M.D.

Professor, Division of Plastic and Reconstructive Surgery, Washington University School of Medicine; Attending Surgeon, Barnes Hospital, St. Louis
Chapter 117. Nerve Injuries: Primary Repair and Reconstruction

Ernest K. Manders, M.D.

Professor, Division of Plastic and Reconstructive Surgery, Pennsylvania State University College of Medicine; Chief, Department of Surgery, The Pennsylvania State University Hospital and The Milton S. Hershey Medical Center, Hershey, Pennsylvania
Chapter 15. Reconstruction Using Soft Tissue Expansion

Paul N. Manson, M.D.

Professor and Chairman, Division of Plastic Surgery, Johns Hopkins University School of Medicine; Director, Department of Plastic Surgery, The Maryland Institute of Emergency Medical Services Systems, Baltimore
Chapter 83. Fractures of the Orbit and Nasoethmoidal Bones

Saeed Marefat, M.D.

Attending Surgeon, Department of Plastic Surgery, Suburban Hospital, Bethesda, Maryland
Chapter 157. Body Contouring with Suction-Assisted Lipectomy

Daniel Marchac, M.D.

Professor, College de Medicine des Hopitaux de Paris; Director, Craniofacial Center, Hopital Necker Enfants Malades, Paris
Chapter 36. Craniosynostosis and Craniofacial Dysostosis

Bernard L. Markowitz, M.D.

Assistant Professor, Department of Surgery, University of California, Los Angeles, UCLA School of Medicine, Los Angeles; Chief, Division of Plastic and Reconstructive Surgery, Olive View Medical Center, Sylmar, California
Chapter 83. Fractures of the Orbit and Nasoethmoidal Bones

Michael A. Marschall, M.D.

Assistant Professor, Department of Surgery, University of Illinois College of Medicine; Attending Surgeon, Cook County Hospital, Chicago
Chapter 8. The Omentum in Reconstructive Surgery
Chapter 102. Pressure Sores

Stephanie F. Marschall, M.D.

Assistant Professor, Department of Dermatology, Rush Medical College of Rush University; Assistant Attending Physician, Department of Dermatology, Rush-Presbyterian-St. Luke's Medical Center, Chicago
Chapter 19. Benign Skin Tumors

Timothy J. Marten, M.D.

Attending Physician, Department of Plastic Surgery, California Pacific Medical Center, San Francisco
Chapter 135. Facial Rejuvenation: Facelift

Alan Matarasso, M.D.

Clinical Assistant Professor, Department of Plastic and Reconstructive Surgery, Albert Einstein College of Medicine of Yeshiva University, Bronx; Assistant Attending Surgeon, Department of Plastic Surgery, Manhattan Eye, Ear, Throat Hospital, New York
Chapter 156. Abdominal Contour Operations

Stephen J. Mathes, M.D.

Professor, Department of Surgery, University of California, San Francisco, School of Medicine; Head, Division of Plastic and Reconstructive Surgery, The Medical Center at the University of California, San Francisco
Chapter 68.   *Oral and Pharyngeal Reconstruction with Transposition Flaps*

Hani S. Matloub, M.D.

Associate Professor, Department of Surgery, Medical College of Wisconsin; Attending Surgeon, Froedtert Memorial Lutheran Hospital, Milwaukee, Wisconsin
Chapter 11.   *Flexor Tendon Grafting*
Chapter 70.   *Reconstruction of the Mandible and the Floor of the Mouth*

W. Earle Matory, Jr., M.D.

Assistant Professor, Department of Surgery, University of Massachusetts Medical School; Attending Surgeon, Department of Plastic and Reconstructive Surgery, University of Massachusetts Medical Center, Worcester, Massachusetts
Chapter 148.   *Aesthetic Facial Surgery in African-Americans*

G. Patrick Maxwell, M.D.

Assistant Clinical Professor, Division of Plastic Surgery, Vanderbilt University School of Medicine; Director, the Institute for Aesthetic and Reconstructive Surgery, Mid-State Baptist Hospital, Nashville, Tennessee
Chapter 97.   *Delayed Breast Reconstruction with Autogenous Tissue*

Dennis E. McDonnell, M.D.

Associate Professor, Department of Surgery, Medical College of Georgia School of Medicine, Augusta, Georgia
Chapter 91.   *Meningomyelocele*

Peter McKinney, M.D.

Professor of Clinical Surgery, Division of Plastic Surgery, Northwestern University Medical School; Attending Surgeon, Northwestern Memorial Hospital, Chicago
Chapter 146.   *Correction of Difficult Nasal Deformities*

N. Bradly Meland, M.D.

Associate Professor of Plastic Surgery, Mayo Medical School, Rochester, Minnesota; Consultant, Plastic Surgery, Mayo Clinic, Scottsdale, Arizona
Chapter 93.   *Intrathoracic Transposition of Soft Tissue*
Chapter 101.   *Reconstruction of Hip and Pelvic Defects*

David Mendes, M.D.

Director, Cleft Palate/Craniofacial Center, St. Luke's/Roosevelt Hospital Center, New York
Chapter 89.   *Traumatic Deformities and Reconstruction of the Temporomandibular Joint*

Frederick J. Menick, M.D.

Clinical Faculty, Department of Surgery, University of Arizona College of Medicine; Chief, Division of Plastic Surgery, Tucson Veterans Administration Hospital, Tucson, Arizona
Chapter 60.   *Principles of Facial Reconstruction*
Chapter 62.   *Reconstruction of the Nose*

Dennis Mess, M.D.

Clinical Associate Professor, Department of Orthopedics, University of Illinois College of Medicine; Attending Surgeon, University of Illinois Hospital, Chicago
Chapter 127.   *Lower Extremity Trauma: Principles of Evaluation and Early Management*

Rodolphe Meyer, M.D.

Former Associate Professor, Department of Plastic and Reconstructive Surgery, University Hospital of Lausanne, Lausanne, Switzerland
Chapter 147.   *Secondary Rhinoplasty*

Michael J. Miller, M.D.

Assistant Professor, Division of Plastic and Reconstructive Surgery, University of Texas Medical School at Houston; Attending Surgeon, Reconstructive Plastic Surgery Service, The University of Texas M. D. Anderson Cancer Center, Houston
Chapter 69.   *Oral and Pharyngeal Reconstruction with Free Tissue Transfer*

Daniel C. Mills II, M.D.

Chief, Department of Plastic Surgery, South Coast Medical Center, South Laguna, California
Chapter 143.   *Ancillary Procedures for Facial Rejuvenation*

Roger C. Mixter, M.D.

Clinical Assistant Professor, Division of Plastic Surgery, University of Wisconsin Medical School, Madison; Medical Director, Center for Plastic Surgery, Mercy Hospital, Janesville, Wisconsin
Chapter 47.   Sphincter Pharyngoplasty

Stan J. Monstrey, M.D.

Associate Professor, Department of Plastic Surgery, University Hospital, Gent, Belgium
Chapter 132.   Leg Ulcers

Daniel C. Morello, M.D.

Attending Surgeon, White Plains Hospital, White Plains, and Northern Westchester Hospital, Mount Kisco, New York
Chapter 152.   Inferior Pedicle Breast Reduction

Prakash C. Mullick, M.D., Ph.D.

Visiting Fellow in Plastic Surgery, University of Pittsburgh School of Medicine and VA Medical Center, Pittsburgh
Chapter 132.   Leg Ulcers

Thomas A. Mustoe, M.D.

Professor and Chief, Division of Plastic and Reconstructive Surgery, Northwestern University Medical School; Chief, Division of Plastic Surgery, Northwestern Memorial Hospital, Chicago
Chapter 1.   Wound Healing

Foad Nahai, M.D.

Associate Professor, Department of Surgery, Emory University School of Medicine; Attending Surgeon, Emory University Hospital, Atlanta
Chapter 128.   Lower Extremity Reconstruction: Management of Soft Tissue Defects

Frank A. Nesi, M.D.

Assistant Clinical Professor, Department of Ophthalmology, Wayne State University School of Medicine, Detroit; Chief, Oculoplastics Service, William Beaumont Hospital, Royal Oak, Michigan
Chapter 79.   Correction of Traumatic Ptosis of the Eyelid and Reconstruction of the Lacrimal System

David T. Netscher, M.D.

Assistant Professor, Division of Plastic Surgery, Baylor College of Medicine; Attending Staff, Veteran's Administration Medical Center, Houston
Chapter 3.   Scar Revision
Chapter 20.   Premalignant Skin Tumors, Basal Cell Carcinoma, and Squamous Cell Carcinoma

M. Haskell Newman, M.D.

Clinical Associate Professor, Section of Plastic and Reconstructive Surgery, University of Michigan Medical School, Ann Arbor, Michigan
Chapter 80.   Fractures of the Frontal Sinus

Mark Nissenbaum, M.D.

Associate Professor of Orthopedics, Temple University School of Medicine, Philadelphia; Director of Hand Surgery, Abington Memorial Hospital, Abington, Pennsylvania
Chapter 105.   Hand-Skin Incisions

James Thomas Nolan, M.D.

Clinical Assistant Professor, Division of Plastic Surgery, Oregon Health Sciences University School of Medicine; Private Practice, Portland, Oregon
Chapter 105.   Hand-Skin Incisions

R. Barrett Noone, M.D.

Clinical Professor, Department of Surgery, University of Pennsylvania School of Medicine, Philadelphia; Chief, Service of Plastic Surgery, Bryn Mawr Hospital, Bryn Mawr, Pennsylvania
Chapter 95.   Immediate Reconstruction of the Breast After Mastectomy

M. Samuel Noordhoff, M.D.

Professor, Department of Surgery, Chang Gung Medical College; Chairman, Division of Plastic Surgery, Chang Gung Memorial Hospital, Taipei, Taiwan
Chapter 41.   Bilateral Cleft Lip

Jerry E. Nye, M.D.

Clinical Instructor, Division of Plastic and Reconstructive Surgery, Oregon Health Sciences University School of Medicine; Attending Physician, Good Samaritan Medical Center, Portland, Oregon
Chapter 105.   Hand-Skin Incisions

† Bernard McC. O'Brien, M.D.

Director, Microsurgery Research Centre, St. Vincent's Hospital, Victoria, Australia
Chapter 24.   Lymphedema

Alfonso Oliva, M.D.

Assistant Clinical Professor, Division of Plastic and Reconstructive Surgery, University of California, San Francisco, School of Medicine; Attending Surgeon, Department of Microsurgical Replantation and Transplantation, Davies Medical Center, San Francisco
Chapter 75.   Facial Reanimation
Chapter 122.   Toe-to-Hand Transplantation

Douglas K. Ousterhout, M.D., D.D.S.

Clinical Professor, Division of Plastic Surgery, University of California, San Francisco, School of Medicine; Attending Plastic Surgeon, Davies Medical Center, San Francisco
Chapter 39.   Hemifacial Microsomia

John Q. Owsley, M.D.

Clinical Professor, Division of Plastic Surgery, University of California, San Francisco, School of Medicine; Active Staff, Davies Medical Center, San Francisco
Chapter 136.   Facial Rejuvenation in Men

Clayton R. Perry, M.D.

Associate Professor, Division of Orthopedic Surgery, Washington University School of Medicine; Director, Division of Orthopedic Surgery, St. Louis Regional Medical Center, St. Louis
Chapter 129.   Lower Extremity Reconstruction: Management of Bony Defects

Richard J. L. Phillips, M.D.

Assistant Professor, Department of Surgery, Wayne State University School of Medicine; Associate Director, Section of Plastic and Reconstructive Surgery, Children's Hospital of Michigan, Detroit
Chapter 81.   Fractures of the Zygoma

John W. Polley, M.D.

Assistant Professor, Departments of Surgery and Pediatrics, University of Illinois College of Medicine; Attending Plastic Surgeon, University of Illinois Hospital and Cook County Hospital, Chicago
Chapter 9.   Bone Grafts
Chapter 97.   Delayed Breast Reconstruction with Autogenous Tissue

Beatriz H. Porras-Reyes, M.D.

Fellow in Plastic and Reconstructive Surgery, Washington University School of Medicine, St. Louis
Chapter 1.   Wound Healing

† Joseph L. Posch, M.D.

Clinical Professor of Surgery, Division of Plastic and Reconstructive Surgery, Wayne State University School of Medicine, Detroit
Chapter 107.   Tumors of the Hand

Jeffrey C. Posnick, D.M.D., M.D.

Associate Professor, Department of Medicine, Georgetown University School of Medicine; Co-Director, Division of Plastic Surgery, Georgetown University Medical Center, Washington
Chapter 50.   The Correction of Secondary Skeletal Deformities in Adolescent Patients with Cleft Lip and Palate

† Deceased.

Mark S. Potenza, M.D.

Resident, Division of Plastic and Reconstructive Surgery, University of North Carolina at Chapel Hill School of Medicine; Resident, Department of Plastic and Reconstructive Surgery, The University of North Carolina Hospitals, Chapel Hill, North Carolina
Chapter 7. *Tissue Transfer: Fat, Dermal, Muscle, Cartilage, and Fascial Grafts*

Christopher D. Prevel, M.D.

Assistant Professor, Division of Plastic and Reconstructive Surgery, Indiana University School of Medicine; Director, Microsurgery Laboratory, Indiana University Medical Center, Indianapolis
Chapter 11. *Flexor Tendon Grafting*

Allen M. Putterman, M.D.

Professor, Department of Ophthalmology, University of Illinois College of Medicine; Senior Attending and Director of Oculoplastic Surgery, Department of Ophthalmology, Michael Reese Hospital and Medical Center, Chicago
Chapter 56. *Congenital Ptosis of the Eyelid*

Sai S. Ramasastry, M.D.

Associate Professor, Department of Surgery, University of Illinois College of Medicine; Attending Plastic Surgeon, University of Illinois Hospital and Cook County Hospital, Chicago
Chapter 59. *Reconstruction of Defects of the Scalp and Skull*
Chapter 132. *Leg Ulcers*

Oscar M. Ramirez, M.D.

Clinical Assistant Professor, Division of Plastic Surgery, Johns Hopkins University School of Medicine; Attending Plastic Surgeon, Greater Baltimore Medical Center and Franklin Square Hospital Center, Baltimore
Chapter 137. *Facial Rejuvenation: Subperiosteal Facelift*

Riley S. Rees, M.D.

Associate Professor, Department of Plastic and Reconstructive Surgery, University of Michigan Medical School; Chief, Plastic Surgery Section, Veterans Administration Medical Center, Ann Arbor, Michigan
Chapter 72. *Cancer of the Larynx*

Dominique Renier, M.D.

Chapter 36. *Craniosynostosis and Craniofacial Dysostosis*

David J. Reisberg, D.D.S.

Assistant Professor, Department of Pediatrics, University of Illinois College of Medicine; Director, Maxillofacial Prosthetics, University of Illinois Hospital, Chicago
Chapter 54. *Prosthetic Management for Patients with Cleft Lip and Palate*
Chapter 73. *Prosthetic Rehabilitation After Operations for Cancer of the Head and Neck*

Bruno Ristow, M.D.

Chief, Department of Plastic Surgery, Pacific Presbyterian Medical Center, San Francisco
Chapter 139. *Transconjunctival Blepharoplasty*
Chapter 140. *Forehead-Lifts*

June K. Robinson, M.D.

Associate Professor, Department of Dermatology and Surgery, Northwestern University Medical School; Attending Physician, Department of Dermatology and Surgery, Northwestern Memorial Hospital, Chicago
Chapter 21. *Principles of Mohs Micrographic Surgery*

Martin C. Robson, M.D.

Professor, Department of Surgery, University of South Florida; Chief, Bay Pines Surgical Service, VAMC, Tampa, Florida
Chapter 30. *Electrical and Chemical Injuries*

Rod J. Rohrich, M.D.

Professor and Chairman, Division of Plastic Surgery, University of Texas Southwestern Medical Center at Dallas; Chief of Plastic Surgery, Parkland Memorial Medical Center, Dallas
Chapter 78. *Primary Repair and Secondary Reconstruction of Facial Soft Tissue Injuries*

Harvey M. Rosen, M.D., D.M.D.

Clinical Associate Professor, Department of Surgery, University of Pennsylvania School of Medicine; Chief, Section of Plastic Surgery, Pennsylvania Hospital, Philadelphia
Chapter 10. Bone Substitutes

R. Bruce Ross, D.D.S., M.Sc., F.R.C.D.

Professor, Department of Orthodontics, University of Toronto School of Medicine; Dental Orthodontist, Hospital for Sick Children, Toronto
Chapter 34. The Clinical Use of Cephalometrics

Robert L. Ruberg, M.D.

Professor and Director, Division of Plastic Surgery, Ohio State University College of Medicine; Director, Burn Unit, Ohio State University Hospitals, Columbus, Ohio
Chapter 27. Burn Wounds: Excision and Grafting

Ross Rudolph, M.D.

Associate Clinical Professor, Division of Plastic Surgery, University of California, San Diego, School of Medicine, San Diego; Head, Division of Plastic and Reconstructive Surgery, Hospital of the Scripps Clinic, La Jolla, California
Chapter 31. Radiation Injuries

Robert C. Russell, M.D.

Professor and Chief, Department of Microsurgery and Research, Southern Illinois University School of Medicine, Springfield, Illinois
Chapter 118. Amputations: Revascularization and Replantation

H. F. Sailer, M.D., D.D.S.

Professor and Chairman, Department of Surgery, Zurich University; Attending Surgeon, Department of Craniomaxillofacial Surgery, University Hospital, Zurich, Switzerland
Chapter 38. Mandibulofacial Dysostosis

Kenneth E. Salyer, M.D.

Founding Chairman and Director, Humana Advanced Surgical Institutes, Dallas
Chapter 42. Primary Correction of the Nasal Deformity Associated with Cleft Lip

James R. Sanger, M.D.

Associate Professor, Department of Surgery, Medical College of Wisconsin; Attending Surgeon, Froedtert Memorial Lutheran Hospital, Milwaukee
Chapter 11. Flexor Tendon Grafting
Chapter 70. Reconstruction of the Mandible and the Floor of the Mouth

Luis R. Scheker, M.D.

Assistant Clinical Professor, Division of Plastic and Reconstructive Surgery, University of Louisville School of Medicine, Louisville, Kentucky
Chapter 120. Salvage of a Mutilated Hand

Robert R. Schenck, M.D.

Associate Professor, Departments of Plastic and Orthopedic Surgery, Rush Medical College of Rush University; Director, Section of Hand Surgery, Rush-Presbyterian-St. Luke's Medical Center, Chicago
Chapter 110. Fingernail and Fingertip Injuries

James D. Schlenker, M.D.

Clinical Professor, Department of Surgery, University of Illinois College of Medicine, Chicago
Chapter 109. Initial Evaluation and Management of Hand Injuries

Richard C. Schultz, M.D.

Clinical Professor of Surgery, University of Illinois College of Medicine; Associate in Surgery, University of Chicago Pritzker School of Medicine, Chicago; Senior Attending Plastic Surgeon, Lutheran General Hospital, Park Ridge, Illinois
Chapter 87. Facial Fractures in Children and Adolescents

Alan E. Seyfer, M.D.

Professor, Department of Surgery, Oregon Health Sciences University School of Medicine; Chief, Division of Plastic and Reconstructive Surgery, University Hospital, Portland, Oregon
Chapter 90. Congenital Anomalies of the Chest Wall
Chapter 91. Meningomyelocele

Kenneth C. Shestak, M.D.

Assistant Professor of Surgery, University of Pittsburgh Medical Center; Attending Surgeon, Magee-Women's Hospital, Pittsburgh
Chapter 59.   Reconstruction of Defects of the Scalp and Skull
Chapter 132.   Leg Ulcers

John D. Siddens, D.O.

Clinical Faculty, Department of Ophthalmology, University of South Carolina School of Medicine, Columbia, South Carolina
Chapter 79.   Correction of Traumatic Ptosis of the Eyelid and Reconstruction of the Lacrimal System

Bonnie E. Smith, Ph.D.

Associate Professor, Departments of Otolaryngology Pediatrics, University of Illinois College of Medicine, Chicago
Chapter 45.   Velopharyngeal Insufficiency

David J. Smith, Jr., M.D.

Section Head, Department of Plastic and Reconstructive Surgery, University of Michigan Medical Center, Ann Arbor, Michigan
Chapter 29.   Reconstruction of Burn Deformities of the Extremities and Trunk

Lawrence M. Solomon, M.D.

Professor and Head, Department of Dermatology, University of Illinois College of Medicine, Chicago
Chapter 19.   Benign Skin Tumors

Mark P. Solomon, M.D.

Associate Professor, Department of Surgery, Medical College of Pennsylvania; Co-Chief, Department of Plastic Surgery, Medical College Hospitals, Philadelphia, Pennsylvania
Chapter 74.   Tumors of the Salivary Glands

Scott L. Spear, M.D.

Professor and Chief, Division of Plastic Surgery, Georgetown University Medical Center, Washington
Chapter 151.   Augmentation Mammaplasty

D. G. Spigos, M.D.

Professor and Chairman, Department of Radiology, Ohio State University College of Medicine, Columbus, Ohio
Chapter 77.   Radiologic Evaluation of Maxillofacial Trauma

Melvin Spira, D.D.S., M.D.

Professor and Chairman, Division of Plastic Surgery, Baylor College of Medicine; Chief, Department of Plastic Surgery, The Methodist Hospital, Houston
Chapter 20.   Premalignant Skin Tumors, Basal Cell Carcinoma, and Squamous Cell Carcinoma

Samuel Stal, M.D.

Associate Professor, Department of Surgery, Baylor College of Medicine; Chief, Plastic Surgery Services, Texas Children's Hospital, Houston
Chapter 3.   Scar Revision

Hans U. Steinau, M.D., Ph.D.

Head, Department of Surgery and Burn Unit, Ruhr University; Attending Physician, University Hospital, Bochum, Germany
Chapter 131.   Reconstruction and Rehabilitation of the Mutilated Foot

Thomas R. Stevenson, M.D.

Professor and Chief, Division of Plastic Surgery, University of California, Davis, School of Medicine, Davis, California
Chapter 130.   Chronic Osteomyelitis

Miroslaw F. Stranc, M.D.

Professor, Department of Surgery, University of Manitoba Faculty of Medicine; Head, Department of Plastic Surgery, Victoria General Hospital, Winnipeg, Manitoba, Canada
Chapter 63.   Reconstruction of the Lips

James W. Strickland, M.D.

Clinical Professor, Department of Orthopaedic Surgery, Indiana University School of Medicine; Chief, Section of Hand Surgery, St. Vincent's Hospital, Indianapolis
Chapter 114.   Late Flexor Tendon Reconstruction and Tendon Grafting

Walter G. Sullivan, M.D.

Associate Professor, Department of Surgery, Wayne State University School of Medicine; Chief, Division of Plastic and Reconstructive Surgery, Children's Hospital of Michigan and Harper-Grace Hospitals, Detroit
Chapter 81.   Fractures of the Zygoma

William M. Swartz, M.D.

Associate Clinical Professor, Department of Surgery, University of Pittsburgh School of Medicine; Private Practice, Shadyside Hospital, Pittsburgh
Chapter 69.   Oral and Pharyngeal Reconstruction with Free Tissue Transfer

John S. Taras, M.D.

Clinical Instructor, Department of Orthopaedic Surgery, Jefferson Medical College of Thomas Jefferson University; Attending Staff, Thomas Jefferson University Hospital, Philadelphia
Chapter 113.   Acute Flexor Tendon Injuries

Bahman Teimourian, M.D.

Clinical Professor, Division of Plastic Surgery, Georgetown University School of Medicine, Washington; Chairman, Department of Surgery, Suburban Hospital, Bethesda, Maryland
Chapter 157.   Body Contouring with Suction-Assisted Lipectomy

Hugh G. Thomson, M.D.

Professor of Surgery, University of Toronto Faculty of Medicine; Attending Surgeon, Division of Plastic Surgery, Hospital for Sick Children, Toronto
Chapter 23.   Vascular Malformations

Bryant A. Toth, M.D.

Assistant Clinical Professor, Department of Surgery, University of California, San Francisco, School of Medicine; Attending Physician, California Pacific Medical Center, San Francisco, and Chief, Division of Plastic Surgery, Children's Hospital and Medical Center, Oakland, California
Chapter 18.   Three-Dimensional Imaging: An Adjunct to Craniomaxillofacial Reconstruction

William C. Trier, M.D.

Consultant, Division of Plastic Surgery, University of Washington School of Medicine; Attending Plastic Surgeon, Children's Hospital and Medical Center, Seattle
Chapter 46.   Pharyngeal Flaps for the Correction of Velopharyngeal Insufficiency

Joseph Upton, M.D.

Clinical Associate Professor, Department of Surgery, Harvard Medical School; Attending Surgeon, Division of Plastic Surgery, Children's Hospital and Beth Israel Hospital, Boston
Chapter 106.   Congenital Anomalies of the Hand

J. C. van der Meulen, M.D.

Erasmus University Rotterdam, University Hospital Rotterdam, Rotterdam, Holland
Chapter 35.   The Classification and Management of Facial Clefts

Karin Vargervik, D.D.S.

Adjunct Professor, Department of Surgery, and Professor, Department of Growth and Development, University of California, San Francisco, School of Medicine; Director, Center for Craniofacial Anomalies, University of California, San Francisco
Chapter 39.   Hemifacial Microsomia

Henry C. Vasconez, M.D.

Associate Professor, Division of Plastic Surgery, University of Kentucky College of Medicine; Chief, Department of Plastic Surgery, Veterans Administration Medical Centers, Lexington, Kentucky
Chapter 4.   Skin Grafts
Chapter 64.   Carcinoma of the Oropharynx

Luis O. Vasconez, M.D.

Professor, Department of Surgery, University of Alabama School of Medicine; Chief, Division of Plastic Surgery, University of Alabama Hospitals, Birmingham, Alabama
Chapter 6.   Skin Flaps, Fasciocutaneous Flaps, and Musculocutaneous Flaps

Michael Paul Vincent, M.D.

Associate Professor of Clinical Surgery, Uniformed Services University of the Health Sciences, F. Edward Hébert School of Medicine; Chief, Plastic Surgery Department, National Naval Medical Center, Bethesda, Maryland
Chapter 142.   Oculoplastic Surgery

Peter A. Vogt, M.D.

Attending Plastic Surgeon, Unity Medical Center, Minneapolis
Chapter 159. Brachioplasty and Brachial Suction-Assisted Lipoplasty

Robert L. Walton, M.D.

Professor, Department of Surgery and Chief, Division of Plastic Surgery, University of Chicago Pritzker School of Medicine, Chicago
Chapter 112. Injuries to the Joints and Ligaments of the Upper Extremity
Chapter 153. The Parenchymal Pedicle Technique for Reduction Mammaplasty

Kevin L. Waltz, M.D.

Fellow, Department of Ophthalmology, Wayne State University School of Medicine, Detroit
Chapter 79. Correction of Traumatic Ptosis of the Eyelid and Reconstruction of the Lacrimal System

Denton Watumull, M.D.

Assistant Professor, Division of Plastic Surgery, University of Texas, Southwestern Medical Center at Dallas, Southwestern Medical School; Attending Physician, Department of Plastic Surgery, Parkland Memorial Medical Center, Dallas
Chapter 78. Primary Repair and Secondary Reconstruction of Facial Soft Tissue Injuries

Jeffrey Weinzweig, M.D.

Fellow, Division of Plastic and Reconstructive Surgery, Mayo Clinic Scottsdale and Maricopa Medical Center, Phoenix
Chapter 2. Basic Principles and Techniques in Plastic Surgery

Norman Weinzweig, M.D.

Assistant Professor, Department of Surgery, University of Illinois College of Medicine; Attending Surgeon, University of Illinois Hospital and Cook County Hospital, Chicago
Chapter 2. Basic Principles and Techniques in Plastic Surgery
Chapter 25. Hidradenitis Suppurativa

Wayde M. Weston, Ph.D.

Research Assistant Professor, Department of Anatomy and Developmental Biology, Jefferson Medical College of Thomas Jefferson University, Philadelphia
Chapter 32. Craniofacial Embryology

Linton A. Whitaker, M.D.

Professor, Department of Surgery, University of Pennsylvania School of Medicine; Chief, Department of Plastic Surgery, Hospital of the University of Pennsylvania, Philadelphia
Chapter 134. Contouring of the Facial Skeleton

Carl N. Williams, Jr., M.D.

Assistant Professor, Department of Surgery, University of Nevada School of Medicine; Chief, Division of Plastic Surgery, University Medical Center, Las Vegas
Chapter 110. Fingernail and Fingertip Injuries

Robert Lee Wilson, M.D.

Clinical Lecturer, Department of Orthopedics, University of Arizona College of Medicine, Tucson; Assistant Chief, Hand Service, Maricopa Medical Center, Phoenix
Chapter 123. Rheumatoid Disease of the Hand and Wrist

S. Anthony Wolfe, M.D.

Clinical Professor, Division of Plastic and Reconstructive Surgery, University of Miami School of Medicine, Miami
Chapter 88. Secondary Reconstruction of Soft Tissue Deformity Associated with Orbital Trauma

Michael J. Yaremchuk, M.D.

Assistant Professor, Department of Surgery, Harvard Medical School; Associate Surgeon, Division of Plastic Surgery, Massachusetts General Hospital, Boston
Chapter 84. Fractures of the Maxilla

V. Leroy Young, M.D.

Professor, Division of Plastic and Reconstructive Surgery, Washington University School of Medicine; Attending Physician, Barnes Hospital, St. Louis
Chapter 125. Wrist Pain

N. John Yousif, M.D.

Associate Professor, Department of Surgery, Medical College of Wisconsin; Attending Surgeon, Froedtert Memorial Lutheran Hospital, Milwaukee
Chapter 11. Flexor Tendon Grafting
Chapter 70. Reconstruction of the Mandible and the Floor of the Mouth

Elvin G. Zook, M.D.

Professor and Chairman, Department of Plastic Surgery, Southern Illinois University School of Medicine, Springfield, Illinois
Chapter 115. Extensor Tendon Injuries

Ronald M. Zuker, M.D.

Associate Professor, Department of Surgery, University of Toronto Faculty of Medicine; Head, Division of Plastic Surgery, Hospital for Sick Children, Toronto
Chapter 58. Facial Reanimation: Cross-Face Nerve Grafting and Muscle Transplantation

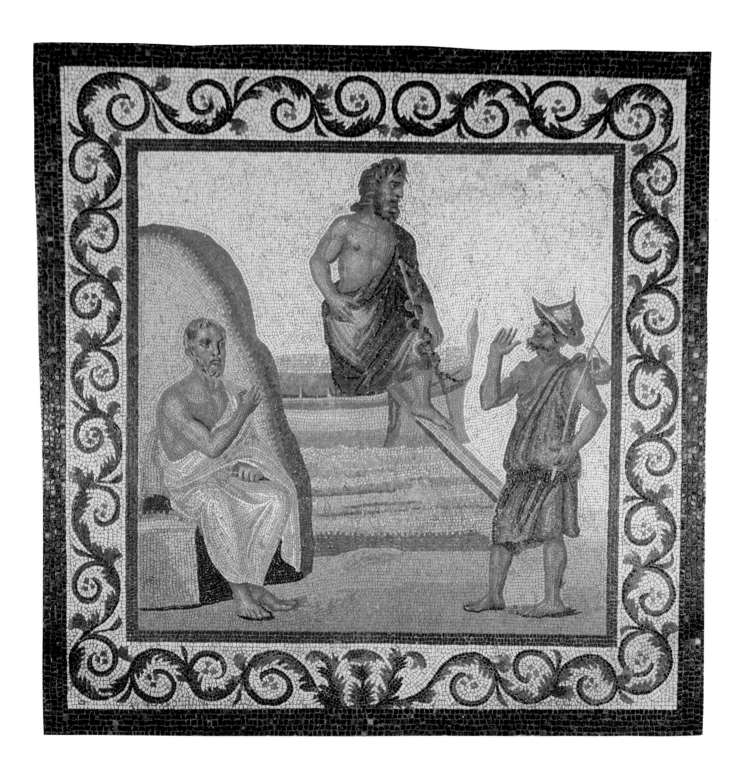

*Asclepius arriving in Cos. Hippocrates sits on the
right as a citizen of the island (left) welcomes the
god of medicine. Mosaic from a Roman villa, 2nd
to 3rd century A.D.. Cos Archaeologic Museum.
Cos, Greece. Reprinted with permission.*

Ὁ βίος βραχύς, ἡ δὲ τέχνη μακρή, ὁ δὲ καιρὸς ὀξύς, ἡ δὲ πεῖρα σφαλερή, ἡ δὲ κρίσις χαλεπή. δεῖ δὲ οὐ μόνον ἑωυτὸν παρέχειν τὰ δέοντα ποιέοντα, ἀλλὰ καὶ τὸν νοσέοντα καὶ τοὺς παρεόντας καὶ τὰ ἔξωθεν.

Ἱπποκράτης: ΑΦΟΡΙΣΜΟΙ

Life is short, the Art long, opportunity fleeting, experiment treacherous, judgment difficult. The physician must be ready, not only to do his duty himself, but also to secure the co-operation of the patient, of the attendants and of externals.

— Hippocrates: APHORISMS

I

General Principles and Techniques

Notice

The indications and dosages of all drugs in this book have been recommended in the medical literature and conform to the practices of the general medical community. The medications described do not necessarily have specific approval by the Food and Drug Administration for use in the diseases and dosages for which they are recommended. The package insert for each drug should be consulted for use and dosage as approved by the FDA. Because standards for usage change, it is advisable to keep abreast of revised recommendations, particularly those concerning new drugs.

1

Wound Healing

Beatriz H. Porras-Reyes   Thomas A. Mustoe

Repair is a natural reaction to injury that results in restoration of tissue integrity. This process occurs in all organs and systems of the body and constitutes the keystone on which surgery is founded. The optimal management of wounds has been a challenge throughout history. The introduction of antibiotics at the beginning of this century provided the first major advance in wound management toward prevention and treatment of bacterial wound contamination. During the past decade the understanding of the mechanism of wound healing has increased dramatically. The eruption of new knowledge from the fields of molecular and cellular biology and recent bioengineering advances may well improve the wound-healing process to a spectacular degree, making available growth-stimulating agents, new dressing materials, and energy from electrical fields—all powerful tools to manipulate the wound healing process. Rational wound management demands a detailed knowledge of the physiology of wound repair. This chapter focuses on the basic principles of wound healing with special emphasis on adequate management, healing difficulties, and complications such as hypertrophic scars and keloids. Special attention is de-

voted to agents that augment healing such as growth factors, electrical charges, and hyperbaric oxygen. Herein we relate biologic and physiologic features of wound healing with clinical aspects and with findings of current research.

Biology of Normal Wound Healing

Acute Inflammatory Phase

Injury alters the homeostatic state of tissue, resulting in an activated sequence of events that compose the acute inflammatory phase. (The sequence of events is illustrated in Figure 1-1.) This inflammatory response involves both a vascular and a cellular reaction. Tissue trauma and local bleeding result in activation of Hageman factor (XII) with initiation of the clotting cascade. The complement and kinin cascades are also activated. They release chemotactic and vasoactive mediators, which induce a transient arteriolar vasoconstriction that lasts for a few minutes and is followed by active vasodilatation secondary to local synthesis of vasodilator prostaglandins. An increase in vascular permeability also is present because

of the action of bradykinin, histamine, and serotonin, which contract endothelial cells resulting in the formation of intercellular gaps causing leakage of fluid and macromolecules into the interstitium. With endothelial injury, platelets adhere to the subendothelial surface stimulated by the exposed collagen of the basement membrane and the thrombin generated by the clotting cascade. Platelet activation generates both thromboxane A_2 (TXA$_2$), which contributes to the initial vasoconstrictive phase, and adenosine diphosphate (ADP), which facilitates aggregation of additional platelets in the growing clot. Several proteins are released when activated platelets discharge their alpha granules, including fibrinogen, fibronectin, platelet factor 4, transforming growth factor–beta (TGF-β), and platelet-derived growth factor (PDGF).

Mediators released by blood coagulation, complement pathways, and platelets induce the influx of inflammatory cells. The neutrophil is the first cell at the scene, protecting against infection by phagocytizing and killing microorganisms and lysing devitalized tissue. The scavenger function of the neutrophils depends on an adequate oxygen supply to produce free

3

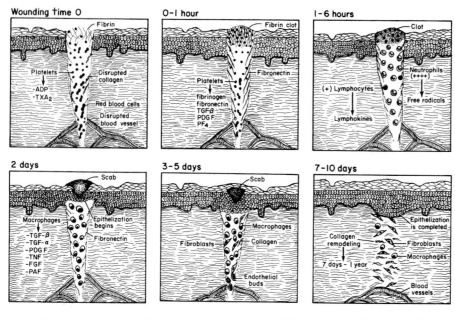

Fig. 1-1. Schematic progression of the process of wound repair. ADP = adenosine diphosphate; TXA$_2$ = thromboxane A$_2$; TGF = transforming growth factor; PDGF = platelet-derived growth factor; PF$_4$ = platelet factor 4; TNF = tumor necrosis factor; FGF = fibroblast growth factor; PAF = platelet-activating factor.

Table 1-1. Selected growth factors of wound healing

Factor	Source	Target	Role
TGF-β	All cells	All cells	Fibrosis Proliferation
TGF-α	Platelets Keratinocytes Macrophages	Epithelial cells Fibroblasts Endothelial cells	Proliferation
PDGF	Platelets Macrophages Fibroblasts Endothelial cells Smooth muscle cells	Neutrophils Macrophages Fibroblasts Smooth muscle cells	Chemotaxis Proliferation Collagenase synthesis
FGF	Macrophages Fibroblasts Endothelial cells	Endothelial cells Epithelial cells Fibroblasts Chondroblasts	Proliferation Chemotaxis Angiogenesis
EGF	Platelets Macrophages Keratinocytes	Epithelial cells Endothelial cells Fibroblasts	Proliferation Chemotaxis
IGF-I/Sm-c	Fibroblasts	Fibroblasts Endothelial cells	Cell replication Collagen synthesis
IL-1	Macrophages	Fibroblasts Neutrophils	Proliferation Collagenase synthesis Chemotaxis

TGF-β = transforming growth factor–beta; TGF-α = transforming growth factor–alpha; PDGF = platelet-derived growth factor; FGF = fibroblast growth factor; EGF = epidermal growth factor; IGF-I/Sm-c = insulin-like growth factor-I/somatomedin-C; IL-1 = interleukin-1.

oxygen radicals, which induce formation of chemotactic lipids from arachidonic acid by additional neutrophils and increase vascular permeability. Neutrophils last only a few hours. After they digest bacteria and necrotic tissue, the neutrophils die and liberate their intracellular content to form part of the wound exudate. Lymphocytes arrive next. The lymphocytes produce lymphokines, which have differing effects on vascular endothelial cells. Studies indicate that two populations of T cells are implicated in wound healing. The first is the population bearing the all-T-cell marker (OKT-11), which appears to be required for successful repair, as shown by the impairment caused by its depletion. The second population, the T-suppressor/cytotoxic subset, appears to play a counterregulatory role in wound healing; depletion of these cells enhances wound breaking strength.

As the number of wound neutrophils begins to decline, the macrophage population increases, replacing the neutrophil as the predominant phagocyte. Although the role of the macrophages once was believed to be exclusively phagocytic, in the last 20 years evidence has demonstrated their central role in wound healing. It is known that macrophages actively participate in at least three aspects of tissue remodeling; they are a source of (1) growth factors for fibroblasts and other mesenchymal cells; (2) angiogenic factors involved in neovascularization of the healing wound; and (3) factors that modulate the production of proteins in the connective tissue matrix by other cells within the local environment. Activated wound macrophages release multiple cytokines (Table 1-1). A partial list includes TGF-β, PDGF, interleukin-1 (IL-1), transforming growth factor–alpha (TGF-α), tumor necrosis factor (TNF), platelet-activating factor (PAF), and fibroblast growth factor (FGF).

Cellular Proliferation

Cellular proliferation involves fibroblast proliferation and angiogenesis.

Fibroblast Proliferation

Fibroblasts become the predominant cells by the end of the first week of healing. They originate from nearby connective tissue cells. The stimulus for subsequent fibroblast mitosis, proliferation, and collagen synthesis appears to be growth factors. The fibroblasts migrate into the wound, forming adhesive contact with the fibrin strands from the initial wound clot and with collagen fibers and fibronectin. The fibroblast activity depends on the adequacy of the local oxygen supply. The fibroblasts proliferate and migrate along the fibronectin, crossing the wound and establishing a lattice for collagen synthesis.

Angiogenesis

Angiogenesis is required to restore the blood flow. The wound surface is relatively ischemic, and healing cannot be competent until sufficient blood flow is reinstalled to allow transfer of oxygen and nutrients. Angiogenesis becomes prominent by approximately the fourth day postinjury and is stimulated at least in part by angiogenic factors secreted by macrophages. These factors exhibit a chemoattractant effect for mesothelial and endothelial cells. Once endothelial cells proliferate, they form capillary buds at the wound surface. Tissue plasminogen activator and collagenase originate from the capillary buds, allowing cellular invasion into surrounding poorly vascularized tissue. The buds build a network of loops that join other buds to form a new capillary bed. Red cells and plasma begin to circulate into the new microvessels. Depending on the metabolic requirements of the wound, the new capillaries remodel, regressing with time after healing as evidenced by a decrease in the erythema of the scar.

Epithelization

Epithelization begins within hours after injury with the movement of epithelial cells from the edge of the tissue across the defect, after activation by growth factors released from platelets and, later, macrophages. The epithelial cells at the wound edge lose their apical basal polarity and extend pseudopodia from their free basolateral side into the wound. Once a single layer of cells has migrated, additional layers develop from mitotic division of the epidermal cells. The epithelization process depends on the size of the defect, nutrient supply, number of remaining basal cells, and wound milieu.

Matrix Formation

Collagen

Collagen is the ultimate product of fibroblasts; its presence results in the development of wound strength. The stimulus for the fibroblast to produce collagen consists of a combination of a high tissue lactate level, adequate oxygen levels, and growth factors, especially TGF-β released from macrophages and platelets. The fundamental unit of polymerized collagen is tropocollagen. This unit has a high content of proline and lysine, which subsequently are hydroxylated and converted into alpha chains. This hydroxylation is the most important step in intracellular collagen synthesis and requires oxygen, alpha-ketoglutarate, iron, and vitamin C. Once formed the alpha chains interact and intertwine to form a triple helix called procollagen, which is glycosylated, secreted from the fibroblasts into the extracellular milieu, and assembled into collagen fibers by subsequent polymerization and cross linking. The rate of collagen synthesis is maximal in the first 2 weeks, and collagen deposition reaches a maximum within 3 to 4 weeks. The type of collagen deposited at the wound site differs with time. In the first hours types IV and V are predominant, whereas type III is noted at 24 hours. By 60 hours type I is predominant, and moderate amounts of types III and IV are still present.

Fibronectin

Fibronectin is produced by a variety of cells, including fibroblasts, endothelial cells, and platelets. During the formation of granulation tissue, fibronectin provides a provisional substratum for the migration and ingrowth of cells, binding macromolecules including collagen, fibrin, heparin, and proteoglycans. Fibronectin also acts as a template for collagen deposition and plays a role in matrix formation. This protein additionally contributes to the debridement of wounds and later remodeling—it has been shown to possess opsonic activity for macrophages and fibroblasts.

Ground Substance

Ground substance is composed of glycosaminoglycans, proteoglycans, and mucoproteins produced by fibroblasts and other mesenchymal cells with the addition of water and electrolytes. Proteoglycans are the major components. The ground substance acts to support and allow organization of the newly made collagen and cells.

Collagen Remodeling

Collagen remodeling, the last phase of the repair process, begins approximately 3 weeks after injury and may persist for months to years. During remodeling of scar tissue, new collagen fibers are laid down and others are digested and removed. The wound remodeling is the result of increased collagen cross linking, the breaking down of excess collagen by collagenase, and regression in wound vascularity. Collagenase, a zinc-containing metalloprotease, is the major enzyme responsible for degrading collagen types I, II, and III. This enzyme cleaves the mature collagen molecule across all alpha helical chains and yields products that are suitable for further cleavage by a variety of other proteases. It has been determined that fibroblasts and macrophages are the sources of collagenase during the repair of healing. The collagenase activity and the process of continued collagen deposition are in equilibrium with remodeling; there is no final net gain in collagen.

Wound Contraction

In the process of wound contraction, a full-thickness wound is gradually covered by peripheral skin that moves toward the center of the defect. It is important to emphasize that contraction involves movement of existing tissue at the wound edge, not formation of new tissue. Previously it was thought that contraction was caused by shortening of collagen fibers or by actin fibers in myofibroblasts. Today it is known that contraction is mediated by fibroblasts moving along collagen fibers, causing the collagen fibers to move together. Although some fibroblasts morphologically become myofibroblasts with very visible actin filaments, all fibroblasts can participate in this process. For wound contraction to proceed normally, therefore, the integrity of the cell mass immediately underlying the wound margins must be preserved. The process continues for weeks to months and can lead to pathologic contractures. Humans are "tight-skinned," meaning the skin adheres to underlying skeletal muscle. Although contraction is important, much healing, especially in chronic scarring and

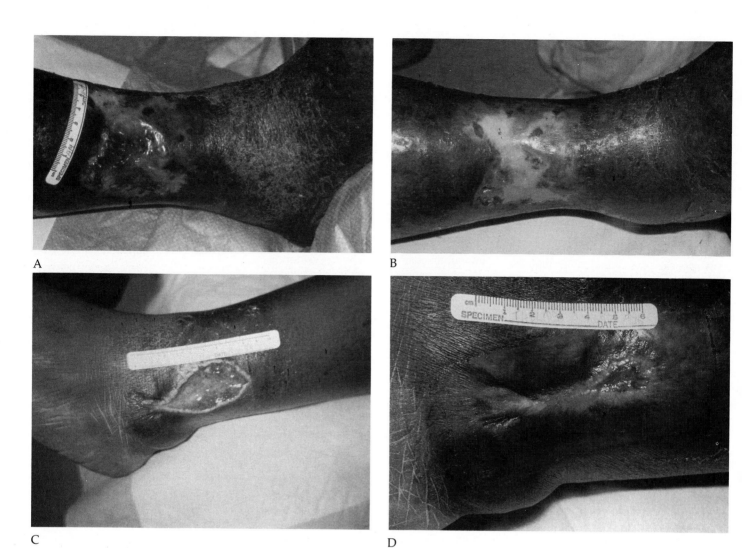

A

B

C

D

Fig. 1-2A. Patient with open wound on leg.
B. The same wound after healing without
contraction. C. Patient with open wound on leg.
D. The same wound after healing with
contraction. (From S.T. Ahn, W.W. Monafo, and
T.A. Mustoe. Topical silicone gel: A new
treatment for hypertrophic scars. Surgery 106:
781, 1989. Reproduced with permission.)

in the lower leg, is caused by reepitheli-zation over a noncontracting wound. Healing with and without contraction is illustrated in Figure 1-2.

Wound Strength

The concept of wound strength was in-troduced to aid in the evaluation of the progress and adequacy of both clinical and experimental repair. The two most common measures of wound strength in tissues are tensile strength and breaking strength. *Tensile strength* is a measure of load applied per unit of cross-sectional area (kg/mm^2). *Breaking strength* is a mea-sure of the force required to break a wound without regard to its dimensions. In the first 3 days after wounding, the gain in tensile strength is caused by the fibrin clot that fills the wound cavity. From days 3 to 30, the gain in tensile strength correlates with the rate of col-lagen synthesis. At 2 weeks, tensile

strength is approximately 10 percent of the final tensile strength achieved; it in-creases to about 25 percent by weeks 3 to 4. After this period the production of col-lagen decreases, but the tensile strength continues to increase. The increasing strength over time is the result of further cross linking and remodeling of collagen. After several months the wound reaches 70 to 80 percent of normal skin strength (Fig. 1-3) but is never as strong as un-wounded skin; therefore, the choice of suture for closure is critical. At one week the strength of an incision is less than 5 percent that of unwounded skin. At 2 to 3 weeks, however (the time in which polyglactin 910, polyglycolic acid, and polyglyconate lose their tensile strength), the wounds are still very weak, and if there is any tension the scars spread. Studies have demonstrated a lack of ben-efit to using dermal polyglycolic acid su-tures compared to cutaneous sutures

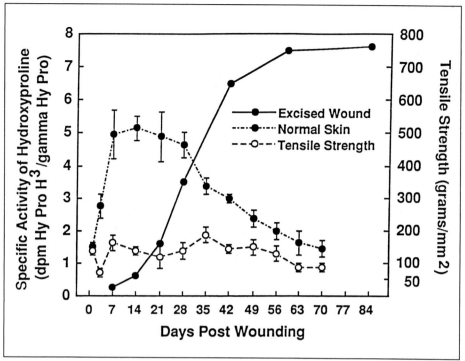

Fig. 1-3. *Comparison of new collagen deposition and tensile strength in skin wounds in rats. Relation of the rate of collagen synthesis to the tensile strength of skin wounds in rats. (From J.W. Madden and E.E. Peacock, Jr. Surgery 64:288, 1968; Tensile strength curve taken from S.M. Levenson, et al. The healing of rat skin wounds. Ann. Surg. 161:293, 1965. Reproduced with permission.)*

alone. There is, however, some advantage to using polydioxanone (PDS), which retains its tensile strength for up to 6 weeks. A subcuticular monofilament left for 6 months results in the narrowest scars.

Growth Factors

A polypeptide growth factor is an agent promoting cell proliferation that interacts with an external receptor to prepare the cell for DNA synthesis and division. Growth factors are also chemoattractants that recruit macrophages and fibroblasts for the injured area. Almost all growth factors are named after the target cell or source that led to their discovery. These polypeptides are produced by different cells and have different targets, resulting in different actions (see Table 1-1). The action of growth factors on cells is mediated by cell surface receptors that show high affinity binding. The growth factors contribute to the initiation, expression, and termination of the inflammatory response.

Basic Principles
Surgical Technique

Surgical technique is an important and controllable factor that has a major influence on wound healing. Minimal scar formation and maximal camouflage are most likely to result when incisions are made parallel to the skin tension lines described by Kraisi and Conway. Persistent inflammation—whether caused by delayed healing, as in deep second-degree burns not grafted; secondary to irritation or infection, as in pierced earlobes; or caused by hematoma that has produced capsular contractures after breast augmentation—leads to increased scarring. Thus meticulous hemostasis, gentle handling of tissue, and judicious use of buried sutures cannot be overemphasized. Electrocoagulation, although useful, causes a zone of necrosis beyond the site of coagulation. The bipolar cautery delivers current only between the two tips; it is often favored because the zone of necrosis is smaller after the more precise delivery of current.

Obliteration of dead space is achieved more effectively by suction drains than by multiple buried sutures.

Blood Supply

Impairment of the blood supply with resulting tissue hypoxia causes severe impairment of healing even if not sufficient to cause tissue necrosis. Neutrophil function is impaired, leading to greatly increased susceptibility to infection. Local perfusion can decrease because of excessive skin tension, constricting sutures, or local infection and is probably at least as common a problem as inadequate flap blood supply.

Sutures

The selection of suture material and the placement of sutures determine the quality of subsequent repair. All suture material is foreign to the tissue and evokes an inflammatory reaction, even if it is monofilamentous, in the zone of necrosis around the suture. One should use as little suture material as possible, therefore, to close a wound. Studies in animals and humans have shown that an intense and prolonged tissue reaction to sutures can lead to delayed wound healing, infection, and dehiscence. Other than evoking an inflammatory response, however, no sutures available today affect the normal progress of healing. Suture selection should be based on the biologic healing properties of the tissue, the physical and biologic properties of the suture material, and the condition of the wound being closed. Today there are many suture materials available for wound closure.

Polyglycolic Acid

Polyglycolic acid (Dexon) is a synthetic absorbable suture. The material produces a low tissue reactivity and is absorbed by hydrolysis. Animal studies have demonstrated that polyglycolic acid is absorbed completely in 90 to 120 days, but tensile strength half-life is only 2 weeks. Polyglycolic acid sutures should not be used in wounds with bacterial contamination, because the braided configuration of the suture may potentiate infection. Studies have shown that scar widening is just as great with polyglycolic acid as with cutaneous sutures alone removed at 7 days; therefore, a subcuticular closure has no advantage over skin sutures that are removed before suture tracks form.

Polyglactin

Polyglactin (Vicryl) is another synthetic suture with a braided configuration that produces a low tissue reactivity. Polyglactin is absorbed in 60 to 90 days and maintains its tensile strength for about 2 weeks. Polyglycolic acid and polyglactin are useful, because of their relative lack of reactivity, for lining up dermis, but they do "spit" with inflammation and have the potential for scar formation. Because they do not prevent scar widening, however, their use as buried sutures should not be indiscriminate.

Polydioxanone

Polydioxanone (PDS) is a monofilamentous absorbable suture that is absorbed by hydrolysis and is minimally reactive. Studies in animals have demonstrated that the suture is absorbed in 120 to 180 days. The material retains considerable breaking strength for 6 weeks and therefore is useful as a buried cutaneous suture in unwounded skin, allowing widening to occur. Because polydioxanone is a monofilamentous suture, there is less affinity for bacteria. Because the sutures are so slowly absorbed, suture spitting is a problem.

Polyglyconate

Polyglyconate (Maxon), another monofilamentous suture absorbed after 180 days, has the same advantages as polydioxanone but retains its tensile strength for only about 3 weeks.

Polypropylene

A monofilamentous nonabsorbable suture with minimal inflammatory reaction, polypropylene, e.g., Prolene, is an ideal suture for a running intradermal stitch because it slides well and can be removed easily.

Staples

During the last few years, staples have been used widely in cutaneous operations. The advantage is speed. In addition, animal studies have demonstrated that staples induce less inflammatory response than sutures and that stapled and sutured wounds have similar mechanical strength for up to 21 days. If the skin edges are coapted carefully and the staples are removed before leaving marks, the scar can be equivalent to all but the most precisely coapted sutured incision.

Optimal wound closure involves meticulous tissue coaptation, minimization of trauma to tissue and of foreign bodies, and prevention of hematoma through obliteration of dead space. The last is accomplished best by suction drains or passive drains. Use of dermal sutures should be kept to a minimum for proper tissue coaptation unless they are needed to provide prolonged dermal support, in these instances the appropriate suture material is important.

Impaired Wound Healing

Irradiation

The detrimental effects of ionizing radiation on skin and wound healing have been observed clinically and experimentally. These effects appear to be caused by injury to DNA produced by high-energy electrons. Rapidly dividing cells are the ones most affected. Radiation is thought to prevent mitotic division and conversion of mesenchymal cells into fibroblasts. In experimental animals, a loss of wound breaking strength of more than 50 percent is seen after electron beam surface radiation is used. The acute effects are equivalent to those of a clinical therapeutic dose. Over time, the radiation effect leads to fibrosis with decreased vascularity and resultant tissue hypoxia. Wounds in irradiated tissue can be extraordinarily difficult to treat.

Immunosuppression

Bone marrow suppression, most often caused by chemotherapeutic agents, can produce increased susceptibility to wound infection if the neutrophils are suppressed. Slow healing caused by a drop in circulating monocytes coincides with poor nutrition owing to the gastrointestinal effects of the drugs. Experimentally, multiple agents that cause bone marrow suppression decrease healing, but within 2 or 3 weeks after chemotherapy, there is no wound healing deficit. Clinically if the bone marrow is recovering, healing should be affected minimally.

Steroids

Adrenocortical steroids have immunosuppressive and anti-inflammatory properties and are well established as agents that inhibit wound healing. Steroids produce a marked decrease in the inflammatory phase by inhibiting release of arachidonic acid products, inhibiting macrophage migration, and altering neutrophil function. Additionally these agents inhibit the synthesis of procollagen by fibroblasts and delay wound contraction. Lymphocytic T-cell function is also altered by steroids, affecting cell-mediated immunity. Systemic steroids reduce the tensile strength of closed wounds, retard epithelization and angiogenesis, and interfere with wound contraction. Patients chronically taking steroids have a considerably thinner dermis than normal, with less collagen, and their healing is greatly impaired, requiring extra measures to prevent wound dehiscence.

Malnutrition

Although wounds are high priority areas for available nutrients, any element of malnutrition or severe stress producing a catabolic state negatively affects the healing process. Recent weight loss of 10 percent or more of body mass increases wound complications.

Protein Deficiency

Protein deficiency prolongs the inflammatory phase and fibroplasia and adversely affects angiogenesis, matrix formation, and wound remodeling. Clinically a patient with a plasma albumin level less than 3.0 g/dl, indicating malnutrition, is at greatly increased risk for wound breakdown; elective operations such as pressure closure should be delayed until an adequate nutritional balance is achieved. Although malnutrition is important to diagnose, there are no single reliable studies. Albumin level is a good indicator of malnutrition but does not drop quickly in acute catabolic states and is slow to rise after nutritional recovery. Serum transferrin levels also can be useful, as can skinfold measurements, but they also are not diagnostic.

Vitamins

Some vitamins play a role in the repair process. Vitamin A appears to be necessary for the stimulation of fibroplasia, collagen cross linking, and epithelization. In animals, vitamin A reverses the wound deficit induced by glucocorticoids by restoring the inflammatory process. It may be useful clinically in this situation or in patients with a depressed inflammatory response, used either topically or systemically; however, there are no conclusive data from studies in humans. Vitamin C is a cofactor in the hydroxylation of lysine and proline in collagen synthesis. It also is required for neutrophil superoxide production and killing of bacteria. Deficiencies of these vitamins affect the specific steps in the processes in which they are required. Clinically scurvy is not seen, except in rare cases. The role of vitamin E remains unclear.

Essential Fatty Acids

Delayed wound healing has been demonstrated in patients receiving long-term essential fatty acid–free, fat-free intravenous nutrition. Rectification of the fatty acid deficiency results in prompt healing, demonstrating a role for essential fatty acids in wound healing.

Zinc

Zinc is a cofactor in a large number of enzyme systems, including RNA and DNA polymerase, which are involved in protein synthesis and, consequently, in wound healing. Serum zinc levels lower than 100 mg/deciliter are related to impaired healing. Rectification of this deficiency results in normal healing. Zinc deficiency as a cause of impaired healing is uncommon, however, unless there is general malnutrition.

Copper

Copper is indispensable for the production of covalent cross linking of collagen fibrils. A copper deficiency produces healing impairment, although this state is rarely seen clinically. The overall nutritional status and recent food intake have a great influence on the final outcome of wound healing.

Aging

Studies have consistently shown that most instances of wound dehiscence occur in older patients. There are age-dependent differences in wound healing that cause a suboptimal response in the elderly. The inflammatory response declines with age, which unquestionably causes some of the alteration in healing. The proliferative phase maturation and remodeling of collagen also are modified with age. Events begin later, proceed more slowly, and often do not reach the level they would if the patient were younger. Hypertrophic scarring is virtually unknown in the elderly, and multiple studies have documented in vitro

the decreased proliferative capacity of dermal fibroblasts and epithelial cells in the aged. Although the decreased proliferation leads to good scars, healing is sometimes dramatically depressed because of malnutrition or other risk factors. Sutures must be left in much longer, but suture marks are not a problem because of the decreased epithelial proliferation along suture tracks.

Ischemia

Even moderate ischemia, experimentally compatible with tissue survival, produces not only severe impairment in granulation tissue and extracellular matrix synthesis but also a dramatic increase in susceptibility to infection, owing to neutrophil dependence on oxygen for its bactericidal effects. Examples of conditions that can cause local ischemia and hypoxia include atherosclerosis, diabetes, vasculitis, excessive fibrosis in chronic ulcers, connective tissue disorders, and irradiation. In considering an operation for a nonhealing ulcer, the first question should be: Is the local tissue oxygenation adequate to support healing? Doppler ultrasonography, tissue oximetry, and angiography all can be helpful, but the judgment is often clinical.

Agents to Augment Healing

Historically no pharmacologic agents have been available to speed wound repair. The recent understanding of the biochemical and physiologic aspects of wound healing has initiated a new phase in the management of this process. The availability of agents to manipulate wound healing is the most important recent advance in this field.

Growth Factors

The discovery of growth factors in the wound healing environment, the understanding of their role, their purification, and now their availability have brought about the possibility of using them to augment wound repair. PDGF and TGF-β are both present in large amounts in macrophages and platelets. Interest has centered on these two factors and on epidermal growth factor (EGF) and fibroblast growth factor (FGF). Growth factors have been shown by different mechanisms to influence positively the process of wound

healing. TGF-β accelerates normal and reverses deficient incisional wound repair. This growth factor has multiple effects, such as in vivo stimulation of granulation tissue synthesis and extracellular matrix synthesis, and inhibition of matrix degradation. In addition, TGF-β stimulates the synthesis of other growth factors. Studies in rats have demonstrated that the tensile strength of incisional wounds treated locally with TGF-β is increased. TGF-β reverses the deficit in wound healing induced in lathyritic rats treated with glucocorticoids, doxorubicin hydrochloride (Adriamycin), and total body irradiation.

PDGF is a potent chemoattractant for neutrophils, monocytes, and fibroblasts. It stimulates the synthesis of fibronectin, collagenase, and additional growth factors in vitro and accelerates reepithelization and formation of granulation tissue in vivo. The topical application of PDGF to incisional wounds in rats causes a striking cellular influx soon after wounding and an increase in tensile strength beginning 5 days after wounding that lasts for more than 7 weeks. PDGF also reverses the deficit in wound healing of rats with streptozotocin-induced diabetes mellitus, surface irradiation, and lathyrism. EGF is a chemotactic and mitogenic factor. Studies in animals demonstrated acceleration of the rate of epidermal repair after topical application of EGF. In human donors, skin graft sites have been demonstrated to heal 2 days faster than sites on controls. This factor has been shown to reverse the glucocorticoid-induced inhibition of wound healing. FGF is a potent mitogen for endothelial cells and angiogenic factor. When injected into incisional wounds on rats, FGF increases the tensile strength and enhances vascularity and deposition of collagen. Recent studies demonstrated that FGF reverses the incisional healing impairment in rats with streptozotocin-induced diabetes mellitus (STZ-DM). TGF-α is a mitogenic factor that, like EGF, accelerates epidermal repair. Clinical trials are planned for TGF-β, PDGF, and EGF.

The therapeutic potential for using growth factors to improve normal and impaired wound healing is immense. The synergism that may be obtained by combining different growth factors will provide critical and integral management of wound healing problems.

Growth Hormone

Growth hormone (GH) is an anabolic hormone that influences the wound repair process. Methionyl–human growth hormone (met-hGH), a synthetic protein that is biologically equipotent with pituitary-derived hGH, has been used in animals. Intramuscular application of this compound enhances wound breaking strength in healthy rats. Studies in humans have demonstrated that the systemic administration of met-hGH augments wound healing. It appears that the action of GH is mediated by somatomedins. The somatomedins represent a family of growth hormone–dependent, insulin-like growth factors (IGFs) that stimulate replication of human fibroblasts in vitro. Patients who have suffered severe trauma or burns and elderly patients have decreased spontaneous secretion of GH. Administration of growth hormone could benefit these patients dramatically.

Electrical Charges

It has been known for a number of years that the wound healing environment possesses electrical potentials. During the first days after wounding, the electrical potentials over the wound are positive. They become negatively charged after the fourth day of healing and remain negative until healing is complete. Electrical stimulation in various forms has been shown to enhance the healing of wounds in both humans and animals, but these findings are controversial. Although the mechanism by which electrotherapy stimulates healing is unknown, in vitro studies have shown that electrical currents influence the migration and proliferation of fibroblasts and increase the expression of receptors for TGF-β on human dermal fibroblasts. Recently electromagnetic effects in tissue repair have been evaluated in animals by the application of charged beads directly to the wound, to produce an electromagnetic field. It was shown that positively charged beads increase the tensile strength of wounds. The mechanisms by which electrical fields influence would repair are likely to be related to the recruitment of macrophages, which then promote healing, releasing cytokines. This postulate is based on the fact that a variety of cell types react to a charged environment in vitro, including macrophages, which migrate toward the anode. The application of positively charged particles in normal and impaired wounds constitutes a new strategy to speed wound repair.

Arginine

The amino acid arginine has been shown recently to be an essential nutrient for healing and survival in injured rats. Studies performed in animals have demonstrated that dietary supplementation of arginine accelerates wound tissue repair. The addition of supplemental arginine to the diet of wounded animals increases collagen deposition and augments tensile strength of healing skin incisions. Recently it has been demonstrated that dietary supplementation with arginine increases the accumulation of collagen in wounded human skin. Although the exact mechanism by which arginine enhances collagen production is not known, several hypotheses have been formulated. Arginine from ornithine production is a metabolic precursor for proline and hydroxyproline and in that manner stimulates collagen production. Acting as a secretagogue on the pituitary gland, arginine stimulates the growth hormone, which has been shown to enhance wound healing. Whatever the mechanism by which arginine promotes wound healing, the final pathway involves increased collagen production.

Vitamin A

Retinoids have been associated with wound healing. For example, it has been demonstrated that vitamin A deficiency retards wound repair. Although it is known that vitamin A stimulates various aspects of wound repair, such as inflammation, fibrosis, and collagen synthesis, the exact mechanism is not fully understood. Animal studies have demonstrated that local or systemic administration of vitamin A makes wounds stronger and increases the deposition of collagen. Specifically, retinoid stimulates wound healing retarded by anti-inflammatory steroids, diabetes, and irradiation.

Zinc

Several studies have indicated that wound healing is impaired when serum zinc levels are low and that restoration of normal levels restores the wound healing rate. Animal studies suggest that zinc has a favorable effect on the inflammatory phase of the wound healing process; acts as a cofactor for collagenase, the enzyme responsible for regulation of collagenolysis; and is involved directly in protein synthesis as a cofactor for at least 18 other metalloenzymes. An observational study in humans showed that oral zinc therapy can accelerate wound healing in patients with corticosteroid-related delays in wound healing. It has been demonstrated that zinc is absorbed from excisional wounds when applied topically. Experiments have indicated that topically absorbed zinc from wounds promotes wound healing in both zinc-deficient and zinc-sufficient rats.

Hyperbaric Oxygen

The clinical usefulness of hyperbaric oxygen is unproved despite its widespread use. Animal studies that attempted to demonstrate the beneficial effects of this therapy have had contradictory results. The mechanism of action of hyperbaric oxygen therapy is believed to be through the delivery of dissolved oxygen to hypoxic tissue. Oxygen increases the ability of neutrophils to phagocytize bacteria and to promote fibroblast proliferation, collagen synthesis, and neovascularization. Possible variables in the treatment include the interval between the operation and the beginning of treatment, the duration of each exposure, the frequency of the atmospheric pressure administered, and the overall duration of treatment. Up until now the values of these variables have been empirically chosen. Supplemental oxygen therapy is used to improve healing of wounds associated with an ischemic environment.

Excessive Scarring

A functional and aesthetically pleasing scar is the goal of all plastic surgeons. The normal consequence of the wound healing process, the scar, depends on the equilibrium between synthesis and degradation of collagen. When this equilibrium is shifted toward collagen synthesis, the end result is a greater accumulation of collagen, which initiates excessive scarring. Keloids and hypertrophic scars (HS) are benign overgrowths of scar tissue that represent different presentations in the spectrum of abnormal scarring. Keloids grow beyond the borders of the original wound and infrequently resolve spontaneously, whereas HS remain within the original boundaries and tend to regress partially.

Etiology

The lack of an animal model on which excessive scarring can be reproduced and studied represents a formidable difficulty for the elucidation of the causes of this pathologic process. The information available has been obtained from descriptions of scarring in humans. Although a specific causative factor has not been identified, there are several postulates regarding abnormal scarring.

Ischemia
Lactate produced during ischemia stimulates fibroblasts to synthesize collagen. Opposing this theory, however, is the fact that ischemia usually does not cause keloid formation. Most keloids occur in wounds that cannot be demonstrated to cause scarring, and ischemia depresses normal healing.

Mechanical Forces
Studies have demonstrated an increase in the production of collagen by fibroblasts under tension. Because keloids are often situated in areas of elevated skin tension, it is possible that these mechanical forces stimulate an excessive production of collagen in the area. Unfavorable to this theory is the high incidence of development of keloids localized in the earlobe, indicating the presence of other causative factors.

Immunologic Factors
Studies regarding the immunologic status of patients prone to keloids are controversial. Levels of immunoglobulins have been reported to be high, normal, or low in these patients, giving insufficient support to this postulate.

Mast Cell Involvement
Alteration in the distribution of mast cells throughout the dermis of keloids and the itching referred to by patients with keloids suggests an increased release of histamine by these cells, which is known to stimulate fibroblast replication.

Hormones
Epidemiologic studies have reported that keloid formation is prevalent during normal rapid growth stages, such as puberty and pregnancy, in which there are high levels of circulating hormones, and in abnormal growth states, such as acromegaly, in which there are high levels of GH. The high incidence of keloid formation among the black population, the absence of keloids in albinos, and the favorable clinical response to corticosteroid therapy support a possible role for melanocyte-stimulating hormone (MSH) in the genesis of keloids.

Growth Factor
Available information on the role of growth factors in the genesis of keloids is limited. Requirements for polypeptide growth factors appear to be abnormal in keloids.

In conclusion, there is more than one triggering factor in the formation of keloids. The proliferation of theories indicates our lack of understanding of the etiology of this process, which is undoubtedly multifactorial.

Features of Keloids and Hypertrophic Scars

Keloids
Ultrastructurally keloids are more disorganized than HS. Keloids have inadequately formed collagen bundles that have irregular fibers haphazardly connected. Keloids have broad eosinophilic refractile collagen fibers organized in swirls. Early lesions contain a rich, vascularized stroma and profuse mucinous material with mild acanthosis in the epidermis. Late lesions are more hyalinized and present less vasculature; epidermal atrophy may be present. Fibroblast density and activity are increased in keloids, but true myofibroblasts are not present in this lesion.

Hypertrophic Scars
Hypertrophic scars have less mucinous material and fewer eosinophilic collagen fibers than do keloids. They contain collagen bundles that run parallel to the epithelial surface and have loosely arranged, shortened, and fragmented wavy fibers.

Chemical analysis of collagen has demonstrated that proline and hydroxyproline activity is more prominent in keloids and HS than in unscarred skin, suggesting an increased rate of collagen biosynthesis. The presence of alpha-1-antitrypsin and alpha-2-macroglobulin has been demonstrated in the interstitial spaces of abnormal scars. The second inhibits collagenase, which is the most important enzyme in collagen degradation.

Most normal skin collagen is type I. There is a greater proportion of type III collagen in keloids and HS, suggesting a failure of normal scar maturation. Activity levels of lysine oxidase, which is the cross-linking enzyme, is increased in keloids and HS. All the features that differentiate keloids from HS give little insight into the etiology of either, which is probably multifactorial.

Treatment

No single therapeutic method has been effective consistently in the treatment of keloids and HS. A combination of treatments is the most accepted approach.

Surgery
Surgical treatment of excessive scarring begins with prevention. Good surgical technique with rapid healing and reduction of inflammation (minimizing foreign bodies and tissue necrosis in suture) and considering all the fundamental principles is absolutely essential to prevent abnormal scarring.

Keloids. Surgical therapy alone is futile because of the high recurrence rate (55 to 100%). Surgical intervention in conjunction with other treatments, however, most often steroid injection, usually is successful. The main role of surgical treatment is to remove the affected area, rendering the skin more amenable to adjuvant therapy. Intralesional excision is recommended to avoid extension of the scar beyond the confines of the original wound.

Hypertrophic Scars. In contrast to keloids, HS often respond well to surgical treatment alone. The objective of excisional scar revision is to redirect the scar along the resting skin tension lines. Postoperative occlusion with silicone gel may prove to be useful.

Laser Therapy
Early studies of laser therapy showed encouraging anecdotal results, but later reports show a success rate of less than 30 percent. The use of laser therapy for either keloids or HS cannot be supported.

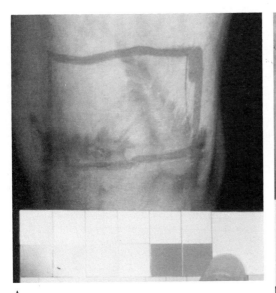

A

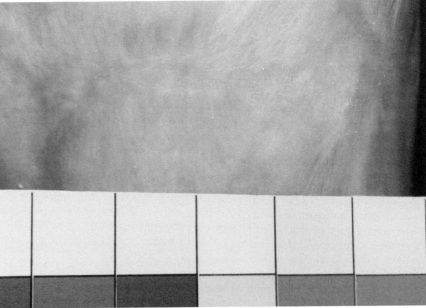

B

Fig. 1-4. Treatment of a popliteal scar for 8 months with elastic compression without improvement. A. Before treatment. B. Two months after treatment. (From S.T. Ahn, W.W. Monafo, and T.A. Mustoe. Arch. Surg. 126:499, 1991. Copyright 1991, American Medical Association. Reproduced with permission.)

Pressure

Pressure, which is known to cause thinning of the dermis, is an accepted noninvasive, adjunctive, and prophylactic treatment. Although the mechanism is poorly understood, it is well known that the body responds to mechanical forces with directed collagen synthesis, which presumably occurs in soft tissue and bone, perhaps by secondarily generated electrical fields. Most reports agree that the pressure necessary to exceed the inherent capillary pressure is at least 24 mmHg. The pressure should not be discontinued for more than 3 hours per day and should be maintained for 6 months to 2 years. Both keloids and HS respond to this therapy, especially after surgical excision. Natural examples are often seen of reduction in scar hypertrophy under a belt or bra strap, giving credence to the importance of pressure.

Radiation

Radiation has no role in benign HS. The potential problem of late development of malignant tumors has limited the use of radiation except as a last resort for the most disfiguring keloids. Most effective in the early phases of healing, radiation acts by limiting the proliferative capacity of local fibroblasts. Radiation accompanied by a surgical procedure is more effective than radiation alone. The recommended total dose varies from 250 to 2000 rad, repeated over a week's time for up to a year. Studies advocating the use of radiation are hampered by a lack of long-term follow-up data. It is possible that ra-

diation merely delays the reappearance of keloids.

Steroids

It is well known that corticosteroids inhibit wound healing. Causing decreased collagen production and increased collagen degradation, intralesional steroids are the first line of treatment of keloids and in responsive lesions can obviate the need for surgical intervention. The suggested dosage of steroids varies depending on the patient's age and the size of the lesion. Injections are repeated once a month for 4 to 6 months. The most common side effects are atrophy, depigmentation, and telangiectasia, all reversible. Success rates vary depending on the age of the patient and the duration of the scar. Lesions present for less than 2 years respond better than older lesions.

Retinoic Acid

Anecdotal reports claim improvement of wounds after the topical application of retinoic acid. Although this is a promising drug, its current use is investigational.

Silicone Gel

The use of silicone gel is a new, effective strategy for the treatment of HS. Initial

studies demonstrated the efficacy of sheets of silicone gel in the treatment of HS (Figs. 1-4 to 1-6) and healing of surgical incisions. In contrast, efficacy in the treatment of keloids has not been clearly established. The mechanism of action of silicone gel is unknown, but the roles of pressure, temperature, and oxygen transmission have been ruled out. It is thought that the gel reduces the inflammation and, possibly, secondary edema. Silicone gel has been approved by the United States Food and Drug Administration for clinical use on healed burn scars. The indications for treatment, such as age and race of patient, scar location, age of scar, incisional treatment, use in keloids, or use in association with other methods of treatment of scar hypertrophy, are still investigational.

Beta-aminopropionitrile Fumarate

Beta-aminopropionitrile fumarate (BAPN) interferes with normal collagen intramolecular and intermolecular cross linking, making the collagen more susceptible to the action of collagenase. BAPN has been used in clinical trials in conjunction with a surgical procedure and colchicine with good results. Because of its gener-

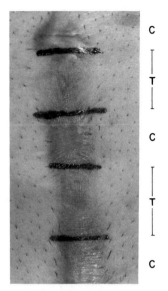

Fig. 1-5. Abdominal incision scar treated with silicone gel for 2 months. T = treated areas; C = control, nontreated areas. (From S.T. Ahn, W.W. Monafo, and T.A. Mustoe. Arch. Surg. 126:499, 1991. Copyright 1991, American Medical Association. Reproduced with permission.)

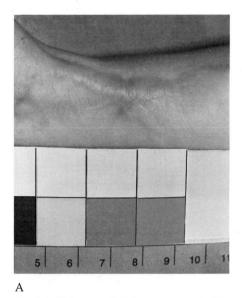 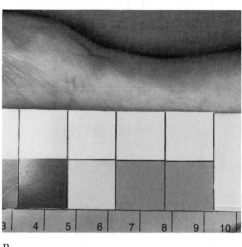

A B

Fig. 1-6. Wrist scar. A. Before treatment. B. Three months after treatment.

alized effects on collagen, long-term use of systemic BAPN is certainly not the solution to abnormal scarring.

Other Treatments

Other therapeutic agents have been proposed for the treatment of excessive scarring. They include interferon alpha-2b, zinc oxide, colchicine, penicillamine, antihistamines, and tetrahydroquinone; all require further investigation.

Fetal Healing

Clinical and experimental evidence has demonstrated that a fetus reacts to injury differently from a child or an adult. A midgestation human fetus heals by mesenchymal proliferation without clinically significant inflammatory cell participation but with tissue regeneration, rather than with tissue generation and scar formation as usually seen in adults. The process is accompanied by major differences in the extracellular matrix in fetal wounds including an increase in hyaluronic acid in fetuses compared with adults, which may be critical. This glycosaminoglycan is found in high concentration during embryogenesis and whenever rapid tissue

proliferation and regeneration occur. Amniotic fluid contains growth and trophic factors required for fetal development. This fluid might also contribute to the unique ability of a fetus to heal with little inflammation by producing a sterile fluid wound healing milieu. The absence of endogenous immunoglobulins in fetal wounds contrasts strongly with the situation in adult wounds at 12 and 24 hours, confirming earlier observations that fetal wounds heal without an inflammatory response. It has been demonstrated that PDGF increases the inflammatory response, fibroblast recruitment, and collagen deposition in fetal wounds, indicating that growth factors probably play a role in determining the markedly different cellular and extracellular events of fetal compared to adult wound repair. Unlocking the mechanisms by which fetal wounds heal by regeneration rather than scar formation is potentially of great importance for understanding wound healing and scar formation and reaching a goal of scarless healing.

Suggested Reading

Ahn, S.T., Monafo, W.W., and Mustoe, T.A. Topical silicone gel: A new treatment for hypertrophic scars. Surgery 106:781, 1989.

Bourne, R.B., Bitar, H., and Andreae, P.R. In-vivo comparison of four absorbable sutures: Vicryl, Dexon Plus, Maxon and PDS. Can. J. Surg. 31:43, 1988.

Clark, R.A.F., and Henson, P.M. (Eds.). The Molecular and Cellular Biology of Wound Repair. New York: Plenum, 1988.

Cromack, D.T., Porras-Reyes, B., and Mustoe, T.A. Current concepts in wound healing: Growth factors and macrophage interaction. J. Trauma. 30(12 Suppl.):S129, 1990.

Eaglstein, W.H. Wound healing and aging. Clin. Geriatr. Med. 5:183, 1989.

Khouri, R.K., and Mustoe, T.A. Trends in the treatment of hypertrophic scar. Adv. Plast. Reconstr. Surg. 8:129, 1992.

Longaker, M.T., Harrison, M.R., Crombleholme, T.M., et al. Studies in fetal wound healing. I. A factor in fetal serum that stimulates deposition of hyaluronic acid. J. Pediatr. Surg. 24:789, 1989.

Madden, J.W., and Peacock, E.E. Studies on the biology of collagen during wound healing. I. Rate of collagen synthesis and deposition in cutaneous wounds of the rat. Surgery 64:288, 1968.

Mustoe, T.A., Pierce, G.F., Thomason, A., et al. Accelerated healing of incisional wounds in rats induced by transforming growth factor-β. Science 237:1333, 1987.

Peacock, E.E. Wound Repair (3rd ed.). Philadelphia: Saunders, 1972.

Peacock, E.E., and Cohen, I.K. Wound Healing. In J.G. McCarthy (Ed.), Plastic Surgery. Philadelphia: Saunders, 1990. Pp. 161–185.

Rudolph, R., and Miller, S.H. (Eds.). Wound Healing. Clinics in Plastic Surgery. Vol. 17, no. 3. Philadelphia: Saunders, 1990.

2

Basic Principles and Techniques in Plastic Surgery

Norman Weinzweig   Jeffrey Weinzweig

Surgery, trauma, and infection disrupt normal anatomy causing impairment of form and function secondary to scarring. Scarless healing is a phenomenon unique to the fetus; clinical and experimental work by Harrison, Siebert, and others has demonstrated that fetal wounds heal rapidly and without scar formation. Wound healing in newborn infants and adults, however, causes scarring regardless of the cause of the wound or the surgical technique applied for repair.

The final appearance of a scar depends on a number of intrinsic and extrinsic factors. These factors include the age and race of the patient; the mechanism, location, type, and extent of injury; the tendency toward keloid formation and hypertrophic scarring; the inherent healing ability of the patient; and the mechanical factors of repair and reconstruction. Although some of these factors are beyond the surgeon's control, most of them can be influenced by appropriate planning, adherence to surgical principles and techniques, and effective postoperative management.

Mastery of these principles and techniques is critical if favorable surgical re-sults are to be achieved. Thorough knowledge of the biochemistry and the dynamics of wound healing, the physiology of tissue blood supply, the design of wound closure, the quality of the reparative tissues, and the bacteriologic management of wound contamination and infection are all essential for the surgeon.

Local and Regional Anesthesia

A large number of plastic surgical procedures, from simple excisional biopsies to aesthetic procedures, can be safely and efficaciously performed with the patient under local or regional anesthesia with or without sedation. The specific sensory nerves are anesthetized either by direct injection of a local anesthetic drug into the cutaneous and subcutaneous tissues at the operative site or by a regional block. The plastic surgeon should be familiar with the various anesthetic agents and their applications.

Dilute solutions of local anesthetic agents are effective because they are injected at their site of action. The drug is usually infiltrated fanwise from two points, one above and one below the operative site. Slow injection through a small-gauge needle minimizes pain. Local concentrations are therefore several orders of magnitude greater than the plasma concentrations after absorption. This allows relative safety when the drug is properly injected in the correct dose. There is a potential danger, however, if the drug is injected intravenously or an overdose is administered.

Even when large volumes of the anesthetic agent are required, the risk of toxicity is not high, especially if a vasoconstrictor such as epinephrine is used. Epinephrine is often combined with local anesthetic agents to improve anesthetic efficacy, increase the duration of anesthesia, and lessen systemic toxicity, while reducing bleeding during dissection through its vasoconstrictive effect. For any major infiltration, the epinephrine concentration should not exceed 1:200,000 to avoid severe vasoconstriction with possible local or even systemic effects. Epinephrine causes local vasoconstriction, slowing absorption with a reduction in peak concentration between 20 and 50 percent. One should allow 7 to 12

Table 2-1. Drug properties and dosages of the most commonly used local anesthetic agents

Drug	Brand name (manufacturer)	Onset	Duration (hours)	Maximal dose	Applications
Amides					
Lidocaine (lignocaine)	Xylocaine (Astra)	Rapid	1–2	300 mg or 4 mg/kg (500 mg or 7 mg/kg)*	All forms of regional anesthesia Topical anesthesia as 4%–10% solution
Mepivacaine	Carbocaine (Eastman Kodak)	Rapid	1.5–3	200 mg (300 mg)*	Similar to lidocaine but less toxic and 20% longer acting
Bupivacaine	Marcaine (Sanofi Winthrop)	Slow	4–8	175 mg (250 mg)*	Spinal and regional nerve blocks of long duration Less motor block at concentrations of 0.5% or less
Esters					
Tetracaine	Cetacaine (Cetylite)	Slow	3–10	100 mg or 1.5 mg/kg	Most commonly used in spinal anesthesia and for topical administration in pharynx and tracheobronchial tree
Cocaine	Cocaine (Astra)	Slow	1–2	200 mg or 3 mg/kg	Topical use in the nose and pharynx to decrease bleeding and shrink congested mucous membranes

* Maximal dose with addition of epinephrine.

minutes for the epinephrine to take effect or observe the wound for blanching.

One should avoid using local anesthesia when operating on apprehensive or uncooperative patients, on patients who have reacted unfavorably to the local anesthetic drug in the past, and on children in most instances. General anesthesia is usually recommended for such patients. Vasoconstrictors should not be used in procedures on tissues supplied by end arteries, such as the fingers, toes, ear, nose, and penis, or in operations on patients with systemic problems such as cardiac arrhythmias, hyperthyroidism, or hypertension.

In general, local anesthetic drugs have a common molecular structure and a similar mode of action. The currently available drugs differ with respect to potency, time of onset, duration, and toxicity. The choice of drug should be individualized to the patient's requirements (Table 2-1).

Local anesthetic agents have a three-part structure consisting of an aromatic ring, an intermediate chain, and an amino group. The intermediate chain contains either an ester (—COO—) or an amide (—NHCO—) linkage. Esters and amides differ in their route of metabolism, their chemical stability in solution, and their potential to cause allergic reactions. Esters are relatively unstable. They undergo rapid degradation by hydrolysis in solution and in the plasma by cholinesterase. Thus they have a relatively short shelf life, are difficult to sterilize because heat cannot be used, are relatively nontoxic, and have a brief duration of action. Allergic reactions are much more common with amino esters than with amides, but amides are much more stable than esters and are able to withstand heat and changes in pH. Because they are metabolized in the liver and are not broken down in the plasma, little or no drug is excreted unchanged.

Physiochemical Properties of Local Anesthetic Agents

Local anesthetic drugs produce sensory loss in a specific area of the body by reversibly blocking the propagation of action potentials in nerve fibers. They inhibit sodium conductance in a depolarizing axolemma by specific action on membrane permeability. By preventing the opening of sodium channels, these agents stabilize the nerve membrane, maintaining the fully polarized state and thus blocking nerve propagation. They decrease only the rate and degree of the depolarization phase of the action potential; thus the critical firing threshold of -55 mV is not achieved, and an action potential does not occur.

The intrinsic properties of any local anesthetic agent are based on lipid solubility, protein binding, pKa, diffusibility, and inherent vasodilator activity.

The potency of a local anesthetic drug is directly related to its lipid solubility. Because 90 percent of the axolemma is lipid, a highly lipid-soluble agent penetrates the nerve membrane rapidly and produces nerve blockage at a low concentration.

The duration of action of a local anesthetic agent is determined by its protein-binding characteristics. Because 10 percent of the axolemma is made up of protein, agents that penetrate the nerve membrane and attach firmly to the membrane proteins show prolonged activity.

The time of onset is related to the rate at which the local anesthetic agent diffuses across the nerve membrane. This is determined by the percentage of the drug existing in the uncharged base form. The ratio of uncharged base to charged cation depends on the specific pKa of the drug and the pH of the solution. A low tissue pH causes a high concentration of the charged cationic form, limiting diffusion across the axolemma. This factor explains the failure of local anesthetic agents in the presence of inflammation or infection.

Diffusibility of the local anesthetic agent through connective tissue or non-nervous barriers also affects the speed of onset.

All local anesthetic agents except for cocaine possess vasodilator activity. Vasodilatation increases vascular absorption, thus decreasing the potency and duration of action of a drug.

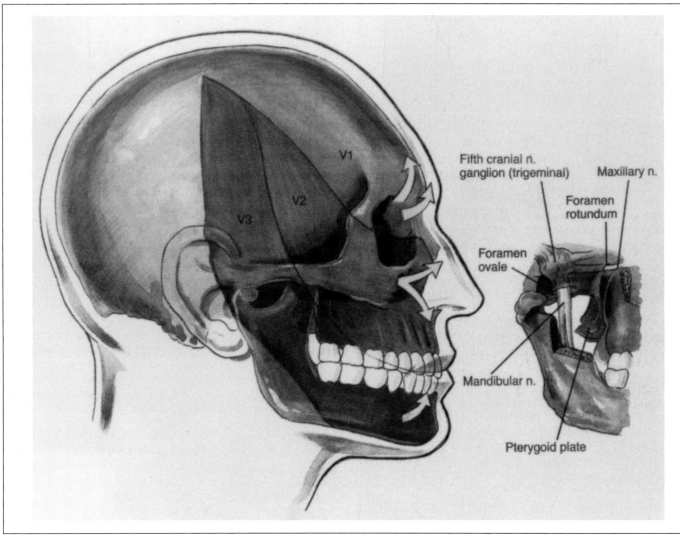

Fig. 2-1. *Fifth cranial nerve ganglion (trigeminal) anatomy—sensory innervation and peripterygoid relationships. (From D.L. Brown [Ed.],* Atlas of Regional Anesthesia. *Philadelphia: W.B. Saunders, 1992. Reproduced with permission.)*

Regional Blocks of the Head and Neck

Regional blocks are used successfully in various areas of the body. The key to success is a knowledge of the anatomy and landmarks of the nerve to be blocked. For the head and neck area, the applications of regional block anesthesia are multiple. A vast variety of procedures are performed with blocks primarily involving branches of the Vth cranial nerve, although the cervical plexus and other nerves are occasionally blocked.

The frontal nerve block (V1) (Fig. 2-1) provides anesthesia of the terminal cutaneous branches of the lateral and medial supraorbital nerves and of the supratrochlear nerve. The supraorbital nerve exits the orbit through the supraorbital foramen, which is palpable at the midportion of the supraorbital rim. Either before or soon after leaving the supraorbital foramen, the nerve divides into its lateral and medial branches. The supraorbital nerve supplies the upper eyelid and conjunctiva; it divides before traveling upward deep to the belly of the frontalis muscle to supply the scalp skin as far posteriorly as the lambdoid suture. The supratrochlear nerve emerges from the medial aspect of the supraorbital rim and courses under the belly of the frontalis muscle to supply sensation to the medial aspect of the forehead, the upper eyelid, the skin of the upper nose, and the conjunctiva.

A supraorbital nerve block is performed by inserting the needle just under the midportion of the eyebrow while palpating the foramen. The needle is directed upward close to the foramen. After aspiration, 2 to 3 ml of 1% lidocaine or 0.25% bupivacaine is injected. The supratrochlear nerve block is performed in a similar way except the needle is inserted

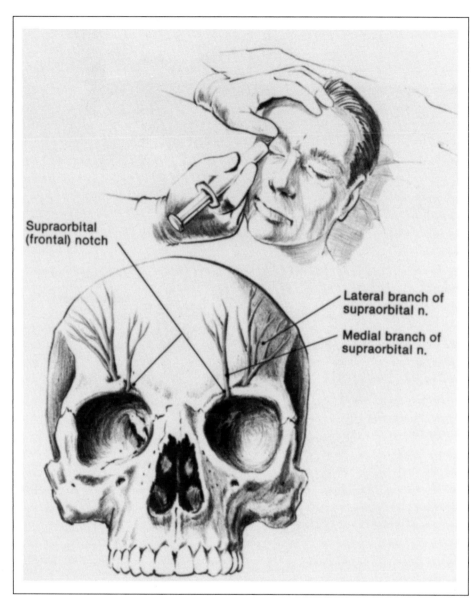

Supraorbital
(frontal) notch

Lateral branch of
supraorbital n.

Medial branch of
supraorbital n.

Fig. 2-2. Supraorbital nerve block. (From J. Katz [Ed.], Atlas of Regional Anesthesia. *[2d Ed.]. Norwalk, Connecticut: Appleton and Lange, 1994. Reproduced with permission.)*

in the medial portion of the orbital rim just lateral to the root of the nose. The terminal branches of both nerves can be blocked by subcutaneous infiltration of a local anesthetic agent in a horizontal line 2 cm above the eyebrow extending from the lateral orbital rim to the midline.

The infraorbital nerve (V2) (Fig. 2-2) exits the infraorbital foramen to supply the lower eyelid, ala, cheek, and upper lip and the mucous membranes lining the cheek and upper lip. The infraorbital nerve block may be approached by the transcutaneous or the transoral route. In the transcutaneous approach, the needle is inserted 1 cm below the lower border of the orbit at its midpoint. The infraorbital foramen usually can be palpated at this point as a notch. In the transoral approach, the needle is inserted into the superior buccal sulcus and directed to the infraorbital foramen as it is palpated with the other hand. Retrograde infiltration of the drug through the infraorbital foramen causes anesthesia of the incisor, canine, and premolar teeth, including the surrounding gums (supplied by the anterior alveolar nerves).

The mandibular nerve proper (V3) (Fig. 2-3) can be blocked transcutaneously as it exits the foramen ovale. This block anesthetizes the lower face and jaw. More often, however, the terminal divisions of the mandibular nerve are blocked. The mandibular nerve block is performed by placing the needle at a point 0.5 cm below the zygomatic arch midway between the condylar fossa and coronoid process, advancing it at right angles to the skin until the pterygoid plate is contacted, and redirecting the needle posteriorly at 20° until paresthesias are elicited. The anesthetized nerves include the buccal, auriculotemporal, lingual, inferior alveolar, and mental nerves.

The inferior alveolar nerve block causes anesthesia of the lower teeth and the skin over the anterior jaw and lower lip, including the mucosa, supplied by the mental nerve. This block is performed by directing the syringe from the premolar teeth of the opposite side to contact the lingual side of the ramus 1 cm above the occlusal surfaces of the molar teeth. The needle is advanced 1.5 to 2 cm until bone is contacted. The needle is withdrawn 1 to 2 mm, and 2 to 3 ml of a local anesthetic agent is injected. This block is usually performed in conjunction with a

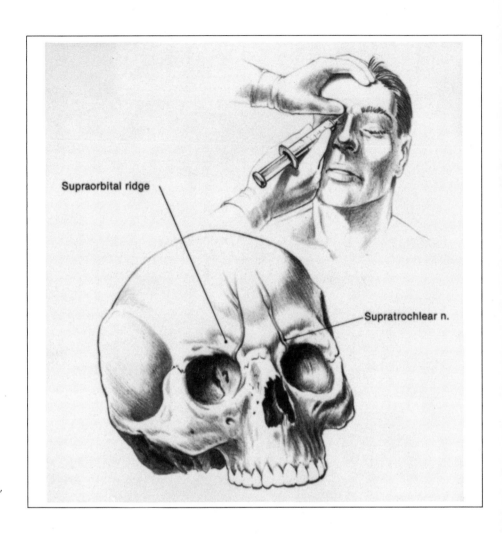

Supraorbital ridge

Supratrochlear n.

Fig. 2-3. Supratrochlear nerve block. (From J. Katz [Ed.], Atlas of Regional Anesthesia. [2d Ed.]. Norwalk, Connecticut: Appleton and Lange, 1994. Reproduced with permission.)

lingual nerve block. After the inferior alveolar nerve is blocked, the needle is withdrawn 5 mm, and an additional 0.5 ml of local anesthetic is injected. This anesthetizes the floor of the mouth, the lingual surface of the lower gums, and the anterior two-thirds of the tongue.

The mental nerve provides sensory innervation to the lower lip and skin of the anterior jaw. This nerve can be blocked transcutaneously or transorally as it emerges from the mental foramen (Fig. 2-4). The mental foramen is palpated just posterior to the first premolar tooth 1 cm below the gum line. It is important to deposit local anesthetic agents outside the mental foramen. Care should be taken to avoid entering the foramen because this can cause nerve damage with hyperesthesias or prolonged anesthesia of the lower lip. The mental nerve block also

anesthetizes the incisor, canine, and premolar teeth because some of the injected agent travels in a retrograde manner to reach the inferior alveolar nerve.

Topical Anesthesia of the Mucous Membranes

The local anesthetic agents available for topical anesthesia of the mucous membranes of the nose, mouth, and conjunctiva include lidocaine 4% solution for use as a spray, lidocaine 10% as aerosol, and cocaine 5 to 10%. Generally, plasma concentrations are one-half to one-third those achieved with a similar intravenous dose of the drug because absorption from mucous membranes is slow and incomplete. Additionally, most of the local anesthetic agent is removed from the site of application, for example, by wiping of tears containing the drug. Richly vascularized

areas such as the nasal mucosa, however, facilitate rapid absorption and higher blood levels, allowing toxic symptoms to occur at lower doses.

Cocaine, the first local anesthetic drug to be discovered, is the only naturally occurring one in clinical use today. Cocaine is a unique compound; it has strong anesthetic actions and powerful vasoconstrictive effects It is an unusual ester-linked agent metabolized both in the blood and, to a lesser degree, in the liver. The metabolites of cocaine are almost entirely excreted in the urine. Cocaine is useful only topically, but in topical use it has unequaled vasoconstrictor activity, decreasing bleeding and shrinking congested mucous membranes.

Calculation of a safe dose of cocaine is confusing because of the peculiar vaso-

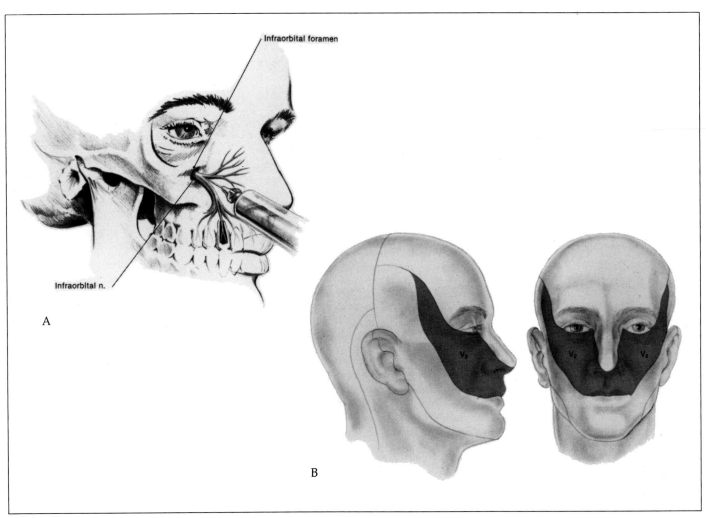

A

B

Fig. 2-4A. Infraorbital nerve block. The infraorbital nerve block exits the infraorbital foramen to supply sensation to the face. B. Sensory distribution of infraorbital nerve. (Part A from J. Katz [Ed.], Atlas of Regional Anesthesia. [2d Ed.]. Norwalk, Connecticut: Appleton and Lange, 1994. Reproduced with permission; and Part B from D.L. Brown [Ed.], Atlas of Regional Anesthesia. Philadelphia: W.B. Saunders, 1992. Reproduced with permission.)

constrictive actions of the drug, which limit systemic absorption. The most important factors for determining cocaine absorption are the method and site of administration. For example, the application of a 300-mg dose of cocaine in crystalline solution to the nasal septum may be safe, but applying the same dose as a 4% spray to the nasopharynx or laryngobronchial tree would probably result in a toxic reaction.

Cocaine overdose promotes massive adrenergic stimulation of the central nervous, cardiovascular, and respiratory systems. The addition of epinephrine to cocaine to form the solution known as "cocaine mud" enhances its sympathomimetic effect and toxicity, and its use should be condemned. Treatment of cocaine overdose requires immediate attention. Arrhythmias and tachycardia should be managed with propranolol,

whereas symptoms of central nervous system (CNS) toxicity such as seizures are best managed with diazepam.

Toxicity

Because local anesthesia affects the sodium channels in nerve membranes, toxic reactions occur in organs with excitable membranes, particularly the brain and myocardium. The brain is more susceptible to toxicity than the myocardium, and all the early signs and symptoms of toxicity are attributed to the CNS. Major myocardial toxicity is seen only with excessive plasma concentrations. It is critical that the surgeon using potentially toxic doses of local anesthetic agents be capable of recognizing and treating any toxic reactions.

Systemic toxicity of local anesthetic agents depends on the chemical structure of the specific drug, the total dose administered, the vascularity of the site of injection, the speed of injection, and the presence or absence of epinephrine. The balance between drug absorption, distribution, and elimination is upset. Different drugs possess different relative toxicities. More vascular sites allow more rapid drug absorption. The most common cause of toxicity, however, is unintentional intravenous injection. A drug overdose is the most common cause of death.

The signs and symptoms of CNS toxicity parallel the serum concentration of the anesthetic agent. This dose-related spectrum of cerebral effects follows a classic increasing order of severity:

1. Circumoral and tongue numbness, metallic taste
2. Lightheadedness
3. Tinnitus
4. Visual disturbances (diplopia, nystagmus)
5. Anxiety, slurring of speech, irrational behavior
6. Muscle twitching
7. Convulsions (grand mal)
8. Unconsciousness
9. Coma
10. Respiratory arrest
11. CNS depression

Myocardial toxicity may cause hypotension, bradycardia, and, eventually, cardiac standstill. The mechanisms of action include slowing of myocardial conduction, myocardial depression, and peripheral vasodilatation. The effect is usually seen clinically only after injection of two to four times the convulsant dose.

Problems with local anesthetic toxicity can be prevented by observing several simple rules.

1. Always use the recommended dose.
2. Before injecting the drug, aspirate the area with the needle in position to prevent intravenous injection.
3. When a local anesthetic contains epinephrine, intravenous injection produces a brief tachycardia 30 to 45 seconds after injection. Watch for this signal.
4. When administering large quantities of local anesthesia, give drugs of low toxicity slowly in several small aliquots.
5. Maintain continuous verbal communication with the patient during drug

administration. It provides the earliest clues to CNS toxicity.
6. Watch for minor symptoms, which can be seen before the drug is entirely given.

Before a local anesthetic agent is injected, all necessary resuscitation equipment and drugs should be available. As soon as toxicity is recognized, one should proceed with the ABCs of resuscitation—establish and maintain a clear *airway;* give oxygen to prevent hypoxia (*breathing*); and administer intravenous fluids and drugs for hypotension and bradycardia (*circulation*). If convulsions occur and they persist for more than 20 seconds, an anticonvulsant such as diazepam, 5 to 20 mg, or thiopental, 50 to 100 mg, should be given intravenously.

Suturing Skin Wounds

Surgical wound closure should be harmonious with biologic events, such as fibroplasia, epithelization, wound contraction, bacterial balance, and host defense mechanisms. It is important to consider each suture a foreign material that evokes a tissue inflammatory reaction, which can cause delayed wound healing, infection, or dehiscence. All suture materials, including the absorbable and nonabsorbable monofilaments, incite some degree of inflammatory response, and one must be discriminating in the selection and placement of suture material. The selection of suture material should be based on the healing properties and requirements of the involved tissue, the biologic and physical properties of the suture material, the location on the body, and patient considerations.

Suture Material

The choice of suture material is critical in the early stages of wound healing because the suture is primarily responsible for "keeping the wound together." In the first 3 to 4 days after wounding, the tensile strength of the skin increases as fibrin clot fills the wound cavity. One week after wounding the tensile strength of the skin is less than 5 percent that of unwounded skin; it is 10 percent after 2 weeks, 25 percent after 4 weeks, and 40 percent after 6 weeks, never achieving more than 70 to 80 percent of normal unwounded tensile strength. Thus the use of absorbable der-

mal sutures, such as polyglactin 910, polyglycolic acid, and polyglyconate, which lose their tensile strength in the first several weeks, when wounds are still very weak, can cause spreading and even dehiscence of wounds. In fact, studies show no significant improvement with dermal sutures over cutaneous sutures alone. The finest scars are seen when a subcuticular monofilament suture material is left in place for several weeks or even months.

Skin margins should always be everted and approximated without tension. After a knot is tied, the suture appears pear-shaped in cross section with raised borders. The everted skin edges gradually flatten to produce a level surface. It is important to place the suture so that the wound edges just touch each other. Postoperative edema produces additional tension with resultant strangulation of tissue and ischemia, leading to necrosis. A layered closure with subcuticular sutures should be performed with knots tied snugly but not so tight as to cause strangulation of tissue by necrosis.

There are many different methods of skin suturing. These include simple interrupted, vertical and horizontal mattress, continuous subcuticular, half-buried horizontal mattress, and continuous over-and-over suturing (Fig. 2-5). Simple interrupted sutures are inserted so that the needle enters and exits the tissue at the same angle, grasping identical amounts of tissue to approximate the wound margins exactly. Vertical mattress sutures produce excellent eversion of the skin edges. Horizontal mattress sutures provide good approximation of the skin edges with some eversion. They usually cause more skin ischemia than either simple interrupted or vertical mattress sutures. Subcuticular or intradermal continuous sutures eliminate the need for interrupted skin sutures, avoid suture marks on the skin, and produce the most favorable scar. These continuous sutures should be left in place for several weeks. Polypropylene is most commonly used for this purpose because it produces little inflammatory reaction, maintains its tensile strength, and can be removed easily. Half-buried mattress sutures are especially useful for closing V-shaped wounds or approximating skin edges of different textures and thicknesses. Using these sutures often prevents the necrosis of the tip

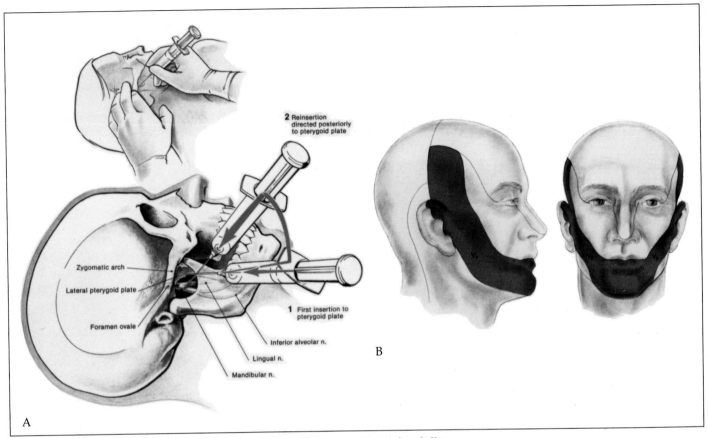

A

Fig. 2-5A. Mandibular nerve block. B. Sensory distribution of mandibular nerve. (Part A from J. Katz [Ed.], Atlas of Regional Anesthesia. [2d Ed.]. Norwalk, Connecticut: Appleton and Lange, 1994. Reproduced with permission; and Part B from D.L. Brown [Ed.], Atlas of Regional Anesthesia. Philadelphia: W.B. Saunders, 1992. Reproduced with permission.)

of the V that occurs with simple interrupted sutures. When the buried portion of the suture is placed within the dermis of the flap, ischemia and damage to the overlying skin are avoided. Continuous over-and-over sutures are most often used in closure of scalp wounds, where they can be rapidly performed and are hemostatic. Last, immobilization of the wound is as important in soft tissue healing as it is in bone healing; it can be achieved with sterile adhesive strips, tapes, collodion, or even plaster splints.

Different types of suture material are currently available for wound closure. These suture materials can be classified as natural or synthetic, absorbable or nonabsorbable, and braided or monofilament. Additional classification takes into consideration the time of absorption, amount of tissue reaction, and tensile strength (Table 2-2).

Absorbable suture material includes catgut, polyglactin 910, polyglycolic acid, polydioxanone, polyglyconate, and silk.

Catgut is derived from the submucosal layer of sheep intestine. It evokes a moderate tissue reaction and is digested by the body's proteolytic enzymes within 60 days. Tensile strength is rapidly lost within 7 to 10 days. Chromization of the catgut suture slightly prolongs the time to loss of tensile strength and digestion. The main uses of catgut sutures include ligation of superficial vessels and closure of tissues that heal rapidly, such as the oral mucosa. Catgut also may be used in situations in which one does not want to remove the sutures, such as wounds of small children or a nipple-areolar inset after breast reduction. However, the use of catgut may incite more tissue reaction than desired.

Polyglactin 910 and polyglycolic acid are synthetic materials that behave similarly. They produce low tissue reactivity and are completely absorbed by hydrolysis within 90 days. Tensile strength is 60 to 70 percent at 2 weeks and is lost at 1 month. Both materials are useful as in-

tradermal sutures because of their low reactivity, but one should be discriminating about using them for buried sutures. They have a tendency to "spit" with inflammation. When polyglactin 910 and polyglycolic acid are used as cutaneous sutures, scar widening may occur. The sutures should be removed 7 days after placement, before sinus tracts form. The braided configuration of these materials may potentiate infection; therefore, these materials should not be used in wounds with bacterial contamination.

Polydioxanone (PDS) is a synthetic absorbable monofilament suture that is minimally reactive and absorbed by hydrolysis over 6 to 9 months. Because of this very slow absorption, "spitting" is a considerable problem. Because the material is a monofilament, there is less affinity for bacterial seeding. This suture material maintains its tensile strength considerably better than the materials previously mentioned. Fifty percent of its original strength remains 4 weeks after suture

Table 2-2. Types of suture materials

Suture	Type	Raw material	Tensile strength	Absorption	Tissue reaction
Catgut	Plain	Submucosal layer of sheep intestine; serosal layer in cattle; flexor tendon	Lost within 7–10 days	Digested by body proteolytic enzymes within 60 days	Moderate
Catgut	Chromic	As above. Treated by chromization to resist digestion by body tissues	Lost within 3–4 weeks	Digested by body enzymes within 90 days	Moderate (less than plain catgut)
Polyglactin 910	Braided	Polymer of glycolic acid	60% remains after 2 weeks 30% remains after 3 weeks Lost within 1 month	Minimal until day 40. Absorbed by slow hydrolysis. Complete in 60–90 days	Mild
Polyglycolic acid	Braided	Polymer of glycolic acid	Lost within 30 days	Complete digestion within 90 days	Mild
Polydioxanone	Monofilament	Polyester filament	70% remains after 2 weeks 50% remains after 4 weeks 25% remains after 6 weeks Lost within 1 year	Minimal until day 90. Absorbed by slow hydrolysis. Complete digestion within 6–9 months	Mild
Silk	Braided	Natural protein spun by silkworm	Lost within 1 year	Complete by 2 years	Moderate
Nylon	Monofilament	Polyamide polymer	Loses 15–20% per year	Degrades at 15–20% per year	Very low
Nylon	Braided	Polyamide polymer	Loses 15–20% per year	Degrades at 15–20% per year	Very low
Polyester	Braided	Polyester polyethylene terephthalate coated with polybutylate	Indefinite	Nonabsorbable; encapsulated in body tissues	Minimal
Polypropylene	Monofilament	Polymer of propylene filament	Indefinite	Nonabsorbable; encapsulated in body tissues	Minimal transient acute inflammation

placement, and 25 percent remains 6 weeks after placement. Polydioxanone completely loses its strength one year after the operation. Polygluconate is an absorbable monofilament suture with the qualities and advantages of PDS; however, it retains its tensile strength for only 3 to 4 weeks.

The nonabsorbable monofilament (nylon and polypropylene) and braided (nylon and polyester) suture materials cause minimal inflammatory reaction, slide well, and can be removed easily, thus providing an ideal running intradermal stitch. Polypropylene appears to maintain its tensile strength better than nylon, which loses approximately 15 to 20 percent of its original strength per year.

Staples provide less inflammatory reaction than sutures, have similar strength up to 21 days, and leave a similar ap-

pearance to sutured wounds when removed by one week after the operation. Large wounds can be closed faster and more expeditiously with staples. Staples are useful for procedures such as large flaps, abdominoplasty, mammoplasty, and skin grafting. One must remember, however, to remove the staples early to avoid permanent suture marks.

The formation of permanent suture marks depends on the length of time a skin suture remains in place, the tension on the wound margins, the region of the body, the presence of infection, and the tendency of the patient for hypertrophic scarring or keloid formation. The most critical factors in avoiding suture marks in the skin are tension-free closure and early removal of sutures. These two factors are far more important than either the size or the type of suture material. Generally sutures left in place for 14 days

cause severe scarring with cross hatching. Wounds from which sutures are removed within 7 days produce a fine linear scar. Wound closure with a running dermal pullout suture provides an optimal scar without interfering with the development of tensile strength. The finest sutures for any given wound should be used. Sutures should be removed at different times from different areas of the body. This period ranges from 3 to 5 days for the face to 10 to 14 days for the limbs.

Elective Surgical Wounds

The quest for the optimal scar is a formidable one. The ultimate goal sought by the plastic surgeon is a fine, flat, concealed linear scar lying within or parallel to a skin wrinkle or natural skin line, a contour junction, or a relaxed skin tension line. There should be no irregularity in contour or distortions of adjacent an-

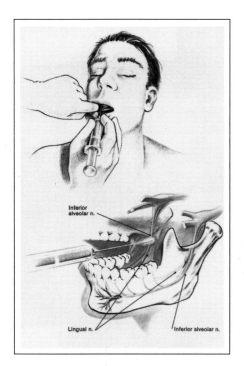

Fig. 2-6. The lingual nerve block is usually performed in conjunction with the inferior alveolar nerve block. (From J. Katz [Ed.], Atlas of Regional Anesthesia. *[2d Ed.]. Norwalk, Connecticut: Appleton and Lange, 1994. Reproduced with permission.)*

atomic units or landmarks. Changes in pigmentation should be avoided.

Elastic fibers within the dermis maintain the skin in a state of constant tension. This fact can be appreciated by the gaping of wounds made by incising the dermis or by the immediate contraction of skin grafts as they are removed from the donor site. Langer, in 1861, demonstrated that puncturing the skin of cadavers with a rounded sharp object made elliptic holes produced by the tension of the skin. He stated that human skin was less distensible in the direction of the lines of tension than across them. The use of the Langer lines has the following shortcomings: (1) Some tension lines were found to run across natural creases, wrinkles, and flexion lines; (2) the lines exist in excised skin; and (3) they do not correlate with the direction of orientation of dermal collagen fiber. Nonetheless, the Langer lines serve as a useful guide in the planning and design of skin excisions.

Scars are least conspicuous when they follow any skin line, preferably a wrinkle or natural skin line, a contour line, or a line

of dependency (Fig. 2-6). Relaxed skin tension lines, also known as wrinkle lines, natural skin lines, lines of facial expression, or lines of minimal tension, lie perpendicular to the long axis of the underlying facial muscles. They are accentuated by contraction of the muscles, as by smiling, frowning, grimacing, puckering the lips, or closing the eyes tightly. On the face, wrinkle lines or lines of facial expression develop in a predictable pattern with age. At about the age of 30 years, upper eyelid redundancy and the fine, lateral orbital laugh lines known as crow's feet develop. By the age of 40 years, periorbital and nasolabial folds deepen and glabellar and forehead wrinkles occur. Wrinkling in the neck and drooping of the tip of the nose appear between the ages of 50 and 60 years. With progressive aging, the facial skin becomes thinner and the wrinkles more prominent. These changes are accompanied by wasting of adipose tissue in the temporal and buccal regions. Wrinkle lines in other parts of the body can be seen by flexing and extending that part of the body.

Scars placed within relaxed skin tension lines or parallel to them are subjected to

minimal tension during the period of healing because they are not subjected to the intermittent pull of the subjacent muscles. Contour lines occur at the junction of body planes, such as the juncture of the nose with the cheek, the juncture of the cheek with the neck skin in the submandibular region, and the inframammary fold. Lines of dependency occur in older people as a result of the effects of gravity on the loose skin and fatty tissue. Jowl lines and "turkey gobbler" folds in the neck are classic lines of dependency. Cross-hatching patterns in the face are caused by the intersection of the lines of dependency and the lines of facial expression.

Principles of Wound Closure

Skin lesions may be removed by elliptic, wedge, or circular excisions. Most skin lesions are removed by a simple elliptic excision with the long axis of the ellipse on or paralleling a wrinkle or natural skin line, a contour line, or a line of dependency (Fig. 2-7). The ellipse may be lenticular and have angular or rounded

Fig. 2-7. The mental nerve can be anesthetized transcutaneously or transorally as it exits the mental foramen. (From J. Katz [Ed.], Atlas of Regional Anesthesia. *[2d Ed.]. Norwalk, Connecticut: Appleton and Lange, 1994. Reproduced with permission.)*

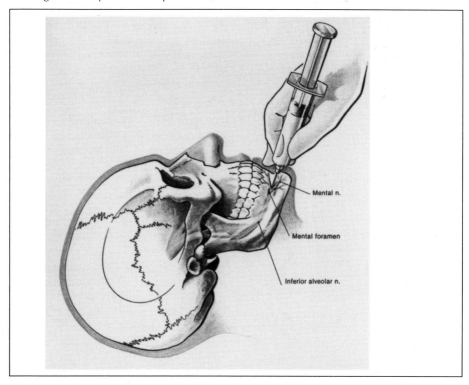

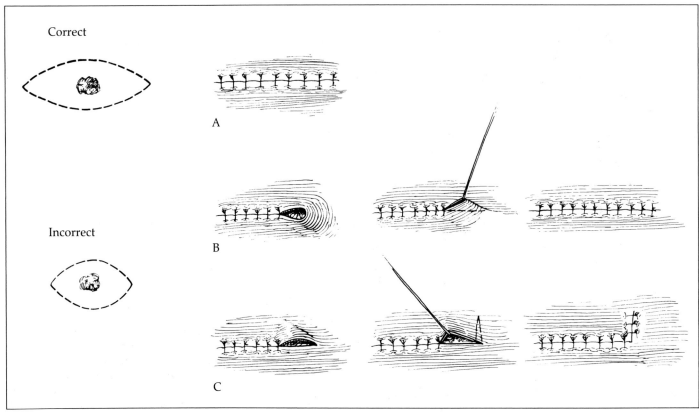

Correct

Incorrect

A

B

C

Fig. 2-8A. *Ideally an ellipse should be planned so that the long axis is about four times longer than the short axis. Dog-ears form at the ends of a closed wound when either the ellipse is made too short or one side of the ellipse is longer than the other. The dog-ear may be corrected by either fusiform extension of the elliptic excision (B) or a short, right-angle incision at the end of the ellipse with removal of the redundant skin (C).*

edges. Ideally, the long axis should be four times longer than the short axis. If this ratio becomes smaller, bunching of excess skin causes a dog-ear. Dog-ears occur when there is a considerable discrepancy between the two sides, one side approaching a semicircle and the other almost a straight line. Dog-ears may flatten over time, but it is best to excise them primarily. There are two methods for eliminating a dog-ear. (1) If the elliptic excision is too short, one can either lengthen the ellipse to include the excess tissue or excise the redundant tissue as two tiny triangles. (2) If the dog-ear has occurred because one side of the incision is longer than the other, one can correct the problem by making a short right-angle or 45° incision at the end of the ellipse (Fig. 2-8).

Large lesions can be removed by multiple serial excisions. The principle takes into account the viscoelastic properties of skin and use of the creep and stress relaxation phenomenon. It has been especially use-

ful for improvement of male pattern baldness by excision of the non-hair-bearing areas of the scalp. With the introduction of soft tissue expansion, however, the technique of serial excision has become less popular.

Wedge excisions are performed primarily for lesions occurring on the free margins of the ears, lips, eyelids, or nostrils. Lesions of the lip can be excised as either triangles or as pentagonal wedges. Excision of lesions occurring in these locations as a pentagon often causes less contracture and shortening along the longitudinal axis of the incision and a more favorable scar than does excising the lesion as a triangle (Fig. 2-9). Closure of circular defects can be performed by a skin graft, by sliding V-Y subcutaneous pedicle flaps, or by hatchet-type transposition or rotation flaps (Fig. 2-10).

Fig. 2-9. *Wedge excision of lesions on free margins of the lip, the rim of the nostril, and the lower eyelids.*

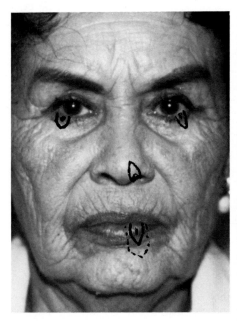

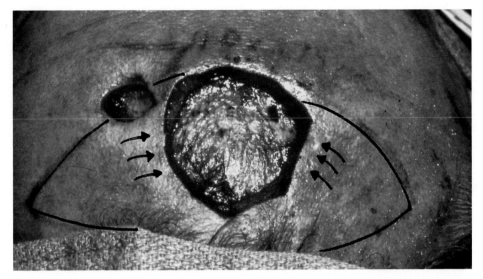

A

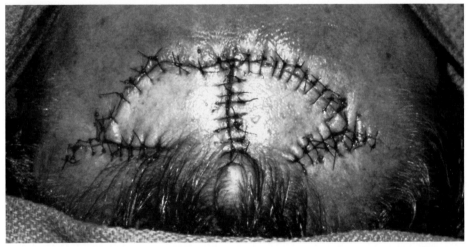

B

Fig. 2-10A. Defect following excision of 4.0-cm by 3.75-cm basal cell carcinoma of the forehead. B. Closure of circular defect with bilateral hatchet-type flaps.

Special Techniques in Plastic Surgery

Borges has written extensively about the optimal placement of incisions, the reasons for noticeable, unattractive scars, and a systematic approach to the management of unfavorable scars. Analysis of any scar should include diagnosis, location, length, width, orientation, contour irregularities, pigmentation, distortion of anatomic landmarks, quality of the adjacent tissue, and loss of local tissue. The characteristics most strongly influencing the appearance of a scar are its direction with respect to the relaxed skin tension lines, its uninterrupted length, and differences in contour from the surrounding tissue. The prime objectives of excisional scar revision, including simple elliptic excision, Z-plasty, and W-plasty, are to reorient the scar, to divide the scar into smaller segments, and to make the scar level and consistent with the adjacent tissue.

Z-Plasty

Z-plasty is one of the most effective and widely used techniques in plastic surgery. Referred to by Limberg as *converging triangular flaps*, the Z-plasty is a technique by which two triangular flaps on two planes are interdigitated without stress, strain, or other biomechanical effects. Each flap is transposed into the defect left by the other flap, resulting in a gain in length along the common limb of the Z, which is especially useful in the treatment of contractures, and a change in the direction of the common limb of the Z, useful in the management of facial scars (Fig. 2-11).

This method is effective in increasing length along a selected axis, breaking up a straight scar, obliterating or creating a web or cleft, and shifting topographic features. It is a precise procedure the theory and practice of which must be fully understood for proper application. Borges emphasizes that Z-plasty and other techniques generally should not be used in the primary treatment of traumatic wounds unless the wound approximates the ideal surgical incision. He argues that it is often extremely difficult to determine what may be viable tissue in the acute setting; the incidence of infection or hematoma is higher after a traumatic laceration than after an elective scar revision; and the patient has not yet had an opportunity to evaluate the primarily closed scar.

Planning is critical and is based not only on geometric principles but also on the biomechanical features of the involved tissue. A Z-plasty cannot be performed in mathematic isolation; one must consider the viscoelastic properties of the skin. A Z-plasty consists of a central limb, which usually lies within the scar or line of contracture, and two limbs positioned so that they resemble a Z. These limbs should be of equal length because the skin flaps must fit together in their transposed position. The angles of the Z can vary from 30 to 90°. A classic Z-plasty contains angles of 60° (see Fig. 2-11).

The central limb, oriented along the line of contracture, is usually under considerable tension. After release or division of this contracture, the shape of the parallelogram immediately changes with spontaneous flap transposition and lengthening along the line of the central limb, or the contractural diagonal. This increase in length along the contractural diagonal is gained at the expense of the transverse diagonal. Essentially, the short contractural diagonal is lengthened so that it approximates the transverse diagonal, and

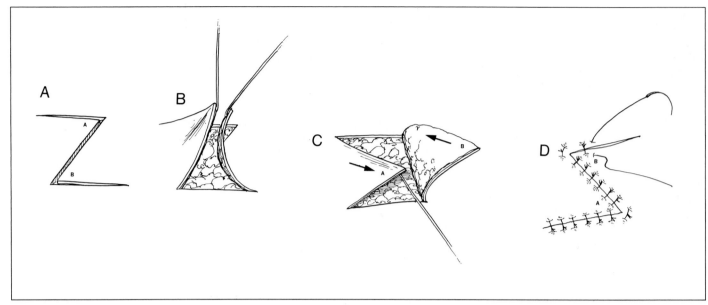

Fig. 2-11. Classic Z-plasty using 60° angles. Flaps A and B are elevated (A, B) and interposed (C) without tension. Limbs of the Z-plasty follow the lines of relaxed skin tension. Half-buried horizontal mattress sutures are placed in the flap edges (D).

the transverse diagonal is shortened so that it equals the contractural diagonal, the absolute increase in length being equal to the difference between the two diagonals. Lengthening is related to the difference between the long and short axes of the parallelogram formed by the Z. The wider the angles of the triangular flaps, the greater is the difference between the long and short diagonals and thus the greater is the lengthening. In designing a Z-plasty, one must be certain that sufficient laxity is available transversely to achieve the appropriate lengthening perpendicular to it. The limbs of the Z-plasty should follow the relaxed skin tension lines.

The critical determinations in construction of the Z are angle size and limb length. The angle size determines the percentage increase in length. The limb length controls the absolute increase in limb length. As the angle size increases, so does the amount of lengthening. With a 30° angle, there is an expected 25 percent increase in length; with a 45° angle, a 50 percent increase in limb length; with a 60° angle, a 75 percent increase in limb length; with a 75° angle, a 100 percent increase in limb length; and with a 90°

angle, a 120 percent increase in limb length. The values for the increases in length are theoretical and cannot be applied clinically with accuracy, but they do provide a good approximation of the actual lengthening. Generally, the actual increase in length is slightly less than the theoretical one.

Angles considerably less than 60° do not achieve any useful lengthening, defeating the purpose of the Z-plasty and causing flap narrowing with concomitant compromise of the blood supply of the flap. Angles much greater than 60° produce extreme tension on the surrounding tissues because there is limited tissue for transverse shortening and the flaps cannot be readily transposed. Therefore, a 60° angle is used most commonly in Z-plasties.

Limb length controls the actual increase in length in proportion to the original length. The longer the length of the central limb, the greater is the actual increase in length for a given angle. The length of the limbs is limited by the amount of tissue that can be brought in from the sides regardless of the length of the contracture. Because 60° is the best angle to use, limb length is the major variable in clinical practice.

Multiple Z-plasties facilitate reduction in the amount of transverse shortening without greatly affecting the amount of lengthening. Whereas a similar amount of lengthening can be achieved by a single Z-plasty and multiple Z-plasties in which

the central limbs add up to that of a single Z-plasty, there is less transverse shortening when multiple Z-plasties are used. The lateral tension is reduced and is more equally distributed over the entire length of the central limbs. Thus there appear to be advantages to multiple Z-plasties over a single Z-plasty, especially when there is insufficient tissue for a larger Z. Multiple Z-plasties of facial scars often result in cosmetically superior scars.

A four-flap Z-plasty is extremely effective in correcting contractures of the thumb-index web space (Fig. 2-12) and axillary contractures. First, a 90°, 90° or 120°, 120° angle Z-plasty is designed. The two-flap Z-plasty is converted into a four-flap Z-plasty by bisecting the angles, producing flaps with angles of 45° or 60°. This allows a greater gain in length (124%) with less tension on the flaps.

The combination of a five-flap V-Y advancement and Z-plasty or double-opposing Z-plasty is especially effective for releasing contractures of concave regions of the body, including the medial canthal region and the dorsum of the interdigital web spaces. The hypertrophic scars need not be excised but can be incised. The size of the Z-plasty flaps can be diminished when the vascularity of the flaps is precarious, as in burn contractures. Double-opposing Z-plasties with small flaps are as effective in the release of burn scar contractures as a single Z-plasty with larger flaps. They are most effective in inter-

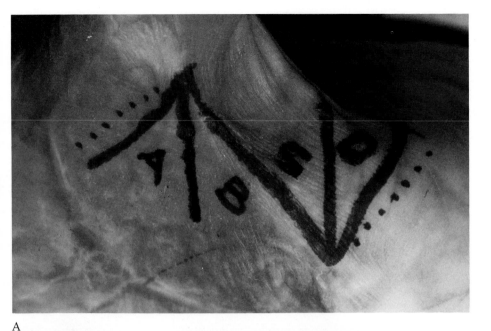

A

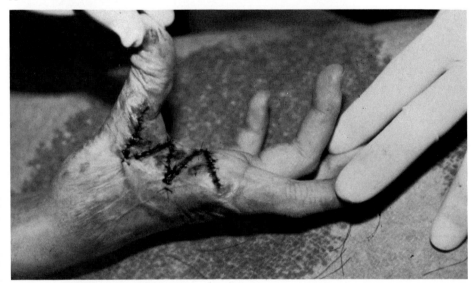

B

Fig. 2-12. Four-flap Z-plasty. This technique is useful in the release of contractures, including those of the thumb-index web space. A. Design of a four-flap Z-plasty. B. Flaps are interposed with release of the contracture.

W-Plasty

The W-plasty is another method of reorienting the direction of a linear scar by breaking it up so that most of it lies in the direction of the RSTL. The linear scar is excised as multiple small triangles lying in all directions. This serves to detract attention from the more obvious linear scar. Templates can be used to assist in designing the W-plasty. Triangles of equal size are outlined on either side of the scar. The tip of the triangle on one side is placed at the midpoint of the base of the opposing triangle on the contralateral side. At the ends of the scar, the triangles excised should be smaller and the limbs of the W tapered. For curved scars, the angles on the inner aspect of the curve should be more acute than the angles on the outer aspect of the curve. The tips of the triangles should be sutured with a three-corner stitch to prevent necrosis of the tips of the flaps.

The main disadvantage of the W-plasty is that it does not lengthen a contracted linear scar; a Z-plasty should be used for this purpose. The W-plasty increases rather than decreases the tension in the area of the scar because of the necessary sacrifice of tissue. The W-plasty should be used only when there is an abundance of tissue adjacent to the scar. The most common applications for a W-plasty are in facial scars perpendicular to or nearly perpendicular to the RSTL, such as horizontal scars across the cheek, lower lip, or chin. A W-plasty is most useful in "trapdoor" scars of the face, in which it allows interdigitation of lymphedematous and normal tissue bordering the scar and excision of constriction bands of the limbs. The W-plasty does not displace anatomic landmarks because there is no transposition of tissue. Despite popularity among some surgeons, the W-plasty is limited in use and may worsen a scar if not appropriately used.

V-Y Advancement

The V-Y advancement technique allows forward advancement of a triangular flap (V) without any rotation or lateral movement. The resulting defect is closed in a Y configuration. The skin actually advanced is the skin on either side of the V (Fig. 2-14). This technique is extremely useful in lengthening the nasal columella, in correcting a whistle deformity of the lip, and in various other mucosal flaps.

rupting scar contractures in which the anatomic position of the contracture does not allow use of large flaps. The central flap is advanced in a V-Y configuration, and the two Z-plasties on each side of the central flap are transposed (Fig. 2-13).

Another variation in the application of the Z-plasty is the interdigitation of triangles of unequal size. The classic descriptions and applications of the Z-plasty are predicated on the design of equal limbs and therefore of equal triangles. In burn scars in which there is nonuniform scarring, one side of the central segment being loose and the other side contracted, and resection of scar tissue is not indicated, a half-Z technique is used. This procedure is useful for lengthening the short side. The Z-flap on the scarred side is elongated to provide greater mobility. The vascularity of the Z-plasty flaps also can be increased, especially in burn-scarred tissue, by curving the limbs in an S configuration, thus broadening the flaps.

Fig. 2-13. Combination five-flap V-Y advancement and Z-plasty, or double-opposing Z-plasty. This technique is effective in the correction of a burn scar contracture.

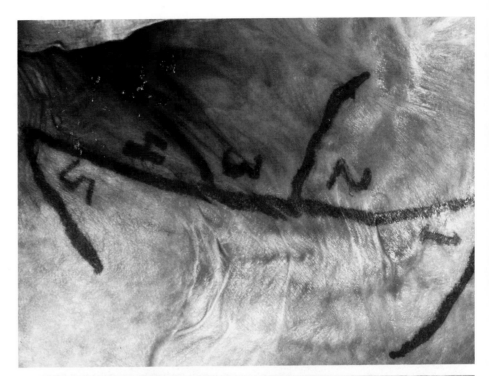

Inset of the V-shaped tip of the flap can be performed using the corner, or three-point, suture popularized by McGregor.

V-Y advancement flaps are occasionally used in serial arrangement to release linear scar contractures, such as those seen in Dupuytren disease. The advancement obtained is perpendicular to the longitudinal axis of the scar contracture. The maximal length of the straight limb of the Y is determined by the amount of lateral skin laxity but does not usually exceed one-third the length of the side. The theoretical gain in length is 1.4 times the length of the straight limb of the Y. Generally, one uses a Z-plasty rather than a V-Y advancement to obtain lengthening.

Rhomboid Flaps

The rhombic flap was originally described by Alexander Limberg of Leningrad in 1946 after extensive geometric analysis and experimentation with paper models. The Limberg, or rhombic, flap is a combination rotation and transposition flap that borrows adjacent loose skin for coverage of a rhombic defect. A rhombus is an equilateral parallelogram with acute angles of 60° and obtuse angles of 120°, long and short diagonals perpendicular to each other, and a short diagonal equal in length to each side of the rhombus. The flap is designed as an extension of the short diagonal opposite either of the two 120° angles of the rhombus. The short diagonal is extended by a distance equal to its length. From this point, a line of equal

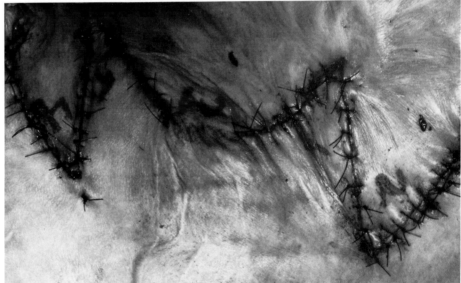

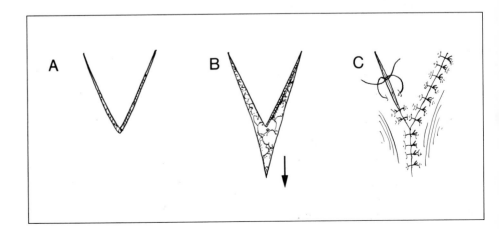

Fig. 2-14. V-Y advancement technique. The central V is advanced forward, and the defect is closed in a Y configuration.

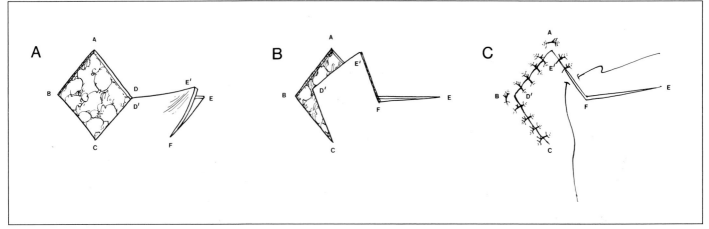

Fig. 2-15. Rhombic flap. A. Design. B. Elevation of flap with wide undermining of the base to allow rotation and advancement. C. Resultant suture lines.

length is drawn at a 60° angle parallel to either side of the rhombus (Fig. 2-15).

Four types of Limberg flaps are possible for any rhombic defect. In choosing the best of the four, consideration must be given to the direction of loose skin, where the final scars will lie with respect to the relaxed skin tension lines, the location of anatomic landmarks to prevent their distortion, and the quality of the surrounding skin. The skin must be lax for direct closure of the wound edges. Laxity can be tested simply by pinching the adjacent skin between the thumb and fingers. This loose skin should lie along the extension of the short diagonal. The short diagonal of the rhombic flap should be placed parallel to or within the relaxed skin tension

lines to minimize tension, make the best use of the available tissue, and achieve the most acceptable donor-site scar. Care must be taken in choosing the best of the four flap possibilities to avoid distortion of facial features such as the eyelids, nostrils, lips, eyebrows, or hairline.

Lesions should not be excised in rhombic shapes but in circles or other shapes. After the lesion is excised, the surgeon draws a rhombus that encompasses the defect. Thus the options for flap design expand dramatically. The adjacent skin is pinched to determine the locations of skin laxity in relation to the relaxed skin tension lines and anatomic landmarks. The surgeon selects the best flap by taking

into account all the foregoing factors. A local anesthetic agent is infiltrated into the areas of dissection, and the flap is incised and elevated.

It is critical to undermine widely beneath the base of the flap to allow the flap to fall into position in the rhombic defect without tension. The initial sutures are placed in the four corners of the defect. Small dog-ears commonly occur at the bases of the flap and the area of donor-site closure. It is best to leave them alone because any attempt to remove them may compromise flap vascularity. In addition, the dog-ears have a tendency to flatten out and improve in a relatively short period of time (Fig. 2-16).

Fig. 2-16A. Design of planned excision of basal cell carcinoma of the nose. B. Excision of lesion and elevation of rhombic flap. C. Final appearance of suture lines.

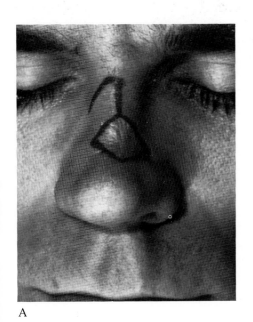

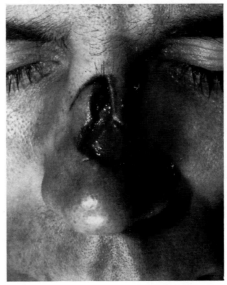

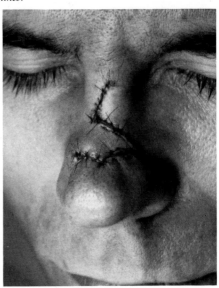

A

B

C

The Dufourmentel flap is a variation of the rhombic flap in which the angles differ from the standard 60° and 120° angles in the Limberg flap. The Dufourmentel flap is useful for coverage of a defect in the shape of a rhomboid rather than a rhombus. Although the two terms often are used interchangeably, a rhomboid differs from a rhombus in several important respects. A rhomboid is a parallelogram, but it has acute angles of various degrees; only its opposite sides are equal in length; its diagonals are not perpendicular to each other and are not equal in length; and the diagonals are not necessarily equal in length to the sides of the parallelogram. The Dufourmental flap may be used for angles of up to 90°. Planning for this flap is complex. It is often more efficacious to convert the defect into one with angles of 60° and 120°.

Fig. 2-17. Appearance of syndactyly scars at one month (A) and at 2 years (B) of age. The scar has matured.

Factors Influencing the Healing of Surgical Wounds

Age

Scarless healing occurs only in the fetus. The prolonged presence of hyaluronic acid and its associated binding proteins in the fetus provides a privileged environment for scarless healing. The deposition of collagen (predominantly type III) and the process of matrix reorganization in fetal wounds proceeds in a much more efficient manner than in the postnatal period. During the first 3 months of life, scars often heal as fine lines. During childhood, however, scars remain erythematous and hypertrophic for prolonged periods of time, slowly improving during adolescence and adulthood. Childhood is probably the worst time for wound healing. The reasons for this may be speculated on but are essentially unknown. A scar usually looks its worst between 2 weeks and 2 months after an injury. Scar maturation takes 9 to 24 months, and one hopes that a flat, white scar will result. The surgeon should await scar maturation before proceeding with scar revision, except when the orientation of the scar mandates early revision. Patience is a virtue for the patient, the patient's family, and the surgeon in this setting (Fig. 2-17).

Race

Keloid formation and hypertrophic scarring show a predilection for young, dark-skinned people. These abnormal scarring processes are histologically indistinguishable; diagnosis is based on the clinical features and the patient's history.

Keloids show a strong familial association with autosomal recessive or autosomal dominant inheritance. They usually occur between the ages of 10 and 30 years, much more commonly in blacks than in Caucasians. Keloids contain excessive amounts of collagen that extends beyond the borders of the scar bed. Keloids most commonly occur on the earlobes, face, and anterior chest. They rarely improve with time and may worsen postoperatively. Keloids can best be managed by a combination of intrakeloidal surgical excision with adjunctive intraoperative steroid injection into the wound edges, followed by postoperative prolonged pressure and, in severe instances, irradiation.

Hypertrophic scars, on the other hand, show less of a familial tendency, less relation to race, and an equal sex ratio. They are most commonly found in young, dark-skinned people. In contrast to keloids, hypertrophic scars contain excess collagen that remains localized within the borders of the scar bed. Hypertrophic scars most commonly occur across flexor surfaces and usually improve with time.

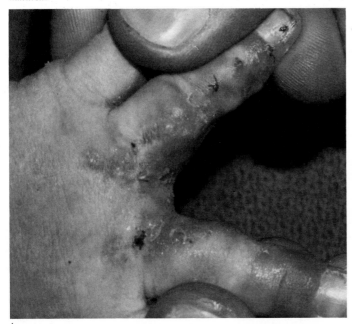

A

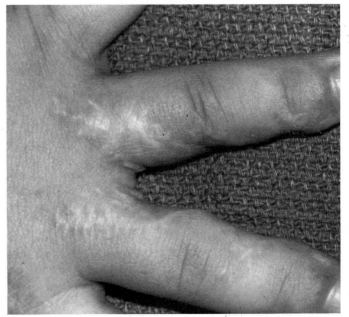

B

Additional improvement can be achieved with pressure, steroid injections, and possibly irradiation.

Location

Particular areas of the body have a strong predilection for hypertrophic scarring, whereas other areas heal with a fine-line scar. The sternal region, deltoid area, and back (trunk and limbs except for the palms and soles) usually heal with a thick, exuberant, butterfly-shaped hypertrophic scar or keloid under otherwise optimal circumstances. The face, eyelids, palm, vermilion, and mucous membranes, on the other hand, heal inconspicuously. Scars adjacent to anatomic landmarks such as the eyebrows, lips, or nose require special techniques to prevent the distortion of these anatomic structures.

Type of Skin

Patients with thick, oily skin containing hypertrophied glands often heal with noticeable, depressed scars. These scars most commonly occur over the lobule of the nose, on the upper cheek, and on the forehead. Single-layer monofilament closure can minimize the development of epithelial inclusion cysts, which are a common problem for some patients.

Skin Disorders

Numerous genetic disorders affect wound healing. Patients with the Ehlers-Danlos syndrome, or cutis hyperelastica, usually demonstrate impaired healing abilities because of abnormal cross linking of collagen. Some forms of this rare autosomal dominant disorder (other than type II, which is sex-linked) are characterized by increased skin elasticity, fragility, and tendency to bruising. The skin generally heals poorly, slowly, and with wide scars. This disease is often diagnosed in early childhood but decreases in severity with aging. Cutis laxa, attributed to a nonfunctional elastase inhibitor or premature degeneration of elastic fibers, presents the opposite picture to that of Ehlers-Danlos syndrome. Beginning in the neonatal period, the defective elastic tissues demonstrate progressive laxity resulting in drooping of all the body skin. Infants frequently have aneurysms, pneumothoraces, emphysema, and hernias, but wound healing problems have not been reported.

Epidermolysis bullosa is characterized by an unusual susceptibility of the skin to mechanical stress. Shearing of the skin occurs after minor frictional trauma. Management includes prevention of frictional trauma by skin lubrication and use of flotation mattresses. Established wounds are treated with protective nonadherent dressings and silver sulfadiazine.

Pseudoxanthoma elasticum, most commonly inherited as an autosomal recessive trait, is characterized by increased collagen degradation and calcium and fat deposition on the elastic fibers. This condition produces skin with a pebbled appearance consisting of small yellowish papules and extreme laxity with no elastic rebound. These skin changes are most marked in the groin, axilla, and neck. Surgical treatment usually is excision of the redundant skin. Wound healing proceeds more slowly than usual and worsens with age.

Management of Soft Tissue Injuries

The acute management of any soft tissue wound must be individualized. Although all these wounds are by definition "contaminated," a number of factors influence how they are managed. The classic "6-hour golden period" makes little biologic sense. A plastic surgeon must consider the specific clinical situation in deciding whether to close the wound or to leave it open (Table 2-3).

Table 2-3. Management of acute soft tissue injuries

Debride and irrigate devitalized tissue
Cleanse wound and traumatic tattoos
Remove any foreign body
Obtain meticulous hemostasis
Obliterate any dead space
Handle tissues gently
Use atraumatic technique
Avoid tension in wound closure
Use buried sutures judiciously
Leave contaminated wounds open

Knowledge of the mechanism of injury is critical to wound management. A thorough understanding of the pathophysiology of the specific type of wounding facilitates effective therapeutic intervention. The roles of tetanus prophylaxis and antibiotics should be appreciated by anyone treating wounds and are not discussed in this chapter. It is vital to ascertain whether the injury was inflicted by a dog, cat, or human bite; whether it occurred in a kitchen or on a farm; how long ago the injury occurred; and what the offending agent was, such as extravasation of doxorubicin hydrochloride (Adriamycin) as opposed to saline, or a burn caused by lye as opposed to hydrofluoric acid.

Linear and stellate lacerations, avulsion injuries, and soft tissue losses all are managed by similar basic principles and guidelines. The sine qua non of treatment of an acutely contaminated wound is sharp debridement and irrigation. The purposes of sharp debridement are to convert a contaminated wound into a clean wound that can be closed primarily; to reorient skin lacerations or avulsions; and to discard devitalized, necrotic tissue. Debridement facilitates the removal of clot, debris, and necrotic tissue and is mandatory for wound closure. After debridement, the wound edges are freshened and trimmed perpendicularly to prevent a step-off deformity. Intermittent high-pressure irrigation with several liters of saline solution using either the pulsatile jet lavage or a 60-ml syringe fitted with a 19-gauge needle is an important adjunct to sharp debridement. The mechanical action of the irrigant, rather than its chemical composition, is important for the removal of particulate matter. However, one should avoid opening up new tissue planes or extensions of the lacerations into normal tissue. Bacterial homeostasis must be re-established. Following this, wound closure may proceed as for a clean wound. When in doubt, we prefer to leave the wound open and proceed with delayed wound closure. Inadequate debridement might lead to additional soft tissue necrosis, possible infection, and unacceptable scarring.

Sharp debridement or wound excision should be planned with functional and aesthetic considerations in mind and should coincide, if possible, with the RSTL. In areas that have an excellent blood supply, such as the face, debridement should be conservative. It is critical to maintain anatomic landmarks, such as the eyebrow, the eyelid, or the vermilion border of the lip, because these structures can never be replaced; furthermore, they guide the surgeon to proper tissue alignment.

Direct closure of semicircular lacerations or U-shaped flaps tends to produce a trapdoor deformity with "pin-cushioning" secondary to contraction of the linear scar centripetally, with edema caused by disruption of the lymphatics and veins. Despite some reports to the contrary, we believe an immediate Z-plasty should not be performed in the emergency room. As advocated by Borges, these lacerations should be revised secondarily as necessary. The risk of infection or hematoma after repair of traumatic lacerations is greater than after elective scar revision. Also, the patient may be unhappy with the resultant zigzag scar without the opportunity to compare it to the trapdoor or other deformity.

Most civilian traumatic wounds can be closed primarily after adequate debridement. On the other hand, heavily contaminated wounds, such as those following farm injuries, human bites, or blast injuries, are usually treated in an open manner. Similarly, when a delay in definitive wound management is anticipated, the wound should be irrigated and debrided, the edges trimmed perpendicular to the skin and loosely approximated, and the wound covered with gauze moistened with saline solution. A minimal number of buried sutures should be placed because the addition of a foreign body to a wound increases the chance for infection; monofilament is safer than braided material. Tapes or sterile adhesive strips may be applied as necessary. A second-look operation should be performed 24 to 48 hours after the first one if there is any doubt as to the establishment of infection. Closure should be delayed until additional debridement is done and repeated quantitative cultures with less than 10^5 bacteria per gram of tissue are obtained.

A variety of topical agents are available for skin antisepsis, including quaternary ammonium salts, povidone-iodine solu-

tion, hydrogen peroxide, and isopropyl alcohol. These antiseptic agents should be used strictly for cleansing the surrounding skin and not on the wounds themselves; the agents are generally toxic to cells, inhibit or retard wound healing, and might be absorbed, with systemic effects. Wounds should be irrigated with saline solution. A scrub brush may be used to remove dirt buried in the dermis and to prevent permanent tattooing beneath the new skin surface.

Meticulous hemostasis must be achieved before the wound is closed. Collection of blood beneath skin flaps promotes the release of oxygen free radicals with possible flap ischemia. Any dead space must be obliterated. Atraumatic technique is critical in achieving a fine scar. Tissues must be handled gently, care being taken to avoid a crush injury. Sharp knives and scissors and proper-size needles and suture materials are important. Skin hooks are far less traumatic to skin edges and subcutaneous tissue than are toothed forceps. Atraumatic manipulation of tiny flaps with skin hooks optimizes flap survival. Tension must be avoided because it causes tissue necrosis. The destruction of cells and vessels provides a good culture medium for bacteria, leading to inflammation, infection, and excessive scar formation. Skin undermining may relieve tension. Frequent irrigation of exposed tissues prevents the desiccation promoted by room heat and by overhead operating room lamps.

Drains should be placed judiciously for therapeutic and prophylactic reasons. They can be passive drains, such as Penrose drains, or suction drains. Passive drains are used to establish a tract or path of least resistance to the outside. They may be used for evacuation of infected materials that are too viscous to pass through the tubular suction drains or in small wounds with a limited amount of drainage. Suction drains are used to remove large amounts of fluid. Beneath large skin flaps, they facilitate apposition of tissue surfaces, obliterating any potential dead space and promoting rapid adherence and healing. Closed suction drains pose less of a risk of retrograde infection than passive drains.

Infection

We do not live in a germ-free environment, even in the absence of clinical infection. Some degree of contamination always exists in soft tissue wounds. The appearance of clinically significant infection depends on the delicate equilibrium between host resistance (defense mechanisms) and bacterial inoculum. An impairment in this equilibrium causes a clinical infection. It is not the mere presence of bacterial organisms in the wound but the level of bacterial growth that is critical in the management of a contaminated or infected soft tissue wound. Krizek and Robson demonstrated clinically and experimentally that a bacterial inoculum of greater than 100,000 organisms per gram of tissue is necessary for most bacterial species for wound infection and, potentially, invasive sepsis to take place.

To make the definitive diagnosis of infection, one must observe (1) purulent material draining from the wound, (2) cellulitis or inflammation spreading beyond the area of injury, (3) quantitative cultures demonstrating greater than 100,000 organisms per gram of tissue, or (4) the presence of beta-hemolytic streptococci. Quantitative bacteriologic cultures provide an objective end point in the management of soft tissue wounds. Bacterial counts less than 100,000 per gram of tissue in the absence of beta-hemolytic streptococci allow successful direct closure, skin graft take, or flap application. Qualitative bacteriologic study is extremely important to determine species and sensitivities.

All traumatic injuries cause contaminated wounds. Bacteria can be readily demonstrated in culture. One study reported that 20 percent of these wounds have more than 100,000 organisms per gram of tissue. The mechanism of injury is critical; the bacterial inoculum from a knife laceration differs from that of a crushing punch press injury, which differs from that of a human bite. (Saliva contains 1,000,000 to 10,000,000 organisms per milliliter.)

Additional factors to be considered in the management of traumatic wounds include the operative time; the time since the injury, known as the "golden period"; the location of the wound with respect to blood supply; and the amount of debris or foreign body in the wound.

In the acute setting, prophylactic systemic antibiotics can decrease the risk of postoperative wound infection; however, they must be delivered before bacteria invade the tissues. Adequate serum levels must be obtained within 4 hours from the time of injury to be effective. Usually, an antibiotic is chosen empirically on the basis of the anticipated pathogens.

Suggested Reading

Borges, A.F. *Elective Incisions and Scar Revision.* Boston: Little, Brown, 1973.

Borges, A.F. Choosing the correct Limberg flap. *Plast. Reconstr. Surg.* 62:542, 1978.

Borges, A.F. W-plasty. *Ann. Plast. Surg.* 3:153, 1979.

Harrison, M.R., et al. Successful repair in utero of a fetal diaphragmatic hernia after removal of herniated viscera from the left thorax. *N. Engl. J. Med.* 322:1582, 1990.

Krizek, T.J., Koss, N., and Robson, M.C. The current use of prophylactic antibiotics in plastic and reconstructive surgery. *Plast. Reconstr. Surg.* 55:21, 1973.

Limberg, A. *The Planning of Local Plastic Operations on the Body Surface: Theory and Practice.* Translated by S.A. Wolfe. Lexington, Mass.: Collamore Press, D.C. Heath & Co., 1984.

McGregor, I.A. The Z-plasty. *Br. J. Plast. Surg.* 19:82, 1966.

McGregor, I.A. *Fundamental Techniques in Plastic Surgery and Their Surgical Applications* (7th ed.). Edinburgh: Churchill Livingstone, 1980.

Peacock, E.E. *Wound Repair* (3rd ed.). Philadelphia: Saunders, 1984.

Scott, D.B. *Techniques of Regional Anaesthesia.* East Norwalk, Conn.: Appleton & Lange/ Mediglobe, 1989.

Siebert, J.W., et al. Fetal wound healing: A biochemical study of scarless healing. *Plast. Reconstr. Surg.* 85:495, 1990.

Smith, J.W., and Aston, S.J. *Grabb and Smith's Plastic Surgery* (4th ed.). Boston: Little, Brown, 1991.

3

Scar Revision

Maher Anous   David T. Netscher   Samuel Stal

"Doctor, can you do something about this scar?" This frequently asked question should raise more questions in the mind of a plastic surgeon preparing to present the patient with a logical solution. Dealing with scars requires observation and organization. In this chapter, we present a simplified scheme for dealing with patients requesting scar revision.

Scar revision may be requested for several reasons:

Aesthetics. Unsightly facial scars, post-traumatic alopecia, and pigmentation disturbances prompt patients to seek scar revision.
Instability. Unstable scars are a source of great annoyance to patients because of continuous breakdown. Furthermore, chronically irritated scars can lead to the development of scar carcinomas.
Function. Scars crossing joints or adhering to underlying structures might impair function. Those close to the eyelids or oral commissure can lead to ectropion and exposure.
Pain. Painful scars contain neuromas.

Consultation with the patient should be divided into three parts: (1) the history of the scar, (2) scar examination and analysis, and (3) the proposed treatment.

History of the Scar

It is important for the treating physician to understand why an ugly scar has formed. Some factors are beyond the control of the plastic surgeon. In other instances problems can be averted at the time of the surgical revision, resulting in a better scar. Physicians examining scars should ask themselves the following question: Is this scar patient-related, wound-related, or physician-related?

Causes Intrinsic to the Patient

Idiopathy. Some patients are prone to development of keloidal scars.
Genetics. In patients with Ehlers-Danlos syndrome, for example (Fig. 3-1), the elasticity of the skin hinders optimal scar formation.
Patient's age. Patients in the first and second decades of life tend to have a prolonged scar maturation phase.

Causes Related to the Original Wound

Anatomic location. Scars located in the "three terrible triangles" (that is, the presternal region and both deltoid areas) frequently undergo hypertrophy.
Road tattooing (Fig. 3-2). Particulate matter may become embedded in the tissues at the time of a road accident. Irritation of the tissues may lead to hypertrophic scarring.
Tissue loss at original injury. This situation leads to closure of the wound under tension and a tendency toward a wider scar.
Wounds crossing flexion creases or lines of tension. Tensile forces acting across a healing scar may widen it.
Circular and trapdoor wounds (Fig. 3-3). These scars collect edematous fluids, resulting in prolonged maturation.
Wound adherence to underlying structures. Adherence results in a tensile force on the healing scar.

Causes Related to Initial Wound Management

Poor attention to technical details
Excessive tension at the time of closure
Wound allowed to heal by secondary intention

Taking the history of the scar can be translated into four simple questions: (1) How old is the scar? (2) How did the wound

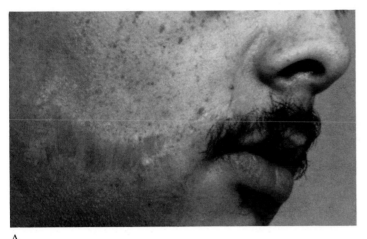

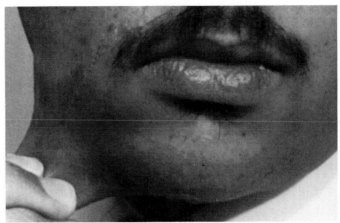

A

B

Fig. 3-1A. Wide scar of the right cheek on a patient with Ehlers-Danlos syndrome. B. Ehlers-Danlos syndrome. Note the skin laxity.

Fig. 3-2. Road tattoos of the columella and right nostril margin.

Fig. 3-3. Trapdoor scar. Note the raised margins of the scar and the puffy appearance of the tissues.

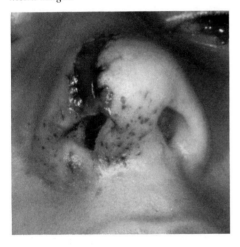

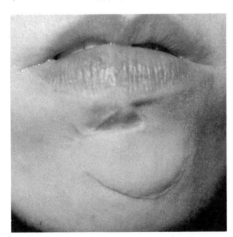

How Did the Wound Occur?

The production of the original wound generally determines the outcome of scar revision. An unsightly scar that results from a controlled surgical incision carries a worse prognosis after scar revision than one produced by blunt injury with soft tissue loss. By producing conditions for optimal tissue healing, the physician can hope for better results after revision in instances of blunt injury.

How Did the Scar Heal?

The physician inquires about events that may have adversely affected the healing of the wound, thus leading to an unsightly scar. Of particular importance is a history of infection or hematomas with their attendant negative influence on healing. Also, the physician should ask about a history of allergies to either a suture material or a topical agent. Finally, whether wounds heal primarily by secondary intention is of utmost importance in explaining the outcome. It is only by avoiding the factors believed to be responsible for the unacceptable initial result that a physician can expect improvement through subsequent scar revision.

Has the Scar Been Revised?

This aspect is pertinent mainly to hypertrophic scars and keloids. To expect an ugly scar to improve after the third or fourth surgical excision using the same

occur? (3) How did the scar heal? and (4) Has the scar been revised?

How Old Is the Scar?

This is the key question because the age of the scar determines the optimal time for scar revision. Part of the established dogma of plastic surgery is that scars should be between 6 and 12 months old before a revision is considered. This arbitrary length of time was determined by observing the changing appearance of wounds over a period of time until their maturation. The time interval, however, is not cast in stone. We have observed scars that have remained raised and erythematous 18 months after the initial in-

jury. It is generally safe to assume that scars improve with time up to the second year after injury, after which they remain stable. This observation does not mean that scar revision should not be completed before this amount of time has elapsed. The age of the scar is simply a rough guide for the physician to use in determining the revision strategy. If all other aspects of the scar are optimal, it is safe to wait for final scar maturation before contemplating revision. On the other hand, if other aspects of the wound fall outside the accepted norm (e.g., wounds perpendicular to the relaxed skin tension lines), it is acceptable to revise the scar before it matures.

surgical technique and without the introduction of an adjunctive treatment for wound healing is wishful thinking on the part of the patient and physician.

The history taking should not occupy more than 5 minutes of the consultation time. By the end of this time, however, the physician should have formed a preliminary opinion regarding the feasibility and timing of the revision and, possibly, of its eventual outcome.

Contraindications Based on History

The history may uncover conditions that preclude scar revision.

Scars in Children
If all other conditions are optimal, scar revision for aesthetic reasons in children should be delayed until the age of full maturation (14 to 16 years for girls and 15 to 17 years for boys). Scars in children and young adolescents have a prolonged maturation phase. Also, scars tend to widen with body growth. Age, however, is not an absolute contraindication to scar revision.

Multiple Previous Manipulations
A multiply recurring keloid is not expected to abate after a conventional excision. Adjunctive modalities of wound manipulation should be introduced in such a situation.

Ongoing Disease
Any local skin condition or systemic disease should be under control before scar revision.

Unrealistic Expectations
This is the only absolute contraindication to scar revision.

Examination of the Scar

After completing a thorough history, the physician enters the examination inclined toward either intervention or abstinence. The examination of the wound not only helps in the final decision but also enables the physician to choose a surgical method if a revision is warranted. The six important aspects to look for include (1) scar location, (2) evidence of scar maturation, (3) physical characteristics of the scar, (4)

relation of the scar to anatomic landmarks, (5) relation of the scar to relaxed skin tension lines (RSTL), and (6) relation of the scar to wrinkle lines.

Scar Location

This is the most important factor in scar analysis. Scars falling within the so-called terrible triangles (both shoulders and the sternum region) tend to recur as widened hypertrophic and keloidal scars. The excessive skin tension caused by the pull of the chest musculature, in scars on the sternum, or by the dependent position of the upper extremity, in scars on the shoulder, is responsible for such unsatisfactory healing. Other areas of potential problems include the lateral submandibular regions and joint flexure areas.

Evidence of Scar Maturation

On a cellular level, a mature scar is one in which hyaluronic acid has been replaced by chondroitin-4-sulfate with increased linearity and cross linking of its collagen bundles and with a dominance of type 1 collagen. The tensile strength of such a scar is 80 percent of the original preinjury level. Clinically a mature scar is one that has lost its hyperemic and raised appearance, has taken on color matching, and has flattened. Usually such a scar is no longer itchy. A mature scar is expected to change very little, if at all, except in a growing child. In children, the length and width of scars are expected to change commensurately with body growth.

Physical Characteristics

Length
According to Borges, the length of a scar can be defined as the uninterrupted distance of a straight scar. Because incisions tend to heal from side to side but contract from end to end, a long, uninterrupted scar has a tendency to bowstring owing to the uninterrupted pull of tension. The aim of surgical treatment in this instance is to break the scar into multiple segments to interrupt the tension forces.

Width
Large wounds that are allowed to heal by granulation and contraction leave wide scars in their transverse diameters. Wide scars also occur in burn wounds covering large surface areas that are allowed to re-

epithelize spontaneously. In such instances, the techniques of linear scar revision are inapplicable. Other methods should be sought.

Type
Hypertrophic and keloidal scars differ considerably from normal scars in their potential for recurrence after revision. The techniques of revision should be modified, and adjunctive methods should supplement the surgical treatment.

Relation to Anatomic Landmarks

The proximity of scars to important anatomic landmarks plays an important role in the choice of revision method. If an operation is contemplated, the design of the flaps should take into account the distortion of adjacent topography. Scars in the middle of the forehead or cheek do not impose revision dilemmas to the surgeon equal to those of scars adjacent to the ala of the nose, the eyebrow, or the vermilion border of the lip.

Relation to Relaxed Skin Tension Lines

The best way to understand the concept of the RSTL (Fig. 3-4) is to study the example of the frontalis muscle. The frontalis is a vertically directed muscle that on contraction approximates the brows to the front of the hairline. The muscle performs well, moving like an accordion, because its tissues are lax along vertical lines parallel to muscle fibers. This excess of tissues in the vertical axis mandates a degree of tightness along a horizontal axis. Thus the forehead is tight from side to side. The facial skin can be thought of as a tight piece of cowhide stretched between two parallel poles, much like a drum. Cutting the cowhide with a knife in the direction of maximal stretch does not result in separation of the edges; however, incising it perpendicular to the axis of maximal stretch results in immediate gaping. The direction of maximal stretch is called the *relaxed skin tension line*. Incision along this line (horizontally in the wrinkle line of the forehead) does not result in wound separation because maximal skin laxity is present in a plane perpendicular to the line. Furthermore, the excessive tension from side to side along

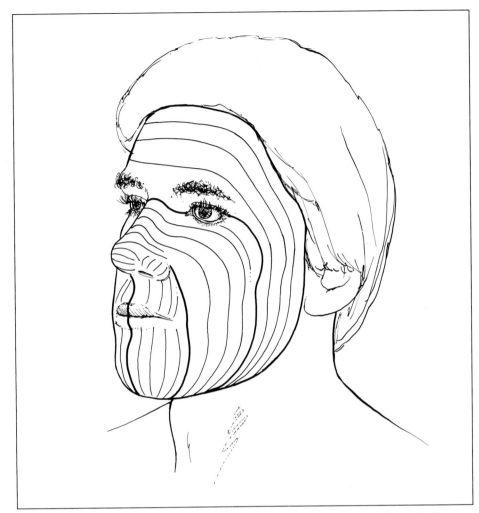

Fig. 3-4. Relaxed skin tension lines. Note that the directions might not correspond to the wrinkle lines.

the RSTL approximates the edges of the wound together. On the other hand, any incision at a right angle to the RSTL results in immediate edge separation, which accounts for widened or hypertrophic scars in the clinical setting.

The physician must envision the direction of the RSTL in relation to the scar. The easiest way is to pinch the skin between the index finger and the thumb to relax it, making ridges and furrows. The RSTL are located when these ridges and furrows are formed easily and in a parallel manner. Once the directions of the RSTL are found, the surgeon pinches the skin at a right angle and compares the resulting ridges and furrows. These should be much fewer in number and more difficult to produce. The surgeon always strives to direct the scar in the direction of the RSTL during a revision.

Relation to Wrinkle Lines

RSTL coincide with facial wrinkle lines in most instances. The surgeon, however, should be aware of the following areas in which the two do not overlap:

1. *Glabella.* Frown lines are vertical, and RSTL are horizontal.
2. *Lower lip.* Wrinkle lines are horizontal, and RSTL are vertical.
3. *Lateral palpebral commissure.* Wrinkle lines are fanned out, and RSTL are oblique.

Contraindications Based on Examination

Findings at the time of the physical examination that preclude scar revision include immature scars, recurrent hypertro-

phic scars and keloids (provided other factors are favorable), recurrent scars in unfavorable locations, and ongoing regional skin conditions, such as acne.

Algorithm

Based on the history and physical examination of the patient, a plastic surgeon should be able to place the scar into an algorithm that dictates the attitude to adopt (Fig. 3-5).

Methods of Scar Revision

There are several surgical options for dealing with scars, each with specific indications regarding scar characteristics or anatomic conditions.

Fusiform Scar Revision

Fusiform scar revision is the oldest and most frequently used method. The scar is incorporated within a fusiform segment of tissue to be excised, and the closure is effected by direct approximation of the skin borders. This technique is indicated only for the revision of unsightly scars that fall within the RSTL. Of course, the surgical conditions that resulted in the unsightly scar should be avoided during revision. The extremities of the ellipse should be incised last to maintain maximal tension at the time of incision of the upper and lower central segments, enabling a clean vertical cut. It is imperative in designing the long axis of the fusiform incision that the axis follow the RSTL and not the direction of the scar. This ensures a tension-free approximation of the edges with minimal undermining. If the scar does not follow the RSTL, another technique of scar revision is in order.

The Z-Plasty

A Z-plasty (Fig. 3-6) entails the transposition of two adjacent triangular flaps using a Z-shaped incision. Although this technique triples the size of the original healed incision, it can improve the appearance of the scar by (1) breaking it into smaller components, (2) relaxing the skin in the direction of the original scar by borrowing lax tissues from a direction perpendicular to it, (3) changing the direction of the scar to lie within the RSTL, and (4) weakening the depressive forces of the

Fig. 3-5. Algorithm for decision making regarding scar revision.

History

Is this scar patient-, wound- or physician-related?

How old is the scar?
How did the wound occur?
How did the scar heal?
Has the scar been revised?

Precluding conditions   No precluding conditions

Examination

Location
Maturation
Characteristics   ⎤ Length
Landmarks   ⎬ Width
Relaxed skin tension lines   Type
Wrinkles   ⎦

Precluding conditions   No precluding conditions

Treatment

Fig. 3-6A. Burn scar, right hand. Note inability to abduct the thumb fully. B. Burn scar, right hand. Proposed release of thumb web contracture. C. Burn scar, right hand. Z-flaps transposed. D. Burn scar, right hand. One year after release, with good thumb abduction and flexion.

A
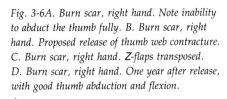

B
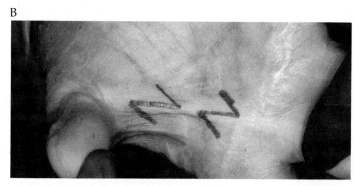

C
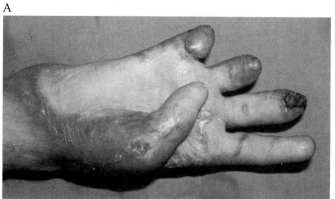

D
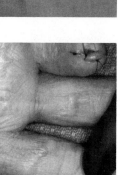
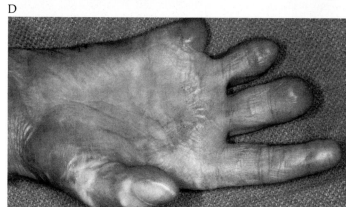

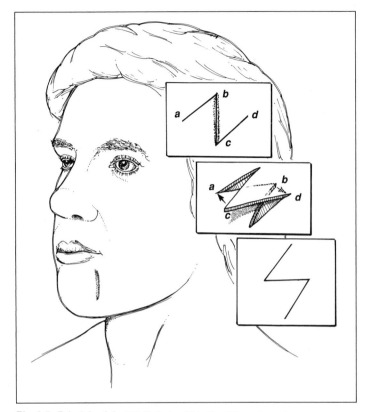

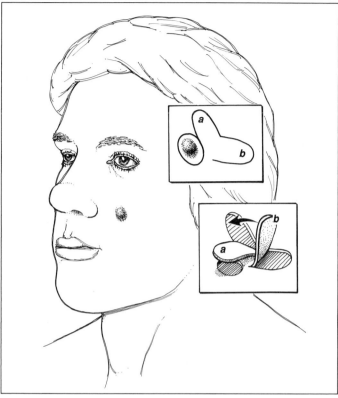

Fig. 3-7. *Principle of the 60° Z-plasty. Note the 90° reorientation of the central scar.*

Fig. 3-8. *Irregular Z-plasty. The bilobal flap.*

scar by breaking the continuity between the skin and the underlying tissue.

Z-plasty in its simplest form consists of three equal limbs and two equal angles of 60° each (Fig. 3-7). The central limb overlies the scar, and the two peripheral ones are parallel to each other. This design is intended to allow a 75 percent increase in length in the direction of the central limb (thus the scar) by adding tissues from the adjacent lax areas. To better understand the Z-plasty, one must consider its components.

Angles

The theoretical percentage gain in the central limb length increases as the angles of the Z-plasty increase. Angles of 30° allow a 25 percent gain in length, whereas angles of 90° allow a 125 percent gain. The more gain there is, the better, except that angles exceeding 75° have a greater propensity for dog-ear formation. Gain in central limb length is, in theory, controlled by the angles between the Z-plasty limbs. In addition to the size of the angles, it is the availability and elasticity of lateral tissues that determine the net gain.

Limbs

There are three limbs to a Z-plasty: the central limb and the two peripheral ones. All limbs are equal in length, and the two peripheral ones are parallel to each other if the angles of the Z-plasty are the same. It is worthwhile to remember that in the 60° Z-plasty, at each angle the central limb is transposed 90°. This 90° transposition of the central limb can be accomplished only with the 60–60 angle Z-plasty. One should always remember where the scar lies in relation to the RSTL and plan the peripheral limb positions in a manner that is compatible with an aesthetic result.

Variations of the Z-Plasty

Whereas it is conventional to have a single Z-plasty with equal limb length and angles, variations call for a Z-plasty with unequal limbs, unequal angles, and multiple components. An example of a Z-plasty with unequal angles is the nasolabial flap (Fig. 3-8); here the angle at the tip of the flap is usually smaller than the angle at the fulcrum of rotation, which might approximate 90°. The main pur-

pose of a Z-plasty with unequal angles is tissue replacement, not lengthening. Examples of a Z-plasty with unequal limbs are some flaps used for nipple reconstruction, such as the skate flap or the double opposing tab flaps. The limbs in these flaps, unlike those in classic Z-flap, which have straight limbs, are curvilinear and approach the appearance of an S-plasty. Finally, multiple Z-plasties give a greater increase in length with less lateral skin distortion (Fig. 3-9).

The W-Plasty

When it became apparent that the indiscriminate use of the Z-plasty for all scars could lead to an undesirable reorientation of tissues (e.g., the reorientation of a portion of the eyebrow), a technique that breaks the continuity of straight scars but without tissue rotation was sought. The W-plasty (Fig. 3-10) was thus born, an operation aimed at breaking up the bolstering effect of straight scars by redirecting tension forces. In its simplest form, the W-plasty comprises a series of small incisions linked at sharp angles and situated

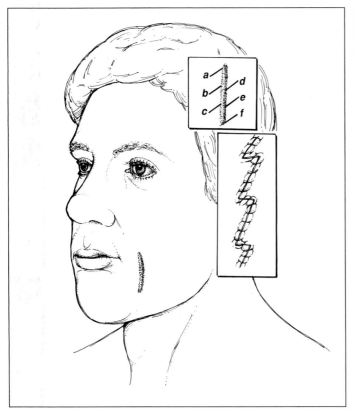

Fig. 3-9. Multiple **Z**-plasties. Note the lengthening of the scar.

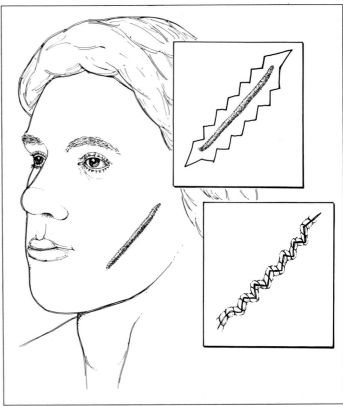

Fig. 3-10. **W**-plasty. Note the effect on total scar length.

Fig. 3-11. Geometric broken line closure. Note the mirror-image configuration on both sides of the design.

on both sides of the scar to be excised. The W-plasty limbs usually measure 5.5 mm, and the angles between these limbs are usually 55°. The number of limbs depends on the length of the scar to be excised. The most common indication for a W-plasty is a facial scar that has more than a 35° inclination from a RSTL on the temple, forehead, eyebrow, cheek, nose, or chin. Scars on the eyelids, lips, and nasolabial folds are better served with a Z-plasty. A W-plasty is rarely used other than on the face and should not be used on small scars or scars that are less than 35° from RSTL.

Geometric Broken Line Closure

Geometric broken line closure (GBLC) (Fig. 3-11) is based on the concept of making the scar irregular to accomplish camouflaging. This irregularity is produced by a series of random and irregular incisions on one side of the scar interposed with mirror-image incisions on the opposite side. The idea is to render the scar pattern so unpredictable (unlike the W-plasty) that the untrained eye cannot see

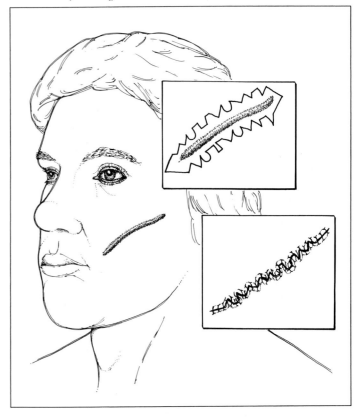

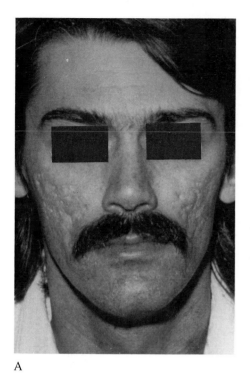
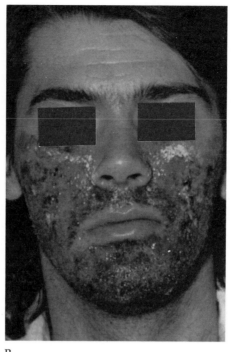
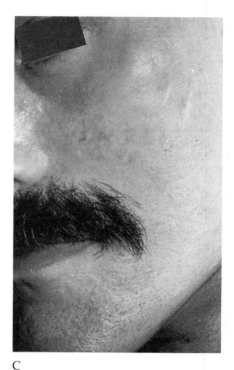

A B C

Fig. 3-12A. Acne scars, both cheeks. No active acne present. B. Acne scars directly after dermabrasion. The entire aesthetic unit is dermabraded. C. Acne scars one year after dermabrasion. Good final result.

it. Geometric broken line closure has not been uniformly accepted, however, especially because the best result is obtained after multiple episodes of dermabrasion of the resulting scar. The technique is also time consuming.

Dermabrasion

In dermabrasion (Fig. 3-12) the superficial layers of the skin down to the interface between the papillary and reticular dermis are removed with a rapidly rotating round or pear-shaped wheel (dermabrader), allowing the skin to resurface in a more homogeneous pattern. Although dermabrasion can be used for different forms of scars and skin conditions (actinic and seborrheic keratoses, rhinophyma, chloasma, and epidermal nevi, among others), the most common indication is acne scarring. Dermabrasion is best suited for fair-skinned people, because dark repigmentation is difficult to predict and usually inconsistent. It is important to inquire about medical conditions precluding the use of this technique, such as active herpes simplex, vitiligo, collagen vascular diseases, and recent intake of oral contraceptives (because of their melanogenic effect).

Dermabrasion is well suited for acne scars because it produces a leveling of the edges of the crater and thus a good blending with surrounding tissues. Additionally, healing of the abraded epidermis and dermis by fibrosis in the center of the crater raises the depressed area and flattens its surface. The most commonly used equipment is a motor- or air-driven unit with an attached diamond fraise or wire brush. It is best to choose a wheel that is at least 4 mm wide because smaller wheels tend to burrow into the skin. The technique is usually carried out under local anesthesia with the patient premedicated with meperidine or diazepam. Regional blocks are preferred to local infiltration anesthesia because local agents distort the skin surface. Skin refrigerants may be used, depending on the surgeon's experience. The advantage of the use of skin refrigerants is that hardened skin lends itself easily to dermabrasion. It is advisable to paint the area to be dermabraded with gentian violet to outline the margins and delineate the center of the crater. Dermabrasion is performed in the painted areas until all the purple coloration disappears. It is best to dermabrade an entire anatomic unit rather than an isolated patch of skin. After the procedure,

a single layer of nonadherent petrolatum gauze integrated with an antibiotic ointment is used on the dermabraded surfaces. The fine mesh gauze is removed during the first postoperative visit 24 hours after the procedure. At this time the patient is instructed to use petrolatum ointment on the surgical area to lessen the pain. The patient is encouraged to use common sense in keeping the area clean until the eschar separates.

Dermabrasion is not an innocuous procedure; it can lead to multiple complications ranging from pigmentary inconsistencies to scarring.

Skin Grafting, Flaps, and Soft Tissue Expansion

Occasionally the local conditions of a scar do not allow the use of conventional techniques for revision. The need for additional tissues to resurface a scarred area depends on the length and width of the scar, the conditions in the anatomic area to be resurfaced, and the aesthetic and functional goals. Most wide scars resulting from burns can be resurfaced adequately with skin grafts. The choice of a donor site depends on the surface area of the scarred tissues, the desired texture of

A

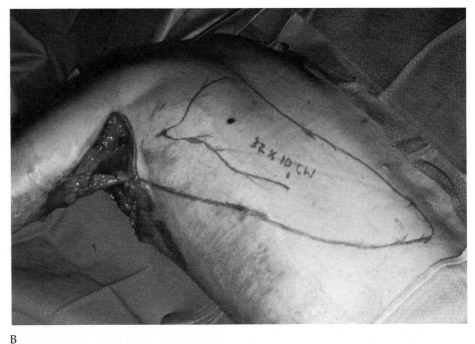

B

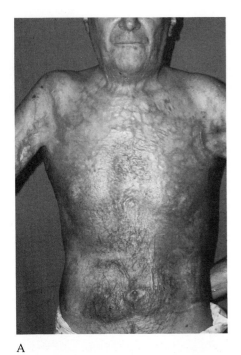

C

D

Fig. 3-13A. Burn wound of chest and both axillae. Note the inability to abduct both arms. B. Design of parascapular flap for release of scar contracture of left axilla. C. Rotation of left parascapular flap and skin grafting of donor defect. D. Procedure performed bilaterally. Final result with good arm abduction.

the final, healed skin (e.g., thin as in the eyelids), and, most important, especially in facial scars, the color match between donor and recipient areas. The scalp and supraclavicular areas are preferred donor sites because of their color compatibility with facial skin. Of course, skin grafts, especially thin ones, are known to contract and thus are likely to scar, especially at their periphery. The application of pressure garments is beneficial in keeping healed skin grafts pliable.

When the recipient site is unsuitable for the "take" of a skin graft or when bulkier tissue is needed for an aesthetic or functional problem, such as across a joint, a local or regional flap, if available, is used (Fig. 3-13). These flaps can be random or pedicled, cutaneous, fasciocutaneous, musculocutaneous, or myoosteocutaneous depending on the elements needed for wound resurfacing. The design, rotational axis, and composition of these flaps are governed mostly by the surgeon's experience and artistic sense.

Microsurgical techniques have added a new dimension to the art of reconstructive surgery. Composite tissues from distant areas of the body can now be transferred to accomplish the specific goals of anatomic recontouring, functional restoration, or aesthetic resurfacing.

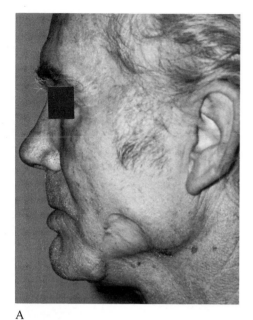

A

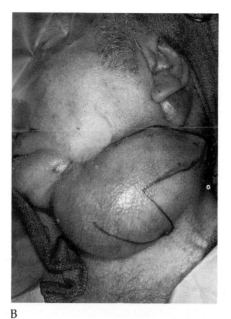

B

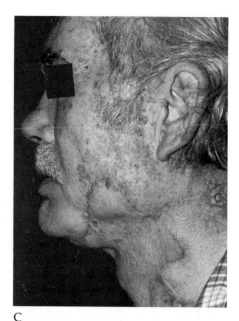

C

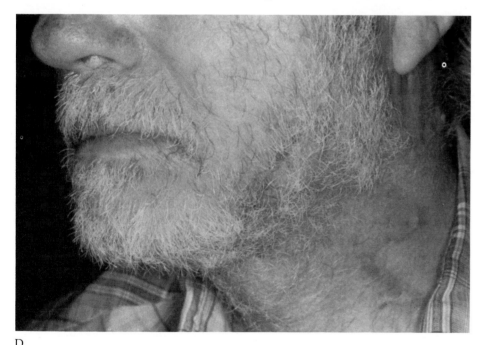

D

Fig. 3-14A. Unaesthetic appearance of skin graft of the left lower cheek after wide excision for basal cell carcinoma. B. Soft tissue expansion of left neck. C. One month after excision of skin graft and rotation of expanded neck skin. D. Final appearance, one year after scar revision.

Soft tissue expansion (Fig. 3-14), introduced in the mid-1970s, has allowed the direct transfer of expanded adjacent skin into the area of a scar. This procedure has the distinct advantages of simplicity, reliability, and the use of like tissue in scar revision. Great caution, has to be exercised, however, when introducing a soft tissue expander into the vicinity of a scar. The expansion of scarred tissues, intentionally or unintentionally, carries the risk of wound dehiscence and expander exposure. Although the idea itself is simple,

the choice of expander shape, size, and location requires a degree of expertise. When soft tissue expanders are used for the purpose of scar revision, the results obtained are often satisfactory.

Keloids and Hypertrophic Scars

Keloids and hypertrophic scars are not the same. Although it may be difficult to distinguish the two, Peacock simplified

the issue by stating that a hypertrophic scar usually remains within the confines of the injury, whereas a keloid extends beyond the borders of the original wound (Fig. 3-15). Such a distinction is not always easy to make, especially if the patient presents soon after the occurrence of an injury. Most hypertrophic scars flatten and lighten with maturity; such regression does not occur in keloids. At a cellular level, an equilibrium is reached in normal scars between the rate of collagen formation and destruction; no such equilibrium occurs in keloidal scars, in which the rate of collagen formation is much higher than the rate of destruction.

Hypertrophic scars seem to be influenced by the type of injury and its location. Wounds in areas of tension more often than not heal by hypertrophic scar for-

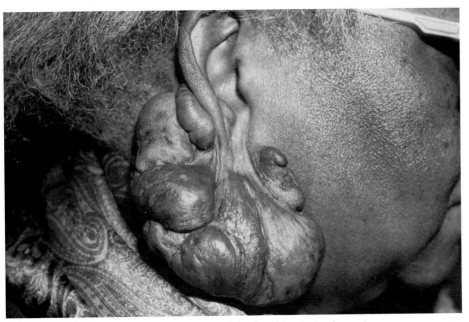

Fig. 3-15. *Long-standing keloid of right earlobe resulting from lobe piercing for earrings.*

Pressure appears to be an additional beneficial adjunctive mode in the postoperative management of revised keloids and hypertrophic scars. In the form of pressure garments or digital manipulation, pressure seems to help in the reorientation of collagen bundles deposited in the wounds. The method appears effective when pressure is applied for a prolonged period of time in healing wounds.

Other methods of wound manipulation remain within the realm of experimentation. Agents inhibiting the cross linking of collagen (D-penicillamine and beta-aminopropionitrile) have shown promise, but there are no conclusive results regarding decreased recurrence of surgically revised keloids.

mation. Keloids, on the other hand, seem to be genetically determined and are more frequent in dark-skinned people. Thus it appears that the greater the activity of melanocyte-stimulating hormone (MSH), the higher the incidence of keloidal scar formation. This relation might explain the favorable effect of steroids on keloidal scars, because steroids inhibit MSH output.

To the patient, the diagnosis of a hypertrophic scar carries a different connotation from that of a keloid regarding prognosis and treatment. Because hypertrophic scars flatten and blend with time, their surgical revision, if the pitfalls of the original injury management are avoided, is expected to yield an improved result. On the other hand, a keloid is expected to proceed unabated during the healing phase, does not regress, and frequently recurs after surgical excision. Accordingly, the patient has to be cautioned about the possibility of recurrence, which remains quite high after keloidal scar revision when only conventional methods of treatment are used.

The guiding principle behind hypertrophic scar revision is the avoidance of tension. Thus the judicious use of tissue rearrangement techniques is strongly favored. On the other hand, the aim of revisional surgery for keloids is to avoid opening additional planes of dissection to minimize tissue reaction and to control collagen metabolism. For this reason intralesional or systemic steroids are often used, sometimes preoperatively. A mixture of triamcinolone acetonide (Kenalog 40), 40 mg/milliliter and lidocaine 2% with 1:100,000 epinephrine is usually used. To be effective, the injection is given within the substance of the keloid and usually under a moderate amount of pressure. A revisional operation is performed 3 months after the injection. Ideally the margins of excision are within the confines of the lesion to protect virgin tissues. The patient is followed postoperatively. At the first sign of recurrence, additional steroid injections are given. Of course, it is possible for the physician to anticipate such a recurrence and inject steroids "prophylactically" after the wound is healed. This injection is repeated at 3- to 6-week intervals. An alternative method of collagen synthesis control is the postoperative use of radiation therapy. It appears that judicious doses of radiation (from 300 to 2000 rad) decrease the rate of collagen synthesis by inducing microvascular changes in the irradiated bed. There is little agreement, however, on the dose and mode of delivery of radiation therapy in the treatment of keloids.

Suggested Reading

Borges, A.F. Scar prognosis of wounds. *Br. J. Plast. Surg.* 13:47, 1960.

Borges, A.F. W-shaped incisions. *Int. Surg.* 48:580, 1967.

Borges, A.F. *Elective Incisions and Scar Revision.* Boston, Little, Brown, 1973.

Borges, A.F. Zig-zag incisions for improved exposure and scarring. *Clin. Orthop.* 145:202, 1979.

Borges, A.F. Relaxed skin tension lines (RSTL) versus other skin lines. *Plast. Reconstr. Surg.* 73:144, 1984.

Borges, A.F., and Alexander, J.E. Relaxed skin tension lines, Z-plasties on scars, and fusiform excision of lesions. *Br. J. Plast. Surg.* 15:242, 1962.

Furnas, D.W., and Fisher, G.W. The Z-plasty: Biomechanics and mathematics. *Br. J. Plast. Surg.* 24:144, 1971.

Limberg, A.A. Design of Local Flaps. In T. Gibson (Ed.), *Modern Trends in Plastic Surgery.* London: Butterworth, 1966.

McGregor, I.A. The theoretical basis of Z-plasty. *Br. J. Plast. Surg.* 9:256, 1957.

Peacock, E.E. Biologic basis for the treatment of keloids and hypertrophic scars. *Southern Med. J.* 63:755, 1970.

Peacock, E.E. Pharmacologic control of surface scarring in human beings. *Ann. Surg.* 193:592, 1981.

Thomas, J.R., and Holt, G.R. *Facial Scars: Incision, Revision and Camouflage.* St. Louis, Mosby, 1989.

Tissue Transfer

4

Skin Grafts

Henry C. Vasconez

A skin graft is a portion of skin of variable thickness that is transplanted to the body to cover an area devoid of cutaneous surface. The graft is totally detached from its blood supply at the donor site and receives all its nourishment from the site to which it has been transplanted, the recipient site. Although skin-grafting attempts were reported sporadically in the early nineteenth century, the technique did not come into widespread use until after Reverdin reported his experience to the Imperial Society of Surgery of Paris in 1869. His technique, using thin "epidermic grafts," was more successful than those of his predecessors, in which the thickness of the skin was not considered important. Since Reverdin's time, the medical profession has developed several types of grafts, different means of harvesting the skin, various ways of preparing the graft and wound, and techniques that enhance graft take. These aspects, as well as the proper selection of grafts and sites and the indications for grafting, are discussed in this chapter.

The skin is the largest organ of the body by virtue of its surface area. Because the skin is in direct communication with the outside environment, its biologic and mechanical properties serve to protect and maintain the delicate homeostasis of the organism. In dealing with wound healing problems, skin grafting offers the surgeon a method of regaining skin continuity. Skin grafting is just one technique within a spectrum of solutions that includes primary closure, contracture, and coverage with various forms of flaps. Because it is usually simple and effective, skin grafting should be included in the decision tree for most wound problems.

The most common and successful form of skin transplantation involves taking a piece of skin from one part of a patient's body and immediately placing it on another, skin-deficient part (autograft). The other transplantation options require taking skin from another person (allograft, homograft) or from an animal of another species (xenograft, heterograft). Skin also can be harvested, divided into its cellular components, and, by special culturing techniques, made to grow in sheets of unlimited supply (cultured autografts or allografts). Active investigation is proceeding to develop further these and other biologic and synthetic skin substitutes.

Classification of Grafts

Skin grafts can be classified according to their source, or origin, and according to their physical characteristics, especially thickness.

Source

The autograft, which poses no immunologic impediment to graft take, is the most successful type of graft. Because identical twins have the same genotype, grafting between them (isograft) is equally successful. Allografts and, to a greater extent, xenografts, serve only temporary roles in wound coverage because of their immunogenic potential. These grafts can be helpful for patients with extensive burns. Because patients with burns tend to be immunosuppressed, they have a less intense rejection reaction, allowing the grafts to provide a good biologic barrier, thereby protecting the wound from desiccation and contamination.

Skin Thickness

Grafts are classified according to skin thickness into (1) split-, or partial-thickness, grafts and (2) full-thickness grafts. The difference between split-thickness

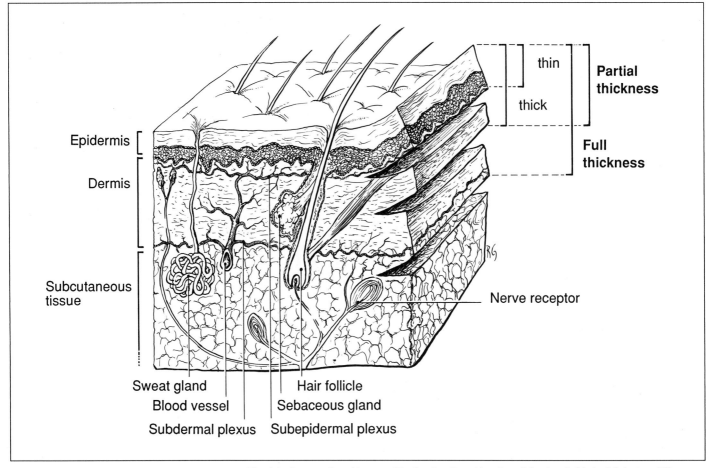

Epidermis

Dermis

Subcutaneous
tissue

thin

thick

**Partial
thickness**

**Full
thickness**

Nerve receptor

Sweat gland
Blood vessel
Subdermal plexus

Hair follicle
Sebaceous gland
Subepidermal plexus

Fig. 4-1. Cross section of human skin showing the epidermis and the dermis (derived from two different germ layers). The relative thickness of skin grafts is shown. The greater the thickness of the graft, the more characteristics of normal skin it will provide. Note the skin appendages, including sebaceous and sweat glands, multiple nerve receptors, hair follicles, and a rich vascular network. When full-thickness grafts are taken, the donor site loses the potential of regenerating skin.

and full-thickness grafts lies in the amount of dermis present. A full-thickness graft contains the entire epidermal and dermal layers, whereas a split-thickness graft contains the epidermis and part of the dermis. Split-thickness grafts are subdivided additionally into thin and thick split-thickness grafts.

Skin thickness varies widely, depending on the region from which the skin is harvested and the age of the patient. Skin from regions such as the trunk, palms, and soles of the feet can provide very thick split-thickness grafts, whereas skin from the eyelids or the retroauricular areas yields relatively thin full-thickness grafts. When selecting appropriate donor sites for skin graft harvesting, these regional differences in skin thickness must be considered. Skin thickness also depends on the age of the patient. Children and older adults tend to have thinner skin.

Anatomy

The skin is a bilaminar organ embryologically derived from two different germ layers (Fig. 4-1). The epidermis, thinner and more superficial, is composed of stratified squamous epithelium derived from surface ectoderm. The dermis, which lies deeper and is derived from the mesenchyme, is composed of vascular, dense connective tissue. The cells of the epidermis arise from the basal layer, or *stratum germinativum*, and gradually migrate to the surface and flake away through keratinization and desquamation. Keratin is a protein that gives the outer skin its protective characteristics against noxious stimuli. The basal layer, as its name implies, lies at the junction between the epidermis and the dermis and in close contact with the dermal blood supply. During fetal life, melanoblasts

migrate from the neural crest to the dermal-epidermal junction, where they differentiate into melanocytes. Melanocytes, in turn, produce melanin, which is distributed to the epidermal cells and imparts a characteristic pigmentation to the skin. The dermis is divided into a thin, more superficial layer called the papillary dermis and a thicker, reticular dermis rich in dense collagen bundles. The dermis contains various cells, collagen and elastic fibers, and ground substance, which provide its tensile strength and flexibility. Vessels, nerves, and skin appendages are present in the reticular dermis.

Skin Appendages

Sweat Glands
The two types of sweat glands, the apocrine and the more numerous eccrine, are distinguished by the manner and content of their secretion. Present in the deep der-

mis and subcutaneous tissue, these glands are important in providing lubrication to the skin and in regulating heat. Skin grafts are temporarily or permanently devoid of these glands and, therefore, require the application of creams or ointments to prevent drying or cracking of the skin.

Hair Follicles

Hair follicles are intradermal, epithelial invaginations associated with sebaceous glands and smooth-muscle bundles called erector pili. The presence of hair and hair follicles must be considered in skin grafting. Both full-thickness and thicker split-thickness grafts retain their hair-bearing characteristics on transplantation. In children, donor sites that appear hairless at the time of grafting may have considerable hair growth in later life. Hair grows at a particular angle to the skin, and this angle should be kept in mind when grafting hair-bearing skin to sites such as the eyebrows or the scalp.

Sebaceous Glands

Sebaceous glands are derived from the pilosebaceous unit and are commonly associated with hair follicles. Exceptions include the sebaceous glands of the lip, prepuce, labia minora, and eyelids (meibomian glands). Sebaceous glands secrete a lipid-rich product that serves to lubricate the hair and skin.

Blood Supply to the Skin

Blood is supplied to the skin from the large branches of the aorta that course through the muscles and perforate the skin either directly or through intermuscular septa in conjunction with the fascial plexus. These cutaneous arteries and veins form both a deep and a superficial plexus of the skin with a rich communication. The subdermal plexus, lying beneath the skin in the subcutaneous tissue, is the larger, deeper network. The more superficial subepidermal, or subpapillary, plexus is located near the junction of the reticular and papillary dermis. Blood flow and temperature control are regulated by the opening and closing of vascular shunts and by the degree of vasodilatation. Vasodilatation is mediated by the hypothalamus and the sympathetic nervous system.

Lymphatic Supply to the Skin

Lymphatics are numerous throughout the dermis; they arise in the papillary layer and form plexuses that parallel the blood vessels. Lymphatic circulation is usually established by the fourth or fifth day after graft placement. Its importance in skin grafting is largely undetermined, but it may have a role in the early elimination of postgraft edema.

Nerve Supply to the Skin

The skin is supplied with deeper myelinated nerve fibers, more superficial unmyelinated fibers, and free receptors. Adrenergic and cholinergic fibers control glandular and smooth-muscle function. Specialized sensory fibers in the skin mediate pressure, temperature, touch, pain, itch, and other sensations. Anatomically distinct end-receptor organs that respond individually or in concert to relay these specific sensations have been isolated.

Graft Take and Healing

An understanding of the biology of graft take and healing is necessary before the ideal graft can be selected. Grafts take by plasmatic imbibition and revascularization. Before these two processes can occur, however, the graft must adhere to the recipient bed. Immediately after a skin graft is placed on the recipient bed, a fibrin network provides a scaffold for the necessary graft adherence. The contraction of this fibrin network pulls the graft into closer apposition to the bed. Cellular and humoral elements that invade this site provide for the nourishment and the eventual healing of the graft. Exogenous fibrin glue, a mixture of fibrinogen-rich cryoprecipitate and a calcium thrombin solution, has been used to affix skin grafts to the recipient bed and has been shown both experimentally and clinically to improve graft take and survival. Fibrin glue enhances strength of adherence and seems to provide a better medium for the processes involved in graft healing.

Plasmatic Imbibition

During the first 48 to 72 hours, the graft becomes engorged with plasmatic fluid by means of diffusion and is thus kept alive. This edema, which causes the graft to increase by as much as 50 percent of its original weight, resolves as the blood and lymphatic vessels regain function. The duration of this phase depends on the thickness of the graft. Split grafts tolerate longer periods of plasmatic imbibition than do full-thickness grafts. The status of the recipient bed is also important. A poorly vascularized bed requires a longer period of plasmatic imbibition before the graft is revascularized.

Revascularization of the Graft

The mode by which skin grafts are revascularized is still a subject of controversy. Two theories have been proposed, and it is possible that both methods occur concomitantly. According to one theory, the source of revascularization is inosculation, that is, the "kissing," or anastomosis, of patent graft vessels with the vessels of the recipient bed. This process may occur as early as the second day after grafting. According to the second theory, neovascularization, that is, a new vessel ingrowth from the recipient bed into the graft vascular channels or into the dermis itself, is a decisive factor in reestablishing vascular supply. Growth of these new vessels is thought to be directed by angiogenic factors. Bidirectional circulation can be restored within 4 to 7 days. Here again, the thickness of the graft and the status of the recipient bed play a crucial role. Inadequate graft revascularization is caused by an insufficient vascular bed, wound contamination, functional defects in the graft vessels, angiogenic control imbalances, or an increased distance or barrier, such as a hematoma or seroma, between the graft and the recipient bed. Lymphatic circulation, which is established by the fifth day, may aid in decompressing the increased graft interstitial fluid.

Graft Innervation

Even though most skin-grafted sites do not regain normal sensation, the sensory pattern of the graft does assume the characteristics of the recipient site. Skin grafted to the fingertips, for example, becomes more sensitive than similar skin grafted to the back. Two-point discrimination is a useful test in evaluating the extent to which a graft has become reinnervated.

Nerve growth from the recipient bed to the graft is similar to the regrowth of blood vessels. Recipient nerves tend to enter the skin graft from the periphery and the base, following the empty neurilemmal sheaths. Nerves also are able to make new paths into the grafts, but only for a short distance. All nerve structures in the skin graft degenerate except for the Schwann tube cells. Although split-thickness grafts achieve a faster return of sensation, full-thickness grafts achieve a better and more complete innervation. Pain sensation is recovered first, followed by the other sensations. In the hand—in particular, the fingertips—sensation in the graft is very important. When these areas are grafted, use of similar nonglabrous skin tends to give the best results, possibly because this skin is rich in nerve fibers, sheaths, and receptors. A split-thickness or full-thickness graft from the palm of the hand or the sole of the foot serves as a good graft for fingertip injuries or avulsions.

Sweat and Sebaceous Gland Function

Full-thickness skin grafts regain sweat and sebaceous gland function much faster and more completely than do split-thickness grafts. Sweat glands, found deep in the dermis or even in the subcutaneous tissue, seem to correlate their activity with nerve regeneration and acquire the characteristics of the recipient site. Sebaceous glands, closely associated with hair follicles, are under hormonal control. Usually the thicker the graft, the better these glands regain normal function. Until function of the sebaceous glands is resumed, the skin graft must be lubricated to avoid desiccation, cracking, and infection of the graft.

Contraction of the Graft

Two forms of contraction can occur in association with skin grafting. Primary contraction, an elastic recoil of the skin caused by retractile forces, occurs as soon as the graft is harvested. Secondary contraction, a longer process, is probably caused by a combination of skin graft and host bed contraction.

Specialized, contractile fibroblasts, known as *myofibroblasts*, cause wound contraction. Myofibroblasts can be active over a period of several weeks. The amount of dermal component in the skin graft,

however, appears to inhibit wound contraction by suppressing the life cycle of the myofibroblasts. Full-thickness grafts with a full complement of dermis, therefore, maximally inhibit contraction of the wound, whereas split-thickness skin graft sites tend to shrink much more. The greatest amount of contraction occurs in open granulating wounds that are left for secondary wound closure. Full-thickness or thicker split-thickness grafts are indicated on the face, over joints, and in the digits, in great part because of their degree of control of wound contraction.

Pigmentation of the Graft

Hyperpigmentation of the skin graft is variable and depends on the amount of pigmentation present in the donor site. In general, split-thickness grafts darken more than full-thickness grafts. Care should be taken when choosing the donor site and thickness of a skin graft, especially when grafting to highly visible areas such as the face. Full-thickness grafts from the neck and the supraclavicular and retroauricular areas are good matches for facial grafting and maintain their blush tint. Sun exposure soon after grafting tends to hyperpigment the graft site. Patients are therefore advised to protect these areas with clothing or appropriate sunscreen for up to 6 months. Dermabrasion, chemical peeling, or cosmetics may be necessary in instances of undesired hyperpigmentation.

Hyperpigmentation of thin skin grafts can be a desirable result at times, for example, in nipple-areolar reconstruction. Skin taken from the abdomen or chest as a thin graft darkens with time. Skin from the labia minora has been used, but this may pigment too much. Tattooing techniques are now available to augment or decrease skin pigment discrepancies.

Indications and Graft Selection

A better understanding of the structure and the biologic behavior of skin grafts enables the surgeon to use the ideal graft and select the optimal donor site. In solving a wound management problem, the alternatives to skin grafting must be considered. These alternatives include primary closure, secondary contraction of the wound, and flap coverage, either by

rotation advancement flaps or by free tissue transfer. Skin grafts are generally used to cover large, open wounds that have adequate vascularity and are not grossly infected. Although a chronic, granulating wound may appear red and beefy, such a wound may harbor a large quotient of bacteria, which will eventually lead to the demise of the skin graft. Quantitative cultures are useful in determining this bacterial count. Animal and clinical studies have shown that the optimal cutoff point is 1×10^5 colonies of bacteria per gram of tissue.

The major advantages of skin grafting are its simplicity and effectiveness. The major disadvantages lie in the aesthetic result and a lack of long-term durability and function. Two main criteria are involved in the selection of a skin graft—the thickness and the donor site.

Skin Graft Thickness

Split-thickness skin grafts, which average between 0.01 and 0.018 inch (0.25 to 0.45 mm) in thickness, are easily harvested by an assortment of manual or power-driven dermatomes. The primary advantage of split-thickness grafts is that they take more successfully. Thin split-thickness grafts take better than thick split-thickness grafts, but, in the long term, the skin of the thicker grafts looks more normal. Full-thickness grafts, because of their complete dermal component, provide not only much more normal skin characteristics but also less contraction of the wound. Full-thickness grafts also provide better sensation and flexibility of the skin and a more aesthetic appearance. Their disadvantage is that they do not take as reliably as split-thickness skin grafts. Full-thickness grafts require a wound bed with excellent vascularity and relatively little contamination. A full-thickness graft is an excellent choice for a small, clean face wound that cannot be closed primarily. Such a graft is not suitable for a larger, contaminated wound on the trunk or lower extremities. A very large wound or a history of tobacco abuse or radiation damage to the wound is also a contraindication to the use of full-thickness grafts.

Donor Site

In extreme situations, such as extensive burns, a donor site may be located wherever skin is intact. For most patients, however, the proper selection of a donor

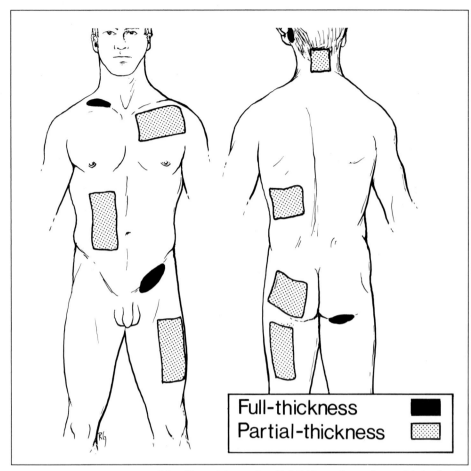

Fig. 4-2. Common donor sites used for skin graft harvesting. Full-thickness donor sites need to be closed primarily. Partial-thickness sites epithelize over time, leaving a large scar.

site requires careful thought (Fig. 4-2). First, due consideration must be given to the needs of the area to be grafted. These needs include quality, thickness, pigmentation, and hair-bearing characteristics of the skin at the donor site. Second, donor site deformity should be weighed. This deformity could include visibility of the scar and functional harvesting across joints, over bony prominences, or from sites that will be exposed to later actinic or occupational hazards.

Split-thickness skin grafts can be harvested from almost any area. When thin grafts are used, they commonly leave a donor-site scar that is visible but not deforming. To avoid evidence of scarring, however, grafts can be harvested successfully from hidden areas such as the proximal thighs, buttock region, and nape of the neck. Thick split-thickness skin grafts can be obtained from the back or thighs. Because grafts from the palm

and the sole of the foot reinnervate well, these areas can provide a source of split-thickness grafts for neighboring nonglabrous sites, especially in the hand and fingertips. On rare occasions, scalp skin can be a source of split-thickness grafts. A thin graft (0.010 inch or less) leaves the hair follicles in the donor scalp and avoids hair growth in the recipient bed.

The surface area of the donor site can be increased by infiltration with saline solution or local anesthetics. This technique is also useful in smoothing out irregular surfaces for easier harvesting.

Full-thickness grafts are usually harvested from areas of thin skin, and the donor defect is closed primarily. Postauricular full-thickness grafts are very popular because they provide thin, blush-zone skin suitable for facial grafting from a place where the scars remain hidden. Blush zones contain a rich vascularity and are found in the supraclavicular neck and

facial regions. Because older adults tend to have much redundant skin, the neck and supraclavicular regions are good sources for full-thickness grafts in these patients. In infants and children, the groin and intergluteal crease are common sources of full-thickness grafts. Excess fat is usually removed from these full-thickness grafts to improve the take.

Skin from external genitalia has been used for grafting. For example, labial skin has been used in areolar reconstruction, but the darker pigmentation acquired from this donor site is somewhat unreliable. In reduction of gigantomastia, nipple areolar grafting is successful and can yield satisfactory results with little scarring. My associates and I do not recommend nipple areolar grafting in mastectomies for cancer.

Harvesting the Graft

The tools for attaining grafts include freehand knives or scalpels, manual drum dermatomes, and air-driven or electric-powered dermatomes. Full-thickness grafts are usually obtained with a scalpel, and the donor defect is closed primarily. On occasion a full-thickness sheet graft can be obtained with an appropriate dermatome and the donor defect covered with a split-thickness skin graft. Split-thickness skin grafts are usually obtained with drum or powered dermatomes set at the desired thickness (Figs. 4-3 to 4-5). Care must be taken to check the distance between the blade and the instrument to avoid accidents. (A No. 15 Bard Parker scalpel blade approximates the thickness of a 0.015-inch split-thickness skin graft and is an appropriate tool.) The air-driven or electric dermatomes are effective instruments in obtaining split-thickness grafts rapidly over large surfaces. To avoid irregularities, a routine check of all working parts should be made before the graft is harvested. Depending on the thickness desired, power dermatomes also can be used for tangential excision of burn wounds or pigmented nevi.

Before a skin graft is harvested with a dermatome, superficial grease and residue should be removed carefully from the donor site. Lubrication with mineral oil may be necessary, although I usually prefer not to use it. Keys to successful use of the dermatome include placing the blade parallel or slightly at an angle to the skin; applying gentle, constant pressure on the

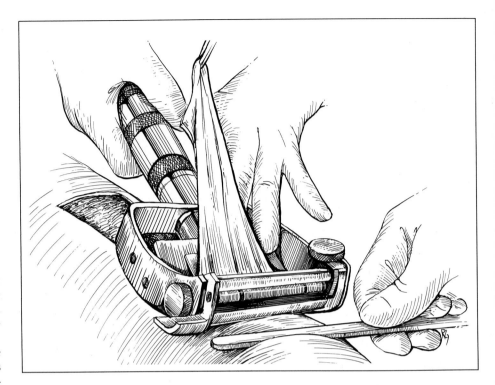

Fig. 4-3. Split-thickness skin grafts are taken conveniently with power-driven dermatomes. Proper calibration, preparation of the skin, and countertraction are important for routinely successful skin graft harvesting.

skin; and having an assistant apply countertension on the skin to be harvested.

The drum dermatome, best exemplified by the Reese, is a precision instrument that can yield relatively small, but uniform, grafts. It contains a sharp blade with a convex surface and a series of templates of varying thickness. The drum dermatome can harvest good grafts, although time is required to master its use. A small, battery-operated dermatome with a disposable head and a thickness premeasured at 0.015 inch is also effective. Freehand blades or instruments include the Humby or Cobbett knife and the smaller Goulian or Weck knife. These blades are useful in the tangential excision of burn wounds. They are not as precise as the aforementioned dermatomes in obtaining uniform thickness, but with proper use they can be effective in harvesting grafts.

Preparation of the Graft

Once it is harvested, the skin graft should be placed on the recipient bed as soon as possible. Split-thickness grafts may be placed as sheets or as mesh grafts of varying proportions. The mesh skin graft currently used was first described by Tanner in 1964 as a method of expanding skin grafts. Depending on the ratio used, a skin graft can be expanded to several times its original surface area. The most commonly used expansion ratio is 1:1.5, which increases the surface area by 50 percent. A mesh graft is much easier to adapt to irregular surfaces and excess fluid can seep through the interstices of the graft, improving the eventual take; however, inadequate hemostasis of the recipient bed or excessive weeping from the wound can endanger the survival even of mesh grafts. Mesh grafts should be avoided on the face, over joint surfaces, and in other areas where excessive contracture is undesirable.

The graft is placed on the recipient bed and fixed with sutures or metal staples. I find metal staples easy to use and to remove after graft take. In children and infants, I use absorbable suture material.

In split- and full-thickness sheet grafts, I recommend "pie crust" incisions that provide for drainage yet heal with minimal scarring. The use of bolsters or stents is recommended in areas that are difficult to bandage or dress. They are also useful in areas such as the eyelids, the back and shoulder, and the neck, where graft immobilization may be difficult. Often the need for bolsters and stents can be eliminated by spraying fibrin glue onto the recipient bed, where it forms an interface to which the skin graft is applied. Studies have shown that exogenous fibrin glue enhances the native fibrin network to ensure adherence, facilitate healing, and provide for a medium through which sterilization of the wound can take place. The glue is also useful both in immobilizing grafts and in providing hemostasis. Simple and fast methods of preparing autologous fibrin glue are available and desirable.

Preparation of the Wound

Preparation of the wound before grafting is important to maximize graft survival. A review and understanding of the causes of graft failure allows the surgeon to provide for an optimal recipient bed. The causes of graft failure are:

1. Inadequate vascularity of the recipient bed
2. Inadequate interface between the skin graft and the recipient bed (hematoma, seroma)
3. Contamination or infection
4. Inadequate immobilization of the graft

The first three causes can be controlled by proper preparation of the wound. If the recipient bed presents an avascular or hypovascular surface, graft take will be limited. In severe radiation damage or chronic scarring, little can be done, and flap closure is indicated. When bone cartilage, tendon, or nerve structures are exposed, flap coverage also may be the most appropriate treatment. In some situations, the bone can be burred-down to viable capillaries, and skin grafts will take on this surface. The bed also can be debrided down to healthier vascular tissue to provide a better recipient bed. Adequate hemostasis must be ensured to avoid hematoma or excess fluid collection between the graft and the host bed, because these factors lead to eventual graft slough. The meshing or pie crusting of the graft can help avoid this problem but cannot guarantee against it.

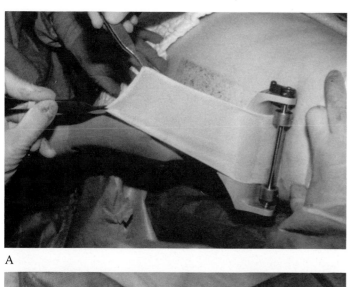

A

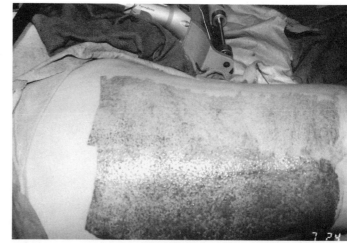

B

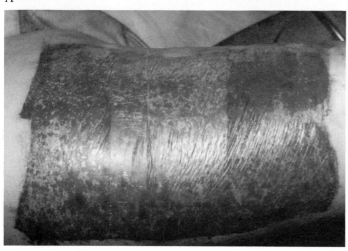

C

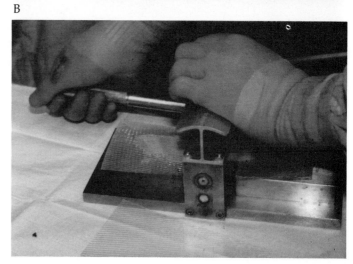

D

Fig. 4-4A. A split-thickness skin graft is harvested. B. The donor site is treated with topical, epinephrine-soaked sponges. C. The donor site is covered with a bio-occlusive transparent dressing that remains until the site heals. D. The skin graft is meshed with a template proportioned 1:1.5. E. The meshed split-thickness graft is applied, using fibrin glue for fixation.

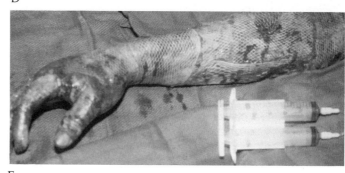

E

Fig. 4-5. A small, disposable, battery-operated dermatome can be used for harvesting of small skin or mucosal grafts.

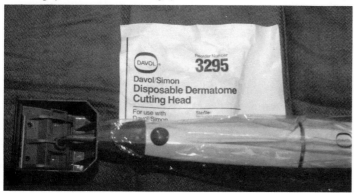

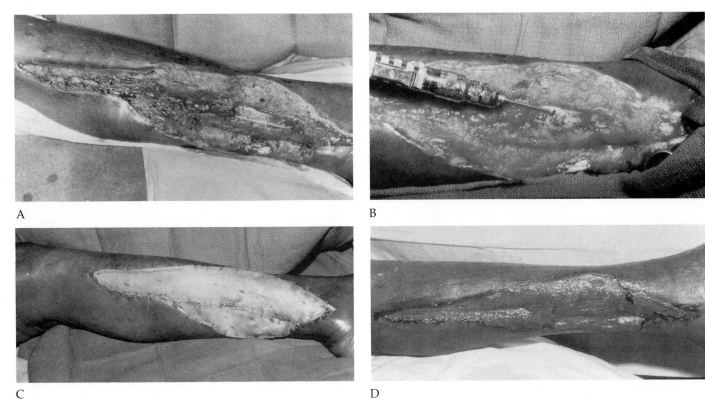

Fig. 4-6A. A 61-year-old patient with peripheral vascular disease after a distal bypass operation. She presented with an open wound and exposed bone. B. Initial debridement of the wound included burring of the fibula down to bleeding tissue. C. A homograft was placed initially to prepare the wound and evaluate it for suitability of autografting. D. Three weeks after the autograft was placed, there was a contracting, well-healed wound.

Infection, especially of contaminated wounds, is a common cause of partial or total graft failure. Surgical debridement of a contaminated wound, such as that found in burn injury, is necessary. All unhealthy, necrotic, and chronic-granulation tissue also must be removed. Use of a biologic dressing such as homograft or xenograft reliably predicts whether or not the wound will eventually take an autogenous skin graft. These biologic dressings also reduce pain and fluid loss through the wound and may in fact enhance the vascularity of the recipient bed. I give perioperative doses of antibiotics to patients receiving skin grafts to eliminate surface contaminants, in particular *Streptococcus*, which can "eat up" a graft within 24 hours.

Once the wound bed has been prepared properly, the graft is placed and fixed with a combination of exogenous fibrin glue, sutures, or staples (Figs. 4-6 to 4-8). A tie-over bolus or stent dressing may be used in areas that are mobile or difficult to bandage. The graft usually is left undisturbed for a period of 5 days, after which the dressing is taken down and wet-to-wet dressings are applied for 2 or 3 more days. When the skin graft is stable and adherent, antibiotic ointment or another mild lubricating agent is used. In some contaminated wounds, I choose to remove the dressing earlier, especially if there is drainage or an increasingly foul smell. Failure to respond to these signs may place the entire graft at risk. On occasion, I treat these contaminated wounds by placing one layer of coarse mesh gauze over the skin graft. The gauze dressing is fixed with collodion so that it will not be removed inadvertently. When using this modified open technique, I usually begin to apply wet-to-wet dressings 4 to 6 hours after the initial grafting to help eliminate any serous or purulent drainage that may accrue in the early postoperative period.

When using the closed technique, I place petrolatum gauze over the skin graft. The petrolatum is covered with soaked cotton balls and gauze, and a circumferential or bolus pressure dressing is applied.

Other Types of Grafts

In addition to the more popular split-thickness and full-thickness autologous skin grafts, other types of autogenic and allogenic grafts and synthetic and semi-synthetic skin substitutes can be used as biologic dressings for the temporary coverage of various wounds.

Composite Grafts

Composite grafts contain two or more types of tissue such as skin with adipose tissue and cartilage. These grafts take by means of a bridging phenomenon from the periphery that ultimately leads to revascularization. For this reason, composite grafts must be small; the maximal safe size is about 1.5 cm in diameter. The recipient bed must be well vascularized

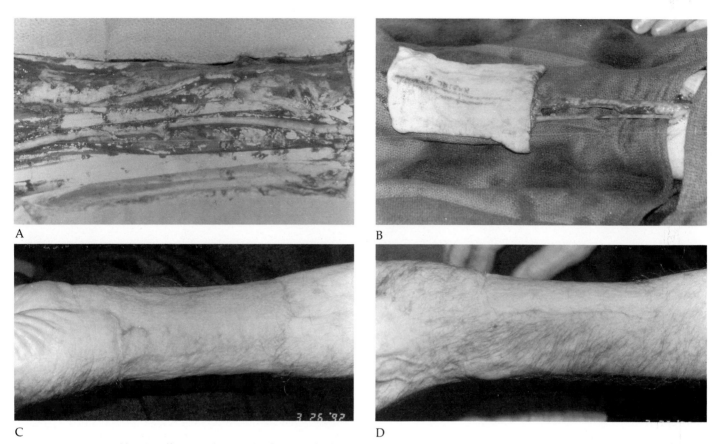

A

B

C

D

Fig. 4-7A. An 83-year-old patient after extensive resection for naso-orbital maxillary cancer. The site of the resection required coverage with a radial forearm free flap. The forearm defect was large and a reverse saphenous vein graft was used to reconstruct the radial artery. Care was taken to preserve the paratenon of the forearm tendons. B. The radial forearm flap before division of the pedicle. C and D. The donor site has healed well after 3 months. The patient, who is a violinist, has resumed his normal activity.

and, at times, can be enhanced to improve healing. A common composite graft is an ear helix wedge used to replace the nasal ala. Skin and cartilage from the ear or septal mucosal cartilage grafts can be used to reconstruct defects in the eyelids.

Dermal Fat Grafts

Dermal fat grafts consist of varying thicknesses of dermis and fat that are buried to provide bulk and contour. Their main problem is resorption, the amount of which depends on the vascularity of the recipient bed. Infection secondary to fat necrosis also may be a problem. The fat in these grafts tends to survive a little better than do injected free fat cells. The donor site defect is similar to that in full-thickness grafts.

Allografts

Allografts (homografts) are sections of skin from a genetically different donor. Human allografts are usually obtained from skin banks that harvest skin from cadaveric donors and maintain it below −60°C (−76°F). Allograft material has been tested for hepatitis, HIV, and syphilis. When needed, it is thawed in a warm bath (37°C [98.6°F]) and used within one hour of thawing. These grafts are used frequently as biologic dressings for extensive burn wounds for which autograft material is scarce. Vascular changes in allografts are identical to those in autografts until a rejection phenomenon takes place, usually 7 to 10 days after placement. Because they are typically immunosuppressed, patients with extensive burns have a considerably delayed rejection

process. A combination of autograft and allograft can be used in these patients to provide faster and more favorable conditions for burn wound healing. The allograft also can be used as a biologic test to predict the success or failure of the future autograft. While on the wound, the allograft enhances vascularity, relieves pain, decreases water loss, and makes dressing care much easier.

Xenografts

Xenografts are portions of skin taken from an animal of a different species. Porcine skin is the type used most commonly in the clinical setting. It has the same indications as allografts but demonstrates little or no vascularization and therefore is effective for only 2 to 3 days. Whether porcine skin produces a clinically signif-

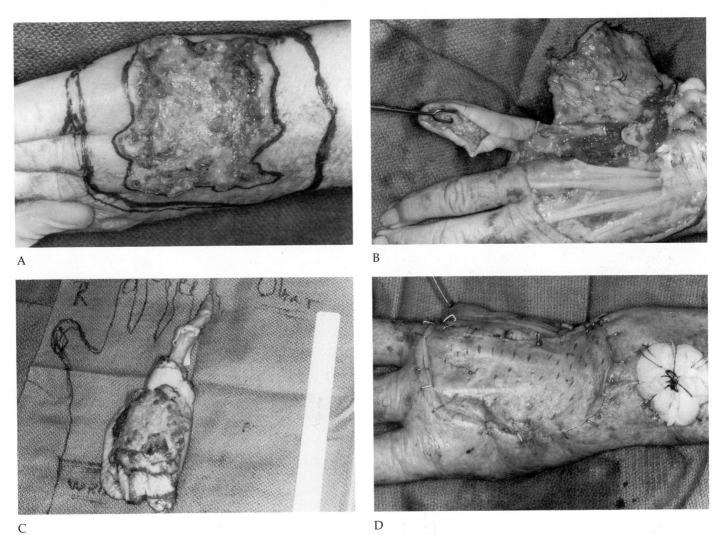

A .... B

C .... D

Fig. 4-8A. A 67-year-old farmer with extensive squamous cell cancer on the dorsum of his right (dominant) hand. No evidence of regional or distant metastasis was found. B and C. Wide excision of the ulcerated mass included removal of the little finger to the metacarpocarpal joint, preserving a volar fillet flap of the finger. D. A nonmeshed, thick, partial-thickness graft was placed to allow fluid to escape. Note the areas of pie crusting. E. Ulnar view with fillet flap inset. F and G. Three months after the operation, the site has healed with no evidence of disease.

icant rejection phenomenon is still a matter of controversy. Porcine xenografts are about five to six times less expensive than human allografts, but they are also considerably less effective.

Cultured Epithelial Grafts

Cultured epithelial grafts were first shown to be successful in vitro by Ronwall and Green and first used clinically by Gallico and associates in 1984. The technique has allowed the successful treatment of extensive, potentially fatal burns with autologous material. When a 1-cm section of normal skin is properly prepared and cultured, an unlimited supply of autologous epithelial sheet grafts is available at approximately 3 weeks. Because of their thin, fragile nature, cultured grafts take only 40 to 65 percent of the time. Their lack of a dermal component restricts adherence and attachment of underlying tissue, reducing the long-term durability of the graft. Some authors report the development of a neodermis 2 to 3 years after epithelial grafting, but oth-

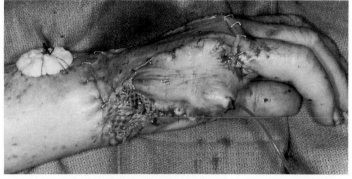

E

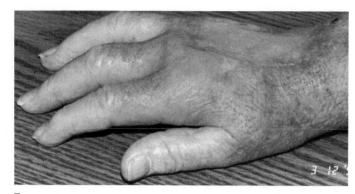

F

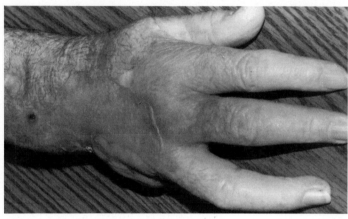

G

ers report neodermal development to be incomplete or inconsistent. Work is also being done on the development of dermal substitutes that can be used as a temporary dressing or that may be combined with conventional or cultured autografts. A combination of an epidermal-dermal skin substitute holds the greatest promise, at present, for future success.

Donor Site Healing

The donor site is important to the success of the skin grafting procedure. Difficulty or complete lack of healing in the donor site can produce a problem that is worse than the original wound. Full-thickness grafts usually are closed primarily except when they are extensive and need to be skin grafted themselves. The donor site for the split-thickness graft heals secondarily to epithelization from adnexal structures in the dermis, that is, hair follicles, sweat glands, and sebaceous glands.

After a split-thickness skin graft is harvested, punctate bleeding occurs from the subepidermal plexus, and hemostasis is obtained by pressure or the use of agents such as epinephrine (1:50,000) or thrombin spray. During the ensuing 7 to 14 days, when healing takes place, a variety of dressings can be placed on the donor site. Moist dressings have been shown to enhance epithelization and tend to be less painful for the patient. We have used a semipermeable transparent dressing such as a transparent bio-occlusive dressing, such as Opsite or Tegaderm with good patient acceptance. Leakage of fluid can lead to infection, which is fortunately rare and can be easily managed. Xeroform or petrolatum gauze also can be placed on the wound. The gauze forms a dry, scablike cover that is initially more painful but can be removed after healing has occurred. Thin split-thickness skin grafts usually leave reasonably good scars, whereas the thicker split-thickness grafts tend to produce hypertrophic scarring in some patients.

Suggested Reading

Cohen, I.K., Diegelmann, R.F., and Lindblad, W.J. (Eds.). Wound Healing: Biochemical and Clinical Aspects. Philadelphia: Saunders, 1992.

Gallico, G.G., III. Biologic skin substitutes. Clin. Plast. Surg. 17:519, 1990.

Rudolph, R., and Ballantyne, D.L., Jr. Skin Grafts. In J.G. McCarthy (Ed.), Plastic Surgery. Philadelphia: Saunders, 1990. Pp. 221–274.

Smahel, J. The healing of skin grafts. Clin. Plast. Surg. 4:409, 1977.

Swain, S.F. Skin grafts. Vet. Clin. North Am. 20: 147, 1990.

Tanner, J.C., Vandeput, J. and Olley, J.F. The mesh skin graft. Plast. Reconstr. Surg. 34:287, 1964.

5

Flaps: Physiology, Principles of Design, and Pitfalls

B. George H. Lamberty   Ciaran Healy

In the field of plastic surgery, a *flap* is understood to be a piece of skin and subcutaneous tissue nourished by arteries and veins that enter it at its base, or pedicle. The word *flap* is now used to refer to a variety of reconstructive techniques using skin and other tissues. These range from the basic pedicled transposition flap, to island flaps, to the more complex free flap. *Graft* is a horticultural term describing the insertion of a shoot into a slit of another stock to allow the sap of one to circulate with the other, thereby nourishing the graft. In plastic surgery, a graft is a free transfer of tissue that relies entirely on the blood supply at the recipient site for nourishment. The essential difference between a free flap and a graft is that a free flap, although transferred by microvascular surgery, is still nourished by its own vascular pedicle, which has been transferred from one site to another.

History of Flaps

The evolution of flaps may be divided into three periods.

In the early period, which culminated in the 1950s, flaps were confined to skin and subcutaneous fat. The earliest written record of an operation involving a flap describes a distally based, pedicled random pattern flap from the upper arm. This flap was used for reconstructive rhinoplasty by Tagliacozzi in the sixteenth century. The use of a pedicled forehead flap for rhinoplasty by the Kanghiara family as early as 1440 is less well documented. Work in the nineteenth century was dominated by von Graefe (1818), Mutter (1843), Dieffenbach (1845), and Gersuny (1887), among others.

Modern plastic surgical techniques of flap transfer are attributed to Gillies and Filatov, whose articles describing the tube pedicle flap were published between 1917 and 1920. All the flaps used by Gillies and Filatov, whether tubed or untubed, are now recognized to be random pattern skin flaps. These flaps could be safely raised only in a 1:1 or 2:1 length-breadth ratio. An increase in the length-breadth ratio of these flaps could be achieved only by the delay phenomenon.

The second period extended from the 1950s to the late 1960s, with a proliferation of new flaps related mainly to head and neck reconstruction. McGregor and Jackson's publication describing axial pattern skin flaps dominated the later part of this period. The axial pattern allowed long length-breadth ratio flaps to be raised primarily and nourished by a named artery and vein, which ran in the long axis of the flap. The muscle flap was first described by Ger in 1968.

The third period, extending through the 1970s and 1980s, saw rapid proliferation in the number of flaps described. This success was based on a wider knowledge of the anatomy of the blood supply to the skin and led to the use of the musculocutaneous flap. The 1980s saw the discovery and evolution of fasciocutaneous flaps.

The anatomic renaissance of the 1970s and 1980s should not eclipse the work of the great anatomists of the past. Manchot's work reemerged in the 1960s, and Salmon's work was recognized in the English literature during the 1980s. The discovery of axial pattern, musculocutaneous, and fasciocutaneous flaps coincided with the development of the technique of microvascular anastomosis. Pioneered by Buncke, Taylor, and others, these two disciplines were united to produce the technique of microvascular free tissue transfer. This advance allowed many of the local and distant pedicled flaps then in use to be transferred as free flaps.

Design of Flaps

The area from which a flap is raised is termed the *donor site* or *secondary defect* and the area of inset is termed the *primary defect*.

The design of a flap involves planning its donor site, shape, size, and constituent parts. The constituent parts may include skin, subcutaneous fat, deep fascia, muscle, tendon, bone, nerves, and, of course, blood vessels. The donor defect may be closed directly or with the use of a skin graft or another flap.

The skin of the proximal portion of the flap that remains attached to the donor site is called the base or pedicle. The vascular supply of the flap runs in its pedicle, which may include skin, subcutaneous fat, deep fascia, and muscle.

The flap may be inset directly into a local primary defect, or there may be an area of intact skin between its base and the primary defect. This area is bridged by a portion of the flap, which can be tubed on itself to reduce infection. The bridging section of the flap, which constitutes its pedicle, may be deepithelized and tunneled subcutaneously, thereby making an island of the flap.

When the vascular supply of the flap can be dissected back to a distinct arterial and venous network, these networks alone may act as its pedicle. When the vessels making up the pedicle are suitable for microvascular anastomosis, the flap may be transferred as a free flap.

Random pattern flaps are not based on a specific vascular supply. They are designed within the limits of length-to-breadth ratios that depend on anatomic location. On the richly vascularized face, the ratio is 5:1. With decreasing vascularity the ratio declines, reaching 1:1 on the lower limb. The fasciocutaneous and musculocutaneous perforators form the vascular supply to these flaps.

The pivot point is the center of the arc around which the flap moves during its transfer. This point is planned to avoid tension on the flap as a whole and on the vascular pedicle. When the pedicle of a flap is reduced to its vascular hilus, this constitutes its pivot point. It is essential in designing all flaps to avoid tension on the vascular pedicle.

The size of a flap, although limited by the extent of the blood supply on which it is based, must be sufficient to fill the primary defect, and the pedicle length must be sufficient to avoid tension. Compromising flap size to facilitate direct closure of the donor site risks breakdown and flap failure.

Pedicled Flaps

Local Flaps

Local flaps are used to close primary defects adjacent to the donor site (Fig. 5-1). The types of movement involved are advancement, rotation, transposition, and interpolation. The predominant type of movement is referred to when describing the flap.

Advancement Flap

The simplest form of advancement flap is direct wound closure. The direct advancement of a flap may be facilitated by excising a triangle of skin (Bürow triangle) at each side of its base as shown in Figure 5-1A. A more complex local advancement flap is the V to Y advancement flap.

Transposition Flap

A transposition flap moves laterally about its pivot point, which lies opposite the apex of the primary defect at the base of the flap, as shown in Figure 5-1B. The donor site is usually grafted, but direct closure may be obtained when local tissue laxity allows. Factors such as this may dictate the orientation of the flap design. Transposition of the flap results in some loss of length, which is compensated for by a design in which the flap is longer than the side of the triangulated primary defect. Failure to compensate in this way may result in a line of tension along the flap, requiring a back-cut to avoid vascular compromise.

Rotation Flap

A rotation flap is part of the arc of a circle of which the primary defect is a triangular segment; both the flap and the primary defect combine to make up a half-circle as shown in Figure 5-1C. The arc of the rotation flap is made as large as possible to enable the donor defect to be closed primarily by distributing the tension equally along the suture line. When unacceptable tension occurs during the direct closure of the donor site, a back-cut may be added

along the diameter of the flap to facilitate closure of the donor defect. The pivot point of the rotation flap lies halfway between the apex of the primary defect and the end of the flap. To avoid tension in the flap, the distance between the pivot point and any point along the flap tip must not be less than the distance between the pivot point and its destination in the primary defect.

In planning transposition and rotation flaps, it is important to triangulate the primary defect. The two sides of the triangle should be longer than its base, which lies opposite that of the flap.

Island Flap

The pedicle of an island flap is reduced to its subcutaneous component, which includes its vascular supply. This supply may consist of a series of vessels within the subcutaneous tissue or a single artery and vein. The cutaneous nerve supply to the skin flap may be included in its pedicle as in the Littler neurovascular island flap used in thumb reconstruction (Fig. 5-2).

Rhomboid Flap

The shape of a local flap may be defined by geometric configurations, as in the rhomboid transposition flap shown in Figure 5-3. For a defect of this shape, there are four possible rhomboid flaps that border it. The flap chosen is the one in which the defect can be closed directly using local tissue laxity.

Distant Flaps

Distant flaps are transferred to primary defects at some distance from the donor site. In general they are transposition flaps in which the donor and recipient sites may be approximated to allow the flap to be inset. Examples include the pedicled groin flap for covering hand defects (Fig. 5-4) and the cross-finger flap (Fig. 5-5).

Microvascular Free Flaps

In a microvascular free flap, the block of tissue is supplied by a pedicle that is reduced to its vascular components alone. These components are divided from their parent vessels at the donor site and anastomosed to appropriate vessels at the recipient site using microsurgical techniques.

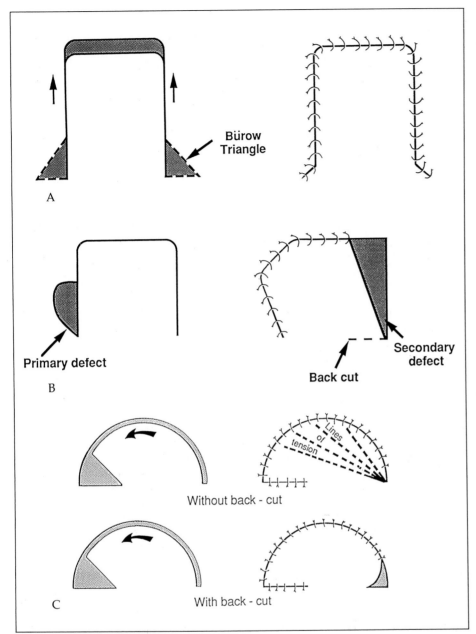

Bürow
Triangle

A

Primary defect

B

Without back - cut

With back - cut

Lines
of
tension

Secondary
defect

Back cut

C

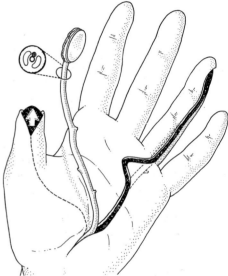

Fig. 5-1. Examples of local flaps. A. Movement of the advancement flap may be facilitated by excision of the Bürow triangles on either side of the flap base. B. The transposition flap moves about the pivot point, which lies at the flap base opposite the apex of the triangulated primary defect. A back-cut at the base may be required to correct a line of tension in the flap. C. The base of the triangulated primary defect forms part of the arc of the rotation flap. A back-cut may be required at the flap base, opposite the primary defect, to facilitate primary closure of the secondary defect and to correct a line of tension across the flap.

Fig. 5-2. The pedicle of the Littler neurovascular digital pulp island flap, containing the ulnar digital artery, digital vein, and digital nerve. The resulting sensate island flap may be tunneled subcutaneously to reconstruct the distal thumb pulp.

Fig. 5-3. Rhomboid-shaped transposition flap. The flap is located about the primary defect in a way that facilitates direct closure of the secondary defect using local tissue laxity.

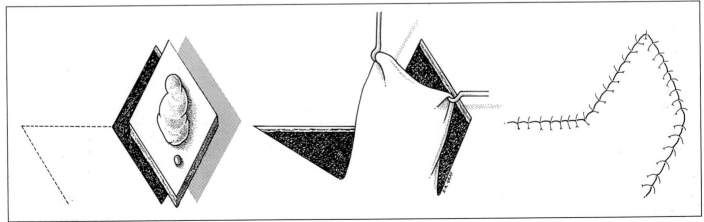

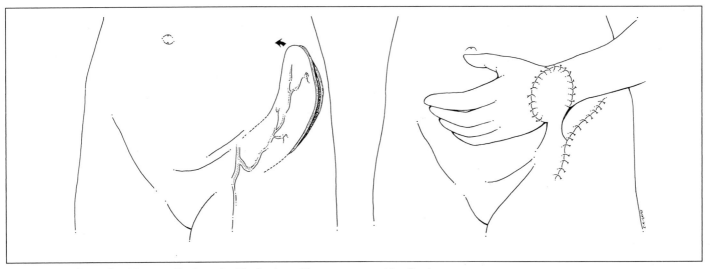

Fig. 5-4. Groin flap with axial pattern blood supply. The flap is used here as a transposition flap for a recipient site on the dorsum of the hand.

Fig. 5-5. Cross-finger transposition flap inset into a defect on the volar aspect of the approximated thumb.

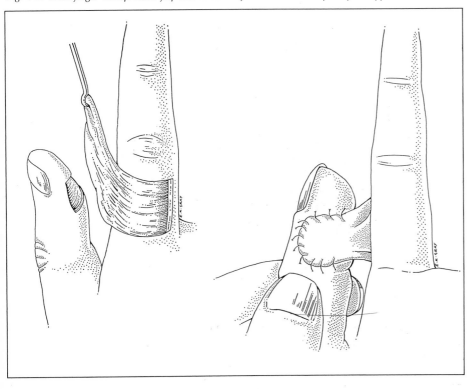

Refinements of Flap Design

According to recipient site requirements, the flap may be raised to include bone, motor-innervated muscle, sensory-innervated skin, or vascularized nerve. The skin may be raised in two paddles to cover intraoral and skin defects simultaneously. The flap donor site may be enlarged by previous tissue expansion, allowing a larger flap than normal to be raised. Such flaps are custom designed to meet the requirements of each patient.

Vascular Basis of Flaps

For a flap system to survive requires adequate arterial input and venous drainage, which communicate by microcirculation within the flap. This is the vascular basis common to all flaps, whether skin, muscle, musculocutaneous, or fasciocutaneous. Three vessel systems supply the skin—direct vessels, musculocutaneous vessels, and fasciocutaneous vessels.

Macrocirculation

The arteries going directly to skin, particularly of fasciocutaneous origin, have variously been termed direct, septocutaneous, fasciocutaneous perforators, fascial perforators, and conductor vessels.

Fig. 5-6. Cutaneous arteries with their anatomic, dynamic, and potential territories. (From G.C. Cormack and B.G.H. Lamberty. The Arterial Anatomy of Skin Flaps. *2nd ed. London: Churchill Livingstone, 1986. Reproduced with permission.)*

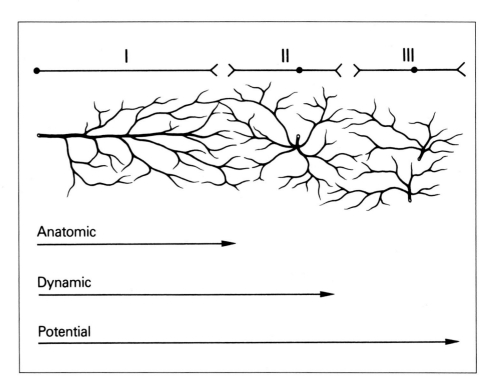

Fig. 5-6. Cutaneous arteries with their anatomic, dynamic, and potential territories. (From G.C. Cormack and B.G.H. Lamberty. The Arterial Anatomy of Skin Flaps. *2nd ed. London: Churchill Livingstone, 1986. Reproduced with permission.)*

The cutaneous arteries supply three types of territories (Fig. 5-6). The *anatomic territory* of an artery can be dissected out macroscopically. The *dynamic territory* of an artery is an extension to its anatomic territory. It depends on the arteriolar anastomoses of the arteries with neighboring vessels. In vivo the direction of blood flow is variable, going from areas of high to low pressure. The pressure gradient across an arteriolar anastomosis is altered when one of the adjoining arteries is ligated. A flap may therefore be raised to include the length of its specific arterial supply extended by a random pattern flap, which incorporates its dynamic territory. This system was first proposed by McGregor and Morgan in 1973 in relation to the deltopectoral flap.

The *potential territory* of an artery is brought into play when the artery is isolated in continuity with the territory of an adjacent artery. The anatomic and dynamic territories of the artery increase when blood is forced into the territory of the adjacent isolated artery because of the pressure gradient. This concept applies to both the direct and the fasciocutaneous systems. From clinical experience the potential territory of an artery usually extends only as far as the territory of its third consecutive neighboring perforator.

The aforedescribed classification of cutaneous vessel territories, although generally accepted, has been called into question by Taylor's group. These authors classify vessels into those going directly to the skin and those that pass indirectly to it through feeding vessels to other structures such as muscle. Taylor and associates describe the source arteries to the skin and underlying tissues as supplying territories termed *angiosomes*. These arteries are reported to follow the connective tissue framework with direct branches to the skin from branches sup-

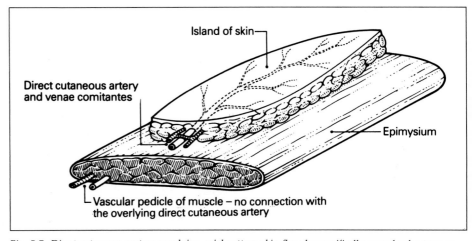

Fig. 5-7. Direct cutaneous system supplying axial pattern skin flaps by specifically named subcutaneous vessels. (From G.C. Cormack and B.G.H. Lamberty. The Arterial Anatomy of Skin Flaps. *2nd ed. London: Churchill Livingstone, 1986. Reproduced with permission.)*

plying the underlying tissues. In keeping with standard anatomic nomenclature, it is preferable to describe these vessels as *trunk* arteries, which arborize in a similar manner to the branches of a tree. Similarly the term *source* is more appropriately applied to the venous system, in which smaller tributaries drain into larger ones.

Types of Flaps

On the basis of the present understanding of blood supply to the skin, three generic types of flaps are accepted—skin flaps, muscle and musculocutaneous flaps, and fascial and fasciocutaneous flaps.

Skin Flaps

The direct cutaneous system of vessels that supplies skin flaps is illustrated in Figure 5-7. Specific named arteries and veins run in the subcutaneous fat parallel to the skin; they are confined to specific anatomic locations, mainly in the head and neck. Those in the trunk include the deltopectoral and the groin flaps based, respectively, on the anterior intercostal

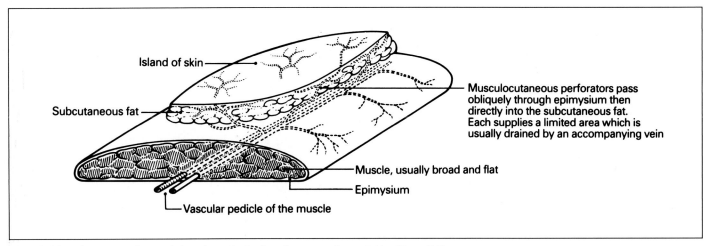

Fig. 5-8. Musculocutaneous flap consisting of muscle, fascia, subcutaneous fat, and skin. (From G.C. Cormack and B.G.H. Lamberty. The Arterial Anatomy of Skin Flaps. *2nd ed. London: Churchill Livingstone, 1986. Reproduced with permission.)*

perforators from the internal thoracic artery and the superficial circumflex iliac artery. These flaps are termed *axial pattern flaps,* and their shape is defined by the pattern of their vascular supply, which may be mapped out using Doppler ultrasonography. In addition to being raised as pedicled or island flaps, these can be used as free flaps.

The random pattern flaps are now recognized to be based on musculocutaneous or fasciocutaneous perforators feeding into the flap base. The original concept of the random pattern flap as having an undetermined vascular supply has led Caplan to describe these as flaps "for the anatomically destitute."

Musculocutaneous Flaps

The constituents of musculocutaneous flaps include muscle, fascia, subcutaneous fat, and skin as illustrated in Figure 5-8. Flaps incorporating vascularized muscle are effective in preventing and controlling infection in the recipient site, particularly in osteomyelitis. Despite this advantage, the donor muscle chosen should be functionally expendable. When the muscle bulk is adequate, a portion of the innervated muscle may be left to preserve its original function.

Mathes and Nahai's classification of the macroscopic arterial supply to muscle and musculocutaneous flaps (Fig. 5-9 and Table 5-1) incorporates the following:

The arterial trunks supplying the muscle
The site of entry of the vascular pedicle into the muscle
The number of independent arterial trunks that enter the muscle
The intramuscular anastomoses among the independent arteries of supply
The size and anastomotic connections among the independent arteries

The skin and subcutaneous tissue of an island musculocutaneous flap are supplied by secondary terminal perforating branches running vertically from the underlying muscle arteries. The skin paddle cannot overlap beyond the underlying muscle edge by more than 3 cm because the supplying branches do not ramify with one another as do those in the fasciocutaneous system. The number of musculocutaneous perforators available and their distribution define the limit of the skin paddle size and shape. The point of entry of the vascular supply of the muscle constitutes the pedicle of an island musculocutaneous flap. This is the pivot point of the flap, around which it rotates through an arc. When the vessels are suitable for anastomosis, the flap may be transferred as a free flap.

The base of a pedicled musculocutaneous flap is supplied by musculocutaneous or fasciocutaneous perforators in a manner similar to the supply of a random pattern flap. The musculocutaneous perforators supplying a pedicled musculocutaneous flap run through the base of the flap.

Fasciocutaneous Flaps

The fasciocutaneous perforators arise from regional arteries and pass along fascial septa between adjacent muscles, as illustrated in Figure 5-10. On reaching the deep fascia, they fan out to form a plexus within and on it; branches from this deep fascial plexus supply the overlying skin. The fasciocutaneous flap, called the "super flap" by Pontèn's team, is raised to include the deep fascia with the overlying skin. The anastomoses among the fasciocutaneous perforators within the deep fascial plexus have a preferred directional axiality, use of which enables a greater length-breadth ratio in the fasciocutaneous flap than in the traditional random pattern skin flap. Although similar in effect to the axial pattern flap, the fasciocutaneous flap has a different vascular anatomy.

Knowledge of the direction of orientation of the fascial plexus, the fasciocutaneous perforators, and the fascial septum with its supplying artery is required when planning a fasciocutaneous flap. Cadaveric injection studies in the lower limb (Fig. 5-11) have shown that the fasciocutaneous perforators and their fascial plexus orientation lie in the longitudinal axis. This relation is illustrated by a photomicrograph of the fascial plexus arising from the fasciocutaneous perforators running in the lateral intermuscular septum of the leg (Fig. 5-12). This anatomic arrangement suggests that a higher length-

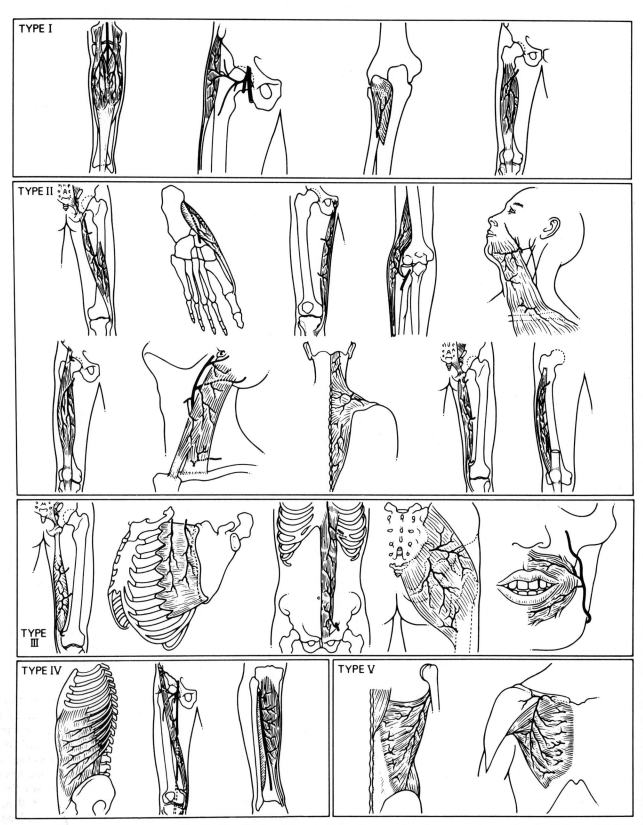

TYPE I

TYPE II

TYPE III

TYPE IV   TYPE V

Fig. 5-9. Classification of the arterial supply of muscle and musculocutaneous flaps by Mathes and Nahai. (From G.C. Cormack and B.G.H. Lamberty. The Arterial Anatomy of Skin Flaps. *2nd ed. London: Churchill Livingstone, 1986. Reproduced with permission.)*

Table 5-1. Classification of the vascular anatomy of muscles

Type I	*One vascular pedicle*

Gastrocnemius
Tensor fasciae latae
Anconeus
Vastus intermedius

Type II	*One dominant vascular pedicle usually entering close to the origin or insertion of the muscle, with additional smaller vascular pedicles entering the muscle belly*

Abductor digiti minimi	Peroneus longus	Sternocleidomastoid
Abductor hallucis	Peroneus brevis	Temporalis
Biceps femoris	Platysma	Trapezius
Brachioradialis	Rectus femoris	Vastus lateralis
Flexor digitorum brevis	Semitendinosus	
Gracilis	Soleus	

Type III	*Two vascular pedicles, each arising from a separate regional artery (except orbicularis oris)*

Gluteus maximus
Rectus abdominis
Serratus anterior
Semimembranosus
Orbicularis oris

Type IV	*Multiple pedicles of similar size*

Flexor digitorum longus	Extensor digitorum longus
Extensor hallucis longus	Flexor hallucis longus
Vastus medialis	Sartorius
External oblique	Tibialis anterior

Type V	*One dominant vascular pedicle and several smaller secondary segmental vascular pedicles*

Pectoralis major
Latissimus dorsi

Source: From G.C. Cormack and B.G.H. Lamberty, *The Arterial Anatomy of Skin Flaps* (2nd ed.), London, Churchill Livingstone, 1986. Reproduced with permission.

breadth ratio would be possible when the fasciocutaneous flap is raised longitudinally; this hypothesis has been supported by clinical findings.

Cormack and Lamberty's classification of the fasciocutaneous system of flaps into types A to D, illustrated in Figure 5-13, is based principally on vascular anatomy.

The type A flap is supplied by multiple fasciocutaneous perforators, which enter at its base and run the longitudinal length of the flap. The flap may be proximally or distally based and the skin removed from its base to make an island flap.

The type B flap is based on a single fasciocutaneous perforator, which also may be isolated as an island flap. This flap type may be transferred as a free flap in areas where the vessels are suitable for microvascular anastomoses.

The type C flap is based on small multiple fasciocutaneous perforators running along a fascial septum. The supplying artery is raised in continuity with the fascial septum and fasciocutaneous flap. The flap can be based distally or proximally as either a pedicled or a free flap.

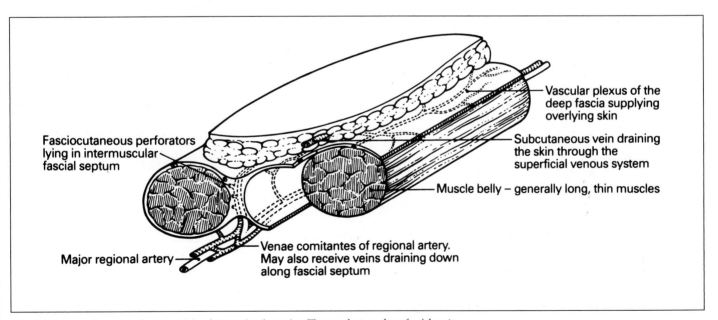

Fig. 5-10. *Fasciocutaneous perforators arising from regional arteries. The vessels pass along fascial septa between adjacent muscles to the overlying skin. (From G.C. Cormack and B.G.H. Lamberty.* The Arterial Anatomy of Skin Flaps. *2nd ed. London: Churchill Livingstone, 1986. Reproduced with permission.)*

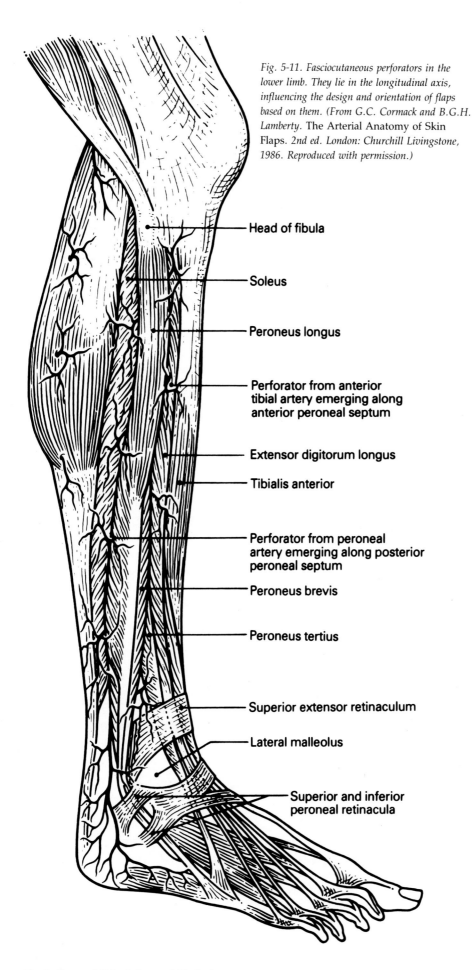

Fig. 5-11. Fasciocutaneous perforators in the lower limb. They lie in the longitudinal axis, influencing the design and orientation of flaps based on them. (From G.C. Cormack and B.G.H. Lamberty. The Arterial Anatomy of Skin Flaps. 2nd ed. London: Churchill Livingstone, 1986. Reproduced with permission.)

— Head of fibula

— Soleus

— Peroneus longus

— Perforator from anterior tibial artery emerging along anterior peroneal septum

— Extensor digitorum longus

— Tibialis anterior

— Perforator from peroneal artery emerging along posterior peroneal septum

— Peroneus brevis

— Peroneus tertius

— Superior extensor retinaculum

— Lateral malleolus

— Superior and inferior peroneal retinacula

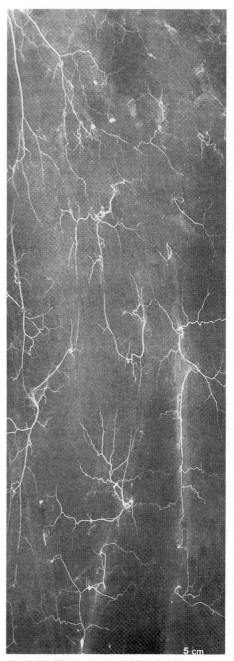

Fig. 5-12. Photomicrograph of the fascial plexus arising from the fasciocutaneous perforators running in the lateral intermuscular septum of the leg. Their longitudinal axial arrangement influences the design and orientation of flaps based on them. (From G.C. Cormack and B.G.H. Lamberty. The Arterial Anatomy of Skin Flaps. 2nd ed. London: Churchill Livingstone, 1986. Reproduced with permission.)

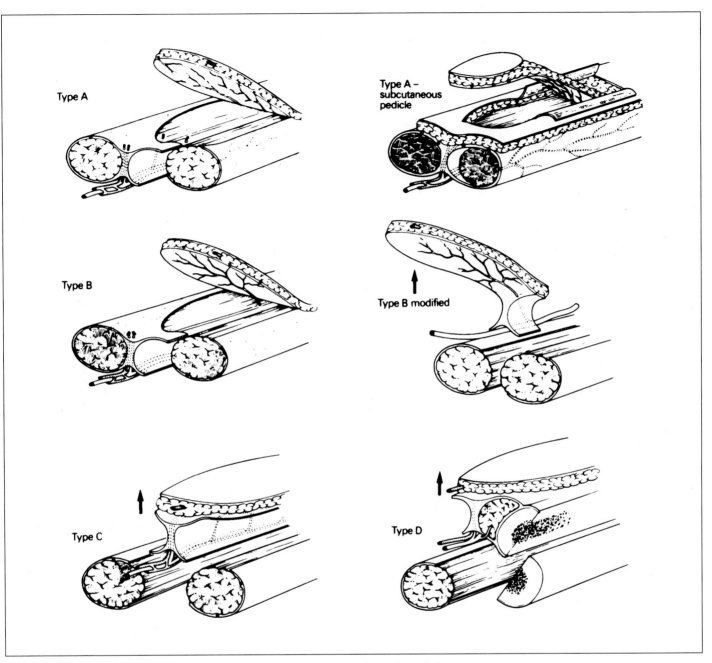

Type A

Type A – subcutaneous pedicle

Type B

Type B modified

Type C

Type D

Fig. 5-13. Classification of the fasciocutaneous system of flaps by Cormack and Lamberty. (From G.C. Cormack and B.G.H. Lamberty. The Arterial Anatomy of Skin Flaps. *2nd ed. London: Churchill Livingstone, 1986. Reproduced with permission.)*

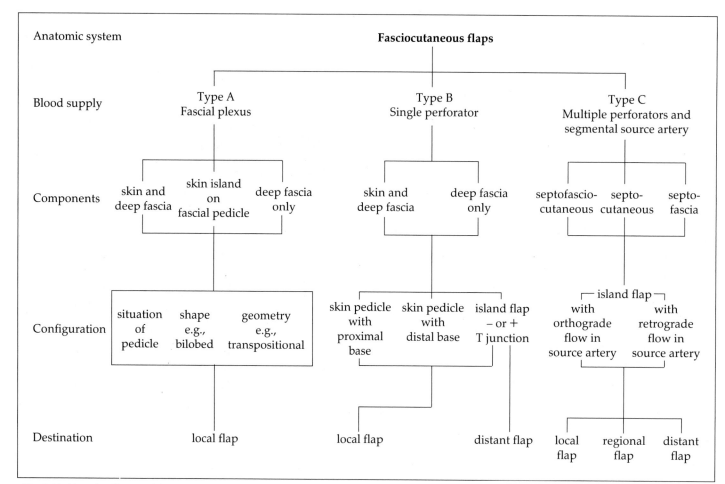

Anatomic system	**Fasciocutaneous flaps**		
Blood supply	Type A Fascial plexus	Type B Single perforator	Type C Multiple perforators and segmental source artery
Components	skin and deep fascia / skin island on fascial pedicle / deep fascia only	skin and deep fascia / deep fascia only	septofascio-cutaneous / septo-cutaneous / septo-fascia
Configuration	situation of pedicle / shape e.g., bilobed / geometry e.g., transpositional	skin pedicle with proximal base / skin pedicle with distal base / island flap – or + T junction	island flap — with orthograde flow in source artery / with retrograde flow in source artery
Destination	local flap	local flap / distant flap	local flap / regional flap / distant flap

Fig. 5-14. New classification of fasciocutaneous flaps incorporating their clinical applications. Included are the flap component tissues, vascular anatomy, configuration, and destination of the flap.

The type D flap is an osteomyocutaneous flap. It is similar to type C with the addition of a portion of adjacent muscle and underlying bone. This flap also can be based proximally or distally as either a pedicled or a free flap.

Subsequent clinical experience has led to a new classification of fasciocutaneous flaps that incorporates their clinical applications. This new system, presented in Figure 5-14, includes the component tissues of the flap, with details of its vascular anatomy, configuration, and destination. This system will be of value in compiling comparable data on the clinical use of these flaps for audit and research purposes.

Venous Drainage of Flaps

Despite the difficulties posed by the presence of valves within the venous system, Taylor's group carried out a comprehen-sive injection study of the architecture of the venous system in the integument and the underlying deep tissues. They found a series of valveless veins linking adjacent valved venous territories, which allowed equilibration of pressure throughout the tissues. These "oscillating" veins corresponded with the choke arteries, which define the angiosomes of the arterial territories, whose corresponding venous territories were called *venosomes*. The venous architecture was found to be arranged in a continuous network of arcades within the connective tissue framework of the body, closely mirroring the arterial system in all but the limbs. Here an additional system of longitudinal channels runs subdermally, although there are channels (venae comitantes) that correspond to the arterial trunks and provide venous drainage from island flaps.

The venous drainage from flaps is by subcutaneous veins or the venae comitantes of the supplying artery. The venous valves do not appear to prevent flow in the opposite direction when flaps are based distally. It has been suggested that in raising the flap the veins are denervated, resulting in incompetence of their valves. Alternatively the incompetence may be caused by the reversal in the pressure gradient across the valve and the opening up of alternative channels that bypass the venous valves.

First described by Baek and associates in 1985, the venous island flap remains controversial. These authors reported experimental evidence that a flap isolated on a venous supply could be perfused sufficiently to survive. They found that the interstitial fluid pressure was subatmospheric. The authors suggested that this pressure maintained the patency of the capillary bed despite the closure of the arterioles. The arteriolar shunting mechanism caused to and fro motion in the venous capillary bed, and this motion was suggested to be sufficient to nourish a flap with only a venous input. Similar experiments were repeated by Thatte and Thatte in 1987, who also reported the clinical use of a cephalic venous flap. It may well be, however, that small fasciocutaneous arterial perforators were included within the fatty cuff of the venous pedicle.

Much work remains to be done regarding the venous systems of flaps. New techniques are constantly being proposed such as the arterialization of venous flaps. Reports of the clinical use of such flaps have appeared, but the flaps have not been widely used.

Microcirculation

In considering the microcirculation of flaps, it is convenient to study first the structure and, following that, physiologic control.

Structural Organization

The microcirculatory bed begins with arterioles with a diameter of less than 300 μ and progresses through terminal arterioles, precapillary sphincters, capillaries, postcapillary venules, collecting venules, and muscular venules with a diameter of up to 300 μ.

Arterioles

Arterioles are derived from the terminal vessels of the direct cutaneous, fasciocutaneous, and musculocutaneous sys-

tems and retain muscle in their walls. They run in the subcutaneous tissue decreasing in intraluminal diameter to 30 μ. As they do so they branch into terminal arterioles that measure 10 to 30 μ and form the subdermal plexus.

Precapillary Sphincter

The precapillary sphincter is the last point of control of blood flow into the capillary network. The luminal diameter decreases from 30 to 10 μ over this segment. The vessel wall contains innervated smooth muscle.

Capillaries

Capillaries have an internal diameter of 3 to 7 μ. They consist of endothelium, basal lamina, and pericytes. On the basis of the type of endothelium present, four types of capillaries are recognized: continuous thick endothelium, continuous thin endothelium, fenestrated thin endothelium, and discontinuous endothelium.

Postcapillary Venules

At this point the luminal diameter begins to increase from 8 to 30 μ, and fibroblasts are seen in the vessel walls. It is this fragment of the capillary bed that is affected by inflammation and allergic reactions and from which fluid diffuses into the tissue spaces.

Collecting Venules

The postcapillary venules coalesce to form vessels approximately 50 μ in diameter. Pericytes and smooth muscle cells begin to appear, although their function is not entirely understood.

Arteriovenous Anastomoses

Arteriovenous anastomoses are normally occurring shunts that connect the arterial and venous sides of the circulation proximal to the capillary network. In the skin these are approximately 50 μ in diameter. There may be little demarcation between the arterial and venous segments or,

more commonly, an intermediate segment of smooth muscle fibers and thickened adventitia. Modified muscle cells in this glomus have a rich nerve plexus around them, enabling contraction or dilatation in response to either nerve or chemical stimulation. Blood shunting through these arteriovenous anastomoses bypasses the capillary bed. By applying Poiseuille's equation, if we accept that intraluminal pressure remains constant, the flow within vessels of even length is proportional to the fourth power of the radius of each vessel. An arteriovenous anastomosis 50 μ in diameter (that is, five times that of the capillary) would have a flow rate 600 times greater than that of a capillary.

The components of the microcirculatory system are distributed in the form of layered vascular arcades in the superficial, middle, and deep dermal plexuses, which lie at the junction of the dermis and subcutaneous tissue. The components and principal functions of these plexuses are listed in Table 5-2.

The density of the vascular arcades varies in different parts of the body. An example is the greater density of the reticular dermis of the face compared with any other region. The horizontal flow along these multiple plexuses at the level of the deep dermis may explain the greater reliability of flaps on the face. These plexuses are involved in the response of the skin to wound healing. They undergo changes during aging and are affected by radiation and burns. They also form new vessels during skin expansion and are subject to congenital malformations such as hemangiomas.

All these factors, which influence the vascular anatomy, together with growth of new vessels in response to injury, highlight an important aspect of flap circulation that has received little attention. The lymphatic system, consisting of lymphatic capillaries, collecting lymphatics,

Table 5-2. Layers of the vascular arcade

Layer	Structure	Function
Superficial plexus	Arterial and venous	Heat exchange and nutrition
Middle plexus	Mainly venous	Heat exchange and defense mechanisms
Deep plexus	Arterial and venous	Heat conservation and shunting

Source: From G.C. Cormack and B.G.H. Lamberty, *The Arterial Anatomy of Skin Flaps* (2nd ed.), London, Churchill Livingstone, 1986. Reproduced with permission.

and lymph trunks, also is involved in the microcirculation of skin flaps. When the flaps are raised, particularly island flaps, these channels are interrupted, possibly contributing to edema in the flap.

Physiologic Organization

The function of the dermal microcirculation includes thermoregulation, blood storage, defense mechanisms, blood flow, and transcapillary fluid exchange. The last two are of greatest relevance to flap physiology.

Control of Blood Flow

Blood flow to the skin is largely determined by thermoregulatory requirements. At ambient temperatures, approximately one-half the total skin blood flow is distributed to the hands, feet, and head. These are the regions with the highest numbers of arteriovenous anastomoses and therefore have the greatest potential for varying blood flow.

The tone in the vessel walls of the arteriovenous anastomoses is set by an intrinsic mechanism whereby smooth muscle cells in the vessel wall are partially constricted in response to distention. This is the myogenic control theory. The constriction may be facilitated or antagonized by neural, hormonal, chemical, and thermal response. It plays a role in the regulation of skin blood flow and is probably the explanation for return of vascular resistance after sympathectomy.

Neural control is affected by cardiovascular homeostatic reflexes that depend on atrial volume receptors and carotid sinus pressure receptors. These, together with factors such as exercise, pain, and the thermoregulatory mechanisms of the hypothalamus, interact at the level of the medulla. It is from here that the efferent sympathetic alpha vasoconstrictor fibers and beta vasodilator fibers arise. They affect the myogenic tone by release of norepinephrine at the smooth muscle motor end plates of the blood vessels. The norepinephrine causes an increase in the cytoplasmic calcium levels, leading to contraction of the blood vessel. The result of beta-adrenergic activity is the opposite; hyperpolarization is caused by a reduction in cytoplasmic calcium leading to dilatation of the blood vessel.

Temperature Effects

Body temperature regulation is a major function of skin circulation and is under both neuronal and hormonal control. The local temperature has a direct effect on the control of skin circulation. At ambient temperature, the blood flow of the skin is greater than required metabolically. By reduction of skin blood flow through decreased skin temperature, body heat is conserved.

Increasing the ambient temperature causes the thermoregulatory hypothalamic centers to inhibit the discharge of sympathetic vasoconstrictor fibers. This results in dilatation of the arteriovenous shunts, mainly in the face, hands, and feet. The increased blood flow through the skin results in heat loss through conduction, radiation, and evaporation.

If temperature control is not achieved in this way, a hormonal mechanism comes into play. Sweat gland activity is stimulated in areas in which there are usually few arteriovenous shunts but where the vascular tone is high in a resting state. Kinin formation induces increased vasodilatation, leading to increased blood flow to the sweat glands. The increased blood flow increases sweat secretion; the sweat evaporates because of the raised skin temperature. The latent heat of evaporation is extracted from the blood as it flows through the skin.

Local direct cooling of the skin is detected by skin temperature receptors. These in turn activate a local vasoconstrictor reflex. Cooling acts directly on the smooth muscle in vessel walls, slowing the sodium pump and depolarizing the cell. Contraction is caused in turn by calcium entering the cell. Local cooling also prolongs the vasoconstrictor effect of the norepinephrine released locally by slowing its metabolic breakdown.

When a flap is raised, its temperature falls, resulting in a decrease in its blood flow of up to 30 percent. It is controversial whether the cooling of a flap has a beneficial effect through reduction of metabolism or entirely the opposite effect in reducing the blood flow to the flap.

Local Injury

Local injury causes local vessel spasm, which is independent of innervation. The spasm appears to be a direct response of smooth muscle to injury. When a vessel wall is pricked with a pin, for example, a localized circumferential spasm occurs. The circumferential spasm goes beyond the area of the direct damage to the muscle cells that results from the pinprick. This suggests that depolarization spreads locally from one cell to another. If a vessel is more severely crushed, there is longitudinal spread of the vasoconstriction. The mechanism here also appears to be a widespread depolarization caused by crossing of the cell membranes by extracellular calcium.

Leakage of blood around a damaged vessel may affect the vessel directly because of vasoconstrictor agents. The most notable agent is serotonin, which is released from aggregating platelets, but norepinephrine and epinephrine also have been implicated, as has thromboxane A_2.

Viscosity

The suspended erythrocytes in blood prevent it from behaving as a simple fluid. In vivo the viscosity of blood changes with flow velocity. High velocity is associated with an increased shear rate and a reduced viscosity. Axial streaming occurs in large vessels: As the shear rate increases, the red cells lie with their long axes parallel to the direction of flow only in that part of the stream where the flow rate is highest. There is no streaming at low shear rates, and frequent collisions between cells cause rouleau formation.

In vivo with a normal hematocrit level and normal flow rates, viscosity is of relatively minimal importance. With a low flow rate, the viscosity in the postcapillary bed rises above that in the precapillary bed. This is because the flow rate is lower in small veins than in small arteries because of the difference in the size of the total cross-sectional area. The increase in postcapillary resistance raises the capillary pressure, causing additional fluid loss from the capillaries. This in turn leads to increased sludging, blocking of capillaries, and tissue hypoxia, resulting in acidosis and damage to capillary endothelium, causing further aggregation of erythrocytes. The situation is exacerbated when it coincides with altered blood composition as, for example, in shock.

Other factors that affect blood viscosity are cold and an increased hematocrit level. Agents that reduce plasma fibrinogen levels reduce blood viscosity. Both the fibrinogen component of plasma viscosity and fibrinogen-mediated red-cell aggregation are reduced. Pentoxifylline inhibits platelet aggregation, as does heparin. Dextran also appears to have an effect on rouleau formation.

Delay Phenomenon

When a pedicled flap is raised in two stages, separated by a period of about 2 weeks, a greater length-breadth ratio is achieved than when the flap is raised in one stage only. This differential is known as the delay phenomenon. Theories that attempt to explain the delay phenomenon are based on the sympathetic system and other factors.

The sympathectomy resulting from raising the flap causes vasodilatation, which may be involved in this phenomenon. Another theory is that the hyperadrenergic state that occurs when a flap is raised causes initial vasoconstriction, which if prolonged would lead to flap necrosis. The hyperadrenergic state persists for approximately 18 to 36 hours, after which recovery occurs in a few days. When the flap subsequently is raised again, there is no longer a hyperadrenergic state at the second stage, and vasoconstriction does not occur.

Factors independent of sympathetic system changes may increase flap vascularity over a longer period than does the recovery of the hyperadrenergic state. These factors include regression of inflammation caused by the initial trauma of the operation and effects of unknown vasodilators on smooth muscle, possibly prostaglandin E. Finally, there may be changes in the vascular pattern such that the axiality of the vascular bed becomes aligned in the long axis of the flap. This situation is akin to that discussed earlier in relation to the fasciocutaneous system and the dynamic and potential territories of arteries. It is not known whether these events occur because of the opening up of longitudinal channels or because of an increase in the tissue vascularity. Certainly in tissue expansion there is an increase in vascularity.

Pharmacologic Manipulation of Flaps

Because the delay phenomenon may be caused in part by a hyperadrenergic state following partial sympathectomy, attempts have been made to simulate it using drugs.

Adrenergic Block

Guanethidine acts on postganglionic sympathetic nerve fibers by reducing the release of norepinephrine.

Alpha-Adrenoreceptor Block

Phenoxybenzamine should in theory increase flap survival, but experimental work has been equivocal, and there is little evidence of a beneficial effect on flap survival. There is some evidence that phentolamine and thymoxamine improve flap survival.

Depletion of Norepinephrine

Reserpine blocks the uptake of norepinephrine into storage granules and leads to a gradual depletion of norepinephrine stores in adrenergic nerve endings. The effect of reserpine on flaps remains equivocal.

Beta-Adrenoreceptor Stimulators

Beta-adrenoreceptors cause vasodilatation of blood vessels in skeletal muscle, but in the walls of skin blood vessels most of the adrenergic receptors are of the alpha type. Isoxsuprine may work as a beta-agonist but also may have the direct effect of relaxing vascular smooth muscle wall. There is little evidence to suggest that it increases flap survival.

Beta-Adrenoreceptor Blockers

Propranolol antagonizes the metabolic acceleration caused by sympathetic stimulation.

Free Radicals

Free radicals are produced during the metabolism of oxygen. Cells are protected from the destructive effects of free radicals by scavenging mechanisms consisting of enzymatic control systems, metal chelators, and antioxidants. Allopurinol is a xanthine oxidase inhibitor, and it is known that ischemia triggers the conversion of xanthine dehydrogenase to the oxygen radical, producing xanthine oxidase. Drugs such as allopurinol may therefore have a role in reducing the effects of injury caused by tissue ischemia.

Factors Affecting Choice of Flap

In choosing the appropriate flap for a defect, the requirements at the recipient site must be taken into account. For example, it must be determined whether vascularized bone, nerve, or tendon is required. In addition to this decision, the donor defect resulting from the flap chosen must be borne in mind. For example, it may not be advisable to include a segment of the radius with a radial forearm flap in a manual worker in view of the risk of subsequent fracture of the radius.

The survival of a flap depends on the reliability of its blood supply, both venous drainage and arterial input. The reliability of free flaps improves with increasing vessel caliber and reduction in the length of the vascular pedicle. The flaps that best satisfy these requirements are the radial forearm flap, the latissimus dorsi flap, and the transverse rectus abdominis flap. Free flaps have additional recipient site requirements that influence the clinician's choice of flap. Previous injury to the site, as from radiation therapy or trauma, may compromise a local vascular anastomosis. Such compromise may necessitate a long flap vascular pedicle or require interpositional reversed vein grafts to allow anastomoses to healthy vessels.

The patient's physical, psychological, and socioeconomic circumstances have bearing on the type of flap chosen. The number of operative procedures involved, the patient's ability to tolerate and comply with the requirements of the treatment, and his or her expectations of the functional and aesthetic outcome are all important.

Morbidity

The usual complications common to all operations may occur with flap surgery; however, some problems are of particular importance in relation to flaps.

Donor Site Repair

Wound dehiscence or skin graft failure may occur. When the vascular anatomy is disrupted, it may give rise to distal ischemic problems, as, for example, in a radial forearm flap in which the ulnar artery–to–radial artery anastomoses are inadequate. When bone is included in a flap, subsequent donor site fractures are not uncommon. The donor site may give a poor cosmetic result because of hypertrophic scarring, skin graft discoloration, or an obvious contour defect.

Recipient Site

Problems at the recipient site are related mainly to failure of the flap, either partial or complete. The immediate causes of such failure may be inappropriate flap design, tension on the vascular pedicle, hematoma formation, or thrombosis of the vascular anastomosis. The failure usually is caused by a technical error or by recipient vessel disease.

It is essential that the pedicles of all flaps be protected from tension or undue kinking, which disrupts the vascular supply. The venous drainage is the first to be affected, giving rise to engorgement of the flap with subsequent thrombosis of the vein and artery. In addition to designing the flap with a view toward avoiding tension on the vascular pedicle, splinting together of the donor and recipient sites may be required.

In flap surgery, the physician should aim to reconstruct the primary defect with a flap consisting of the appropriate tissue to provide the optimal functional and cosmetic result. In doing so, the donor site chosen should be repaired in a way that avoids morbidity.

Suggested Reading

Cormack, G.C., and Lamberty, B.G.H. *The Arterial Anatomy of Skin Flaps.* London: Churchill Livingstone, 1986.

Healy, C., et al. Focusable Doppler ultrasound in mapping dorsal hand flaps. *Br. J. Plast. Surg.* 43:296, 1990.

Mathes, S.J., and Nahai, F. *Clinical Atlas of Muscle and Musculocutaneous Flaps.* St. Louis: Mosby, 1979.

Mathes, S.J., and Nahai, F. *Clinical Applications for Muscle and Musculocutaneous Flaps.* St. Louis: Mosby, 1982.

McCraw, J.B., and Arnold, P.G. *McCraw and Arnold's Atlas of Muscle and Musculocutaneous Flaps.* Norfolk: Hampton, 1986.

Morain, W.D. Introduction. In C. Manchot, *The Cutaneous Arteries of the Human Body.* New York: Springer, 1983.

Taylor, G.I., Caddy, C.M., Watterson, P.A., Crock, J.G. The venous territories (venosomes) of the human body: Experimental study and clinical implications. *Plast. Reconstr. Surg.* 86: 185, 1990.

Taylor, G.I., and Palmer, J.H. The vascular territories (angiosomes) of the body: Experimental study and clinical applications. *Br. J. Plast. Surg.* 40:113, 1987.

Taylor, G.I., and Tempest, M., *Michel Salmon: Arteries of the Skin.* London: Taylor and Tempest, 1988.

Tobin, G.R. *Clinics in Plastic Surgery: Refinements in Flap Reconstruction.* Philadelphia: Saunders, 1990.

6

Skin Flaps, Fasciocutaneous Flaps, and Musculocutaneous Flaps

Luis O. Vasconez   Mabel Gamboa-Bobadilla   Michael P. Bentley

The plastic surgical literature during the past two decades has presented an enormous amount of information about flaps. This knowledge has enabled surgeons to reconstruct defects in a predictable and safe manner through the design and use of flaps in areas of the body where there is a known blood supply and a safe arc of rotation.

The traditional teaching was to achieve solutions in the form of a reconstructive ladder. The schema emphasized simplicity of a procedure as the most important determinant in flap selection. For example, one would progress from primary wound closure to a skin graft, to a local flap, to a distant flap, and finally to a free flap. Forgoing tradition, our group now approaches each patient requesting reconstruction intent on using the flap that can provide optimal functional and aesthetic results. We approach a defect with creativity rather than a preconceived solution. Although a deltopectoral or pectoralis flap provides good results for most defects remaining after tumor extirpation in the oral cavity and hypopharynx, there are new techniques that provide improved results with other flaps, such as a thin and pliable radial forearm fasciocutaneous flap or a free jejunal flap.

Flaps usually are categorized as random cutaneous, arterial cutaneous, fasciocutaneous, musculocutaneous, or muscle flaps. Each of these types has a different blood supply and arc of rotation. With our current knowledge of wound healing and tissue transfer, we use the specific type of tissue indicated for the defect being treated. For example, when there is traumatic skin loss, skin is necessary; for osteoradionecrosis, muscle or omentum is used; and for osteomyelitis or infected wounds, muscle is used.

Basic Principles of Flap Surgery

Wound Preparation

Wound physiology and pathophysiology are beyond the scope of this chapter. It should be emphasized, however, that wound preparation is extremely important for the success of any flap procedure. Although muscle flaps are known to promote the decontamination of minimally infected wounds, their capabilities are limited in grossly infected wounds. Wound preparation before coverage with flaps is a prerequisite for success in such situations. If quantitative wound cultures are obtained, a reasonable effort should be made to obtain a preoperative bacteriologic count of less than 10^5 bacteria per gram of tissue. The accuracy of quantitative wound cultures is unpredictable, however. Such cultures are also economically infeasible, adding another operative procedure to the patient's care. We have opted instead for aggressive preoperative and intraoperative debridement; topical care is of lesser importance. We use enzymatic degradation and various topical "gels and powders" with much less frequency. Thus the mainstay of preoperative wound preparation is surgical debridement followed by application of either a dilute 0.1 strength Dakin solution for grossly infected wounds or normal saline wet-to-dry dressing changes.

Choice of Flaps

Numerous choices exist for closing a wound. The surgical challenge is to select the optimal method. Multiple factors, including donor site morbidity, operative complexity, recipient site requirements, and other patient-related factors, must be balanced. These considerations must be weighed in an aggregate manner because no single factor ordinarily has overriding importance. Contributory factors include durability, morbidity, and functional and aesthetic considerations. These factors help to illustrate the limitations of the so-called reconstructive ladder approach referred to earlier. There are many times when a musculocutaneous flap may require a longer convalescence than a skin graft, which is simpler but may produce vastly inferior results. A free flap to the low distal third of the tibia may be more complex than a local or fasciocutaneous flap, but often it prevents multiple operations, lessens morbidity, and shortens the time for healing and rehabilitation.

Some wounds require single-tissue reconstruction, whereas others require composite and complex tissue transfers to achieve both a functional and an aesthetic result. For example, in the facial region a resection of a large skin tumor often causes a single-tissue defect (skin), whereas removal of an intraoral squamous cell tumor can produce a compound defect requiring oral lining and bone or a composite defect requiring oral lining, bone, and skin for reconstruction.

Size and Arc of Rotation

A foremost consideration in flap surgery is whether or not the proposed flap will cover the defect. Coverage depends on the axis of the dominant vasculature and the expected size of the muscle, skin, or musculocutaneous flap. Anatomic constants dictate precisely the extent of flap excursion. This knowledge can be obtained only through anatomic studies, cadaveric dissections, and extensive operative experience. Scarring caused by injury or infection and the normal contractibility and tension of muscle, however, result in a shorter arc of rotation in live patients than in cadavers.

Vascular Supply

The location and dominance of the vasculature are the anatomic and physiologic keystones of flap surgery. Present anatomic knowledge demonstrates that the blood supply to the skin is multifactorial. The sources include distinct arteries that course under the skin and supply it. Examples include the superficial temporal artery and the dorsalis pedis artery supplying the forehead and the dorsum of the foot, respectively. These flaps have been called *axial flaps*. The demonstration that the overlying skin remains alive as long as the underlying muscle and the major vascular supply are maintained intact indicates that the skin is supplied from vessels that emanate from the muscle and perforate the fascia toward the skin. This anatomic observation is the basis for the successful use of *musculocutaneous flaps* and for the design of a large variety of such flaps on many areas of the body.

A third source of blood to the skin is in the septocutaneous vessels that perforate the fascia and course superficially to it. These vessels could be direct branches from the major arteries or segmental branches from larger arteries that course through the intermuscular septum, perforate the fascia, and arborize on top of it to supply the skin. This variable vasculature is the basis for *fasciocutaneous* flaps. There may be other sources of blood supply and, more important, the same segment of skin may be supplied from multiple sources in such a way that if one vessel is destroyed or ligated, the overlying skin remains alive. The multifactorial source of the blood supply is important to remember and helps in the understanding and design of successful flaps based on a reliable supply of blood.

Donor Site

Donor site considerations and morbidity are pivotal in the choice of a flap. Problems range from bothersome seromas of a latissimus dorsi flap to the potential for exsanguinating hemorrhage associated with harvest of the gluteus maximus muscle with unintentional avulsion of the superior gluteal artery and resultant retroperitoneal hemorrhage. The functions of each muscle should be known before each reconstructive procedure, and the functional deficits from the loss of a muscle should be taken into consideration before a reconstructive plan is formulated. The reconstructive benefits should always be individualized and weighed against the specific functional deficits when any reconstructive procedure is designed.

Sensation

Most local, random, or arterial cutaneous flaps maintain a portion of their original sensation from the surrounding area or are able to achieve protective sensation after a period of time. Muscle flaps maintain some pressure sensibility. Most island musculocutaneous flaps contain nei-ther deep nor superficial sensibility because the segmental nerves are distant from the island vessels and are sacrificed in the process of flap elevation. Deep pressure sensibility that persists in a muscle flap may be adequate to provide a durable surface for walking or for the protection of a skin graft. It has been noted that the gastrocnemius and soleus muscle flaps are able to maintain surface tactile sensibility. The tensor fasciae latae and external oblique musculocutaneous flaps are unusual in that they sometimes maintain the integrity of their nerve supply after flap elevation and may have subsequent normal sensation. The use of random cutaneous flaps to cover larger defects has decreased dramatically with the advent of more reliable methods, but their value in resurfacing smaller defects, especially on the face, remains.

Types of Flaps
Arterial Cutaneous Flaps

Axial or arterial flaps have been used for several decades. They have been mastered only recently, however; they now are designed to include a specific artery within their pedicle as well as venous drainage through associated subcutaneous veins and venae comitantes. Bakamjian in 1965 first described his deltopectoral flap. This flap was of impressive length and could be raised based on perforators of the internal mammary artery. This deltopectoral flap has been used extensively in the reconstruction of defects of the head and neck. Its use has led to an understanding of the principles of the axial flap and the description of several other arterial cutaneous flaps, such as the groin flap based on the superficial circumflex artery and the lateral thoracic flap based on the intercostal perforators. With the description of the septocutaneous arteries, which are branches of major arteries passing through the intermuscular septa, many advances have been made in designing useful flaps for a multitude of reconstructive problems.

The design of skin flaps based on the septocutaneous vessels begins with localization of the penetration of the vessel through the fascia. A retrograde dissection is performed to follow the vascular pedicle until a major artery with sufficient diameter for microanastomosis is encountered or enough length for the pedicle rotation of the flap is obtained. Examples of such flaps include the scapular flap, the parascapular flap, the groin flap, and multiple lower extremity flaps.

Fasciocutaneous Flaps

The fasciocutaneous flap includes the skin, subcutaneous tissue, and underlying fascia, which may be distinct from the fascia investing the muscle. The sources of blood supply to the fasciocutaneous flap are varied and may include a perforating vessel from the underlying muscle, septocutaneous vessels, or direct longitudinal vessels coursing on top of the fascia. Cadaveric dissection and clinical experience have demonstrated a number of territories of safe fasciocutaneous flaps. The blood supply has not been completely delineated in some of these territories. The septocutaneous vessels that supply some of the fasciocutaneous flaps are seen especially in the lower leg, with branches from the three major arteries of the leg (peroneal, anterior tibial, and posterior tibial) coursing along the intermuscular septa to perforate the fascia and supply the overlying subcutaneous tissue and skin. Each septocutaneous artery supplies a segment of overlying skin and arborizes on top of the fascia to form an anastomosis of the adjacent superior and inferior vessels at the subcutaneous plane. When one of these vessels is maintained intact, a pedicled flap based superiorly or inferiorly can be designed. An island design also is possible.

Muscle Flaps

A muscle flap consists of muscle that has been detached from its normal origin or insertion and transposed to another location. The flap may remain attached to its intact blood supply by its vascular pedicle or may be completely detached and transferred as a microvascular free muscle flap. The muscle flaps used most frequently today involve the rectus abdominis, pectoralis, latissimus dorsi, and gastrocnemius muscles.

Musculocutaneous Flaps

A musculocutaneous flap is a composite of muscle and overlying skin and subcutaneous tissue. The muscle is the carrier for the skin and provides blood through its perforators. Most muscles have several vascular pedicles; the dominant vascular pedicle is capable of providing nutritional support to a large segment of muscle when adjacent vascular pedicles are ligated. The point of entry of the dominant vascular pedicle into the muscle is pivotal for rotation and thus determines the mobility and transfer of the flap. This point is the so-called axis of rotation. The exact reach of the arc of rotation varies with the person's build and in general is greater for thinner people. Several authors have attempted classifications for muscle and musculocutaneous flaps. The understanding of skin and muscular vascular anatomy is evolving and so is the need for a better classification system. Mathes and Nahai in 1981 reported on one of the earlier systems based on the following anatomic variables:

1. A regional source of arterial pedicle entering the muscle
2. The size of the pedicles
3. The number of pedicles
4. The location in relation to origin and insertion
5. The angiographic patterns of muscular vasculature

These authors defined five patterns of muscle circulation based on these variables.

Bonnel in 1985 described a newer classification based on two criteria—the type of main arterial pedicle penetrating the muscle and the presence or absence of intramuscular anastomotic accessory arteries or osteoperiosteal anastomotic arteries. Although this classification adds further detail to the understanding of vascular anatomy as does the classification of Mathes and Nahai, both are cumbersome to memorize. These classifications are often restrictive as knowledge expands, and they do not provide major clinical benefit for practicing plastic surgeons.

We provide examples of each of the types of flaps and describe their specific uses. We place special emphasis on avoidance of complications and selection of appropriate flaps for specific defects. Wound problems and their solutions using a variety of flaps are described to illustrate the points we have emphasized regarding techniques and the avoidance of complications.

Techniques of Flap Use

Skin Flaps

Scapular and parascapular flaps, because of their pliability, lack of hair, and good color match, offer a satisfactory solution for coverage of any skin defect, whether small or large, in most regions of the body but particularly in the head and neck area, specifically the face (Table 6-1). With microvascular transfer these flaps also may be used on the upper extremity, including the hand, and on the lower extremity. Local rotational flap coverage of the posterior shoulder or the axilla has also proved beneficial with these flaps.

Indications

A combination of the parascapular flap and the latissimus dorsi muscle with inclusion of the border of the scapula when needed provides a composite flap that can be used in the most complex of reconstructions, including a one-stage mandibular reconstruction with multiple soft tissue defects of the head and neck. These flaps are easily accessible, and a two-team operative approach can be used because patients may be placed in a lateral decubitus position to allow easy access to the recipient area and adequate exposure for the flap dissection. Dissection of the flap causes no functional morbidity because no major muscular groups are disturbed, and the donor site may be closed primarily.

Anatomy

After several anatomic dissections of the scapular region, Dos Santos illustrated a cutaneous branch of the circumflex scapular artery, which he named the *cutaneous scapular artery*. The cutaneous scapular artery is the direct blood supply to the cutaneous vascular territory over a large area of the scapular region. Through injection studies it was demonstrated that the skin area supplied by the cutaneous scapular artery is 10 cm in its longest vertical dimension and 13 cm in its longest horizontal dimension. The superior limit is the scapular spine, and the inferior limit is 3 cm above the angle of the scapula. The medial extent is 2 cm from the vertebral column, and the lateral extent is the posterior axillary line. The pedicle arises at the subscapular artery from the axillary artery and gives off the circumflex scap-

Table 6-1. Skin flaps

Most commonly used flaps	Blood supply	Indications	Advantages	Disadvantages	Donor site morbidity
Scapular and parascapular	Cutaneous scapular artery Descending scapular artery (branch of circumflex scapular artery)	Satisfactory coverage of skin defect on shoulder and axilla With microvascular transfer, useful on head and neck, hand, and lower extremity In reconstruction requiring an osseous component (there are multiple branches of the circumflex scapular artery to the lateral border of the scapula in its superior portion)	Pliable Hairless Good color match Easy accessibility	Change of position of patient to harvest: prone, lateral, decubitus	No functional morbidity Closed primarily
Abdominal skin flaps	Superiorly based: intercostal, local epigastric perforators Inferiorly based: periumbilical perforators from the rectus abdominis muscle	Useful in defect of hand	Stable Pliable Hairless	Second operation needed to inset skin flap	Minimal difficulty Closed primarily

ular artery, which egresses through the omotricipital space. At this point the circumflex scapular artery gives origin to the cutaneous scapular artery and the descending scapular artery; the second is the artery supplying the parascapular flap. With a parascapular flap design, the upper edge of the flap is outlined at the line of the emergence of the pedicle, with the lower edge as far as 25 to 30 cm from the upper edge. The main axis of the pedicle is the lateral border of the scapula. The width of the flap that has proved to be consistent with direct closure of the resultant defect is about 15 cm, with wide variations ranging from 6 to 20 cm (Fig. 6-1).

Technique of Flap Dissection

Important projecting points such as the scapular spine, the lateral border, and the inferior angle of the scapula, in addition to the muscles that border the triangular space, are marked on the skin. The patient is either in a prone or in a lateral

decubitus position. The arm is abducted or adducted depending on the operative procedure. The flap is marked as scapular or parascapular and, occasionally, as a combined parascapular and scapular flap. At this point the skin flap is incised, undermined, and reflected caudally through an avascular plane encountered between the subcutaneous tissue and the fascia of the infraspinatus muscle.

With the flap caudally reflected, the cutaneous scapular artery is instantly identified within the subcutaneous tissue. The dissection subsequently proceeds toward the triangular space bordered by three muscles: the teres major, inferiorly; the teres minor, superiorly; and the long head of the triceps, laterally. Here the cutaneous scapular artery joins the circumflex scapular artery, and the main vascular pedicle is formed. The second elliptical skin incision is made at a superior point, and the flap is freed from the underlying fascia in its entirety to allow easier dis-

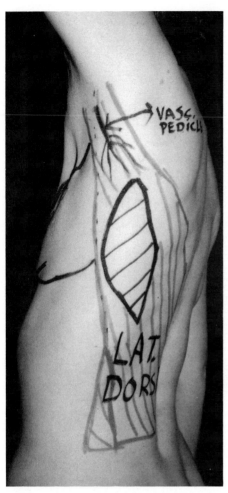

Fig. 6-1. Outline of a parascapular flap.

section of the pedicle into the inner part of the triangular space. The pedicle may be followed all the way to its origin from the axillary artery if additional length is needed. The parascapular flap has a longitudinal orientation with regard to the lateral border of the scapula and may be dissected in a similar manner, beginning inferiorly after the flap is marked elliptically. The deep plane of dissection is suprafascial and moves superiorly to incorporate the descending branch of the cutaneous scapular artery. This dissection is followed into the omotricipital space, as in the scapular flap.

As the pedicle is dissected proximally, an S-shaped extension of the incision into the axilla may be necessary. A good example is the parascapular flap, which we have come to use as our first-line flap for closure of large axillary defects. The flap can be left on its vascular pedicle and rotated into the defect with minimal difficulty (Fig. 6-2). Adequate debridement is

carried out, as always, and the wound is thoroughly irrigated with a dilute povidone-iodine solution before the flap is inset. Insetting is a two-layer process with a monofilamentous suture in the subdermis and nylon in the skin. In flaps that require an osseous component, there are multiple branches of the circumflex scapular artery to the lateral border of the scapula in its superior portion. These branches originally supply the periosteum and the muscle to which they attach. The pedicle length from the bone edge to the axillary artery varies from 4 to 6 cm, and beginning at the scapular border, the pedicle to the overlying skin paddle measures approximately 3 cm. The importance of this vascular anatomy is in demonstrating that the skin paddle has an independent vascular pedicle from the bone flap, thereby allowing multiple degrees of freedom in the spatial positioning needed in complex reconstructions of the head and neck.

Abdominal Skin Flaps

Cutaneous defects of the upper extremity usually can be repaired with skin grafts or local skin flaps. When these two methods are not indicated, flaps from a distant site are necessary. Lower chest wall flaps and upper abdominal flaps offer the advantage of allowing elevation of the hand at the time of their initial application unlike flaps located on the lower abdomen. Skin flaps from the anterior chest wall and abdominal wall are bounded by the xiphoid superiorly, the region of the umbilicus inferiorly, and the midaxillary line laterally. Consideration must be given to the defect on the hand being addressed—whether it is situated closer to the ulna or the radius and whether it is over the dorsal or palmar surface of the hand. The skin flaps in the regions of the anterolateral chest wall and the upper abdomen should be approximately 8 cm wide and 12 to 15 cm long. These flaps can easily be transposed to digits, palms, the dorsum of hands, and, occasionally, wrists.

The blood supply for an inferiorly based flap comes primarily from the rich periumbilical perforators through the underlying rectus abdominis muscle. These perforators arborize above the level of the Scarpa fascia. A superiorly based upper abdominal and lower chest wall flap may be based on intercostal and local epigastric perforators, allowing their bases to be oriented laterally, superiorly, or medially

as needed to conform with the resurfacing requirements of the extremity. These donor sites may be closed primarily with minimal difficulty. With proper dressings the flap can be stabilized to prevent obstruction of venous return at the base. The flaps should be raised in a subcutaneous plane, or just to the depth of the Scarpa fascia, and not in the relatively avascular plane overlying the deep fascia. These sites provide stable, pliable, relatively hairless coverage for upper extremity defects and if well inset can be divided in 10 to 14 days (Fig. 6-3).

Fasciocutaneous Flaps

The most commonly used fasciocutaneous flaps are described in Table 6-2.

Medial Plantar Flap

Several neurovascular flaps from the toes have been designed for coverage of the heel. Their disadvantage, however, has been the extensive dissection required and the sacrifice of one or several toes. Muscle flaps have been used as well, including the flexor digitorum brevis with split-thickness skin grafts, which have the disadvantage of limited sensibility in a weight-bearing area. With the use of the medial plantar artery in an axial pattern flap with sensation provided by the cutaneous branches of the digital branches of the medial plantar nerve, it is now possible to provide stable sensate flap coverage for the weight-bearing portion of the sole of the foot and heel.

Anatomy. The medial plantar artery originates from the posterior tibial artery, which divides into the medial and lateral plantar arteries deep to the origin of the abductor hallucis muscle. The medial plantar artery lies between the abductor hallucis and the flexor hallucis brevis. It is quite small compared with the lateral plantar artery and divides into small digital branches that accompany the common digital branches of the medial plantar nerve. Although the flap is theoretically an axial pattern flap, the small cutaneous arterial branches may be damaged unintentionally. The medial plantar nerve is the larger of two branches of the tibial nerve and also arises beneath the abductor hallucis. It runs with the artery between the abductor and the flexor digitorum brevis muscles. Cadaveric dissections have shown that a cutaneous branch can be separated from each digital nerve,

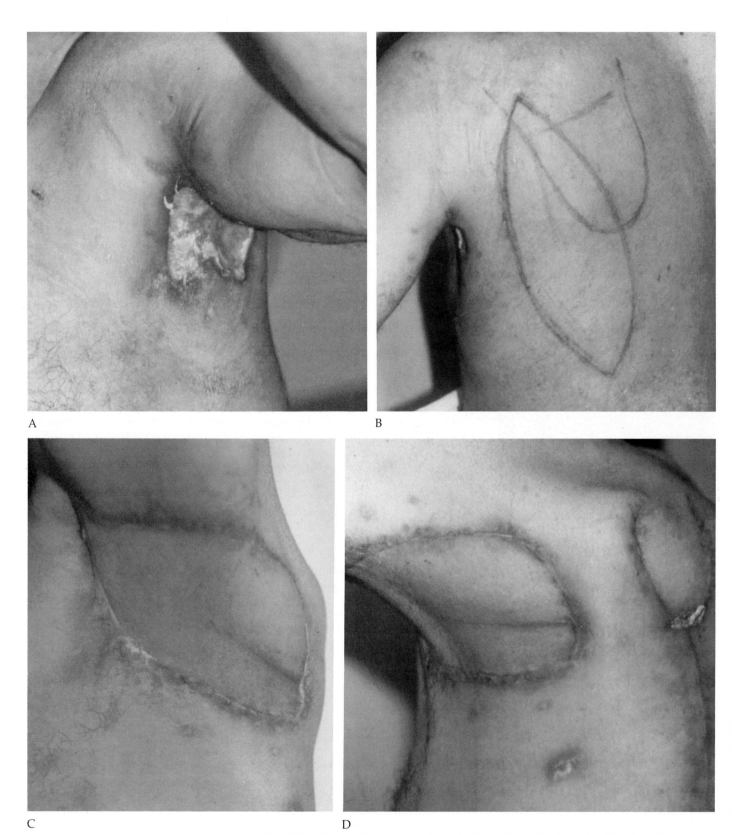

A

B

C

D

Fig. 6-2A. A 62-year-old man after excision of axillary hidradenitis of the left axilla. Wound dehiscence and infection followed primary closure. Considerable axillary contracture is present. B. Outline of parascapular flap. C. Two months after radical debridement, release of axillary contracture and closure with a parascapular flap. D. Parascapular flap 5 months postoperatively. A portion of the flap was deepithelized and tunneled under healthy skin. Donor site was closed primarily.

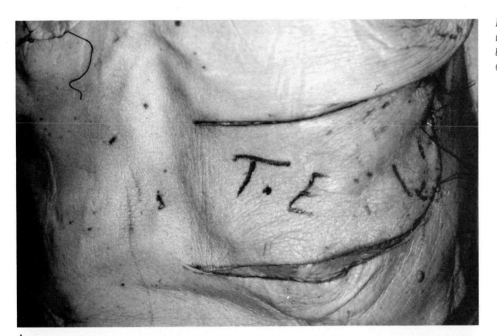

A

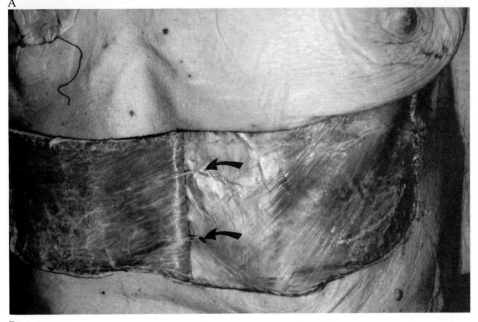

B

Fig. 6-3A. Anatomic dissection showing thoracoepigastric skin flap. B. The blood supply is based on perforators from the epigastric arcade (arrows).

is dissected to the base of the flap. To complete the proximal dissection and allow the flap to be rotated, the attachments of the plantar fascia must be divided.

In clinical application the flap offers another option for the coverage of heel defects and has the advantage of bringing in sensibility if sensation is present in the donor skin. The donor site can be covered with a split-thickness skin graft with minimal deficit in a non-weight-bearing area of the foot (Fig. 6-4).

Fasciocutaneous Flaps of the Lower Extremity

Fasciocutaneous flaps of the lower extremity can be based on the septocutaneous vessels. Each of the three arteries from the trifurcation of the popliteal artery runs in a longitudinal course toward the foot. Each vessel delivers segmental branches that travel through the intermuscular septum, perforate the overlying fascia, arborize on top of it, and supply the overlying skin. The arborizing vessels anastomose freely with the ones from above and below. In this way, the skin and fascia on the medial aspect of the leg are supplied by the posterior tibial artery, on the anterolateral aspect by the anterior tibial artery, and posteriorly by the peroneal artery. Each of these septocutaneous vessels supplies a territory of skin and fascia that is probably 10 to 15 cm in length and that can be transposed for reconstructive purposes. As long as one

and the separation can be continued proximally from the medial plantar nerve fasciculi as far as the base of the flap by using loupe magnification.

Operative Technique. Under tourniquet control a skin incision is outlined and made and the plantar fascia is identified. The longitudinal bands of the plantar fascia, which is included with the flap, are identified distally and divided. The digital neurovascular bundles are identified and dissected proximally. The medial branch

to the big toe should be identified before the medial and lateral skin incisions are deepened. Next, the cutaneous nerve branches are separated from the digital nerve branches. More proximally, the cutaneous nerve branches are separated from the fascicles of the medial plantar nerve. Branches to adjacent muscles can be preserved. The digital artery branches that accompany the common digital nerves are identified and divided at the tip of the flap. They are kept intact in the flap. Proximally, the medial plantar artery

Table 6-2. Fasciocutaneous flaps

Most commonly used flaps	Blood supply	Indications	Advantages	Disadvantages	Donor site morbidity
Radial forearm flap	Radial artery Venous return by two venae comitantes and subcutaneous forearm veins, which drain into the cephalic basilic, and median antecubital veins	Useful for head and neck, especially intraoral reconstruction Elbow, hand, penis, urethral reconstructions	Thin Pliable Hairless The medial and lateral antebrachial cutaneous nerves may be anastomosed if a sensate flap is desired Can be used as a composite osseofasciocutaneous flap	Ligation of the radial artery	Non-mesh, split-thickness skin graft used to cover the defect Aesthetically unacceptable donor site Fracture of radius has been reported when flap is used as osteocutaneous flap
Medial plantar flap	Axial pattern flap Blood supply originates in the medial plantar artery. (Nerve supply is medial plantar branch of tibial nerve)	Plantar defects caused by diabetes, trauma, tumors, and breakdown in patients with anesthetic plantar surfaces	Able to provide sensate flap coverage for weight-bearing portion of sole of foot and for heel defects	Difficult dissection	Covered with a split-thickness skin graft with minimal deficit in a non-weight-bearing area of the foot
Fasciocutaneous flaps of the lower extremity	Medial: posterior tibial vessels Anterolateral: anterior tibial vessels Posterior: lateral peroneal vessels	Soft tissue defects in lower extremity, caused by trauma	Flap can be designed with proximal or distal base and converted to an island or used as a turnover flap	Requires surgical or Doppler determination of lowest septocutaneous perforator	Covered with meshed split-thickness skin graft Donor site may be aesthetically unacceptable
Neurovascular pudendal-thigh fasciocutaneous flaps	Three to four vessels located within 5 cm of the perineum as afferent vessels to the suprafascial vascular plexus of the medial thigh	Reconstruction of vagina Closure of difficult perineal wounds and fistulas after irradiation Reconstruction of scrotum, penis Partial or total reconstruction in vaginal atresia	Durable, less bulky, and potentially sensate alternative to the gracilis musculocutaneous flap for vaginal and perineal reconstruction	Anterior part of the flap may be denervated in the process of elevation	Donor scar well hidden

septocutaneous vessel remains intact, the particular territory is versatile and viable. The flap can be designed with a proximal or distal base and converted to an island or used as a turnover flap. The most distal subcutaneous vessel arises approximately 10 cm above the medial or lateral malleolus. This anatomic limitation is responsible for the variable success of flaps used for coverage of the ankle and Achilles tendon.

Anatomy. According to their origin, septocutaneous vessels form three groups:

medial, from the posterior tibial vessels; anterolateral, from the anterior tibial vessels; and posterolateral, from the peroneal vessels.

The medial septocutaneous vessels are enclosed in the deep transverse fascial septum of the leg that separates the soleus and gastrocnemius muscular compartment from the deep muscular compartment of the posterior leg. Four or five of the septocutaneous vessels are found on the medial aspect of the leg. They most frequently are present at the following levels above the tip of the medial malleo-

lus: 9 to 12 cm, 17 to 19 cm, and 22 to 24 cm. The arteries with larger diameters in this region are found in the middle third of the leg and are about 1.5 mm in diameter. The posterolateral septocutaneous vessels originate from the peroneal arteries and veins. They run through the posterior intermuscular septum, first passing between the fibula and the flexor hallucis longus muscle and then between the soleus and peroneus longus muscles. There are three to five of them and their external diameters are 0.4 to 1.3 mm. The larger of these vessels tends to be at either end of the fibula.

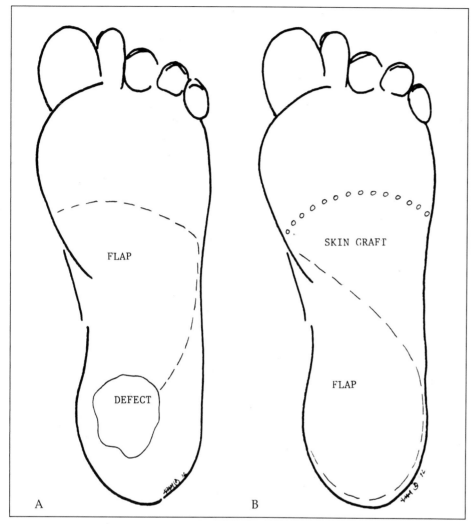

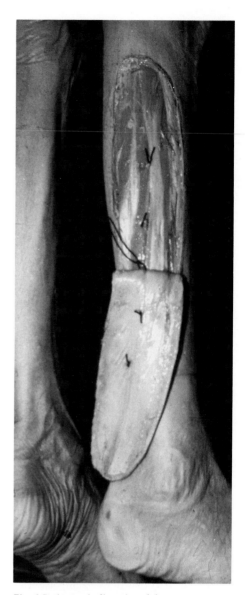

Fig. 6-4A. Large heel defect with plantar flap design. B. Flap is rotated into place and the donor defect is skin grafted.

Fig. 6-5. Anatomic dissection of the fasciocutaneous flaps of the lower extremity showing the segmental septocutaneous branches, which perforate the overlying fascia.

The anterolateral septocutaneous arteries originate from the anterior tibial vessels. There are six to ten of these vessels, and their diameters are 0.3 to 0.8 mm. The anterolateral and posterolateral septocutaneous perforators originate at variable levels; we have not found a fixed point at which the vessel always originates. There is a remarkable area of intercommunication between the systems depending on the anterior and posterior tibial trunks. This area is found at the level of the periosteum covering the anterior aspect of the tibia. This configuration allows rather large fasciocutaneous flaps of the lower extremity to be constructed; they can be based either distally or proximally (Fig. 6-5).

Operative Technique. The arc of rotation of a fasciocutaneous flap is often quite extensive. We prefer longitudinal incisions along the axis of the leg, and every effort is made to avoid tension. Before making the incision one must remember not to touch or disturb the circulation between the fascia and the skin; the incision goes through the skin, fat, and fascia in continuity. Hooks are used in the fascia and not in the skin to prevent shearing when handling the flap. The incision is best made in an area where the fascia is easily identified. The dissection from the underlying muscle is usually quite easy; this portion of the procedure is amenable to finger dissection. The intermuscular septum should be divided

from the distal portion of the flap with utmost attention to preserving a segment of septum continuous with the base of the flap—often a septocutaneous vessel is included there. This step may be essential for flap survival. It is often necessary to perform a back-cut in the fascia only to allow lengthening of the flap and to facilitate rotation. A delay procedure is not necessary with these flaps. If deemed necessary, suction drains may be used for a period of 24 to 48 hours; however, these drains often are not employed. The secondary donor defect is covered with a meshed split-thickness skin graft.

The flap can be used after tumor excision and in posttraumatic soft tissue defects. It has also been used successfully in places where osteosynthetic material is exposed in combination with bone grafting; it can be used in chronic osteomyelitis, pressure sores, and even in postphlebitic ulcers. The operative technique is simple, short, and safe, and should be one of the first considered when reconstructing defects of the lower extremity.

Neurovascular Pudendal-Thigh Fasciocutaneous Flaps

Many attempts have been made to reconstruct the vagina, usually with mixed results ranging from a nonphysiologic angle of the neovagina to total flap necrosis and a wound healing problem. A new technique of vaginal reconstruction has been proposed by Wee and Joseph. Their preliminary experience demonstrates that the flap is reliable and simple and that stents or dilators are not needed. The reconstructed vagina has a natural angle for intercourse and is sensate, and the donor scars in the groin are well hidden.

Anatomy. By a process of "capture" of adjacent territory of the deep external pudendal artery, the posterior labial arteries extend to the femoral triangle. This is the vascular basis of the pudendal-thigh flap—it is nourished by this direct cutaneous system of arteries. The deep fascia and the epimysium over the proximal part of the adductor muscles underlying the flap should be included in the flap to prevent injury to the direct cutaneous arteries when the flap is elevated. The veins closely follow the arterial supply. The posterior part of the pudendal-thigh flap retains its innervation from the posterior labial branches of the pudendal nerve and from the perineal rami of the posterior cutaneous nerve of the thigh when it is elevated. The anterior part of the flap near the medial corner of the femoral triangle may be denervated in the process of elevation; if so, sensation would be retained only in the lower part of the reconstructed vagina (Fig. 6-6).

Operative Technique. On the basis of the anatomic findings, a skin flap measuring 15 × 6 cm with its posterior skin margin at the level of the posterior end of the introitus is raised as a skin island based on a subcutaneous pedicle supplied by the posterior labial arteries. It is trans-

posed through 70° to meet a similar flap from the opposite side to form a cul-de-sac in the midline. By raising a flap at the deep fascia of the thigh and including the epimysium of the adductor muscles, an additional barrier is made that prevents unintentional damage to the neurovascular structures in the flap. The flap is horn-shaped with the flare of the horn at its base. It is planned for placement lateral to the hair-bearing area of the labia majora and centered on the crease of the groin. The donor site can be closed directly with minimal undermining.

For elevation of the flap, the patient is placed in a lithotomy position with the legs in stirrups. The incision, beginning at the tip of the flap, is deepened through the skin and subcutaneous tissue down to the deep fascia on two sides, except for the posterior margin of the flap. The subfascial plane is developed, raising the epimysium of the adductor muscles with the deep fascia. The deep fascia is tacked to the skin flap to prevent shearing, and the flap is elevated until the posterior skin margin is reached. At the posterior skin margin, the incision is made through the dermis to the subcutaneous tissue to a depth of approximately 1 to 1.5 cm and undermined in a plane parallel to the skin for a distance of about 4 cm posteriorly. This allows 70° to 90° of transposition of the flap to enable it to meet a similar flap from the opposite side near the midline. The posterior skin margin of the flap can thus be sutured to the labia minora, which is achieved by elevating the labia off the pubic ramus and the perineal membrane. The flaps are then tunneled under the labia. The posterior suture line, where both flaps meet, is completed first with the flaps everted through the introitus. The tip of the cul-de-sac is invaginated and anchored to the curve of the sacrum in the totally exenterated pelvis with nonabsorbable sutures between the flap and the periosteum of the sacrum. The opening of the vagina is sutured to the mucocutaneous edge of the labia minora. The cavity is drained, and the patient is encouraged to keep the legs adducted to allow healing. The lower part of the flap can be seen through the introitus for monitoring of circulation (see Fig. 6-6).

The advantages of this procedure are that it is simple and can be completed in 2 to 2½ hours with minimal blood loss. The

Fig. 6-6A. Pudendal-thigh flap design and diagrammatic representation of the blood supply. B. Diagrammatic representation of the pudendal-thigh flap. C. Pudendal-thigh flaps raised bilaterally. D. Pudendal-thigh flaps sutured together to make a tube. E. The flaps are sutured to their opposites and to the mucocutaneous junction of the labia minora. The donor sites are closed directly. (Parts A, B from J.T.K. Wee and B.T. Joseph. A new technique of vaginal reconstruction using neurovascular pudendal-thigh flaps: A preliminary report. Plast. Reconstr. Surg. 83:701, 1989. Reproduced with permission.)

blood supply of the flaps is reliable, which leads to early wound healing. The angle of inclination of the vagina is physiologic and natural, and the linear scars of the donor sites are well hidden in the groin crease and perineum. The vagina is sensate, retaining the same innervation of the erogenous zone as the perineum and upper thigh. In addition, this flap may be used for closure of difficult perineal wounds and fistulas, especially after irradiation. It may be used to reconstruct the scrotum or the penis in men. It also has been used for partial or total reconstruction in children with vaginal atresia.

Musculocutaneous Flaps

The most commonly used musculocutaneous flaps are described in Table 6-3.

Trapezius Musculocutaneous Flaps

The trapezius muscle is the basis for both muscle and musculocutaneous flaps that we have found useful in reconstructing defects of the head, neck, and upper back. Its location frequently makes it the flap of choice for defects in the occipital and posterior cervical regions.

Anatomy

The muscle can be separated into three functional parts. The most important, the upper occipital and cervical parts act to elevate the shoulder, holding it in a normal postural position by continuous tonic contraction. Because this action is not shared by any other muscles, the loss of innervation of the trapezius or functional loss of its upper portion results in the shoulder drop deformity. Selective loss of the middle and inferior fibers has no clin-

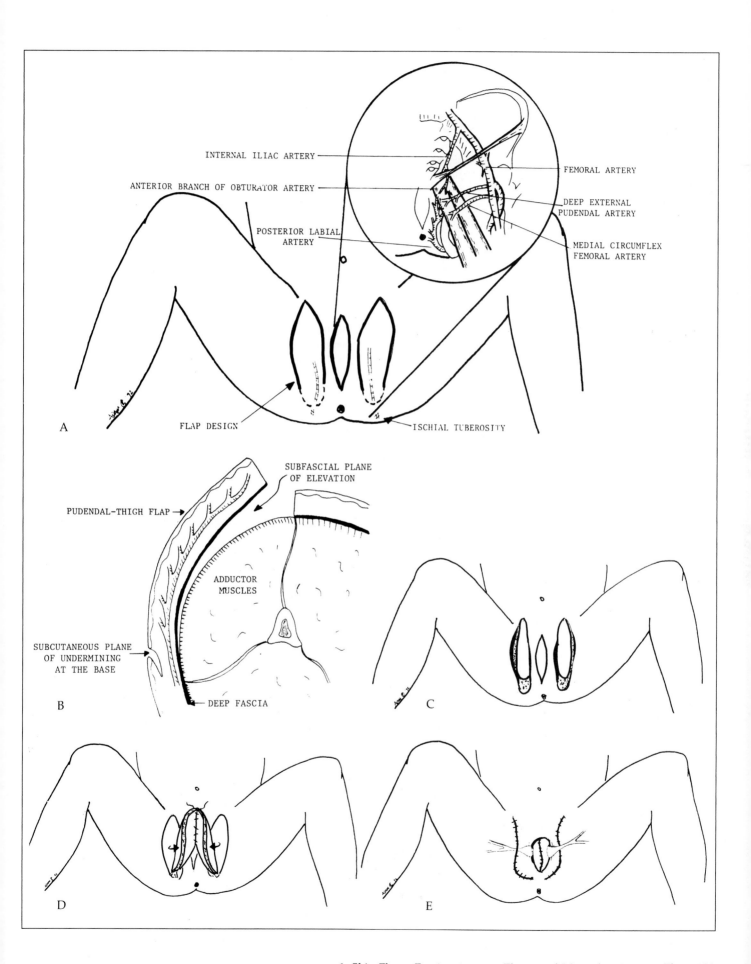

INTERNAL ILIAC ARTERY

ANTERIOR BRANCH OF OBTURATOR ARTERY

POSTERIOR LABIAL ARTERY

FEMORAL ARTERY

DEEP EXTERNAL PUDENDAL ARTERY

MEDIAL CIRCUMFLEX FEMORAL ARTERY

FLAP DESIGN

ISCHIAL TUBEROSITY

A

SUBFASCIAL PLANE OF ELEVATION

PUDENDAL-THIGH FLAP

ADDUCTOR MUSCLES

SUBCUTANEOUS PLANE OF UNDERMINING AT THE BASE

DEEP FASCIA

B

C

D

E

Table 6-3. Musculocutaneous flaps

Most commonly used flaps	Blood supply	Indications	Advantages	Disadvantages	Donor site morbidity
Transverse rectus abdominis (TRAM) flap	Perforating vessels from superior and inferior epigastric system	Based superiorly: Breast reconstruction Sternal wound infection Chest wall ulcers after irradiation Based inferiorly: Pelvic, perineal, superior thigh, and groin defects With microsurgical technique, can be transferred to distant sites	Formidable size Donor site closed aesthetically as an abdominoplasty	Potential hernia of the abdominal wall	Closed primarily Long abdominal scar
Trapezius musculocutaneous flap	Transverse cervical artery. (Most useful flap is based on the descending branch)	Reconstruction of the head, neck, and upper back, especially in occipital and posterior cervical defects	Flap is based on the middle and inferior portion of the trapezius to avoid loss of function to superior fibers and thus maintain proper shoulder position	In irradiated neck or after radical neck dissection, the transverse cervical artery may be surgically absent	Closed primarily

ically significant sequelae because the functions of these fibers are shared by other muscle groups. The vascular supply is made up of a dominant pedicle, consisting of the transverse cervical artery and vein, which courses between the sternocleidomastoid and the scalene muscles crossing the anterior margin of the trapezius and entering the deep surface of the muscle at the base of the neck (Fig. 6-7). The vasculature subsequently divides into ascending and descending branches, which form the basis for the separate superior and inferior musculocutaneous flaps. The ascending branch courses along the deep surface of the muscle between the spine and the scapulae supplying musculocutaneous perforators to the overlying skin. The ascending branch, which may arise occasionally as a separate branch from the thyrocervical trunk, courses laterally on the deep surface of the superior portion of the muscle, giving perforating vessels to the overlying skin just posterior to the clavicle. The average length of the dominant pedicle is 4 cm. Minor pedicles include a branch of the occipital artery, which supplies the superomedial portion of the muscle. Several remaining minor pedicles arise from the

posterior intercostal arteries and veins that enter the muscle along the midline adjacent to the cervical and thoracic vertebral bodies.

The nerve supply to the trapezius muscle consists of the spinal accessory nerve, which enters the deep surface of the muscle approximately 5 cm above the clavicle. The spinal accessory nerve is the primary motor nerve; cervical nerves III and IV provide sensory fibers.

The entire cutaneous territory of the trapezius muscle measures 34 × 28 cm, which includes several centimeters superiorly and inferiorly beyond the muscle fibers. These cutaneous perforators are located throughout the muscle surface, but the largest and most consistent perforators occur along the medial aspect 2 to 3 cm from the midline.

The vertically oriented posterior flap, based on the descending branch of the dominant artery with a vertical skin island located between the spine and the scapula, has proved most useful in our clinical experience. We have taken this flap as a musculocutaneous flap, attempting to avoid loss of function to superior fibers and thus to maintain proper shoul-

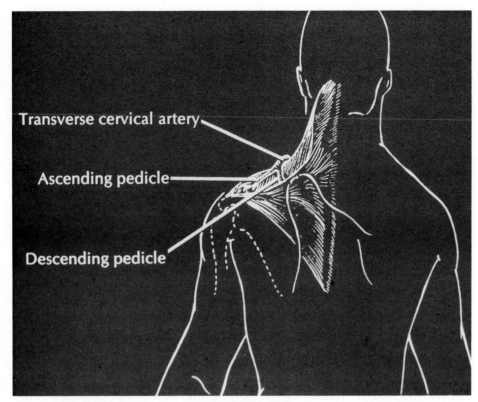

Fig. 6-7. Vascular supply of the trapezius musculocutaneous flap.

der position. The flap is based on the middle and inferior portions of the trapezius muscle, with the skin island located between the scapula and the spine. The skin dimensions may be up to 25 × 8 cm extending as much as 5 cm below the inferior border of the scapula. The arc of rotation of this flap extends to the shoulder, upper third of the posterior scalp, and the lateral neck. We begin raising the flap from inferior to superior positions (that is, distal to proximal). The flap incision is deepened to the level of the upper fibers of the latissimus dorsi muscle, which are left intact. When it is identified, the inferior border of the trapezius muscle is elevated, with the flap dividing its vertebral origin. At the level of the scapula, special care must be taken to avoid raising the rhomboid muscles with the flap, which would lead beneath the scapula. The descending branch of the transverse cervical artery is visualized on the undersurface of the trapezius muscle. The muscle is divided at the lateral edge of the skin paddle, with care taken to preserve the uppermost fibers between the skull and the clavicle, which as mentioned before are responsible for shoulder elevation.

The donor defect almost always can be closed primarily. Debulking or division of the muscle pedicle, if needed, can be done after a period of 3 to 4 weeks. An additional note of caution is given regarding patients who have had irradiation to the neck, which may have damaged the transverse cervical artery, and especially patients who have had either modified or radical neck dissections, which frequently ablate the pedicle. If doubt exists regarding the patency of the pedicle, an arteriogram or Doppler study should be obtained (Fig. 6-8).

Transverse Rectus Abdominis Musculocutaneous Flap

The transverse rectus abdominis musculocutaneous (TRAM) flap, based on the superior epigastric artery, is one of the most elegantly designed musculocutaneous flaps. It has become the mainstay of autogenous tissue breast reconstruction. Since its initial description for breast reconstruction, this flap has been used additionally for reconstructive problems of the chest wall such as sternal wound infections, chest wall ulcers after irradiation, and defects after tumor extirpation.

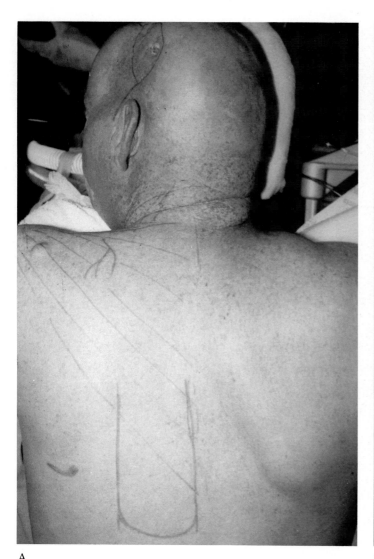

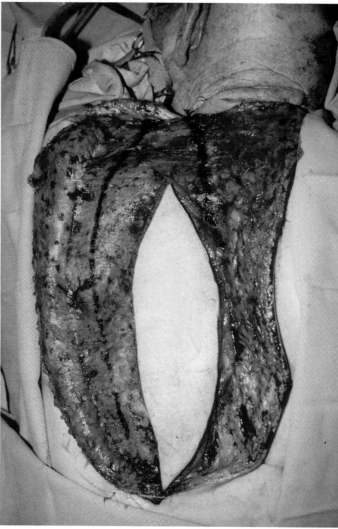

A   B

Fig. 6-8A. Male patient with temporoparietal defect. A vertically oriented posterior flap based on the descending branch was designed. B. The flap based on the middle and inferior portion of the trapezius muscle, with the skin island located between the scapula and the spine. C. Lateral view of the trapezius musculocutaneous flap covering the temporoparietal defect before debulking of the muscle pedicle. D. The donor defect closed primarily.

(See Chap. 97 for a detailed description of anatomy and flap dissection.)

This flap also may be based inferiorly for coverage of large pelvic and perineal defects and of defects of the superior thigh and groin. Furthermore, this flap can be used as a free vascularized tissue transfer for the coverage of defects in the head and neck area with considerable tissue deficiency (Fig. 6-9). These flaps can provide a generous amount of well-vascularized skin and fat to obliterate residual cavities and correct unsightly contour deformities.

Conclusion

An extensive body of knowledge of the blood supply to different types of flaps is now well established. Selection of the most appropriate flap is based primarily on clinical judgment, a detailed knowledge of the anatomy, and the surgeon's personal experience. Advances in microsurgery have facilitated the transfer of flaps, and microsurgical transference of flaps is probably as safe as any other flap procedure we perform. Technical errors decrease as the team develops experi-

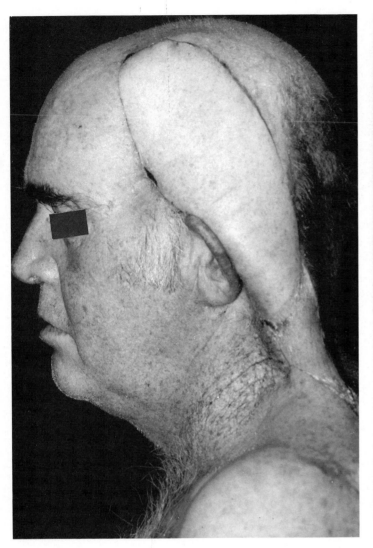

C

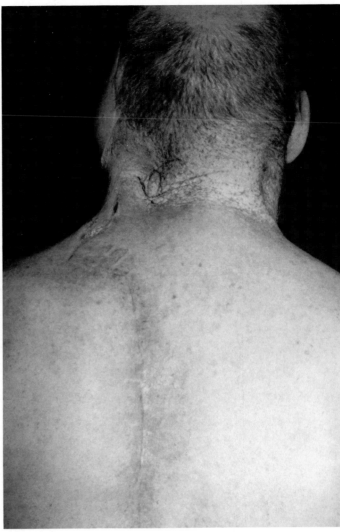

D

ence. The time is past when a flap was outlined and on occasion "delayed" in the hope that the blood supply would be sufficient for a successful transfer. At present, for every flap that is developed, the surgeon should have a good knowledge of the blood supply and of the limitations on length and arc of rotation. If a local flap would be pushed beyond the limits of certain success, it is probably better to design another flap that can be transferred by microvascular surgery.

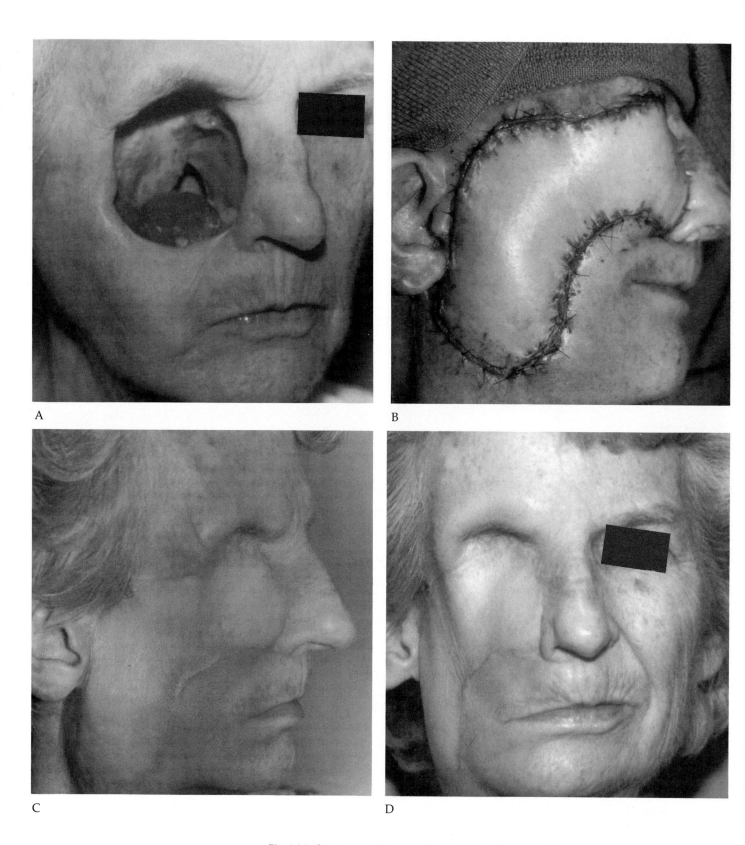

A

B

C

D

Fig. 6-9A. *Seventy-year-old woman after partial maxillectomy and postoperative radiation with recurrence. B. After insetting of transverse rectus abdominis musculocutaneous (TRAM) flap to obturate palatal, nasal, and orbital defects. C. Postoperative view after 5 months. D. Postoperative view after 5 months. (From G.E. Peters and J.C. Grotting. Free flap reconstruction of large head and neck defects in the elderly.* J. Microsurg. *10:325, 1989. Reproduced with permission.)*

Suggested Reading

Bakamjian, V.Y., Long, M., and Rigg, B. Experience with the medially based deltopectoral flap in reconstructive surgery of the head and neck. *Br. J. Plast. Surg.* 24:174, 1971.

Bonnel, F. New concepts on the arterial vascularization of skin and muscle. *Plast. Reconstr. Surg.* 75:552, 1985.

Carriquiry, C., Costa, M.A., and Vasconez, L.O. An anatomic study of the septocutaneous vessels of the leg. *Plast. Reconstr. Surg.* 76:354, 1985.

Gould, J.S. Management of soft-tissue loss on the plantar aspect of the foot. *Instr. Course Lect.* 39:121, 1990.

Maruyama, Y. Ascending scapular flap and its use for the treatment of axillary burn scar contracture. *Br. J. Plast. Surg.* 44:97, 1991.

Mathes, S.T., and Nahai, F. Classification of the vascular anatomy of muscles: Experimental and clinical correlation. *Plast. Reconstr. Surg.* 67: 177, 1981.

McCraw, J.B., Magee, W.P., Jr., and Kalwaic, H. Uses of the trapezius and sternocleidomastoid myocutaneous flap in head and neck surgery. *Plast. Reconstr. Surg.* 65:16, 1980.

Netterville, J.L., and Wood, D.E. The lower trapezius flap: Vascular anatomy and surgical technique. *Arch. Otolaryngol. Head Neck Surg.* 117:73, 1991.

Strauch, B., Vasconez, L.O., and Hall-Findley, E.J. *Grabb's Encyclopedia of Flaps.* Boston: Little, Brown, 1990.

Wee, J.T. Reconstruction of the lower leg and foot with the reverse-pedicled anterior tibial flap: Preliminary report of a new fasciocutaneous flap. *Br. J. Plast. Surg.* 39:327, 1986.

Wee, J.T., and Joseph, V.T. A new technique of vaginal reconstruction using neurovascular pudendal thigh flaps: A preliminary report. *Plast. Reconstr. Surg.* 83:701, 1989.

7

Tissue Transfer: Fat, Dermal, Muscle, Cartilage, and Fascial Grafts

W. Thomas Lawrence   Mark S. Potenza

Grafts of fat, dermis, muscle, cartilage, and fascia have found many aesthetic and reconstructive uses through the years. These grafts have been used essentially in all surgical specialties. Early in the history of reconstructive surgery, the indications for grafts were broader than they are now. In many circumstances, the effectiveness of grafts was limited by partial or total resorption, the amount of resorption varying with the graft material. Today flaps and prostheses more reliably meet many reconstructive needs previously met by grafts. In this chapter, each type of graft will be discussed in terms of its biology (Table 7-1) and its past and present uses.

Fat Grafts

Fat is a mesenchymal tissue consisting primarily of adipocytes arranged in lobules. When nutrition is adequate, adipocytes are characterized by lipid within their cytoplasm. This lipid is used as an energy source by the body, and it becomes depleted in times of starvation. Fibroblasts, blood vessels, and nerves also are found within fat, although fat has many fewer blood vessels running through it than do other tissues such as muscle. Fat is not normally an extremely dynamic tissue. The number of fat cells in the body rarely changes after puberty unless there are massive weight changes. Tissues in different anatomic areas are predestined to contain a particular quantity of fat, and they retain these characteristics when transferred as flaps or grafts.

Theoretically fat grafts can be harvested from any fat-containing part of the body. As in most grafts, however, donor sites that are relatively concealed and that contain an abundance of graftable tissue are preferred. The abdomen, buttocks, and thighs are the most commonly used donor sites for fat grafts. The traditional

Table 7-1. Characteristics of graft materials

Graft material	Tissue characteristics	Common donor sites	Anticipated resorption
Fat	Primarily adipocytes	Abdomen Buttock Thigh	High (50% or more)
Dermis	Fibroblasts in collagenous matrix	Abdomen Buttock Thigh	Moderate (<50%)
Fascia	Fibroblasts in dense collagenous matrix	TFL Temporalis	Limited (<20%)
Muscle	Primarily muscle cells	None	Extensive (near 100%)
Cartilage	Chondrocytes in matrix of collagen and chondroitin sulfate	Ear Septum Costal cartilage	Limited (<20%)

Key: TFL = tensor fasciae latae.

method of harvesting fat for grafting has been to make an incision or raise a small flap and to excise fat sharply from the subcutaneous tissue layer. A separate incision at the recipient site is used for graft placement and positioning. Some surgeons have aspirated fat for grafting with either a liposuction cannula or a syringe. When a technique of aspiration is used, the fat generally is reinjected into the recipient site. Although these methods initially were approached with enthusiasm, lack of reproducible success and experimental support have dampened interest in them.

Fat grafts are infiltrated with neutrophils, macrophages, lymphocytes, and eosinophils soon after placement, and this inflammatory response persists for months. Revascularization of the graft is noted histologically as early as 4 days after grafting and is followed quickly by granulation tissue formation and evidence of fibroblast proliferation. Fibroblasts generate a capsule of fibrous tissue around the surviving fat, which gradually thins during the first 8 months after grafting. Although little degeneration of fat is evident during the first few days after grafting, phagocytosis of fat cells by inflammatory cells is histologically evident by 10 days after grafting. Phagocytic cells containing lipid can be seen for months in the graft site. After 10 months, the graft reaches its final, mature form with a thin fibrous capsule surrounding persisting fat cells. Cystic cavities are interspersed between more cellular areas in the graft. Although the surviving cells are most likely those originally transferred, they may be derivatives of undifferentiated mesenchymal cells known as *preadipocytes* transferred with the graft. Proponents of this "preadipocyte theory" suggest that the originally transferred cells die and that the normally dormant preadipocytes differentiate into mature fat cells because of the ischemic stimulus of grafting.

Under unfavorable conditions such as infection or excessive trauma, no fat cells of any kind survive at the graft site, and the transferred fat is replaced by fibrous tissue. Fat allografts are similarly resorbed and have no clinical indications at this time.

Many techniques have been developed to limit graft resorption. Surgeons realized early on the importance of meticulous surgical technique. Absolute hemostasis,

careful harvesting, and gentle handling of the fat maximize graft survival. The graft preferably is not sutured; instead it is immobilized carefully for at least 10 days after placement. It has also been suggested that fat grafts from lean people survive better than those from obese people, and preoperative weight loss has been encouraged for patients undergoing fat grafting. There have been contradictory recommendations regarding graft size. Some surgeons recommend the use of small grafts and others state that larger grafts are preferred. Ellenbogen attempted to increase graft viability in small (6 to 8 mm in diameter) grafts by incubating them in insulin before transfer and treating the patients with vitamin E for 6 months after grafting. Experimental studies suggest that both insulin and vitamin E retard degeneration of fat cells. Although some or all of these methods may be helpful, none can completely prevent partial graft resorption. Overcorrection is routinely used to optimize results with fat grafts.

Uses of Fat Grafts

Fat grafting has been used in a variety of clinical situations. Fat grafts have been used for correction of soft tissue depressions resulting from trauma, surgical procedures, and congenital malformations in all parts of the body, particularly the face. In the past, fat grafts were used for extensive deformities such as hemifacial atrophy (Romberg disease) and chest deformities resulting from Poland syndrome. The microvascular transfer of fat or dermal-fat flaps has supplanted free fat grafting as the method of choice for Romberg disease. In Poland syndrome, muscle transfers and custom-made polymeric silicone (Silastic) implants have been found to be more reliable than free fat grafting for precise anatomic reconstructions. Fat grafts are still used for less extensive contour irregularities in all parts of the body, however. Smaller grafts are used by some surgeons for the correction of prominent folds and wrinkles in the aging face.

The first breast reconstruction, performed in 1895 by Czerny, consisted of a free fat graft from the buttock to the chest. Fat grafting also has been used for breast augmentation and testicular replacement. The high rate of resorption, however, has led to the abandonment of free fat graft-

ing for these indications. Polymeric silicone implants are the method of choice for breast augmentation and testicular replacement, and flaps or implants are used more commonly for breast reconstruction.

Fat grafts have been used to fill potential spaces caused by disease or ablative operations, for example, to fill bony defects resulting from osteomyelitis, intrapleural defects after pulmonary resections, and orbital defects caused by enucleation. They have been used to fill the frontal sinus after removal of the mucosal lining to treat trauma or chronic sinusitis. Other uses are to fill intracranial, postmastoidectomy, and postparotidectomy defects. Because fat grafts fare poorly in infected sites, they no longer are used in the presence of infection. Either local or microvascularly transferred muscle flaps are used more commonly for filling defects caused by osteomyelitis or pulmonary disease. Because the brain expands to fill potential intracranial spaces, fat grafts are rarely used in this setting. Fat or dermal-fat grafts are still sometimes used for orbital defects and frontal sinus obliteration, although some surgeons prefer other graft materials or flaps.

Fat grafts have been used as tissue buffers to prevent formation or reformation of adhesions in a variety of circumstances. They can be placed under adherent scars after surgical release to prevent readhesion. They are used successfully to prevent the adherence of overlying muscle to lumbar dura after spinal operations. Another use has been to prevent reankylosis of joints after surgical release, although other autogenous grafts or flaps or polymeric silicone spacers are used more commonly today. In the past fat grafts were used to limit adhesions to nerves after neurolysis and to tendons after tenolysis, but fat-containing flaps are more reliable and are used more commonly. Fat grafts were also used unsuccessfully in the past as a means of limiting peritoneal adhesions.

Fat grafts have been used as autogenous hemostatic plugs for parenchymal injuries to the kidney or liver. Rarely used for this purpose anymore, they have been supplanted by synthetic collagen products. Fat grafts were also transplanted into the posterior pharynx for the treatment of velopharyngeal incompetence; this unreliable treatment has been supplanted by pharyngeal flaps or pharyngoplasties.

Dermal Grafts

Because fat grafts have been plagued continually by resorption and fragility, surgeons began to transfer dermis, often in conjunction with fat, to decrease resorption and make the graft easier to manipulate. Dermal and dermal-fat grafts are definitely easier to handle than fat grafts and resist resorption better, although the reason for this is not entirely understood.

To harvest a dermal or dermal-fat graft, a thin split-thickness skin graft is harvested initially from the dermis in the chosen donor area. Dermis or dermis and fat are excised sharply. In most instances, the fascia underlying the fat is left intact. The graft is transferred to the desired site, and the donor site is closed with the thin superficial skin graft that was harvested initially. Smaller grafts may be harvested in an elliptic design so that the donor site may be closed by direct wound approximation (Fig. 7-1). The most common donor sites for dermal-fat grafts are the same as for fat grafts—the abdomen, thighs, and buttocks.

When dermis is included with fat, the cellular response to the transplant is increased, although the response to dermal-fat grafts is otherwise similar to the response to fat grafts. When examined over time, the sebaceous glands disappear within 2 weeks and the hair follicles in 2 to 8 weeks, whereas sweat glands seem to persist. The end result is normal-appearing dermis with sweat glands. Dermis appears to maintain bulk and structure when examined over time.

Uses of Dermal Grafts

Because the use of dermal-fat grafts grew out of the use of fat grafts, it is difficult to separate discussions of the two materials. Fat and dermal-fat grafts have been used by different surgeons for many of the same purposes. Dermis, like fat, has been used primarily to provide bulk to deficient areas. Dermal-fat grafts are still indicated for the correction of small contour irregularities and as a buffer layer to prevent the adhesion of scar to underlying tissue. Dermal grafts have been used without fat to provide more bulk to the nasal dorsum in patients with saddle nose

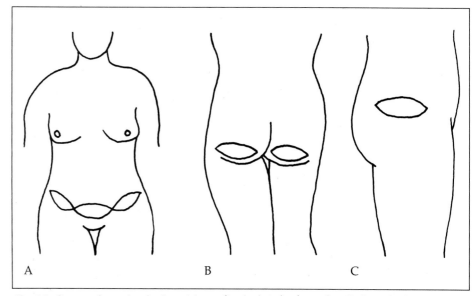

Fig. 7-1. Common donor sites for dermal-fat grafts. A. Anterior donor sites. B. Posterior donor sites. C. Lateral donor site.

deformity, although bone or cartilage is used more commonly at this time.

Dermal grafts have been used to provide an additional layer of coverage to wounds in highly traumatized areas such as pressure sores and pretibial wounds. Hynes proposed harvesting dermis from an area, applying it upside down to a wound, allowing the graft to take and granulate, and overgrafting the dermis. Although sometimes successful, this approach is currently used rarely and has been supplanted by musculocutaneous and other flaps, which provide improved blood supply and tissue bulk.

Dermal grafts have been placed subcutaneously in the neck after radical neck dissections as a protective layer for the carotid artery. The incidence of carotid artery blowout is decreased in patients undergoing postradiation radical neck dissections if dermal grafts are placed as a secondary layer over that artery. Because musculocutaneous flaps provide better coverage and protection for the carotid artery than do grafts, the more frequent use of such flaps has limited the use of the dermal grafting technique.

An additional area in which dermal grafts may be used is intraorally. Skin grafts intraorally have been hampered by contraction and by their nonmucoid characteristics. Deeper dermis limits wound

contraction more effectively than superficial dermis when transferred as a graft. When deep dermal grafts are placed intraorally, the mucosa regenerates and appears more normal than that provided by standard skin grafts.

Dermis has been used as a replacement for fascia or ligaments in a variety of clinical situations. Dermal grafts have been used for hernial and diaphragmatic repairs, although currently fascia or prosthetic materials are used more commonly. Another use for dermis has been to reinforce repairs of the temporomandibular joints, knees, fingers, and elbows after various surgical procedures. Dermis is rarely used for any of these purposes today. Dermal grafts are used after excision of extensive chordee that requires excision of the Buck fascia and the tunica albuginea. Dermal grafts also have been placed between the rectum and the vaginal wall to correct rectoceles. Muscle or musculocutaneous flaps are generally preferred for vaginal reconstructive purposes.

Dermal grafts have been used as weights for the upper eyelid in instances of proptosis and as a replacement for dura. Gold is more commonly used today in proptotic eyelids. Dermis also has been used successfully to prevent refusion after release of ankylosed temporomandibular joints.

Muscle Grafts

Muscle is a unique mesenchymal tissue in that it can contract when stimulated. It is primarily a cellular structure consisting of muscle cells and a few fibroblasts in a limited extracellular matrix. Under normal circumstances the number of muscle cells in the body does not change with time, although the size of the cells changes with muscular activity.

Experimental and clinical results with free muscle grafts have been contradictory and confusing. Muscle cells have a limited ability to tolerate ischemia as functional units. When most grafts are evaluated over time, it is noted that the grafts are revascularized but the muscle cells have died. Fibroblasts within the muscle survive and proliferate and replace the muscle with a diminished quantity of fibrous tissue. The result is similar whether the muscle is transferred into a muscle cell environment or into some alternative environment. Various investigators have attempted to prevent fibrosis with electrical stimulation, but these efforts have been unsuccessful.

Experimental studies evaluating the transfer of small muscles (less than 4 g) in rats or cats have provided different results. In these studies, viable, functional muscle cells survive grafting, especially in younger animals. It is postulated that dormant stem cells, known as *satellite cells*, at the edge of the muscle are better able to survive an ischemic interval than traditional muscle cells. These satellite cells appear identical to muscle cells under light microscopy, although they can be distinguished under the electron microscope. It is believed that the inner muscle cells degenerate and the outer satellite cells survive and regenerate muscle. These findings are similar to results of studies using tissue culture, in which muscle cells can survive and even contract after transplantation.

Noel Thompson is the only author who has reported the successful functional transfer of free muscle grafts in a human. He transferred the extensor digitorum brevis to the face 2 weeks after denervation to correct a deficiency in orbital closure caused by facial palsy. He believed the 2-week interval after denervation conditioned the muscle to ischemia. When transferred to the face, the muscle belly was placed in apposition to the functional contralateral orbicularis oculi. The tendons were tunneled into the paralyzed side of the face to produce orbital closure. Thompson described the process of neurotization by which nerves grew from the functional orbicularis into the muscle graft and contributed to function in the transferred muscle. Noone has repeated his success in transplanting functional nonvascularized muscles in a human.

Uses of Muscle Grafts

Nonvascularized muscles currently have limited usefulness. They can be used as autogenous hemostatic sponges for bleeding surfaces and to reinforce suture lines in the parenchyma of liver and kidney, although they are not commonly used for these purposes. They also can be used to fill potential spaces, such as in the frontal sinus, in a manner similar to fat.

Cartilage Grafts

Cartilage is a mesenchymally derived dense tissue that consists of cartilage cells (chondrocytes) surrounded by an extracellular matrix. The extracellular matrix consists primarily of type II collagen and glycosaminoglycans. The type II collagen in the matrix is relatively unique to cartilage. The primary glycosaminoglycan found in cartilaginous matrix is chondroitin sulfate. Cartilage, like cornea and epidermis, lacks an inherent blood supply, and under normal circumstances the tissue survives with nutrients supplied through diffusion from the surrounding perichondrium. Chondrocytes normally are not very active metabolically, and there is little ongoing remodeling in cartilage. There are three types of cartilage: hyaline cartilage, elastic cartilage, and fibrocartilage. The differences among the types of cartilage lie in the extracellular matrix; the chondrocytes in all types of cartilage are similar. Costal cartilage, nasal septum, and alar cartilage are examples of hyaline cartilage. The cartilage of the external ear, ear canal, and eustachian tube is elastic cartilage, characterized by elastic fibers within the matrix. Fibrocartilage is found in the interarticular areas of the knee and between the vertebrae. The three types of cartilage respond similarly when transferred as grafts.

Fresh autogenous cartilage is preferred for grafting. The primary sources of cartilage for grafting are the costal margin, the septum, and the ear (Fig. 7-2). The harvesting of costal cartilage grafts requires a fairly extensive procedure with a lower thoracic incision and the risk of pneumothorax. Septal grafts generally are harvested through a submucous resection. Although a substantial amount of cartilage can be obtained, and L strut of cartilage approximately 1 cm wide must be maintained as suggested by the dotted line in Figure 7-2B. Overzealous resections may result in a saddle nose deformity. Auricular grafts can be harvested successfully from several portions of the ear, including the concha, the helical rim, and the helical crus. Reasonably large conchal grafts can be harvested, producing only a limited deformity.

As stated, cartilage is avascular, and the relatively quiescent chondrocytes are sheltered from surrounding tissues by a matrix that is immunologically nonreactive. An immune response is generated to homologous cartilage only when chondrocytes are exposed because of the nature of the graft or because of breakdown of the matrix by inflammatory cells or fibroblasts. These facts have generated interest in the clinical usefulness of both fresh and preserved homologous cartilage grafts. Cartilage specimens preserved by freeze drying or treatment with 70% alcohol survive in a manner similar to fresh homologous cartilage; thus preserved grafts are used routinely both for convenience and to limit disease transmission. All homologous grafts induce a more intense inflammatory response than does autogenous cartilage, and they are surrounded by a thicker connective tissue capsule. Homologous cartilage is resorbed to a greater degree than autogenous cartilage, and autogenous cartilage is preferred in most instances. Formalin-fixed xenografts also have been used in the past, although they resorb even more than homologous grafts. The resorption process is prolonged, however, and early results can be good.

Heat treatment of both autogenous and homologous cartilage has been used to decrease the inherent tendency of cartilage to bend. Heat kills the chondrocytes and denatures the matrix, causing the graft to be resorbed. For this reason, it is used rarely.

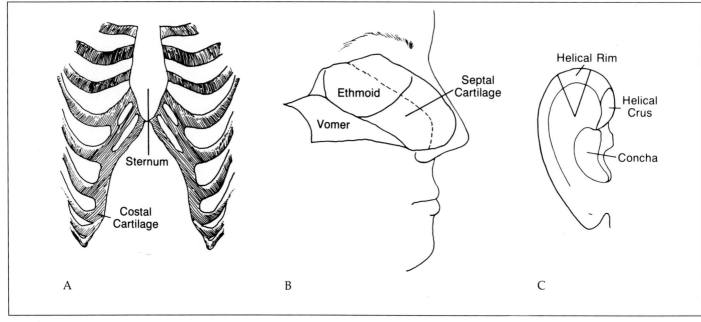

Fig. 7-2. Common donor sites for cartilage grafts. A. Costal cartilage. B. Septal cartilage. C. Auricular cartilage.

After transfer, cartilage cells survive by osmosis. They can survive in any well-vascularized recipient site and maintain cartilaginous characteristics. Transplanted autogenous cartilage elicits only a limited inflammatory response, which dissipates relatively quickly. After 2 months, no sign of inflammation is generally noted. There is also a limited fibro-blastic and angiogenic response, which results in a connective tissue capsule that serves, to a certain extent, as perichondrium. Initially the capsule is thick, although it thins with time. The chondrocytes survive, as does the durable extracellular matrix. The cells continue to function and maintain the extracellular matrix with its hyaline, fibrocartilage, or elastic characteristics. Occasionally a portion of the cartilage is replaced by either bone or fibrous tissue and becomes vascularized. This process occurs more often in younger than in older people. It may be related to infection or hematoma formation around the graft.

Placing cartilage in either a cartilaginous or noncartilaginous milieu does not affect survival. Cartilage does not require functional stress to retain its bulk as bone does. In animals, embryonic cartilage grafts may grow. Some authors have suggested the same may be true in humans, especially if perichondrium is included

with the graft, although this theory is not universally accepted.

Cartilage can be used to provide form and rigidity, unlike fat, dermis, and muscle, or it can be morseled or diced to provide a less rigid reconstructive material. It has the advantage over bone that it can be carved easily. The disadvantages of cartilage are that it can warp and that it cannot bear weight as bone can.

Uses of Cartilage Grafts

Cartilage grafts have been and still are used for many purposes. The rigidity and firmness of cartilage can be used to advantage in many ways. Cartilage grafts often are used for structural augmentation. For many years, cartilage grafts have been used to correct saddle nose deformities. Septal, alar, and auricular cartilages are used most commonly for limited abnormalities. More extreme deformities generally require costal cartilage. In auricular reconstruction for microtia, cartilage grafts are used to replace the relatively rigid internal structure of the ear. Costal cartilage is generally used for this purpose. Cartilage grafts also have been used to provide structural rigidity to the trachea and eyelid. They have been used similarly to maintain the patency of fallopian tubes.

Cartilage grafts also can be used as onlay-type grafts to correct traumatic, congenital, or surgically induced facial deformities, although bone is probably used more commonly. An alternative method of correcting contour deformities is to apply diced cartilage, which subsequently is surrounded by fibrous tissue. This technique was used to correct deformities in the frontal area, although the method is not commonly used today. Cartilage grafts also have been used to provide contour to areas that require it. They have been used in the correction of inverted nipples and to form pseudo-Montgomery glands in reconstructed areolae.

Diced cartilage has been placed in molds and buried in tissue to allow reformation of cartilage into ear- or riblike structures. Structure is generally not well maintained after mold removal and transplantation, however. Diced cartilage also has been used in the past as a way of providing added structure to hernial and myelo-meningocele closures. All these uses of diced cartilage have been supplanted by other methods.

Cartilage grafts have been used as spacers to maintain mobility after excision of ankylosed temporomandibular joints in a manner similar to dermal and fascial grafts. They have been used as replacements for the stapes of the middle ear after stapedectomy.

Fascial Grafts

Fascia is a tough mesenchymal tissue consisting of fibroblasts interspersed in a dense matrix. The matrix is made up of type I collagen and glycosaminoglycans, both of which are synthesized by fibroblasts. Fascia is extremely strong, having a tensile strength of 7000 pounds per square inch. It provides support for underlying muscles throughout the body, and in the hand and foot, compartmentalizes tendinous and other structures to facilitate their isolated functions.

Autologous fascia is the preferred graft material. In the past both homologous and preserved ox fascia were used, but both are resorbed with time. In some circumstances, the fibrosis generated by nonautologous fascia yielded a functional result, although good results were not predictable enough to warrant its recommendation. Fascia has occasionally been transferred with fat to limit the resorption of fat, although its effectiveness in that situation is not well documented.

The most common donor site is the tensor fasciae latae (TFL). A large, thick piece of fascia can be harvested from the TFL with limited morbidity. The fascia can be harvested through a longitudinal incision on the lateral thigh. Elevation of superior and inferior flaps allows exposure of as much of the fascia as desired. If a strip wider than 10 to 15 mm is harvested, the underlying muscle herniates through the fascial defect after graft harvesting, although this defect improves with time. A fasciae latae stripper allows excision of the fascia through a limited distal incision in the lateral thigh. When this instrument is used, two longitudinal parallel cuts are made while the fascia is held taut with an instrument. The fascia is severed proximally, allowing removal of a fascial strip. Temporalis fascia has also been used as a graft and as a flap as well. It is generally harvested through a vertical temporal incision within the hairline (Fig. 7-3).

Transplanted fascia elicits an early, mild inflammatory response that dissipates after 3 weeks. The graft becomes edematous soon after transplantation and remains so until about the sixth day. When the graft is examined over time, revascularization is evident beginning at 3 days. By 15 to 18 days, transplanted fascia is surrounded by a thin film of capillaries

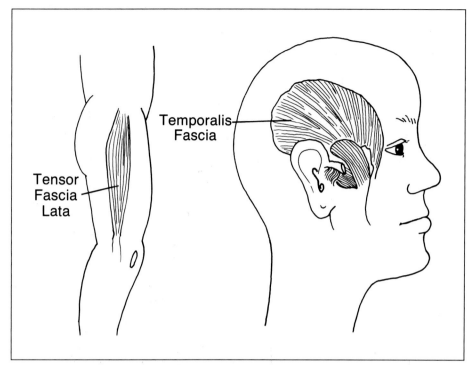

Fig. 7-3. Common donor sites for fascial grafts. Left, tensor fascia lata. Right, temporalis fascia.

and fibroblasts, which is initially relatively thick but subsequently becomes thinner. The fibroblasts of transplanted fascia generally survive, and the extracellular matrix remains relatively unchanged. In experimental models, fascia has been observed to maintain size if not weight.

Uses of Fascial Grafts

Fascial grafts have been used for a variety of purposes including, in the past, many inappropriate purposes. For example, fascia was used to line the stomach and bladder, and in both circumstances it broke down. These attempts emphasized that fascia needs to be buried in tissue to be effective and that it is generally not a good replacement for tissues that are normally lined by mucosa. It has been effective in closing tracheal and urethral defects in isolated instances, however.

Fascial grafts have been used in a manner similar to fat and dermal-fat grafts for tissue augmentation and for protection against readhesion of adherent scars. Fascia, like dermis, has been used as a protective layer for the carotid artery after radical neck dissection, as a dural substitute, and as a spacer to limit readhesion of ankylosed structures such as the tem-

poromandibular joint after surgical release. It also has been used to block tissue ingrowth into a particular area. For example, fascial grafts have been placed in the subcutaneous layer in patients with Frey syndrome to limit symptoms. Although these attempts were sometimes effective, fascial grafts have no particular advantage in such settings, and they are rarely used for these purposes today.

Fascial grafts have been used as "natural sutures" and as grafts for chest or abdominal wall repairs. Experience with fascial grafts for these purposes demonstrated the importance of the alignment of collagen fibers within the graft. When used as suture, the graft must be taken in line with the fibers for the graft to maintain strength. This use of fascia as suture has been obviated for the most part by newer synthetic sutures. When used for chest or abdominal wall reconstruction, fascial grafts are limited by their tendency to separate when stress is applied perpendicular to the direction of their fibers. To overcome this problem, two layers of fascia may be used, with the fibers oriented at 90° to each other.

Fascial grafts also have been used as structural supports, such as in patients with facial palsy. Fasciae latae strips have been used in a static manner to suspend lax facial structures; they have also been used to extend either temporalis or masseter muscle transfers to provide motion for the paralyzed face. These grafts have been used to suspend the upper eyelid to the frontalis muscle in patients with severe eyelid ptosis. In a somewhat similar way, fascial grafts have been used as tendon and ligament substitutes; examples include the extensor tendons in the hand and ligaments around the knee and shoulder. Fascia is still used at times for all of these purposes.

Fascial grafts have been used for a variety of other functions. They were used to make a pseudosheath to fill gaps for nerves and ureters; however, nerve grafts are currently preferred to fascial sheaths for the treatment of nerve defects, and ureteral defects are treated more reliably by other methods. Fascial grafts have been used as a method of reinforcing the liver when sewing defects. Although potentially helpful, fascial grafts are not generally necessary in this setting. Fascial grafts have also been used for tympanic membrane reconstruction with some success.

Conclusion

Plastic surgery is a field undergoing constant evolution. The changing role of grafts in aesthetic and reconstructive surgery mirrors this evolutionary process. Early plastic surgeons had few reconstructive techniques to rely on other than grafts, and grafts of various sorts were used for a wide variety of purposes. With time it became apparent that grafts were unsuitable for some of these purposes, and improved alternative techniques made grafting a second choice of reconstructive method for others. Grafts remain the procedure of choice for some purposes, however. Although the indications for fat, dermal, muscle, cartilage, and fascial grafts are changing, understanding the biology of each of the materials allows their effective and appropriate use.

Suggested Reading

Billings, E., Jr., and May, J.W. Historical review and present status of free fat autotransplantation in plastic and reconstructive surgery. *Plast. Reconstr. Surg.* 83:368, 1989.

Cedars, M.G., et al. The microscopic morphology of orthotopic free muscle grafts in rabbits. *Plast. Reconstr. Surg.* 72:179, 1983.

Duncan, M.J., Thomson, H.G., and Mancer, J.F.K. Free cartilage grafts: The role of perichondrium. *Plast. Reconstr. Surg.* 73:916, 1983.

Ellenbogen, R. Free autogenous pearl fat grafts in the face: A preliminary report of a rediscovered technique. *Ann. Plast. Surg.* 16:179, 1986.

Hynes, W. The reversed dermis graft. *Br. J. Plast. Surg.* 7:97, 1954.

Miller, T.A. Temporalis fascia grafts for facial and nasal contour augmentation. *Plast. Reconstr. Surg.* 81:524, 1988.

Peer, L.A. *Transplantation of Tissues,* Vol. 1. Baltimore: Williams & Wilkins, 1959.

Peer, L.A. *Transplantation of Tissues,* Vol. 2. Baltimore: Williams & Wilkins, 1959.

Schultz, E., et al. Survival of satellite cells in whole muscle transplants. *Anat. Rec.* 222:12, 1988.

Thompson, N. A review of autogenous skeletal muscle grafts and their clinical applications. *Clin. Plast. Surg.* 1:349, 1974.

8

The Omentum in Reconstructive Surgery

Michael A. Marschall   Elias G. Gikas   Mimis Cohen

The greater omentum is a fatty, vascular double layer of peritoneum attached to the greater curvature of the stomach and the transverse colon. It spreads as an apron and covers the small intestine and colon. Its rich vascular supply with extensive lymphatics makes it a useful structure in the defense against intraabdominal infections.

An initial surgical use of the omentum was described by Drummond and Morrison in 1896 when they attempted to shunt blood from the portal to the systemic circulation. Since that time, the omentum has proved to be useful in strengthening visceral repairs, protecting anastomotic sites, and filling potential dead spaces. There are numerous extraabdominal uses for the omentum, including revascularization of the myocardium, increasing blood flow to ischemic brain, and relief of chronic lymphedema of the extremities. In plastic and reconstructive surgery, the omentum has been used as a pedicled flap in the management of chest wall defects. Microsurgical techniques additionally enhance the reconstructive usefulness of the omentum as a free flap to cover defects in various areas of the body.

Anatomy and Embryology

The omentum is a syncytium of blood vessels, fat, and lymphatics. It originates embryologically as a mesentery between the stomach and the posterior abdominal wall. This double peritoneal structure rotates with the stomach and ultimately shifts to the left to lie horizontally. Toward the middle of intrauterine life, the posterior surface fuses with the serosal layer of the transverse colon extending from the hepatic to the splenic flexure. This relatively avascular fusion plane is important during operative dissection because it tends to be more defined around the splenic flexure, making separation easier to initiate at this area. The double peritoneal layer encloses a rich network that includes blood vessels, lymphatics, varying amounts of fat, and macrophages.

The omental blood supply comes from the right and left gastroepiploic arteries, which are branches of the right gastroduodenal and splenic arteries, respectively (Fig. 8-1). The gastroepiploic vessels form an arch that is complete in most instances. Branching marginal and central

vessels extend from the gastroepiploic arcade in a generally predictable pattern.

Three major vessels extend vertically lengthwise along the omentum. They are the right, middle, and left omental arteries. The middle omental artery bifurcates terminally and joins the other two, forming a distal arcade. Valveless veins accompany the arteries and drain into the portal circulation. Because anatomic variants have been recognized, the individual anatomy should be studied carefully before vascular division to facilitate lengthening and ensure viability (Fig. 8-2).

Contraindications to omental transfer noted preoperatively include a history of abdominal procedures, particularly if an inflammatory process was present. In addition, portal hypertension, cirrhosis, active peptic ulcer disease, or other gastric or splenic disease precludes the procedure. Generalized debility and cachexia render the omentum thin and of little use, as does overt omental involvement with carcinoma.

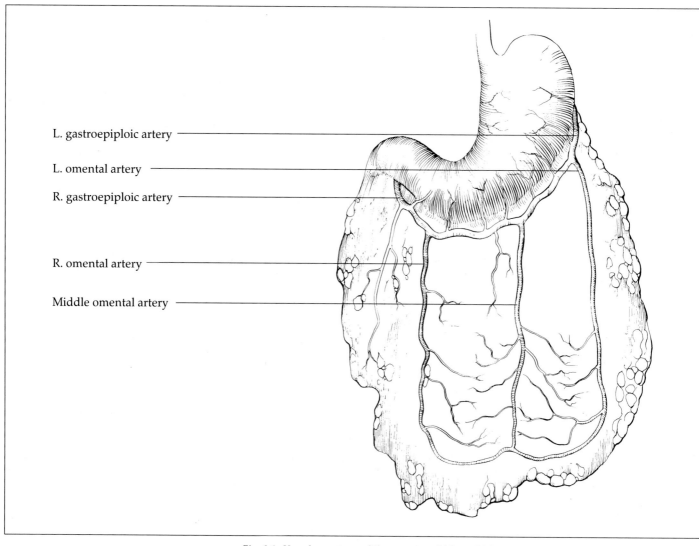

L. gastroepiploic artery

L. omental artery

R. gastroepiploic artery

R. omental artery

Middle omental artery

Fig. 8-1. Vascular anatomy of the omentum. Right and left gastroepiploic arteries with distal arcade structure including right, left, and middle omental arteries.

Operative Technique

Before omental transfer, the patient should have a limited intestinal preparation to facilitate abdominal dissection. Before the flap is harvested, the recipient site should have the appropriate surgical preparation or debridement. In refractory wounds, particularly chronic chest wounds caused by radiation after mastectomy, a preoperative marginal biopsy may be indicated to rule out intercurrent malignant tumors.

Placement of the abdominal incision depends largely on the surgeon's preference; an upper abdominal transverse or a midline approach is usually used. We

favor a short, upper midline incision for most patients, although previous scars may dictate an alternative incision. After a laparotomy and manual exploration of the abdominal contents to identify gross pathology, the omentum and transverse colon are delivered from the abdominal cavity. The arterial anatomy and the size and quality of the omentum, are assessed, with close attention to the bulk and vascularity.

We start omental dissection by separating the omentum from the transverse colon. This dissection is most expediently carried out from left to right. Small vessels should be ligated carefully. The use of electrocautery is avoided to minimize in-

Fig. 8-2. Anatomic variants and lengthening options of the omentum. A. Distal bifurcation of middle omental artery. B. High bifurcation of middle omental artery. C. Midlength bifurcation of middle omental artery. D. Absent middle omental artery. (Adapted from E.S. Alday and H.S. Goldsmith. Surgical technique for omental lengthening based on arterial anatomy. Surg. Gynecol. Obstet. 135:103, 1972.)

jury to the delicate omental vasculature and the serosa of the transverse colon. Overzealous traction along the splenic attachments should also be avoided to prevent splenic bleeding or rupture. Identification of the middle colic artery is important to avoid accidental dissection or disruption. Any tears in the mesocolon

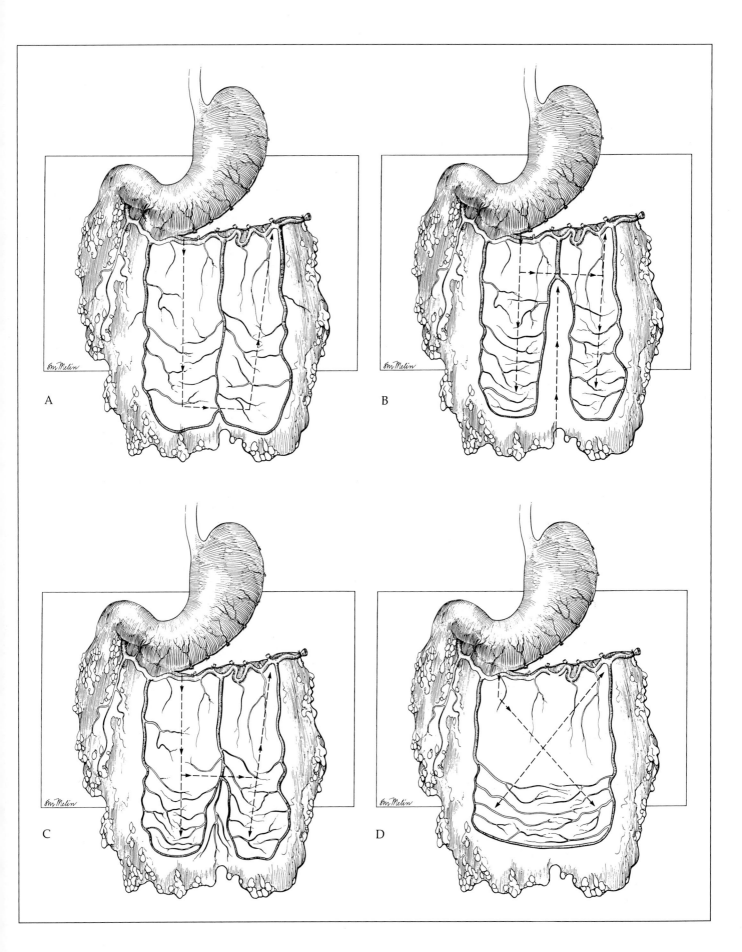

A

B

C

D

should be repaired to prevent subsequent herniation.

After complete separation of the omentum from the transverse colon, attention is turned to dissection from the greater curvature of the stomach. The plane of dissection is between the gastroepiploic arcade and the gastric wall with careful clamping, division, and ligation of all short gastric vessels. Extreme caution is needed during this phase to avoid including the gastric wall in any clamp or ligature, which might result in subsequent necrosis and gastric perforation. The omentum is fully skeletonized on the right and left gastroepiploic vessels and may be pedicled on either vessel, depending on the reconstructive needs. When performing a free tissue transfer, we prefer to use the right gastroepiploic artery for the anastomosis because its luminal diameter is generally larger than that of the left artery, ranging from 1.5 to 2.0 mm.

Pedicle length can be increased by additional proximal skeletonization toward the arterial axis. Effective flap length can be increased by specific lengthening techniques. Arterial anatomic variants are possible, and the omentum should be studied carefully before any vascular division is attempted. When an intact pedicle is maintained, lengthening can extend coverage as far cephalad as the head and neck or as far distally as the lower extremity.

Depending on whether the omentum is used as a pedicled transposition flap or as a free microvascular transfer flap, additional counterincisions and tunneling may be necessary. The omentum can be brought into the anterior mediastinum and chest through the cephalic portion of a midline incision or through the diaphragm to the right of the falciform ligament. For pedicled transfer to the lower extremity, similar tunneling is required with exteriorization over the inguinal ligament. Abdominal closure around the pedicle should be done carefully to avoid potential hernial formation or possible pedicle strangulation. Kinking, torsion, or compression of the pedicle should be avoided, and clinical monitoring of the omental circulation during mobilization and inset of the flap is essential. In addition, torsion, kinking, or compression of the duodenum or stomach should be prevented by careful assessment of the

position of the pedicle during flap transfer.

Draining the abdominal cavity is unnecessary, but drains might be required in the area of subcutaneous dissection or tunneling. Abdominal closure is done in a routine manner, and a nasogastric tube is maintained for 24 to 48 hours postoperatively for decompression of any resulting ileus. If there is a need for coverage of the omentum with a split-thickness skin graft, this is done without delay along with the omental transposition. The skin graft is meshed, applied directly over the omentum, and secured with absorbable sutures, with attention to avoiding injury to the underlying vessels. An absorptive dressing without a stent is applied to absorb the relatively large amount of serous transudate. This drainage seals after a few days as epithelization is completed.

Applications

The omental flap fills a wide variety of reconstructive needs and has diverse applications in a variety of clinical conditions. It has been used successfully for coverage of large thoracic defects in the midline or the lateral chest and for the treatment of lymphedema or vascular insufficiency of the upper and lower extremities. With the advent of microsurgery, applications of the omental flaps have been greatly extended, with free flap transfers based on either gastroepiploic vessel.

As a reconstructive tissue, the omentum has unique properties that make it particularly applicable in some circumstances. It can be spread to cover a large surface area with thin, well-vascularized tissue and immediately skin grafted. This property is particularly advantageous in scalp reconstruction. Skin graft adherence and take over of the omentum, when this graft is applied immediately after flap transfer, has been excellent in all our patients (Fig. 8-3). The omentum has a unique pliability that allows for folding and filling of defects or dead spaces, such as the orbit, sinuses, pleural space, mediastinum, pelvis, and large bony cavities after debridement of osteomyelitis. The intrinsic immune capabilities of the omentum ensure good flap coverage for contaminated wounds, and its rich blood

supply makes it useful for coverage of wounds that occur after radiation therapy.

The omentum has been used as a free vascularized transfer for the reconstruction of hemifacial atrophy. Its pliability and vascular arcade pattern allow exact tailoring and filling of the tissue deficit. Omentum shows little tendency to atrophy as muscle does, but large weight swings of the patient may alter its volume and clinically change its configuration.

Most wounds of the anterior chest wall and virtually all mediastinal wounds can be covered with omentum based on either gastroepiploic vessel. Transfer on a single pedicle additionally increases its arc of transposition, allowing coverage of lateral and even posterior chest wall defects. The omentum has been used successfully for closure of large chest wounds secondary to radionecrosis after debridement of all necrotic tissue. The improved regional vascularity after omental flap transfer and the additional lymphatic drainage intrinsic to the omentum offer an advantage over local tissue closure in such instances (see Chap. 92).

An additional application of the omental flap has been in the reconstruction of traumatic defects of the lower extremity using a microvascular transfer. The omentum provides stable wound coverage and obliterates any residual cavities. Furthermore, the great length of the omental pedicle, with or without additional lengthening, allows coverage of distal defects without the need for venous grafts. All anastomoses are performed well out of the zone of injury with relatively large-caliber vessels and without venous grafts, thus reducing operative time and microvascular complications (Fig. 8-4).

Fig. 8-3. Omental free flap for scalp reconstruction with immediate skin grafting. A. Preoperative defect following Mohs micrographic excision of basal cell carcinoma. B. Omental flap in place after anastomosis with temporal vessels. C and D. Healing 9 months after the reconstructive procedure.

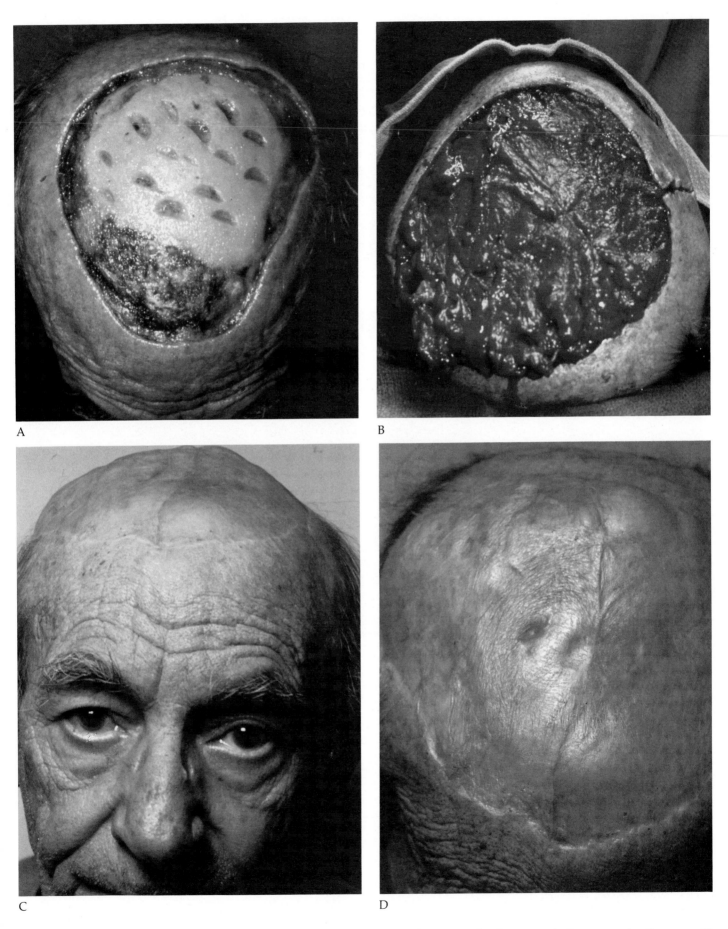

A

B

C

D

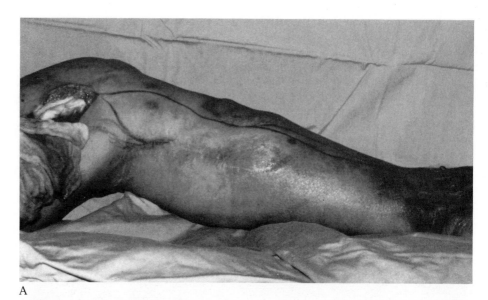

A

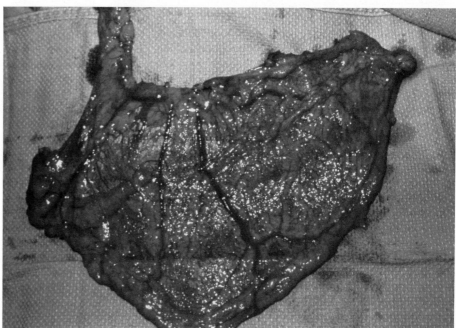

B

Fig. 8-4. Omental free flap for chronic venous stasis ulcer of lower extremity after trauma to the knee and distal venous insufficiency. A. Preoperative defect (femoral vessel has been exposed). B. Flap before transfer based on right gastroepiploic vessels. C. Flap transfer with anastomoses to superficial femoral artery and vena comitans. Area of venous insufficiency is bypassed with lengthened omental flap. A skin graft was immediately applied over the omentum. D. Healed wound 6 months postoperatively.

Disadvantages

Despite the distinct advantages of the omentum as a flap in reconstructive surgery, there are some clear disadvantages to its use. A laparotomy is necessary for flap harvest with all the attendant complications of that procedure. The possibility of splenic, gastric, or colonic injury is present, although such injuries are unusual when operative technique is meticulous and dissection is careful. Obstructive sequelae of torsion, compression, adhesions, or intra-abdominal or incisional

hernia can also occur. The risk of seeding the abdominal cavity when using the omentum to cover an infected median sternotomy or chest wound is a possibility, although probably more theoretical than real. There was no intra-abdominal infection in any of the 14 instances of infected median sternotomy wound we managed with omental flaps.

With advances in reconstructive surgery and the availability of muscle, musculocutaneous, or fasciocutaneous flaps, the omentum is no longer a first consideration in the management of difficult prob-

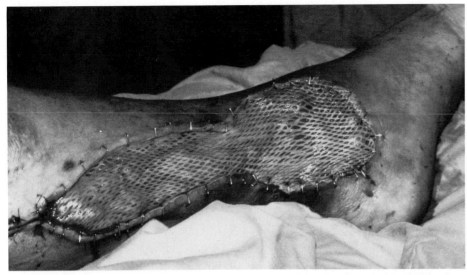

C

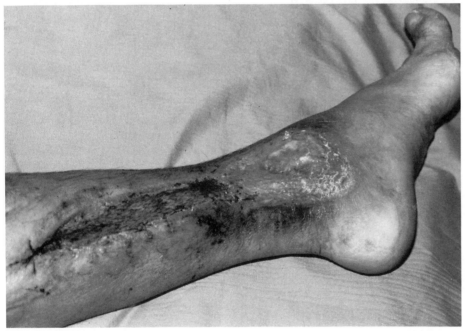

D

lems outside the abdominal cavity. In selected circumstances, however, it remains a good alternative flap if planned and executed with care.

Conclusion

The omentum provides a relatively large amount of well-vascularized, pliable, and easily obtainable tissue suitable for a wide variety of reconstructive needs. It can be transferred reliably, and it can be extended when used as a microvascular free transpositional flap. The unique properties of the omentum, including its vascularity, pliability, large potential surface area, and lymphatic infection-fighting capabilities, make it a flap of high regard for closure of difficult thoracic and mediastinal wounds. Most patients tolerate well omental harvesting and transfer, with little added morbidity. Patients ultimately receive stable and durable wound coverage when other flaps are unavailable or unsuitable for the task.

Suggested Reading

Alday, E.S., and Goldsmith, H.S. Surgical technique for omental lengthening based on arterial anatomy. *Surg. Gynecol. Obstet.* 135:103, 1972.

Arnold, P.G., and Irons, G.B. The greater omentum: Extensions in transposition and free transfer. *Plast. Reconstr. Surg.* 67:169, 1981.

Casten, D., and Alday, E. Omental transfer for revascularization of the extremities. *Surg. Gynecol. Obstet.* 132:301, 1971.

Goldsmith, H.S., Kiely, A., and Randall, H. Protection of intrathoracic esophageal anastomoses by omentum. *Surgery* 63:464, 1968.

Jurkiewicz, M.J., and Arnold, P.G. The omentum: An account of its use in the reconstruction of the chest wall. *Ann. Surg.* 185:548, 1977.

Jurkiewicz, M.J., and Nahai, F. The omentum: Its use as a free vascularized graft for reconstruction of the head and neck. *Ann. Surg.* 195:756, 1982.

Liebermann-Meffert, D., and White, H. (Eds.). *The Greater Omentum.* Berlin: Springer, 1983.

McLean, D., and Buncke, H. Autotransplant of omentum to a large scalp defect with microsurgical revascularization. *Plast. Reconstr. Surg.* 49:268, 1972.

Ohtsuka, H., Torigai, K., and Itoh, M. Free omental transfer to the lower limbs. *Ann. Plast. Surg.* 4:70, 1980.

Shaw, W., and Hildago, D. Omentum Free Flaps. In W. Shaw and D. Hildago (Eds.), *Microsurgery in Trauma.* Mount Kisco, N.Y.: Futura, 1987.

9

Bone Grafts

John W. Polley

The past few decades have witnessed a dramatic change in the availability and use of bone grafts in plastic surgery. Much of our current sophistication in the use of bone grafts has resulted from the development of craniomaxillofacial surgery and microsurgery. The coronal incision unveiled an enormous bony donor site. Successful subperiosteal bony exposure, osteotomies, recontouring, and repositioning of large segments of the cranial vault and facial skeleton opened the door to radical and creative techniques for managing difficult craniofacial deformities. With these new techniques came an increased need for bone grafts. Similarly, with advances in microsurgery came the ability to transfer large segments of bone with an intact vascular supply. These techniques have led to a new clinical understanding of bony anatomy. Research in bone physiology and biomechanics has promoted advances in osteoconduction, osteoinduction, bone substitutes, and rigid fixation techniques.

This chapter discusses the current understanding of bone graft physiology and repair and reviews the autogenous bone grafts most commonly used in plastic surgery today.

Anatomy of Bone
Macroscopic Assessment

Bone is strong, withstanding tensile forces of 12,500 pounds per square inch and compressive forces of 7000 pounds per square inch. It is by no means static, however; its shape and volume change markedly in response to functional and physiologic influences. The dynamic nature of bone was recognized by Wolff in 1864 and is now described in "Wolff's law." Bone is composed of two types of osseous tissue, *cortical* and *cancellous*. Cortical bone is dense and makes up the exterior surfaces of bone; cancellous bone is spongy in consistency, made up of a latticework of trabeculae. The difference between cortical and cancellous bone lies in the size and number of spaces within.

Bone is enclosed, except at articular surfaces, in a fibrous membrane, or periosteum. The periosteum transmits blood, lymphatic vessels, and nerves to the outer surfaces of bone. It consists of two closely united layers, an outer layer made up chiefly of collagenous tissues and an inner layer, or *cambium*, made up of finer, more elastic tissues. In immature bone the periosteum is thick, vascular, and ad-

herent to bone. The cambium contains osteoblasts, the cells responsible for the ossification process on the exterior surface of immature bone. In mature bone the periosteum is thinner and less vascular, with a reduced number of osteoblasts in the cambium. The inner cortical surface of long bones is lined with an inner vascular membrane called the *endosteum*.

Bone marrow fills the cavities in cancellous bone. Yellow marrow predominates in the larger cavities of long bones, consisting of fat cells and primitive blood cells. Red marrow predominates in flat bones and at the articular ends of long bones. Red marrow consists of primitive blood cells that produce leukocytes and erythrocytes.

The blood supply to cortical bone is derived largely from small periosteal vessels, which penetrate minute orifices in the bone. Cancellous bone is vascularized by larger, less numerous vessels that perforate the cortical bone and distribute to the trabecular cavities. Most long bones have a large nutrient artery that enters the marrow space near the center of the body of the bone and represents the dominant arterial supply to the inner cancellous bone and marrow cells. In flat bones, numerous veins and small arteries penetrate the cortical surfaces to supply abundant blood flow. Small lymphatics and nerves accompany the veins and arteries of bone.

Microanatomy

The primary structural unit of cortical bone, the osteon, or haversian system, consists of concentric rings of bony tissue (lamellae) arranged around a central canal called the haversian canal. Each canal contains one or two blood vessels, lymphatics, and nerve filaments. Within a haversian system are numerous small spaces or lacunas, which are occupied by osteocytes. Minute channels, or canaliculi, crisscross the haversian system, connecting lacunas with lacunas and lacunas with the haversian canals. Within the canaliculi run the cytoplasmic extensions of osteocytes. In thin, flat bones and in the trabecular walls of cancellous bone, the haversian canals and their concentric systems are absent. Instead, the canaliculi open into the spaces of the cancellous tissue, which serve a purpose similar to that of haversian canals.

Osteocytes, osteoblasts, and osteoclasts are the three cell types characteristic to bone. Osteoblasts are the cells that actively lay down bone matrix. They are derived from a progenitor bone cell line and are able to begin or cease organic matrix production depending on local conditions. With mineralization of the surrounding organic bony matrix, osteoblasts become entrapped in their surrounding space, or lacuna, and become osteocytes. With resorption of the surrounding matrix, an osteocyte can revert to being a matrix-producing osteoblast.

Osteoclasts are found on the surfaces of resorbing bone and are known to be the mediators of the process of bone resorption. Osteoclasts are large, multinucleated cells, believed to be derived from lymphoid cell lines.

Bone Healing
Healing of Fractures

Bone is unique among body tissues in its ability to regenerate itself completely after injury. Following fracture, skeletal function is compromised, and the goal of any treatment is to achieve solid union of the fractured segments. Many factors, both physiologic and mechanical, influence the process of fracture healing. At a microscopic level the oxygen concentration, amount of tension, and relative dynamic motion between the fracture segments causing tissue deformation or strain all play important roles in the mechanism of fracture repair.

In spontaneous bone healing of long-bone fractures, relative dynamic motion produces strain between the fracture segments that inhibits direct bone formation. In an effort to reduce interfragmentary strain, a callus of scar tissue forms around the fractured segment. As this callus gradually increases in diameter, it reduces the dynamic motion and strain at the fracture site, producing an environment conducive for bone formation. In addition, with spontaneous bone healing, resorption at the fracture surfaces occurs, increasing the size of the fracture gap, which further decreases strain within the fracture. As rigidity at the fracture site increases, interfragmentary strain decreases, and the rigidity or stiffness of the tissues between the fractured segments increases. Over time, the tissues between the fractured segments change from connective tissue, to cartilage, and finally to bone. The same histologic sequence has been demonstrated for the repair of membranous bone fractures.

In primary bone healing, the rigidity and compressive nature of the splinting device reduces strain at the fracture site and reduces the size of the fracture gap itself. The biomechanical advantages of rigid internal fixation allow primary bone healing across the fracture gap, eliminating the need for callus and for the connective tissue and cartilaginous stages of bone healing found in spontaneous healing. Close approximation of bony segments also is important for osteoinduction.

Incorporation of Bone Grafts

Successful bone graft repair depends on a number of interdependent variables. Processes such as the proliferation of osteoprogenitor cells and their differentiation into osteoblasts, osteoconduction, osteoinduction, and appropriate biomechanical stimulation of the graft all play key roles in the incorporation of the graft into a viable new bony complex. Underlying these processes is a technically well-executed bone grafting procedure. Albee, in 1915, described the basic tenets of surgery essential to the success of all bone grafting procedures. These included (1) ensuring sufficient blood supply to the graft from the recipient site; (2) appropriate fixation of bone grafts; (3) optimization of the biomechanical environment of the bone graft; and (4) meticulous intraoperative tissue technique. These principles are well accepted to this day.

Contribution of Host and Graft to Healing

The successful incorporation of a bone graft results from a contribution from both host cells and viable cells within the graft. The relative contribution from each cell type is variable, but failure to transplant viable cells impedes graft incorporation. Viable graft cells may be derived from the periosteum, endosteum, cortical bone, or marrow.

Cells from the periosteum can survive transplantation and contribute to bone formation. Cells forming the cambium in particular are capable of osteogenesis, and delayed union and decreased callous formation in long bones can occur with extensive denudation of the periosteum. The periosteum may contribute up to 25 percent of new bone formation, and the use of periosteal grafting as "boneless" bone grafts, described by Skoog, is well documented.

With cortical bone grafts some osteocytes or endothelial cells of the bone may survive, but the quantity of bone produced by these cells is generally quite small.

The endosteal and marrow cells in a bone graft are known to be revascularized readily and to survive transplantation. The exact role each plays in osteogenesis is uncertain, but it is known that together they can contribute up to 50 percent of the new bone produced in a bone graft. The hemopoietic cells of the marrow are not believed to contribute to bone formation.

The periosteal, cortical, endosteal, and marrow cells from the host contribute to the incorporation of the bone graft in a manner similar to the cells from the graft. Generally the host contribution is dominant because of its intact cytologic and vascular elements.

Osteoconduction

Osteoconduction is the process of capillary and perivascular tissue ingrowth from the host recipient bed into the graft. This ingrowth of tissues includes osteoprogenitor cells, which differentiate into osteoblasts and produce bone. The process initially follows canaliculi and marrow spaces, and the ingrowth gradually replaces the areas in which original bone graft is resorbed. Osteoconduction occurs more rapidly in viable bone grafts, and it is enhanced by osteoinductive processes.

Osteoinduction

Induction is the process by which one tissue acts on another to induce cellular differentiation. Bone has this ability through a component known as bone morphogenic protein (BMP). The process of bone formation by BMP-induced cell differentiation was recognized by Urist when he stimulated bone formation from transplanted demineralized bone matrix in the anterior chamber of the eye in rats. Human BMP is a polypeptide with a molecular weight of 17,500 and is associated with two other proteins of lower molecular weight. Bone morphogenic protein constitutes only 0.001 percent of cortical bone but is active in very small concentrations and is readily available in large quantities from large bones.

Bone morphogenic protein acts by irreversibly inducing the differentiation of perivascular mesenchyme-like cells (pericytes) into osteoprogenitor cells. These cells, acted on by various bone-derived growth factors, stimulate chondrogenesis, which is followed soon afterward by osteogenesis.

The clinical applications of BMP in plastic surgery should prove exciting.

Remodeling of Bone

Investigators in the middle of the twentieth century observed that when forces were applied to bone, measurable electrical charges were produced. These charges were called stress-generated potentials and were found to be independent of cell viability. Further investigations revealed bioelectric potentials, which depended on tissue viability. Bone under compression was found to develop a negative charge, whereas bone subjected to tensile forces had a positive electrical charge. Since the time of these findings, the ability of small electrical currents to stimulate bone formation has been demonstrated. When periosteum in the region of a cathode is electrically stimulated, osteoprogenitor cells proliferate from the cambium. In areas of bone growth, electronegative charges are found, whereas in areas of bone that are inactive in terms of growth, the charges are neutral or slightly positive.

Using these findings, Moss and others have postulated models of bone growth and remodeling that describe skeletal development based on the functional sum of soft tissue forces on the involved bone. These theories have been tested clinically, with some success, through the use of mechanical orthopedic appliances stimulating soft tissue forces in attempts to induce bone formation.

Autografts

Cancellous Bone Grafts

Cancellous grafts are used to bridge defects or provide additional bulk to bone. Initially they offer little structural support. The revascularization of cancellous grafts may begin within hours of grafting and is complete within the first 2 weeks. As the vascular invasion of the graft proceeds, primitive mesenchymal cells (from host and graft) differentiate into osteoblasts, which begin to lay down osteoid around grafted nonviable bone. Later the entrapped, nonviable bone is resorbed gradually and replaced with new bone. Thus initially there is an increase in the radiodensity of cancellous grafts, which is followed by a decrease and another increase as the final new bone is deposited. In time a cancellous graft is completely replaced with new, viable bone.

Cortical Bone Grafts

The histologic difference between cortical and cancellous graft repair is in the rate of revascularization of the graft. Cortical grafts are revascularized at a slower rate, with initial blood vessel penetration of the graft at about one week. Complete revascularization usually does not occur until 6 to 8 weeks after grafting. This slower revascularization period is attributed to cortical bone structure, which requires osteoclastic resorption in most areas before vascular penetration.

Repair of cortical bone is first initiated by osteoclast resorption. The resorption increases up to the sixth week after grafting and gradually declines to near-normal levels at one year. The formation of new bone by osteoblastic activity begins approximately 2 weeks after grafting and continues through the first 6 months. This creeping substitution phenomenon progresses along the haversian systems of cortical bone. Bone that has not undergone resorption can be sealed off by the deposition of bone around it and may remain unaltered after the catabolic and anabolic stages of repair have been completed at 6 to 12 months. Thus cortical bone grafts tend to remain admixtures of necrotic and viable bone after complete repair.

Mechanical Strength of Bone Grafts

The strength of a bone graft correlates with the healing process. It has been demonstrated that the mechanical strength of bone is not affected by its viability. In cancellous grafts, strength initially increases with the addition of new bone and returns to normal as the necrotic bone is replaced with viable bone. With the initial dominance of osteoclastic activity in cortical bone grafts, the porosity of the graft increases and the strength decreases immediately after grafting. Cortical bone grafts weaken by approximately 30 percent at 6 weeks to 6 months after grafting. Twelve to eighteen months after grafting, a successful cortical graft regains its normal mechanical strength.

Onlay Bone Grafts

The information reviewed thus far has been derived mostly from work done with inlay bone grafting. In plastic surgery, however, onlay grafting is frequently used, primarily in the craniomaxillofacial skeleton, with the emphasis on changing form rather than function. In these situations, both clinical and experimental results have shown that the maintenance of bone graft volume can be unpredictable: The resorption rates are as high as 80 percent or greater.

A critical factor in obtaining long-term maintenance of onlay bone graft volume is the method of fixation used to secure the graft to the recipient site. As was discussed under the section Healing of Fractures, a gap in a fracture site does not heal directly when subjected to dynamic motion. Even in a small gap, motion produces strain between the segments, resulting in resorption at the fracture site. Elimination of motion through static compression across a bony gap produces biomechanical stability, eliminating interfragmentary strain and allowing direct or primary bone healing across the gap. Static compression is obtained with rigid fixation techniques, using metal screws or plates.

Using lag screw fixation for onlay bone grafts, Phillips and Rahn eliminated interfragmentary strain with onlay grafting and showed that volume maintenance of the grafts was far superior than found in grafts with no fixation, regardless of the nature of the bone used.

Other factors have been hypothesized to affect the amount of resorption of onlay bone grafts, including the nature of the recipient site and the type of bone used. Aside from fixation, the factor that seems most important in survival of onlay bone is the biologic limitation of the recipient area in terms of soft tissue coverage, tension, and muscular activity.

Vascularized Bone Grafts

With the development of microvascular surgical techniques and increased knowledge of bony anatomy, bone grafts from various sites can be transferred with an intact blood supply. Vascularized bone grafts have proved to be advantageous in clinical settings in which nonvascularized bone grafts have been unsatisfactory.

When vascularized bone is transferred, the cells of the graft survive fully because their blood supply is only temporarily interrupted. With vascularized bone there is no dead bone matrix that must undergo revascularization through osteoconduction. The healing process is similar to that of simple fracture; the time of bone graft incorporation is reduced by months.

Because the transferred bone brings its own blood supply, vascularized grafts can survive regardless of length of bone and in scarred or irradiated recipient sites with poor vascularity. These bone grafts are more successful than nonvascularized grafts in nutritionally depleted patients and in areas of high bacterial contamination such as the oral cavity.

Vascularized bone grafts maintain their mechanical strength and undergo less resorption using nonrigid fixation techniques than do nonvascularized bone grafts. In addition, it has been shown that vascularized bone transfers of epiphysis and membranous bone can maintain the ability to grow in animals with immature skeletons.

Autogenous Graft Donor Sites

Bone graft donor sites are selected on the basis of a number of variables. The reconstructive requirements and nature of the recipient site dictate the quantity and type of bone graft needed and whether or not the graft should carry its own vascular pedicle. Donor site morbidity and the age and sex of the patient are also important factors in donor site selection (Tables 9-1 and 9-2).

Ilium

Nonvascularized Grafts

The ilium is frequently used as a donor site because of its ready availability and ample supply of both cancellous and cortical bone. The anterior half of the iliac crest, beginning at the anterior superior iliac spine, supplies the thickest portion of bone (1.5 cm), including a generous layer of cancellous bone between the inner and outer cortical plates. Cancellous, corticocancellous, or full-thickness iliac grafts can be harvested relatively

Table 9-1. Common free bone grafts

Graft type	Advantages	Disadvantages
Ilium	Large quantity of cortical and cancellous bone	Donor site morbidity
Cranium	Large quantity of cortical bone Low donor site morbidity Various harvesting techniques	Bone brittle in adults Minimal cancellous bone
Rib	Large quantity of bone Malleable bone	Limited cancellous bone More difficult to fix rigidly
Tibia	Limited bone quantity	Donor site morbidity

Table 9-2. Common vascularized bone grafts

Vascularized graft type	Arterial supply	Advantages	Disadvantages
Ilium	Deep circumflex iliac	Large vessel (3 mm) Long pedicle (6 cm) Large quantity bone can be harvested	Bulky with limited skin component Donor site morbidity, especially with crest removal
Rib	Posterior intercostal Anterior intercostal	Posterior vessel (2 mm) Long posterior vessel (5 cm)	Small anterior vessel Donor site morbidity Skin island limited Rib offers limited bony volume
Fibula	Peroneal	Excellent bone length Long pedicle (8 cm) Dependable skin island	Bone diameter limited to size of fibula
Radius	Radial	Large vessel (3 mm) Large pedicle (6 cm) Reliable skin island	Donor site morbidity Limited bony volume

simply with the donor site defect well camouflaged; however, the potential morbidity from harvesting these grafts should not be taken lightly. Possible sequelae include pain, bleeding, ileus, donor site defects, postoperative limping, and thigh dysesthesia from injury to the lateral femoral cutaneous nerve.

The incision should parallel the natural skin lines over the iliac crest, which run in a transverse direction. Oblique or vertical incisions paralleling the crest run perpendicular to the natural skin lines, often leaving a wide, unsightly scar. The transverse skin incision begins 1.5 to 2.0 cm above the anterior superior spine and extends laterally. The scar should not be placed directly over the crest, to avoid local irritation, tenderness, and pain. The skin is retracted in a rostral-caudal direction, and the periosteum over the crest is exposed. Subperiosteal dissection of the medial cortical surface along the iliac fossa is readily performed to give wide bony exposure. Similar exposure of the lateral cortical surface can be performed with a bit more difficulty in adults because the external lip of the crest and the gluteal lines form a much more textured surface than does the smooth iliac fossa. Cutting through the lateral musculature also increases postoperative pain.

In adult patients in whom cancellous bone only is needed, the periosteum is left on the cortical bone and two vertical bony cuts along the inner cortex are joined by a cut along the internal lip of the iliac crest. The inner cortex is hinged medially (Fig. 9-1) to expose abundant cancellous bone, which can be harvested in strips or blocks as needed. For smaller amounts of cancellous bone, an inner cortical window can be made and the cancellous bone removed through this exposure. Similar techniques can be used for the lateral cortex; unless the exposure is absolutely needed, however, medial dissection and exposure are preferred because of the higher morbidity associated with lateral dissection.

Cortical-cancellous and full-thickness iliac grafts can be harvested by hand or power tools, preserving a 1- to 2-cm bridge of the crest to prevent cosmetic deformity (Fig. 9-2). This preserved bridge of crest bone can be removed if needed for exposure and fixed back into place at the end of the procedure.

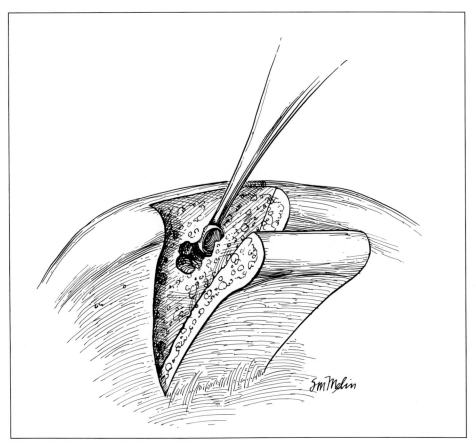

Fig. 9-1. Iliac crest removal and replacement for harvesting of a large corticocancellous graft in an adult.

In children, the crest of the ilium is covered by cartilage, which overlies the ossified body of the bone. Very thick at birth, this cartilaginous layer measures approximately 1 cm at 10 years of age and completely ossifies in the third decade of life. Harvesting of iliac bone in children is approached through medial cortical exposure and an inner cortical window, preserving the cartilaginous ossification at the center of the crest. The skin incision is as already described; whenever possible, the left ilium should be used so that the scar cannot be mistaken for an appendectomy scar. Cancellous or corticocancellous bone is harvested as needed with osteotomes and curettes. The incision must be closed in layers, approximating the periosteum as well as possible, the Scarpa fascia, and the skin.

The lateral femoral cutaneous nerve courses in a retroperitoneal direction over the medial aspect of the iliac muscle and leaves the pelvis just below the attach-

ment of the inguinal ligament to the anterior superior iliac spine. This course is variable, however, and the nerve sometimes exits right over the anterior spine itself. Direct or indirect damage to the nerve through aggressive traction can produce permanent paresthesia or anesthesia over the lateral aspect of the thigh.

The rich blood supply of cancellous bone can allow for excessive hematoma formation, particularly if a large dead space is left when a sizable amount of bone is removed. Bone wax or thrombin-soaked gelatin sponge can be used to aid in hemostasis. In sizable bone resections, closed suction drainage of the operative site should be considered. Early ambulation is encouraged to help reduce the period of discomfort.

Vascularized Iliac Bone
The ilium has an extensive internal blood supply based on feeding vessels from the surrounding periosteum. This bone with

its intact periosteal covering can be transferred as a free vascularized graft based on the deep circumflex iliac artery, as described by Taylor. Venous drainage is from the venae comitantes, which usually unite to form a single large vein. This vascular pedicle provides an excellent blood supply to the bone and also supplies the skin immediately overlying the iliac crest. Because of this, groin skin and iliac bone can be raised as a free composite flap.

The surface markings for a standard groin flap are outlined. This includes the anterior superior iliac spine, the pubic tubercle, and the inguinal ligament. The femoral vessels are palpated, and an approximation of the iliac vessels is outlined. The origin of the deep circumflex iliac artery lies approximately 1 cm above the inguinal ligament in the line of the iliac vessels. If a composite flap is needed,

an ellipse of skin over the iliac crest is outlined.

Through the medial incision of the skin ellipse, a direct transinguinal approach to the external iliac artery and vein is made by retracting the contents of the inguinal canal downward and laterally. The origin of the deep circumflex iliac artery and vein lies just lateral to the large inferior epigastric artery. With this approach, the deep circumflex iliac pedicle is followed laterally through the transversalis fascia and into the musculature on the medial border of the iliac bone.

From the lateral portion of the skin island, dissection is carried through the tensor fasciae latae and the attachment of the gluteal muscles to reach the outer plate of the iliac bone. With both sides of the bone exposed, the predetermined segment of

bone is removed with the vascular pedicle. Care must be taken to keep the attached iliac muscle and vessels on the medial aspect. The vascular pedicle for this flap averages at least 6 cm and the arterial and venous diameters are in the 3-mm range.

Rib

Nonvascularized Rib Grafts

The ribs offer a large amount of relatively easily accessible bone. A rib consists of two cortical surfaces surrounding a well-formed marrow space containing cancellous bone. It can be readily split, allowing an increased surface area. Rib is not as dense as ilium and calvarium and can be shaped more easily to fit various defects. Because of its increased porosity, however, wires and screws more readily tear through this bone; thus delicate tech-

Fig. 9-2. Iliac cancellous bone harvesting by inner cortical hinge technique.

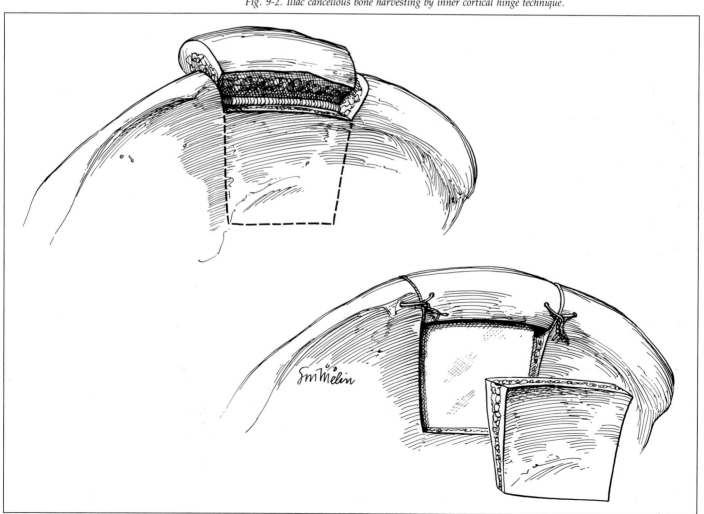

nique is needed when fixation is applied. Using a washer with screw fixation in rib is helpful. It is often stated that rib is the ideal donor site for children because when the periosteum is preserved a new rib is generated. The quality of the regenerated bone, however, can be disappointing.

When a small amount of rib is needed, the scar can be camouflaged by placing the incision just above the inframammary crease, beginning at the midthoracic line and running laterally for approximately 5 cm. Through this incision, a 10- to 15-cm rib segment can be readily resected from the sixth or seventh rib. If a large amount of bone is needed, the patient can be placed in the lateral decubitus position and a standard posterolateral thoracotomy incision performed. Through this exposure, up to four full-length ribs can be harvested. Alternate ribs should be left intact when this much harvesting is planned to prevent instability of the chest wall.

After the skin incision, dissection is carried through subcutaneous tissue and the Scarpa fascia down to the periosteum. When the posterolateral approach is used, the latissimus dorsi muscle must be transected and the trapezius muscle retracted to allow complete rib exposure. The periosteum is incised and the rib is circumferentially dissected in a subperiosteal plane (Fig. 9-3). I prefer using a periosteal elevator for the entire subperiosteal dissection, although Doyan rib strippers also can be used. Once the rib is removed, the periosteum should be meticulously approximated with an absorbable running suture. Muscle and fascial layers are subsequently closed, followed by closure of the skin. Before closure, the wound should be filled with saline solution and the lungs expanded with positive pressure to check for parietal pleural leaks. If a puncture occurs, a catheter should be placed and the wound closed under positive pressure. With the lungs fully expanded, the catheter can be removed at the completion of wound closure.

Vascularized Rib Grafts

The dominant vascular pedicle to the ribs is from the posterior intercostal artery and vein. The posterior intercostal artery originates halfway between corresponding ribs passing upward to the lower border of the superior rib. The medial dorsal branch of the posterior intercostal artery should be preserved because it supplies blood to the spinal cord. Just lateral to this dorsal artery, the nutrient artery of the rib can be included in the flap to augment blood supply to the flap. An island of skin directly overlying the rib can be taken with the flap, although venous drainage of the skin paddle can be tenuous. When skin is included, a subcutaneous vein should be identified and preserved, if possible.

When only rib is to be taken as a graft, an incision over the rib is made. The latissimus dorsi and serratus posterior muscles are divided as needed for exposure, and the intercostal muscles are divided similarly along the upper border of the rib. Dissection is continued posteriorly toward the angle of the rib. As the angle is approached, the vascular pedicle exits the subcostal groove, passing downward separately from the rib. The rib should be sectioned as far posteriorly as possible and the pedicle harvested between the dorsal and nutrient branch of the posterior intercostal artery. At this level, the vessel diameter is approximately 2 mm and a 4- to 5-cm vascular pedicle length usually can be achieved.

Vascularized rib grafts also can be raised by an anterior approach based on the anterior intercostal vessels, a branch of the internal thoracic vessels. This flap has found less application because of the limitation in vessel size and donor site morbidity. Anterior rib also can be raised in continuity with the overlying pectoralis major muscle as an osteomyocutaneous flap.

Calvarium

Nonvascularized Grafts

The calvarium offers a vast supply of membranous bone. The postoperative morbidity from harvesting calvarial bone should be low, and the donor incision is beautifully hidden in the hair. When a craniofacial procedure is undertaken with a coronal incision, a second prepared field or incision is not needed for the donor site.

The thickness of the calvarium in adults varies from 4 to 12 mm depending on the individual and the specific region of the calvarium. The calvarium in adults has an inner and outer cortical layer with a thin layer of cancellous bone, or diploë, separating them. The inner and outer cortical layers can be separated through the diploetic space, effectively doubling the surface area of bone and decreasing its thickness to that of each cortex. In children younger than 6 or 7 years, the cortical plates are thinner and a functional diploetic layer may not yet exist. In this situation, successfully splitting the calvarial bone can be extremely difficult.

The two most common methods of harvesting calvarial bone both involve splitting the inner and outer cortex through the diploë. In the first technique, the outer cortex is split from the inner in situ (Fig. 9-4). With a bur, a trough of bone is removed down to the diploetic layer circumferentially around the area of the graft. An osteotome and mallet are used to separate the outer cortical layer along the plane of the diploë. The outer edge of the trough is burred down so that a "step-off" cannot be palpated through the scalp. The ideal location for harvesting split cranial bone grafts is the parietal bone. This bone is generally thick, with an adequate diploë. The midline should be avoided to prevent accidental injury to the sagittal sinus. In situ split grafts tend to be smaller because harvesting large grafts with this technique increases the risk of fracturing the graft or removing full-thickness bone. In the second technique, used when large amounts of bone graft are needed, bone is removed through a full craniotomy (Fig. 9-5). The craniotomy is often performed with the aid of a neurosurgeon. Once the full-thickness cranial bone is procured, it can be split on a sterile work surface with power or hand instruments. The outer portion is used to reconstruct the donor defect and the inner cortex is used as the graft.

Other methods can be used to harvest calvarial bone. Bone dust can be collected by low-speed burring of the outer cortex. Shavings of the outer cortex can be obtained with the use of a sharp osteotome.

Vascularized Calvarial Grafts

Pure vascularized bone flaps are not routinely used because the relatively inaccessible middle meningeal artery is the dominant vascular supply to most of the calvarium. However, bone grafts from the calvarium have been transferred on a number of soft tissue pedicles. The most

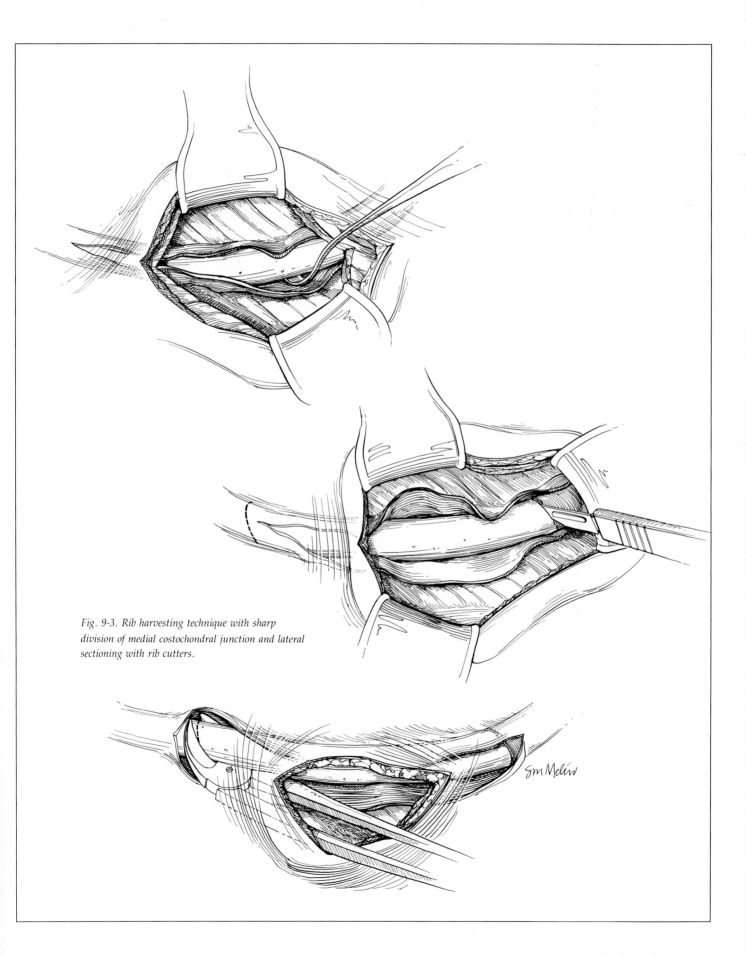

Fig. 9-3. Rib harvesting technique with sharp division of medial costochondral junction and lateral sectioning with rib cutters.

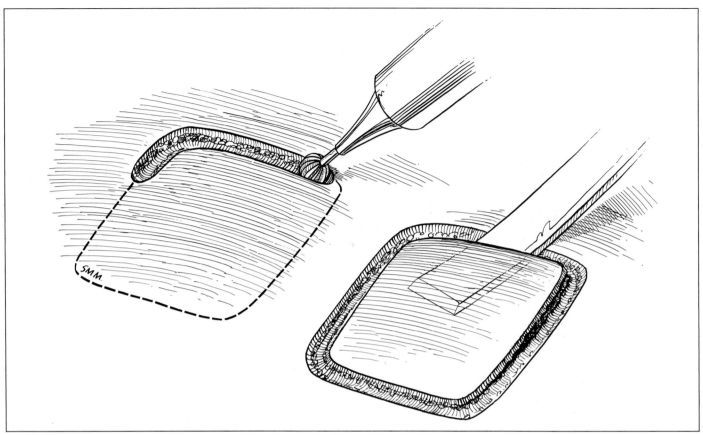

Fig. 9-4. Split cranial bone graft harvesting technique.

Fig. 9-5. Full-thickness cranial bone harvesting with splitting of graft.

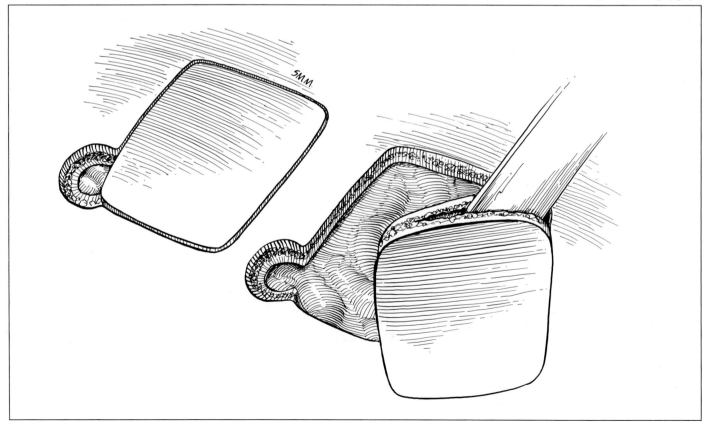

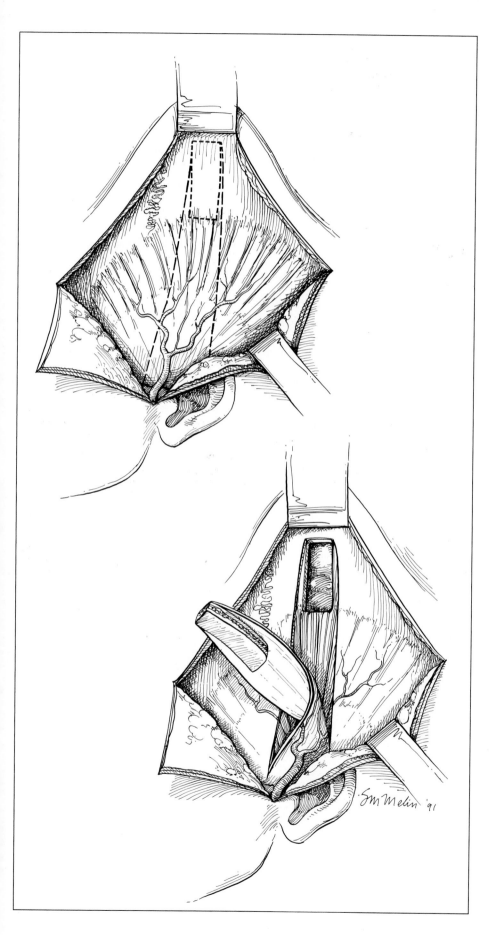

Fig. 9-6. Pedicled vascularized cranial bone graft based on the superficial temporal vessels.

commonly performed pedicle transfer of calvarial bone is based on the superficial temporal artery and vein and the deep temporal vessels through the galea (superficial musculoaponeurotic system, SMAS) over the temporalis musculature (Fig. 9-6). Split outer cortical bone, located posterior to the coronal suture and above the superior temporal line, is harvested on a pedicle of periosteum and galea with or without deep temporal fascia and temporalis muscle. The skin dissection must be performed in the subfollicular plane to avoid damage to the delicate vasculature overlying the galea. Loupe magnification, bipolar cauterization, and traction sutures greatly aid in this dissection. Pedicled bone harvested in this manner is usually used in reconstructing the superior and lateral orbits, the zygomatic complex, and even the mandible.

Lower Extremity

Tibia

The tibia once was used as a source for bone grafts. The unsightly donor scar, the morbidity associated with an overzealous harvest, and the development of more suitable donor areas has placed the tibia low on the list of potential donor sites.

Fibula

The fibula is used commonly as a free vascularized bone flap based on the peroneal artery. The nutrient artery to the fibula enters the medial surface of the bone just above its midpoint. Venous drainage is by the venae comitantes, and the vascular pedicle length can measure more than 8 cm.

Skin can be included as an osteocutaneous flap. Vasculature to the skin pedicle depends on the peroneal intermuscular septum as in a fasciocutaneous flap.

With the patient's knee flexed, the fibula is readily palpated and a line is drawn from the head of the fibula to the lateral malleolus. The incision is made and dissection is carried down to the fibula between the peroneal and soleal musculature. The midportion of the fibula generally is used to maintain integrity of the bone at the knee and ankle joints. After exposure of the bone, early division of the length of bone required allows for easy preservation of a cuff of tibialis posterior and flexor hallucis longus musculature, which includes the peroneal vessel. The peroneal pedicle can be dissected superiorly up to the trifurcation of the popliteal fossa. When an ellipse of skin is to be included in the flap, a generous segment of deep fascia based over the bone, including the peroneal intermuscular septum, needs to be preserved.

Radial Forearm Flap

The radial artery lies in the intermuscular septum dividing the flexor and extensor compartments of the forearm. This intermuscular septum attaches to the periosteum of the radius distal to the pronator teres. The subcutaneous location of the artery in the forearm allows for ready access and, in combination with preservation of the intermuscular septum, provides for a generous blood supply to the underlying radius. Venous drainage is supplied by a vena comitans accompanying the artery. The radial forearm flap allows for a large amount of skin and subcutaneous tissue to be transferred in addition to bone.

The subcutaneous path of the artery is outlined, as is the skin island for the flap. The margins of the skin island are incised and carried down to deep fascia. This deep fascia is elevated in a plane directly off the muscle bellies and tendons of the forearm. Care must be taken to preserve the peritenon of the tendons to allow for

skin graft reconstruction at the donor site. The attachment of the intermuscular septum to the periosteum of the radius must be preserved to allow for bone in the flap. Up to 8 to 10 cm of radius can be harvested with this flap between the insertion of the pronator teres proximally and the brachioradialis distally. Less than half of the cross section of radius should be harvested to avoid subsequent fracture. Because of this limitation, a large quantity of bone is generally not available.

The Future

Although autogenous bone grafts currently are considered the material of choice for most reconstructive procedures, all the techniques for harvesting bone grafts discussed in this chapter may become of historical interest only within the next decade or so. With the development and availability of sophisticated synthetic or alloplastic bone substitutes and osteoinductive compounds, surgeons will be able to pull from the shelf a readily available and reliable source of bone graft material in any size or shape. The "antiquated" and crude method of harvesting bone from patients will live only in the lectures of older surgeons conducting floor rounds and early morning conferences.

Suggested Reading

Albrektsson, T. Repair of bone grafts: Histological investigation. *Scand. J. Plast. Reconstr. Surg.* 14:1, 1980.

Anderson, L.D. Compression plate fixation and the effect of different types of internal fixation on fracture healing. *J. Bone Surg.* 47:1, 1965.

Burchardt, H. Biology of bone graft repair. *Clin. Orthop.* 174:28, 1983.

Daniel, R.K. Mandibular reconstruction with free tissue transfers. *Ann. Plast. Surg.* 1:346, 1978.

Hieple, K.G., Chase, S.W., and Herndon, C.H. A comparative study of the healing process following different types of bone transplantation. *J. Bone Joint Surg.* 47A:1593, 1963.

Perren, S.M. Physical and biological aspects of fracture healing with special reference to internal fixation. *Clin. Orthop.* 138:175, 1979.

Phillips, J.H., and Rahn, B.A. Fixation effects on membranous and endochondral onlay bone-graft resorption. *Plast. Reconstr. Surg.* 82: 872, 1988.

Pollack, S.R. Bioelectrical properties of bone: Endogenous electrical signals. *Orthop. Clin. North Am.* 15:3, 1984.

Pollack, S.R., Townsend, P., and Corlett, R. Superiority of the deep circumflex iliac vessels as the supply of free groin flaps: Clinical work. *Plast. Reconstr. Surg.* 64:745, 1979.

Taylor, G.I., Townsend, P., and Corlett, R. Superiority of the deep circumflex iliac vessels as the supply for free groin flaps: Clinical work. *Plast. Reconstr. Surg.* 64:745, 1979b.

Urist, M.R., et al. Bone induction principle. *Clin. Orthop.* 53:243, 1967.

Webster, M.H.C., and Soutar, D.S. *Practical Guide to Tissue Transfer.* London: Butterworth, 1986.

10

Bone Substitutes

Harvey M. Rosen

There is little doubt that autogenous bone is the material of choice for any osseous reconstruction. Unfortunately, autogenous bone has some disadvantages, including donor site morbidity and the inevitable resorption of bone grafts when used in an onlay manner. Although the use of cranial bone grafts in the craniofacial region has lessened this potential, it certainly has not eliminated the problem of resorption. The greatest disadvantage of autogenous bone, however, is its limited supply. For all these reasons, the search continues for alloplastic materials that can serve as bone substitutes.

Currently available alternatives to bone grafts include sintered and porous tricalcium phosphate and hydroxyapatite, calcium sulfate (plaster of paris), various synthetic polymers, and metallic prostheses. Although used extensively for altering the surface topography of the maxillofacial skeleton, synthetic polymers such as block silicone and polytetrafluoroethylene (PTFE)-graphite (Proplast) cannot be considered bone substitutes because they represent foreign material that becomes encapsulated and therefore has no healing capabilities. As a result, the applicability of these materials remains extremely limited. The same liability applies to metallic prostheses;

with the exception of joint reconstruction, metal has no role as a material for replacement of bone. In the past, plaster of paris was used for cranial reconstruction, but because it degrades quickly, it is of historical interest only. Only the calcium phosphates remain as legitimate clinical bone substitutes. Of these, porous hydroxyapatite in block form has been used most widely by plastic and reconstructive surgeons.

General Considerations

The de novo manufacture of synthetic implants with the physical properties required to promote bone ingrowth has proved unsuccessful because of the unique porous structure of bone. As a result, researchers have looked to nature and have discovered that certain corals from the genus *Porites* secrete a calcium carbonate exoskeleton remarkably similar to human bone, i.e., a skeletal structure with an average pore size of 200 μ that is completely interconnected. Interconnectivity is critical to the performance of any porous implant because it is isolated or dead-end pockets (incomplete interconnectivity) that limit vascular support to ingrowing tissues.

It remains for the manufacturer to convert this calcium carbonate skeleton to hydroxyapatite through a hydrothermal exchange reaction replacing the carbonate with phosphate. The result is a material that has the porous anatomy of bone and a chemical composition identical to that of the largest constituent of human bone, i.e., hydroxyapatite. The material is supplied in both granular and block form; the blocks are available in several shapes and sizes.

Coralline-derived, porous hydroxyapatite has been used in many clinical situations, including the grafting of periodontal defects, posttraumatic long-bone defects, and augmentation of the alveolar ridge. Its greatest uses by plastic and reconstructive surgeons have been to augment the surface contour of the maxillofacial region and as an interpositional bone graft substitute in orthognathic surgery.

Clinical Considerations

The various biomechanical properties of porous block hydroxyapatite, including its compressive strength and relative brittleness, favor its use in the craniomaxillofacial region as opposed to the long bones of the extremities. Of the various

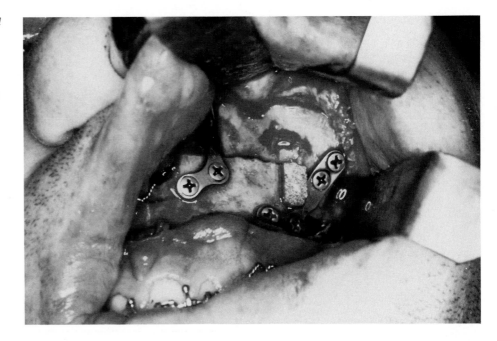

Fig. 10-1. Blocks of porous hydroxyapatite wedged into lateral osteotomy gaps to promote stability in extensive Le Fort I advancements. (From H.M. Rosen. Porous block hydroxyapatite as an interpositional bone graft substitute in orthognathic surgery. Plast. Reconstr. Surg. *83: 985, 1989. Reproduced with permission.)*

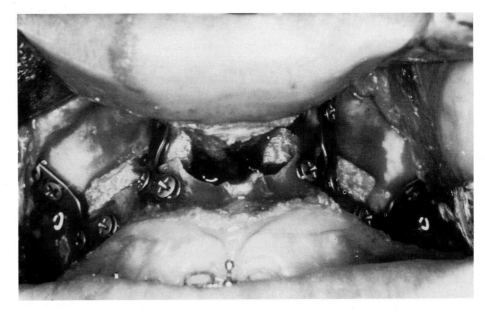

Fig. 10-2. Blocks of porous hydroxyapatite inserted into anterolateral maxillary osteotomy gap and lateral nasal wall after vertical lengthening of the maxilla. (From H.M. Rosen. Porous block hydroxyapatite as an interpositional bone graft substitute in orthognathic surgery. Plast. Reconstr. Surg. *83:985, 1989. Reproduced with permission.)*

areas of the craniomaxillofacial region, it has been used most extensively in the middle and lower face. To date hydroxyapatite has been used sparingly in the upper face and cranial vault because of the relative thinness of the soft tissues covering these areas and because of concern regarding future growth in children. Accordingly orthognathic surgery and aesthetic skeletal surgery of the middle and lower face have become the primary settings for use of block hydroxyapatite.

In orthognathic surgery, hydroxyapatite has been used primarily as an interposi-

tional bone graft substitute in circumstances in which large osteotomy gaps have been surgically produced. Because of the potential for skeletal instability, these gaps otherwise would have been grafted with autogenous bone. The availability of hydroxyapatite in block form has reduced operating time, eliminated donor site morbidity, and enhanced skeletal stability because of its favorable biomechanical properties. The three basic indications for hydroxyapatite in orthognathic surgery are (1) extensive maxillary advancements in which blocks of hydroxyapatite are wedged into the result-

ing anterolateral maxillary osteotomy gaps (Fig. 10-1); (2) vertical elongation of the maxilla, unassociated with clinically significant sagittal movement, that results in large osteotomy gaps in the anterolateral maxillary wall and lateral nasal wall; blocks of hydroxyapatite are placed in these gaps (Fig. 10-2); and (3) extensive transverse expansions of the maxilla with blocks placed in the osteotomy of the nasal floor (Fig. 10-3).

In aesthetic operations on the facial skeleton, block hydroxyapatite is used in both an inlay and an onlay manner. Interpo-

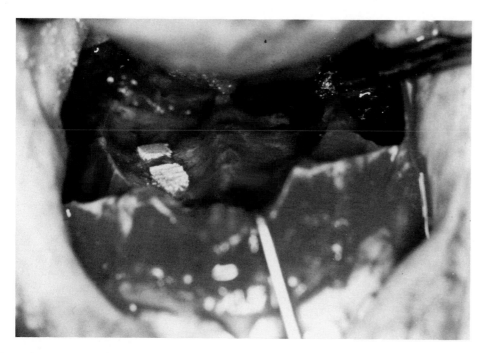

Fig. 10-3. Blocks of porous hydroxyapatite placed into osteotomy defect of nasal floor resulting from transverse expansion of the maxilla. (From H.M. Rosen. Porous block hydroxyapatite as an interpositional bone graft substitute in orthognathic surgery. Plast. Reconstr. Surg. 83: 985, 1989. Reproduced with permission.)

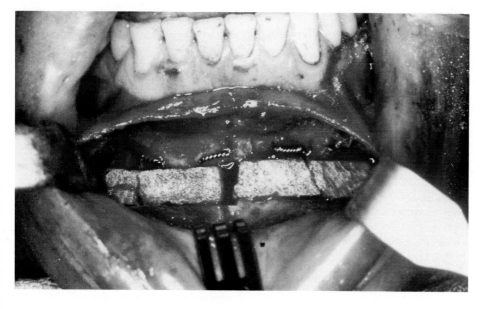

Fig. 10-4. Blocks of porous hydroxyapatite inserted into osteotomy gap of the anterior mandible to elongate the chin vertically. (From H.M. Rosen. Porous block hydroxyapatite as an interpositional bone graft substitute in orthognathic surgery. Plast. Reconstr. Surg. 83: 985, 1989. Reproduced with permission.)

sitional placement of block hydroxyapatite into osteotomy gaps of the anterior mandible has expanded the versatility of the standard osseous genioplasty to enable surgeons to elongate the chin vertically without resorting to harvesting of autogenous bone grafts (Fig. 10-4). Block hydroxyapatite also has been used in an onlay manner over the anterolateral maxillary-zygomatic and anterior symphyseal regions to augment these areas of the maxillofacial skeleton.

Extreme care is required in the handling of hydroxyapatite because of its brittle nature. It cannot be wedged or forced into position because of its tendency to crack. If the material is not carved to an exact negative contour of the area of desired augmentation, there is a high probability that it will fracture.

The cutting of blocks and their subsequent contouring are performed with dental burs. Once the block is completely carved, copious irrigation with saline solution is performed to clear its pores of debris. Insertion into antibiotic solution has not been found to be necessary. Fixation in an osteotomy gap relies on friction with no direct fixation. Single lag screw fixation is suggested when blocks are placed in an onlay manner over the facial skeleton (Fig. 10-5). Screws should not be tightened excessively for fear of cracking the implant block.

Reported complication rates of the use of porous hydroxyapatite in large clinical series have been acceptably low, in the range of 4 to 10 percent. Most complications have been related to an inadequate soft tissue covering for the implant. That is, when placed in areas where the soft tissue has been traumatized, is exceedingly thin, or is poorly vascularized, the implant usually becomes exposed, with subsequent infection and extrusion. In-

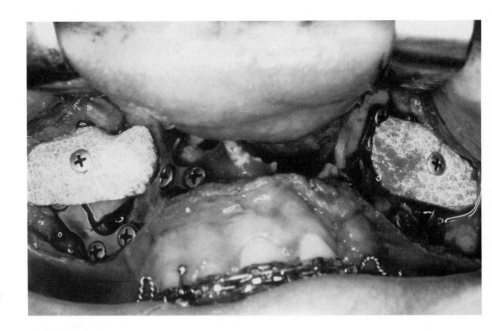

Fig. 10-5. Blocks of porous hydroxyapatite placed in an onlay manner over anterior maxilla for additional augmentation of the midface after maxillary advancement. Blocks are immobilized in place with single lag screw.

fection, therefore, is directly related to deficient soft tissue coverage. Accordingly implants should not be used to augment the nasal spine or paranasal region. Nor should they be placed in an onlay manner over the anterior mandible close to the buccal sulcus. Exposure of the implant in these areas is likely to occur secondarily to the breakdown of the suture line. Problems also are likely to occur when the graft is placed in an onlay manner in areas of healthy but thin soft tissue coverage, such as the upper face and nasal dorsum. When the implant is covered with adequate, healthy soft tissue, however, and there is a secure soft tissue closure, the incidence of complications, particularly infection, has been remarkably low. This is true despite transoral placement of the implant into osteotomy gaps adjacent to open paranasal sinuses and is undoubtedly related to the rapid ingrowth of tissue into the implant block.

Biologic and Mechanical Properties of Hydroxyapatite

Porous block hydroxyapatite has many biomechanical properties that make its use in the craniomaxillofacial region practical. As previously mentioned, dry implant blocks are extremely brittle but gain rapidly in torsional and compressive strength as the implant pores are invaded, first by fibrovascular tissue and

then by bone. The ultimate compressive strength has been estimated to be approximately 25 percent that of cortical bone, which far exceeds masticatory forces generated in the human maxillofacial skeleton. The ultimate torsional strength of the ingrown implant block has been reported to be approximately 50 to 60 percent that of human cortical bone. Loss of volume of the implant material is minimal—less than 2 percent within 2 years. Stress shielding does not appear to be a consideration, because the elastic modulus of ingrown hydroxyapatite has been shown to approximate that of human bone. As a result, there is no histologic evidence of host bone resorption adjacent to the implant block.

These biomechanical properties favor the use of hydroxyapatite as an interpositional bone graft substitute. Rigid fixation should be used with hydroxyapatite when the material is placed in maxillary osteotomy defects to allow time for tissue ingrowth to occur so that the strength of the material can increase before it is subjected to masticatory loads. The high compressive strength of the implant, coupled with its low rate of biodegradation and lack of host bone resorption, is responsible for the improved stability observed in maxillary advancement and maxillary vertical lengthening procedures.

Histologic studies of patients receiving implants of porous hydroxyapatite help

explain its aforementioned mechanical attributes. Fibrovascular tissue rapidly invades the implant pores within 1 to 2 weeks, and by 2 months there is evidence of bone deposition along the walls of the implant pores. Holmes demonstrated mean bone volumes of approximately 20 percent. Bone deposition within the implant is always accompanied by osteoid (Fig. 10-6), which is indicative of ongoing production of bone and a high degree of metabolic activity within the implant pores. This degree of cellular activity can take place only in the presence of an abundant blood supply. Gross in vivo examination of previously implanted blocks confirms the extensive vascular supply of ingrown hydroxyapatite (Fig. 10-7). Although the extent of bone deposition does not correlate well with the time from implantation, only specimens harvested after long intervals postoperatively (more than 11 months) demonstrate almost complete replacement of the implant pores with bone (Fig. 10-8). Histologic examination of the bone-implant interface consistently reveals a direct osseous union between implant and bone (Fig. 10-9) with no intervening fibrous tissue. In addition, no evidence of resorption of host bone can be demonstrated at the bone-implant interface (Fig. 10-10). It is only in the unusual instance of a fibrous union that lack of bone deposition has been observed within the implant block. That is, this material is osteoconductive only; it has no osteoinductive capabilities.

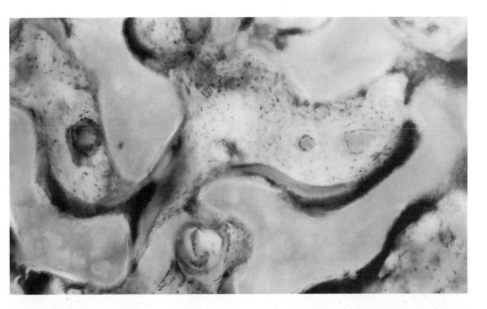

Fig. 10-6. Photomicrograph of center of implant block harvested 3 months after implantation. Bone is deposited against the implant wall followed by deposition of osteoid. The remainder of the implant pore is filled with fibrovascular tissue. Villanueva Goldner trichrome stain, 40×. (From H.M. Rosen and M.M. McFarland. The biologic behavior of hydroxyapatite implanted into the maxillofacial skeleton. Plast. Reconstr. Surg. 85: 718, 1990. Reproduced with permission.)

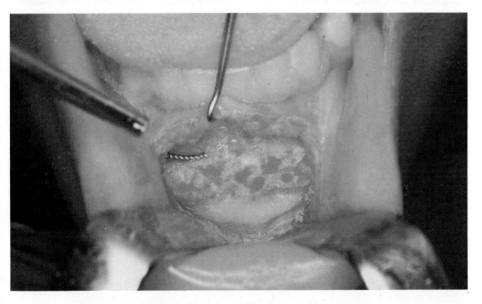

Fig. 10-7. Implant blocks placed in osteotomy gap of anterior mandible 12 months earlier. Note punctate bleeding from implant block when cut. (From H.M. Rosen and M.M. McFarland. The biologic behavior of hydroxyapatite implanted into the maxillofacial skeleton. Plast. Reconstr. Surg. 85:718, 1990. Reproduced with permission.)

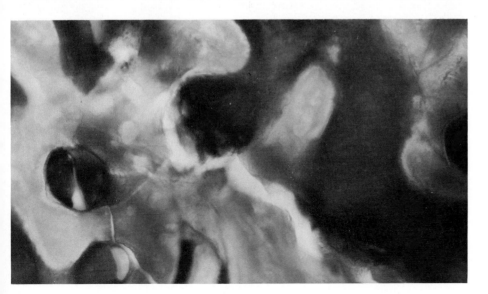

Fig. 10-8. Late biopsy specimen harvested 12 months after implantation demonstrating almost complete obliteration of the implant pores with bone. Note the persistent presence of osteoid. Villanueva Goldner trichrome stain, 40×. (From H.M. Rosen and M.M. McFarland. The biologic behavior of hydroxyapatite implanted into the maxillofacial skeleton. Plast. Reconstr. Surg. 85: 718, 1990. Reproduced with permission.)

Fig. 10-9. A composite bone-implant specimen with bone on left and implant on right. Note the direct osseous union of bone to implant. There is no intervening fibrous tissue. Villanueva Goldner trichrome stain, 10×. (From H.M. Rosen and M.M. McFarland. The biologic behavior of hydroxyapatite implanted into the maxillofacial skeleton. Plast. Reconstr. Surg. 85:718, 1990. Reproduced with permission.)

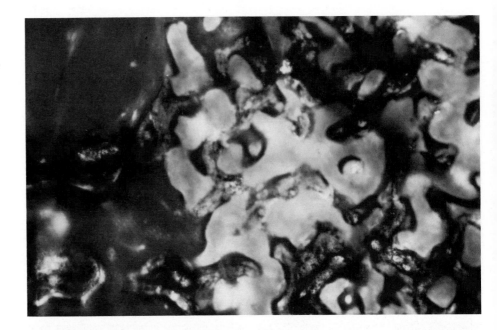

Fig. 10-10. High-power photomicrograph of bone-implant interface seen in Fig. 10-9. No osteoclast or remodeling activity can be identified at the bone-implant interface. Villanueva Goldner trichrome stain, 40×. (From H.M. Rosen and M.M. McFarland. The biologic behavior of hydroxyapatite implanted into the maxillofacial skeleton. Plast. Reconstr. Surg. 85:718, 1990. Reproduced with permission.)

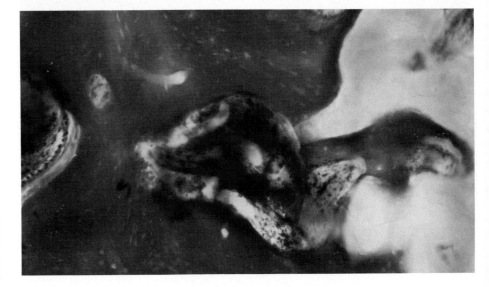

Patients examined radiographically up to 39 months after receiving an implant demonstrate no change in the appearance of the implant block. The blocks remain well visualized with no loss of marginal discreteness or radiodensity (Fig. 10-11). This unchanged roentgenographic appearance supports the relative lack of resorption of this implant material.

As previously mentioned, the remarkably low rate of clinical infection associated with the use of this implant material is thought to be related to the rapid establishment of a vascular network throughout the implant block. Instances in which infection has occurred in contiguous tissue have not necessitated removal of the implant despite its being in direct communication with the infection. This clinical impression—that previously vascularized implants resist established infection in adjacent tissue—has been supported by experimental data.

Future Considerations

The future appears promising for the continued development of bone substitutes. Materials most likely will involve a combination of osteoinductive peptides with a carrier of either nonresorbable material, such as porous, block hydroxyapatite, or a resorbable material, such as polylactide coglycolide. This advancement will allow the synthesis of specific bone replacements that have both osteoinductive and osteoconductive properties. If necessary, this material can be vascularized at an initial stage and transferred on a vascular pedicle so that placement in a contaminated area will become feasible. The clinical applications for synthetic bone substitutes are limitless.

Suggested Reading

Bernard, S.L., and Picha, G.L. The use of coralline hydroxyapatite in a "biocomposite" free flap. Plast. Reconstr. Surg. 87:106, 1991.

Bucholz, R.W., Holmes, R.E., and Mooney, V. Synthetic Hydroxyapatite as a Bone Graft Substitute in Traumatic Defects of Long Bones. In Transactions of the 53rd Annual Meeting of Orthopaedic Surgeons, 1986. P. 149.

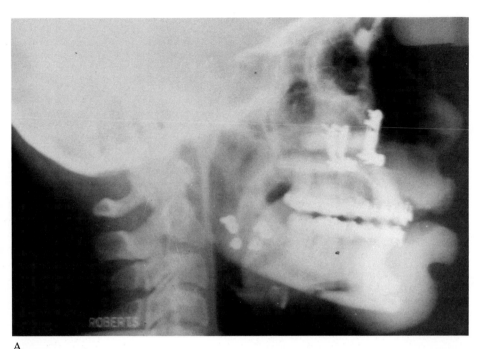

A

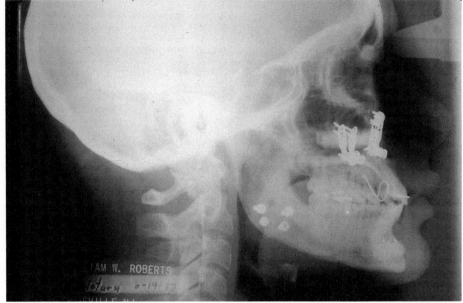

B

Fig. 10-11. Roentgenographic appearance of implant blocks placed in anterolateral maxillary wall and anterior mandible to elongate the maxilla and chin vertically. A. Appearance 24 hours after implantation. B. Appearance 28 months later. Note that there is no loss of radiodensity or marginal discreteness of the implant blocks. (From H.M. Rosen and M.M. McFarland. The biologic behavior of hydroxyapatite implanted into the maxillofacial skeleton. Plast. Reconstr. Surg. 85: 718, 1990. Reproduced with permission.)

bone induction and potential application in craniofacial surgery. J. Craniofac. Surg. 1:154, 1990.

Piecuch, J.F. Augmentation of the atrophic edentulous ridge with porous replamineform hydroxyapatite. Dent. Clin. North Am. 30:291, 1986.

Rosen, H.M. Surgical correction of the vertically deficient chin. Plast. Reconstr. Surg. 82: 247, 1988.

Rosen, H.M. Porous, block hydroxyapatite as an interpositional bone graft substitute in orthognathic surgery. Plast. Reconstr. Surg. 83: 985, 1989.

Rosen, H.M. Definitive surgical correction of vertical maxillary deficiency. Plast. Reconstr. Surg. 85:215, 1990.

Rosen, H.M., and McFarland, M.M. The biologic behavior of hydroxyapatite implanted into the maxillofacial skeleton. Plast. Reconstr. Surg. 85:715, 1990.

Salyer, K.E., Ubinas, E.E., and Snively, J.L. Porous hydroxyapatite as an onlay graft in maxillofacial surgery. Plast. Surg. Forum 8:61, 1985.

Tessier, P. Autogenous bone grafts taken from the calvarium for facial and cranial applications. Clin. Plast. Surg. 9:531, 1982.

Torgalkar, A.M. A resonance frequency technique to determine elastic modulus of hydroxyapatite. J. Biomed. Mater. Res. 13:907, 1979.

Wardrop, R.W., and Wolford, L.M. Maxillary stability following downgraft and/or advancement procedures with stabilization using rigid fixation and porous block hydroxyapatite implants. J. Oral Maxillofac. Surg. 47:336, 1989.

White, E., and Shors, E. Biomaterial aspects of Interpore 200 porous hydroxyapatite. Dent. Clin. North Am. 30:49, 1986.

Wolford, L.M., Wardrop, R.W., and Hartog, J.M. Coralline, porous, hydroxyapatite as a bone graft substitute in orthognathic surgery. J. Oral Maxillofac. Surg. 45:1034, 1987.

Zins, J.E., and Whitaker, L.A. Membranous versus endochondral bone autografts: Implications for craniofacial reconstruction. Surg. Forum 30:521, 1979.

Hollinger, J.O. Preliminary report on the osteogenic potential of a biodegradable copolymer of polylactide and polyglycolide. J. Biomed. Mater. Res. 17:71, 1983.

Holmes, R.E. Bone regeneration within a coralline hydroxyapatite implant. Plast. Reconstr. Surg. 63:626, 1979.

Holmes, R.E., Wardrop, R.W., and Wolford, L.M. Hydroxyapatite as a bone graft substitute in orthognathic surgery: Histologic and histometric findings. J. Oral Maxillofac. Surg. 46:661, 1988.

Jackson, I.T., et al. Update on cranial bone grafts in craniofacial surgery. Ann. Plast. Surg. 18:37, 1987.

Kenney, E.B., et al. The use of porous hydroxyapatite implant in periodontal defects. J. Periodontol. 56:82, 1985.

Laurie, J.W., et al. Donor site morbidity after harvesting rib and iliac bone. Plast. Reconstr. Surg. 73:933, 1984.

Marden, L.J., Reddi, A.H., and Hollinger, J.O. Growth and differentiation factors: Role in

11

Flexor Tendon Grafting

Hani S. Matloub   Christopher D. Prevel   N. John Yousif   James R. Sanger

Tendon Anatomy

Proximally attached muscles connected by tendinous cords to mobile units, or bones, move the hand. The surrounding supportive components (palmar bursa, tendon sheath, vincula, and synovial fluid) provide nutrition, a smooth gliding surface, and a mechanism for efficient translation of linear muscle contraction into angular motion. Tendon consists of both cellular and extracellular components. The cellular elements are the tenocytes, epitenon cells, and endotenon cells. The extracellular components include collagen, ground substance, and elastin fibers.

Cellular Components

The epitenon cells line the outer surface of the tendon. Their projection between the tendon bundles is the endotenon (Fig. 11-1). Tenocytes are considered to be immature fibroblasts that reside within the primary tendon bundles. They are relatively inactive and serve primarily in a maintenance role. When the tendon is injured, the tenocyte may assist the epitenon cells in the intrinsic mechanism of tendon healing.

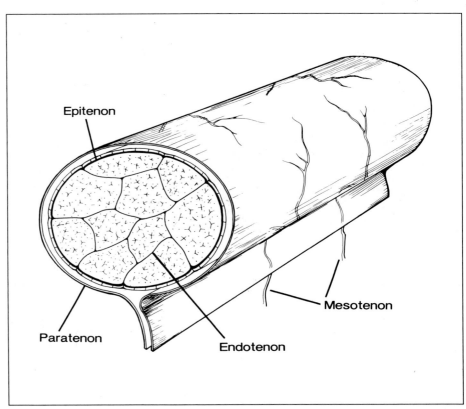

Fig. 11-1. Cross section of a tendon showing the paratenon, which surrounds and covers the tendon outside the fibro-osseous sheath. The vessels reach the tendon through the mesotenon. The epitenon cells line the outer surface of the tendon; their projection between the tendon bundles is the endotenon.

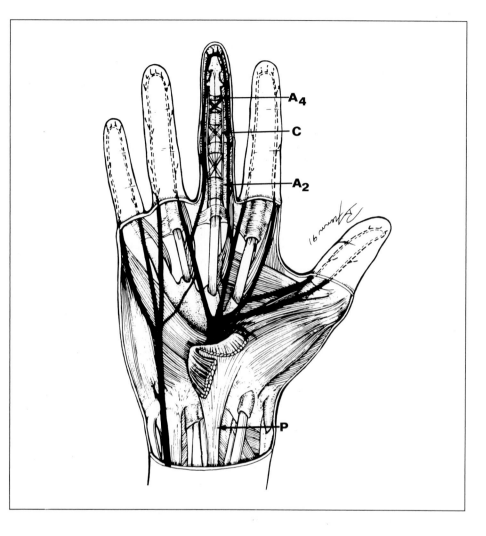

Fig. 11-2. The tendon sheath of the middle finger, which extends from the distal palmar crease to the midportion of the distal phalanx. Condensations of the sheath form five annular and three cruciate pulleys. A_2 and A_4 = annular pulleys 2 and 4. C = one of the cruciate pulleys. P = palmaris longus tendon.

the tendon to move back and forth while maintaining perfusion.

Tendon Sheath

The tendon sheath consists of condensed fibrous tissue and is found on the flexor side of the hand, usually extending from the level of the distal palmar crease (overlying the head of the metacarpal) to the middle portion of the distal phalanges. It is lined by a parietal layer of cells, which assists in gliding and nutrition by the production of synovial fluid (Fig. 11-2).

The flexor sheath has five annular pulleys, labeled A1 through A5, and three cruciate pulleys, C1 through C3 (see Fig. 11-2). This system provides the mechanism for efficient transmission of muscle force throughout the normal arc of motion by maintaining tendon proximity to the underlying bone. In cadaveric studies, preservation of the A2 and A4 pulleys retained more than 90 percent of the mechanical function of the sheath.

Tendon Blood Supply

The vascular supply of a tendon takes both intratendinous and extratendinous routes. The extratendinous blood supply may reach the tendon through the mesotenon, the vincula, or the bony insertion.

The mesotenon (see Fig. 11-1), an extension of the paratenon, provides cover for a segmental vascular supply through filamentous extensions from the tendon bed into the hilus, or deep surface, of the tendon. The vincula provides a mesentery-like mesotenon within the fibro-osseous sheath. At the level of the bony insertion, small vessels perfuse the terminal portion of the tendon.

The intratendinous blood supply parallels the collagenous fibers of the tendon and

Extracellular Components

The extracellular components are mainly collagen, ground substance, and elastin fibers. Type I collagen makes up 70 percent of the dry weight of the tendon. The rough endoplasmic reticulum of the fibroblast synthesizes tropocollagen, the collagen molecule precursor, which is converted to molecular collagen. The collagen fibers are grouped into increasingly larger numbers as filaments, fibrils, fibers, and fascicles, and ultimately make up the tendon. The remaining extracellular structures serve in a supporting role.

The ground substance is mainly glycosaminoglycan, which mechanically lubricates the movement of fibrils and fibers during deformation. Elastin fibers are present within the tendon and are responsible for the cushioning effect at the fascicular level.

Adjacent Structures

Adjacent structures involved in tendon function include the gliding mechanism and the nerve and blood supply. The gliding surface is composed of the paratenon, the tendon surface, the epitenon, and the synovial sheath. The paratenon is a loose, multilayered areolar tissue that surrounds and covers the tendon outside the fibro-osseous sheath. It contains a semifluid substance that assists in gliding and in tendon nutrition. This multilayered structure provides a barrier against the surrounding structures, protecting the tendon and providing additional nutritional support via a vascular capillary network (see Fig. 11-1).

The vessels reach the tendons covered by a portion of the paratenon called the mesotenon. The mesotenon resembles an umbilical cord the length of which allows is prevalent on the dorsal aspect of the tendon. Within the flexor tendon sheath, consistent areas of vascular paucity have been noted, and in these areas nutrition is derived from the synovial fluid.

Tendon Nutrition

It is believed that tendons receive their nutrition through a combined system including contributions from the extratendinous and intratendinous blood supply and from the diffusion of nutrients in the surrounding synovial fluid. Many studies have tried to isolate the contribution of each of these systems. Although in the absence of one system, the other may be able to take over a portion of tendon nutrition, it is not clear which system is more important physiologically.

Nutrition of a tendon graft also combines perfusion from the adjacent vascular supply with diffusion from the surrounding fluid. Adhesions produce vascular pathways that reach the tendon graft, and the synovial fluid bathes the graft to assist in survival of the graft. The importance of each and their importance to the tendon are subjects of ongoing research.

Physiology of Tendon Healing

During the healing process a tendon graft must form stable, strong connections both to the distal structure, be it bone or tendon, and to the existing proximal tendon. The graft must revascularize to maintain its viability, and its movement must be smooth and unrestricted.

The process of tendon healing progresses through the typical phases of wound healing, including a cellular phase, a collagen synthesis phase, and a final remodeling phase.

Initially a hematogenous clot is formed at the repair sites. Fibrous material and granulation tissue containing macrocytes and inflammatory cells are drawn to the area. Epitenon cells from the surface of the tendon proliferate and colonize the repair site. These cells change their form to look more like fibroblasts. These fibroblasts, over a period of several weeks, strengthen the repair by producing collagen as early as the sixth day after injury.

While the production of collagen continues, revascularization of the tendon progresses. This process occurs most likely through formation of adhesions to the surrounding tissue. Healing subsequently passes to the remodeling phase, in which both the distal and proximal repairs gain strength through the cross linking of the collagen. Peritendinous adhesions lose strength and allow some amount of gliding.

Controversy exists regarding the origin of the repairing cells within the site of the tendon injury. The question is whether cells within the repair site originate from the tendon or from fibroblasts found within the surrounding tissue. The issue remains under investigation.

Revascularization of the Graft

Survival of the tendon graft within its transplanted bed requires a vascular supply. This vasculature may be derived from direct anastomosis with vessels in the bed or from ingrowth of capillaries and the production of a new vascular network. Eiken and Lundborg in 1983 demonstrated that tendon grafts in a sheath revascularize by ingrowth of capillaries and the establishment of a new vascular network in the absence of clinically significant adhesions. Tendon grafts outside the sheath showed revascularization by direct anastomosis to the surrounding bed.

Tendon Grafting

Lexer in 1912 described the first use of tendon grafts for operations on the flexor tendons. Because of inconsistent and often poor results with primary tendon repair in the first half of the twentieth century, Sterling Bunnell advocated delayed flexor tendon grafting for zone II flexor tendon injuries. Improved results were achieved with the use of a tendon graft because the repair was undertaken outside the confinements of zone II (Fig. 11-3).

Indications for Single-Stage Tendon Grafting

Although primary repair of tendon lacerations is now the treatment of choice,

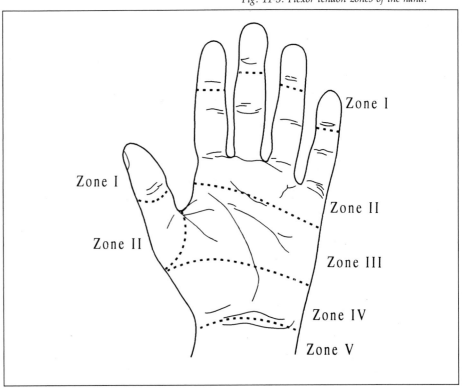

Fig. 11-3. Flexor tendon zones of the hand.

Zone I

Zone I

Zone II

Zone II

Zone III

Zone IV

Zone V

there are several settings in which results are routinely improved with the use of single- or two-stage tendon grafts. Single-stage tendon grafting is indicated when segmental tendon loss results in excessive tension on the repair. Tension predisposes to both joint contracture and tendon rupture. In addition, overadvancement of a flexor tendon may cause a quadriga effect, adversely influencing the function of adjacent digits.

Late presentation of a tendon disruption with secondary shortening of the muscle fibers may be another indication for single-stage tendon grafting. Also, if the quality of the tendon is poor after tenolysis, replacement with a tendon graft may be indicated.

Staged Tendon Reconstruction

Although a variety of methods have been used to decrease tendon graft adhesions in a poor vascular bed, the concept of a multiple-stage reconstruction has proved useful. In this technique, a pseudosheath is induced by placement of a polymeric silicone rod in the proposed bed. The first successful use of a silicone tendon rod for the formation of a pseudosheath was reported by Hunter in 1965; multiple reports have followed during the past 20 years. A staged reconstruction of the flexor tendon involves initial placement of a silicone rod as a temporary spacer while an adequate bed is produced, a pulley system is reconstructed, or soft tissue coverage is obtained. These events are followed by the exchange of the silicone rod for an autogenous tendon graft.

Indications for Staged Tendon Reconstruction

A staged reconstruction is required when, because of the mechanism of injury, severe postoperative scarring is the predicted outcome. Included may be situations in which underlying fractures are exposed, repair of the pulley system is required, or a pseudosheath, promoted by the silicone rod, is deemed advantageous.

Tendon Graft Donor Sites and Harvest Technique

Multiple donor sites for the tendon graft are available. The sites from the upper extremity include the tendons of the pal-maris longus, the flexor digitorum superficialis, the extensor indicis proprius, and the extensor digiti quinti proprius muscles. Donor sites from the lower extremity include the tendons of the plantaris and the extensor digitorum longus muscles. Because of the ease of harvesting and the quality of the harvested tendon, the palmaris longus and plantaris tendons are the preferred sites. When longer lengths of flexor tendon grafts are necessary, the plantaris and extensor digitorum longus tendons are suitable.

Palmaris Longus

The presence of the palmaris longus (see Fig. 11-2) may be assessed easily by palpation of the tendon at the level of the wrist crease while the hand is cupped. Many variations exist in the anatomy of the palmaris longus. In as many as 20 percent of patients, the tendon is absent. It may present as a complete cord from origin to insertion. The anatomy may be reversed and a tendon may be present at the origin, ending as a fleshy muscle inserting in the palm. It also may present as multiple tendons at its insertion.

The proximity of the tendon to the median nerve at the wrist requires special attention during harvesting. The graft may be harvested by one of two techniques. In the first, the tendon is identified at the proximal wrist crease through a small transverse incision. The distal tendon is sectioned and the proximal end passed through a tendon stripper, which is advanced proximally in the subcutaneous plane along the course of the tendon. As the stripper reaches the muscle belly, the muscle gives way against the distal pull on the end of the tendon, and the tendon is released. The second method is to expose the tendon at the level of the wrist and tent it upward. Successive small transverse incisions are made along the length of the palpable tendon proximally, which is cut at the musculotendinous junction.

Plantaris

The plantaris is a small muscle whose distal tendon is located deep to the medial aspect of the Achilles tendon at the ankle. Unlike the palmaris, its presence may not be confirmed preoperatively. The plantaris has been noted to be absent in as many as 19 percent of dissections, and if it is absent on one side it has only a 30 percent chance of being present on the other side.

The harvesting technique for the plantaris tendon begins with a 4-cm transverse incision carried anteriorly and medially to the Achilles tendon at the level of the medial malleolus. The plantaris tendon is identified along the medial border of the Achilles tendon near its insertion using blunt dissection and is separated from the surrounding tissue. The tendon is divided distally and a core suture placed at its base. The suture and proximal end of the plantaris tendon are passed through the tendon stripper, which is advanced proximally and parallel to the tibia in a twisting manner while proximal tension is maintained on the plantaris tendon (Fig. 11-4). To facilitate harvest of the graft, the knee should be placed in full extension.

Fig. 11-4. The distal end of the plantaris tendon has been cut and passed through the tendon stripper. With a twisting motion, the tendon stripper is advanced proximally to detach the plantaris from its muscle belly.

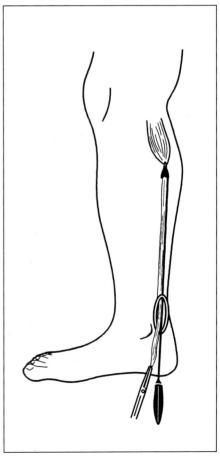

Extensor Digitorum Longus

The extensor digitorum longus muscle arises from the proximal part of the anterior compartment. It divides into four slips, which pass below the extensor retinaculum at the dorsal aspect of the foot. The extensor digitorum brevis tendon joins the tendons of these muscles at the lateral aspects over the metatarsophalangeal joints.

These tendons may be removed either by serial transverse incisions along the course of the tendons or by one long, curved incision over the dorsal aspect of the foot. The branches of the superficial peroneal nerve are in close approximation to these tendons, and special attention must be paid to avoid injuring this nerve.

Flexor Digitorum Superficialis

The muscle belly of the flexor digitorum superficialis (FDS) arises in the proximal two-thirds of the forearm and divides into four slips just proximal to the carpal canal. It passes through the canal and inserts after decussation around the flexor profundus on the proximal base of the middle phalanx.

The desired tendon may be removed using two incisions. One is placed just distal to the distal palmar crease over the metacarpal of the desired tendon. The tendon is identified, retracted proximally, and transected. A slip of distal tendon should be left in place distally at its insertion to prevent a hyperextension deformity. The proximal portion of the tendon can be retrieved by an incision at the level of the distal forearm.

Pulley Reconstruction

If the annular pulleys are inadequate, they can be reconstructed using three common techniques: (1) The Bunnell-Strickland method uses a single loop of free tendon graft, as well as a single interweave with six sutures. (2) The Weilby pulley uses a flexor tendon graft in a shoelace-like pattern woven into the flexor tendon sheath remnants, as described by Kleinert and Bennett. (3) The Lister pulley reconstruction uses a 10-mm width of extensor retinaculum at the A2 and A4 pulley sites, passing above the extensor mechanism for one pulley and between the extensor mechanism and bone for the second pulley. All three pulley techniques are depicted in Figure 11-5.

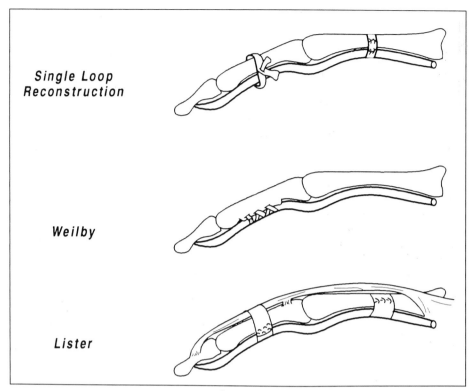

Single Loop Reconstruction

Weilby

Lister

Fig. 11-5. Various methods of pulley reconstruction.

Single-Stage Flexor Tendon Grafting

Technique

Exposure of the flexor fibro-osseous sheath for tendon grafting can be achieved through the existing incision, a zigzag Bruner incision, or a combination of both. Care is taken to identify and preserve the neurovascular bundles bilaterally. All intact annular pulleys should be retained. At a minimum, the A2 and A4 pulleys are required for adequate function. The presence of the A3 pulley is desirable, and if this pulley is not present, reconstruction is advised.

Remnants of the remaining flexor tendons are removed, leaving, when present, a 1-cm stump of the profundus tendon distally to allow suture of the tendon graft and enough FDS tendon proximal to the proximal interphalangeal (PIP) joint to prevent the late formation of a recurvatum deformity. One slip of the FDS tendon may be sutured to the A2 pulley to achieve a similar effect.

Either the profundus or the superficialis muscle may be used as the proximal motor unit. The decision to attach the tendon graft either in zone III or in zone V depends on the free excursion of the proximal muscle and the absence of limiting scar across zone IV (carpal tunnel). The profundus tendon is more commonly used for the motor unit of the tendon graft because of its longer range of muscle excursion. When the profundus tendon is used, the lumbrical muscle should be separated from the proximal tendon unit to prevent development of the lumbrical plus deformity.

If the decision is made to attach the graft to the flexor digitorum profundus (FDP) tendon in zone III, the FDP tendon may be resected and allowed to retract to the wrist. If attachment is to be in zone V, a similar evaluation of the proximal musculotendinous unit is performed, and the graft is attached to the best available site.

The flexor tendon graft can be passed through an intact pulley system in one of several ways. After placement of a core suture into the graft, either a silicone rod or a No. 8 French red rubber catheter is passed through the flexor sheath and sutured to the graft. The catheter is pulled back through the sheath, pulling the flexor tendon graft into place.

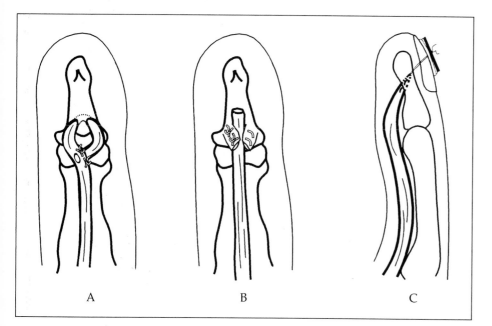

A   B   C

Fig. 11-6. Several techniques for distal tendon graft tenorrhaphy, including the transverse tunnel (A), tendon-to-tendon juncture (B), and modified Tinel technique using a pullout wire (C).

Fig. 11-7. Tendon graft interwoven to the proximal tendon. The excess tendon has been trimmed and removed, and a fishmouth has been made at the end of the proximal motor unit around the tendon graft.

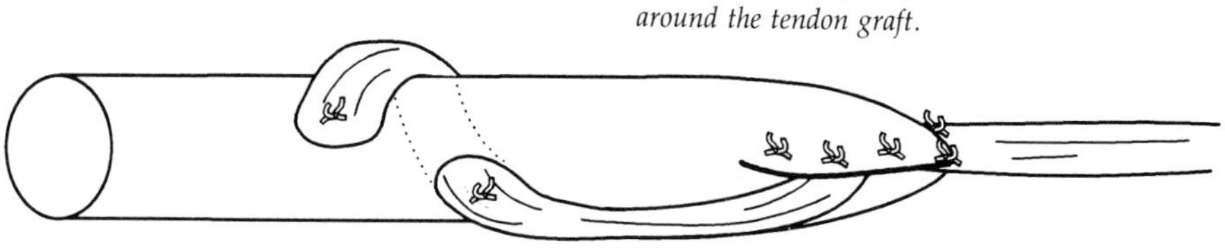

Initial fixation of the graft distally allows easier adjustment of final tension on the repair. Several techniques have been reported for distal flexor tendon graft tenorrhaphy (Fig. 11-6). These include the transverse tunnel, tendon-to-tendon juncture, and the modified Bunnell technique.

We prefer the modified Bunnell technique, in which the residual stump of the profundus tendon is elevated from the underlying periosteum of the distal phalanx (Fig. 11-6). With an osteotome, a portion of the bony cortex just proximal to the insertion of the FDP tendon is removed. Two Keith needles are drilled parallel to each other through the osteotomy site, exiting at the distal nail bed dorsally. A modified Kessler suture is placed in the distal end of the tendon graft using 4-0 stainless steel wire. The two ends of the wire are threaded through the loops of the Keith needles, which are passed distally such that the tendon graft is pulled snugly against the medullary canal of the distal phalanx. The wire suture is pulled taut, passed through a small plastic button, and twisted into place. The distal remnant of the profundus stump is sutured to the tendon graft with figure-of-eight sutures of 4-0 braided nonabsorbable suture.

Traction is placed on the tendon graft proximally to test the full excursion of the metacarpophalangeal (MP) and interphalangeal (IP) joints, the integrity of the pul-

ley system, and the strength of the distal tenorrhaphy. If resistance is encountered, the A2, A3, and A4 pulleys must be individually checked for sites of stricture. If, on the other hand, laxity or the tendency to bowstring is noted, reconstruction of the pulleys is indicated.

The preferred technique for the proximal tenorrhaphy is the Pulvertaft tendon weave. Setting the appropriate tension of the repair is of paramount importance. With the wrist placed in a neutral position, appropriate tension should bring the digit to approximately 15° greater total flexion than the normal cascade. This is achieved by placing a needle through the palmar skin and tendon to achieve fixation of the digit in the appropriate position. Next the distal end of the tendon motor unit is pulled out to determine the range of motor excursion. The midpoint of the motor excursion is determined, and a needle is placed through the proximal forearm skin into the musculotendinous unit to maintain it at the proper length. Thus with the digit in the proper degree of flexion and the motor unit at the proper length, a Pulvertaft tendon weave is constructed, weaving the distal tendon graft into the proximal tendon motor unit. The weave is held in place with figure-of-eight

sutures of 4-0 braided nonabsorbable suture. The excess tendon graft is removed and a fishmouth is made at the end of the proximal motor unit around the tendon graft (Fig. 11-7). The tension at the repair is checked again by extending and flexing the wrist to observe the effect of tenodesis of the tendon graft on the motion of the digit. Excessive flexion of the digit may predispose to a flexion contracture deformity, and too little flexion may cause an increase in total length of the tendon unit and thus a decrease in the total active range of motion.

Postoperative Care

The postoperative management of tendon grafts should be no different from that following primary repair of lacerated flexor tendons. One may choose the Duran and Houser controlled passive motion technique or the Kleinert technique of early active motion by rubber bands. Some surgeons prefer to immobilize the digits for 3 to 4 weeks after grafting. We prefer to splint the hand and wrist immediately after the operation, placing the wrist in 20° of flexion, the MP joint in 50° of flexion, and the IP joints in full extension. A program of early passive motion is initiated with the dorsal splint in place.

The patient is instructed to perform repeated passive flexion and extension of each IP joint and composite passive flexion and extension of the MP, PIP, and distal interphalangeal (DIP) joints for 4 weeks. In the fifth and sixth weeks, active and passive flexion and active extension exercises may be initiated with a dorsal block splint. The splint is removed during the sixth week, and strengthening exercises are started 8 weeks postoperatively. Normal activity is allowed 10 to 12 weeks after the operation.

Complications

Complications include joint contracture, flexor tendon adhesions, rupture of the tendon graft at the proximal and distal tenorrhaphy sites, infection, recurvatum deformity of the PIP joint, the lumbrical plus deformity, and the bowstring effect caused by the absence, rupture, or inadequate reconstruction of the pulleys. The problems of tendon rupture and the bowstring effect are often technique-related. The recurvatum deformity results from a lack of balance between the flexor tendon and the extensor mechanism, with the PIP joint in a position of hyperextension and the DIP joint in flexion. As previously mentioned, this deformity can be prevented at the time of the operation by the use of a distal FDS tendon slip through the A2 pulley. The lumbrical plus deformity described by Parkes occurs in the index and middle fingers. It is caused by a tendon graft that is longer than necessary and retraction of the lumbrical muscles. This deformity can be prevented by separating the proximal tendon motor unit from the lumbrical muscle at the time of the operation.

Two-Stage Repair

In the two-stage technique, the flexor tendons are excised, a silicone tendon rod is placed, and the annular pulleys are reconstructed (Fig. 11-8). The tendon rod is attached distally to a 1-cm cuff of profundus tendon and is unattached proximally. In joint contractures, capsulotomies are performed simultaneously. The digit subsequently undergoes a postoperative passive range-of-motion protocol. Approximately 8 to 16 weeks after tendon rod placement, in the presence of supple, soft tissue and joints, an adequate pseudosheath forms, which allows removal of the tendon rod and placement of a tendon

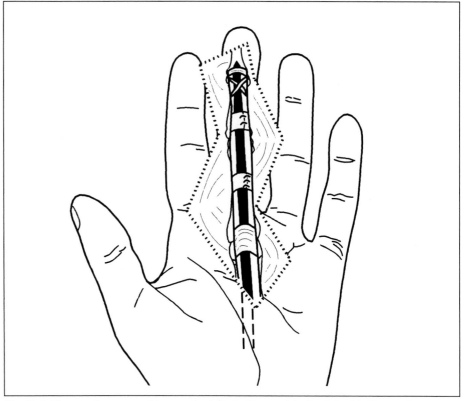

Fig. 11-8. Flexor tendons removed from tendon bed. A silicone rod is placed. In this diagram the A1 pulley is intact, and the A2 and A3 pulleys have been reconstructed.

graft. Although Hunter and others reported the use of a permanent active tendon implant in a one-stage technique, most authors recommend a two-stage tendon reconstruction.

Suggested Reading

Duran, R.J., and Houser, R.G. Problems in the Management of Flexor Tendon Injuries in Zones I and II. In J.W. Strickland and J.B. Steichen (Eds.), *Difficult Problems in Hand Surgery*. St. Louis: Mosby, 1982. Pp. 86–93.

Hunter, J.H., and Aulicino, P.L. Salvage of the Scarred Tendon Systems, Utilizing the Hand Hunter Tendon Implant. In J.E. Flynn (Ed.), *Hand Surgery* (3rd ed.). Baltimore: Williams & Wilkins, 1982. Pp. 265–293.

Hunter, J.M., and Cook, J.F. The Pulley System: Rationale for Reconstruction. In J.W. Strickland and J.B. Steichen (Eds.), *Difficult Problems in Hand Surgery*. St. Louis: Mosby, 1982. Pp. 94–102.

Hunter, J.M., et al. Tendon Reconstruction with Implants. In R. Tubiana (Ed.), *The Hand*. Philadelphia: Saunders, 1988. Vol. 3, Pp. 255–279.

Lister, G.D. Flexor Tendon. In J.W. May and J.W. Littler (Eds.), *Plastic Surgery: The Hand*. Philadelphia: Harcourt Brace Jovanovich, 1990. Vol. 7, Pp. 4516–4564.

Pulvertaft, R.G. Flexor Tendon Grafting. In J.E. Flynn (Ed.), *Hand Surgery* (3rd ed.). Baltimore: Williams & Wilkins, 1982. Pp. 265–293.

Schneider, L.H. Secondary Procedures in Flexor Tendon Surgery. *Flexor Tendon Injuries*. Boston: Little, Brown, 1985. Pp. 77–109.

Schneider, L.H., and Hunter, J.M. Flexor Tendons: Late Reconstruction. In D.P. Green (Ed.), *Operative Hand Surgery* (2nd ed.). New York: Churchill Livingstone, 1988. Pp. 1969–2044.

Strickland, J.W. Functional Recovery after Flexor Tendon Severance in the Finger: The State of the Art. In J.W. Strickland and J.B. Steichen (Eds.), *Difficult Problems in Hand Surgery*. St. Louis: Mosby, 1982. Pp. 73–85.

Strickland, J.W. Flexor tendon injuries. *Orthop. Rev.* 15:632, 701, 1986; 16:18, 78, 137, 1987.

Tubiana, R. Flexor Tendon Grafts in the Hand. In R. Tubiana (Ed.), *The Hand*. Philadelphia: Saunders, 1988. Vol. 3, Pp. 217–243.

Widstrom, C.J., et al. A mechanical study of six pulley reconstruction techniques. Part I. Mechanical effectiveness. *J. Hand Surg.* 14A: 821, 1989.

12

Nerve Grafting

Warren C. Breidenbach   Waqar Aziz

Philipeaux and Vulpian performed the first experimental nerve grafts in 1870 by using a segment of the lingual nerve to bridge a defect in the hypoglossal nerve. Sporadic attempts at clinical nerve grafting followed. In 1919 Platt reported a series of 20 nerve grafts, all with poor results. This report gave rise to considerable pessimism about the procedure, and nerve grafting subsequently was avoided at all costs. Primary repair was advocated, even if extraordinary measures were necessary to close the nerve gap.

In 1972 Millesi published experimental evidence that nerve repair under tension leads to increased fibrosis. He speculated that better results could be obtained with nerve grafting if tension were avoided at the repair sites. This concept of tension-free nerve grafts formed the basis of his interfascicular nerve technique. Subsequent clinical studies by Millesi confirmed that nerve grafting was a viable technique when performed in this manner. That tension is associated not only with increased fibrosis at the repair site but also with poor axonal regeneration was subsequently confirmed by a separate study. In this study Millesi found that the conduction velocities and amplitudes of evoked responses were poor across ex-

cessively long nerve grafts or moderately stretched repair sites. These studies led to the fundamental principle of nerve grafting—that axonal regeneration is better across two tension-free repair sites than across one site under tension.

Grading of Nerve Injury

There are several ways to classify a nerve injury. A classification proposed by Seddon in 1943 is based on experience gained in World War II. Seddon divided nerve lesions into three categories: *Neurapraxia* entailed a conduction block without any anatomic lesion; *axonotmesis*, the next in severity, was a loss of continuity of the axons at the level of the injury, with preservation of the endoneurial sheaths but with distal wallerian degeneration; *neurotmesis* entailed complete loss of continuity of the nerve and permanent loss of function.

Sunderland introduced a more comprehensive classification in 1951, which not only encompassed the three grades of Seddon but defined intermediate grades between axonotmesis and neurotmesis.

Grade I

Local conduction block with local myelin damage occurs in grade I. The damage is reversible within a variable period from a few weeks to months. Axonal continuity is preserved, and there is no accompanying wallerian degeneration. The functional involvement is confined to motion and proprioception. Some sympathetic function may be preserved. This grade corresponds with Seddon's neurapraxia.

Grade II

A loss of nerve conduction occurs at the level of the injury and in the distal segment in grade II. At the cellular level, axonal discontinuity is accompanied by distal wallerian degeneration. Because the endoneurial sheaths are preserved, however, recovery depends on proximal axonal regeneration. Because axonal orientation is preserved, reinnervation of the end organs may be expected following a time period based on the level of injury. This grade corresponds with Seddon's axonotmesis.

Grade III

A loss of axonal continuity as well as continuity of the endoneurial sheath occurs in grade III. The perineurial sheath is intact. As a result, axonal regeneration may be disrupted depending on scarring and on the extent of the injury. Chances of malorientation of axons are greater, and surgical intervention may be required if recovery is not satisfactory.

Grade IV

This injury results in loss in continuity of the endoneurial and perineurial sheaths and axons. The only structure preserved and contributing to the continuity of the nerve is the epineurium. If left unrepaired, this injury may result in a neuroma in continuity with poor or no functional return. Surgical therapy is required for any meaningful recovery.

Grade V

This grade entails the complete transection of the nerve. Surgical therapy is required to obtain good results. Grades III, IV, and V all correspond to the neurotmesis of Seddon's classification.

Physiologic Events Following Nerve Injury

After the transection of a peripheral nerve, several changes ensue that can be categorized broadly as mechanical and biologic. The mechanical changes involve nerve elasticity. The peripheral nerve has inherent elasticity by virtue of which immediate retraction of the nerve ends occurs after the nerve is divided. The gap resulting from these elastic forces varies according to the level of injury and the nerve involved. Gaps without nerve tissue loss can be closed easily by coaptation immediately after the injury has occurred. The situation changes in long-standing gaps because the nerve loses its inherent elasticity owing to fibrosis. The nerve gap becomes fixed, making delayed repair more difficult.

Biologic changes in the nerve are initiated by transection. Nerve transection results in a series of sequential events that are different in the proximal and distal nerve segments. In the proximal segment, retrograde axonal degeneration progresses for one or two nodes of Ranvier. Along with this process, changes take place in the parent cell body. These two physiologic facts are often overlooked by the cli-

nician. The "die-back" of the proximal nerve may be great after traction injuries, whereas the extent of parent cell body changes may influence nerve regeneration.

In addition to the proximal effects, biologic changes also affect the distal segment. In an uninjured nerve, axoplasmic flow carries substances from the cell body to the nerve end and vice versa. Neurotropic factors that maintain nerve integrity are carried by this transport system. After nerve transection, axoplasmic flow is not suddenly blocked but is reduced gradually. When this flow falls below a critical level, the stimulating effect of neurotropic factors is lost, and Schwann cells become activated. These activated Schwann cells phagocytize the axons and myelin sheath until the nerve is cleared of cellular debris, a process referred to as wallerian degeneration. At this point, the nerve is composed of endoneurium surrounding a core of Schwann cells.

Indications for Nerve Grafting

The indications for nerve grafting depend on the presence of a nerve defect, level of injury, and extent of contamination.

Presence of Nerve Defect

Transection of a nerve results in the elastic retraction of its ends, even when no actual loss of nerve tissue occurs, which produces a nerve gap. Coaptation entails overcoming these physiologic elastic forces. With primary or delayed primary repair (up to 2 weeks), these forces may be overcome easily, and the nerve gap closed. In secondary repair, however, which by definition is carried out weeks after injury, nerve fibrosis may have reduced elasticity, making it difficult if not impossible to close an equivalent distance between the nerve ends. In this situation, the gap has become a nerve defect.

A nerve defect may be secondary to fibrosis of a nerve gap or may result from loss of nerve tissue. The distinction between a nerve gap and a nerve defect is made by evaluating the time from injury and intraoperatively determining nerve elasticity. Most nerve gaps may be repaired primarily. A nerve defect normally requires nerve grafting.

Distinguishing between nerve gap and defect to determine suitability of nerve grafting versus primary repair requires clinical experience. For example, when do the elastic forces of the nerve gap become too great for primary nerve repair? When is the nerve defect so small that nerve grafting is not indicated? The best way to approach these problems clinically is to evaluate nerve elasticity intraoperatively. If the nerve ends may be brought together and held by two 9-0 sutures (10-0 for digital nerves), primary repair should be carried out. If this cannot be accomplished, nerve grafting is indicated regardless of the size of the defect. Nerve grafting may be necessary in defects measuring only 2 to 3 cm, for instance.

Although defining the distinction between nerve gaps and defects is important, clinical evaluation in the operating room determines whether primary repair or a nerve graft is carried out. The elastic forces of the ulnar nerve are so strong, for instance, that even its clean transection at the cubital tunnel produces a large nerve gap. Although nerve grafting is not indicated under these circumstances, primary repair is best achieved after anterior transposition of the nerve.

Nerve gaps or defects may be closed by changing joint position, because flexion or extension (depending on the location of the nerve) automatically shortens the distance between the severed nerve stumps. This procedure is to be condemned, however, because increased tension will be applied across the repair site when joint motion resumes.

Level of Injury

For practical purposes, peripheral nerve injuries can be divided into three categories: those at the brachial plexus level, those between the shoulder and the wrist, and those distal to the wrist. The distinction is based on the distance to the end organs and the changing nature of peripheral nerves. The farther a nerve is from the end organ, the longer regeneration takes and the less likely it is that a good result will occur. A better result can be anticipated for an injury at the wrist than for a similar one at the brachial plexus. Furthermore, motor and sensory fibers are mixed within fascicles proximally but have separated out distally,

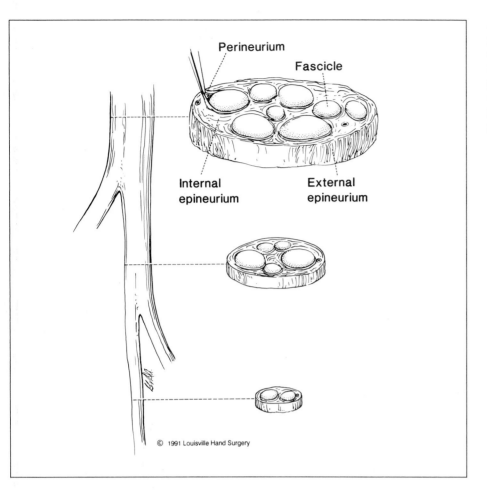

Fig. 12-1. *Peripheral nerve cross sections from proximal to distal. Fascicles continuously separate and combine as they run from proximal to distal in the peripheral nerve. Because of this, the fascicular pattern is different at each level, making it difficult in large defects to know which fascicular groups should be coapted to the nerve graft at each end.*

each into their own fascicles. Also interfascicular exchanges are extensive proximally and diminish distally (Fig. 12-1). Appropriate alignment of motor and sensory fascicles is accordingly more difficult proximally than distally.

Contamination

We believe that in most instances it is possible to convert a contaminated wound of the hand or digit into a clean wound, thus making primary nerve grafting possible. For instance, in revascularization or replantation of a digit, we proceed with primary nerve grafting.

In essence, the hand represents a privileged site where wounds normally can be debrided adequately and primary nerve grafting can be carried out regardless of the severity of the initial contamination. With contaminated wounds involving the arm or forearm, one needs to be more cautious. Conventional teaching advocates delayed primary repair of severely

contaminated wounds and that nerve grafting must be done only after successful closure of the wound. Our group seldom follows this conventional wisdom. We often cover severely contaminated forearm wounds after debridement on the night of injury with free tissue transfers. In spite of this, we normally do not carry out immediate nerve grafting both because of time limitations caused by free tissue transfer and because we must await confirmation of flap viability. We delay nerve grafting under these circumstances but not out of fear of wound contamination.

Associated Injury

Associated injury to the extremity does not necessarily preclude the use of primary nerve grafts. In a patient with multiple trauma for whom the nerve defect is one of many problems, however, the benefits and risks should be assessed individually, with attention to all the factors outlined previously.

Timing of Nerve Grafting

The timing of nerve grafting depends greatly on evaluation of the patient's wound, level of contamination, and associated injuries. Here we address the question of the optimal time to carry out nerve grafting assuming all other factors regarding the wound and patient are equivalent.

Theoretical arguments suggest delaying nerve grafting. To explain our position, we need first to examine primary versus delayed primary nerve repair. For years controversy has existed regarding which type of repair produced the best results. Surgeons who advocated primary nerve repair listed the following advantages: (1) The nerve ends were not fibrosed; (2) no shrinkage occurred with the proximal segment; and (3) immediate repair ensured against loss of time for reinnervation of end organs. Those who advocated delayed primary repair argued that immediately after nerve transection, the proximal nerve undergoes a phase of retrograde wallerian degeneration before axonal sprouting starts. Therefore, the extent of proximal damage cannot be assessed accurately until some time after the initial injury. Furthermore, axonal regeneration through a distal segment that has already undergone wallerian degeneration produces an easier pathway than does one currently undergoing wallerian degeneration.

At the present time, conventional teaching advocates primary repair. In previous decades, however, delayed primary repair was in vogue and again today some experimental evidence supports this approach.

Applying these principles to nerve grafting helps us in terms of the timing of repair. Those who advocate primary nerve repair also advocate early nerve grafting (primary or delayed primary). Those who believe in delayed primary or secondary repair of nerves advocate delaying nerve grafting. The arguments for the timing of nerve grafting are often academic, and in fact timing is dictated much more by the condition of the wound and patient. By this we mean that we have no hesitation about primary nerve grafting in digital replantation. For forearm defects of nerve and soft tissue requiring emergency free tissue transfer, however, we normally delay nerve grafting. We do not believe that the advantages of primary nerve grafting are so clearly established to warrant taking a risk in this situation.

Operative Technique

Although the individual approach and required exposure vary with the nerve involved, some general principles have proved helpful to us.

Exposure

A generous exposure is essential for the assessment of damage, and it is always helpful to approach the area of the lesion by defining the normal anatomy both proximally and distally. Otherwise, in secondary nerve grafting it is easy to lose perspective in the scar tissue. Some authors have expressed the reservation that mobilization of the nerve causes vascular compromise. Experimental work by Lundborg, confirmed by work in our laboratory, however, shows that peripheral nerves have a tremendous vascular reserve and can withstand considerable mobilization without any effect on their intrinsic microcirculation.

Preparation of Nerve Ends

In secondary nerve grafts, the extent of proximal damage is sometimes impossible to determine. We find that a frozen section of the proximal stump after the neuroma is excised helps determine the adequacy of the resection. Experience has shown us time and again that frozen sections result in a more accurate evaluation of the nerve than clinical microscopic evaluation does. After assuming a proximal stump is ready to receive a nerve graft based on evaluation under the microscope, we have discovered that a frozen section from the proximal stump contained few or no axons. Thus clinical evaluation under the microscope has proved inaccurate. Presence of normal architecture and neural tissue in the proximal stump is a primary requirement for the nerve graft. Similarly, excision of the glioma from the distal nerve stump ensures that the distal nerve repair is not being carried out on scar tissue.

Orientation

When the nerve defect is between the shoulder and the wrist, it most commonly involves a mixed (sensory and motor) nerve. This entails the additional problem of orienting the nerve graft properly so that axonal loss is kept to a minimum by avoiding sensory-motor mismatch. After the nerve has been adequately exposed and its ends prepared, the cross section of the nerve ends should be viewed under high magnification using an operating microscope. This evaluation reveals cross-sectional fascicular topography that falls into one of three categories.

Monofascicular

The cross section consists of one big fascicle. In this situation sensory-motor mixing is more diffuse, making adequate alignment of graft sections problematic. Dissection may produce false groups of fascicles.

Oligofascicular

The nerve cross section shows several large fascicles. In this situation interfascicular nerve grafting can be achieved by gentle dissection. If the distal and proximal architecture are comparable in the number of groups and their arrangement, interfascicular nerve grafting can be performed with a reasonable degree of accuracy.

Polyfascicular

Numerous fascicles are present with proportionately more connective tissue than neural tissue. This type can be subdivided additionally into two subcategories: In *polyfascicular nerves with a group arrangement*, the several fascicles are located closely enough to make a group, thus making it possible to perform dissection and separate these groups from each other. In this situation it is possible to do a group-fascicular nerve graft. In *polyfascicular nerves without a group arrangement*, multiple fascicles are present without a specific pattern. This situation makes correct graft alignment difficult.

Fascicular Identification

Intraoperative identification of motor and sensory fascicles is one of the challenges in operations on the peripheral nerves. At our center we have used intraoperative electrophysiologic studies including awake stimulation, radiobioassay for acetylcholinesterase activity, and histochemical staining techniques to assess whether the fascicle is sensory or motor. We have occasionally used all three techniques simultaneously only to find some (although not large) differences among the methods in identifying sensory and motor fascicles, calling into question the sensitivity and specificity of these methods. This issue is still being worked out in our experimental and clinical studies. It should be noted, however, that we regularly use one or more of these techniques.

The distal stump poses a problem, especially in patients with long-standing injuries. Histochemical staining techniques do not provide satisfactory differentiation, even when performed as close to the injury as 5 days afterward. The fascicles of the distal stump can be identified by anatomic dissection under high magnification, in which the known motor and sensory branches are dissected back to the nerve end. This method has serious limitations, including changing fascicular pattern, crossovers, and trauma caused by extensive interfascicular dissection. It can be used over short distances only. Its most likely application is in identifying the motor branch of the median nerve when performing nerve grafting at the level of the distal forearm.

When using awake stimulation for sensory and motor identification, it is important to use the lowest amplitude and duration of the stimulus discernible by the patient. Otherwise, the jumping of the stimuli across fascicles may make precise localization by the patient difficult. Although this technique sounds complicated, it is simple when performed with a neurologist who has the appropriate equipment. A machine that can vary the duration and amplitude of stimulation and record the compound action potential is brought into the operating room. The initial dissection is done with the patient under Bier block and followed by release of the tourniquet. Local infiltration is used around the edge of the wound to avoid wound pain. Lidocaine should not be allowed to come in contact with the nerve because that would result in conduction block. While the neurologist varies the amplitude and duration of stimulation, the surgeon applies the stimulating electrode to the fascicle in question. The patient, who has had a Bier block and thus is awake, can tell you if he or she feels a stimulus, indicating the fascicle is sensory, or does not feel a stimulus, indicating the fascicle is motor. Before stimulating the first fascicle, the amplitude and duration are lowered to a point at which the patient feels nothing. Both are increased slowly until the patient feels something. This level of stimulation is used to test each of the fascicles.

For histochemical staining we use Kanaya's modification of the Karnovsky method (Fig. 12-2). The processing time required by this technique is less than one hour. Because histochemical and radiobioassay methods depend on acetylcholinesterase activity, their usefulness in identifying the sensory and motor distribution in the distal nerve end in longstanding injuries may be compromised. From about 5 days following injury, however, the staining of the distal nerve stumps is unsatisfactory.

Identifying Normal Nerve Tissue

The nerve lesions most commonly treated with nerve grafts are categorized as polyfascicular with group arrangement. These lesions present an optimal situation for interfascicular nerve grafting. The proximal and distal nerve stumps are prepared as described earlier. The proximal neuroma is resected, and the epineurium is incised to identify the group fascicles present within the nerve segment. Interfascicular dissection separates the nerve into groups of fascicles. Similar dissection is carried out distally after the glioma is resected.

At this point the patient has a nerve defect with the proximal and distal stumps separated into group fascicles. The nerve graft should be positioned in such a man-

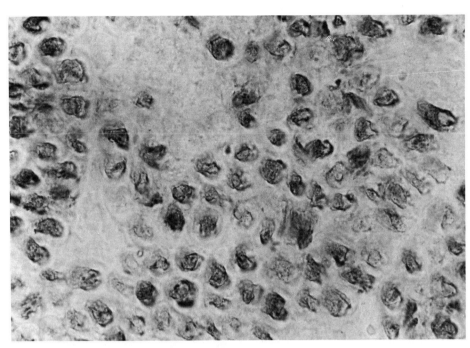

Fig. 12-2. Histochemical staining of human nerve using the Karnovsky method as modified by Kanaya. Motor axons stain dark using this technique (magnification ×250).

ner that it connects the appropriate group fascicle proximally with its counterpart distally, as determined by sensory and motor identification (discussed previously).

Although the procedure appears cleancut when described on paper, the reality is far different. First of all, we often find that our arbitrary separation of the nerve into group fascicles may lead us to group sensory and motor fascicles together proximally in a way that does not correspond to the distal pattern. Furthermore, the nerve graft often does not correspond with the size of the fascicular group. The nerve graft is usually larger than one group fascicle, requiring the placement of two group fascicles into the end of one nerve graft. Finally, the matching areas of the nerve and nerve graft proximally may not be equivalent to the matching areas distally. All the group fascicles may line up well with the cross-sectional area presented by the proximal nerve graft, but distally, where the nerve is smaller, the area of the nerve graft may exceed that of the distal nerve stump, leading to loss of axons. All these problems can be overcome only with accurate intraoperative planning and meticulous attention to detail. Even in ideal nerve graft repairs, im-

perfections may result from these problems.

The foregoing discussion describes nerve grafting for polyfascicular nerves with group arrangement. In monofascicular, oligofascicular, or polyfascicular nerves without group arrangement, the situation is more difficult. Often motor and sensory identification techniques are not useful because the two components are mixed throughout the nerve; therefore, the best method of properly aligning the nerve graft between proximal and distal segments is to evaluate the structural configurations apparent under the microscope. For example, a large epineurial vessel or one predominant fascicle may give the surgeon a point of reference.

Harvesting the Sural Nerve

The sural nerve can be harvested by stepcut or open techniques. The open technique involves an incision from the ankle to the popliteal fossa that completely exposes the nerve. The advantage of this technique is that it allows direct visualization of the nerve with no traction. The disadvantage is that it leaves a long and often unsightly scar.

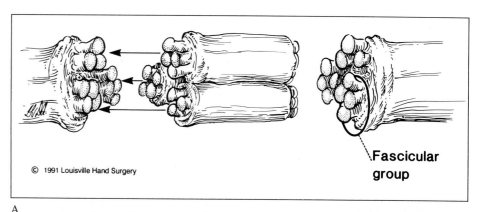

Fig. 12-3. Group fascicular nerve grafting. A. The size of the nerve graft usually does not match the size of the fascicular group. B. Note the whiteness typical of the conventional nerve graft. A vascularized nerve graft, because it is transferred with its blood supply, would appear similar in color to the proximal and distal nerve stumps to which it is coapted. (Courtesy Thomas W. Wolff, M.D.)

© 1991 Louisville Hand Surgery

Fascicular group

A

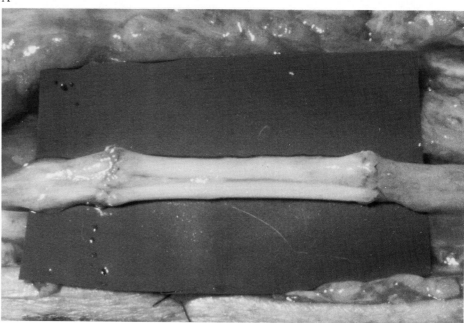

B

The step-cut technique makes multiple step cuts (approximately four) from ankle to popliteal fossa. The nerve is removed by dissection along its length through these step cuts. An alternative to this technique is to use a vein stripper, stripping the nerve to a point at which resistance is felt and then making a step cut. The disadvantage of these techniques is that they apply tension to the sural nerve, which theoretically can produce internal damage to the nerve. The techniques do leave a better scar on the leg, however.

We use the vein stripper through multiple step cuts to obtain the sural nerve. Under no condition is tension applied to the nerve. If the vein stripper does not advance easily, a step cut is made. In this manner, we believe we can avoid the complication of tension injury to the nerve. Sometimes the whole nerve can be removed with only one or two step cuts. Usually, besides the opening incision, at least one step cut is necessary at the mid-calf level where the lateral sural nerve joins the medial sural nerve.

Coaptation

A decision must be made whether fascicular or group fascicular grafting will be carried out. The first aligns each individual fascicle with a cable graft, whereas the second aligns a group fascicle with an individual cable graft. With group fascicular nerve grafting, groups of fascicles must be identified and the external epineurium removed, leaving a small amount of internal epineurium surrounding each fascicle (Fig. 12-3A and B). The nerve graft is aligned with the group fascicle, and the suture is placed through the internal epineurium of both group fascicle and nerve graft. In fascicular nerve grafting, both external and internal epineurium are removed, and the fascicle is aligned with

the nerve graft. The suture is placed through the perineurium.

Theoretically fascicular nerve grafting should give better alignment, but it is time consuming and technically difficult. Also this technique requires the placement of a suture through the perineurium, violating the endoneurial space and requiring a larger number of sutures than group fascicular nerve grafting does. Because the result could be increased perineurial scarring, we consistently use group fascicular nerve grafting as described by Millesi.

Group fascicular repair is accomplished by aligning the nerve graft with the appropriate group fascicles. A 10-0 nylon suture is placed through the epineurium of the graft and the internal epineurium

of the group fascicle. The nerve graft is placed with the adjacent joint in extension, so that the length of the graft is appropriate even under conditions of maximal extension. Wound closure is carried out with care that there is no tension.

Postoperative Care
Splinting

All nerve injuries require postoperative splinting. Ideally splinting should completely immobilize the repair site and include one joint above and one below the site of injury. That procedure is not often followed, however, because injuries of associated structures require appropriate modification of the splinting regimen. Also, the more distant the nerve repair site and nerve graft lie from a joint, the less likely that the joint needs to be immobilized.

When deciding which splint to apply, it must be ascertained whether motion of the joint will apply tension across the nerve repair site. This task is best accomplished by intraoperative evaluation of motion of the joint while visualizing the nerve graft repair sites. For example, a nerve graft of the median nerve at the level of the midforearm probably requires immobilization of the wrist only. Nerve repair at the level of the distal carpal tunnel, however, may require immobilization of both the wrist and metacarpophalangeal joints.

The situation is complicated by associated injuries. In secondary repair of a nerve, a nerve defect is made that often needs to be reconstructed with a nerve graft. The associated tendons, however, are caught in scar and need tenolysis. After tenolysis, mobilization is necessary, but the nerve graft requires immobilization. An intraoperative decision needs to be made by visualization of the nerve repair site while taking the joints to be mobilized through their full range of motion to assess the stress that would be placed across the repair site if tenolysis were done. It may not be possible to move the patient as vigorously as one would wish; the result could be that the tendons would scar down again if tenolysis were done. The patient should be warned of this possibility preoperatively.

In all situations in which there is a dilemma requiring the choice between mobilization to avoid adhesions of the tendons and immobilization for the nerve, we protect the nerve. In a later procedure, we carry out tenolysis. Tenolysis done after nerve grafting has the advantage of allowing a second look at the nerve repair site to determine whether neurolysis is necessary to enhance return of function.

Two considerations must be kept in mind when deciding on postoperative splinting. First, the length of time a nerve graft needs to be splinted is not established. We always splint for a minimum of 10 days to 2 weeks and often extend the time to 3 weeks. The duration varies depending on the position of the nerve graft in relation to the mobile joints and how much tension the joints are going to apply across the site of nerve repair. For median

nerve gaps reconstructed at the level of the wrist, for instance, we immobilize the wrist for 3 weeks.

Second, and contrary to the first consideration, immobilization may be deleterious to final nerve outcome. Although immobilization avoids disruption of the nerve repair site, it also allows adhesions to form between the nerve and surrounding tissues. During normal motion of the extremity, nerves glide through a range of motion and have an excursion; although it is less than that of tendons, an excursion is definitely present. Leaving the nerve graft immobilized may increase adhesions, resulting in postoperative scarring and decreased nerve return. It is necessary to balance the duration of splinting to protect the repair site with the necessity for restoring motion before the nerve becomes firmly scarred to the surrounding structures.

Finally, long-term splinting may be necessary while awaiting nerve return. For example, after ulnar nerve reconstruction an anticlaw splint should be used, and after high radial nerve repairs outrigger and cock-up splints may be necessary.

Follow-Up Care

After nerve grafting, return of nerve function is evaluated, first by monitoring the advance of the Tinel sign, and second by monitoring the return of sensory and motor function. Both the meaning of the Tinel sign and the exact method of evaluating it are important. Always using a reflex hammer (to make the percussing instrument a constant), we percuss starting proximally to the injury site and progress distally until paresthesias are felt. These sensations indicate a positive Tinel sign and normally correspond to the proximal graft repair site. We subsequently use the hammer to percuss, starting distally at the fingertips and progressing proximally. The site where the first paresthesias are felt is referred to as a negative Tinel sign, or distal Tinel sign, and represents the most distal advancement of the regenerating axon. Measuring the distance from the proximal to the distal Tinel sign and dividing by the number of postoperative days gives a measurement of axon regeneration. This figure should be approximately 1 mm/day. Sometimes there is a lag period of weeks or even

months, depending on the type of injury, before the onset of nerve regeneration.

The rate of axon regeneration and the position of the distal Tinel sign should be used to estimate returning nerve function. One cannot anticipate return of motor or sensory function until the distal Tinel sign reaches the appropriate motor or sensory end organ. Furthermore, a distal Tinel sign may stop, indicating that axons are not advancing. This situation is sometimes seen at the distal nerve graft repair site if it becomes accidentally disrupted or is too scarred.

Unfortunately the arrival of the distal Tinel sign at the appropriate end organ does not guarantee reinnervation. The Tinel sign probably results from stimulation of the small regenerating axons that carry painful sensation. Larger fibers, which lag behind the small fibers, are necessary for return of motor and sensory function. Thus the small fibers may arrive at the distal end organ, but because of the inherent problems of nerve grafting, the large fibers do not follow.

Monitoring the advancing Tinel sign and calculating the rate of axonal regeneration helps the surgeon make two decisions. First, a poorly advancing Tinel sign indicates that poor return of function is likely and other alternatives such as regrafting or tendon transfers may be necessary. Second, when the advancing Tinel sign reaches the motor or sensory end organ, physical therapy should be initiated.

Controversies
Allografting

One of the limiting factors in nerve grafting is the availability of a donor nerve. With large sciatic nerve defects, for example, it is difficult if not impossible to find sufficient donor nerve. If donor nerves could be transplanted from another person (allograft), it is possible large nerve defects could be reconstructed.

Theoretically nerve allograft reconstruction should function as follows. The nerve defect would be reconstructed with the allograft, which is immunologically different from the recipient. The recipient host would be immunosuppressed immediately on the start of reconstruction. The nerve allograft would undergo wallerian degeneration, leaving only supporting nerve structures to be recognized as foreign material. The patient would continue immunosuppression until the host axons had grown through the foreign nerve graft. At this point, immunosuppression could be stopped. Theoretically the axons would continue to survive, and the support structures would be removed by the immune response and replaced by the host. At the present time, studies in animals are being conducted in several laboratories to see if such a sequence of events is plausible.

Vascularized Nerve Grafting

In the nerve grafting referred to in this chapter, the nerve is moved without its blood supply (conventional nerve graft). The bed must be well vascularized in the recipient site so that vessels may rapidly grow into the nerve graft. A period of ischemia occurs before revascularization of the nerve graft, however. This period of ischemia may damage Schwann cells and increase intraneural fibrosis. These problems could be avoided if the nerve graft were moved with its blood supply—a so-called vascularized nerve graft. This term is a misnomer, although it is ingrained in the literature. The nerve moved with its blood supply is in reality a free flap, not a graft.

Considerable experimental and clinical work has been done on vascularized nerve grafting. It now seems clear that these grafts are indicated in a badly scarred bed, because a conventional nerve graft will not revascularize in such a bed. Whether vascularized nerve grafts should be used to reconstruct nerve defects in a well-vascularized bed is still controversial.

Nerve Conduits

Sometimes it is necessary to sacrifice a donor nerve to reconstruct a small nerve defect. Sacrifice of the donor nerve could be avoided if an artificial conduit were placed to guide the regenerating axons. Intense research is going on to find such a conduit. Some authors have advocated the use of veins, whereas others have advocated the use of synthetic absorbable material. Attempts have been made to place nerve growth factor or cultured Schwann cells in the conduits to increase

nerve regeneration. This work is still experimental, although the long-term implications are that nerve grafts may be reconstructed from synthetic material or from tissue that is more readily available than nerves.

Muscle Autografts

Skeletal muscle, with its parallel fibers, has a structure of tubular basement membranes similar to that found in peripheral nerves. Experimental work in nonhuman primates has used muscle grafts from the same animal to repair nerve defects. These muscle autografts are frozen, thawed, tailored so that they have the same size and shape as the segment of nerve they are replacing, and sutured into the defect. Although axons were found to grow quickly through the tubular basement membranes, the extent of myelination seemed to be less than that found after conventional nerve grafting. Used to repair digital nerves in a small series of patients, muscle autografts have yielded good results. This procedure still must be considered investigational, however.

Conclusion

Since the report of Millesi in 1972, nerve grafting has been accepted as a method of reconstructing peripheral nerve defects. The reader should now understand how to use the microscope for appropriate intraoperative identification techniques, harvest a donor nerve, and reconstruct a nerve defect with interfascicular nerve grafting. The reader should be aware, however, that even when these techniques are used, the results of nerve grafting are less than optimal. For this reason, peripheral nerve grafting remains one of the great challenges to be solved in the future. Through the work on allografting, vascularized nerve grafts, nerve conduits, autografts, or some unforeseen discovery, we hope to be able to reconstruct nerve defects with results that approach normal function.

Suggested Reading

Bonney, G., et al. Experience with vascularized nerve grafts. In J.K. Terzis (Ed.), *Microreconstruction of Nerve Injuries*. Philadelphia: Saunders, 1986. Pp. 403–414.

Breidenbach, W.C., and Terzis, J.K. The blood supply of vascularized nerve grafts. *J. Reconstr. Microsurg.* 3:43, 1986.

Engel, J., et al. Choline acetyltransferase for differentiation between human motor and sensory nerve fibers. *Ann. Plast. Surg.* 4:5, 1980.

Ganel, A., Engel, J., and Rimon, S. Intraoperative identification of peripheral nerve fascicle: Use of a new rapid biochemical assay technique. *Orthop. Rev.* 15:669, 1986.

Gaul, J.S. Electrical fascicle identification as an adjunct to nerve repair. *Hand Clin.* 2:4, 1986.

Gruber, H., and Zenkur, W. Acetylcholinesterase: Histochemical differentiation between motor and sensory nerve fibers. *Brain Res.* 51: 207, 1973.

Jabeley, M.E., Wallace, W.H., and Heckler, F.R. Internal topography of major nerves of the forearm and hand: A current view. *J. Hand Surg.* 5:1, 1980.

Kanaya, F., et al. Sensory and motor fiber differentiation with Karnovsky staining. *J. Hand Surg.* 16:851, 1991.

Millesi, H. Interfascicular nerve grafting. *Orthop. Clin. North Am.* 12:287, 1981.

Millesi, H. The nerve gap: Theory and clinical practice. *Hand Clin.* 2:651, 1987.

Millesi, H., Berger, A., and Meissl, G. Experimentelle untersuchungen zur heilung durchtrennter peripherer nerven. *Chir. Plast.* 1:174, 1972.

Millesi, H., and Meissl, G. Consequences of tension at the suture site. In A. Gorio, H. Millesi, and S. Mingrino (Eds.), Post-traumatic peripheral nerve regeneration: Experimental basis and clinical implications. New York: Raven Press, 1981. P. 277.

Sunderland, S. The interneural topography of the radial, median, and ulnar nerves. *Brain* 68: 243, 1945.

Sunderland, S. A classification of peripheral nerve injuries producing loss of function. *Brain* 74:491, 1951.

Taylor, G.I., and Ham, F.J. The free vascularized nerve graft: A further experimental and clinical application of microvascular techniques. *Plast. Reconstr. Surg.* 57:413, 1976.

Terzis, J., Faibisoff, B., and Williams, H.B. The nerve gap: Suture under tension vs. graft. *Plast. Reconstr. Surg.* 56:166, 1975.

Williams, H.B., and Jabaley, M.E. The importance of internal anatomy of the peripheral nerves to nerve repair in the forearm and hand. *Hand Clin.* 2:689, 1986.

Special Techniques

13

Principles of Craniomaxillofacial Surgery

Ian T. Jackson

Craniofacial surgery is a logical extension of maxillofacial surgery. In 1950 Sir Harold Gillies performed a Le Fort III osteotomy for a patient with Crouzon deformity. According to an eyewitness, Gillies's assistant, Stewart Harrison, declared that the operation was too dangerous and that he would never do another. Gillies remained true to his word, and he must have impressed his assistant because Harrison also avoided this area of plastic surgery. It was left to Paul Tessier to make the "breakthrough," literally, into the cranium, and thus in the mid-1960s craniofacial surgery was born. Initially it was the surgical treatment of deformities, but with time the principles of craniofacial surgery have been applied to the treatment of trauma, both the acute incident and the subsequent deformity, and to tumors involving the base of the skull. A totally unexpected development has been the introduction of the craniofacial philosophy into aesthetic surgery. It is these extensions into areas other than deformities that will be most useful to the field of plastic surgery. The theme of this chapter is safety—how to prevent complications and how to give patients the best possible treatment in light of present options and experience.

The Craniofacial Team

To perform the procedures of craniofacial surgery, a well-integrated, complete, and harmonious team is essential. The team consists of many specialist surgeons—a plastic surgeon, a neurosurgeon, a maxillofacial surgeon, an ophthalmic surgeon, an otorhinolaryngologic surgeon, and a neuro-otologic surgeon; dental specialists—a pedodontist, an orthodontist (adult and pediatric), and a prosthodontist; medical specialists—a pediatrician, a geneticist, and an internist; intensive care specialists (adult and pediatric); a speech pathologist; a medical social worker; a photographer; a dietician; and nursing specialists—intensive care nurses, office nurses, ward nurses, and operating room nurses. Without this type of organization, the complex investigations and operative procedures that these patients require cannot be coordinated and performed in an efficient and safe manner.

General Principles
The Timing of Craniofacial Procedures

The decision regarding when a craniofacial intervention should be performed always leads to a great deal of heated discussion. To contemplate and execute early surgical intervention requires a good reason. Early release of craniosynostosis to relieve intracranial pressure and to allow the growing brain to contribute to cranial development is without question a justifiable procedure (Fig. 13-1). With early midface advancement, the ground is less stable. If the eyes require early advancement for protection, there is no question about performing the procedure. To improve the airway is a poor reason because an improvement is unlikely to result. To prevent psychological upset is a dubious reason—the parents are frequently affected psychologically, the child surprisingly rarely, unless the defect is severe. Severe deformities such as a cleft nose or clefts of the face and eyelids are valid indications. Severe maxillary retrusion is an indication, but it has to be accepted that a maxilla with little or no growth potential is being advanced,

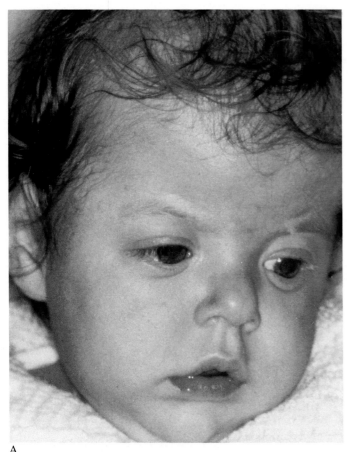

A

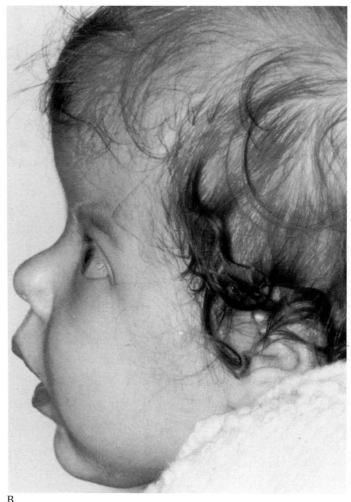

B

Fig. 13-1. *Early release of bilateral craniosynostosis. A, B. Three-month-old child with Crouzon syndrome showing retrusion of frontal and supraorbital areas. C, D. Postoperative result 10 years after correction by frontal advancement with advancement of supraorbital rims and lateral orbital walls using the free-floating forehead technique. E. Serial roentgenograms show the spontaneous advancement of the floating forehead.*

Fig. 13-2. *Early correction of hypertelorism. A C-shaped osteotomy based cranially is used to correct hypertelorism at an early stage. This eliminates injury to tooth buds lying close to the orbital floor.*

and in virtually every patient a high Le Fort I advancement will be necessary later.

Although early correction of hypertelorism may be desirable unless the somewhat fragile C type of osteotomy is designed, the orbits cannot be moved together because of the tooth buds, which lie just under the infraorbital rim (Fig. 13-2). It is better to allow the teeth to descend in the maxilla and later perform the standard osteotomy.

It is helpful to determine, regarding early surgical intervention, how much retardation of growth would be caused by plate fixation. Although the experimental evidence is mixed, it appears that the bone may grow forward, leaving the plate in its original position.

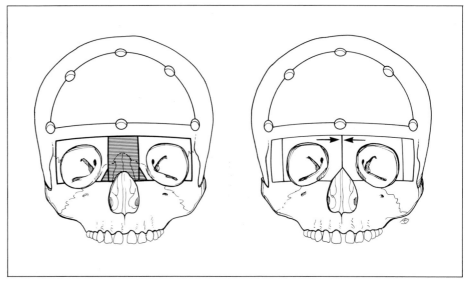

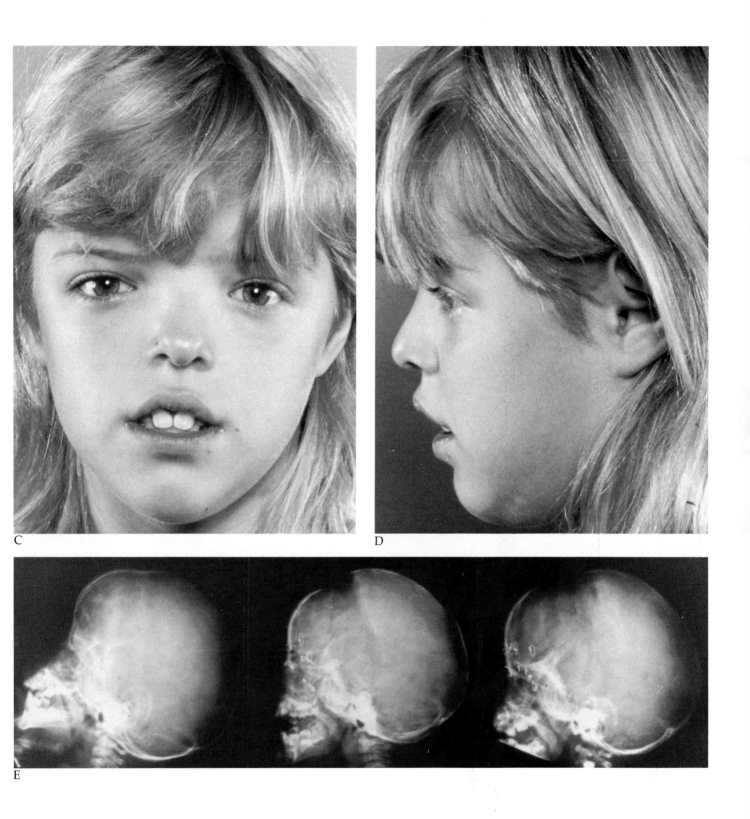

C

D

E

Airway Management

Airway management, another bone of contention, depends greatly on the experience of the surgeon, the anesthesiologist, and the nursing staff. It is interesting to note that in a department inexperienced in dealing with clefts, many of the so-called Pierre Robin babies have tracheostomies and gastrostomies. When the nurses are experienced, there is rarely a need to resort to these drastic and complication-prone maneuvers.

When the maxilla is being moved and intermaxillary fixation is being established, a nasal endotracheal tube is passed; in virtually all other situations an oral tube is inserted. The fiberoptic endoscope has made all the difference in intubation even of patients with difficult deformities such as Treacher Collins syndrome and severe hemifacial microsomia. Rarely in the past did experienced surgeons find it necessary to use tracheostomies; now tracheostomies are almost never used except in emergency situations.

The anesthesiologist and surgeon must be aware of two potential problems during an operation. First, the tube may become displaced unless the surgeon allows for advancement in Le Fort II and III osteotomies. The second problem is that the septal osteotomy in the Le Fort II and III procedures could traumatize the tube. Cut tubes have been reported, which must result from lack of anatomic knowledge combined with carelessness. It should not happen. In the postoperative phase the situation has been made infinitely safer by the use of plates and screws. Intermaxillary fixation can be omitted, and if any relapse occurs the fixation can be replaced later when the potential airway problem has resolved. The endotracheal airway can be left in situ for as long as 10 to 14 days as required; patient tolerance is remarkably good.

Three-dimensional Computed Tomographic Imaging

The technology of imaging is evolving and improving rapidly. In combination with the Biodynamics Research Unit of the Mayo Clinic, I began to use specially designed software (ANALYZE) in 1984; I have progressed to ANALYZE V. The main aim of this software is interaction between the surgeon and the computed tomographic (CT) images produced to allow calculation of distance, area, and volume. In addition, the CT images can be oriented correctly using the Oblique portion of the program. The program also provides the opportunity to perform a mock operation. Exact models of bony defects can be made, but they are of little value in craniofacial surgery at the present time. In the future the value of this technique may be immense.

The CT slices are 1.5 mm thick and are stacked into a three-dimensional image, which is relayed to a Sun workstation for display on a screen. With the correct type of printer, hard copy can be provided, which is used in the operating room, for patient education, for resident education, and to give the referring doctor insight into the plans for reconstruction. In addition to the functions already mentioned, deficiencies or overgrowths in instances of asymmetry can be demonstrated accurately by a technique of mirror imaging, in which the abnormal side is overlaid by the normal side. From this demonstration the osteotomies or onlay bone grafts can be planned. An additional, useful feature is the ability to measure and display the shape and volume of a soft tissue defect. This feature has become important; we know from investigations that the galea vascularized from the superficial temporal vessels can provide 25 to 30 cc of soft tissue for cheek reconstruction. Any volume deficit greater than this amount requires free tissue transfer.

Three-dimensional imaging is most useful in post-traumatic deformities and in complex and rare congenital anomalies. It can provide information about the position and shape of some tumors (Fig. 13-3). There is no indication for the use of this imaging technique as a routine investigation.

Basic Techniques
Coronal Flap

The coronal flap becomes a daily procedure for the craniofacial surgeon and must be performed correctly. The incision is made from ear to ear. Its inferior extension in the preauricular region depends on the extent of the face to be exposed and should be placed as for a standard face-lift. The direction of the hair is examined and the incision is made in that direction to minimize trauma to the hair follicles. After infiltration with 0.5% lidocaine, 1:400,000 epinephrine, and hyaluronidase, the incision is made in stages of 4 to 5 cm. Raney clips are placed over the front edge of the incision, which is augmented with a folded sponge, and Dandy forceps are placed posteriorly on the galea at regular intervals. In this way there is little or no blood loss at this point in the procedure (Fig. 13-4).

The flap is raised above the periosteum down to within 1 to 2 cm of the supraorbital rim; the periosteum is incised transversely at this point. The subperiosteal dissection is continued downward, over the supraorbital rims, and along the orbital roof. When the supraorbital nerves and vessels course through a small foramen, the roof of the foramen is cut with a fine osteotome and is removed. Laterally, with a Farabeuf periosteal elevator, the innominate, or subgaleal, fascia is swept off the deep temporal fascia. From the face side, a finger is placed on the lateral orbital rim. When this structure is located, a vertical incision is made through the periosteum of the rim, which is elevated over the lateral rim to be continued under the periorbita. The dissection proceeds down to the zygomatic arch, where the periosteum is incised along its upper edge.

It is now possible to elevate the periosteum over the anterior face of the maxilla down to the gingival attachment inferiorly and to the pyriform aperture medially; the floor of the orbit and the infraorbital rim can be exposed. In the midline the periosteum and the galea of the flap are incised vertically. The edges of this incision are spread apart with a scissors, and a great increase in exposure is obtained. The periosteum is now elevated down to the edge of the pyriform aperture, and the nasal mucosa can be dissected from the undersurface of the nasal bones. The medial wall of the orbit is dissected subperiosteally and meets the inferior dissection from the lateral side. This maneuver is also done over the maxilla. The medial canthal ligament may or may not be detached.

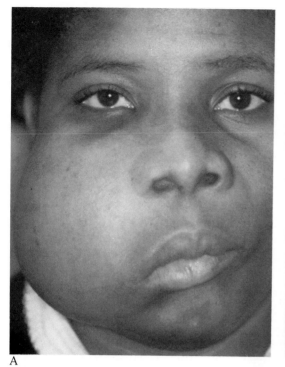

A

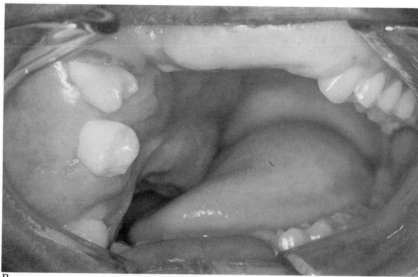

B

Fig. 13-3. Three-dimensional CT imaging. A. Patient with multiple recurrent fibrous dysplasia of right maxilla transgressing the midline. B. Intraoral aspect of the tumor. C. The fibrous dysplasia appears green; the oblique program has been used to return to the original CT scan and have an accurate estimation of tumor extension in the axial, sagittal, and coronal planes.

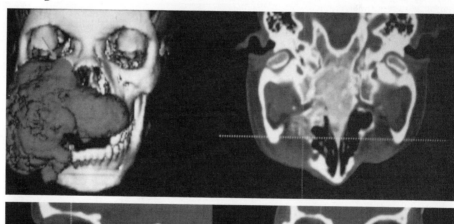

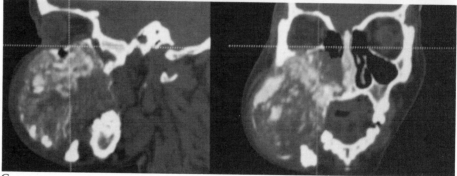

C

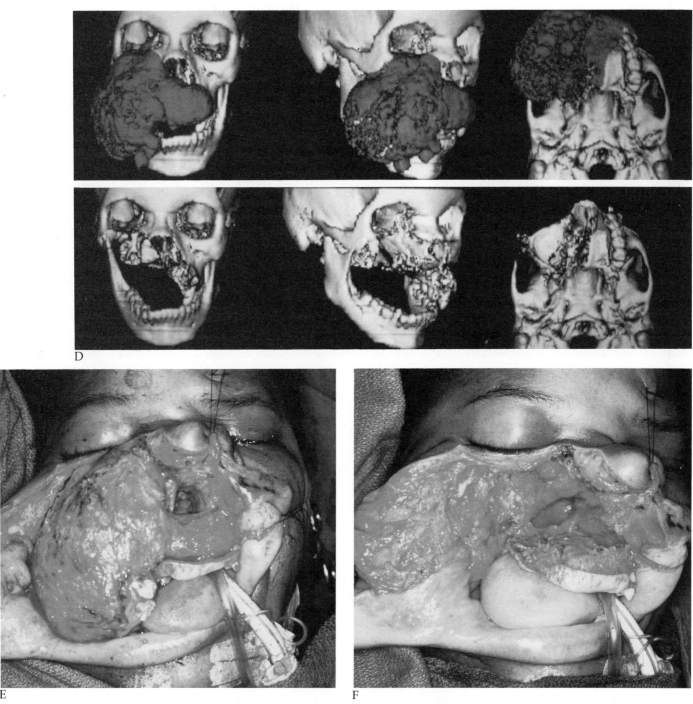

Fig. 13-3. (Continued) D. The tumor may be viewed from any aspect by manipulation on the computer workstation screen. A simulated resection of the lesion has been performed, as illustrated on the lower row of reformatted images. E. Approach through a Weber-Fergusson incision, which gave excellent exposure of the lesion. F. Resection has been completed. G. Postoperative results, 6 months after the operation.

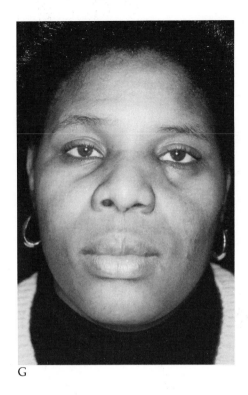

G

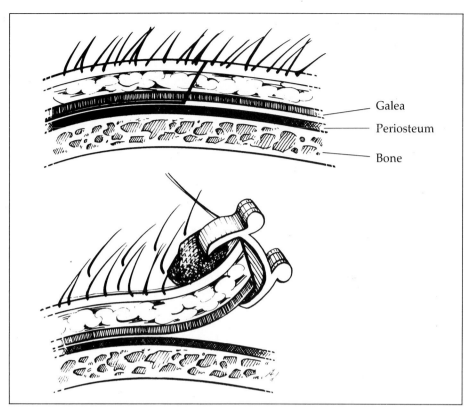

Galea

Periosteum

Bone

Fig. 13-4. Coronal flap illustrating correct application of Raney clips to the anterior edge of the coronal incision. Note that the scalp is protected with gauze under the teeth of the Raney clip.

Management of the Temporalis Muscle

Management of the temporalis muscle is part of the craniofacial procedure and should not be left to the neurosurgeon. The pericranium is incised in the sagittal line and along the edge of the coronal incision. A Farabeuf elevator and irrigation are used to elevate the pericranium down to the temporal crest. The muscle is stripped off the temporal bone, the lateral orbital wall, and the lateral orbital rim as required.

When the procedure is completed, the temporalis muscle is returned to the fossa. When the fossa is altered in either size or position, as in correction of Crouzon syndrome or hypertelorism, the muscle position must be changed. The muscle is mobilized by a vertical incision through the deep temporal fascia in the posterior area; this allows the muscle to be shifted as required. Holes are drilled in the zygomatic arch, the lateral orbital rim, and the temporal crest. Through these holes the muscle is sutured into the correct position with nonabsorbable material. In the

lateral orbital wall it is especially important to advance the muscle in such a way that it comes to lie in the concavity behind the lateral edge of the rim; otherwise a visible hollow will occur when the postoperative swelling resolves. If stretching of the muscle is required, the deep temporal fascia is incised vertically with multiple parallel incisions (Fig. 13-5).

Plate and Screw Fixation

Although they have been used on the facial skeleton for the past 25 years, plates and screws only recently have become standard in craniofacial surgery. There is now a plethora of designs: miniplates, microplates, intermediate plates, compression plates, and self-tapping and non-self-tapping screws with a variety of screw head designs. Most of these are unnecessary in the upper face. Here the surgeon needs two sizes of plates—microplates and miniplates—and screws with standard heads; even simpler would be a universal intermediate plating set small enough and strong enough for all purposes. The argument regarding various

types of metal is irrelevant. Computed tomography (CT) and magnetic resonance imaging (MRI) can be used with all the available plates, and none need to be removed unless the surgeon has an unusual motive for doing so. Plates and screws greatly speed up procedures, especially if the concept of "side table" assembly is used; in this situation parts of the procedure are performed on the patient while the portions of bone that were removed are reassembled by a colleague on a side table. The finished reconstruction is delivered with the edge plates applied, and thus it can be inserted and stabilized quickly (Fig. 13-6).

The element of stability provided by plates and screws has in many ways been the key to the advancement of techniques in craniofacial surgery. Multiple portions of bone in trauma or skull contouring can be put together accurately, and exposure osteotomies in tumor operations and advancement osteotomies for congenital deformities can be fixed with less chance of relapse. The plates must be applied accurately, or malpositioning of fragments will occur. Onlay bone grafts can be sta-

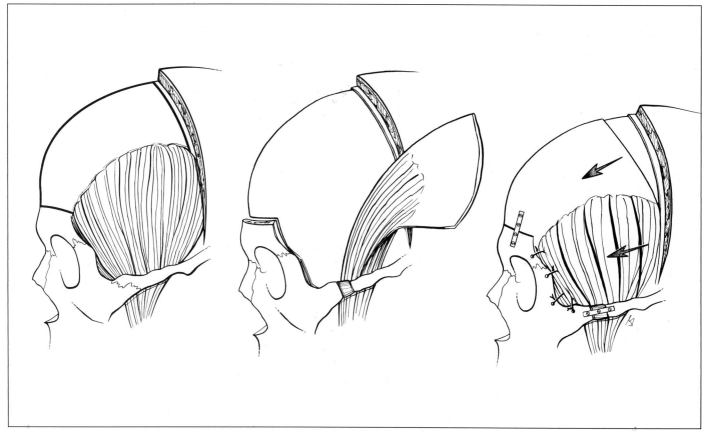

Fig. 13-5. *Reposition of temporalis muscle after orbital advancement. After the orbit has been advanced and fixed, the temporalis muscle is moved forward and sutured to the lateral orbital rim through drill holes. It is important that the muscle be brought behind the rim of the lateral orbital wall; otherwise there will be retraction, and a concavity will appear in this area. Should the muscle be tight, the deep temporal fascia is scored to allow anterior expansion.*

bilized with lag screws and contoured in situ. Inlay bone grafts can be screwed onto an existing plate in the precise anatomic position, as for lateral orbital wall defects. It seems likely that solid fixation and good graft adaptation to underlying bone leads to less resorption. The complications of plates and screws are few; occasionally they may be felt or seen, but rarely do they become infected unless a screw has become loose. Removal is performed as indicated, but this is rare. Usually it is only the involved screw that needs to be removed.

Galeal Frontalis Musculofascial Flap

The galeal frontalis musculofascial flap is based on the supraorbital and supratrochlear vessels; it consists of the frontalis muscle and the galea. The flap can be raised as a broad flap with a bilateral blood supply, as a narrow flap, or as two narrow flaps. The longest possible length of the flap is as yet undetermined. This flap is highly vascularized and has saved the lives of many of our patients by preventing intracranial infection when the cranial base is resected in continuity with the nasopharyngeal area. After it is raised, the flap is placed in the floor of the anterior cranial fossa and is stabilized by sutures through drill holes to the edge of any bony defect (Fig. 13-7). It also has been used successfully to cover free bone grafts in the skull base and medial orbital wall. For the 11 years in which this flap has been used, there have been no serious infections reported resulting from an extradural nasopharyngeal connection.

Fig. 13-6. *Side table assembly. A. Exposure required for resection of extensive meningioma of the sphenoid wing. B. Removed fragments of bone: frontotemporal, supraorbital, lateral orbital wall. C. Side table assembly. D. Reinsertion of reassembled osteotomies.* ▶

Canthopexy

Lateral

The lateral canthal tendon is an indefinite concentration of periorbita that has a close connection to the overlying canthal area. After it has been detached it can be found by trial and error, and picked up with a fine hemostat. When it has been identified, in spite of widespread periorbital freeing, the tendon may not move as much as is necessary. This situation can be improved by releasing the tendon from any tight periorbita inferiorly using sharp pointed scissors.

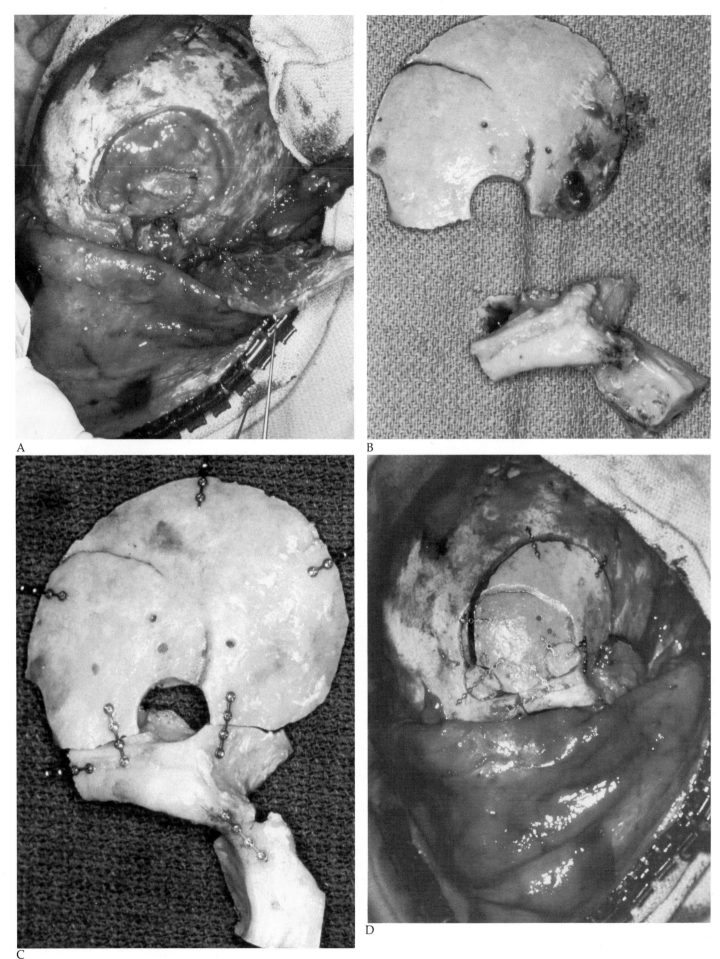

A

B

C

D

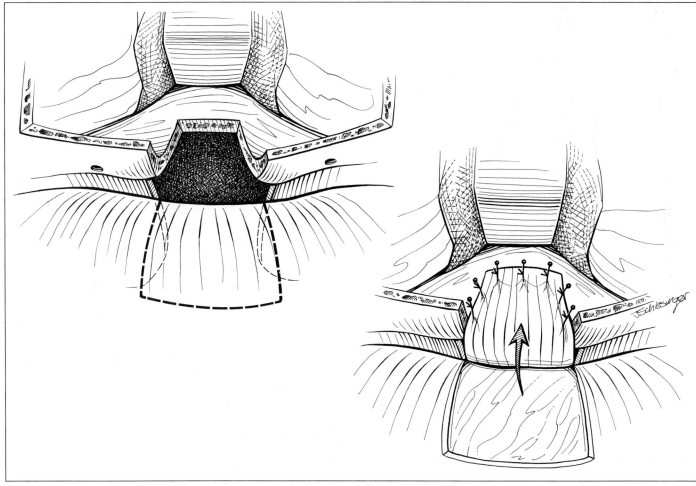

Fig. 13-7. Galeal frontalis musculofascial flap. The raising of the galeal frontalis musculofascial flap is shown, including how it is inserted to close off a defect in the anterior cranial fossa. The flap prevents a nasopharyngeal-extradural connection.

The area of insertion is in the upper third of the lateral orbital wall. Two holes are drilled and a wire cut to a point is passed through one of them; the wire is passed twice through the tendon and tightened (Fig. 13-8A). At this point, by pulling on the wires, the accuracy of the wire placement can be assessed. If the placement is correct, the wire is taken through the second hole and tightened on the outside of the lateral orbital rim, bringing the canthal tendon into its correct position on the medial aspect of the rim. A slight overcorrection in terms of the cranial position of the ligament is planned.

Medial

There have been many problems associated with medial canthopexy, and the results have been variable. The problems have been caused by the traditional method of doing the procedure. Traditionally, the wires have been taken from one medial orbital wall to the other, because there is no solid bone to tighten onto; various types of supporting toggles have been used, including rolled-up wire and bone—a truly unsatisfactory mechanical situation.

The foolproof method is to make a hole for the medial canthal tendon just above and behind the posterior lacrimal crest (see Fig. 13-8B). From the thick bone of the nasal process of the frontal bone, two drill holes are made down to the hole on the medial orbital wall; this is performed bilaterally. A sharp pointed wire is double-looped through the canthal tendon; it is tightened and pulled on to check that the position is correct. A Keith needle is backed through the holes and the wire pulled out; the wire is then tightened onto

the thick frontal bone. This procedure can be performed bilaterally, and if the tendon has been identified accurately, the correction should be successful and permanent. Caution is necessary when the dura dips downward because of a low-lying cribriform plate; the drill or the wire could tear the dura.

Use of the Temporal Galea

The temporal galea is supplied by the superficial temporal vessels. The vascularity is axial until the sagittal suture, but beyond that it becomes random. There is an extensive anterior and posterior vascularization resulting from anastomotic connections with the occipital and frontal vessels. Because of its length and volume and by recruitment from the occipital area, the galea can be used as a filling material in the cheek, a cover for the anterior

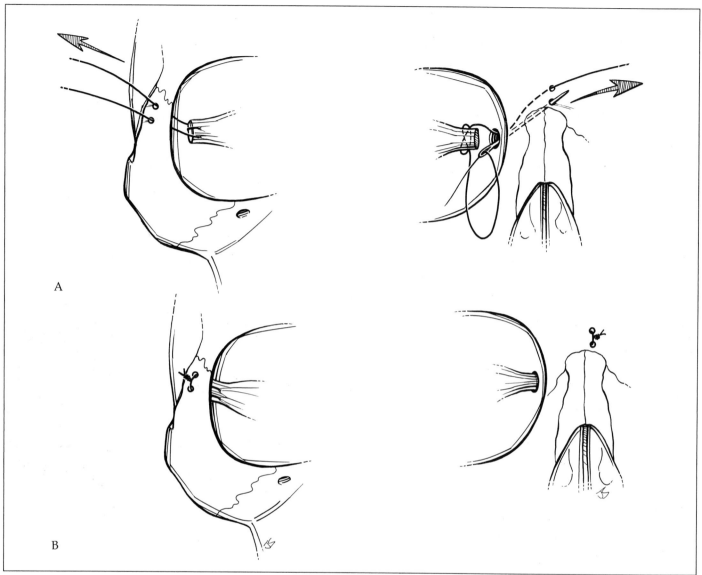

A

B

Fig. 13-8. Lateral and medial canthopexy. A. The important points are the double looping of the wires through the lateral canthal ligament and the positioning of the lateral canthal ligament on the medial aspect of the lateral orbital rim. B. The wire is double-looped through the medial canthal tendon and a Keith needle is placed retrogradely through the drilled tunnels to pick up the wire and bring it out in the glabellar area. The drill holes are placed so that the wire can be tightened onto solid bone and the canthal tendon brought into its position in a drill hole just behind the posterior lacrimal crest.

cranial fossa, and for the orbit, the ear, and the oral cavity. It can carry vascularized cranial bone.

It becomes important to preserve the superficial temporal vessels if there is any possibility of future use of vascularized galea. As in the galeal frontalis musculofascial flap, this material has been used to separate the nasopharynx and the anterior cranial fossa when the galeal frontalis flap has not been available (Fig. 13-9).

Cranial Bone Grafts

Cranial bone is said to show minimal resorption when used as a graft for the facial skeleton—it is membranous bone placed on membranous bone—especially when

rigid fixation is used. Additional advantages are that the donor site is already exposed; thus there is no extra scar and no pain caused by graft harvesting. The disadvantages are that it is hard and unyielding, except in infants, in whom it can be bent. When any portion is infected or exposed, the whole fragment of bone must be removed. There may be serious complications during harvesting, which have not been emphasized enough. Inadvertent full-thickness harvest and dural tears may occur and can be dealt with easily. Eminently more serious complications are brain damage from an osteotome and intracerebral hemorrhage, possibly from the transmitted forces of hammering and unrecognized intradural and extradural bleeding. This bleeding has led to

Fig. 13-9. Use of a temporal galeal flap. A. Patient had a frontal abscess after resection of a tumor of the anterior cranial fossa and destruction of the frontal soft tissue; therefore, a galeal frontalis musculofascial flap was not available. The connection between the extradural space and the nasopharynx can be clearly seen. B. Temporal galeal flap is raised, based on superficial temporal vessels. C. Flap easily comes to the midline of the floor of the anterior cranial fossa. D. The temporal galeal flap is sutured into the floor of the anterior cranial fossa, effectively closing the nasopharyngeal-extradural connection.

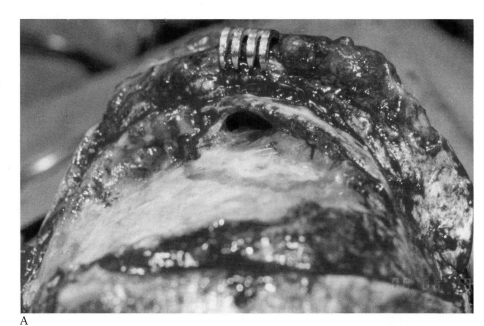

A

hemiplegia, aphasia, and prolonged coma. When these complications occur, the surgeons concerned usually are inexperienced. In my own large series, there have been no serious complications. Harvesting from skull overlying the nondominant hemisphere and over the parietal area is strongly recommended to avoid complications. Any surgeon who wishes to do this procedure should work with a craniofacial surgeon, try the procedure on a cadaver, and initially get some help from a neurosurgeon.

There are four types of cranial grafts—split-thickness, full-thickness, shaving grafts, and bone dust (Fig. 13-10). In thin skulls and when thick bone is required, a split graft should not be used—harvesting is too dangerous. A full-thickness graft is taken using a standard neurosurgical craniotomy technique or by gradually exposing the dura around the edge of the graft with a contouring bur. A split graft is taken by contouring down to the inner table and removing lateral bone; the skull to be taken sits up like an island. This allows an osteotome to be placed at the correct angle, and gentle tapping will allow it to proceed safely through the diploë and produce a good bone graft. Shaving grafts are produced with an osteotome in a manner similar to shaving wood. For those more mechanically minded, an air-driven instrument called a Micro-Impactor (Zimmer/Berger Associates, Inc., 2311 Shelby St. Suite 106, Ann Arbor, MI 48103) can be used. If the pericranium is left on, the grafts curl and provide excellent lining for the orbit. Bone dust is produced using the craniotome. The drill and the dust must be kept cool for osteoblasts to remain viable. Bone

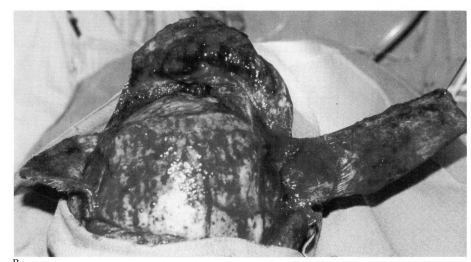

B

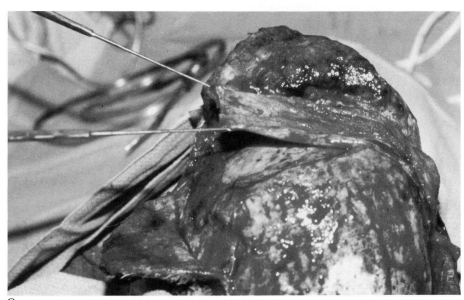

C

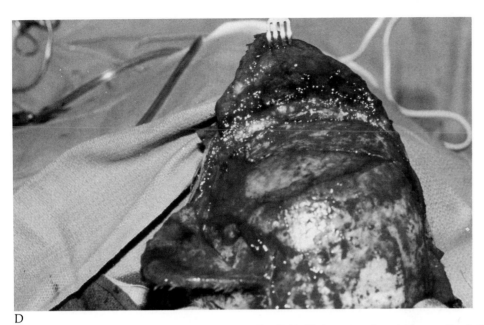

D

Fig. 13-10. *Various types of cranial bone grafts. A. Full-thickness graft may be harvested using bur holes and a drill or a Gigli saw to connect the bur holes and remove the full-thickness slab of cranial bone. B. The craniotome can be used to generate bone dust, which is collected and used to fill defects. C. A split skull graft is prepared by producing a gutter around the desired area of bone and removing bone lateral to that with an air drill. The osteotome must be placed into the diploë in such a way that the inner table is not penetrated. D. Shaving grafts can be taken with the Micro-Impactor or with a curved or straight osteotome.*

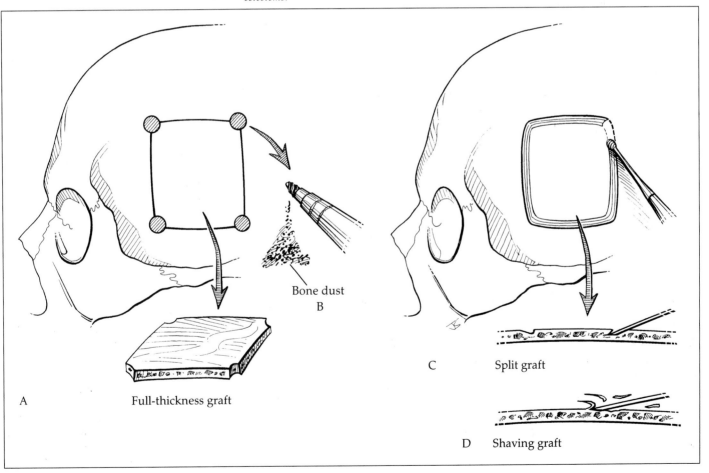

Bone dust
B

A   Full-thickness graft

C   Split graft

D   Shaving graft

dust provides excellent packing material and is frequently used to fill skull defects. Cranial bone is a wonderful material, but a cavalier attitude to its harvest is to be deprecated.

Use of Alloplastic Material

Several alloplastic materials are available. Silicone is virtually never used by bona fide craniofacial surgeons. Polytetrafluoro-ethylene-graphite has been useful in the past when placed deep in the orbit, but the United States Food and Drug Administration has banned this substance. Hydroxyapatite, also is used increasingly in granular form to correct contour defects; however, its use in the solid form at present is somewhat limited to reducing orbital volume. The most useful material is the one that has been around longest, namely, methyl methacrylate. Only the material for hip joint fixation should be used. This substance is practical for onlay contouring and is mainly applied to the frontal skull and temporal area. In the temporal region it is safely placed under the temporalis muscle. The important points in using methyl methacrylate are to have a well-vascularized skin cover and to fix the onlay securely into precarved ridges or holes. When methyl methacrylate is applied carefully, complications are rare, and the result is absolutely satisfactory without resorption.

Craniosynostosis

Premature fusion of the cranial sutures may occur in any location and in any number, ranging from one to all sutures. There is raised intracranial pressure, the severity of which is related to the number of sutures involved. The sequelae of this rise in pressure include visual deterioration, which is beyond dispute, and mental deterioration, which is impossible to prove. In some patients there may be an associated hydrocephalus. Premature fusion occurs, in decreasing frequency: sagittal, coronal (unilateral), coronal (bilateral), metopic, lambdoid sutures, and kleeblattschädel. The reason for surgical intervention in most instances is aesthetic. Occasionally on fundal examination there may be disk swelling or atrophy with or without visual deterioration. Total suture involvement is an indication for surgical treatment in its own right. In-

vestigations include roentgenograms of the face and skull, CT (in some complicated instances three-dimensional (3D) CT is of value), an ophthalmic examination, and a psychological assessment. If possible, the deformity should be measured in relation to a contralateral normal area or to what is considered a "normal" face in bilateral involvement.

Although surgical corrections have been done in children as young as one week, 3 to 6 months is probably the optimal age. It goes without saying that this operation is a joint venture between craniofacial surgeons and neurosurgeons. At times the neurosurgeon decides that the patient should have a shunt placed before any reconstructive procedure is done, because correction of the deformity in the presence of untreated hydrocephalus may result in serious complications.

Sagittal Craniosynostosis (Scaphocephaly)

Sagittal craniosynostosis is often corrected by a neurosurgeon alone, but complex deformities require a team approach. A coronal incision is made in the scalp from ear to ear, and the flaps are peeled anteriorly and posteriorly. A strip of cranium 2 cm wide is taken along the sagittal line, with care taken not to injure the sagittal sinus. This traditional method of suture release may be effective in minor deformities. In most patients it is best to make anterior and posterior coronal craniotomies just behind the coronal and just in front of the lambdoid sutures. Both parietal bones can be pried laterally and loosened, that is, hinged inferiorly. The bones are left loose so that the head can be expanded transversely. When the deformity is more severe, the anterior cranial fossa is narrowed and the upper parts of the orbits are rotated posteriorly; the rotation is maximal in the lateral area. A total correction of this deformity requires a fronto-orbital osteotomy with a midline vertical cut and an anterior rotation of the lateral part of the frontal bone and orbital segments to flatten the forehead and thus widen it and correct the orbital rotation. This part of the operation requires plate and screw fixation (Fig. 13-11). The scalp is closed with or without drains depending on the surgeon's preference. Antibiotics are given during the procedure and for 48 hours afterward. The child leaves the hospital in 4 to 5 days.

Unilateral Coronal Craniosynostosis (Plagiocephaly)

In unilateral coronal craniosynostosis the sphenoid wing is involved, the fronto-supraorbital region is retruded and rotated posteriorly on a medial hinge, and the orbit is misshapen and contracted, as is the temporal fossa. This is a more complex deformity than was first thought, in that more basal sutures such as the sphenozygomatic are also involved, which results in varying degrees of sphenoid wing contracture. The approach is by a coronal flap. The whole frontal bone is removed because there may be protrusion on the contralateral side. The orbit is measured transversely and compared with the normal orbit; it is frequently contracted between 0.5 and 1.0 cm. The supraorbital rim, part of the roof, lateral rim, lateral orbital wall, and a portion of the zygoma are removed as a single segment. If the orbit is contracted, the supraorbital rim and roof are divided in the midline, and a cranial bone graft of the required size is inserted and stabilized with a microplate. When this is done the correction of the rim curvature is adjusted to match that of the other side using a stout wire or long miniplate as a template. When an osteotomy is not necessary, a series of cuts are made in the orbital roof, and the supraorbital rim is shaped with bone benders; again, the use of a template is advised. The orbital segment is placed in position, aligned correctly with the normal side, and fixed with a microplate or wire. A similar fixation is applied at the zygomatic region.

The frontal bone may be handled in two different ways. In mild-to-moderate deformities, it can be turned 180° so that the flat area is under the hair. It is fixed to the frontal area with microplates; there is no other fixation to the posterior stable skull. If there is undue instability, polyglactin 910 sutures can be used to give fixation. The sutures are placed through drill holes in strategic areas. When the deformity is more severe or if the surgeon prefers, the frontal bone may be bent after the cuts have been made in it; again, bone benders are used. Others prefer to cut the skull into pieces, bend them, and reassemble the fragments with microplates to give an ideal frontal area—admirable but time consuming and tedious. The subject of

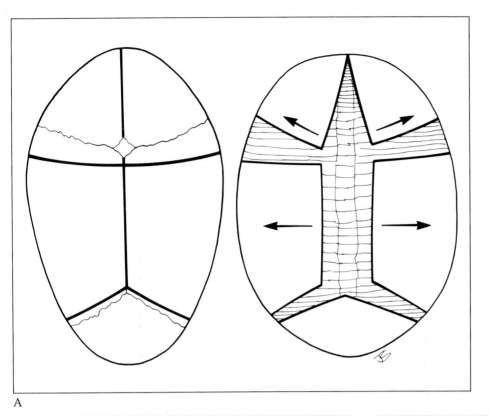

A

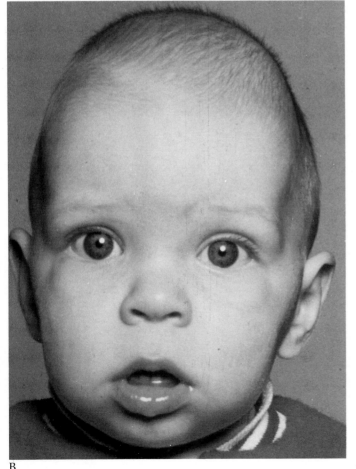

B

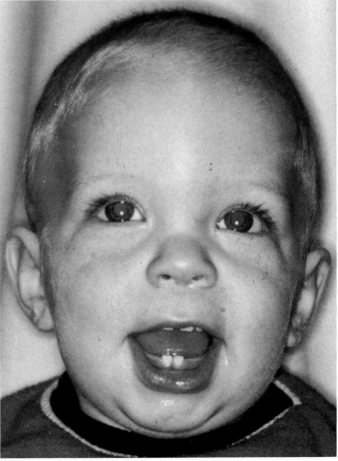

C

Fig. 13-11. Correction of sagittal craniosynostosis. A. Diagram of the expansion of the anterior cranial fossa and derotation of orbits with standard expansion in temporoparietal area. B. Preoperative appearance. C. Postoperative appearance.

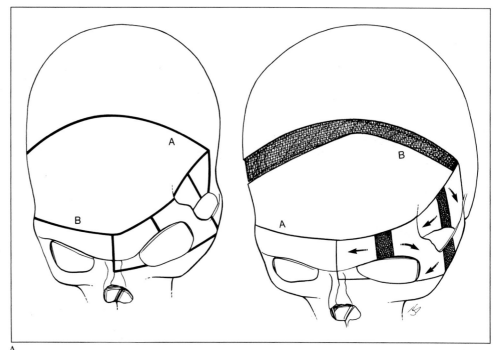

Fig. 13-12. Correction of unilateral coronal craniosynostosis. A. Diagram of the bone cuts made to correct severe unilateral coronal craniosynostosis. The orbit is expanded and advanced to be symmetric with that of the other side. The middle cranial fossa is expanded both anteriorly and laterally to release the sphenoid wing. The frontal bone flap may be reversed to obtain frontal symmetry. This is illustrated by the change in points A and B. B. Preoperative appearance. C. Postoperative appearance.

A

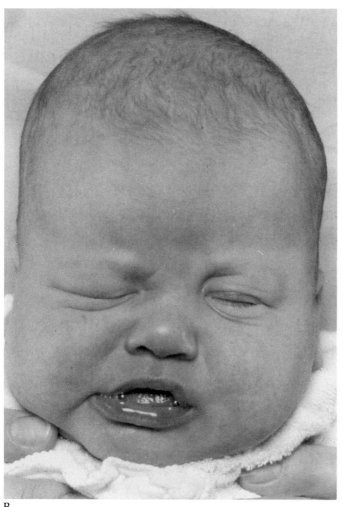

B

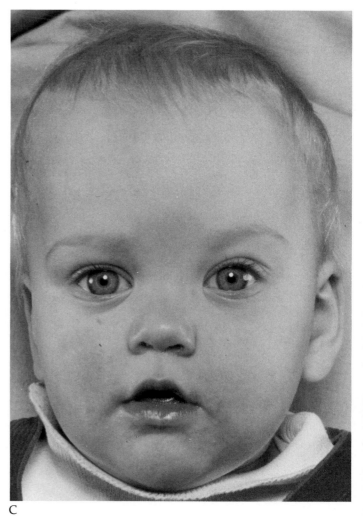

C

posterior stabilization is a matter for debate, and only time will tell which method is correct—at the moment it seems to make little or no difference. Scalp closure is performed in the standard way. Lately there has been more effort to release the basal sutures and to expand the middle cranial fossa to release the constricted temporal fossa. This procedure involves removing the temporal region down to the zygomatic arch. The bone is reshaped correctly by bending or osteotomies and is held in position with microplates and returned to the temporal defect. Basically the bone is released from the constricting forces of the sphenoid wing (Fig. 13-12).

Bilateral Coronal Craniosynostosis (Oxycephaly, Brachycephaly)

Frequently bilateral coronal craniosynostosis is associated with a syndrome such as Crouzon or Apert. In some ways this condition is easier to correct than unilateral coronal craniosynostosis. The flat supraorbital rim and lateral orbital walls are divided with an osteotome and shaped into the desired curvature, as described for the unilateral deformity (Fig. 13-13). This segment is advanced by at least 2 cm and fixed with microplates. When necessary, the shallow lateral orbital walls are rearranged using an anterior vertical osteotomy and moving the walls medially through 90°. It may be possible to effect the correct contour of the forehead by turning the frontal bone around 180° and fixing it to the supraorbital rim with microplates. Because of the anteroposterior reduction of the frontal area, the middle cranial fossa is enlarged laterally. To achieve correction the bulging lateral wall of the middle cranial fossa is removed, reversed, or recontoured by bending or osteotomies and fixed. When this procedure is performed bilaterally, a reduction in the width of the middle cranial fossa of 2 to 2.5 cm is achieved and is permanent (see Fig. 13-13). The midface can be moved forward by modifications of the maxillary osteotomies. This is not difficult to do, but stabilization can be a problem, and the gain, if any, must be weighed against the potential complications. There may or may not be posterior stabilization of the cranio-orbital complex.

Metopic Craniosynostosis (Trigonocephaly)

In metopic craniosynostosis the degree of constriction of the anterior cranial fossa is variable. There is a midline ridge, and the frontal bones and the orbits are rotated laterally; there is hypotelorism. The standard coronal flap approach is used. The frontal bone is removed as are the supraorbital rims and lateral orbital walls. In mild deformities a midline osteotomy is made and the angulation of the frontal bones and orbits is corrected as described for correction of severe scaphocephaly; no attempt is made to address the slight hypotelorism.

In more severe deformities the midline osteotomy is used to widen the anterior cranial fossa and to correct the hypotelorism (Fig. 13-14). The separated bone fragments are fixed with microplates. The central gap may or may not be bone grafted depending on the surgeon's preference. The coronal flap is closed as described previously. Some surgeons have used bone from elsewhere on the skull to reconstruct the forehead; this increases operating time and is unnecessary.

Pansuture Craniosynostosis (Microcephaly)

When all sutures are fused, they are all released, and bone fragments are rearranged or moved as indicated.

Kleeblattschädel

Kleeblattschädel is a complex and variable deformity that requires careful planning with release of involved bone segments for correction. Midface advancement is usually required at a later date.

Isolated Lambdoid Craniosynostosis

Isolated lambdoid craniosynostosis may be unilateral or bilateral, as in coronal craniosynostosis, and is handled in approximately the same way.

Hypertelorism

In hypertelorism the orbits are too far apart. This condition should not be confused with telecanthus, in which the orbits are in the correct position but the medial walls are too far apart. This distinction is important because it prevents an unnecessary orbital shift operation for telecanthus.

The cause of hypertelorism may be a midline cleft, an adjacent cleft, or an encephalocele. There is a true excessive separation of the orbits with enlargement of the ethmoid sinuses. The treatment is to resect the central area and move the orbits together. In clefting deformities the nose is grossly deformed and short, whereas in encephaloceles the nose is often long, as are the medial orbital walls.

Extracranial Approach

An extracranial approach is rarely indicated except in minor deformities. Through a coronal flap approach the orbits and upper maxilla are dissected subperiosteally. The orbital roofs are kept intact. The central nasal segment is resected, and osteotomies are performed on the medial and lateral orbital walls and the orbital floor. The resulting C-shaped orbital osteotomy is moved medially to correct the deformity (Fig. 13-15).

Intracranial Approach

A coronal flap is used for exposure, and the dissection is taken to the zygomatic arch, across the front of the maxilla and around the orbit, totally freeing the orbital contents. The nasal periosteum is freed from the nasal bones and the walls of the pyriform aperture. A frontal craniotomy is performed to allow retraction of the frontal lobes; the central bone is resected with preservation of the nasal mucosa. The contents of the ethmoid sinus and the bone of the anterior cranial fossa floor are resected lateral to the cribriform plates. One osteotomy is made transversely across the frontal area maintaining a frontal bar between the orbit and the frontal defect. The osteotomy is taken into the temporal area down the lateral orbital wall and across the maxilla under the infraorbital nerve to the pyriform aperture. The orbits are mobilized and plated together; the lateral orbital wall is bone grafted and stabilized with plates.

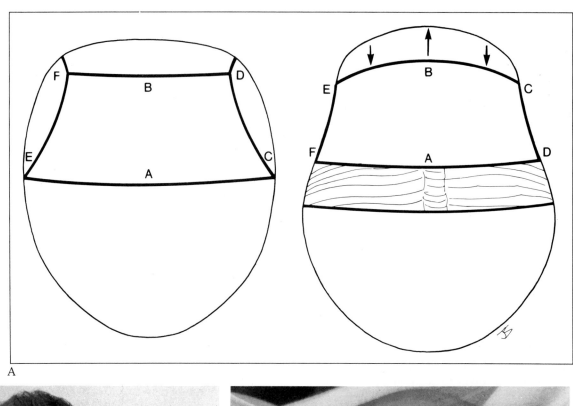

A

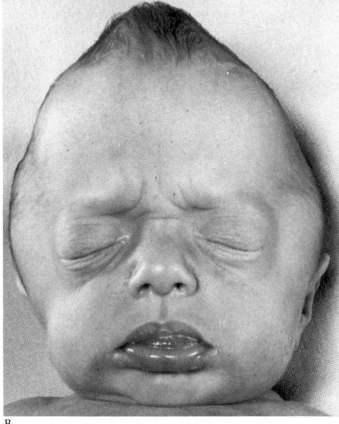

B

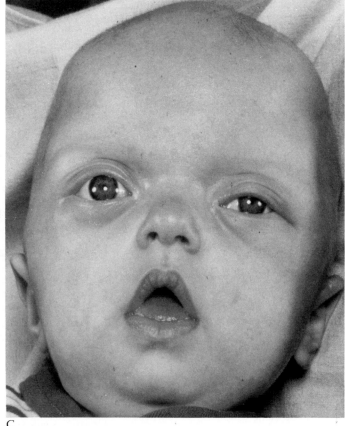

C

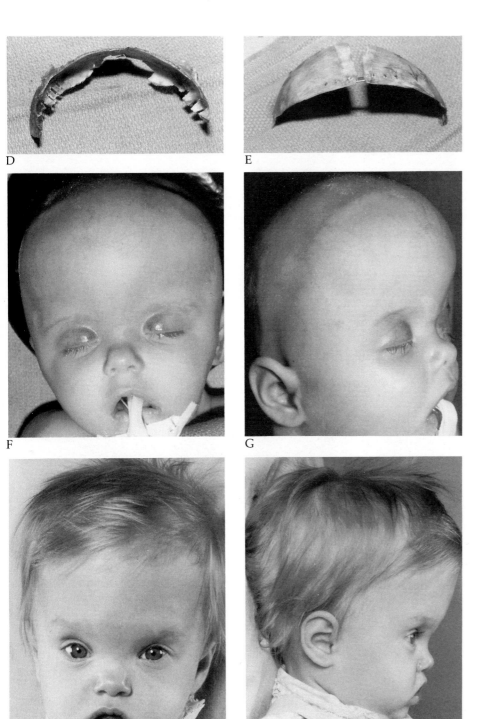

Fig. 13-13. Early correction of bicoronal craniosynostosis. A. Diagram of the advancement of the supraorbital rims and the forehead with a 180° rotation of the expanded temporal bones to produce a reduction in the volume of the middle cranial fossa and a narrowing of the transverse diameter of the skull in this area. This is illustrated by the changes in points C and D and E and F. B. Severe bicoronal craniosynostosis with considerable increase in intertemporal skull width. C. Appearance after fronto-orbital advancement, skull recontouring, and decrease in intertemporal skull width by 180° rotation of temporoparietal area. D. The flattened supraorbital rim can be bent into the correct shape after barrel staving of the sphenoid wings. The barrel staving cuts can be seen clearly on either side of the supraorbital rim before reinsertion. E. The frontal area is rearranged to fit accurately to the supraorbital rim. F, G. Bilateral coronal craniosynostosis with severe constriction of the supraorbital rim. H, I. Correction by method illustrated in D and E.

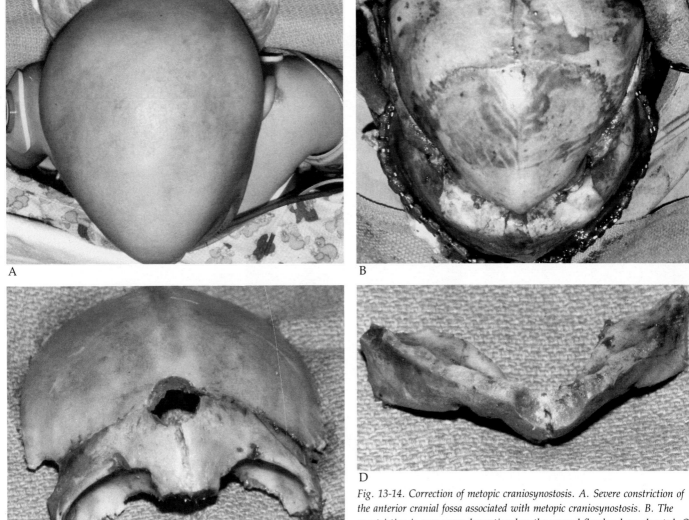

A

B

C

D

Fig. 13-14. Correction of metopic craniosynostosis. A. Severe constriction of the anterior cranial fossa associated with metopic craniosynostosis. B. The constriction is even more dramatic when the coronal flap has been elevated. C. Removed constricted frontal bone and supraorbital rims with lateral walls of the orbit. D. The constriction of the supraorbital rims is clearly seen. E. Osteotomy of supraorbital rims and frontal bones. F. Expansion of anterior cranial fossa by repositioning of the frontal bones, supraorbital rims, and lateral orbital walls. The floating forehead technique was used. G. Preoperative appearance. H. Postoperative result.

The pyriform aperture is enlarged, and the nose is reconstructed with bone grafts and by rearrangement of soft tissue. If there is a connection between the nasal cavity and the extradural space, a galeal frontalis musculofascial flap is inserted. The frontal bone is replaced and the coronal incision is closed (Fig. 13-16).

In instances of hypertelorism in which a vertical bony deficiency in the midline causes a central anterior open bite, the more extensive procedure of facial bipartition is indicated. In this operation, a central wedge of bone based cranially is removed; the palate is split in the midline. Instead of the standard osteotomies for correction of hypertelorism, cuts are made in the lateral orbit and retrotuberosity as for a Le Fort III osteotomy. The two separate halves of the face are mobilized and rotated in a way that corrects the orbital hypertelorism and levels the occlusion (Fig. 13-17). In patients with associated midface retrusion, the maxilla can be advanced. The presence of a cleft lip and palate, either unilateral or bilateral, makes facial bipartition an easier procedure. Asymmetric hypertelorism is corrected using whatever design of osteotomy is indicated; these operations may be complex (Fig. 13-18).

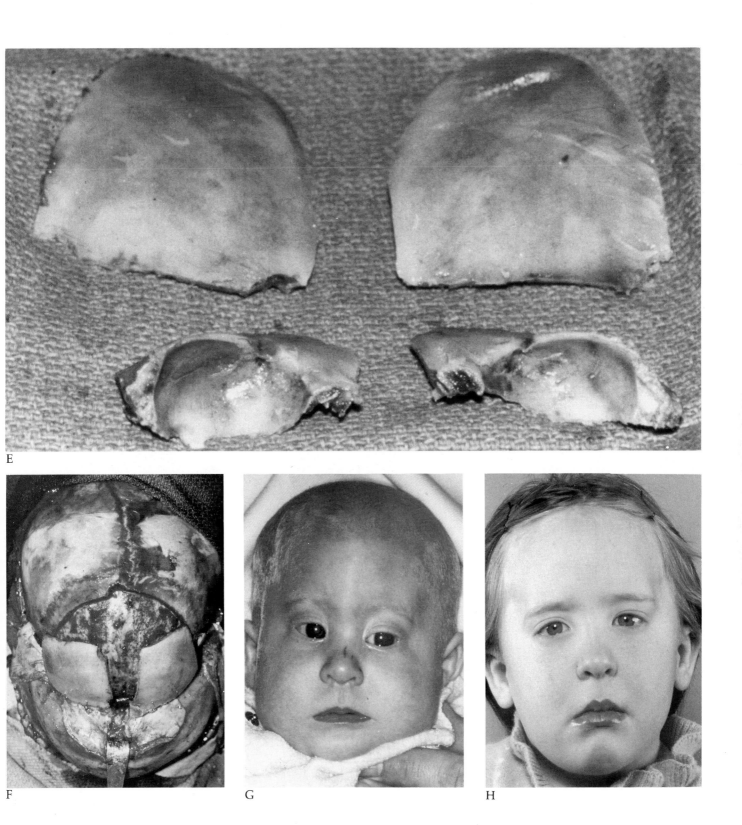

E

F

G

H

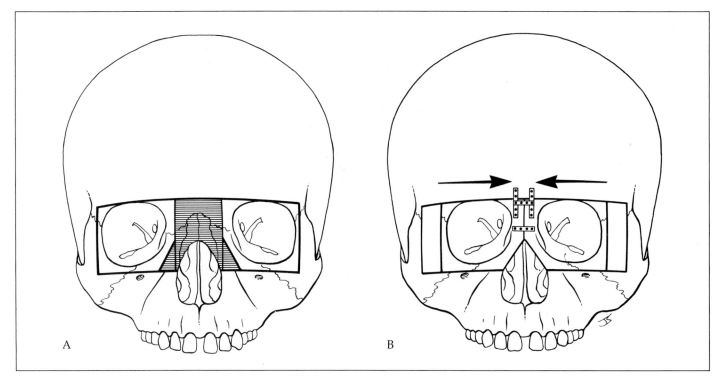

Fig. 13-15. Extracranial approach to hypertelorism. A. A *C*-shaped osteotomy based caudally can be used to move the orbits together once the central segment has been resected. B. Lateral bone grafts inserted.

Fig. 13-16. Intracranial approach to correction of hypertelorism. A. Total orbital shift medially following resection of central segment. A sagittal split of the lateral orbital walls is shown; more commonly, the entire orbital wall is moved medially. B. Symmetric hypertelorism. C. Appearance 23 years after original operation.

A

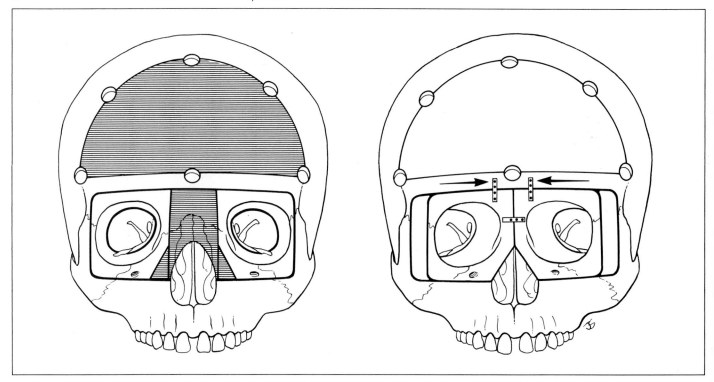

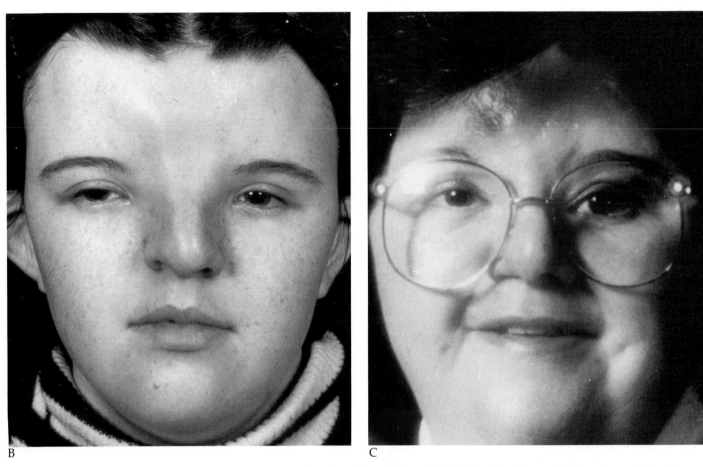

B   C

Fig. 13-17. Correction of hypertelorism with facial bipartition. The method of carrying out the facial bipartition to correct hypertelorism and rotational deformities of the midface and orbits with leveling of the occlusal plane is shown.

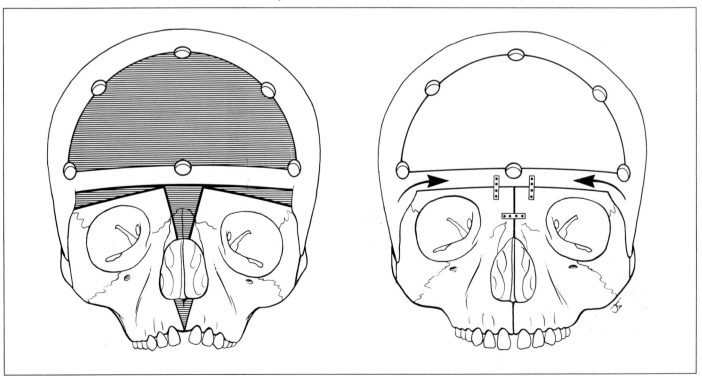

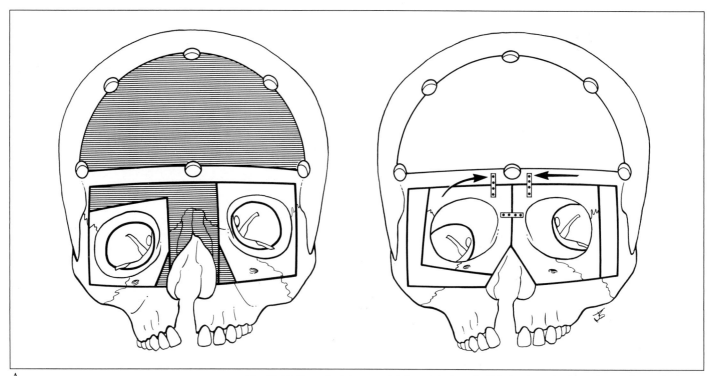

A

Fig. 13-18. Correction of asymmetric hypertelorism. A. Osteotomies and ostectomies may be required to correct asymmetry and rotational defects of an orbit. B. Dystopic and rotated orbit. C. Postoperative result.

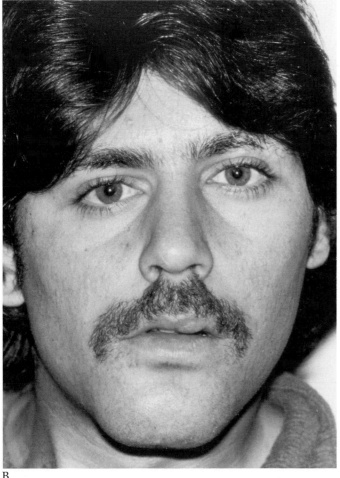

B

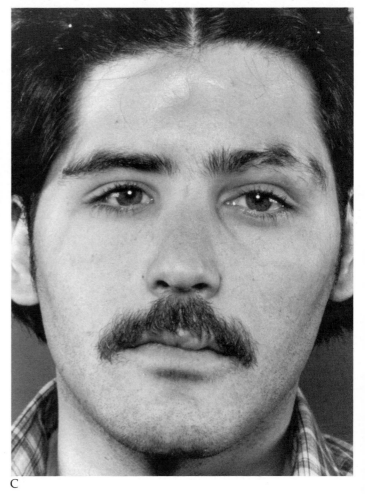

C

Telecanthus

Telecanthus classically occurs with midline frontonasal encephaloceles. The encephalocele comes from the skull base under the nasal process of the frontal bones, depresses the nasal skeleton backward and downward, and pushes the medial orbital walls outward; ethmoid mucoceles can do the same. In mild-to-moderate hypertelorism, telecanthus is the clinically significant deformity. Basically, the facial width looks normal but the intercanthal width is abnormal.

Additional diagnostic help is gained from CT. The scans are reformatted into three dimensions when indicated. This process can be useful when a pathologic condition is present. In addition, the level of the cribriform plate and thus the central extension of the dura can be accurately determined.

Surgical Treatment

The surgical procedure may be extracranial or intracranial. The extracranial approach should be used with caution and only by those with considerable experience. The intracranial method is used when a pathologic condition is the cause of the deformity.

Extracranial Approach

A coronal incision is used, and the frontal, supraorbital, and nasal areas are exposed. The dissection is taken down the medial orbital wall. The lacrimal duct is dissected out, and the attachment of the medial canthal ligament is kept if possible. The lateral wall of the pyriform aperture is dissected subperiosteally to the floor of the nose. The amount of bone to be excised from the midline is drawn out. Although measurements are made, a working rule is to excise everything medial to the medial edge of the lacrimal crest; this gives a bony intercanthal distance of 18 to 20 mm. The osteotomy is marked out with a soft lead pencil. The line goes from the edge of the midline excision horizontally to join the supraorbital rim. Inferiorly the horizontal line is from the lateral pyriform margin to the infraorbital rim. The nasal mucosa is separated from the back of the nasal bones and the lateral walls of the pyriform aperture. With an oscillating saw, the parallel central cuts are made and the bone is removed, leaving the deep portion still attached to the cribriform plate. The superior horizontal cuts, the medial orbital wall cuts, and the horizontal maxillary cuts are made, and the medial orbital wall segments are mobilized. This part must be done carefully because the dura usu-

ally dips down to the upper quarter or third of the osteotomy and may be injured. The central bone and precribriform area are removed with a rongeur. The cartilaginous septum is dissected out submucosally and is excised to give more room intranasally. A small triangle of bone may need to be removed from the pyriform margin inferiorly to increase the pyriform opening. If the medial canthal ligaments have been detached, they are reinserted. The coronal incision is closed in the standard manner (Fig. 13-19).

Intracranial Approach

A coronal flap is used, and the frontonasal area is exposed as before. If possible the craniotomy is minimized to a trephine defect because the smaller the craniotomy, the less bone lost if there is an infection. The central area of bone to be resected is marked out and removed. The osteotomies are performed as before; with these pieces of bone retracted, there is enough exposure to resect the encephalocele or the mucocele. It should be possible to keep the nasal mucosa intact, but any tears should be carefully repaired. Any connection of clinical significance between the nose and the extradural space should be closed off with the vascularized tissue of a galeal frontalis musculofascial flap. The flap is placed into the floor of

Fig. 13-19. Correction of telecanthus. A. Telecanthus corrected by subcranial approach with approximation of the medial orbital walls.

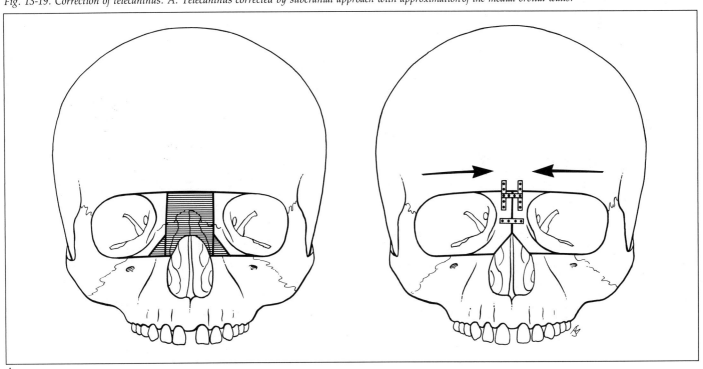

A

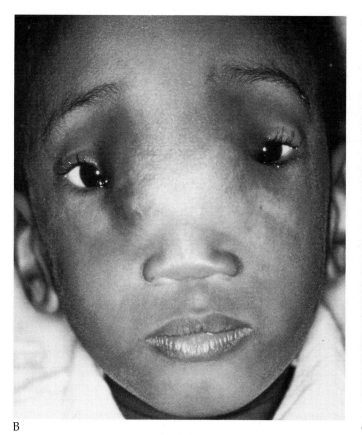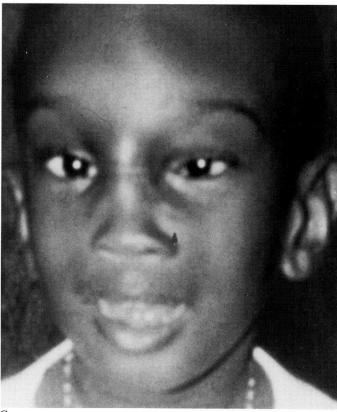

B   C

Fig. 13-19. (Continued) B. Large nasoencephalocele. Although the upper portion was corrected by a cranial approach, the technique illustrated in A was used to correct the telecanthus and nasal shortening. C. Postoperative result.

the anterior cranial fossa covering any connections down into the nose. The osteotomies are made as described previously, moved together, stabilized, and trimmed. The trephine is replaced and is stabilized with either wire or microplates. The coronal flap is closed in the usual way.

Crouzon and Apert Syndromes

In Crouzon and Apert syndromes and associated conditions, midface retrusion, class III dental malocclusion, and shallow orbits are present. Frequently associated brachycephaly and oxycephaly are found. The middle cranial fossae are enlarged in Apert syndrome. In severe instances the eyes are at risk for two reasons—increased intracranial pressure and severe exorbitism.

There are three options in treatment: A Le Fort III advancement osteotomy is indicated when maxillary retrusion is the prominent deformity; a two-stage proce-

dure consisting of a frontal advancement followed by a Le Fort III osteotomy may be done; or a one-stage frontomaxillary advancement, the monobloc procedure, may be performed.

Before any maxillary advancement is done, a plan is developed using a cephalometric tracing, dental study models, and orthodontic treatment to place the upper and lower dentition in a position to achieve optimal dental occlusion after the osteotomy. This treatment may take as long as a year. At the completion of the orthodontic model, an operation is performed and a definitive occlusal splint is made, ensuring accurate positioning of the maxillary teeth at the conclusion of the maxillary osteotomy.

Le Fort III Osteotomy

The approach once again is through the coronal flap with exposure of the orbits, zygomatic arch, temporal fossa and lateral orbital wall, and all of the interior of the orbits (Fig. 13-20). The pterygomaxillary groove is clearly identified. The

nasal bridge line is less extensively exposed. Because the upper portion only is required, depending on the orbital recession, the orbital osteotomy varies. It may begin at the fronto-orbital suture line or midway along the supraorbital rim. The cut is made with an oscillating saw; it continues down the lateral orbital wall to the inferior orbital fissure. A cut is made across the nasal bridge line and down the medial orbital wall. The vertical cuts are joined across the orbital floor using a side-cutting drill and an osteotome, avoiding injury to the infraorbital nerve. With a curved osteotome inserted into the transverse osteotomy on the bridge line, the septum can be separated from the skull base. Care is taken to direct the end of the osteotome anteriorly to avoid damage to the endotracheal tube. A similar curved osteotome is inserted behind the tuberosity, and the tuberosities are disconnected from the pterygoid plates.

To mobilize the maxilla, Rowe disimpaction forceps are placed with one blade on the floor of the nose and one on the palate; two forceps are used. The surgeon

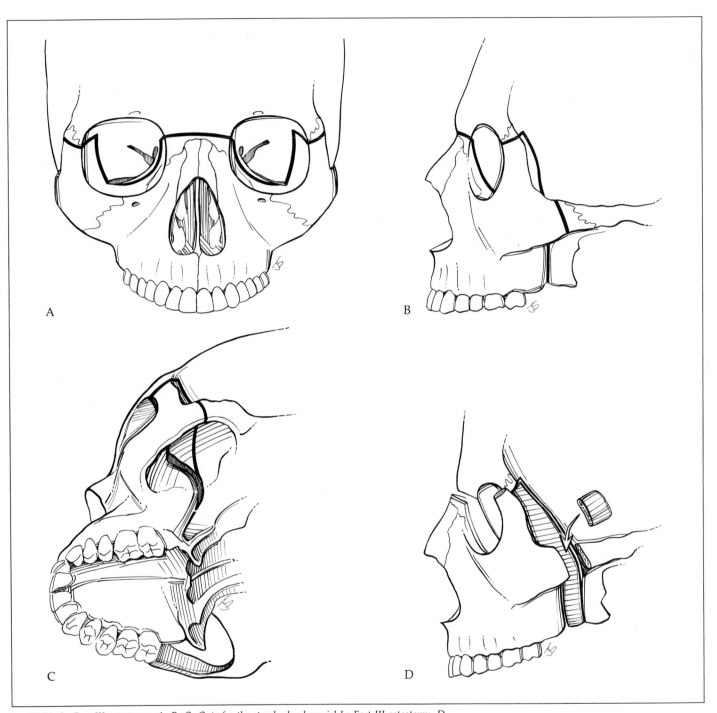

Fig. 13-20. *Le Fort III osteotomy. A, B, C. Cuts for the standard subcranial Le Fort III osteotomy. D. The long iliac crest bone graft is placed from the top of the lateral orbital wall defect to the post-tuberosity region. A bone graft is also inserted into the zygomatic arch.*

stands on a small platform behind the patient's head and breaks the maxilla off the skull base, moving the maxilla from side to side with a component of circular movement to loosen it completely. Tessier maxillary advancement instruments, one in each hand with the blades placed behind the tuberosities, can be used to pull the maxilla forward. It is often necessary to insert a finger behind the tuberosity to break down all adhesions in that area; once this is done, the maxilla should advance easily. At this point the maxillary and mandibular teeth should fit accurately into the occlusal splint, and intermaxillary fixation is applied. Plates are now placed on the zygomatic arch, the lateral orbital wall, and the frontonasal region. Inlay bone grafts are placed in the defects resulting from the advancements; these grafts may be iliac bone or cranial bone and are fixed by screws placed through the plate holes. Frequently the intermaxillary fixation is removed at this time. Bone grafts are placed on the anterior aspect of the hypoplastic maxilla; if possible they are fixed with lag screws. The lateral canthal ligaments and, if indicated, the medial canthal ligaments are reattached in their correct positions. The temporalis muscles are put back into the temporal fossa and are advanced and fixed to compensate for the maxillary advancement. The coronal flap is sutured, and suction drains are inserted in the standard manner. Occasionally when indicated a Le Fort I osteotomy or a mandibular procedure may be combined with the Le Fort III osteotomy.

Two-Stage Craniomaxillary Procedure

When there is frontosupraorbital recession in combination with maxillary retrusion, both the frontal area and the maxillary area need to be advanced. The main reason for doing this in two stages is to avoid any connection between the nasopharynx and the extradural space. Also, the operating time will be shorter and it may be possible to defer maxillary advancement long enough to achieve a permanent correction. The disadvantage is that the eyes may not be fully protected, and the nasomaxillary retrusion will appear to be worse.

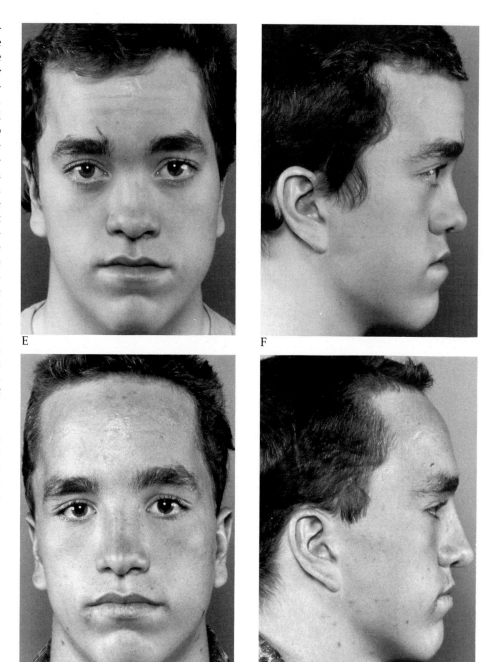

Fig. 13-20. (Continued) E, F. Preoperative appearance of a patient with Crouzon syndrome. G, H. Postoperative appearance.

A standard fronto-orbital advancement of at least 2 cm is performed as described earlier. It may be left to float in an infant, or it may be stabilized. In older children and adults stabilization is achieved with insertion of split skull bone grafts into all defects.

The Le Fort III maxillary advancement is carried out within 6 months in severe deformities and in patients in whom the facial skeleton is fully developed. In mild deformities, while the face is still growing the advancement is delayed as long as possible.

Single-Stage Frontomaxillary Advancement (Monobloc)

The original operation designed by Tessier was a true monobloc. The frontal area was removed as a single segment, and the facial block—total orbits and maxilla—was divided and advanced as a unit. The problem with this operation was that the optic nerves took the whole force of the maxillary manipulation. It is possible to eliminate this problem to a degree by advancing the frontal area, the supraorbital rims, and the maxilla as three distinct sections (Fig. 13-21). The major complication of this procedure still remains, that is, a constant communication between the nasopharynx and the extradural space. Unless this opening is covered with a galeal frontalis musculofascial flap, the incidence of infection and the mortality are unacceptable. In all published series, it is this type of procedure that has the highest rate of clinically significant complications. The procedure does have the advantage of producing a satisfactory profile in one operation, but without experience, care, and an appreciation of the biology of the area, the cost can be too high. In addition, the lower face needs later advancement when the operation is performed on a growing facial skeleton.

Craniofacial Trauma

With the development of craniofacial surgery for the correction of congenital anomalies, it seemed natural that the philosophy and techniques be applied to the treatment of trauma and its sequelae. Once this treatment was available, the management of trauma changed radically and the results improved dramatically. The craniofacial principles that effected this change were exposure, immediate total reconstruction including bone grafting, and supplying vascularized tissue when indicated.

Acute Trauma

In the past acute trauma to the facial skeleton was managed without any exposure whatsoever, the opposite of classic surgical principles. With the advent of the coronal flap, augmented if necessary by lower eyelid incisions, almost all of the facial skeleton can be visualized. If a

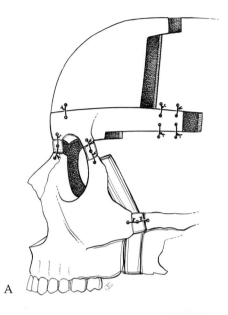

A

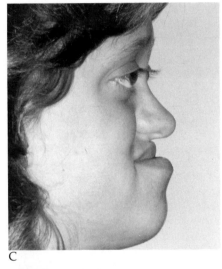

Fig. 13-21. Single-stage frontomaxillary advancement (monobloc procedure). A. The monobloc procedure is not truly a monobloc but a segmental monobloc, which is a contradiction in terms. In this procedure there are separate advancements of the frontal area, the supraorbital rim, and the maxilla. B, C. Severe midface retrusion with supraorbital and frontal retrusion in Crouzon syndrome. D, E. Postoperative result after the monobloc procedure shown in A.

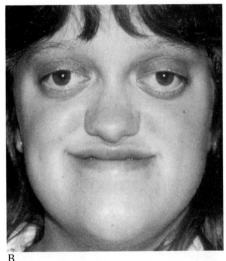

B

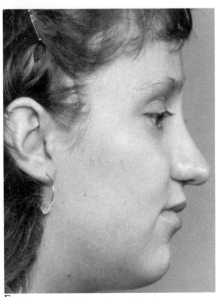

C

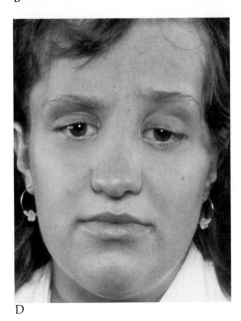

D

E

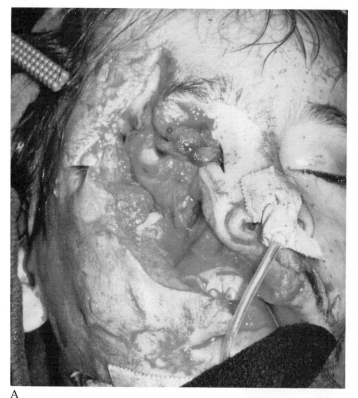

A

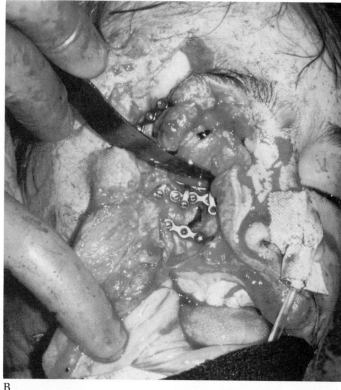

B

horseshoe upper buccal sulcus incision is added, all of the upper facial skeleton can be seen. With this exposure all fractures can be accurately reduced and securely fixed, preferably with plates. If bone is missing, especially in the orbit, it should be replaced with an immediate bone graft from the skull. The orbital area is of particular importance because any increase in orbital volume results in enophthalmos, which is difficult to correct later.

The cranium should always be replaced—to throw away cranial bone is a surgical crime. The frontal sinus, if fractured, should be stripped of mucosa, the irregularities drilled out, and the sinus lined with a well-vascularized galeal frontalis musculofascial flap; any dead space is filled with fragmented cranial bone. All connections to the nasopharynx are closed with the galeal frontalis musculofascial flap. The mandible is always reconstructed and stabilized with a mandibular reconstruction plate. When these techniques are used, infection is negligible and deformity is much reduced, as are enophthalmos and diplopia. To use any other approach is unthinkable (Fig. 13-22).

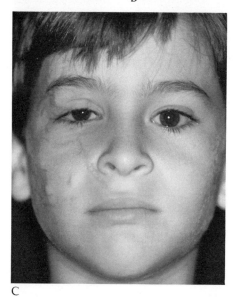

C

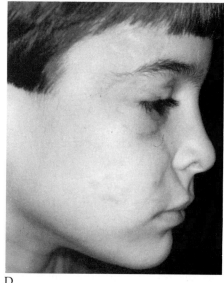

D

Fig. 13-22. Management of acute facial trauma. A. Severe soft tissue and bony injury involving the upper and lower eyelids and right cheek with a complex comminuted fracture of the right orbit and maxilla. B. Fixation with miniplates. An orbital floor titanium mesh implant was used to reconstruct the extensive bony defect. C, D. Result one year after correction. E. Three-dimensional CT scan showing the position of the titanium orbital floor implant. (From I.T. Jackson, Severe orbital floor fractures: Repair with a titanium implant. Eur. J. Plast. Surg. 15:35, 1992. Reproduced with permission.)

Acute Orbito—Zygomatic Fracture orbital plate reconstruction

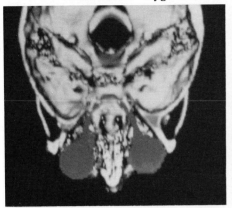
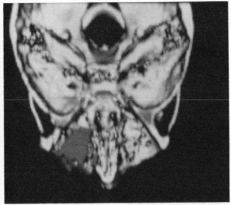

intact bony tale

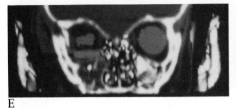
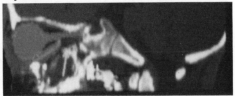

E

Post-Traumatic Deformity

A craniofacial team is continually presented with severe post-traumatic deformities. Each patient is unique, but there is a pattern—missing cranial bone; an unreduced orbitozygomatic or naso-orbitoethmoid fracture, or both; enophthalmos; diplopia; maxillary retrusion; telecanthus; orbital dystopia. The worst scenario is when all these deformities are present in one patient, not an infrequent occurrence.

Analysis and planning using 3D imaging and calling on experience is necessary to achieve good results in these patients. The basic principles include good exposure; osteotomies to correct displaced fractures; onlay bone grafts; reconstitution of the correct orbital volume; correction of soft tissues—the canthi, cheek, and orbital contents; and rigid fixation whenever possible. The bone grafts are usually taken from the skull in either full or split thickness. Any defects into the nasopharynx are closed with galeal frontalis musculofascial flaps. Alloplastic materials are rarely used and only with excellent indications. The most important rule is that the whole deformity must be corrected in one procedure (Fig. 13-23); there is no indication for piecemeal surgery.

The one problem that often defies total correction is diplopia; frequently it is absent in neutral gaze but present at the extremes of eye rotation.

Tumors of the Base of the Skull

All tumors of the upper face have the potential to involve the base of the skull. Failure to appreciate this fact may lead to misdiagnosis and insufficient treatment. These tumors may occur at all ages. Because of the multitude of cellular types in the area of the base of the skull, the variety of nonmalignant and malignant tumors that can occur in this region is extensive.

Excision of these tumors in the past resulted frequently in secondary complications, particularly infection and death, and often was associated with disfigurement. The procedures were difficult to carry out, excision was incomplete even in nonmalignant tumors, and recurrence was frequent. The application of craniofacial principles, knowledge of the complex anatomy, tumor identification, adequate exposure, and accurate reconstruction using vascularized tissue when indicated have eliminated many of the

complications, have reduced residual deformity, and appear to have improved survival rates. Once again, it is important to have as much information as possible about the tumor before treatment is contemplated. One must know if the lesion is primary or recurrent, the tumor type, the size and position of the tumor by CT or MRI, previous treatment, of the possible need for presurgical radiation treatment or chemotherapy, and of the need for embolization in vascular tumors.

Cooperation with a neurosurgeon is paramount—an association should be established within the craniofacial team. Adequate exposure using the standard soft tissue approaches is essential—the coronal flap, the face split, the Weber-Fergusson incision, and the extended temporal preauricular neck incision. The first three are used largely for lesions of the anterior cranial fossa, and the other for exposure of the middle cranial fossa. Bone tumors are resected, and if possible the resected area is reconstructed immediately. Soft tissue tumors frequently require disassembly of the face or exposure osteotomies for adequate visualization and resection. The rule is that whatever bone needs to be removed to expose the tumor to allow for complete and safe excision should be removed. The bone may

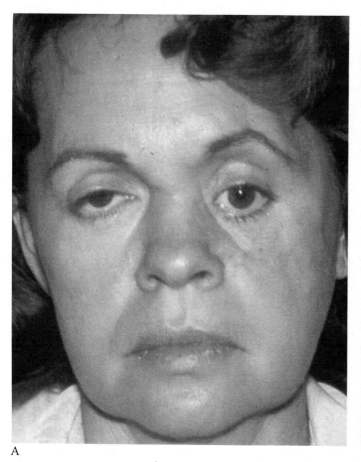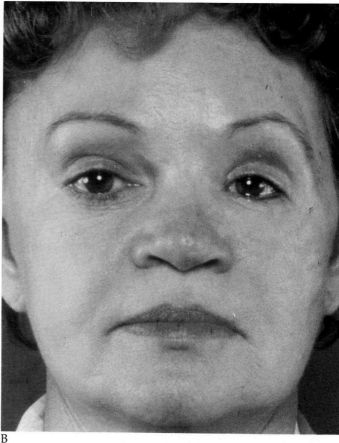

A   B

Fig. 13-23. Management of posttraumatic facial deformity. A. Residual deformity following Le Fort III fracture, left orbitozygomatic fracture, nasal fracture, and left frontal fracture. B. Postoperative result following frontal supraorbital reconstruction. Left orbitozygomatic repositioning, Le Fort I osteotomy, and rhinoplasty are done in a one-stage procedure.

be removed as free segments or pedicled on soft tissue (Fig. 13-24).

In the anterior approach the maxilla can be moved for exposure as in a Le Fort I osteotomy; it even may be split centrally if more exposure is required. In the lateral or temporal approach to the middle cranial fossa, the parotid gland is removed, the facial nerve is preserved, and, again, bone is removed or divided for exposure. While the tumor is being resected, a second team connects the removed bone segments with plates, some of which protrude from the edge of the specimen; this allows for rapid reinsertion (see Fig. 14-6). Frequently in these patients the floor of the anterior cranial fossa and the medial orbital walls have been removed. When they are reconstructed, these regions must be protected on the nasopharyngeal surface with a galeal frontalis musculofascial flap. This is especially im-

portant when there has been a dural repair. In extensive soft tissue resections it may be necessary to use a free vascularized tissue transfer.

Complications: Infection

Of all the complications, apart from death and blindness, which are exceedingly rare, infection is the most feared. Infection may lead to death, meningitis with its possible sequelae, or, most frequently, loss of all bone that was freed from its soft tissue covering. Once its cause is appreciated, this problem can be eliminated almost completely.

The reason for the high incidence of infection in these patients is twofold. First, there is frequently a connection between

the extradural or intradural spaces and the nasopharynx, and second, an intracranial dead space may be associated with that connection. The intracranial nasopharyngeal problem is easily eliminated by the judicious use of the galeal frontalis musculofascial flap whenever this connection is even remotely possible. The possibility of a dead space—as in frontal bone advancement in an adult; delayed frontal bone reconstruction in the presence of scarred, inextensible dura; or after tumor resection with a possible connection down into the nasopharynx—is a potentially lethal situation.

There are two courses of action. The first is to be aggressive and immediately fill the defect with a free tissue transfer, either omentum or a muscle flap anastomosed to temporal or neck vessels. The second is to wait, watching carefully for signs of infection. If the signs do occur,

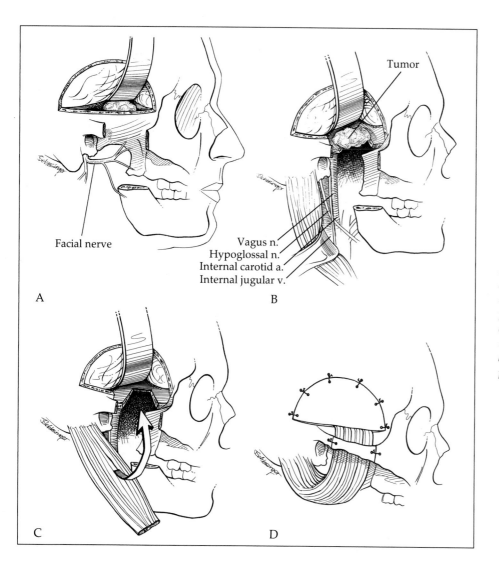

A

Facial nerve

B

Tumor

Vagus n.
Hypoglossal n.
Internal carotid a.
Internal jugular v.

C

D

Fig. 13-24. Lateral (temporal) approach to middle cranial fossa. A. Total parotidectomy is performed. Facial nerve is preserved. Osteotomy is performed to remove as much bone as necessary to provide exposure. This bone is reinserted later or pedicled on soft tissue. The ascending ramus of the mandible and the zygomatic arch have been removed. A temporal craniotomy provides intracranial access. B. The skull base has been removed to expose the tumor lying in relation to the foramen rotundum. C. After resection, vascularized tissue is used if possible to fill in the defect in the floor of the middle cranial fossa, particularly when there has been a dural repair. The sternocleidomastoid muscle has been raised on its superior vascular pedicle. D. Insertion of the sternocleidomastoid muscle into the floor of the anterior cranial fossa with restoration of removed bone. E. Appearance of patient 10 years after petrosectomy for deeply penetrating basal cell carcinoma. F. Three-dimensional computed tomographic scans show defect of the petrous bone after such a resection. Reconstruction with pectoralis major musculocutaneous flap.

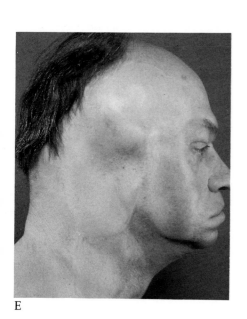

E

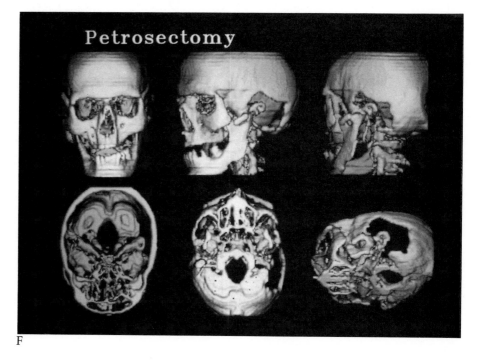

Petrosectomy

F

CT is performed to see if the dead space remains and if there is a fluid level. A free tissue transfer can then be performed, which fills the dead space and provides much-needed vascularity to combat the infection. Antibiotics are of little or no value in this situation. The decision regarding which of these two courses to follow depends on the situation, the experience and judgment of the surgeon, and the ready availability of microsurgical expertise. An additional factor that has been important in reducing the incidence of infection is a drastic reduction in the time required to perform craniofacial operations.

Conclusion

Although we appear to be in a quiet period in craniofacial surgery, advances are still being made in the surgical treatment of tumors of the base of the skull. In addition, the instrumentation and technical aspects of the operations are improving. Three-dimensional imaging has not yet realized its full potential, and the day of constructing "new parts" has yet to come. With time, microsurgery will play a larger part in craniofacial surgery, perhaps in ways as yet not imagined.

Complex deformities cannot be corrected by a single procedure. In hypertelorism, for example, the most challenging area is the nasal deformity, and frequently this cannot be addressed at the initial operation. It has been estimated that correction of an average craniofacial deformity requires at least three operations.

It must be emphasized at the conclusion, as it was at the beginning of the chapter, that safety in this type of surgery is all important. It is too easy to be carried away by the glamor and excitement; we must remember not to harm our patients in any way.

Suggested Reading

Curioni, C., et al. Cranial and craniofacial resections and reconstruction techniques for tumors involving the orbital walls. *Chir. Testa Collo* 1:15, 1984.

David, D.J., and Simpson, D.A. Craniodysostosis. In J.C. Mustardé and I.T. Jackson (Eds.), *Plastic Surgery in Infancy and Childhood*. Edinburgh: Churchill Livingstone, 1988. Pp. 188–207.

Fukuta, K., and Jackson, I.T. Three dimensional imaging in craniofacial surgery: A review of the role of mirror image production. *Eur. J. Plast. Surg.* 13:209, 1990.

Jackson, I.T. Resection of Tumors Involving the Anterior and Middle Cranial Fossa. In H. Dudley, D. Carter, and R.C.G. Russell (Eds.), *Operative Surgery*. London: Butterworth, 1986. Pp. 572–598.

Jackson, I.T. Osteotomies in the Craniofacial Area and Orthognathic Procedures. In H. Dudley, D. Carter, and R.C.G. Russell (Eds.), *Operative Surgery*. London: Butterworth, 1986. Pp. 599–627.

Jackson, I.T. Orbital Hypertelorism. In J.C. Mustardé and I.T. Jackson (Eds.), *Plastic Surgery in Infancy and Childhood*. Edinburgh: Churchill Livingstone, 1988. Pp. 223–252.

Jackson, I.T. Cranial Base Tumors. In J.L. Marsh (Ed.), *Current Therapy in Plastic and Reconstructive Surgery*. Toronto: Decker, 1989. Pp. 389–400.

Jackson, I.T., Adham, M.N., and Marsh, W.R. Use of galeal frontalis myofascial flap in craniofacial surgery. *Plast. Reconstr. Surg.* 77:905, 1986.

Jackson, I.T., and Bite, U. Three-dimensional computed tomographic scanning and major surgical reconstruction of the head and neck. *Mayo Clin. Proc.* 61:546, 1986.

Jackson, I.T., French, D.J., and Tolman, D.E. A system of osseointegrated implants and its application to dental and facial rehabilitation. *Eur. J. Plast. Surg.* 11:1, 1988.

Jackson, I.T., and Shaw, K. Tumors of the Craniofacial Skeleton, Including the Jaws. In J.G. McCarthy (Ed.), *Plastic Surgery*. Philadelphia: Saunders, 1990. Pp. 3336–3411.

Jackson, I.T., et al. *Atlas of Craniomaxillofacial Surgery*. St. Louis: Mosby Year Book, 1982.

Jones, N.F., Sekhar, L.N., and Schramm, V. Free rectus abdominis muscle flap reconstruction of the middle and posterior cranial base. *Plast. Reconstr. Surg.* 78:471, 1986.

Lyons, B.M., and Donald, P.J. Radical surgery for nasal cavity and paranasal sinus tumors. *Otolaryngol. Clin. North Am.* 24:1499, 1991.

Marchac, D., and Renier, D. *Craniofacial Surgery for Craniodysostosis*. Boston: Little, Brown, 1982.

McCarthy, J.G. Craniodysostosis Syndromes: Surgery in Infancy. In J.L. Marsh (Ed.), *Current Therapy in Plastic and Reconstructive Surgery*. Philadelphia: Decker, 1989. Pp. 235–244.

Mustardé, J.C. (Ed.). *Repair and Reconstruction in the Orbital Region*. Edinburgh: Churchill Livingstone, 1991.

Nuss, D.W., et al. Craniofacial disassembly in the management of skull base tumors. *Otolaryngol. Clin. North Am.* 24:1465, 1991.

Shotton, J.C., Schmid, S., and Fisch, U. The infratemporal fossa approach for adenoid cystic carcinoma of the skull base and nasopharynx. *Otolaryngol. Clin. North Am.* 24:1445, 1991.

14

Principles of Rigid Bony Fixation of the Craniofacial Skeleton

Hans-G. Luhr

History

Although use of plates and screws has been reported since 1886, when the Hamburg surgeon Hansmann wrote about his fixation device for fractures of the long bones, these devices were not generally accepted until the 1960s and 1970s. Because of lack of knowledge of the physiology of bone and its biomechanics and because unsuitable implant materials were used, bony fixation with plates and screws frequently led to nonunion or severe bone infection. The use of implant materials that were not resistant to corrosion resulted in the slogan "not too much metal to the bone!" Because of this policy, plates frequently were used that were too weak to withstand muscle traction and weight-bearing forces on the fracture site, which resulted in primary instability of the fracture. Instability, that is, permanent motion of the fracture ends, in open reduction is the main reason for infection and nonunion.

The situation changed when Danis in 1949 advocated his idea of axial compression of the fracture ends. Axial compression leads to a close adaptation and impaction of the fracture ends and increases the degree of rigidity, thus providing the

optimal conditions for fast and economical bone healing. It took another 15 years, however, before the Swiss Association for the Study of Internal Fixation (ASIF) developed the principle of axial compression for clinical use in operations on the limbs; however, the traction devices used in operations on long bones to produce axial pressure could not be applied to the mandible because of its different size and configuration. This realization led to the development of the self-tightening, or automatic, mandibular compression screw (MCS) plate. Vitallium (cobalt-chromium alloy) was used as an implant material because its well-known resistance to corrosion and self-tapping screws made the operation fast and simple. The MCS plate in a simple way guarantees axial compression of the ends of a fracture (Fig. 14-1) with maximal rigidity and optimal adaptation of the fractured bone.

The MCS plate achieves the objective of immediate mobilization of the mandible postoperatively without the need for any intermaxillary fixation. Use of the plate in the treatment of fractures of an edentulous mandible represented great progress compared with interosseous wiring and the need for long-term immobilization of

the jaws by complicated intra- and extraoral appliances and prosthetic splints. Later other types of "dynamic" plates came to be advocated for operations on the limbs with subsequent applications for mandibular fractures. Today the treatment of mandibular fractures by compression osteosynthesis has reached a high standard and is widely accepted; however, the principles of axial compression and bicortical screw fixation compete with Champy's technique, in which smaller, noncompressive miniplates are applied in the so-called tension-band areas of the mandible together with monocortical screw fixation. Champy's technique may not result in the same degree of rigidity as compression plating does when the mandible is mobilized.

Compared with the mandible, the midfacial skeleton consists of thinner bone that is not exposed to as great muscle forces. For this reason, miniaturized bone plates and screws with smaller diameters were developed in the late 1970s and subsequently were applied in midfacial fractures and orthognathic operations. Although the principle of axial compression is a favorite one, it rarely can be applied to the midfacial skeleton, particularly when the maxilla, i.e., the occlusion, is

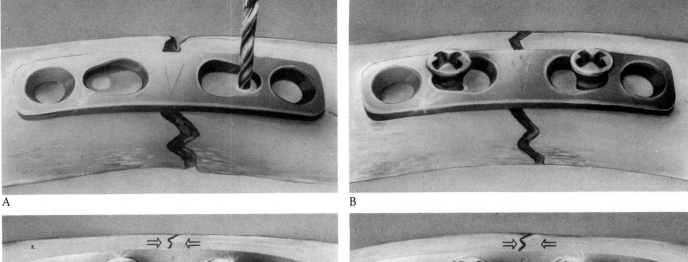

A

B

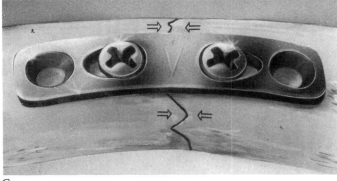

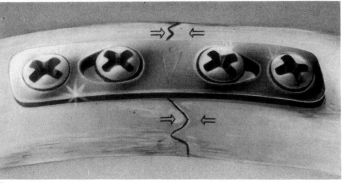

C

D

Fig. 14-1. Mandibular compression screw (MCS) plate. A. The region of the mandible under the small end of the eccentric plate holes is perforated by a surgical drill. B. As long as the compression screws are only partially inserted, the fracture gap is still open. C. During the last phase of screw insertion, the conical screw heads slip into the large end of the holes; thus the fracture ends are pulled together and positioned by high pressure (arrows indicate the direction of pressure forces). D. After the compression process of the active compression screws is completed, the plate is stabilized by two additional screws to secure the fragments against possible rotational stresses.

involved. Axial compression on the thin midfacial bones easily could result in overriding of the tooth-bearing alveolar segment with subsequent shortening in this area, which would result in malocclusion. Noncompressive minifixation plates usually are indicated, therefore, for rigid fixation in the midface.

Unlike interosseous wires or wire suspension, plates and screws allow a three-dimensional rigid fixation of skeletal fragments or segments in various reconstructive procedures on the facial skeleton. Plate and screw systems of different dimensions and functions have been developed for the different sizes and functional requirements of the anatomic regions of the face. It is the art and the science of rigid fixation to select a system of adequate dimensions and to apply the system correctly based on an extensive knowledge of biomechanics and the physiology of bone.

Basic Principles of Plate and Screw Fixation

Low-Speed Drilling

When a hole is drilled into the bone, a reduced drill speed of less than 1000 rpm should be used to avoid heat necrosis of the adjacent bone. Irrigation may not prevent devitalization of the bone at high drill speeds. Devitalized bone around a screw frequently leads to early loosening of the screw and to bone infection. Furthermore, high drill speeds result in wobbling of the drill bit because of centrifugal force, enlarging the drilled hole. Particularly in the thin bones of the maxilla, enlarged drill holes frequently result in stripping of the self-tapping screws.

Continuous Cooling

Continuous irrigation of the drill bit and the adjacent area of the drill hole is strongly recommended to minimize damage to the bone. The bone may be devitalized when the temperature exceeds 47°C (116.6°F).

Self-Tapping Screws

I have used self-tapping screws with a cutting flute (Fig. 14-2) for 20 years without any problems. Self-tapping screws provide a safe anchorage, and screw insertion is fast. Especially in very thin bone such as the maxilla, self-tapping screws show increased holding power compared with pretapped ones. If a screw has been stripped, it can be replaced with a so-called emergency screw, which has a

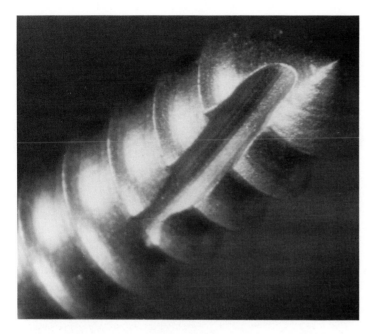

Fig. 14-2. *High-power photograph of a self-tapping Vitallium screw. Each screw is equipped with two cutting flutes. (Only one of the flutes is visible.)*

slightly larger diameter. As a rule two screws should be placed in each segment to protect the osteosynthesis against rotational forces.

Plate Contouring

Plates must be contoured exactly so that they fit passively to the bone surfaces before the screws are inserted. If the plate stands out at one end or the other, the underlying bone segment is pulled toward the plate when the screws are tightened, resulting in undue displacement of the bone segments. To facilitate plate contouring, templates made from a soft, malleable tin alloy are available. The template can be adapted to the bone surface across the fracture or osteotomy line by light finger pressure only. Away from the surgical field, the actual osteosynthesis plate of a corresponding size is contoured duplicating the shape of the template.

Intermaxillary Fixation During the Operation

Although one of the major advantages of rigid fixation is the avoidance of intermaxillary fixation (IMF) postoperatively, it is mandatory to ensure the occlusion during the plate and screw fixation procedure. This is true for fractures in which the dentulous mandible or maxilla is involved as well as for elective osteotomies in orthognathic surgery. Any rigid fixation procedure in which the occlusion is

not stabilized *during* the operation may result in a malocclusion that may be impossible to correct later on. Arch bars and intermaxillary wire loops, usually enforced by acrylic coating, are preferred for this temporary fixation of the occlusion.

Fractures of the Facial Skeleton

Rigid fixation techniques have revolutionized the treatment of facial fractures. The elimination of the need for postoperative IMF in fractures of the jaw is one of the main advantages. It has decreased morbidity and hospital stay and is more comfortable for the patient. In midfacial fractures a three-dimensional stable fixation of skeletal complexes can be achieved by plating techniques as a prerequisite for a facial appearance close to normal after accidents. Surgeons should be familiar with the basic principles already mentioned. Furthermore, they have to realize the different biomechanical conditions in the various anatomic areas of the facial skeleton, which require different dimensions of plates and screws and a variation of techniques.

Mandibular Fractures

Because the mandible is exposed to remarkable muscle and leverage forces, strong plates are needed to immobilize

the fracture site. I prefer Vitallium compression plates (Fig. 14-3) and bicortical screw fixation (Fig. 14-4). Axial compression is the simplest way to achieve rigidity. The plate should be placed as near as possible to the inferior border of the mandible to avoid injury to the alveolar nerve and the roots of the teeth when the screws are inserted. A plate of the proper length should be selected carefully according to the individual fracture pattern. A common mistake is to use a plate that is too short, particularly in oblique fractures, which may result in placing a screw into the fracture gap itself with subsequent instability of the osteosynthesis (see Fig. 14-4). When sagittal oblique fractures are present, even longer plates are needed to avoid screw insertion into the fracture line.

While the occlusion is ensured by IMF, the fracture is exposed by an intraoral incision deep in the vestibule. A broad-pedicled soft tissue flap is preserved at the gingiva while the periosteum is incised nearer to the lower border of the mandible (Fig. 14-5). This technique provides a thick soft tissue cover of the plate and prevents wound dehiscence. The intraoral plating technique is easy in the anterior part of the mandible because drilling and screw insertion can be performed under direct visualization when the lower lip is retracted (Fig. 14-6). Plating is more difficult at the posterior part and at the angle of the mandible. When the fracture

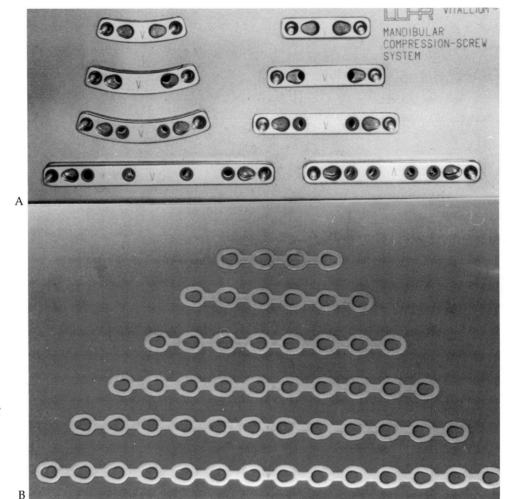

Fig. 14-3. Plates of the Vitallium MCS system. A. Standard MCS plates. B. Three-dimensional MCS plates with specially designed connection bars between the plate holes that allow contouring of plates in all three dimensions of space without deforming the plate holes.

Fig. 14-4A. In rigid fixation of oblique fractures, selection of a plate that is too short causes one of the screws to enter the fracture gap, resulting in primary instability of the osteosynthesis. Instability frequently results in nonunion or infection of the fracture site. B. In oblique fractures a longer plate should be used to make sure that both screws at each of the fracture ends are securely anchored bicortically.

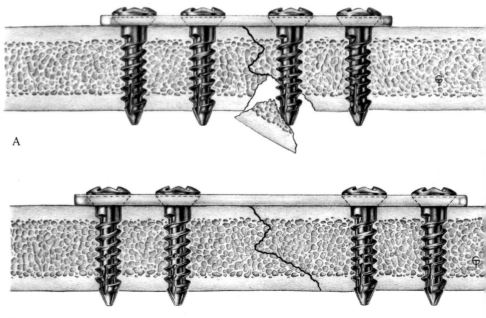

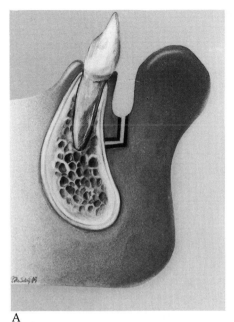 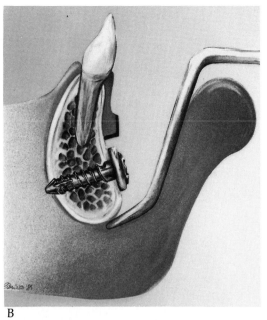 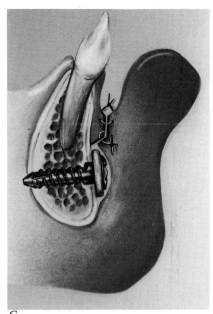

A   B   C

Fig. 14-5. Intraoral rectangular incision to avoid later soft tissue dehiscence. A. First an incision is placed in the vestibule in a vertical direction (about 5 mm deep). Only then is the incision led horizontally, cutting the muscular layer and the periosteum. B. The periosteum is stripped down to the lower border of the mandible, and the plate and screws are placed (bicortical screw fixation). Note that a broad-pedicled soft tissue layer is preserved at the gingiva. Later on it provides a thick soft tissue cover of the plate. C. The incision is closed by two layers of sutures (resorbable ones in the muscle layer) to prevent suture dehiscence and plate exposure.

Fig. 14-6A. Mandibular fracture in the right lateral chin area is exposed by an intraoral incision. Note that during the surgical procedure, the occlusion is ensured by dental splints and intermaxillary wires. B. After the mandibular compression screw plate is adapted precisely to the bone surface by means of bending forceps, drilling and screw insertion in the frontal area can be performed easily. Intermaxillary fixation can be removed immediately after the fracture has been stabilized by a compression plate.

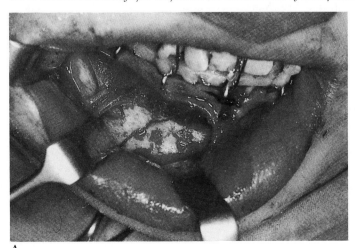 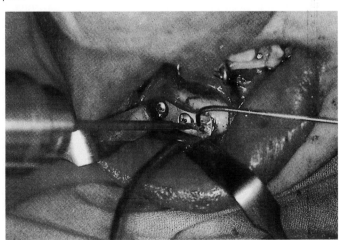

A   B

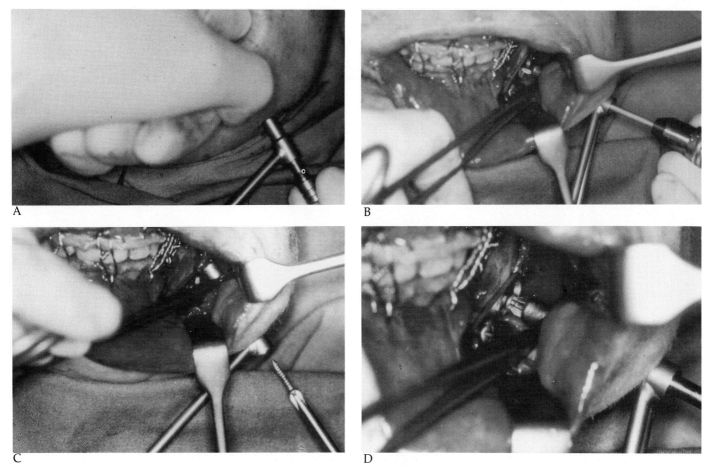

Fig. 14-7A. *The protective sleeve with a mandrel is inserted through the soft tissue canal, which has been opened by blunt dissection. When the outer end of the drill sleeve is visible intraorally, it is fixed by means of special holding forceps. The mandrel is taken out. B. The surgical drill is inserted intraorally through the bore sleeve, and drilling is performed at the desired part of the mandible. The plate must be carefully contoured to the individual bone surface. C. A screw of the desired length is attached to the screwdriver and inserted through the bore sleeve. D. The screw is inserted transbuccally into the predrilled hole, cutting its own threads.*

is exposed by a similar sulcus incision and the plate is contoured, drilling and screw insertion are performed through a protective sleeve that is inserted transbuccally (Fig. 14-7).

The intraoral approach has been used exclusively within the last 10 years because there is no outer scar, no risk of facial nerve damage, and a reduced incidence of bone infection compared with the extraoral route. There are, however, a few instances in which the extraoral approach still is preferred in rigid fixation. Comminuted mandibular fractures need a wide exposure to identify the individual fracture pattern with subsequent stabilization of every segment (Fig. 14-8). The extraoral approach is also preferred in fractures of an extremely atrophied man-

dible (when the height of the mandible is less than 10 mm). In these fractures the periosteum around the fracture line, which is important for nutrition of the sclerotic bone, should be preserved without extensive stripping. This is easier to perform with an extraoral exposure. Also, condylar neck fractures are exposed by extraoral incisions when rigid fixation is indicated. (Most condylar neck fractures are treated nonsurgically.)

Mandibular fractures in children require some deviation from the standard technique. The smaller size of the mandible in infants necessitates the use of plates and screws of reduced dimensions. Vitallium minicompression plates have proved to be successful in these patients (Fig. 14-9). Because any injury to the

tooth buds must be avoided, very short screws—4 or 6 mm long—are used (monocortical screw fixation). When the screws are placed the area of the canines should be avoided because these tooth buds are situated very low, near the mandibular border. Another deviation from the standard regimen in infants is that plates and screws are removed 4 to 5 weeks after plating. There is virtually no indication for plate and screw fixation of condylar fractures in infants. The regional-specific principles of rigid fixation of mandibular fractures can be summarized as follows:

Axial compression
Bicortical screw fixation
Intraoral approach

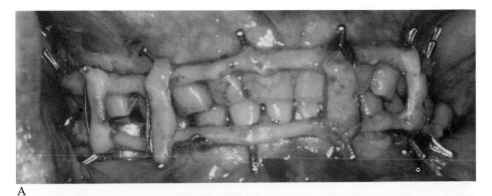

A

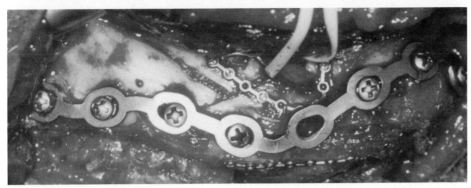

B

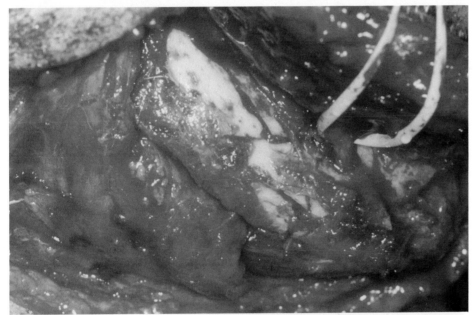

C

Fig. 14-8. Rigid fixation of a comminuted mandibular fracture. A. Arch bars are applied and the occlusion is reestablished and ensured by intermaxillary fixation (IMF). The mandibular-maxillary wire loops are enforced by self-curing acrylic. B. Wide exposure of the fractured area by a submandibular incision. The mental nerve is identified and marked by a rubber loop. The photograph makes it clear that an intraoral incision would not allow identification of the complex fracture pattern and proper fixation of all the fragments. As far as possible epiperiosteal preparation is performed and extensive periosteal stripping is avoided. This technique seems to be the key to avoiding infections in multifragmented mandibular fractures. C. The multiple fragments are pinned together by microplates and screws (as if reassembling a puzzle). The whole fractured area is bridged by a three-dimensional MCS plate, which is contoured individually to stabilize the major segments. Some of the plates are placed on top of the periosteum. D. Roentgenogram 2 days after the operation. There is no IMF, and the mandible can move freely. The lower arch bar is left in place for 4 weeks acting as a tension band supplying additional rigidity to the fracture site. Healing was uneventful.

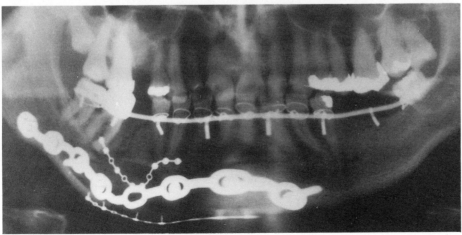

D

Fig. 14-9. Rigid fixation of mandibular fractures in a child. Because of the size of the mandible and tooth buds, different sized plates and screws from those used in adults are required. A. Intraoral exposure of a fracture through the left mental foramen. The occlusion is ensured by IMF and arch bars, which are reinforced by self-curing acrylic. B. The fracture is stabilized by a minicompression plate and fixed by short monocortically placed screws. Note that IMF already is released after placement of plates and screws so that the occlusion can be checked. C. Postoperative roentgenogram shows that no screws are placed in the area of the tooth bud of the left canine (empty plate holes in this area). A second fracture at the right mandibular angle was stabilized by a shorter minicompression plate. There was no IMF postoperatively.

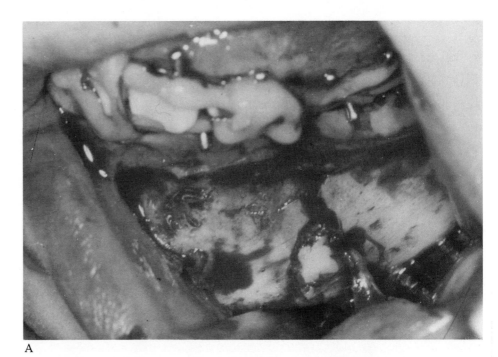

A

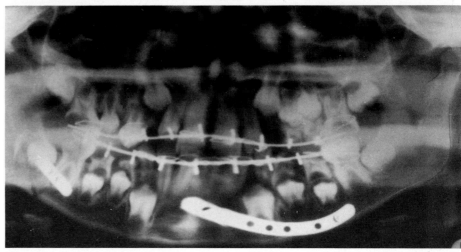

B

C

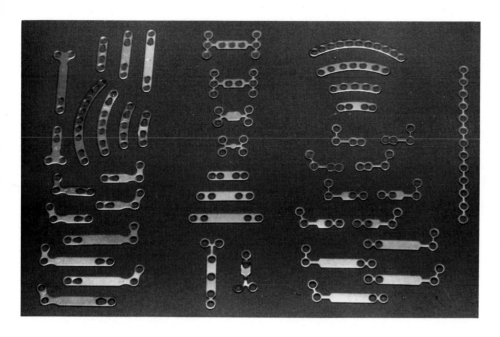

Fig. 14-10. Vitallium miniplates. Left, compression miniplates equipped with the typical eccentric compression holes. (The straight and curved types have two compression holes; L-type and T-type plates have one of these eccentric holes.) Right, selection of minifixation plates (noncompression plates).

Midfacial Fractures

The thinner bones of the midfacial skeleton and their reduced exposure to muscle forces necessitate smaller plates and screws than are used in the mandible. The common systems have screws 2 mm in diameter (or possibly a few that are 1.5 mm in diameter) and a variation of types of plates (Fig. 14-10). Because axial compression on midfacial fractures is not indicated when the maxilla, i.e., the occlusion, is involved, most of the plates are noncompression fixation plates. For rigid fixation of the stronger bones such as the zygoma, however, we prefer compression miniplates to achieve maximal rigidity. The standard technique in fractures of the zygoma is single-point fixation at the frontozygomatic suture (Fig. 14-11). But even in single-point fixation it is mandatory to expose the area of the zygomatic buttress by an intraoral incision. The purpose is to control the result of zygomatic reduction before the plate at the lateral orbit is applied. The visualization of only one fracture line by an eyebrow incision is not sufficient to judge the correct anatomic position of the zygomatic complex. Fractures of the zygoma are quadruple fractures. In some patients additional exposure of the infraorbital rim and even the zygomatic arch is needed. Variations of fixation technique are shown in Figure 14-12.

Fig. 14-11. Single-point fixation of a fractured zygoma at the frontozygomatic suture is the standard procedure. It is presumed that a compression miniplate is used to provide sufficient rigidity. The exposure of the zygomatic buttress is mandatory to make sure that a proper anatomic reduction is achieved.

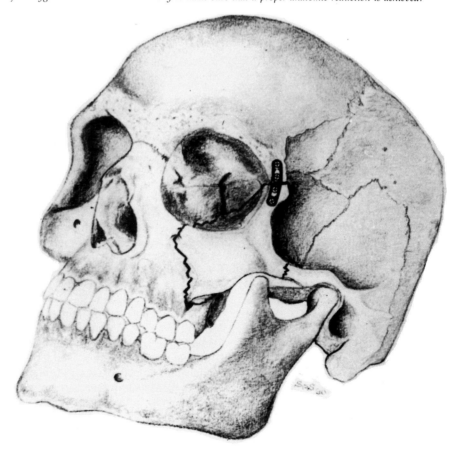

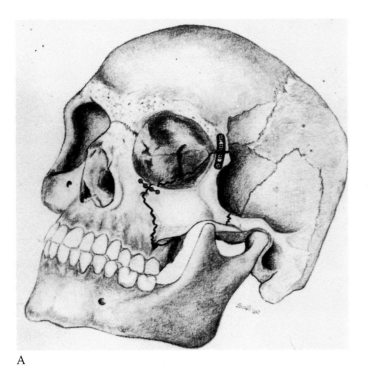

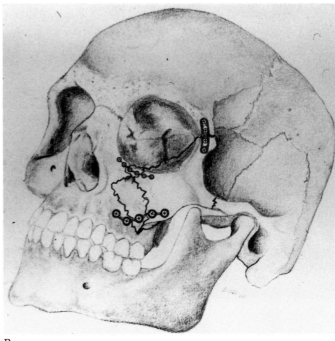

A

B

Fig. 14-12. Fixation technique may be varied in some patients depending on the individual fracture pattern. A. Compression miniplate at the frontozygomatic suture providing the major part of rigidity. An additional microplate with its significantly reduced dimensions is favored at the infraorbital area because it does not interfere with the thin soft tissue cover in this area. B. In comminuted fractures of the zygoma, in addition to the compression miniplate at the frontozygomatic suture, noncompression minifixation plates or microplates have proved to be useful to achieve three-dimensional fixation of all the fragments. Exposure and fixation of the zygomatic arch may be required, particularly in complex midfacial fractures.

Whenever the occlusion is involved, and in every complex midfacial fracture, noncompression minifixation plates are indicated to avoid overriding thin bones with subsequent shortening of the affected areas and the risk of a malocclusion. It is mandatory to ensure the occlusion by arch bars and IMF before plates and screws are applied. Careful contouring of the plate until it fits exactly to the bone is mandatory to avoid displacement of tooth-bearing segments, which would result in a malocclusion. In Le Fort I fractures, four plates are needed. They are placed beside the pyriform apertures and at the zygomatic buttresses (Fig. 14-13). The bone in these areas usually is strong enough to provide a safe screw anchorage. At the extremely thin bone of the lateral sinus walls, however, placement of screws is more difficult and stripping of screws may occur. The fixation of Le Fort II fractures is shown in Figure 14-14.

Rigid fixation of complex midfacial fractures is more difficult. A prerequisite for successful treatment is the wide exposure of all the fractures and their proper anatomic reduction. In this type of facial fracture a combination of soft tissue incisions usually is required. These incisions include the intraoral upper sulcus incision for exposure of the lateral sinus walls and the pyriform aperture, subciliary incisions for the infraorbital area, lateral eyebrow incisions for the lateral orbit, and the bicoronal incision. The bicoronal incision allows good exposure of the frontal bone, the upper nasoethmoidal area, the lateral orbit, and the zygomatic arches. The sequence of treatment is to start with reduction and plate fixation of the upper part of the skeleton, i.e., zygoma including the arch, frontal bone, and nasoethmoidal area. Only when those areas are stabilized is the fixation of the lower maxillary fractures performed.

In maxillary fractures reestablishment of correct facial height is demanded. This is particularly important in complex fractures associated with severe comminution of the walls of the maxillary antrum. These vertical dimensions can be restored more precisely and effectively by plate and screw fixation of the supporting pillars, i.e., the buttresses of the midface, than by interosseous wiring and wire suspension techniques (Fig. 14-15). If more than two of the buttresses are extremely comminuted and bone is missing, bone grafts are necessary for buttress reconstruction.

Besides the stronger bones such as the zygoma and maxilla there are many very thin bones in the midfacial skeleton that are not exposed to any remarkable muscle or masticatory forces. In these areas the common plating systems are too large. A microsystem was developed, therefore,

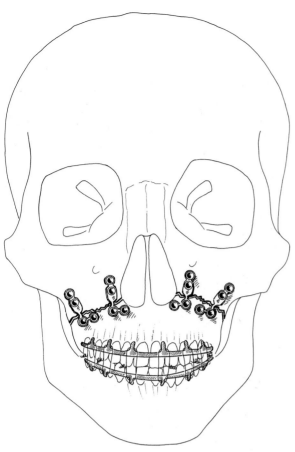

Fig. 14-13. *Principle of rigid fixation in Le Fort I fractures.* L-type *noncompression fixation plates are preferred, but slightly curved plates may be used alternatively. The plates should be placed near the pyriform aperture and at the zygomatic buttress where the bone is strong enough to provide a safe anchorage of screws.*

Fig. 14-14. *Le Fort II fractures usually are stabilized by four fixation plates.*

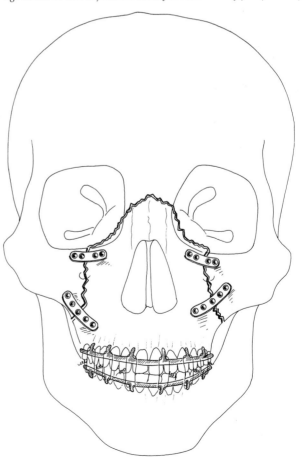

with the remarkably reduced dimensions of 0.8-mm screw diameter and 0.5-mm plate thickness (Fig. 14-16). The microsystem is a supplement to the common plating systems and can be applied in specific areas of the facial skeleton (Fig. 14-17). The advantage is that plates and screws are hardly palpable later, even under thin soft tissue cover. Clinical examples demonstrate the application of the microsystem in nasoethmoidal fractures (Fig. 14-18) and fractures of the walls of the frontal sinus (Fig. 14-19).

The regional-specific principles of rigid fixation of midfacial fractures can be summarized as follows:

Noncompression plates whenever the occlusion is involved and IMF during the operation
Wide exposure of every fracture
Exact plate contouring
Selection of plates of adequate dimension

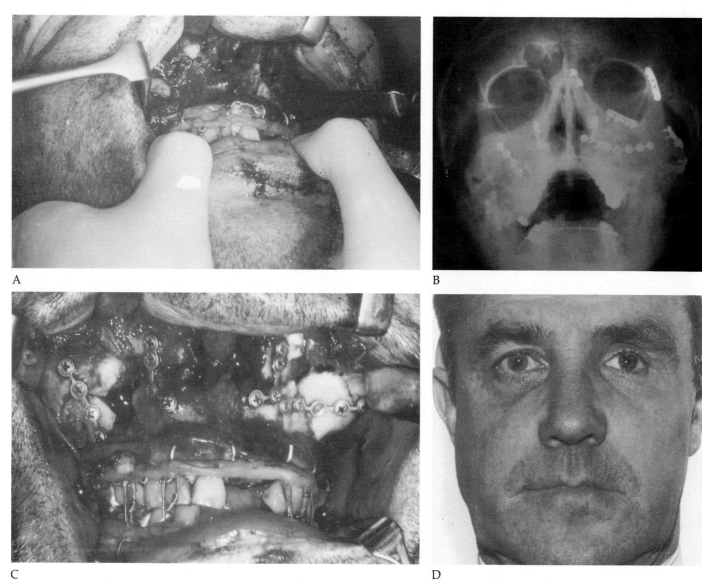

Fig. 14-15. Reestablishment of the correct vertical dimension in comminuted midfacial fractures. A. The comminuted area of the maxilla is exposed, arch bars are applied, and the occlusion is ensured by IMF. (Fractures of the upper third of the facial skeleton, i.e., zygoma, zygomatic arch, and nasoethmoidal area, are already stabilized.) The mandibular-maxillary complex is rotated upward while the assistant applies slight pressure in an upward and forward direction at the mandibular angles to make sure that both the mandibular condyles are seated in the fossa (see also Fig. 14-29). B. The four buttresses are reestablished by plates after multiple bone fragments are repositioned. Intermaxillary fixation is released and the occlusion can be checked. C. Postoperative roentgenogram demonstrates the placement of plates. D. Frontal view of the patient about one year after the accident shows the correct facial height and width. (The patient lost his left eye during the accident; this is an artificial one.)

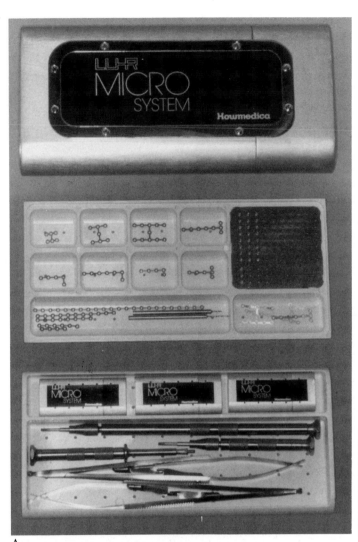

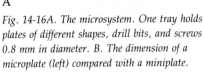

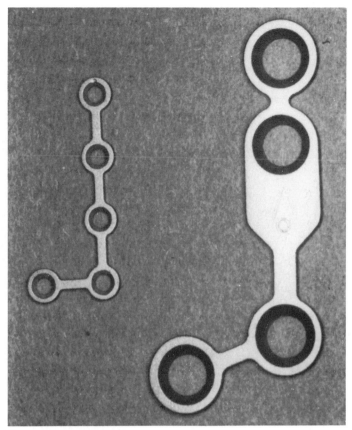

B

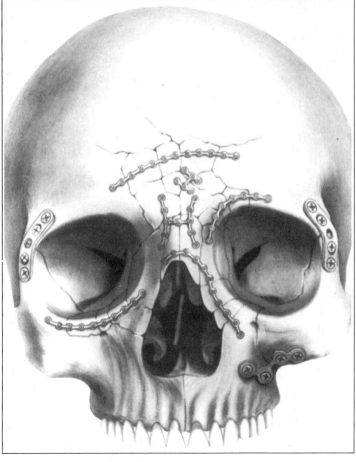

A

Fig. 14-16A. The microsystem. One tray holds plates of different shapes, drill bits, and screws 0.8 mm in diameter. B. The dimension of a microplate (left) compared with a miniplate.

Fig. 14-17. The microsystem is indicated in fractures of the nasoethmoidal bones, the walls of the frontal sinus, and the infraorbital area. The stronger bones, such as the zygoma, which is exposed to remarkable muscle forces, should be stabilized by the stronger miniplates.

14. Principles of Rigid Bony Fixation of the Craniofacial Skeleton **181**

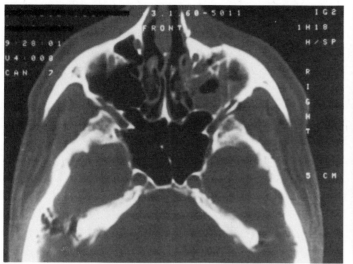

A

Fig. 14-18A. Computed tomogram demonstrates a nasoethmoidal fracture on the right side. B. The fractures were reduced and fixed by multiple microplates. The plates do not interfere with the relatively thin soft tissue cover in this area.

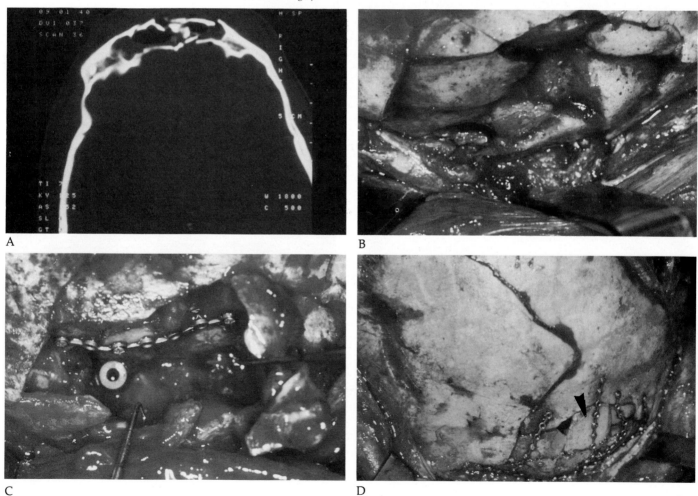

B

Fig. 14-19A. Computed tomogram demonstrating multiple fractures of the anterior and posterior walls of the frontal sinus. B. The frontal area exposed by a coronal incision. C. Multiple bone fragments are temporarily removed or retracted and the sinus is opened. The mucosa is removed and the posterior wall stabilized by a microplate and screws 2 mm long. (There was no dural injury.) The sinus is drained to the nasal cavity (drain in situ). D. Reconstruction of the anterior frontal sinus wall by multiple microplates. Because some bone was missing, a split calvarial graft was placed to cover the remaining defect. Arrow indicates the graft.

A

C

B

D

Mandibular Reconstruction

In discontinuity defects of the mandible following tumor resection (or gunshot injuries) reconstruction of the mandibular arch is required. This is to avoid displacement of the resection stumps because of scar traction and muscle pull. Reconstruction of the arch is particularly indicated in defects of the symphysis to provide a new suspension for the tongue and the larynx, thus avoiding a tracheostomy and a long-lasting tracheostoma. Because of the large leverage forces acting on the resection stumps, a remarkable degree of rigidity is required. This can be achieved by plate and screw fixation systems. I prefer the Vitallium mandibular reconstruction system (MRS), which is based on experience with the MCS system. The self-tapping screws (2.7 mm in diameter), drill bits, and most of the instruments are the same in both the fracture and the reconstruction system. Straight and angled plates 1.5 mm thick are available, including a metal condylar head (Fig. 14-20A). Supplementary plates with bending sections are available (Fig. 14-20B) when in-plane contouring of the plates is required. Because the plates are equipped with a number of eccentric holes, the MRS also can be applied for bone graft fixation with axial compression.

Fig. 14-20. Mandibular reconstruction system (MRS). A. Straight and angled MRS plates are equipped with eccentric plate holes for bone graft fixation with axial compression. A TMJ endoprosthesis (right upper corner) can be connected to all types of angled plates. B. Supplementary MRS plates with bending sections to facilitate plate contouring when in-plane bending is required.

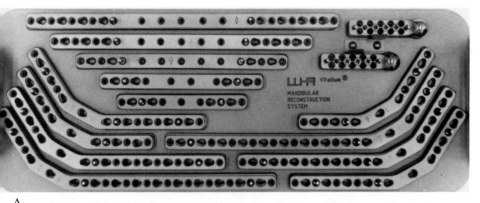

A

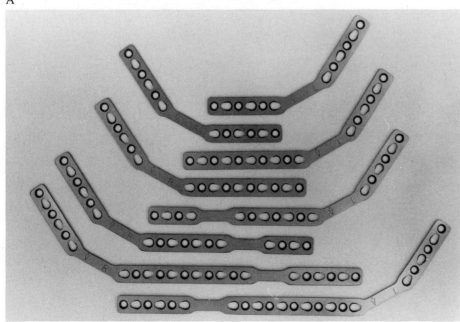

B

Alloplastic Mandibular Reconstruction

In defects following ablative operations for malignant tumors, I prefer alloplastic bridging rather than primary bone grafts. This procedure is fast and does not add much time to the radical tumor resection usually combined with radical neck dissection. Before a plate of proper length and shape is selected, the residual teeth of the mandible are put into correct occlusion to the maxilla using arch bars and IMF. The plate is carefully contoured to the resection stumps. Templates facilitate plate contouring. In alloplastic defects, bridging a minimum of four screws in each of the resection stumps is required to withstand the strong muscle forces. In larger defects the number of screws must be increased because of the increased leverage forces (Fig. 14-21). The intraoral lining is closed by a double layer of sutures and the plate is covered by soft tissue and muscle flaps, which are wrapped around the plate and fixed with resorbable sutures. At the end of the operation IMF is released, and the mandible can move freely. In hemimandibulectomy (Fig. 14-22), an artificial condylar endoprosthesis is connected with one of the angle plates and is positioned into the glenoid fossa (Fig. 14-22B). Its high polished head contacts the articular disk, which is usually preserved in tumor resection. Usually there is no need for an additional fossate prosthesis. (The artificial condylar head is not indicated when the glenoid fossa itself is affected by tumor or infection.) Intermaxillary fixation is mandatory during the operation and in joint replacement. Alloplastic mandibular reconstruction generally is temporary because dentures cannot be worn on top of the plate and late plate exposure to the intraoral lining or skin or a plate fracture cannot always be prevented.

Mandibular Reconstruction with Bone Grafts

A definitive reconstruction of the mandible when discontinuity defects are present is possible only with bone grafts. For malignant tumors I prefer this definitive reconstruction as a secondary procedure usually done 1 or 2 years after the ablative operation, when the patient is found free of tumor recurrence. Primary bone graft reconstruction, however, is performed

Fig. 14-21. Alloplastic bridging of a mandibular defect replacing the ascending ramus (top) and the TMJ. Whereas four screws in each resectional stump is the minimum, the number of screws must be increased in larger defects because they have to withstand the increased leverage forces acting on the plate and the residual mandible.

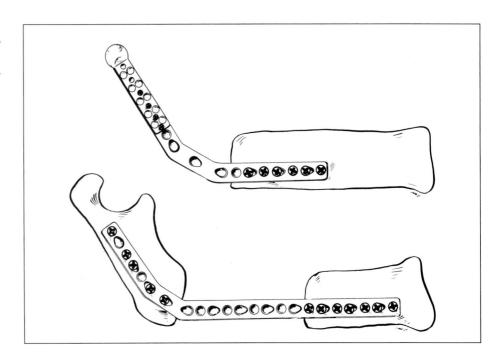

Fig. 14-22. Alloplastic reconstruction and joint replacement after hemimandibulectomy. A. After the right mandible including the condyle is resected because of an osteosarcoma, an MRS plate of adequate length is connected with a ramus joint endoprosthesis. B. The intraoral soft tissue defect is already closed, and the occlusion of the residual teeth is ensured by IMF when the MRS plate is contoured and fixed to the resectional stump by multiple bicortical anchored screws. The artificial condylar head is positioned precisely into the glenoid fossa. The articular disk can be preserved in most instances. C. Postoperatively no IMF is needed. A sufficient mouth opening is achieved; however, a deviation of the mandible toward the affected side is a common finding when the mouth is opened. This is because an artificial joint is a rotation joint only, and the condyle does not glide forward when the mouth is opened extremely wide. D. A satisfactory occlusion.

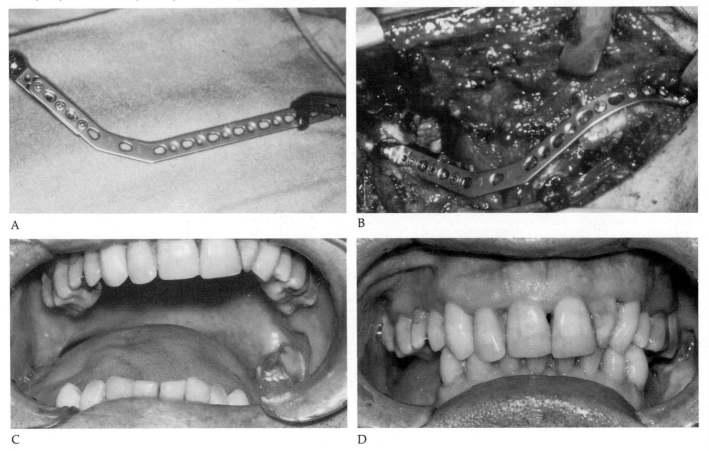

A

B

C

D

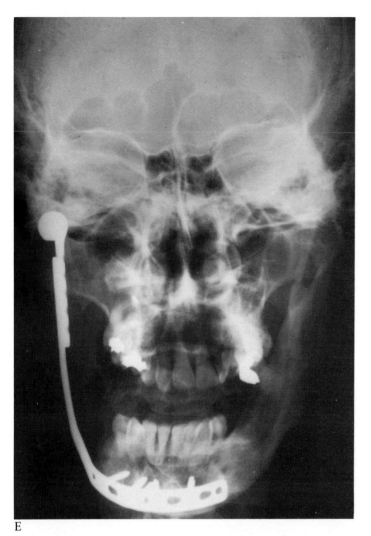
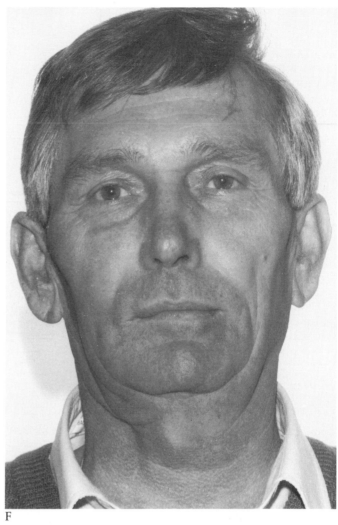

E   F

Fig. 14-22. (Continued) E. Roentgenogram demonstrates the result of reconstruction after hemimandibulectomy. F. There is no major asymmetry after mandibular reconstruction. The artificial joint has functioned without any problems for more than 4 years after the operation.

when discontinuity defects result from removal of benign tumors, such as ameloblastoma and dermatofibroma. A prerequisite for fast and economical bone healing is rigid fixation of the graft to the residual mandibular stumps. This objective is achieved best by axial compression. Axial compression is the simplest way to achieve maximal rigidity. To enlarge the contact surfaces between host bone and graft, a steplike preparation of the resectional stumps is recommended (Fig. 14-23). The outer cortex of the stumps is removed by an oscillating saw in a length of about 1 cm. Both free ends of the graft are trimmed correspondingly. Graft fixation requires a minimum of three screws

in each of the resection stumps. In larger defects the number of screws should be increased because of the greater leverage forces.

For mandibular reconstruction I prefer the corticocancellous iliac graft. Before the graft is harvested, the residual teeth of the mandible must be put in proper occlusal relation to the maxilla and occlusion must be ensured by IMF. Only then can the actual size of the defect be determined and a graft of corresponding length and shape be harvested. When the resectional stumps and the graft are trimmed to a steplike shape at their free ends, the graft is positioned exactly into

the defect. An MRS plate is carefully contoured to the resectional stumps and fixed by multiple screws (Fig. 14-24). Using the eccentric compression holes of the MRS plate, the graft is fixed by axial compression between the stumps. At the end of the operation, IMF is released.

Usually plates and screws do not need to be removed later on when implant materials that are resistant to corrosion (Vitallium, titanium) are used. In bone graft procedures, however, removal of the stabilizing plate and screws is recommended 4 to 6 months after grafting. The purpose is to expose the graft to unlimited functional stress during the period of late bone

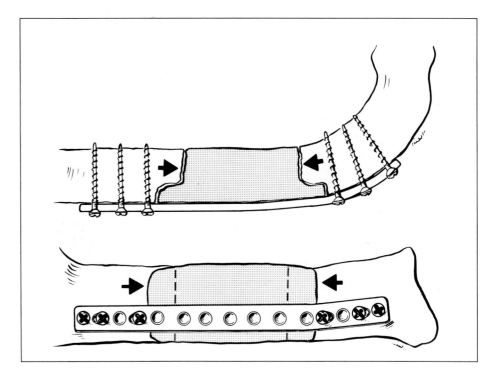

Fig. 14-23. Mandibular reconstruction by a bone graft and graft fixation by an MRS plate. Steplike preparation of the resectional stumps and, correspondingly, of the bone graft is shown. The purpose is to increase the contact surface between the graft and the host bone. Rigid fixation of the graft is achieved by axial compression. Arrows indicate compression forces. In graft fixation a minimum of three screws is recommended in each of the resectional stumps.

Fig. 14-24. Final mandibular reconstruction following mandibular resection and radical neck dissection performed a few years before the reconstruction. A. The free ends of a corticocancellous iliac bone graft are trimmed to a steplike shape. The graft is ready for insertion. B. The graft is wedged precisely into the mandibular defect and rigidly fixed by an MRS plate under axial compression. The occlusion of the residual teeth must be ensured by IMF during this procedure. C. Postoperatively no IMF is needed, and the mandible can move freely. D. Four months after the reconstructive procedure, the stabilizing MRS plate was removed to expose the graft to unlimited functional stress. Roentgenogram demonstrates mandibular reconstruction one year after the plate was removed.

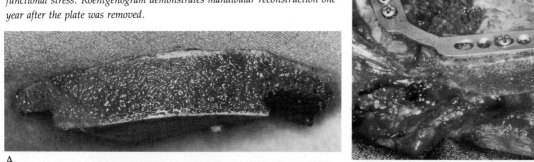

A

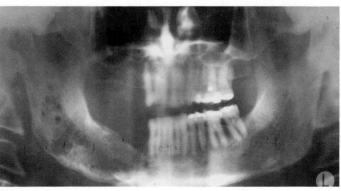

B

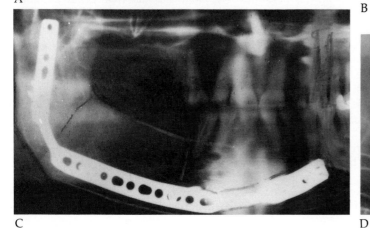

C

D

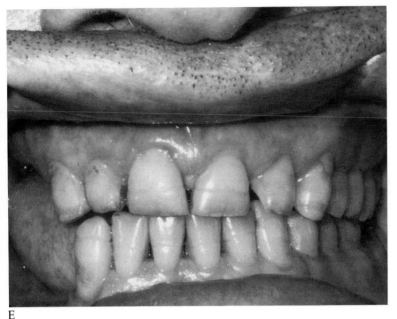

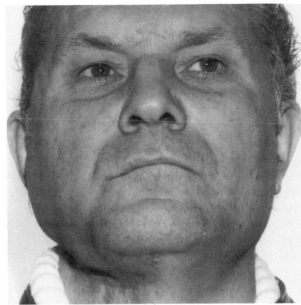

E   F

*Fig. 14-24. (Continued) E, F. A satisfying occlusion and facial symmetry were
achieved. (The asymmetry of the right neck is caused by radical neck dissection.)*

remodeling and to avoid extensive atrophy of the graft. In free, nonvascularized bone grafts, however, 30 percent resorption of the graft (loss of vertical height) should be expected.

The regional-specific principles of rigid fixation in mandibular reconstruction can be summarized as follows:

Alloplastic bridging:

Intermaxillary fixation during plate and screw fixation
A minimum of four screws in each resectional stump
A larger number of screws when extensive defects are bridged

Bone graft fixation:

Intermaxillary fixation before the graft is harvested and during plate fixation
Axial compression
A minimum of three screws in each resectional stump
Plate removal 4 to 6 months after the operation

Rigid Fixation Principles in Orthognathic Surgery

The field of orthognathic surgery has been greatly influenced by rigid fixation techniques. The goal of plate and screw fixation in elective osteotomies is to eliminate the need for IMF in the immediately postoperative period. The avoidance of a long-term IMF, which was required when interosseous wiring was used, makes the operation more comfortable for the patient, may eliminate the need for intensive care, and shortens the hospital stay and overall time of morbidity. Better oral hygiene can be maintained, and orthodontic treatment can start early. In elective displacement osteotomies of the facial skeleton, special principles must be followed when rigid fixation is used. This is necessary to avoid problems, particularly malocclusion.

Mandibular Osteotomies

The sagittal split-ramus osteotomy (SSRO) is the most common surgical procedure for the correction of mandibular deformities. Although most surgeons use bicortical screw fixation of the SSRO (usually three screws are applied in a noncompressive mode), I prefer plate fixation with monocortical screws combined with the so-called temporomandibular joint (TMJ) positioning technique. The maintenance of the TMJ condylar position is one of the key points in orthognathic surgery. This is particularly true when rigid fixation is used. One has to realize that the proximal segment, including the condyle after the mandible has been split, is a free-floating segment (Fig. 14-25). Under general anesthesia and muscle relaxation it easily may be displaced from its original position in the glenoid fossa without being noticed by the surgeon. If the displaced proximal segment is rigidly fixed (in the wrong position) to the distal greater part of the mandible, the condyle will slip back into its original position when IMF is released, resulting in a mal-

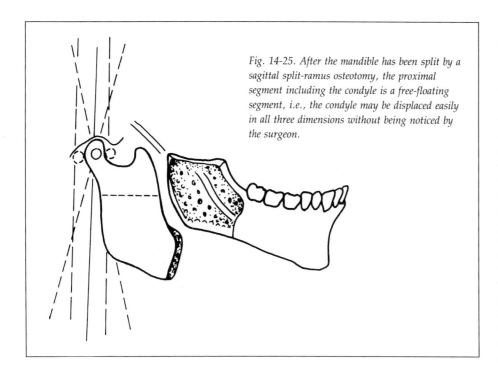

Fig. 14-25. After the mandible has been split by a sagittal split-ramus osteotomy, the proximal segment including the condyle is a free-floating segment, i.e., the condyle may be displaced easily in all three dimensions without being noticed by the surgeon.

occlusion. To avoid condylar displacement (Fig. 14-26), the ascending ramus (proximal segment) is connected by an L-shaped positioning miniplate and four screws to the acrylic occlusal splint before the mandible is split.

The prefabricated splint is a so-called double splint that has on its lower side two lines of tooth impressions. One line represents the preoperative position of the mandible (and simultaneously the centric relation of the condyles). The other line of impressions represents the planned postoperative position. For the splitting procedure, IMF and the splint must be removed. The two screw holes in the splint later serve as reference points when the positioning plate and the screws are reinserted. The teeth of the distal large segment after the mandible is split are indexed into the second line of tooth impressions of the aforementioned splint, and the new occlusion is ensured

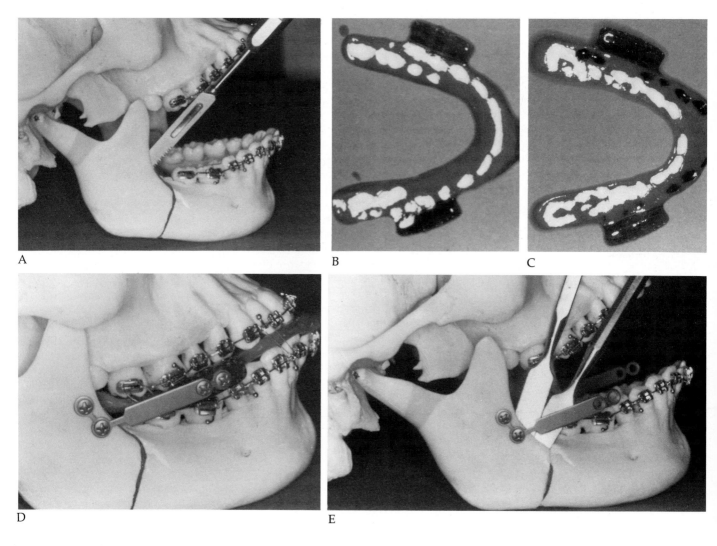

A

B

C

D

E

Fig. 14-26. Temporomandibular joint positioning technique in SSRO. A. Typical bone cuts are performed in SSRO using a reciprocating saw. The mandible has not yet been split. B. A prefabricated acrylic occlusal double splint is used. On its upper side the splint has only one line of tooth impressions, which will be indexed to the maxillary teeth. Note the balconies on both sides of the splint. The "positioning" miniplates will be fixed onto the balconies. C. View of the lower side of the occlusal splint shows two lines of tooth impressions. One line (black) represents the preoperative position of the mandible and simultaneously the centric relation of both the mandibular condyles. (The splint was fabricated in the dental laboratory by transferring a preoperative bite registration of the patient to a semiadjustable dental articulator.) The second line of tooth impressions (white) represents the desired postoperative position of the mandible. D. The double splint is inserted and the (preoperative) occlusion is ensured by intermaxillary wire fixation. The condyles are automatically seated in a centric relation. The ascending rami are connected with the balconies of the acrylic splint by a so-called positioning L-shaped miniplate. Monocortical screws are used at the lateral surface of the ascending ramus. Two screws of the same length are placed at the balcony of the acrylic splint. E. Intermaxillary fixation is released, and the anterior parts of screws and the occlusal splint are temporarily removed when the actual splitting of the mandible is performed. For splitting of the mandible, two thin spatula osteotomes are used, which are alternately driven into the osteotomy gap. F. After the mandible is completely split, the distal tooth-bearing segment is mobilized and the mandibular teeth are indexed into the second line of tooth impressions of the occlusal double splint. The proximal (completely mobile) segment is guided back to its original preoperative position by refixation of the anterior part of the positioning plate to the acrylic balcony of the splint. Two screws are reinserted into the preexisting screw holes of the splint. By this maneuver the preoperative position of both the condyles is reestablished. G. The actual osteosynthesis plate is placed. A noncompression slightly curved miniplate is carefully contoured until it passively lies flush to the bone following the steps and maintaining the gaps between the two segments. The use of a template facilitates the procedure. Monocortical screws 6 mm long are used. H. The frontal view demonstrates both the positioning plates and the contoured osteosynthesis plates in situ. The different sizes and shapes of the gaps and steps between the divided segments, which are maintained by the precisely contoured miniplates, are clearly visible. I. At the end of the operation, the positioning plates and the occlusal splint are removed and IMF is released. (The screw holes at the outer cortex of the proximal segment are visible.) A prefabricated orthodontic wafer is inserted, and light guiding or training elastic bands are applied. J. The elastic bands allow limited motion of the mandible and, together with the wafer, guide the jaw to its new occlusion. During meals (a soft solid diet is recommended), the patient temporarily removes the elastic bands and the wafer; he or she reinserts them later on. The use of these elastic bands usually is recommended for a period of 4 weeks. (SSRO = sagittal split-ramus osteotomy.)

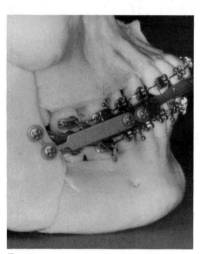

F

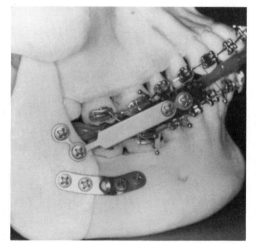

G

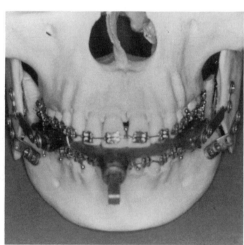

H

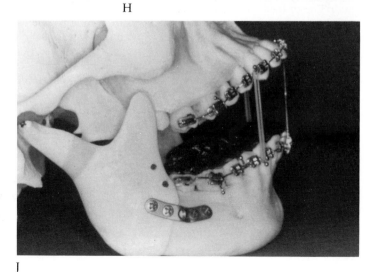

I

J

Fig. 14-27A. Ninety-degree screwdriver for intraoral screw insertion. The instrument consists of a turnable handle (a), which transfers the power to the transmission, and a short screw blade in the screwdriver head (b). The screw-holding device (c) is shown in its retracted position. B. The screwdriver head is shown with the screw-holding device in its advanced position holding a miniscrew ready for screw insertion. (Luhr-Fritzemeier 90° screwdriver, Howmedica, Inc.)

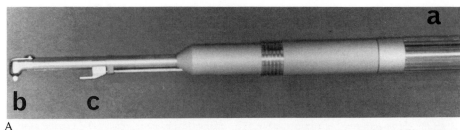

A

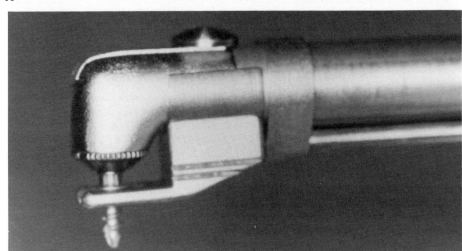

B

by IMF. The positioning plate is fixed again to the splint by reinserting the anterior screws to the already existing screw holes of the splint. By this maneuver the proximal segments including the condyles are situated in the exact preoperative position. Only then is the actual osteosynthesis plate—a noncompression, slightly curved miniplate—contoured crossing the osteotomy line. Usually gaps and steps are present between the segments in sagittal split osteotomies. They must be maintained to avoid condylar displacement. The plate is fixed with short monocortical screws (6 mm long). The intraoral insertion of screws is facilitated using a 90° screwdriver (Fig. 14-27), thus avoiding a transbuccal approach. For predrilling of the bone, any standard 90° dental handpiece can be used.

The positioning plates and IMF are removed and the occlusion is checked. Postoperatively an orthodontic wafer and light guiding or training elastic bands are applied. They guide the mouth and jaw to the new occlusion and adapt the neuromuscular system to the new conditions. The elastic bands can be removed by the patient while he or she eats a soft solid diet and reapplied. The wafer is worn for a period of about 4 weeks. Although monocortical miniplate fixation is not as rigid as bicortical screw fixation, I have never observed a nonunion in a large series of cases.

In two-jaw operations the technique of TMJ positioning is somewhat different. Because the maxilla also changes its position, it cannot serve as a reference to the position of the ascending ramus and the condyle; therefore a skeletal area above the Le Fort I osteotomy line is chosen for the placement of the reference holes (Fig. 14-28).

The regional-specific principles of rigid fixation in sagittal split mandibular osteotomies can be summarized as follows:

Close cooperation with orthodontist
Exact planning based on cephalometric and model studies
Prefabricated occlusal splint
Maintenance of condylar position
Noncompression screw or plate fixation of the osteotomy

Maxillary Osteotomies

Rigid fixation has proved to be particularly useful in Le Fort I osteotomies. The avoidance of intermaxillary fixation post-operatively and the ability to reposition the maxilla in all three dimensions has increased the efficiency of treatment. When the maxilla has been mobilized, it is moved to its planned position by indexing of the maxillary teeth into a prefabricated occlusal splint, and IMF is applied. The maxillary-mandibular complex is rotated upward until good contact is achieved at the osteotomy site. Bony interference is removed with a bur or rongeur. During plate adaptation, the assistant should apply light pressure on the mandibular angle to hold the condyles upward and forward against the posterior slopes of the articular eminences (Fig. 14-29). The purpose is to avoid condylar displacement, which would result in a malocclusion. In elective osteotomies gaps frequently occur between the segments. These gaps should be maintained by bridging them with noncompressive miniplates because close impaction of the bone at the osteotomy site could result in distortion of the tooth-bearing segment and disturbance of the occlusion. Passive adaptation of the plates to the individual

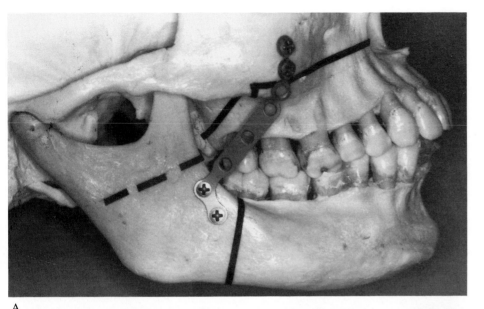

A

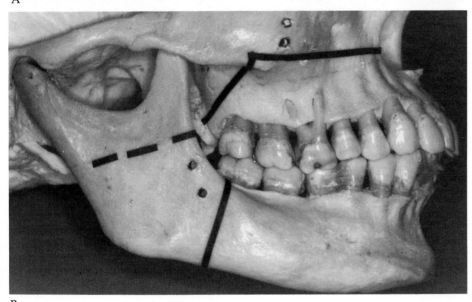

B

Fig. 14-28. *Temporomandibular joint positioning technique in bimaxillary operation. A. At the beginning of the operation, a positioning miniplate (long type) is carefully contoured to the lateral surface of the ascending ramus and to the zygoma well above the planned Le Fort I osteotomy line. The miniplate is fixed by four screws while the occlusion is ensured by a prefabricated occlusal splint and IMF. This situation represents the preoperative condylar position in its centric relation. B. Immediately after the plates have been placed on both sides, plates and screws are removed, leaving four reference holes in the bone for later reinsertion. Intermaxillary fixation is released and the Le Fort I osteotomy is performed. The maxilla is moved to its planned new position and stabilized by four miniplates. The sagittal splitting of the mandible is performed, and the distal segment is moved to its planned position. IMF is applied with a second prefabricated splint. The original position of the proximal segments and the condyles is reestablished by reinsertion of the positioning plates and screws to the preexisting screw holes. Only then are the mandibular osteotomies bridged by osteosynthetic miniplates in the manner described in Fig. 14-26.*

bone contour is another procedure critical for avoiding displacement of tooth-bearing segments (Fig. 14-30). Templates of a soft malleable tin alloy, which can be adapted to the irregular shape of the bone, are particularly helpful when steps are present at the osteotomy site; the templates facilitate contouring of the osteosynthesis plate.

In Le Fort I osteotomies four miniplates are needed. They are placed at both the zygomatic buttresses and beside the pyriform apertures, where the bone is sufficiently strong to provide a safe anchorage for the self-tapping screws. When the maxilla is rigidly fixed, IMF is released and the occlusion is checked. The use of an occlusal splint (orthodontic wafer) and light guiding or training elastic bands is recommended for the first few weeks after the operation. Any other type of midfacial osteotomy may be stabilized by rigid fixation in a similar manner. The regional-specific principles of rigid fixation of elective maxillary osteotomies can be summarized as follows:

Close cooperation with the orthodontist
Cephalometric and model studies
Prefabricated occlusal splints
Exact contouring of noncompression minifixation plates
Avoidance of condylar displacement

Fig. 14-29. During plate and screw fixation, light pressure should be applied in an upward and forward direction on the mandibular angles to make sure that the condyles are passively seated in the fossa. This principle applies to rigid fixation of Le Fort I osteotomies and to Le Fort I fractures.

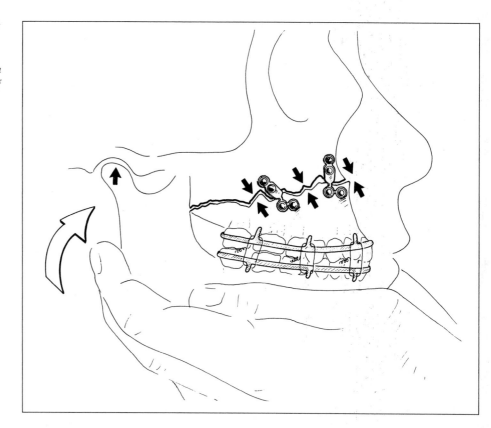

Fig. 14-30A. In rigid fixation of maxillary osteotomies, exact adaptation of the plates to the individual bone contour is critical. The plates must lie passively flush to the bone. B, C. When the plate is not correctly contoured and stands off the bone, the tooth-bearing segment is pulled toward the plate when the screws are tightened. This results in a malocclusion.

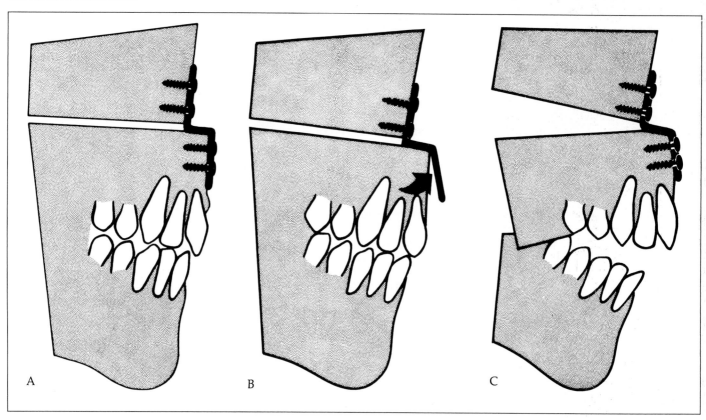

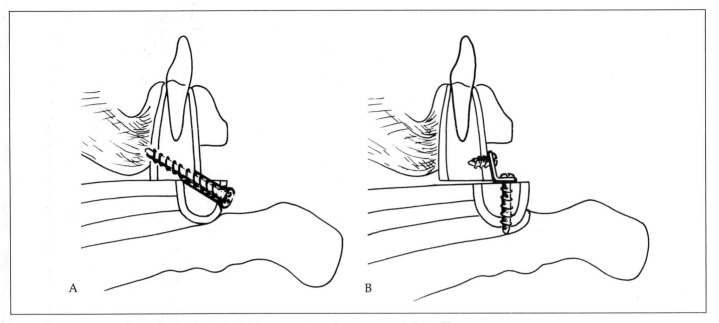

Fig. 14-31A. Lag-screw technique for fixation of the distal segment in an advancement genioplasty. The distal segment is predrilled with the diameter of the screw so that the screw slips through. The screw grips in the proximal segment only. B. Special plating technique for genioplasty fixation. The plate consists of two holes only and is bent to a right angle. The screw inserted in the distal segment must be long enough (usually 12 to 14 mm) to grip in the cortical bone at the lower border of the chin. Only then is a safe anchorage provided (see also Fig. 14-32B).

Genioplasty Fixation Techniques

Rigid fixation offers some advantages over fixation with wires in genioplasty. With the differentiated application of plates and screws, stable fixation of the smaller distal segment in all three dimensions can be achieved. I recommend two different techniques: the lag-screw technique (Fig. 14-31A) and a special plating technique (Fig. 14-31B). In the lag-screw technique the distal segment is predrilled with a special lag-screw drill with exactly the same diameter as the screw. The proximal segment is predrilled with a common drill of a smaller diameter. The screw slips through the outer hole and is anchored in the proximal segment only. When the screw is tightened, the distal segment is pulled toward the proximal one pressing both the bones together. This technique is not recommended when interpositional hydroxyapatite (HA) grafts are used for vertical lengthening of the chin because the hydroxyapatite blocks frequently crack when the lag screws are tightened.

The second fixation technique in genioplasty has proved to be both simple and versatile. Two small segments are cut off from a fragmentation miniplate (Fig. 14-32A); each segment contains two plate holes. The segments are placed about 1 to 2 cm from the midline (Fig. 14-32B). The advantage is that no plates or screws are situated at the mental prominence; thus no implant can be felt by the patient later on. A variation of this technique is shown in extreme advancement genioplasty in Figure 14-33.

Fixation Principles in Craniofacial Reconstruction Procedures

Craniofacial reconstruction includes fixation techniques for reconstruction of the skull following trauma or tumor resection and for craniofacial operations on infants. Plate fixation has proved to be superior to internal wiring because it results in a

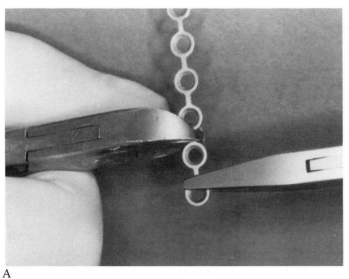

A

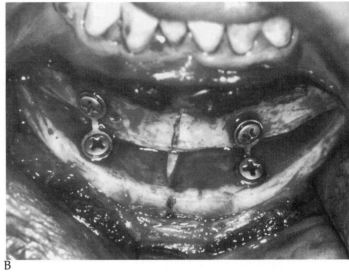

B

Fig. 14-32A. A section of two holes is cut from a fragmentation miniplate using a plate cutter. B. For rigid fixation of the genioplasty segment, two of these two-hole plates are bent to a right angle and placed 1 to 2 cm from the midline. This technique has the advantage that no plate or screw is placed at the prominence of the chin. The patient cannot feel any foreign body later on.

Fig. 14-33. Fixation technique in a two-step 20-mm advancement genioplasty. A. Each of the two lower segments was advanced about 10 mm. Two fragmentation miniplates are carefully contoured to follow the steps. B, C. Preoperative and postoperative profiles after advancement genioplasty.

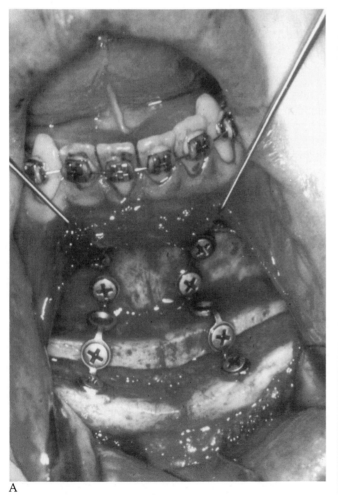

A

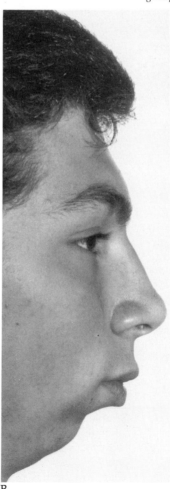

B

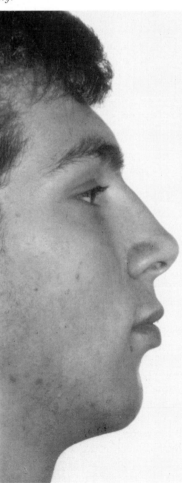

C

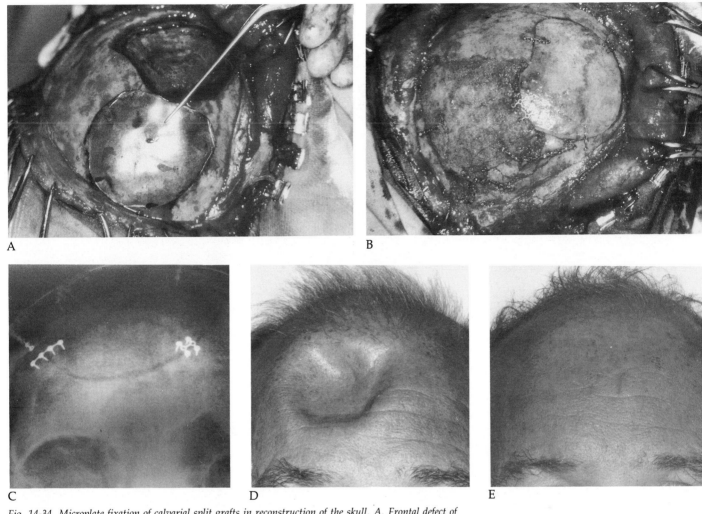

Fig. 14-34. Microplate fixation of calvarial split grafts in reconstruction of the skull. A. Frontal defect of the skull resulting from a gunshot injury is exposed. A lead template representing the size and shape of the defect facilitates harvesting of an appropriate full-thickness calvarial graft by the neurosurgeon. B. After the graft is split, the outer table covers the original defect. The inner table is used to reconstruct the donor site. Graft fixation is achieved by microplates. C. Roentgenogram after skull reconstruction. D. Original frontal skull defect. E. The patient one week after skull reconstruction.

stable, three-dimensional fixation of skeletal segments and bone grafts. The microsystem (see Fig. 14-16) is preferred for these indications; because they are small, the plates and screws are hardly palpable later on. One of the disadvantages of the larger (2-mm diameter screws) minisystems was that the patient could feel the implants, which frequently resulted in complaints; therefore, for reconstruction of the skull I now prefer microplates for graft fixation (Fig. 14-34). As a supplement to the microsystem, a micromesh (Fig. 14-35) is available that can be used for bridging bone defects of the skull or

the orbital walls. One example of the application of the micromesh (Fig. 14-36) shows reconstruction of the orbital roof after resection of a fibrous dysplasia.

Infant craniofacial operations provide an ideal use for modern rigid fixation techniques. Unlike internal wires, plates and screws provide safe and simple fixation of skeletal complexes in all three dimensions without the need for interpositional bone grafts (Fig. 14-37). Because the bones are thin and no great muscle forces act on the skull, very small plates and screws can be used (Figs. 14-38 and 14-39).

The regional-specific principles of rigid fixation in craniofacial reconstruction can be summarized as follows:

Analysis of muscle forces acting on the individual skeletal complex

Selection of plates and screws of adequate dimension

Performing the procedure for the appropriate indications: bone graft fixation in skull reconstruction, reconstruction of the walls of the frontal sinus and the nasoethmoidal area, and infant craniofacial operations

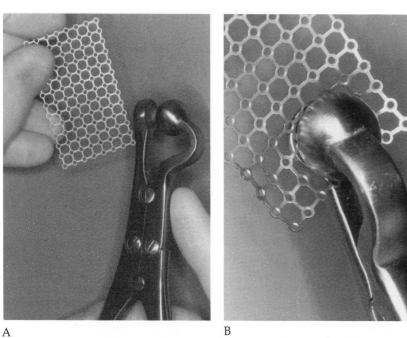

A

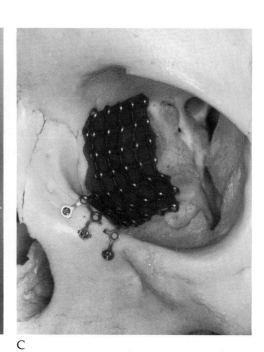

B

C

Fig. 14-35A, B. Micromesh (0.3 mm thickness) and special bending pliers for three-dimensional contouring. C. For bridging of orbital wall defects, an appropriate size and shape is cut out from a standard sheet by a wire cutter and is contoured. Use of a template facilitates the procedure. Note that some connection bars have been cut off for easier contouring of the mesh and fixation with screws outside the orbit.

Fig. 14-36. Micromesh and microplates in reconstruction of the orbital roof and frontal skull. A. Extensive defect of the orbital roof and the frontal skull resulting from resection of a fibrous dysplasia. B. A micromesh fixed by two

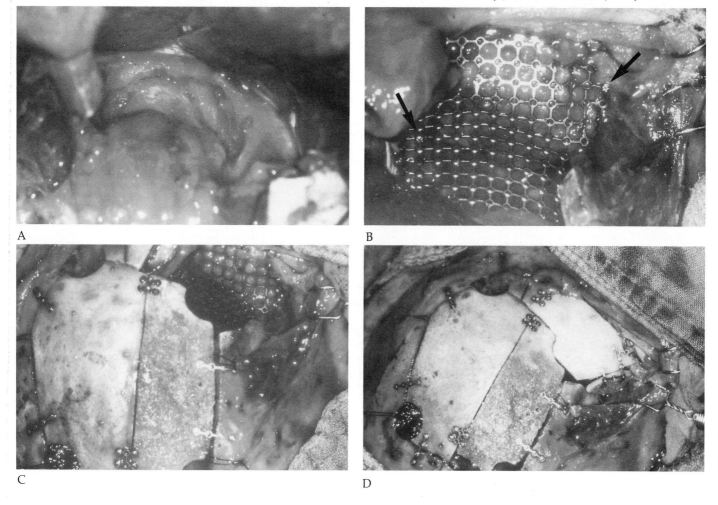

A

B

C

D

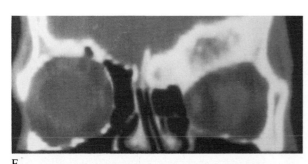

E

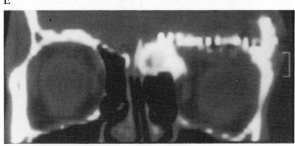

F

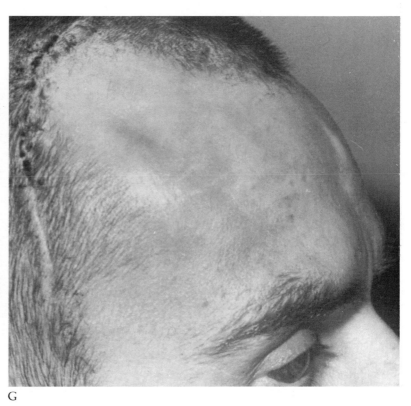

G

microscrews (arrows) covers the orbital roof defect. The mesh was cut from a standard sheet using a template to define the appropriate size and shape. C. After placement of the mesh, the skull is reconstructed by split calvarial grafts, which are stabilized by microplates. D. Final reconstruction of the frontoparietal skull area. E. Computed tomogram demonstrates fibrous dysplasia of the right orbital roof. F. Computed tomogram after resection of the lesion and reconstruction of the orbital roof by micromesh. G. Condition of the patient 2 weeks after reconstruction of the orbital roof and forehead.

Fig. 14-37. Craniofacial operations on infants are another good indication for microplates. Advancement procedures are possible without interpositional bone grafts, and gaps can be maintained.

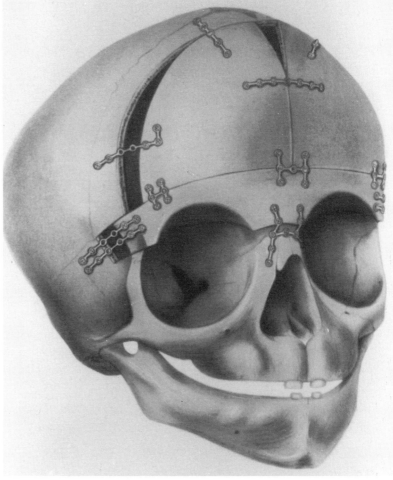

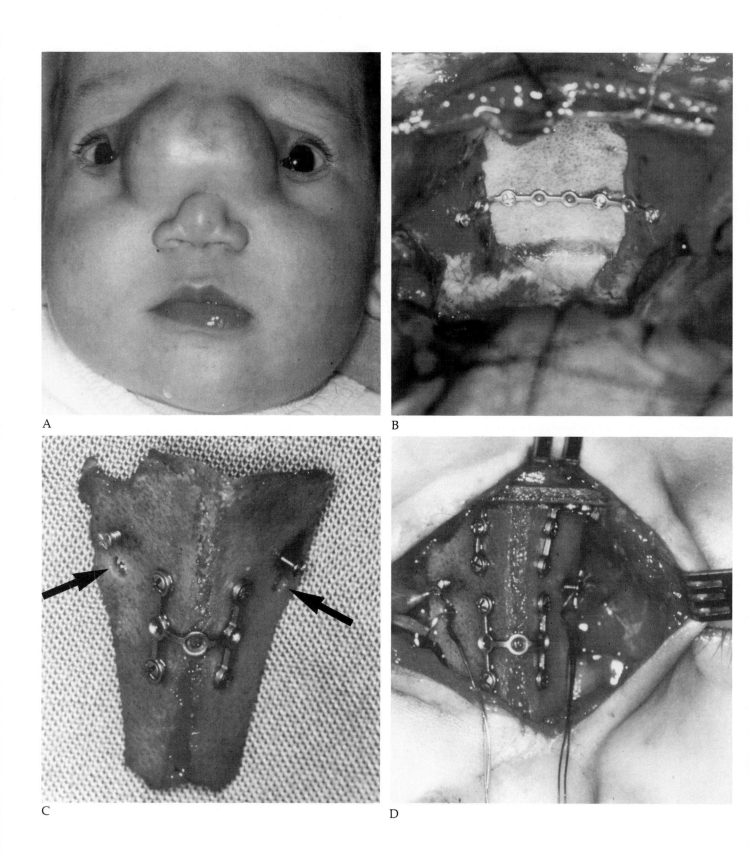

A

B

C

D

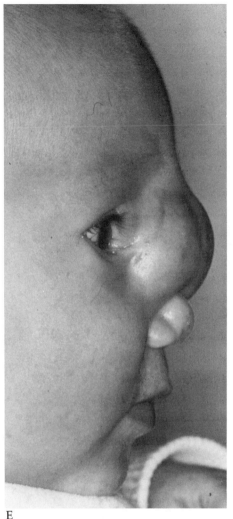

E

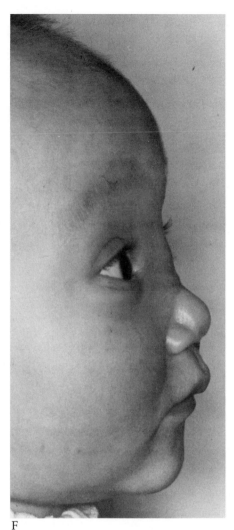

F

Fig. 14-38A. Encephalocele in an 8-month-old baby. B. After removal of the encephalocele by the neurosurgeon, the resulting defect of the anterior cranial fossa was covered by a calvarial bone graft and fixed with a microplate. (The retracted brain shows in the lower part of the photograph.) C. Another calvarial bone graft was greenstick-fractured in the midline to build a rooflike nasal skeleton. An H-type microplate maintained this configuration. Note the large drill holes (arrows) beneath the single screws. The medial canthal ligaments later will be pulled into these holes for medial fixation of the canthi. D. The newly built nasal skeleton is inserted and fixed to the bone graft by two L-shaped plates; the graft previously was placed into the anterior cranial fossa. Two thin wire sutures are fixed to the medial canthal ligaments and guided crosswise through the nasal bone graft. They will be tightened and fixed to each of the single microscrews. E, F. Preoperative and postoperative profiles of the patient.

Suggested Reading

Antonyshy, O., and Gruss, J.S. Complex orbital trauma: The role of rigid fixation and primary bone grafting. *Adv. Ophthalmol. Plast. Reconstr. Surg.* 7:61, 1988.

Ardary, W.C. Plate and screw fixation in the management of mandible fractures. *Clin. Plast. Surg.* 16:61, 1989.

Bell, W.H., Mannai, C., and Luhr, H.G. Art and science of Le Fort I downfracture. *Int. J. Adult Orthod. Orthognath. Surg.* 3:23, 1988.

Gruss, J.S., and Mackinnon, S.E. Complex maxillary fractures: Role of buttress reconstruction and immediate bone grafts. *Plast. Reconstr. Surg.* 78:9, 1986.

Gruss, J.S., and Phillips, J.H. Complex facial trauma: The evolving role of rigid fixation and immediate bone graft reconstruction. *Clin. Plast. Surg.* 16:42, 1989.

Luhr, H.G. Vitallium Luhr systems for reconstructive surgery of the facial skeleton. *Otolaryngol. Clin. North Am.* 20:573, 1987.

Luhr, H.G. A micro-system for cranio-maxillofacial skeletal fixation. *J. Craniomaxillofac. Surg.* 16:312, 1988.

Luhr, H.G. The significance of condylar position using rigid fixation in orthognathic surgery. *Clin. Plast. Surg.* 16:147, 1989.

Luhr, H.G. Indications for use of a microsystem for internal fixation in craniofacial surgery. *J. Craniofac. Surg.* 1:35, 1990.

Luhr, H.G., and Kubein-Meesenburg, D. Rigid skeletal fixation in maxillary osteotomies. *Clin. Plast. Surg.* 16:157, 1989.

Manson, P.N. Management of facial fractures. *Plast. Surg.* 2:1, 1988.

Manson, P.N., et al. Sagittal fractures of the maxilla and palate. *Plast. Reconstr. Surg.* 72:484, 1983.

Markowitz, B.L., and Manson, P.N. Panfacial fractures: Organization of treatment. *Clin. Plast. Surg.* 16:105, 1989.

Munro, I.R. The Luhr fixation system for the craniofacial skeleton. *Clin. Plast. Surg.* 16:41, 1989.

Rosen, H.M. Miniplate fixation of Lefort I osteotomies. *Plast. Reconstr. Surg.* 78:748, 1986.

Schilli, W., Ewers, R., and Niederdellmann, H. Bone fixation with screws and plates in the maxillofacial region. *Int. J. Oral Surg.* 10(Suppl. 1):329, 1981.

Steinhäuser, E.W. Bone screws and plates in orthognathic surgery. *Int. J. Oral Surg.* 11:209, 1982.

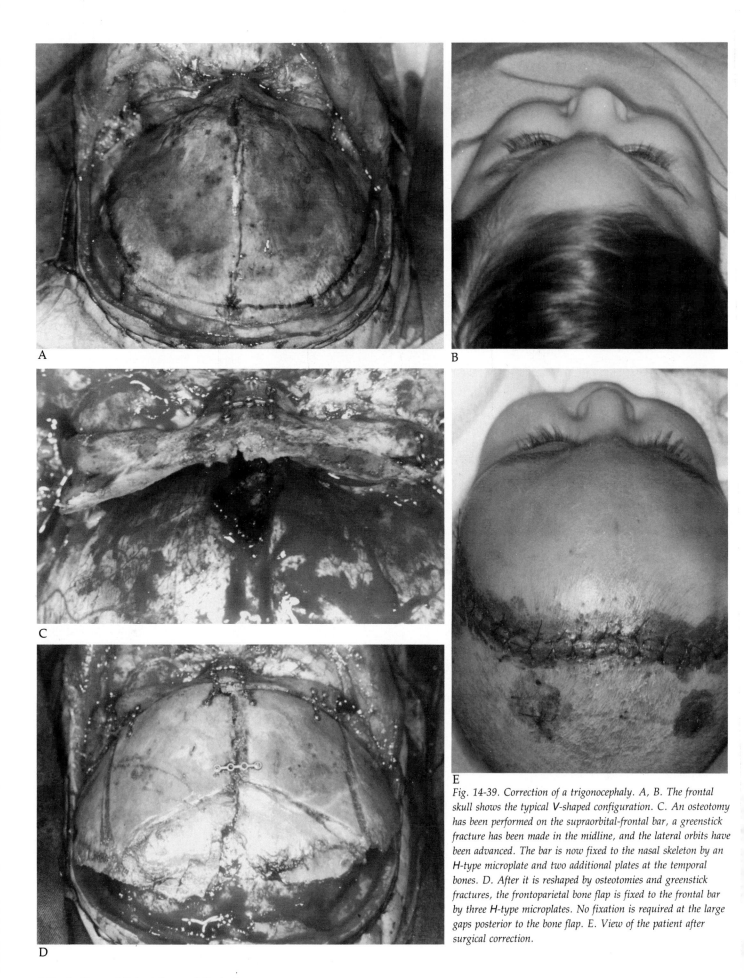

Fig. 14-39. Correction of a trigonocephaly. A, B. The frontal
skull shows the typical *V*-shaped configuration. C. An osteotomy
has been performed on the supraorbital-frontal bar, a greenstick
fracture has been made in the midline, and the lateral orbits have
been advanced. The bar is now fixed to the nasal skeleton by an
H-type microplate and two additional plates at the temporal
bones. D. After it is reshaped by osteotomies and greenstick
fractures, the frontoparietal bone flap is fixed to the frontal bar
by three *H*-type microplates. No fixation is required at the large
gaps posterior to the bone flap. E. View of the patient after
surgical correction.

15

Reconstruction Using Soft Tissue Expansion

Ernest K. Manders

Soft tissue expansion requires the implantation of a silicone elastomer balloon that is filled by the serial injection of sterile isotonic saline solution over a period of weeks to months. The process of inflation of the balloon stretches the overlying soft tissue and induces growth. If given enough time, expansion can provide enormous increases in the soft tissue available for reconstruction of adjacent defects. The chief advantage of using this technique is that it replaces an area of missing skin with almost normal integument. In the scalp, the uniform distribution of hair follicles and hair shafts is restored. No technique today allows such successful restoration of major surface loss as the process of soft tissue expansion.

Tissues that undergo a deliberate, slow expansion provide a durable soft tissue cover. The expanded tissue is typically sensate; its vascularity is preserved and even augmented. Of great importance to both patient and surgeon is the fact that there is no visible donor site defect.

As with any surgical technique, there are limitations, and they should be acknowledged at the outset. Soft tissue expansion is generally not useful for immediate reconstruction after traumatic loss of tissues. The insertion of an expander requires a surgical field that is not colonized by bacteria nor invaded by a malignant tumor. The patient who opts for reconstruction using soft tissue expansion must accept the limitations of time required for expansion, a minimum of two operations, and the transient deformity noted during the late stages of expansion. The deformity usually is easily disguised, except in facial expansion, and the patient can be counseled that the end result is almost always gratifying.

Soft tissue expansion is a versatile technique for the plastic and reconstructive surgeon. The process may be applied in a general way to replace missing integument over almost the entire surface of the body. It may be used in unique ways, as in expanding the forehead to prepare a flap for total nasal reconstruction. Such an expanded flap not only amply covers the reconstructed nasal skeleton but also provides a lining for the reconstructed nose while the donor site defect is closed primarily. Orbital expansion is another example of a newer application of soft tissue expansion that will undoubtedly be used increasingly as more surgeons become familiar with it.

Some regional problems are particularly well handled by soft tissue expansion. Scalp reconstruction is certainly one. The discussion of the technique of expansion begins with a somewhat detailed account of the planning and performance of a simultaneous forehead and scalp reconstruction. The planning, principles, and technical points presented here apply to expansion in other areas of the body. Expansion in other regions will be discussed later in the chapter.

Natural History and Anatomy

The scalp follows the skull in its growth; the skull in turn grows in response to the enlarging brain. In the first year of life, the brain increases in mass approximately 2.5 times, and in the second year of life it increases by one-third again. The scalp ceases enlargement when it is not stretched by the underlying enlarging skull. The potential for growth is not lost, however, and it is this basic biologic process that is exploited in soft tissue expansion.

It is important to realize in planning that children experience some recession of the anterior hairline with growth. Although the anterior hairline pattern and the vertex scalp pattern in girls is stable after late childhood, a boy may proceed to male pattern baldness. All men experience some recession of the anterior hairline as a secondary sex characteristic. All Caucasian men have some hair loss if they have normal endocrine function. This normal loss should be borne in mind by any surgeon planning a scalp reconstruction in a boy or young man. Clearly the defect should be reconstructed so that there will be minimal abnormality should hair loss occur.

The scalp consists of several readily identifiable layers. Beneath the skin and subcutaneous fat is the galea aponeurotica. The areolar layer below the galea affords an avascular plane for easy dissection. Working in this plane minimizes blood loss and does not interrupt the innervation of the scalp. If dissection is extended anteriorly in this plane, the surgeon enters a space beneath the frontalis muscle in the frontal area. Every effort should be made to avoid tearing the pericranium because this tissue has rich vascularity and will bleed. This can be especially important in operations on children.

The surgeon must respect the natural boundaries of the hairline. Unless there is a specific reason to cross the boundary with an expander, such as simultaneous reconstruction of the forehead and anterior hairline with the anterior scalp, the soft tissue expander should be confined to the area of the hair-bearing scalp.

Some attention should be given to the fact that there is a characteristic angulation of hair shafts as they exit from the skin, and this angulation is specific to the region of the scalp where the hair shaft lies. The surgeon should attempt to position the advanced scalp so that the angle of exit of the hair shaft is normal for that region of scalp. This is not always possible, and the result will not be marred greatly by failure to meet this goal. The surgeon should be aware that if the angle of exit cannot be matched to the native angle, the aberrant angle will persist for the life of the patient.

Scars widen, and the patient should be informed of this. Usually, a sagittally oriented incision in the scalp heals with a wider scar than does a coronally oriented incision. The reason is that the coronally

oriented fibers from galea to dermis in effect pull laterally. A coronal incision splits these fibers as one might split fascia in the long axis of its fibers. There is little tendency for the fibers to distract the healing dermis and widen a coronal scar. On the other hand, a sagitally positioned incision widens more because interruption of the scalp architecture allows greater distraction of the dermal edges.

The surgeon also should be aware that some areas are easier to dissect than others. Ease of dissection is a function of the density and adherence of the areolar tissue beneath the galea. The occipital area in an adult, for example, is always more difficult to raise than the frontal and temporal scalp.

Surgical Procedure

I use the example of a large nevus involving the forehead as a model for discussion of the principles involved in planning the treatment of patients by tissue expansion (Fig. 15-1). These principles virtually always apply, regardless of the area of the body being operated on.

The nevus does not involve the frontalis muscle as a traumatic defect might. When faced with a congenital nevus, the surgeon must decide whether to expand the frontalis muscle with the overlying skin or to expand atop the frontalis. It is generally my practice to expand the frontalis muscle only when it is needed for the reconstruction. If this muscle is not needed, I preserve it by expanding on top of it. In that situation the pigmented skin only is replaced—not the native frontalis muscle underlying it.

Counseling the Patient

There are two questions to be answered when beginning to plan a reconstruction with soft tissue expansion. What tissue is available for expansion? and Where do we want the final scar to lie? These questions should be held as paramount during the process of treatment design.

Design is the key to successful treatment. Defects should be surrounded as much as possible. A plan should be made for a large expansion in every patient. The expansion should be widest where there is the need for the greatest advancement. There is rarely a necessity for formation

of complicated flaps. Simple advancement flaps with no back-cuts usually suffice.

The suitability of the patient must be considered. The surgeon should ask what the patient's personal needs are. Can the patient afford the time required for the soft tissue expansion? Will the patient allow a second or even a third expansion if indicated? Are soft tissue expanders readily available? Will the patient cooperate with the requirement of a weekly or biweekly injection? It is important to remember that the transient deformity may be difficult for members of some cultures to accept. The cost of the procedure may be an overriding issue. Not only are two operations required but also the soft tissue expanders, the needles, the sterile saline solution, and possibly travel to the doctor's office impose additional expenses.

One must consider whether the patient is suitable from the standpoint of health. Is the patient in good mental and physical health? Are there any systemic contraindications to implantation of a foreign body, such as depressed immunity? Are there any local contraindications to insertion of the soft tissue expander, such as surface infection or colonized open wounds? Open wounds may be prepared by covering them with an allograft. There also should be no malignant tumors immediately adjacent to the area of expansion. Radiation therapy of more than 5000 cGy should be considered a relative contraindication to expansion.

The patient should be evaluated to determine whether anesthesia is best delivered generally or locally. Direct infiltration of the scalp with or without ring block infiltration is highly effective for major procedures. Operations for male pattern baldness in the entire hair-bearing scalp and much of the forehead can be accomplished easily with local anesthesia. Children, of course, virtually always require general anesthesia to eliminate the risk of inadequate cooperation.

The patient can be counseled that scars widen and that this widening will become visible about one month after the operation. The scar reaches its maximal width by 3 months postoperatively. After that time, a revision can be contemplated if the scalp is lax. Transverse scars at the anterior hairline where the scalp meets the hairless forehead are usually excellent

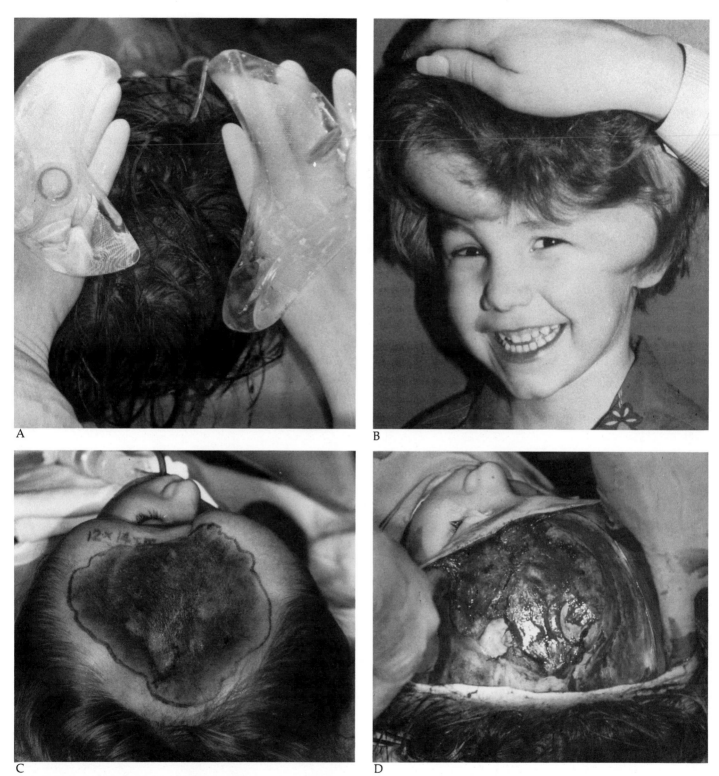

A

B

C

D

Fig. 15-1A. Custom-made croissant slope expanders to be placed under healthy scalp and forehead through an incision within the congenital hairy nevus to be removed. B. Expansion underway. This expansion should be safe and unhurried and should produce minimal discomfort and pain to the patient. C. The extent of the nevus to be removed by advancement of expanded scalp and forehead was 12 cm by 14 cm. The expanded skin has increased enough to provide a tension-free coverage. D. The defect following excision of the nevus and removal of the expanders.

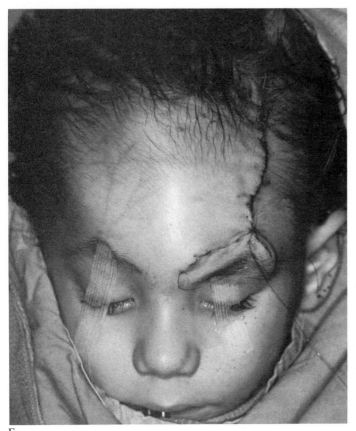

E

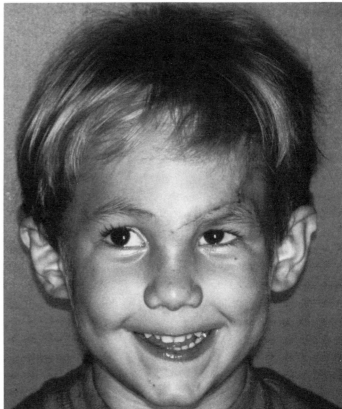

F

Fig. 15-1. (Continued) E. The advancement and closure. Closing the circular defect in a linear manner has slightly lowered the left eyebrow. F. Several months later, after a scar revision to narrow the scar and elevate the left eyebrow. G. Excellent skin distribution with minimal scarring and without residual areas of alopecia.

and are barely distinguishable from the surrounding tissues. When possible, the interface of advanced expanded scalp with the normal forehead should be kept as short as possible.

Choice of Soft Tissue Expander

Soft tissue expanders should be as large as possible. One expander is preferred over two whenever possible. It can be safely said, however, that any required expansion can be accomplished with the appropriate overlapping of available designs. Custom soft tissue expanders of special design and shape do have a role, but few are required. They are advantageous when several expanders would be required to fit an odd-shaped defect; in this situation, a custom expander is cost-effective. The expander is prepared by making an outline of the area to be ex-

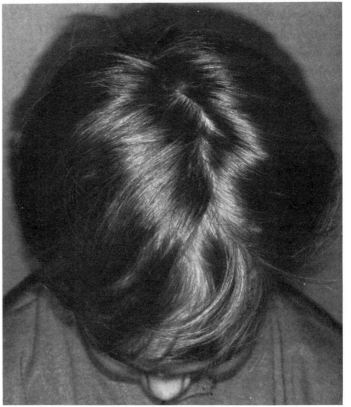

G

panded on exposed x-ray film. The template can be sent to the manufacturer with instructions regarding how redundant the envelope should be. Little redundancy is required for a typical operation.

Surgeons have their preferences, but almost all soft tissue expanders on the market today will do the job required. There is an advantage to the use of high-compliance floppy expanders without stiff backing. These may be folded to fit odd-shaped defects effectively.

Surgeons have preferences regarding the use of integrated versus remote injection ports. The use of expanders with valves integrated into the envelope is especially important in the region of the head and neck. Using an expander with an integrated valve allows rapid insertion without additional dissection to accommodate removal of the remote valve. There is no need to pursue the tedious delivery of the port at the time of removal of the expander. A surgeon who does not have an expander with an integrated port available when placing soft tissue expanders under the scalp can simply place the injection port atop the expander as if it were an integrated port. The envelope must be positioned so that there are no redundant folds to cover the port. Some surgeons have suggested leaving the remote valve outside the skin to facilitate serial injections and expansion, particularly in children. I have not resorted to exiting the injection tubing of a remote port through a subcutaneous tunnel with the port hanging free outside. A buried port is tidier both aesthetically and bacteriologically.

Placement of Soft Tissue Expander

The patient shampoos the night before and the morning of the operation. He or she is positioned on the operating table so that the surgeon may have comfortable access to the scalp to be undermined. The scalp is never shaved. The hair is painted with povidone-iodine, and prophylactic broad-spectrum antibiotics are administered intravenously. The site of the incision is injected with a lidocaine solution containing epinephrine, typically before the scalp is prepared and draped. In the usual operation, incisions are made at the border of the defect. The incision may be entirely within a benign nevus. The incision should be large enough only to allow introduction of the port itself. Two or more incisions may be used when access is facilitated by a broader approach. The bridge of attached scalp between the incisions makes closure more secure, and the danger of suture line dehiscence is minimized.

The surgeon should avoid an additional scar on the scalp. He or she should even resist making additional incisions for placement of an injection port or for removing it later. The incisions themselves should be beveled to avoid injury to the hair follicles lying in the dermis and beneath. If the normal scalp meets a skin graft, the boundary itself can be safely incised and closed in most instances.

With incision of the skin and subcutaneous tissue, the dissection is extended sharply through the galea to the white, loose, areolar plane beneath the galea. Here the scalpel blade is positioned with its back against the pericranium and is swept back and forth with the cutting edge pointing up to elevate the areolar tissue. There should be little or no bleeding. Once a pocket is formed in this manner, the blade is removed from the field and the surgeon inserts his or her finger or a curved Van Buren male urethral sound. The sound is a valuable instrument for dissecting the scalp. After this dissection, a malleable retractor is curved to fit the cranium, passed into the incision, and moved back and forth to ensure that a broad pocket with no intervening bands from pericranium to galea has been prepared. Finger dissection is especially useful in children, but it should be performed carefully to avoid tearing the pericranium.

There are regional differences that are important in making the dissection. The occipital scalp is tightly bound to the pericranium, and in adults it must be elevated sharply down to the level of the nuchal ridge. Care must be shown here; otherwise the bleeding from the occipital arteries can be severe and difficult to control from a distant incision.

The vertex scalp is elevated readily as is the area over the temporalis muscles. Over the temporalis, however, the surgeon must be careful not to bruise the underlying muscle; otherwise the patient will experience considerable pain and prolonged discomfort postoperatively.

As the dissection moves forward to the forehead, the areolar plane enters the subfrontalis plane. If the surgeon wishes to move about the frontalis, the transition must be sought with care, often through a separate and more anterior incision so that the operator can work from the known anterior border of the frontalis muscle posteriorly to a point where the muscle ends and the subgaleal plane can be entered.

Again, the operator should remember that an infant's scalp is much more vulnerable to injury than is an adult's, and when instruments with a long reach are used, attention should be paid to the tension on the wound edges so that there is no tearing of the scalp.

When it appears the pocket has adequate dimension, it is helpful to place a sterile template in the pocket. The template can be prepared of x-ray film and should be traced from the baseplate of the expander intended for use in the pocket. A stock of templates of different styles can easily be prepared from x-ray film if they are not available from manufacturers; after use the templates can be sterilized and saved for future patients. It should be emphasized that the pocket should be large enough to allow full unfurling of the expander by maximal expansion so that the greatest possible area of scalp is expanded.

After irrigation to ensure hemostasis and removal of introduced hair, a closed suction drain is placed in the wound and its tube is tunneled under the adjacent scalp and exited through a stab wound. It is then sewn in place.

The soft tissue expander is inserted with care to avoid introducing hair along with it. It should be noted again that the hair is never shaved. To minimize the chance for introduction of hair, it is possible to sew a drape to the edges of the wound with a 000 nylon suture material. This produces a neat field that is not marred by strands of hair introduced with the expander. The surgeon typically changes gloves and rids them of surface powder before handling the expander. Afterward, additional irrigation with saline solution containing an antibiotic is carried out, and the expander is inserted. All air is removed from the expander before insertion. The port is carefully positioned and, in some instances, it is inserted before the expander; typically it is inserted with it or after it. The expander should be positioned flat so there are no folds. If necessary, a large Van Buren urethral sound can be used to spread out the expander with little danger of injury to its envelope. A trial fill is then carried out. If there is any question in the operator's mind regarding the possibility of perforation of the envelope, the expander should be injected with saline solution containing methylene blue. Inspection of the fluid in the wound and exiting from the drain confirms that there is no leak if the drainage is clear.

After inflation to ensure the expander is fully unfurled and occupies the extent of the pocket desired, the saline solution is removed and the expander is deflated. The deflation aids closure and contributes to the patient's comfort postoperatively.

The closure is accomplished with a running vertical mattress suture or interrupted vertical mattress sutures and a superficial running nylon suture. I use only monofilament nylon. It is often advantageous to close with a malleable retractor in place shielding the expander from the end of the needle. Good lighting, proper assistance, and care are required for a safe, secure closure. In the case of a particularly lax scalp, some sterile saline solution may be left in the expander after the wound is closed. The pressure within the expander should not exceed 20 mmHg. The pressure can be estimated roughly by observing the column of saline solution in the tubing of a conventional butterfly needle connected to the port. If the meniscus is just below the hub of the needle with the tube outstretched, the pressure is 20 mmHg or less.

Postoperative management includes admission for overnight observation and administration of analgesics the night after placement of the soft tissue expander. The drain is typically removed in 1 or 2 days; the patient is instructed to shampoo in the shower on the first postoperative day even if the drain is in place. I administer prophylactic antibiotics for 5 days postoperatively because of the chance that some hair has been introduced with the expander.

Expansion

The skin is prepared with 70% ethanol, and a 23-gauge needle is inserted into the port. When the patient notes that the scalp is beginning to feel tight, the injection is halted. This sensation typically occurs with an internal pressure of 40 to 50 mmHg. Sometimes I measure the pressure with an electronic meter or a manometer. I do so for patients whose reactions I cannot properly gauge, infants, patients undergoing expansion adjacent to muscles such as the frontalis, and patients with an obviously thinning or unstable scalp. One cannot generalize and state that a given volume is added to every patient at every filling. I typically find that filling once a week approaches adding 10 percent of the design volume of the expander per week. The rate of inflation can be increased by about one-third with two injections. I have had no trouble teaching the families and friends of patients how to perform these injections. Home injection has been successful and a great convenience for the patients. Additionally, patients typically have achieved a sense of gratification in helping to manage their own care.

Final Advancement

The planning for the final advancement begins with measurement of the increase in arc length available at that time in the expansion. The operator estimates the width of the base of the expansion or sites directly over the expander. A tape measure is placed from the bottom of the expander across the top of the expanded dome, to the top edge of the tissue expander in the line of intended advancement. By subtracting the base width from the arc length, it is possible to estimate the advancement. This estimate works best when the defect is surrounded, as in a croissant expander or multiple expanders. Clearly the expansion should proceed until there is, at minimum, an increase in arc length equal to the width of the defect to be covered.

The orientation of the final scar should be planned carefully. Local anesthesia often is sufficient for carrying out the advancement because there is less pain, both intraoperatively and postoperatively, than during the time of expander placement. Local anesthetic is injected as before; again, a ring block for the scalp may prove useful for adults undergoing advancement.

The incision is made with attention to avoiding damage to the hair follicles. The reactive capsule around the expander is opened with electrocautery using a rounded blade, not a needle tip, to avoid perforation of the expander. Every effort should be made to remove the soft tissue expander intact. If necessary, the surgeon should deflate the expander before removal by inserting a fine needle into the port valve.

Before any of the nevus or scar is removed, a trial advancement should be carried out. If the planning has been accurate, the results are immediately gratifying.

The bed is prepared by excising the split-thickness skin graft or tumor, removing temporary allografts, and debriding the area. The capsule surrounding the expander is not removed. Capsulotomies are performed, however, when necessary to facilitate mobilization of the expanded tissues. The soft tissue expanders may be deflated and immediately reinserted if a second expansion is required to accomplish the reconstruction. The use of drains should be judicious. Sometimes there is little reason to expect much accumulation of blood and serum. The closure is carried out with meticulous technique. The surgeon must realize that in performing the closure, he or she is preparing a final closure, and the scar will be the final result. Dog-ears should not be excised because they shrink and become inapparent in a matter of days to weeks.

Postoperative Care

The patient's hair may be shampooed on the table, or the patient may shampoo in the shower the next morning. My associates and I simply wrap the patient's head in a terry cloth towel. If a drain was inserted, it is removed on the first or second postoperative day. If additional soft tissue expansion is required, it typically is begun one week after the first expander is removed.

Complications

There are both major and minor complications of soft tissue expansion (Fig. 15-2). Minor complications include problems such as seroma formation, transient alopecia during scalp expansion, postoper-

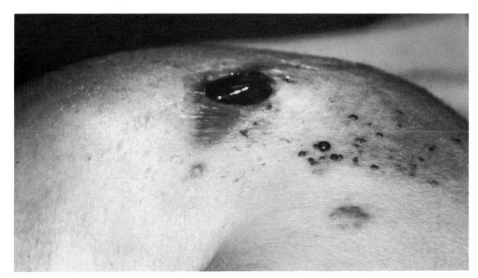

Fig. 15-2. A complication from placing a round expander near a hemangioma. The knuckle of the expander caused an exposure through the placement incision. The fault was in failing to make the pocket large enough, causing the expander to gather and press on the incision. Although it is not ideal to place expanders directly under incisions, it is common to place them next to incisions. Success depends on having a pocket of adequate size.

ative dog-ears at the ends of surgical incisions, and postoperative widening of scars. Seroma formation often can be prevented with the insertion of a drain at the time of expander replacement or treated by aspiration over the injection port. Typically alopecia induced by the pressure of an injection port on the skin or from an overly ambitious inflation schedule clears with time as hair follicles come out of the telogen, or resting phase. Dog-ears may be revised as needed. On the scalp, revision is seldom required. Scars may call for revision depending on their location and final appearance.

Major complications include hematoma, infection, expander exposure or extrusion, and tissue necrosis. Hematoma is not a common complication. The surgeon should approach a hematoma with a careful decision-making process. Typically exploration with evacuation of the hematoma and a search for bleeding points are required. Hematomas should not be evacuated by drains.

Today, few surgeons see expander exposure and extrusion in the absence of infection. Prophylactic antibiotics are commonly used at the time of expander insertion. I have learned to begin postoperative expansion carefully and to observe the tension to which the skin is subjected. As a consequence of a careful

approach, direct disruption of an incision is rare indeed. Breakdown of an incision or drainage from an incision indicates the presence of an infection.

Although it is sometimes possible to salvage an expander that has become exposed and a periexpander infection, this is not usual, especially in the limbs. In the head and neck, however, the area has been salvaged by thorough irrigation of the expander pocket, cleansing and autoclaving of the expanders, drainage, and treatment with appropriate antibiotics. In general, however, the surgeon's action should be conservative, and the expander should be removed and the pocket drained. Although this method slows the process of reconstruction, it is safe for the patient and does not risk a protracted course with potential worsening of the infection. The surgeon should remember that no tissue will be lost, the tissue planes can be opened later, and the reconstruction will be just as successful, although delayed.

One of the greatest problems plaguing the neophyte using soft tissue expansion is inadequate expansion. A surgeon must be prepared to encourage the patient to endure the periodic expansions for as long as it takes to achieve an expansion that provides tissue that allows reconstruction of the defect. As already dis-

cussed, the arc length over the expansion is an important guide for estimation of the amount of tissue available for advancement. This measurement may be conservative in some instances and may provide an overestimate in others, depending on the geometry of the expansion and the extensibility of the tissues. Planning in three dimensions is a necessity. When possible, the wound should be surrounded as indicated previously, and expansions should be large. Careful planning and adequate expansion are prerequisites for successful soft tissue expansion.

Regional Reconstruction
The Face

Good judgment is required when deciding whether or not to use soft tissue expansion in major facial reconstructions (Fig. 15-3). The forehead certainly may be expanded with benefit. Forehead expansions may be combined with scalp expansions. The geometry of expansion, however, often makes forehead reconstruction using expansion a difficult and tedious process. This is because the adjacent landmarks, such as eyebrows and hairline, limit the expansion that can be attained and the advancement that can be effected after expansion. Simple advancements are best whenever possible. Long incisions to unfurl the hemispheric flap before an expansion may be of great value at times, but, if at all possible, scar should be held to a minimum by use of simple advancements. For some patients, a second expansion requiring an extra operation may lead to a smaller scar and an aesthetically superior result.

Defects of the central face generally are best treated by a reverse face-lift. One might ask when to make the decision to use soft tissue expansion as opposed to serial excision. My rule is that if I believe I can reconstruct a defect with three or four serial excisions of the central face, I do serial excisions. Soft tissue expansion in the face is difficult to disguise. Fat atrophy is common. If there is any tension on the closure, there will be distortion of facial features; therefore, it is absolutely essential that an expansion be well designed and planned and that an ample amount of expanded skin be available.

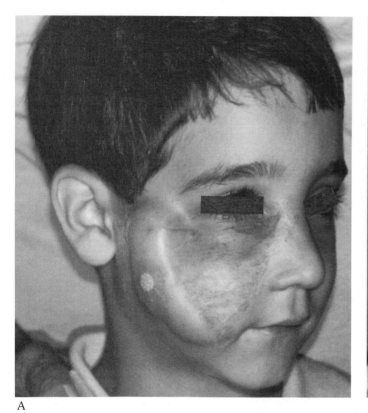

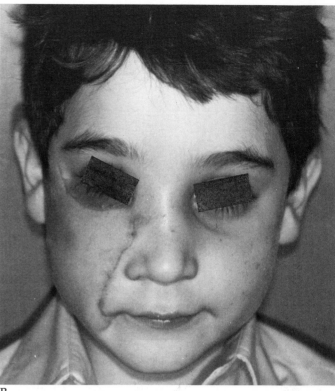

A

B

Fig. 15-3. Cheek expansion. A. This young patient had discolored, scarred skin as a result of a large facial hemangioma that subsequently underwent involution. B. An early photograph after advancement of an expanded right cheek flap. The darker skin of the lower eyelid was later replaced with a full-thickness graft of retroauricular skin.

The surgeon should consider a trial deflation to manipulate the expanded skin flap to determine just how much skin there really is when the tension is released. It is easy to be fooled when looking at a large, tense expansion. The dimensions may indeed be exactly what one needs, but in eagerness to find this result, we often overlook the fact that the skin is not expanded but still under stretch. When the force of the underlying expander is taken away, the skin naturally recoils, the advancement becomes tight, and the ultimate result is distorted by this tension. A surgeon who worries about the possibility of lateral drift of the nasal base, ectropion, or distortion of the position of the oral commissure should not hesitate to deflate the expander and manipulate the expanded skin to determine whether it is time to proceed with the advancement.

Surgeons are now familiar with the strategy of expanding neck skin and carrying such expanded flaps up over the line of the mandible. It should be remembered, however, that this strategy is fraught with difficulty. The extent of expansion is often overestimated because when expanding on the underside of the mandible and over the neck, one is expanding from a concave surface. The expander must be quite large before there is any actual gain in tissue. When the flap is brought up over the line of the mandible, there often is tension after advancement, which distorts facial features and obliterates the line of the mandible and the natural concave line beneath it. If this is the only strategy available, the surgeon should attempt to inset the posterior line of the flap at the anterior edge of the ear, if possible, to avoid an obvious line of scar at the posterior edge of the flap.

An additional concern is potential injury to branches of the facial nerve in central facial expansions. I have never seen apraxia from compression of a facial nerve branch by an expander, but once in opening the capsule to obtain more mobility of the expanded flap, I was surprised to find I had exposed the branches of the facial nerve. I was dissecting more deeply into the face because traction had lifted the soft tissues upward with the flap. If a capsulotomy is contemplated, the surgeon must be careful to perform the procedure so that the deeper structures are not injured.

The Nose

The ability to perform an acceptable nasal reconstruction is the mark of an accomplished plastic surgeon. Soft tissue expansion of the central forehead for construction of an axial pattern flap based on the supratrochlear neurovascular bundle can prove expeditious in the hands of most surgeons (Fig. 15-4). Soft tissue expansion helps in the reconstruction of large nasal defects, but it is not necessary for most nasal defects, even those of large extent. It does, however, offer a reliable, readily reproducible technique for a rel-

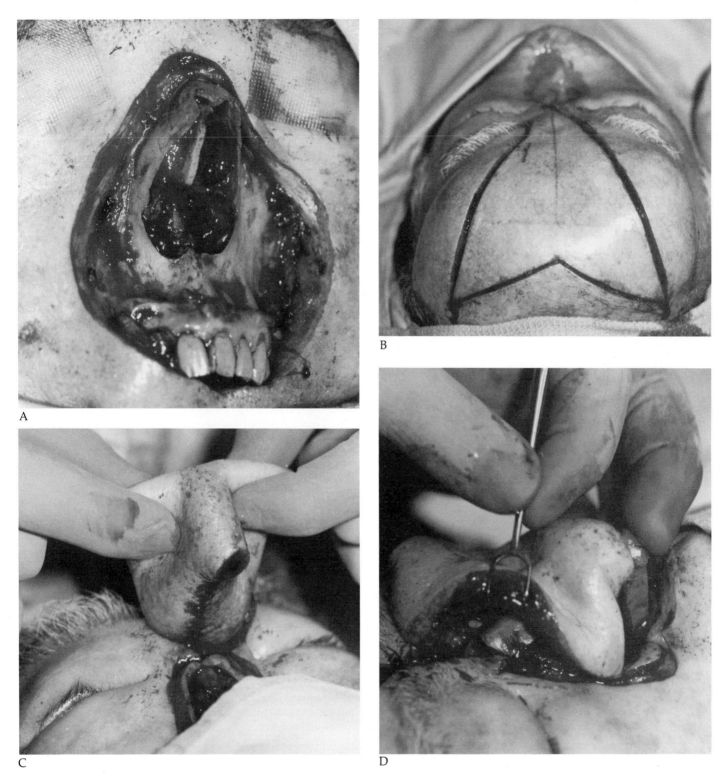

Fig. 15-4. Nasal reconstruction. A. This patient had an extensive basal cell carcinoma requiring rhinectomy and removal of a large portion of the upper lip. B. The expanded forehead flap was designed with extensions to allow coverage of an autogenous cartilage graft within the newly constructed nose. C. The nasal flap is folded with the extensions brought together at the area of the radix. D. The autogenous cartilage graft is inserted and fixed to the facial skeleton. It is about to be fully covered by the expanded forehead flap.

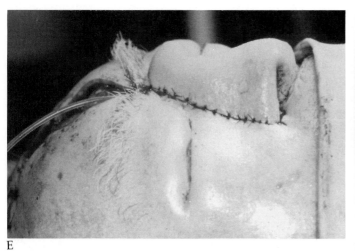

E

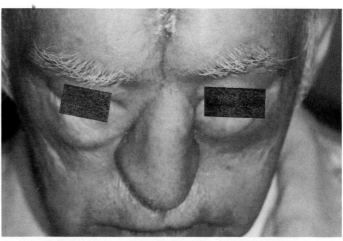

F

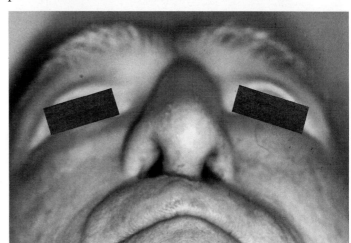

G

Fig. 15-4. (Continued) E. The expanded forehead flap is inset in place. F, G. The result following closure and early healing of the forehead donor site. The patient can breathe through his nose, and the autogenous cartilage support graft is entirely invested by viable forehead skin.

atively inexperienced surgeon. The technique allows closure of the donor site and avoids wound healing by secondary intention. At times, the scar resulting from forehead healing by secondary intention may be undesirable, especially in younger patients. The flap generated easily can be 8.5 to 10.0 cm wide and is a hardy one, having been conditioned by expansion.

The essential point in constructing this flap is the thinning of the distal end of the flap to be folded. The frontalis muscle and capsule can be separated with blunt and sharp dissection from the overlying fat subcutaneous tissue, which contains the vessels nourishing the flap. When folded, a large amount of skin is available to line the nasal reconstruction. The folded flap invests a dorsal strut of cartilage or bone. Cartilage from the conchae may be added to stiffen the alae, although this step usually is not necessary. The technique is straightforward and has much to recommend it.

The Ear

Despite an early wave of enthusiasm in our clinic for reconstruction of microtia using expanded skin, my associates and I have abandoned this technique. We now believe that the standard techniques for reconstruction of microtia are superior. For reconstruction of auricular defects after major trauma, our first choice is a temporoparietal fascial flap turned over an autogenous cartilage graft. This flap is covered by a split-thickness skin graft. Although there may be times when soft tissue expansion is valuable, existing techniques for auricular reconstruction usually are just as good if not superior.

The Neck

The neck may be reconstructed with very large flaps of supraclavicular skin expanded above the top of the shoulder and in the supraclavicular area. The dimen-

sions of the expansion must be impressive. The flap is based over the trapezius muscle at the posterior neck, and when fully expanded, there typically is enough redundant tissue to allow easy closure of the donor defect while a major area of the lateral and anterior neck is reconstructed. This reconstruction also may be carried up onto the face in selected patients. This flap has been highly effective for difficult burn reconstructions. The supraclavicular area is also an excellent site for expansion in preparation for harvesting of full-thickness skin grafts for facial burn reconstruction. Relatively large amounts of full-thickness skin grafts thus become available. The donor site closes easily and the skin has an excellent quality, allowing reconstruction of major defects with most satisfactory results.

The Breast

Reconstruction of the breast has been advanced considerably by soft tissue expan-

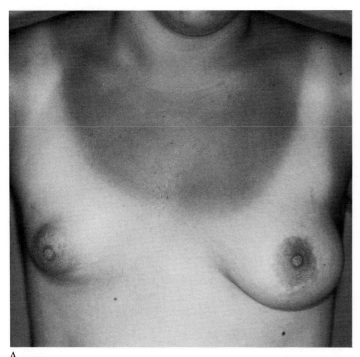
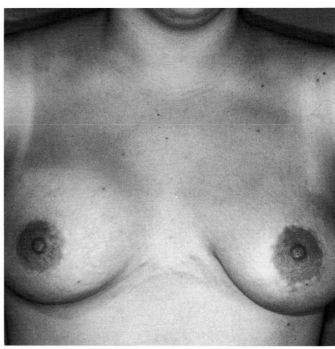

A   B

Fig. 15-5. Hypoplastic breast. A. This young patient had a hypoplastic right breast. B. After a period of expansion and placement of a gel-filled prosthesis, she has an excellent reconstruction with similar volume to and a shape that is aesthetically superior to that of the left breast.

sion (Fig. 15-5). No technique is as good as soft tissue expansion in reconstructing a hypoplastic breast. The soft tissue expander may be placed in a pocket that is not totally covered by muscle. As my experience has grown, I have come to see that the lower pole of the expander is almost never fully covered by muscle, even when attempts have been made to achieve this. In fact, expansion may be aided by deliberately leaving the lower pole of the expander exposed in a subcutaneous position. I place the upper portion of the expander under the pectoralis major muscle. This requires detachment of the portion of the origin of the muscle that starts from the ribs. I do not detach the sternal origin. I make no attempt to cover the lower pole of the expander with serratus anterior and rectus fascia. The resulting expansion is easier and the form superior.

For a young woman with a hypoplastic breast, the expander typically is placed through an axillary incision. It is placed through a subpectoral dissection with release of the origin. The expander can be inflated over several years to match the gradually enlarging normal breast. The patient can see the breast enlarge while the nipple-areolar complex also enlarges and striae develop to match those on the normal breast if they are present there. This procedure results in an excellent form, and when growth is completed it is a simple matter to remove the expander and place a permanent prosthesis in its place.

I have used a variety of expanding devices. At present, I strive to use a device that minimizes expansion in the supraclavicular area and directs expansion toward the inferior pole. At times I have used expanders intended to remain as the permanent breast prosthesis. These are usually firmer than permanent gel-filled prostheses. I reserve the inflatable permanent prosthesis for patients who have B-cup-size breasts and who are fairly thin so that there will be a relatively sharp inframammary fold after expansion. If the patient is heavier, she is more likely to require a second operation for definition of the inframammary fold.

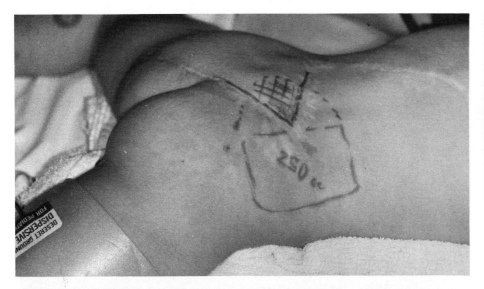

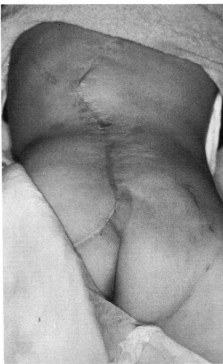

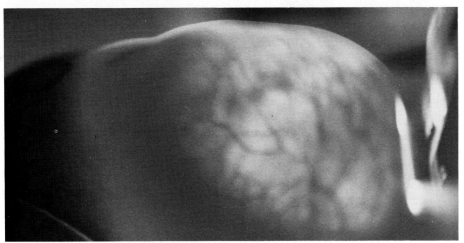

C

Fig. 15-6A. This patient with myelomeningocele requires replacement of unstable skin (cross-hatched area) at the time of elective rhizotomy. Position and size of proposed area of expansion are marked. B. Transillumination of the expanded tissue reveals an impressive vascularity. C. Advancement was successful. Expansion allowed advancement of a healthy well-vascularized flap across the midline, providing stable coverage.

The Trunk

Soft tissue expansion on the trunk is typically straightforward (Fig. 15-6). There is absolutely no contraindication to expanding over the muscular abdominal wall. Expansions here can be highly successful.

The trunk presents relatively large, flat surfaces for expansion. Whenever possible I surround the defect with expanders. In addition, croissant expanders generate flaps of which the dimensions and form are well suited for use on flat surfaces; these expanders frequently are the best shape for expanding over the trunk.

When expanding over the trunk, as in other areas of the body, the surgeon should think about areas of maximal tissue availability and about where the final scars are to lie. (When possible, the scars should be on the patient's sides, where they are less visible.)

The Upper Limbs

Soft tissue expansion over the arms is often highly successful (Fig. 15-7). The hemispheric flap generated by a typical expander is not ideally suited to lie flat on the cylindrical surfaces of the limbs, however. One should keep in mind that the croissant flap is a better geometric shape for reconstruction of defects on flat or cylindrical surfaces. Also, defects should be surrounded whenever possible to minimize the time required for expansion. Scars should be hidden on the inner aspects of the arms, if possible, where they will not be visible. In addition, the sur-

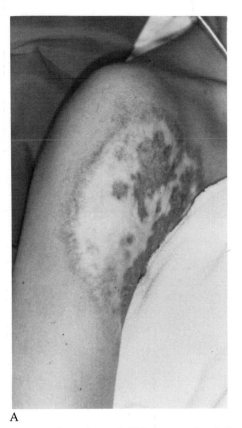 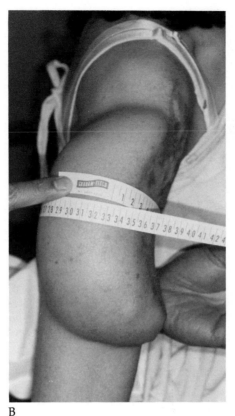 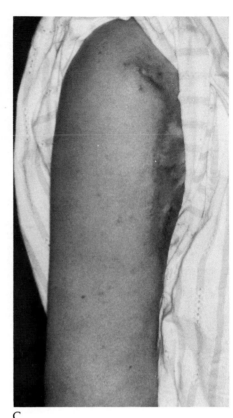

A   B   C

Fig. 15-7. Burn of arm. A. This young patient had an obvious burn scar on her anterior right arm. B. A croissant expander presented the correct expander geometry to allow advancement of the expanded tissue over a cylindrical surface with a minimum of redundant tissue that would have caused dog-ears. C. The final result shows good advancement and coaptation.

geon should remember that it is easier to advance skin transversely than axially on the upper limbs and plan the reconstruction and the positioning of expanders accordingly.

Although skin-grafted fasciotomy defects may appear large, if there has been no loss of skin the defect can be resurfaced in virtually all patients by simple serial excision and advancement of the skin edges. In most instances the closure can be accomplished in one operation; some patients require two simple serial excisions.

I do not use soft tissue expanders for reconstruction of syndactyly; the traditional techniques work well. In addition, I have not had occasion to carry out expansions on the dorsum of the hand. Expansion at the wrist has been an impediment to activity for patients and is quite uncomfortable.

The Lower Limbs

I have found expansion over the legs to be successful down to the distal third of the lower leg (Fig. 15-8). I have not attempted expansion over the feet, but I am aware of unsuccessful attempts. Again, surgeons should plan to surround the defects, and again, croissant expanders provide the ideal geometry. The planning guidelines are similar to those given for soft tissue expansion in the upper limbs.

Often there are substantial depressions in the subcutaneous fat after expansion in the lower limbs. The surgeon should reassure the patient that this appearance will improve with time. If the pressure in the expanders has not been so excessive to result in fat necrosis, the eventual contour will be excellent, resembling the shape before the operation.

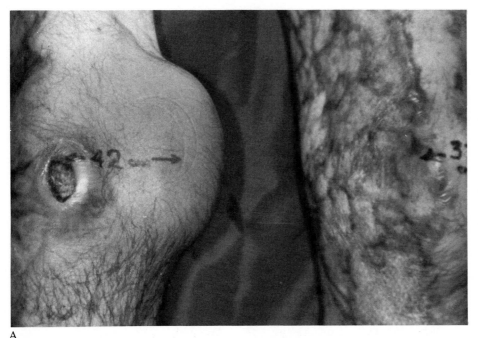

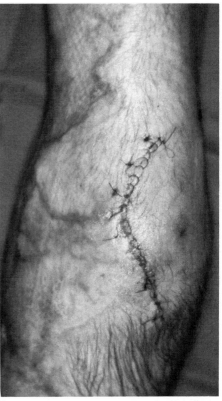

A

Fig. 15-8A. Unstable postburn knee scar managed with tissue expansion. Expansion proceeds until measurement indicates the increase in arc length of expanded tissue will allow advancement and reconstruction of the defect. B. The final result provides coverage with stable, unburned skin from the medial surface of the knee.

B

Other Clinical Uses

Soft tissue expansion can be used to increase the size of distant flaps. I have made expanded buttock flaps for foot and lower leg coverage, expanded cross-leg flaps, and expanded free flaps. Every operation has provided increased vascularity and has eased closing of the donor site defect. For example, the buttock flap can be closed at the line of the inferior gluteal crease. These applications should not be used for every patient but for selected patients when other reconstructive options are not available or have failed.

I have treated a number of patients with neuromas in continuity with the median nerve by expanding the proximal nerve to allow resection of the neuroma and primary coaptation of the normal nerve ends. This experience has been gratifying. At present this technique has limited usefulness because the distal end of the nerve must be tethered securely to allow elongation in response to an underlying expander. Although neuromas in continuity present an opportunity for nerve elongation through expansion, the op-

portunity is not frequently available. Additionally, the nerve must lie superficially enough to allow the expansion process to proceed without interfering with the junction of adjacent anatomic structures.

The orbit has been expanded in infants with microphthalmia or anophthalmia. Neurofibromatosis and congenital glaucoma expanding in the orbit are well known to clinicians. Several groups have expanded the orbits of laboratory animals. I now have a series of patients who have undergone successful orbital expansion. A 6-cc expander is placed inside the orbit and inside the muscle cone if it exists. A crucial point contributing to success is to make a lateral orbitotomy through which the filling tube is passed. The filling tube is subsequently passed through a deep tunnel under the soft tissues and up over the skull, where a separate incision is made to allow formation of a subcutaneous pocket for the remote fill port. Typically only two incisions are required, one in the scalp above and anterior to the ear and the other in the line of the conjunctiva and across the lateral canthus. Both the interior of the orbit and

the lateral orbital wall can be approached through the latter incision, which heals well.

There must be good soft tissue coverage of the expander in the orbit and a careful, leisurely expansion. I proceed with expansion adding approximately 0.5 ml of saline solution per month initially until a bulge is visible beneath the lids. The orbital growth is evident within months and can be followed with periodic computed tomography or magnetic resonance imaging. As one might expect, not only the orbit but also the eyelids increase in size. When adult orbital dimensions have been reached, usually by about the age of 3 years, the expander can be replaced with a permanent spacer, and later an ocular prosthesis can be fitted and inserted under the lids and above the conjunctiva.

Conclusion

Soft tissue expansion is safe and extremely effective. Although there is a period late in the process of expansion when the deformity may be exaggerated by the appearance of the protruding bulge of the expander, this bulge is easily disguised, even in expansions in the head and neck area.

The technique provides tissue that matches the color, thickness, and texture of the surrounding tissues without additional donor-site scars. Ideally the only visible scar should be at the area of flap advancement. Careful planning and execution ensure the best possible functional and aesthetic results and minimize the possibility of complications.

Suggested Reading

Argenta, L.C., Marks, M.W., and Pasyk, K.A. Advances in tissue expansion. *Clin. Plast. Surg.* 12:159, 1985.

Bauer, B.S., and Vicari, F.A. An approach to excision of congenital giant pigmented nevi in infancy and early childhood. *Plast. Reconstr. Surg.* 82:1012, 1988.

Laitung, J.K., Brought, M.D., and Orton, C.I. Scalp expansion flaps. *Br. J. Plast. Surg.* 39:542, 1986.

Leighton, W.D., Johnson, M.L., and Friedland, J.A. Use of the temporary soft-tissue expander in posttraumatic alopecia. *Plast. Reconstr. Surg.* 77:737, 1986.

Leonard, A.G., and Small, J.O. Tissue expansion in the treatment of alopecia. *Br. J. Plast. Surg.* 39:42, 1986.

Manders, E.K., Au, V.K., and Wong, R.K. Scalp expansion for male pattern baldness. *Clin. Plast. Surg.* 14:469, 1987.

Manders, E.K., and Graham, W.P. Alopecia reduction by scalp expansion. *J. Dermatol. Surg. Oncol.* 10:967, 1984.

Manders, E.K., Mottaleb, M.A., and Hetzler, P.T. Soft Tissue Expansion. In J.L. Marsh (Ed.), *Current Therapy in Plastic and Reconstructive Surgery.* Philadelphia: Decker, 1989. Pp. 88–98.

Manders, E.K., et al. Skin expansion to eliminate large scalp defects. *Ann. Plast. Surg.* 12:305, 1984.

Manders, E.K., et al. Soft tissue expansion: Concepts and complications. *Plast. Reconstr. Surg.* 74:493, 1984.

Mottaleb, M., et al. Tissue Expansion. In W.B. Riley (Ed.), *Instructional Courses.* St. Louis: Mosby, 1988. Vol. 1, Pp. 277–304.

Neale, H.W., et al. Complications of controlled tissue expansion in the pediatric burn patient. *Plast. Reconstr. Surg.* 82:840, 1988.

Ortega, M.T., McCauley, R.L., and Robson, M.C. Salvage of an avulsed expanded scalp flap to correct burn alopecia. *South. Med. J.* 83:220, 1990.

Spence, R.J. Clinical use of a tissue expander enhanced transposition flap for face and neck reconstruction. *Ann. Plast. Surg.* 21:58, 1988.

Wieslander, J.B. Repeated tissue expansion in reconstruction of a huge combined scalp-forehead avulsion injury. *Ann. Plast. Surg.* 20:381, 1988.

16

Blunt Suction-Assisted Lipectomy

Gregory P. Hetter

After visiting France in June 1982, I realized that lipolysis was by far the most important advance in body contouring of my professional lifetime (20 years at the time). Whereas most previously written material concerned how to minimize the severe problems attendant on existing operations, lipolysis represents a leap to an entirely different medium. Plastic surgeons already understand much of the anatomy involved, the limitations of the method, and why many aesthetic sequelae occur. Herein I discuss general principles first, followed by lipoplasty of the trunk and limbs, and last, liposculpture of the face and neck.

Curette Techniques

Lipexeresis Schrudde Technique

The term *lipexeresis* was used by Schrudde in the 1960s to describe his technique of removal of fat—blind undermining with long scissors, followed by the use of a sharp uterine curette. Prolonged drainage, lymphorrhea, hematoma, and skin necrosis prevented this technique from gaining many adherents, although Schrudde's published results appeared to be good.

Fischer Technique

The first surgeon to apply suction with a sharp, mechanically driven curette was George Fischer. He used an instrument called a planotome to make a plane in the fat, thus severing the lymph and blood vessels and the retinacula cutis. He then used an electrically driven blade at the tip of the curette attached to suction to snip off globs of fat. The complications were similar to those of lipexeresis. Fischer's efforts were publicized and became known in Europe in 1976 and 1977. Many problems encountered by other surgeons led to limited acceptance of the machinery (which Fischer manufactured and sold) and the technique.

Kesselring Technique

Ulrich Kesselring devised a large-bore instrument with a sharp, back-cutting blade that was introduced after a plane was made with a scissors, much as in the Schrudde technique. Kesselring, however, attached suction to evacuate the fat. He worked deep on the muscle fascia with the blade facing upward to carve away fat toward the surface. Working in the deep fat compartments was an important advance in technique. Kesselring introduced his technique in 1978 and had

performed 36 operations by October 1982. He limited his procedure to *small* amounts of excess fat in the lateral thigh in young women with good skin tone. The results presented in 1982 appeared to be excellent. Later Kesselring adopted the basics of the Illouz technique.

Teimourian Technique

Bahman Teimourian used a technique similar to Kesselring's. He used a scissors for undermining followed by curetting with a modified fascia lata stripper attached to suction. Later, he used the types of instruments Kesselring did as well as others of his own design. Bolder than Kesselring, Teimourian extended his procedure to many areas of the body. He reported a 30 percent complication rate, which characterized all the curette techniques. Teimourian, however, recognized early the value of separate tunnels. His technique subsequently evolved into a cannula technique.

Cannula Technique

In 1976 Illouz heard about the "Italian technique" at a meeting in Mexico. He tried the technique using a blunt Karman cannula attached to a high vacuum. He

Table 16-1. Chronology of subcutaneous fat removal without skin resection

Author	Type	First published	Number of operations	First operation
Schrudde	Manual curette	1972	?	1964
Fischer and Fischer	Mechanized sharp curette with suction	1977	245	1976
Kesselring and Meyer	Sharp curette with suction	1978	?	?
Illouz	Blunt cannula with suction	1980	300	1977
Teimourian and Fischer	Sharp curette with suction	1981	54	1977

used no undermining, no sharp instruments, and—most important—spared most of the structures intervening between the muscle fascia and the skin. This was the vital step that had not been understood previously. It was this maneuver that reduced complications and allowed for the dynamic spread of blunt suction lipectomy (BSL); other surgeons could consistently reproduce the results with a low incidence of complications. Illouz gradually extended his technique to almost every area of the body.

The essence of the technique is that as the cannula is pushed through the deep fat, the mechanical thrust plus the suction avulses fatty globules. A honeycomb pattern results in the fatty tissue, sparing most vessels, nerves, and skin ligaments. When an area is surgically opened for resection of skin after fat extraction, the septa between muscle fascia and skin form a spongelike network. Physicians who have never opened a suctioned area can never truly grasp the mechanics of the procedure.

The chronology of these fat-removal techniques is shown in Table 16-1.

Biochemistry and Histology of Fat: All Fat Is Not the Same

Studies, primarily by French and Swedish investigators, have demonstrated that fat cells (adipocytes) possess two chemical receptors for catecholamines—epinephrine and norepinephrine. The beta-1 receptors are lipolytic and secrete lipase, which causes triglycerides (fat) within the adipocyte to split into fatty acids and glycerol. These substances can then pass the cell membrane into the general circulation, where they are metabolized under normal conditions. It is particularly important to know that fasting or starving and using tobacco or caffeine can cause the release of catecholamines, which activate beta-1 receptors and thus cause lipolysis.

The alpha-2 receptors conversely block lipolysis, yet they are also stimulated by catecholamines. They are antagonists to the beta-1 receptors. These receptors have been found to be particularly prevalent in areas such as the lateral thigh, lower abdomen, and buttocks, the areas often clinically called "diet resistant." Whereas catecholamines induce lipolysis in areas of metabolically active fat with many beta-1 receptors, such as the upper body, breast, and face, the same hormone blocks lipolysis in areas of so-called reserve fat such as the buttocks, thighs, and lower abdomen, where alpha-2 receptors predominate.

The *reserve fat*, a term coined by Illouz, has been shown to be more receptive to glucose than the more superficial active fat. The reserve fat cells are larger and can hypertrophy faster than those of the active fat. Metabolically the reserve fat areas resist weight loss, particularly during fasting or when catecholamines are stimulated by drugs such as amphetamines or their derivatives, but increase easily in the presence of glucose. This research explains the common clinical syndrome seen in a dieting woman who has lost upper body fat (face, shoulders, breasts, and upper abdomen) and in fact appears gaunt, except her outer thighs appear larger after weeks of fasting. Many physicians have been cruel in their ignorance in telling such people that "pushing themselves away from the table" is the only exercise needed. In fact the number and type of receptors appear to form a genetic basis for these problems; the cause does not appear to be acquired habits or upbringing.

Subcutaneous Fascial System

The superficial fascia is an important membrane in some areas of the body, rudimentary in others, and fused with the muscle fascia in most. The fat above the fascia is divided by vertical arches of connective tissue called *retinacula cutis*. These fibers are anchored to the undersurface of the dermis above and the superficial fascia below (Fig. 16-1). The retinacula cutis are somewhat elastic but have limits to their stretch, hence the dimples or *peau d'orange* seen in cellulite during fat hypertrophy. The fat fills in the spaces within this complex honeycomb network of fascial extensions. Here beta-1 receptors predominate.

Beneath the superficial fascia lies the deeper laminar fat (reserve fat of Illouz), where the separations are horizontal rather than vertical and alpha-2 receptors predominate. This configuration is macroscopically clear during abdominoplasty when the incisions for the hypogastric dermolipectomy are carried out (Fig. 16-2).

Within the confines between the superficial fascia and the dermis lie the arcades of capillaries, nerves, and lymphatic vessels. Excessive surgical intervention in this layer leads to destruction of the retinacula cutis, with the probability of surface irregularities and irregular shrinkage, vascular pattern abnormalities, and dysesthesias and hypesthesias. Selective surgical treatment of tethering retinacula cutis can, however, relieve some of the dimples of cellulite.

Topographic Anatomy

Most of the commonly recognized areas of localized fatty deposits are defined by the superficial fascia's enveloping the deposit and fusing with the muscle fascia at the perimeter of the deposit (Fig. 16-3A and B). This fusion is strong and is readily felt when a blunt cannula is passed along the abdominal wall. Laterally the cannula meets real resistance at the point of fusion. When the surgeon punches through this resistance, he or she leaves the subfascial space and enters the subcutaneous space, usually with a divot or dimple as a result.

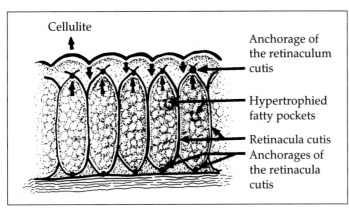

Fig. 16-1. *Illouz' anatomic explanation of the origin of cellulite. The anchor points of the retinacula cutis cause a "chesterfield couch" appearance of the skin surface. (From Y.-G. Illouz and Y.T. De Villers.* Body Sculpturing by Lipoplasty. *New York: Churchill Livingstone, 1989. P. 35. Reproduced with permission.)*

Fig. 16-2. *The horizontal architecture of the deep fat compared with the vertical compartmentalization of the superficial fat. (Redrawn after Illouz.)*

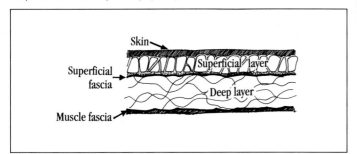

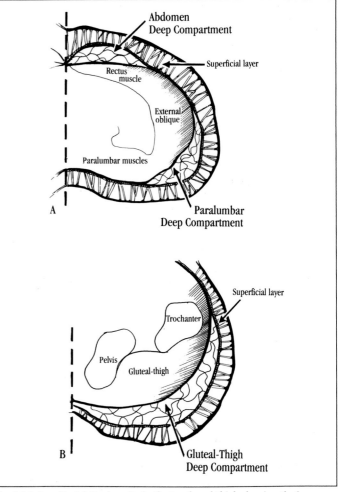

Fig. 16-3. *Localized fatty deposits in the trunk and thigh showing the layers. Note that at the perimeter of the localized deposits, the fascia superficialis fuses with the muscle fascia. (Redrawn after Markman.)*

The most common surgical violation of this fascial fusion is in the lateral thigh, where the superficial fascia fuses with the fascia lata (Fig. 16-4). This is a tough fusion. When the surgeon passes the cannula from the infragluteal crease too far around the curve of the trochanter, he or she punches through the fascia with the resultant extraction of superficial fat and severe surface irregularities.

Other areas of well-defined localized deposits encased in their fascial envelopes are the hypogastrium, the iliac crest, the medial thigh, the medial knee, and the upper posterior arm. Various fascial condensations throughout this system account for the buttock fold (or lack thereof), fatty rolls on the back and flanks, and the submammary fold. I refer to this whole system as the subcutaneous fascial system (SFS). This system is probably more important surgically than the submuscular aponeurotic system (SMAS). This anatomic basis for suction lipectomy is of such importance for successful results that each reader is encouraged to read Illouz' chapter on anatomy in *Lipoplasty: The Theory and Practice of Blunt Suction Lipectomy* and view his cadaver dissections available on videotape from the Lipoplasty Society of North America (Arlington Heights, Ill.).

Physics and Equipment

The physics of pressure has been forgotten by most surgeons. Suffice it to say that there are two ways to move the dislodged fat down the cannula or tube. The first is

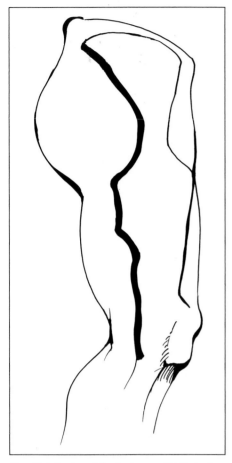

Fig. 16-4. Fusion of the fascia superficialis to the fascia lata. In front of this line only superficial fat is found in the upper thigh. Violating this fusion results in superficial extraction with resultant dents anterior to this line.

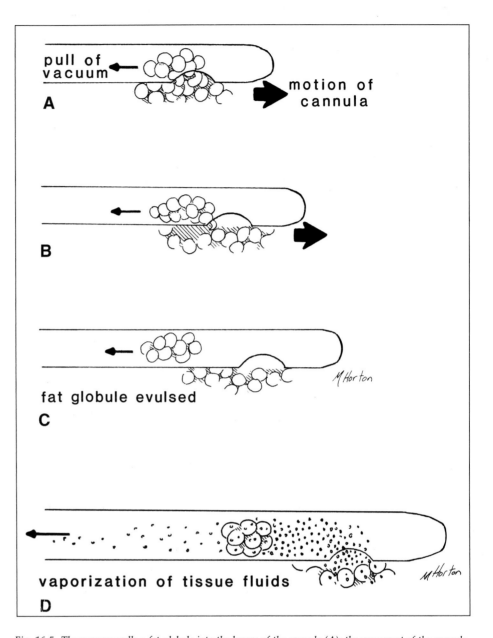

Fig. 16-5. The vacuum pulls a fat globule into the lumen of the cannula (A); the movement of the cannula causes evulsion of the fat globule (B, C), and the vaporization of the tissue fluids provides the motive force that pushes the fragments toward the collection bottle (D).

to have an air line to the tip of the cannula or an open wound where air enters the lumen and carries the fat fragments down the tube. Such systems work with pressures of $\frac{1}{4}$ to $\frac{1}{2}$ atmosphere (190 to 380 mmHg at sea level). The other way is to produce so near to an absolute vacuum that tissue fluids "boil" and the molecules drive the fatty fragments down the cannula or tube (Fig. 16-5) toward the vacuum. At 20°C (68°F) tissue fluids vaporize or "boil" when the remaining pressure in the collection bottle or syringe is less than 17 mmHg. This can be achieved by pulling the plunger of a 50-cc syringe to full extension or by an electromechanical vacuum pump. The latter is the traditional approach and the most common; however, I have removed 700 cc of fat from the flanks and abdomen using syringe-driven suction without difficulty.

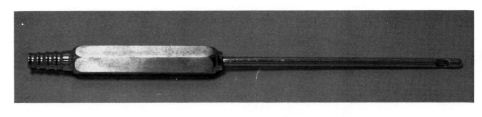

Fig. 16-6. Typical Illouz cannula with a hemispheric head, with the opening back from the tip and well-machined edges to prevent a rasping effect.

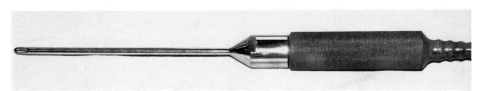

Fig. 16-7. Cobra cannulas have openings at the tip and extract fat quickly. They are useful when an area is flat, without curves, and there is no danger of perforation of a viscus.

Cannulas

Briefly, the following items are important. The cannula should be blunt with the lumen sufficiently far back to avoid removal of subdermal fat (Fig. 16-6). The shortest cannula that can be used to reach the area to be defatted allows for the best control by the surgeon. The finer the caliber, the less the bleeding; the finer the tunnels, the less the subsequent waves or irregularities. In general, 6-mm cannulas are used for body work. For facial and neck areas, I use a 1.5-, a 2.4-, and a 3.8-mm single-hole Illouz cannula. Multihole cannulas extract fat too quickly for my taste.

Small so-called cobra cannulas, which have their lumens near the tip, are useful in fibrous areas such as the epigastrium and the calves. Where the operative plane is fairly level, the risk of subdermal removal is less. Three- to five-millimeter cannulas are common in this style (Fig. 16-7). The finish around the lumens should be smooth and bur-free and should have edges that clearly feel dull to the finger.

Biohazards

Biohazards have not yet been proved with the use of suction pumps; however, vaporization of tissue fluids raises the possibility that bacterial and viral particles may be exhausted into the operating room by any suction pump. It is recommended that a special filter be placed between the collection jar and the pump to reduce this risk. These filters can stop particles larger than 0.3 μ, have a large surface area to allow good airflow, and are reasonably priced. *It is recommended that such filters be used with all machines at all times.* Ideally the exhaust should be vented to the outside roof air after the filter is passed. It is also expedient to have disposable plastic collection jars and disposable tubing, thus avoiding the risks inherent in cleaning blood-contaminated jars and tubing.

Nomenclature

Ambiguous terms should be avoided; the term *hip*, for example, may mean either the lateral pelvic brim or the trochanteric area. Adjacent fatty areas may have different anatomies and hence should be clearly differentiated from one another, e.g., epigastrium lacks the superficial fascia as a discrete membrane, whereas in the hypogastrium the superficial fascia is fully developed and invests the deep fat. Accuracy of description is important, and the recording of amounts removed by discrete area leads to disciplined thinking and hence a chance of improving results.

Figures 16-8 and 16-9 show the correct names of the areas in which aspirative lipoplasty is performed on the torso and limbs. The nomenclature of the face and neck is depicted in Figure 16-10. The fat adjacent to the nasolabial groove is called the *preantral* fat and is attached to the underlying maxillary bone or facial muscles; it has nothing to do with the nasal or labial structures, where there is almost no fat medial to the nasolabial groove.

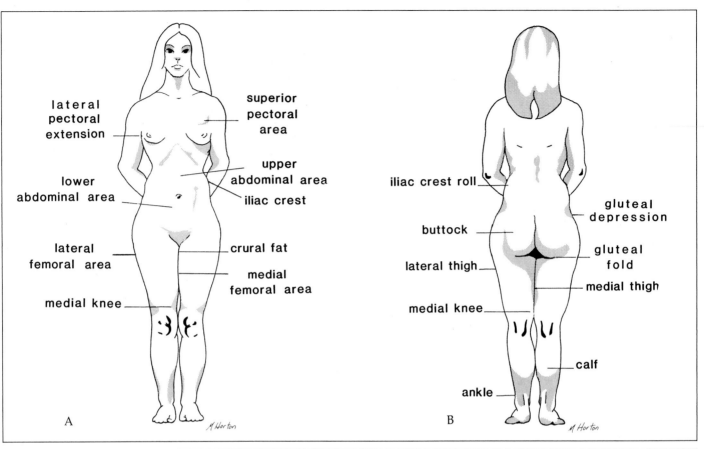

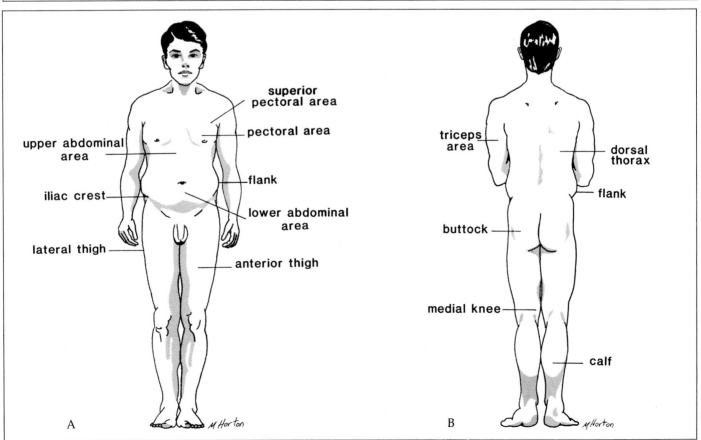

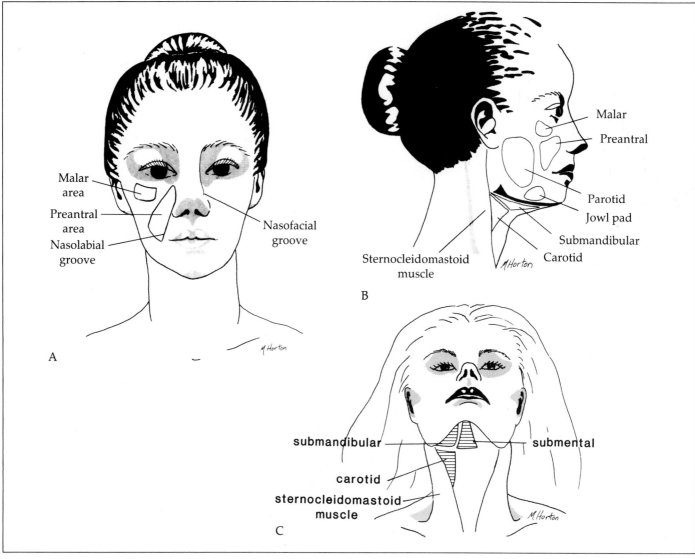

Fig. 16-10A. Anterior view of head and neck. B. Lateral view of head and neck. C. Anterior view of head and neck with head extended on neck.

Harmony and Proportion in the Female Figure

Because 9 of 10 patients inquiring about blunt suction lipectomy in most communities are women, a brief exposition on the artistic values by which female beauty is judged is in order. Standards of form and beauty clearly vary in time and place, yet much remains common in human history. In our ever smaller world, the Greco-Roman ideals of beauty influence cultures in which there is little genetic representation of those ideals in the local population. The desire of Mexican women with flat calves for calf implants

and the desire of Asian women for blepharoplasties to provide a larger upper eyelid are examples of collisions between unrelenting genetics and everchanging cultural values.

The classic proportions are illustrated in Figure 16-11. A work from the 1940s shows the proportions from Greece and Rome that are admired to the present day (Fig. 16-12). Today our ideal is a bit more leptosomatic, but the proportions remain valid for most observers. In Figure 16-13, a free-form sculpture is shown that emphasizes open **S** curves. Again and again in the female form there is the repetition of an open **S** curve, which most observers recognize as beautiful and by which many people find themselves sexually stimu-

lated. Examples of this **S** curve are the epigastric-hypogastric curve (Fig. 16-14A), the thoracolumbosacral curve (Fig. 16-14B), and the flank–iliac crest–thigh curve (Fig. 16-14C).

When the expected troughs of these curves are filled with unexpected fatty bulk, the figure loses its "beauty" and is perceived as unattractive and unstimulating. Epigastric or iliac crest fullness or deficiency of buttock fullness flattens the sinuous curve to a straighter line, and the tension of the line and its beauty disappear. Reconstructing the curves by suction removal of fat (Fig. 16-15) is appreciated as a restoration of the beauty associated with youth.

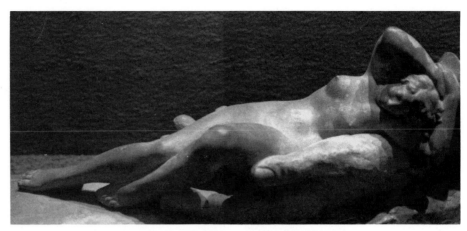

Fig. 16-12. A contemporary Venus. Note the open **S** curve of the flank-hip-thigh.

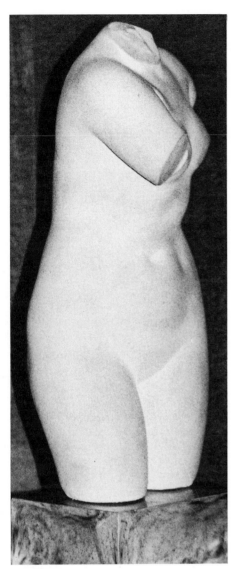

Fig. 16-11. The classic Venus.

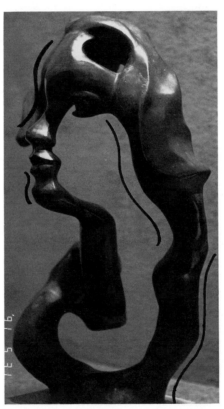

Fig. 16-13. A modern sculpture with abstract elements. Note the repetitive open **S** curves found throughout the forms.

Greco-Roman ideals of facial beauty are seen in the comparison of a Roman head and a twentieth century photographic model (Fig. 16-16). In the oblique view, the prominence of the malar area and the sinuous curve of the cheek are notable. A strong chin prominence, clean jawline, and defined sternocleidomastoid muscle are all important. When fat obliterates the definition of these landmarks, beauty is lost. The removal of this fat reveals the form and harmony of the underlying structure (Fig. 16-17).

The surgeon-sculptor must develop an aesthetic frame of reference. To a great extent, as with all talent, the ability seems to be inborn. It can be refined and de-

veloped, however, by the study of great works of art, especially sculpture. The balance, harmony, and tension of line and form that affect our hearts are easily recognized but not easily described. Study is necessary to achieve refined results in liposculpture surgery.

Photographic Considerations
Trunk and Limbs

The photographs for documenting the status of the patient need to be descriptive of two attributes—form and surface. It is not necessarily true that both are shown by the same photographic technique. The standard views should be taken at 45° steps around an imaginary circle. A 50-mm macroscopic lens on a tripod at the level of the mons pubis at 1.7 meters (5½ ft) documents the body from calves to clavicles. Such photographs taken with consistent background, film, lighting, distance, focus, and patient attire document well the form of the patient. On-camera flash lighting, however, flattens and tends not to show skin surface irregularities.

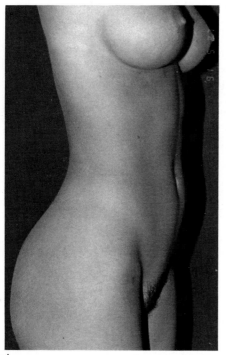

A

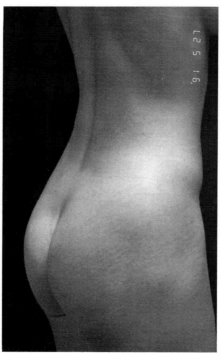

B

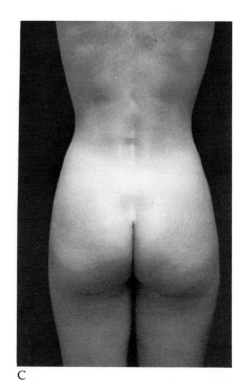

C

*Fig. 16-14A. The epigastric concavity followed by the hypogastric convexity is well shown here. The open **S** line is present. B. The thoracolumbar concavity followed by the sacrogluteal convexity (unspoiled by an iliac crest roll) shows the aesthetic open **S** line. C. The thorax-flank concavity passes into the iliac crest-trochanteric convexity as one continuous uninterrupted curve with a harmonic open **S** line.*

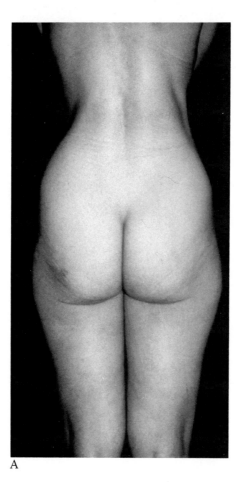

A

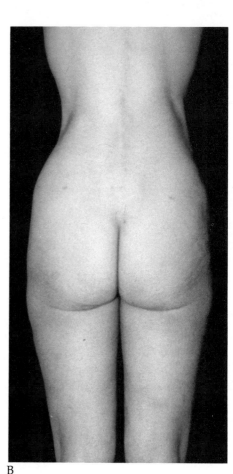

B

*Fig. 16-15A. Preoperative view with both an iliac crest bulge and a lateral thigh bulge giving the "violin deformity" appearance. Note the lack of upper body fat. B. Postoperative view showing the long open **S** curve, which produces a perception of youth and beauty.*

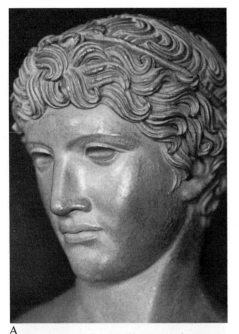

A

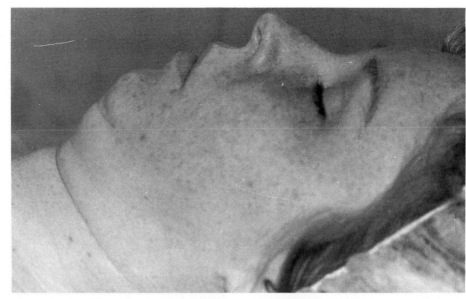

A

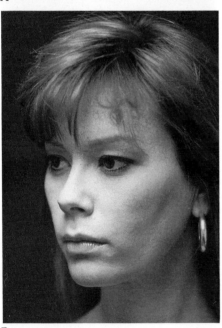

B

Fig. 16-16A. A Roman head illustrates the Greco-Roman aesthetic that has passed down to our time. B. A photographic model of the late twentieth century. Note the similarity of jawline, mentum, cheek plane, malar highlight, and sternocleidomastoid line between the Roman head and the model. (From G.P. Hetter (Ed.). Lipoplasty. *Boston: Little, Brown, 1990. Reproduced with permission.)*

B

Fig. 16-17A. Preoperative view on the operating table of a female patient with fatty cheeks, fatty neck, and retrusive chin. B. Immediately postoperative view of same patient after sculpting of cheeks, fatty extraction in neck, and extended chin implant. (From G.P. Hetter (Ed.). Lipoplasty. *Boston: Little, Brown, 1990. Reproduced with permission.)*

Fig. 16-18A. Preoperative view of 49-year-old patient taken with camera-mounted flash. Note lack of fine detail. Most published pictures are of this kind. B. Ambient light photograph taken moments after the photograph in A shows considerable skin irregularity.

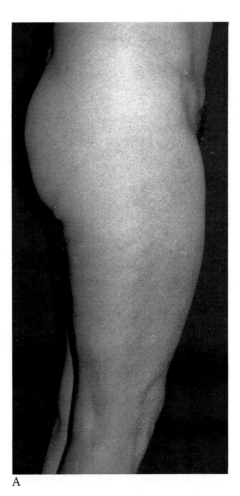
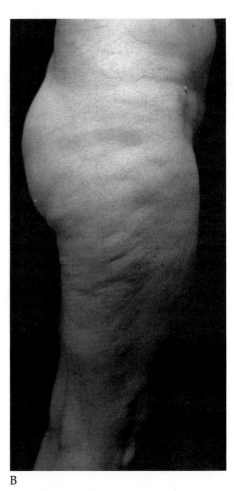

A

B

Most patients have only a faint idea of what they look like from the rear. They pay more attention in the 3 months after an operation to viewing this aspect of their anatomy than they ever did before. I prefer to photograph with no flash but only ambient ceiling light, therefore, to record the surface irregularities that exist before surgical intervention. Such photos shown to the patient during preoperative discussion add a needed note of realism. Figure 16-18A shows a side-mounted flash photograph and Figure 16-18B shows the same patient photographed with ambient ceiling light only. If a surgeon were presented with an ambient light photograph such as Figure 16-18B by a deceptive plaintiff's attorney and had only Figure 16-18A in the patient record, a serious problem of credibility could be developed by the attorney.

Face and Neck

Facial photographs are taken with a 90- to 105-mm lens in the lateral, oblique, anterior, and lateral "reading" positions. The last view is crucial to document what cervicofacial surgery has achieved in the relaxed neck (Fig. 16-19). That is why the reader rarely sees this view published. Instead the reader is given postoperative views with patients stretching their necks as if they were swans.

Patients usually forget how they looked before the operation, undervaluing the improvement brought about by the surgeon's efforts. Preoperative and postoperative photographs can increase their appreciation or decrease their dissatisfaction. The surgeon, on the other hand, usually exaggerates the patient's preoperative condition. A comparison of photographs can serve to establish a more realistic balance for both.

Fig. 16-19A. Preoperative "reading" view before face-lift with suction. This position throws the flaccid soft tissues of the neck into redundant folds. Note camera flash left. B. Postoperative "reading" view shows that improvement in the neck tissues is real even when tissues are relaxed. Note camera flash right, which makes the cheek shadow worse.

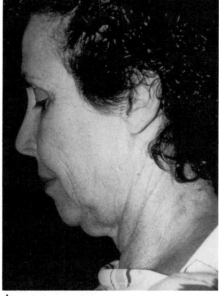
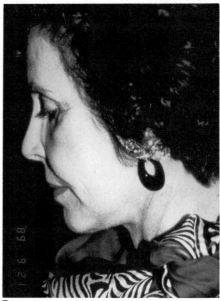

A

B

Patient Evaluation

The patient evaluation is the most important step in the surgeon's procedure. From this process flows the success or failure of the surgeon's practice and the sense of satisfaction as a professional. Wrong choices lead to unsatisfactory results, repeat surgical interventions, nagging patients, and lawsuits. Patient evaluation has four parts: a psychological evaluation, a medical evaluation, a physical evaluation, and an aesthetic evaluation.

Psychological Evaluation

The patient should be evaluated for body image disturbances, including bulimia and anorexia nervosa. Patients who exhibit low self-esteem, marked anxiety, fear, paranoia, or unrealistic expectations are not good candidates for aesthetic surgery.

Low Self-Esteem

Patients who want to be "made over" or who have such turmoil in their lives that they are dissatisfied with their existence have low self-esteem. They respond postoperatively to any disparaging comment from any source with worry and dissatisfaction. Such patients rarely if ever are satisfied and torment their surgeons with requests for revisions and additional surgery. These patients should be told at the first office visit that their expectations are beyond the scope of plastic surgery.

Marked Anxiety

Markedly anxious patients wring their hands, have a "wet" handshake, and appear as if they expect to be scolded. Such patients may have a genetic predisposition to this reaction of their autonomic nervous system. They need constant reassurance from a supportive staff. If they require more reassurance than the surgeon is able or willing to give, they should be asked to seek another surgeon. These patients can be grateful, but they should not be treated by a surgeon who does not have the time or the patience to attend to their worries.

Fear and Paranoia

Some patients seek several plastic surgical consultations. They compare what they have been told, exaggerate the differences, and stir controversy. They attend to exquisite detail to find differences in approach or technique. They ask the same question in different ways to elicit inconsistencies. The surgeon begins to feel on trial. These patients ask to have office routines changed especially for them. They demand that each step in the evaluation be specially structured at a different time, place, or manner from the surgeon's routine. They fight constantly for control of the surgical situation and do not relinquish it to the surgeon. Such patients are dangerous and highly litigious. If the operation is not done their way, they deem the results not good. These patients should be told they cannot be given the results they envision. The surgeon should refuse to operate on such patients.

Unrealistic Expectations

The surgeon must know what he or she can realistically achieve. The appearance the patient desires must be within the capability of the surgeon. Only talent, time, and experience equip the surgeon to make this judgment.

In addition, the surgeon must be assured that the patient is not depending on the surgical procedure to bring about important life changes. A surgeon cannot save a disintegrating marriage or secure a career position for a patient. The patient's motivation for the procedure should be thoroughly discussed. The surgeon should not operate on a patient whose expectations he or she deems unrealistic.

Medical Evaluation

The medical evaluation should rule out a history of thromboembolic disease, bleeding disorders, chronic lung disease, a brittle cardiovascular system, and acute or chronic systemic diseases. The evaluation should include nutritional practices. Many people follow bizarre diets and are chronically malnourished with low iron stores or low albumin levels or both. Others use steroids or diuretics to influence some aspect of their physiology. Taking vitamins in megadosages is common; vitamin E can influence clotting, for example.

Many people today are chronically infected by untreatable viral agents such as hepatitis B and C and human immunodeficiency virus-III (HIV-III), among others. Because the usual technique of blunt suction lipectomy involves suction pumps, which aerosolize tissue fluids, which exhaust into the operating room, it would be imprudent to operate on patients with live virus in their blood and tissue fluids. The testing and exclusion of those who are positive for hepatitis B surface antigen or core antigen or HIV-III antibody reduces considerably the aggregate viral exposure of the operating room staff. Testing does not remove all risk because of the large window between exposure to the virus and registration of positivity. When antigen testing becomes feasible for hepatitis C and HIV-III, these tests should be performed and patients with the viruses excluded until such time as it is proved that the exhaust is not infectious.

The use of sedimentation rate is recommended. This nonspecific test detects cryptic infectious processes and connective tissue diseases. Using the test often prevents the surgeon from operating on someone who is about to become ill and who may perceive the operation as the inciting event. "I never had any trouble until I went to the plastic surgeon," is a refrain most of us have heard. A complete blood count and liver enzyme, sugar, and potassium levels are useful to help rule out common problems.

A thorough history is most important. Unfortunately some patients are not truthful about their medical problems. Special importance should be placed on a pulmonary history to rule out restrictive lung disease. A history of thromboembolic disease together with smoking, being overweight, and using oral contraceptives places the patient at high risk for a pulmonary embolus following blunt suction lipectomy. Such a patient should not be operated on.

Physical Evaluation

A complete physical examination including deep tendon reflexes is useful. An abnormal tendon reflex may be a signal of a spinal disk problem, which may be aggravated when the patient is turned on the operating table. On the basis of the history and physical and laboratory examinations, the surgeon may wish to refer the patient for an ECG, chest roentgenogram, or other studies or to refer the patient for a specialty evaluation.

Aesthetic Evaluation

Ideal Candidate
The ideal candidate for BSL is a young, relatively thin woman or man with a highly localized fatty excess with taut skin (Fig. 16-20).

Average Candidate
The average candidate is 30 to 45 years of age, weighs 5 to 10 pounds over ideal, may have striae from pregnancy or weight fluctuations, and has some degree of skin relaxation (Fig. 16-21). The skin must be evaluated in addition to the fat excess. Usually, BSL will suffice; however, the patient should be informed that subsequent suctionings and an ultimate dermolipectomy may be necessary. Patients in this age group are more difficult to satisfy than younger patients.

Less Than Ideal Candidate
The less than ideal candidate is older than 45 years of age, is more than 20 pounds overweight, or has a history of fluctuating weight with clearly loose skin. Scars, striae, waves, cascading, the beginning of an abdominal apron, buttock ptosis, or a combination of these features is present on examination (Fig. 16-22). Younger patients in this group tend to be critical of their postoperative results, whereas those older than 55 years seem more satisfied. Dermolipectomies combined with BSL are more commonly done. The patient should be aware that the extent of the initial suction may be limited by loose skin. Secondary suctioning, after interim skin contraction, may be required as well as dermolipectomy. The major limitation on the procedure is the condition of the skin.

Pinch Test
It is wise to show the patient by the pinch test where the area of fatty excess is localized and how it differs from surrounding areas. This demonstration is easily understood by patients (Fig. 16-23). The fat of the thigh is palpated above, below, and anterior to the saddlebag, and the area of localized excess is determined. If the area of apparent excess is clearly composed of fat (rather than the trochanter), the area is treatable. Often in men with large beer bellies, pinching the hypogastrium reveals the same amount of fat as there is laterally. There is in fact no substantial localized deep fat, and the bulge is from *intra*-abdominal fat that causes the abdominal wall to bulge forward. Suction of course leads to disappointing results in such patients. This determination of lo-

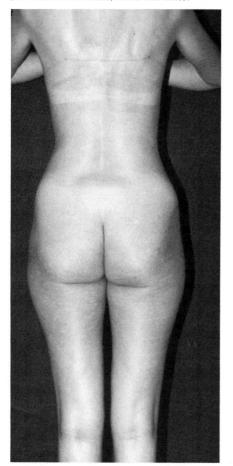

Fig. 16-20. Patient with good skin turgor and highly localized deep fatty excess of lateral thighs (and small crural excess). Note thin limbs.

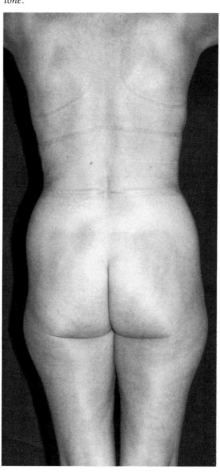

Fig. 16-21. Patient with obvious excesses of iliac crest roll and lateral and medial thighs. Note asymmetry and fat on triceps area of upper arm indicating modest overweight but reasonable skin tone.

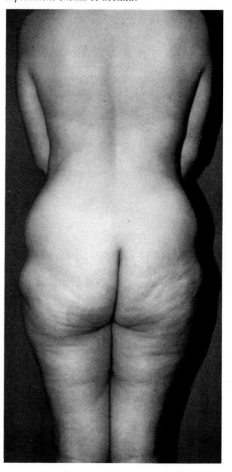

Fig. 16-22. Patient demonstrating striae, relaxed skin, and excess superficial fat deposition. Improvement can be expected but excessive expectations should be avoided.

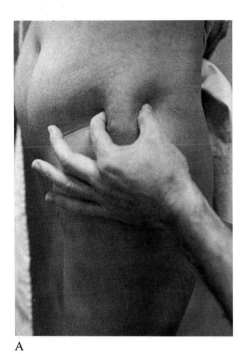

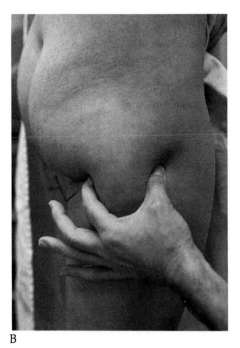

A   B

Fig. 16-23A. Pinch test above the saddlebag area shows the diet-responsive superficial fatty layer to be about 3 cm. B. Pinch test at the saddlebag area shows the fat to be 7 to 8 cm. Subtracting the 3 cm of superficial fat leaves the 4- to 5-cm deep layer, or reserve fat of Illouz. This amount would be removed by the operation.

calized fatty excess demonstrates to the patient two important concepts: (1) Not all fat is to be removed, and (2) what remains is more important than what is removed.

The surgeon must be able to pinch at least one inch of fat to consider removal on the torso. The pinch test doubles the thickness of the underlying skin-fat complex (Fig. 16-24). Generally, excess lateral thighs measure 3 to 4 inches, abdomens 2 to 4 inches, iliac crests 1 to 3 inches, and knees 1 to 2 inches.

Visual inspection is not enough for an aesthetic evaluation. Evaluation of the skin turgor, elasticity, and strength is also important. Striae are a sign of poor skin elasticity. When pinched skin does not instantly return to the normal position, an operation is contraindicated; there is no potential of retraction. Pointing out areas of waves, dimpling (cellulite), and looseness is vitally important. The posterior photographic view needs to be shown to patients as an important part of their aesthetic education, demonstrating what can and, as important, what cannot be done about their concerns.

Fig. 16-24. The "pinch test" doubles the real thickness. (Redrawn after Mladick.)

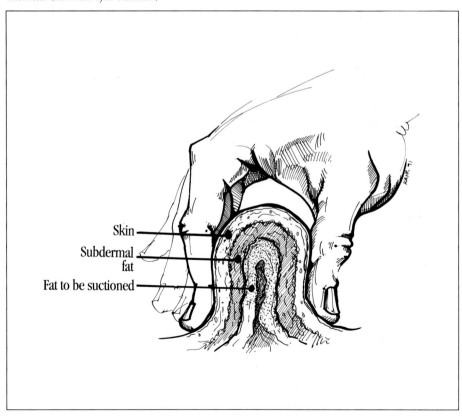

Skin
Subdermal fat
Fat to be suctioned

Informed Consent

The terms the patient must understand in the unprecedented adversarial legal climate of the United States in the late twentieth century are as follows:

1. The surgeon is not God.
2. The two sides of the body or face are not alike.
3. Improvement is possible, but perfection is impossible.
4. Small contour irregularities will always be present.
5. Skin quality, color, and texture will not be improved by the procedure.
6. Follow-up care is limited in time. (There is no open-ended contract.)
7. The fee paid is for the performance of the specific procedure only and does not include reoperations.
8. Additional unforeseen procedures may become necessary and will require additional charges.
9. Additional expenses may be incurred if complications arise. These expenses are the patient's responsibility.
10. The patient has an obligation to return for postoperative photographs to the surgeon's office or to the surgeon's designated photographer.

Anesthesia and Fluid Resuscitation

The most convenient anesthesia for large removals is general anesthesia. Epidural or spinal anesthesia may be used but requires more recovery time. Neuroleptic anesthesia with local application is used by many surgeons in office settings in areas where local medicopolitical or medicolegal constraints limit the use of general anesthesia in offices.

Most anesthesiologists are unaware of the internal burn produced by BSL and the degree of ongoing serum loss over the following 18 to 24 hours. Experience has shown that removal of less than 1500 ml of fat in healthy young adults rarely is associated with problems. As the volume of fat removed increases above 1500 ml and as the size of the body surface area damaged increases above 15 percent, however, the need for autologous blood increases.

Hetter's Rule

Whenever the area of injury exceeds 15 percent, the hemodynamic morbidity rises out of proportion to the additional percentage removed above 15 percent. In such situations, autologous blood transfusion should always be planned. The goal of intraoperative patient care and fluid resuscitation is to maintain levels of albumin, red cell mass, body temperature, and tissue perfusion as near to normal as possible.

Role of Albumin

A low serum albumin level predisposes to a number of chemical disturbances after any severe injury. These pathophysiologic changes appear to be especially applicable to the fatty "crush injury" of suction lipectomy. A low albumin level may be insufficient to bind the free fatty acids released. This situation in turn sets in motion a neutrophil-mediated injury to the lung tissue, resulting in the condition known as "fat embolus syndrome." The characteristics are pulmonary edema, low PO_2, and failure of gas transfer at the alveolar level. Low tissue perfusion caused by hypovolemia may exacerbate this syndrome with a lethal outcome. Any patient

who has an insufficient quantity of or an inappropriate type of intravascular resuscitation after the substantial trauma of extensive suction lipectomy procedures is at risk for this potentially lethal syndrome. Recommendations for resuscitation are shown in Table 16-2.

Table 16-3 shows the approximate percentage of body surface area subjected to the "internal burn" with each area of the body. The palmar surface of the patient's own hand represents 1 percent of the body surface (Fig. 16-25); a quick clinical estimate can be performed. Removal exceeding 20 percent of the body surface area increases risk to an unjustifiable level in an aesthetic operation. An average case of saddlebags, hip rolls, and medial knees can easily exceed 15 percent (9% + 4% + 2% = 15%); this exercise is useful in predicting physiologic injury.

Table 16-3. Approximate percentages of internal burn for common areas of the body

Area	Percentage
Abdomen—upper and lower	5–8
Abdomen with flanks	7–12
Buttock	4–6
Iliac crest roll, bilateral (hip rolls)	2–6
Knees, medial, bilateral	2–3
Thighs, lateral, typical, bilateral	6–12
Thighs, medial, typical, bilateral	2–4

Maintaining Body Temperature

Patients lose heat because of the large area of the body exposed and because of the physical effects of vaporization of tissue fluids. Heat is extracted by the suction process itself. To minimize this loss, the body should be covered as much as possible, an endotracheal humidity trap should be used, and intravenous fluids should be warmed to close to 37°C (98.6°F). The patient's head may be covered with plastic to retain heat. In the recovery period, oxygen should be administered; oxygen consumption may be enormous during the production of body heat by the muscle activity seen clinically as shivering.

Table 16-2. Recommendations for resuscitation

Amount of tissue removed	Amount and type of perioperative fluid replacement
<500 ml	2 L crystalloid
500–1000 ml	3 L crystalloid
1000–1500 ml, <15% body surface area (if >15%, treat as no. 4)	3 L crystalloid plus 1 unit hetastarch before ambulatory discharge
1500–2000 ml, <15% body surface area (if >15%, treat as no. 5)	3 L crystalloid plus 1 unit autologous blood
2000–2500 ml, <15% body surface area (if >15%, treat as no. 6)	3 L crystalloid plus 2 units autologous blood and possible overnight monitoring
2500–3000 ml, >15% body surface area	4 L crystalloid plus 3 or more units autologous blood and probable overnight monitoring in a hospital

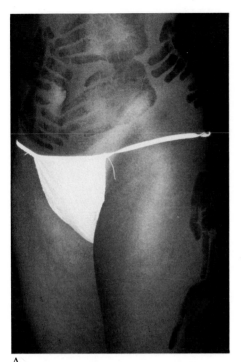

A

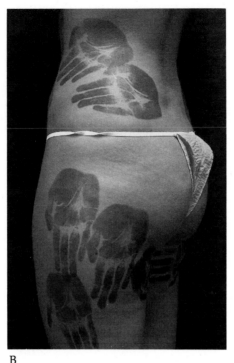

B

Fig. 16-25A. Anterior oblique view with patient's handprints (1% of body surface) on intended areas of suction. The abdomen is 4 percent of the body surface. B. Lateral posterior oblique view shows lateral thigh (3%), medial thigh (1%), and iliac crest (2%). Thus the lateral thighs, medial thighs, iliac crests, and abdomen would be 16 percent of the body surface area, over the safe maximum of 15 percent.

Hypovolemia

Almost all lethal complications of BSL stem from failure to maintain a normal intravascular volume with resultant poor tissue perfusion. In a review of lethal operations in which the end stage was massive infection, acute respiratory distress syndrome, pulmonary embolus, or myocardial infarction, *usually the primary physiologic deficit that was not initially corrected was hypovolemia.*

Autologous blood should be planned for and given to maintain normal homeostatic mechanisms. The surgeon should not delay by adhering to the unrealistic criteria set by nonclinicians for the administration of autologous blood. The patient's intravascular volume should be as close to normal as possible at the end of the operation and for the next 48 hours.

Surgical Technique

There are eight technical steps to be followed to achieve good results:

1. Careful marking of the patient after tactile and visual evaluation
2. Placing the patient in a position that allows full treatment of the area from two directions at right angles to each other
3. Pretreatment with epinephrine
4. Careful pretunneling to establish the extent and proper depth before extraction begins
5. Extraction of fat with the least trauma
6. Cross tunneling and mesh undermining for a smoother result
7. Knowing when to stop by visual and, primarily, tactile evaluation
8. Irrigation of the wound

Marking the Patient

The patient should agree to the area to be treated and the incision sites on the day of the operation so that no misunderstanding can later be claimed. Patients occasionally add or delete an area during this marking. If appropriate, an instant photograph of the markings can be taken to document a change that contradicts earlier office notes. The markings are done with a broad, felt-tipped indelible marking pen. I mark the patient immediately before going to the operating room and obtain the patient's concurrence in front of a nurse who serves as a witness.

Before marking is done, the patient's fatty deposits should be evaluated by both sight and touch with the patient standing. Turning the patient slowly in side lighting and in light from above reveals areas of irregularity, high spots, waviness, and depressions. These areas should be marked and pointed out to the patient.

The areas of claimed fatty excess are also judged by the "pinch test." The areas of excess beyond normal superficial body fat are noted in centimeters. A topographic map of the deformity is marked out. The surgeon decides where maximal extraction should be performed (where plus signs are placed), where crisscrossing should be carried out, and where simple undermining without suction should be done (mesh undermining). Figure 16-26 shows a patient marked to illustrate these concepts.

Fig. 16-26. Topographic markings show the contour. Plus marks show their greatest excess. Minus marks show dimples. Heavy marks show area to extend the gluteal fold.

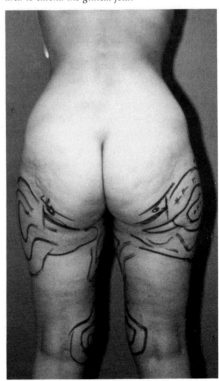

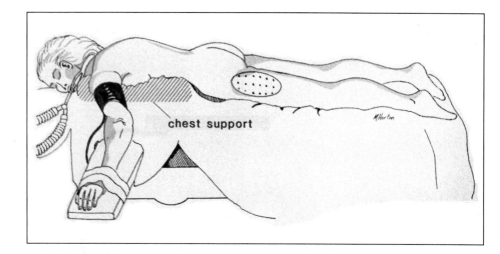

Fig. 16-27. The prone position. Care must be taken while turning; chest support, normal neck posture, and arm and shoulder support must be provided.

Occasional dells or valleys should be noted with minus signs and should be avoided to prevent worsening such areas. When the patient is on the operating table, such an area may no longer appear as a depression because of shifting of the fat. The tactile pinch test probably provides the most information about the thickness and quality of the fat to the surgeon both before and during the procedure. This test should be performed during marking immediately preoperatively. The normal superficial fat (by pinch) varies between 1.5 and 3.0 cm in nonobese people. The areas where there is a deeper layer of fat invested by the superficial fascia may reach 6 to 8 cm in nonobese people. It is usually this deep fat that causes the bulges of the lower abdomen, iliac crest, lateral femoral area, medial thigh, and medial knee.

Before the marking is completed, an appraisal of the surrounding subcutaneous thickness should be made by pinching these tissues as seen in Figure 16-23. If 2 to 3 cm can be pinched above and below a saddlebag, and the localized fatty deposit is 6 to 7 cm, the goal of the extraction process should be to reduce this excess to the level of the surrounding 2- to 3-cm thickness and not more.

Positioning the Patient

For treatment of thoracodorsal rolls, iliac crest rolls, sacral bulge, the buttock, lateral thigh, subgluteal areas, the posterior medial thigh, medial knee, and calves, I turn the patient into the prone position with the chest supported by chest rolls and the arms outstretched as shown in

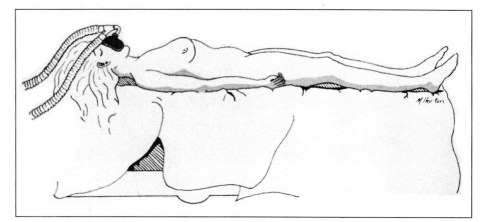

Fig. 16-28. Supine position.

Figure 16-27. Some, but not all, of these areas can be operated on in the lateral decubitus position favored by Mladick, which was developed to allow mask anesthesia and avoid the time and personnel required to turn the patient. The inspection and palpation of bilateral areas during the procedure, the access to near midline structures, and the greater accuracy the prone position affords outweigh for me these practical concerns; therefore, my patients are intubated and placed in the prone position. Great attention must be paid to the placement of the patient on chest rolls, use of a soft mattress, protection of bony prominences, care in turning, and the prevention of brachial plexus injuries. The neck must be placed in the normal postural position to avoid potential pinching of the cervical roots. For the breast, abdomen, flanks, anterior thigh, medial thigh, and suprapatellar areas, I place the patient in the supine position (Fig. 16-28).

Incisions to reach these areas should be as close as possible to the fatty excess. As short a cannula as possible is used to reach the area involved and thus to provide the best control. To reach the epigastrium, for example, I always use two incisions beneath the breasts rather than a long cannula from the hypogastrium (Fig. 16-29). For dorsal rolls, I use paraspinal incisions. Figure 16-30 shows approaches to the back and posterior extensions of the iliac crest fat, which I can treat successfully only with the patient in the supine position.

Pretreatment with Epinephrine

Originally Illouz used a hypotonic solution containing hyaluronidase believing it would make the fat easier to extract. I added epinephrine to this solution in 1982 and demonstrated a considerable reduction in blood loss, as would be antici-

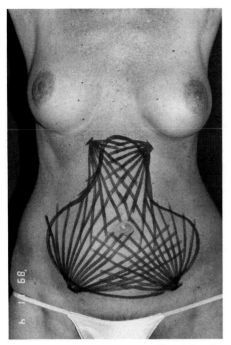

Fig. 16-29. Drawing on a patient illustrating the approach to the epigastrium though two rib margin incisions and to the hypogastrium through two high inguinal incisions, allowing complete crisscrossing of both areas.

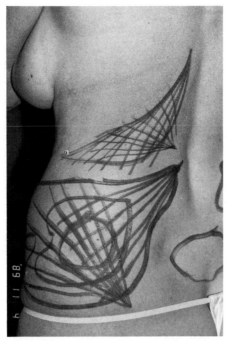

Fig. 16-30. Paraspinal incisions are used to reach the most medial extension of the iliac crest folds and the dorsal rolls. Criss-cross lipoplasty may be used through two paraspinal incisions as shown for a dorsal roll. The iliac crest roll is treated through a more lateral upper buttock port and a paraspinal port.

pated. This work has subsequently been well corroborated by others; nevertheless, there are plastic surgeons who lecture on this procedure who say it makes no difference whether or not epinephrine is given. If so, they should give up epinephrine for their face-lifts as well. Either epinephrine in saline solution in dilutions of 1:500,000 to 1:1,000,000 or dilutions of lidocaine of $\frac{1}{4}$% to $\frac{1}{8}$% with epinephrine 1:400,000 to 1:800,000 may be used. Some surgeons believe the lidocaine reduces postoperative pain and in shorter operations could be of help.

The epinephrine-containing solution is delivered to the areas of intended suction in the deep fatty excess. A long blunt needle with many fine holes is introduced through the suction incision. It can deliver the solution along the fascial plane above the muscle where the vascular perforators come through to the fat and skin. Application in this manner appears to reduce the amount of blood in the fatty aspirate of the lower abdomen, which otherwise can be rather bloody. These blunt needles pass along the tissue planes easily through the incisions that ulti-

mately are used for the cannula. Table 16-4 shows the amounts of epinephrine generally used for various areas.

If epinephrine 1:500,000 is used, about half of the amounts listed in Table 16-4 is needed. Some surgeons believe that instilling large amounts of fluids distorts the tissue and makes it difficult to visually judge the end point of fat extraction. Stronger concentrations of less fluid may be used. Illouz emphasized for many

Table 16-4. Amount of injection of epinephrine in saline 1:1,000,000 injected per area

Area	Amount of epinephrine (ml)
Lateral thigh	100–200
Abdomen	150–300
Iliac crest	75–100
Knee	30–50
Anterior thigh	100–250
Calf	75–200
Face and neck	50–125

years that the use of large amounts of fluid led to accumulation of yellow fat in the collection bottle. Observing his results in 1982 showed this to be true.

Because I determine the end point of my procedures by touch, reaching it when the affected area has been reduced by pinch and roll to the same thickness as the unaffected areas, and because I inject into the deep reserve fat being removed and not the superficial fat, I have never found fluid instillation to be a problem. I routinely use 350 to 500 ml when average amounts of fat are to be removed and more when large amounts are removed.

Pretunneling

Pretunneling is simply passing a cannula that is not connected to suction through the incision into the proper plane. The feel of running through superficial fat where there are many retinacula cutis is "gritty," whereas the deep reserve fat produces an easier, smoother passage. Too pointed a cannula does not give this important information. When suction is applied, the cannula has more resistance to movement, which detracts from this tactile information.

By passing the cannula into the proper plane and developing the plane by regular radiating thrusts, a kind of pseudoplane is developed at or just below the superficial fascia. In the hypogastrium, for example, the edge of the deep fat compartment can be exactly defined as the su-

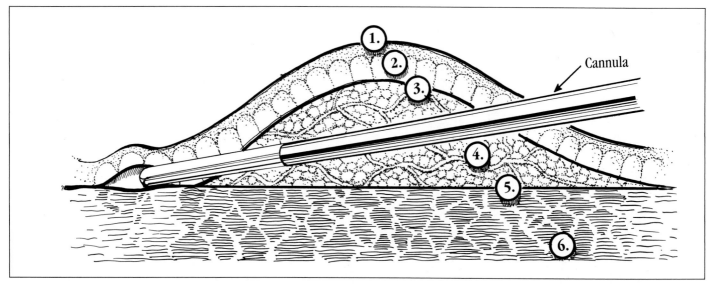

Fig. 16-31. The cannula has punctured the fusion of the superficialis muscle and fascia and has entered the superficial fat. No dimple or divot results from this maneuver if no suction is present. 1. Skin. 2. Superficial fat. 3. Superficial fascia. 4. Deep fat. 5. Muscle fascia. 6. Muscle.

Fig. 16-32A. The hole of the cannula is an adequate distance from the tip to prevent subdermal suction. B. A hole at the tip allows subdermal fat removal. C. A clinical photograph of a superficial fat defect of the lateral thigh caused by passing a "shark mouth" cannula too far laterally from a subgluteal incision.

perficial fascia fuses with the muscle fascia laterally and the easy movement of the cannula stops as it hits this fusion (Fig. 16-31). Similarly, where the superficial fascia of the lateral thigh fuses with the fascia lata, the cannula stops (see Fig. 16-4). A cobra or pointed cannula may not stop as does a hemispherically tipped cannula. Of course, when no suction is attached, a puncture into the superficial fat causes no lasting defect as would happen if suction were attached (Fig. 16-32). Pretunneling is useful in defining the

depth, extent, and character, or "feel," of the fat.

Technique of Extraction

I start at one side of the bulge and work toward the other in a regular, even manner. Using a single-hole No. 6 Illouz blunt cannula, I turn the hole away from the muscle fascia by about 30° in the direction I intend to proceed. I stop after making about 10 to 15 passes or until I can feel that little more fat is forthcoming or the

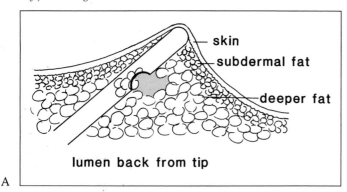

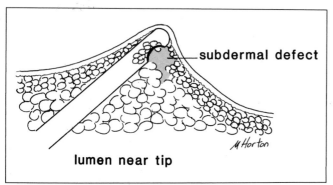

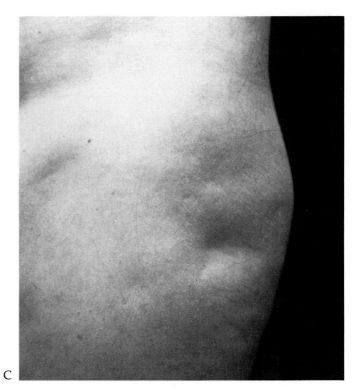

fat becomes bloody. At that point I go on to the next tunnel and so on, over the whole area. Where plus signs indicate more fat to remove, I make a few more passes. The length of the pass is determined by the topographic map. The edge of the deposit is feathered by thrusts of different length or by using a smaller cannula at the periphery.

When removing the cannula, I break suction to avoid overextracting near the entry site. The pinch and roll test is performed regularly throughout the procedure to monitor progress. It should be remembered that what is pinched is two thicknesses of fat.

Cross Tunneling

When about 65 to 70 percent of the extraction is complete, I use a second incision to cross tunnel at right angles to the first tunnels. The remaining 30 to 35 percent of the procedure is completed using both directions. The pinch and roll test is performed often to avoid the unpleasant surprise of an overextracted area. Small lumps or islands of fat can be grasped with the control hand and speared with a small cannula. In this manner any remaining irregularities are extracted.

What is *not* done is as important as what is done. No side-to-side windshield wiper motion is performed. This motion could injure the SFS and the vessels and nerves. The cannula lumen is not turned toward the surface. Persistently overworking a bloody area is not done. Excessive cross tunneling is not done because it may lead to a cavity and then a pseudobursa. Overthinning beyond the normal thickness of surrounding superficial fat is not done.

Mesh Undermining

When extraction is complete, the edges of the extracted area are loosened up simply by passing a very blunt Illouz cannula into the surrounding area *without* suction. This maneuver tends to break up the edge and allow some recontouring of the adjacent tissue. The theory behind such a maneuver is that there are three phases to the improvement seen from BSL: (1) immediate fat cell extraction, (2) subsequent fat cell death, and (3) fibrosis and retraction. Mesh undermining is believed to cause some additional fat cell death at the periphery, which allows a more even transition.

When to Stop

When to stop is the hardest thing to know in all human endeavor. It is a question asked by many who are just beginning a procedure. Several factors influence the decision.

Blood

When it is mostly blood and little or no fat that appears in the tube, it is time to move on to the next tunnel. There are a few patients whose fat seems very fibrous, who bleed a great deal early on, and from whom little fat is obtained. I have no explanation for this. It does not help to persist in the attempted removal.

Lax Skin

When the skin becomes wavy, especially in the lateral thighs or abdomen, it is reasonable to stop. A secondary suction may be done 6 months later, after skin retraction has occurred. To go beyond the ability of the skin to retract risks uneven contraction or sliding of the skin because of a lax SFS.

Pinch and Roll Test

It is important to compare the extracted area to the surrounding normal areas and the evenness within the extracted area. The areas should be uniform as you pinch and roll.

Visual Examination

The areas should be looked over from side to side and from directly above to operating table level to judge the "skyline" view on both sides for symmetry and evenness of contour and silhouette. Small refinements should be made with 4-mm cannulas, or some fat injection may be done by the syringe technique to fill in any areas marked with minus signs.

Cannula Feel

The feel of the passage of the cannula changes as the procedure progresses. The feeling is difficult to describe, but it is grittier because the passage is through fibrous shrouds drawn into the lumen of the cannula rather than through fatty substance.

Aesthetic Sense

Overresections are often done because patients have emphasized that they desired a flat stomach or straight thighs. The natural curves of the body should be

known and respected. If less fat is left over the trochanter than over the surrounding areas, a female patient will appear masculine in the posterior view. More fat can always be removed later, but that which is in the collection jar cannot be reinserted.

Irrigation

In the areas where irrigation can be undertaken easily (iliac crest, calves and ankles, face and neck), it has proved useful. When blood and fatty fragments are removed, both swelling and bruising are reduced and hemosiderin pigmentation is less likely. Saline solution is instilled through a cannula, and a folded towel rolled along the operated area toward the entry sites is used to distribute it.

Common Procedures: Suggestions and Results

Iliac Crest and Dorsal Rolls

The iliac crest roll may be mostly lateral or mostly posterior, high or low, or in between. It may have a large dorsal roll extension (see Fig. 16-30). The bulk of the iliac crest roll is suctioned laterally with a 6-mm single-hole Illouz cannula through a lateral port. Dorsal rolls may be separate from each other and are formed by fibrous elements attaching to deeper structures. Some of these can be extracted accurately *only* with the patient in the prone position. An incision approximately 4 or 5 cm from the midline is made 6 mm in length, and a 4-mm cobra cannula is used for these dorsal rolls or iliac crest extensions and the posterior flank area.

Lateral Thighs

I use single-hole 25-cm, 35-cm, and 6-mm Illouz cannulas. I make one infragluteal incision 3 cm lateral to the ischial tuberosity and an iliac crest incision about 10 to 12 cm from the midline. Both incisions are 8 or 9 mm long and are closed with polyglactin 910 or nylon.

Suction is applied after thorough pretunneling. The first two-thirds of the removal is made through the infragluteal incision and the final third through both incisions. The most anterior portion of the saddle-

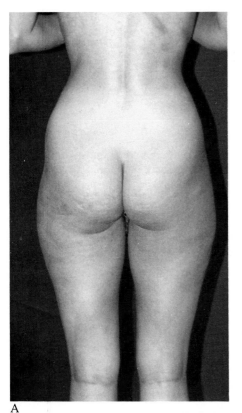

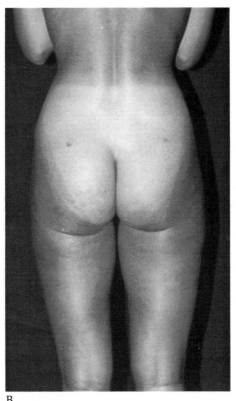

A

B

*Fig. 16-33A. Preoperative posterior view of 31-year-old woman with asymmetric iliac crest excess and large asymmetric lateral thigh deposits. (The excess is greater on the right side.) B. Postoperative view shows better symmetry and the open **S** line from rib cage to midthigh uninterrupted by bulges or waves. The buttock folds have been defatted to accentuate them.*

Anterior Thighs

The suprapatellar fat often hangs over the patella. This fat may be approached from two 5- to 6-mm parapatellar incisions. A criss-cross lipoplasty is carried out with 3- to 4-mm cobra or Illouz cannulas. The inferior anterior thigh is reached from these incisions, and similar 4- to 5-mm cannulas are used. The whole anterior thigh has only superficial fat. It may be debulked from above and below, but great care needs to be exercised to prevent subdermal vascular damage and grooving. Anterior thigh reduction is shown in Figure 16-35.

Knees

The approach to the medial knee may be from the medial popliteal fossa. This fat should come out easily with almost no blood, and a 4- or 6-mm Illouz cannula is a good choice depending on bulk. The inferior hook of fat below the level of the joint is more fibrous and a 4-mm cannula is preferable there.

Abdomen

There are two distinctly different anatomic areas of the abdomen. The *epigastric* fat is more fibrous, bleeds more, and lacks a discrete superficial fascia starting several centimeters above the umbilicus. I make two 7- to 8-mm incisions either beneath the breasts or at the fibrous fat pads overlying the flare of the ribs (see Fig. 16-29). In some people these fat pads are

bag is approached from the iliac crest incision because it is a much straighter approach. The results of trying to curve around the trochanter from the infragluteal incision are illustrated in Figure 16-32C. A typical example of lateral thigh and iliac crest reduction is shown in Figure 16-33.

Medial Thighs

The danger in operating on the medial thigh is overextraction because the skin is thin and fine (in contradistinction to the lateral thigh). I liken it to eyelid skin when explaining this to patients. A posterior infragluteal incision can be combined with an anterior inguinal incision if the patient is to be turned. Cannulas in the 3- to 5-mm range usually are best. The frog-leg position allows approach from above and below. An inguinal incision and a midthigh incision allow a good criss-cross approach, and the incisions need be only 5 to 6 mm long (Fig. 16-34).

Fig. 16-34. Intraoperative photograph shows approach to medial thighs through inguinal port and a small midthigh incision using a relatively short cannula for maximal control.

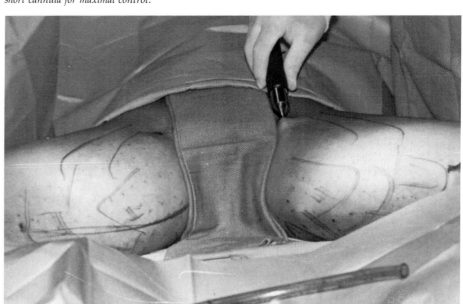

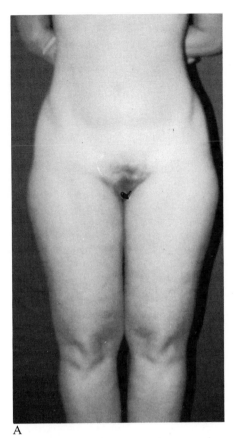
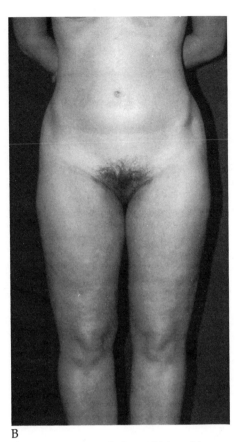

A   B

Fig. 16-35A. Preoperative photograph of a 28-year-old woman showing generally heavy thighs and knees.
B. Postoperative photograph after removal of 1100 ml of fat from each thigh including lateral, medial, and
anterior aspects and the knees. Note improved definition around knee caps.

quite prominent and the patient wants them reduced. Criss-cross lipoplasty is carried out with 4- or 5-mm short cobra cannulas over the whole epigastrium through these two incisions. I am satisfied if I can reduce the pinch test by half; I rarely achieve more. The return of mostly blood rather than a full reduction is often the end point of the operation.

The deep *hypogastric* fat is softer, is less bloody (if adequate suprafascial epinephrine is used), and has a well-demarcated superficial fascia. Extraction here is through two lateral incisions just above the inguinal crease. Pretunneling is performed to delimit the deep compartment. Thereafter, extraction begins laterally, proceeding medially toward the umbilicus. The reduction is to bring the thickness down to that of the surrounding lateral superficial fat (in the hypochrondrium). After the extraction on the other side is performed, criss crossing from the

opposite side is carried out. A variety of cannulas in the 6-mm range are acceptable. I usually use a three-hole version designed for me and an offset blunt cobra, which allows the hand to clear the thigh and mons pubis. Extraction in the superficial fat, if desirable, is best accomplished with 4-mm cannulas. The periumbilical area requires fine reworking with a 4-mm cannula because this fat is more resistant to removal.

Male Flanks

The male flanks lack superficial fascia, and the extraction is from the superficial fat. There are many retinacula cutis. The fat is fibrous and work is difficult. The material extracted is usually bloody. Plenty of epinephrine and a 20-minute wait are useful. Keeping a centimeter of undamaged fat beneath the skin ensures a better result. Several entry sites and short 4- and 5-mm cobra cannulas are my

usual choices. The end point is usually bloody extract and a reduction to half the beginning thickness by pinch and roll. Flanks are not to be confused with an iliac crest deformity in a gynecoid man, which is similar in all respects to dealing with the same deformity in a woman. A typical result of hypogastric and flank suction in a man is shown in Figure 16-36.

Gynecomastia

Gynecomastia responds well to BSL. A periareolar incision is advocated by many, but I find two inframammary incisions best. Illouz or cobra cannulas are useful in 4- to 6-mm sizes. If the tissue is very fibrous, it can be grasped with the control hand like a sausage and speared by the cannula; extraction occurs as the control hand squeezes the tissue around and into the cannula. Criss-cross BSL is necessary for good results.

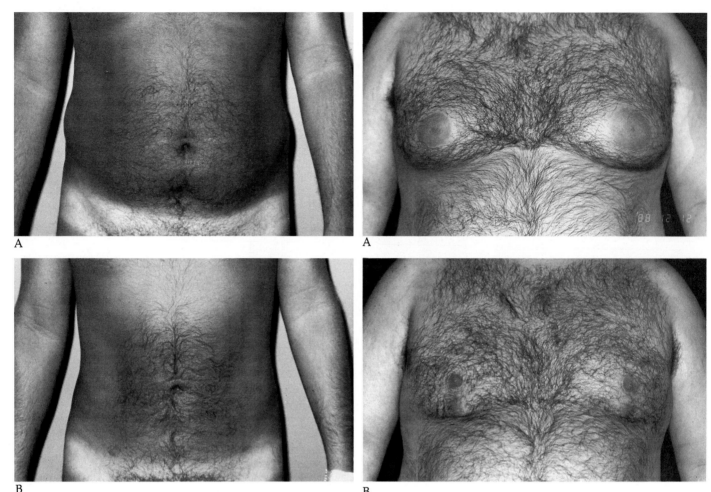

Fig. 16-36A. Preoperative view of typical male flanks with confluent hypogastric excess not amenable to remedy through exercise. B. Postoperative view after suction of flanks and hypogastrium showing more youthful figure.

Fig. 16-37A. Preoperative frontal view of 25-year-old man 5 feet 9 inches tall and weighing 250 pounds. He complained of large breasts from the age of 12 years. B. Postoperative frontal view 3 years after treatment showing results of removal of 300 ml of fat by suction, 200 ml of gland per side by resection, and areolar reduction by the VOQ technique of Regnault.

The glandular component may easily be underestimated, and gland resection through a periareolar incision may become necessary. Sometimes an areolar reduction is also necessary. Little glandular removal is possible by suction alone, although it is often mentioned. A result of suction resection and areolar reduction is shown in Figure 16-37.

Pectoral Fat Pad

Many women seeking augmentation complain of a fatty excess at the junction of the anterior axillary fold and the tail of the breast in the superficial fat. This fat is easily and almost bloodlessly removed by light suctioning (because this fat is loose) with a 4-mm Illouz single-hole cannula through an axillary incision. I use the same transaxillary incision used for the augmentation mammoplasty.

Calves and Ankles

Good results can be achieved in the calves and ankles, but several anatomic constraints need to be understood. Because there is only superficial fat and it is not uniform from high calf to ankle nor circumferentially, careful preoperative evaluation, marking, and planning are necessary. I use at least six entry sites: two on either side of the Achilles tendon, two high on the posterior calf, and usually one low and one high anteriorly. For large amounts of fat, I begin with the offset 6-mm cobra cannula for the thickest areas.

This cannula allows the hand to clear the calcaneus when working through para-Achilles incisions. The extraction is essentially circumferential except for the area above the tibia. I use a 2.5-mm cannula around the anterior ankle. Frequent pinch and roll tests are necessary to control the removal.

Tourniquets may be used as described by Stallings. If they are not used, saline irrigation of the area operated on washes out many fatty fragments and blood. If left behind, the breakdown products cause an increased oncotic pressure with resultant prolonged edema and pain, which adversely affects skin shrinkage and may lead to hemosiderin deposits. Drains may be left in for 24 hours when necessary.

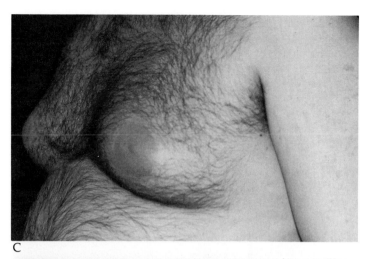

C

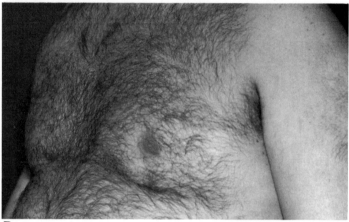

D

Fig. 16-37. (Continued) C. Left oblique preoperative view. D. Left oblique view 3 years postoperatively.

pears to be lasting recontouring. The procedure certainly is not a commercially viable alternative to breast augmentation. Nevertheless, it has potential, as shown in Figure 16-39. It is the only technique available for the filling of iatrogenic divots or grooving. A divot noticed during the operation should be refilled immediately using the SDS. Using fat from the suction bottle is probably not practical. Touchups years later appear to have some benefit.

Treatment of Cellulite

The anatomic basis for cellulite is shown in Figure 16-1. The theory behind the treatment is to cut the restraining retinacula cutis to release a dimple. This treatment has been successful when performed by Gasparoti and Toledo among others. A specially designed crochet hook–like instrument is passed in the subdermal plane with the hook in a vertical direction parallel with the retinacula cutis until the offending retinacula are approached. It is turned perpendicular to the retinacula and advanced sideways to hook and cut the retinacula cutis much as a tree trimmer hooks and cuts branches with a trimming hook. I am cautiously hopeful that this technique will allow improvement in severe dimpling and cellulite; however, a word of caution is needed. Operations in the superficial compartment carry a high risk of surface irregularities. This operation needs to be approached cautiously by surgeons who have worked with those skilled in its application.

Fat Injection

Fat injection remains a controversial subject. My impression is that some long-term benefit results from its use. Illouz and Mladick are doubters. Guerrerosantos and Lewis are believers. I maintain a skeptical viewpoint but use fat injection for postoperative divots and dimples and for filling the gluteal depression on occasion.

The fat is harvested with a syringe-driven system (SDS) (Fig. 16-38). It is washed in Ringer lactate or saline solution and reinjected with the same harvest system in multiple tunnels. Whether the apparent bulk that remains is based on living cells, microcysts, or some other phenomenon that is not understood, there often ap-

Fig. 16-38. A SDS designed by Louis Toledo, M.D. (JMJ Products), for the extraction, washing, and reinjection of fat.

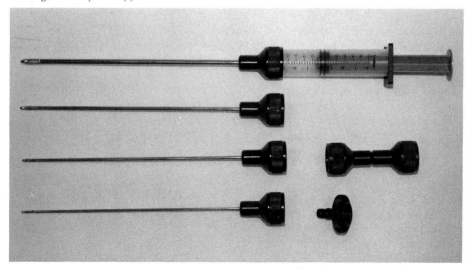

Fig. 16-39A. Preoperative view showing very large iliac crest roll and marked gluteal depression. B. Postoperative view at 15 months showing filling out of gluteal depression by injection of 150 ml of fat per side harvested from the iliac crest with the SDS and injected into multiple tunnels.

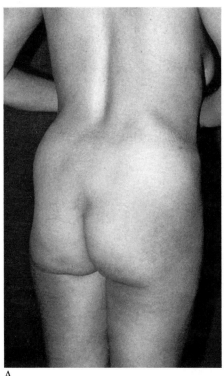

A

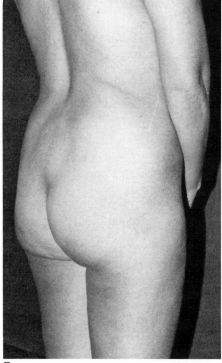

B

Postoperative Care

Fluids

Fluid shifts in BSL of the torso can be large, with massive sequestration in a fourth space. This acute sequestered edema is mobilized, as in a burn patient, after several days. The need for attention to these fluid and hemodynamic shifts is only one reason this procedure should be performed only by surgeons adequately trained in the physiology of shock and trauma. Hypovolemia, oliguria, fat embolism syndrome, shock, renal shutdown, pulmonary embolism, and myocardial infarction may follow injudicious ambulatory discharge of these patients without adequate blood and fluid replacement.

Antibiotics

A cephalosporin should be given intravenously before the start of the operation and continued for 1 or 2 days by mouth. More important, *the barrel of the cannula should never be touched, even with a gloved hand.*

Dressings

Elastic tape is used for the classic dressing of Illouz. To raise a gluteal fold, taping is absolutely necessary. Nonstretch tape should not be placed on the edge of the elastic tape because tape burns arise from the shearing effect of inelastic tapes.

Girdles of various kinds are useful for the abdomen, iliac crest, thighs, buttocks, and knees. The constant mild pressure is believed to reduce edema. Girdles are usually worn for 1 to 2 weeks followed by use of a support pantyhose. The patient should be cautioned about not letting either garment cause constriction around the knee.

Nutrition

Additional amounts of protein, iron, zinc, and vitamin C are recommended during the postoperative phase of 4 to 6 weeks. Recommended levels are protein, 150 g per day (twice normal); vitamin C, 500 to 1000 mg per day (higher in smokers); zinc, 50 to 60 mg per day; and iron, 325 to 650 mg per day as gluconate. Generally patients are asked not to smoke and are encouraged to have a diet rich in seafood, vegetables, and fruits in addition to the supplements.

Physical Therapy

I use massage and ultrasonic therapy. The massage therapist in the office, by the laying on of hands and attentive listening, takes a great burden from the surgeon and nurses. My patients undergo massages for 45 minutes three times a week for 3 weeks beginning on the tenth postoperative day. It appears that early ultrasonic therapy softens areas of hardening, especially on the abdomen. It is also useful on the face for small "knots."

General Convalescence

I recognize five phases in the convalescence of lipoplasty patients. Appropriate nursing and physician support during these phases mitigates problems. The massage therapist is invaluable during phase 3.

1. Bandage phase (days 1 to 7)
2. Fatigue phase (days 7 to 15)
3. Disappointment phase (days 16 to 25)
4. Relief phase (days 26 to 42)
5. Satisfaction phase (after 6 weeks)

The remodeling of the tissues is relatively complete 3 months after the procedure except for the ankles, which may take 6 to 9 months for remodeling. Changes continue for as long as a year as collagen contracture and fatty remodeling progress.

Touch-ups

Every patient is told preoperatively that touch-ups will be discussed 3 to 6 months after the operation. The patient's financial responsibility for the touch-ups should be clear before the first procedure. Fat injection and fine cannula recontouring are usually done 4 to 6 months postoperatively, generally with the SDS technique.

Sequelae

Imperfections commonly seen after BSL include the following:

1. Mild over- or underresection
2. Temporary hypesthesia
3. Mild waviness
4. Occasional minor dent or divot
5. Faint hemosiderin deposits
6. Transient pain
7. Some asymmetry
8. Transient fatigue

These sequelae usually resolve within 3 months, although some areas take longer to resolve than others. In order of rapidity of healing, the areas are the knees, iliac crests, lateral thighs, abdomen, and calves.

Aesthetically Unfavorable Results

The boundary between expected sequelae and unfavorable results aesthetically is hard to define and may vary from one patient to another, depending mainly on the skin condition before the operation. The following are the problems that lead most often to lawsuits claiming malpractice:

1. Grooving of the skin
2. Multiple dents and divots
3. Localized overresections (dishing out)
4. Generalized overresections, such as flat thighs, flat buttocks, skinny thighs, or no remaining iliac crest roll
5. Generalized washboarding
6. Androgynous appearance
7. Buttock ptosis
8. Skin adhesions to muscle fascia
9. Subdermal damage to the vasculature (reticulate pattern)

All these aesthetic problems can be minimized or prevented by careful work and anatomic knowledge. An example of "dishing out" of the lateral buttock, grooving, multiple dents, and divots is shown in Figure 16-40.

Severe Complications

The most common life-threatening medical complications are as follows:

1. Pulmonary embolus
2. Fat embolism syndrome
3. Myocardial infarction
4. Massive infection

5. Viscus perforation, including intestine, spleen, liver, and lung
6. Renal shutdown

Pulmonary embolus and myocardial infarction may be random events; however, postoperative hypovolemia caused by inadequate blood and fluid resuscitation is all too often associated with these complications. The fluid loss continues in the wound for at least 12 to 36 hours, and the intravascular volume may reach its nadir 18 to 24 hours postoperatively.

A word about fat embolism syndrome is in order. Restrictive lung disease such as emphysema and acute restriction of lung excursion caused by abdominal or chest operations and dressings (abdominoplasty with fascial plication or subpectoral augmentation) may predispose to this syndrome. A healthy lung making good excursions is the best prevention. Suction of a large body surface area combined with procedures that limit diaphragmatic

or chest excursion increases the risk, as does a low albumin level. *Fat embolism syndrome* should not be confused with a *fat embolism*, which is generally benign. The treatment of these complications is much more difficult than their prevention. Despite all precautions, however, fat embolism syndrome may appear.

Lesser Complications

Other complications, from lesser to greater frequency, are as follows:

1. Anemia
2. Seroma
3. Hematoma
4. Pseudobursa formation
5. Incision site infection
6. Muscle or muscle fascia damage with persistent pain
7. Sensory nerve damage with persistent dysesthesias or hypesthesias

Fig. 16-40. A patient referred for medicolegal evaluation. She has overextraction, uneven extraction, subdermal extraction, grooving, dents, and divots. Note the extraction in the area of the gluteal depression.

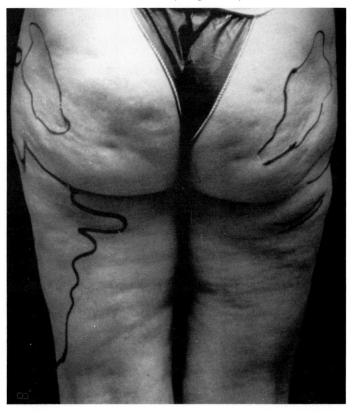

Most severe complications can be traced to violations of the physiologic or anatomic principles of surgery. Most aesthetic complications are caused by a lack of aesthetic perception, a lack of knowledge of the subcutaneous fascial system or of the anatomy of the site, or the use of the wrong cannulas.

Face and Neck Suction

The use of closed aspiration in fat removal from the neck during face-lifts has rapidly gained in popularity. It replaced scissors resection because bleeding seemed to be decreased, and the procedure was much faster to perform. The cannula could be used as a vacuum cleaner after flap elevation. Suction above the mandibular line, especially in the areas medial to the limits of flap elevation near the nasolabial folds, has not gained in popularity as quickly. Closed suction or liposculpture

Fig. 16-41A. Cervicomental angle filled with fat, giving a matronly impression. B. Same drawing as A except empty cervicomental angle and defined mandibular line give a youthful impression.

of the younger fatty face has also gained ground slowly. The margins of error are smaller than in open techniques in which the skin can be advanced. Mistakes can rarely be corrected, a factor that has given pause, understandably, to many careful practitioners.

Aesthetic Ideal

I hope to achieve a clean mandibular line, a well-defined mentum, a flat cheek plane ending in a highlighted malar eminence, a defined sternocleidomastoid element, and an oval face. Fatty faces usually lack these architectural features because the features are hidden by the fat in the lower third of the face and neck as seen in Figure 16-41. I discuss each of the following areas with the patient before the operation:

1. Malar eminence
2. Cheek contour
3. Mentum
4. Mandibular line
5. Cervicomental angle
6. Sternocleidomastoid element

Conceptual Viewpoint

Modern facial rejuvenation must deal with five possible problem areas: (1) tightening the lax face and neck skin envelope; (2) contouring the fatty layer of the cheek, jowl, and neck; (3) positioning the platysma and components of the SMAS; (4) augmenting (or, rarely, reducing) the malar and mental areas; and (5) peeling the face and neck skin for improvements in color, texture, and quality. Each of these areas had or will have a period of heightened interest and activity. In the 1970s it was SMAS and chin augmentation; in the 1980s it was fat aspiration and malar augmentation. I predict that in the 1990s emphasis will be on advances in facial peeling. For younger patients undergoing closed suction, the concern is generally with items 2 and 4 and occasionally item 5.

Diagnosis and Marking

The patient is evaluated in frontal, oblique, lateral, and lateral neck-flexed positions.

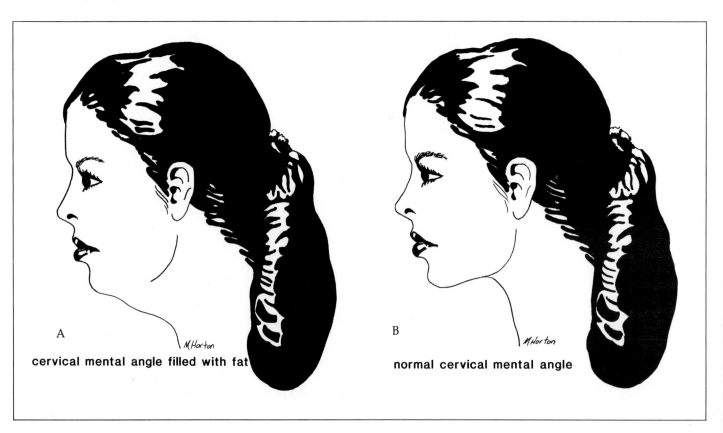

A
cervical mental angle filled with fat

B
normal cervical mental angle

1. The skin envelope is judged for laxity, elasticity, thickness, and volume. If the skin is very loose or the skin envelope is large (large fatty neck), a face-lift with a postauricular incision line needs to be carried out. The incision must be both long and at the hairline to avoid markedly raising the hairline. This incision allows the neck skin to advance parallel with the mandibular line rather than toward the postauricular area, which carries skin creases to an abnormal position.

2. The subcutaneous fat of the neck, cheeks, and jowls is judged by the pinch and roll technique and marked as a careful topographic map on the face and neck (Fig. 16-42). A normal pinch test in a young woman is 6 to 7 mm in the lower cheeks and neck. The submental area is lightly pinched, and the patient is asked to bite hard and tighten the neck muscles. If the fat is preplatysmal, the fat remains in the surgeon's grasp and is easily mobile over the tightened platysma as a mass. If the fat is subplatysmal, the fat slips away as the platysma contracts superficially to it, leaving skin in the examiner's grasp. By subtraction one can estimate the preplatysmal and platysmal plus the subplatysmal fat component. I call this the dynamic test for platysmal fat.

3. The SMAS and platysma muscle are evaluated with attention to slumping of the malar mass off the malar prominence, ptotic preantral mass, flaccid anterior platysma, and bowstringing or asymmetry of the medial platysmal bands. Positive findings need to be addressed by one or more surgical interventions such as malarpexy, SMAS slide, medial band myectomy, or anterior platysmotomies, or platysmoplasties.

4. The malar area and mentum need to be judged for adequacy of contour. A deficient chin is often seen in fatty faces. The deficiency of the geniomandibular groove was identified as an aesthetic problem by Mittelman, who has addressed it by designing a series of implants. Fatty cheeks and jowls often exaggerate this deficiency. Malar implants designed by Terino address deficiencies in the malar area. Submalar implants designed by Binder improve this area. Patients often are unaware of these problem areas. If the deficiency is marked and the patient refuses augmentation, it is better aesthetically not to perform the operation. If the deficiency is modest in dimension, the patient should be encouraged to add the

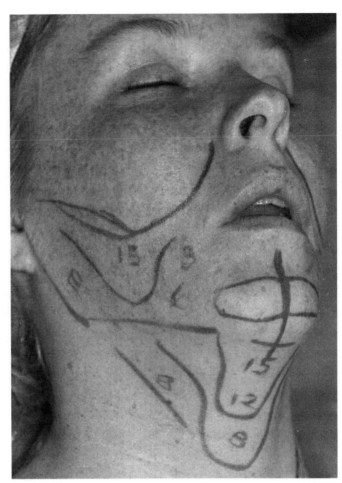

Fig. 16-42. Intraoperative photograph shows topographic marking with "pinch" thickness marked in millimeters. (From G.P. Hetter (Ed.). Lipoplasty. Boston: Little, Brown, 1990. Reproduced with permission.)

augmentation, but it is not necessary for aesthetic reasons to refuse to operate at all if the patient does not want the augmentation.

5. The patient's skin condition is emphasized during the evaluation. Pigmentation irregularities, fine wrinkles, desiccation, sun damage, and loss of glow are pointed out. The patient must understand that the operation will alter the shape, contour, and silhouette of the face but will not greatly alter the color, texture, or quality of the skin. Skin treatment alternatives such as dermabrasion and the various peel alternatives are mentioned. Many patients choose not to treat their skin.

False Indications

Hypertrophy of the masseter muscle, a wide bony mandible, a hyperplastic platysma muscle, and hypertrophy of the fat

pad of Bichat are commonly mistaken indications when only a visual examination is undertaken. Bimanual intraoral palpation is necessary to evaluate fully the fat pad of Bichat. The pinch and roll test should rule out the other false indications. Steroid hypertrophy is a relative contraindication. Cessation of steroids is the treatment when possible.

Integration of Data

Integrating the results of the evaluation is important. When fat is in excess of 6 to 8 mm by pinch and roll, it is removed to that level in indicated areas. Fat alone in patients older than 35 years is rarely the sole problem, however. Sagging jowls usually are a problem of the SMAS. The SMAS correction should be completed before fine tuning with suction. Slumping of the malar fat often can be corrected by a malarpexy or SMAS slide; however,

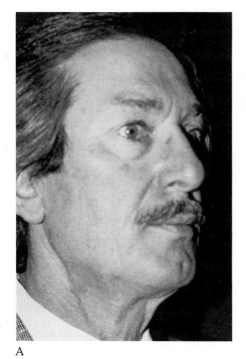

A

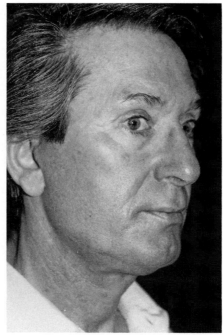

B

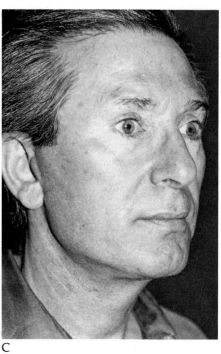

C

Fig. 16-43A. Preoperative photograph of male patient requesting face-lift. B. Postoperative photograph one year later, following SMAS face- and neck-lift and blepharoplasty. Note persisting deep nasolabial folds and some submental fullness. C. Eighteen months later following lysis of subdermal attachments of nasolabial folds and fat grafting, more submental fat removal, and redraping of the cervicofacial skin flap. No further SMAS work was performed. (SMAS = submuscular aponeurotic system.)

malar bone deficiency requires a malar augmentation. Wide undermining and a good skin lift correct mild nasolabial relaxation. A midcheek SMAS undermining procedure with SMAS slide is necessary to correct more severe problems. Deep nasolabial lines respond to subdermal undercutting and fat grafting (Fig. 16-43).

Treatment Plan

Incisions
When much neck skin is to be advanced markedly, the postauricular incision is at the hairline. If the hair is very fine or the sideburn is high or scant, the incision is in front of the sideburn. The submental incision is a curved incision just below the submental crease, and the submental crease is freed in the manner of Connell. When no face-lift is performed, five incisions are made—two sublobular, two alar, and one submental (Fig. 16-44).

Skin Undermining
If the skin is lax, extensive undermining is necessary. If the skin is tight and there is much fat, I complete closed suction

through the five ports. I subsequently undermine as much as necessary to advance the skin envelope. Undermining of the cheek is usually moderate after extensive suction in a fatty face with tight skin. I completely undermine the neck through a submental incision if the platysma is flaccid. A complete anterior platysmoplasty including considerable resection is required in such patients.

Open and Closed Suction
In patients with little or modest fat, I undermine and vacuum the undermined areas with a 6-mm Illouz cannula. The flaps are placed on tension to demonstrate contour. The jowl and cheek medial to the undermining are treated by crisscross lipoplasty through an alar incision (see Fig. 16-44B) and from beneath the flap using 1.5- and 2.4-mm cannulas until recontouring is judged aesthetic. Small resections cause major changes. It is important to stay below the alar-antral-zygomatic line (Fig. 16-45).

In heavy, fatty necks, I pretunnel and suction the entire neck and lower cheek and

jowl with a 3.8-mm cannula. Undermining of the cheeks and neck is then completed (Fig. 16-46). If indicated, an anterior platysmoplasty is completed. There is noticeably less bleeding with this routine. The skin flaps are put on tension to view contour. More suction or more undermining, or both, is performed as required.

Local SMAS Advancement and Platysmal Resection
Cadaveric dissections have shown that the best anterior neck improvement is obtained by an anterior platysmoplasty rather than a posterior platysmal approach. Hence my patients undergo resection of excess anterior platysma muscle and an anterior repair. When the preantral mass is ptotic, I undermine the preparotid SMAS and advance it. If the malar mound is ptotic, a simple malarpexy may suffice. If not, the SMAS can be advanced over the zygomatic arch, which serves to augment the malar area and can lift the nasolabial fold.

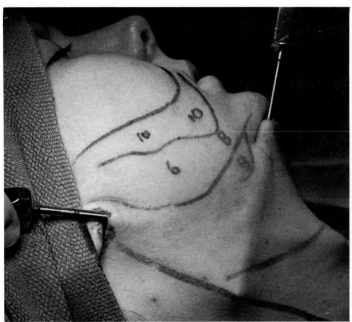

A

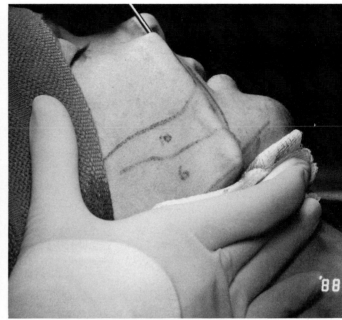

B

Fig. 16-44A. Submental and sublobular incisions allow criss-cross lipoplasty of the whole neck from sternocleidomastoid to sternocleidomastoid. B. The alar incision combined with the sublobular incision allows treatment laterally to the nasolabial folds. (From G.P. Hetter (Ed.). Lipoplasty. Boston: Little, Brown, 1990. Reproduced with permission.)

Fig. 16-45. The alar-antral-zygomatic line is the upper limit of resection.

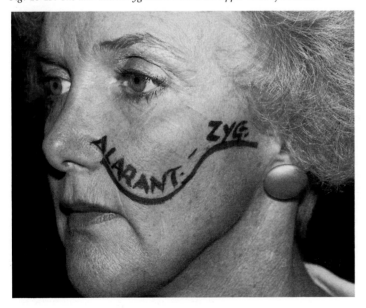

Fig. 16-46. Drawing of an intraoperative photograph showing the tunnels made by the suction process in the preplatysmal space leaving the intervening fibrous septa containing vessels and nerves.

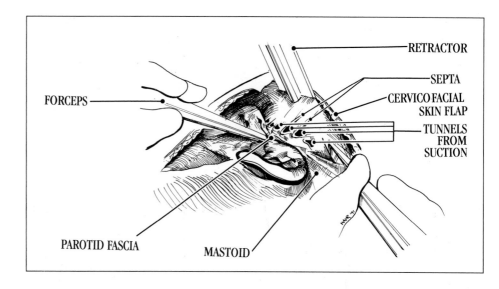

RETRACTOR
SEPTA
CERVICO FACIAL SKIN FLAP
TUNNELS FROM SUCTION
FORCEPS
PAROTID FASCIA
MASTOID

Augmentation

The usual augmentation procedures are done on the mentum, geniomandibular grooves, and malar and submalar areas. The extended chin implant is placed through the submental incision. The elevation is preperiosteal in the central 4 cm and subperiosteal laterally to protect the infraorbital nerve. During face-lifting, malar implants are placed through a blunt incision in the soft tissues over the zygoma anterior to the crossing of the frontal branch of the facial nerve. In closed suction, they are placed subperiosteally through either a blepharoplasty incision or a buccogingival incision depending on the type of implant and ancillary procedures.

Technique

As mentioned, I generally use five ports to perform facial suction both for closed operations and for procedures combined with a face-lift: one submental port, two infralobular ports, and two alar ports. Pretunneling is carried out beneath the dermis with a 3- to 4-mm single-hole Illouz cannula in the areas below the mandibular ramus to the level of the cricoid to define the subdermal neck-lift plane. Suction is applied always with the hole down. The submental port is used to clear fat across the anterior neck. The infralobular ports are used to cross-tunnel and clear fat from the sternocleidomastoid grooves forward. Through these same ports, pretunneling of the cheeks is car-

ried out with a 2- to 3-mm single-hole Illouz cannula. The area of the jowl and lower preantral fat is handled through this port. Four to six strokes in each tunnel are followed by control by the pinch and roll test. The alar port is used to finalize the contour of the fat in the preantral area and just lateral to the nasolabial fold and the jowl. This fat is easily extracted here, and great delicacy is necessary to avoid overextraction. A millimeter or two, just as in a nasal operation, is the difference between aesthetic success and mediocrity or failure (Fig. 16-47).

Suction Beneath the Flap

It is important to leave 2 to 3 mm of fat on the undersurface of the elevated cervicofacial flap to prevent adherence to platysmal or parotid fascia and to prevent injury to the blood supply of the skin. Open suction is performed with a 6-mm single-hole Illouz cannula, which acts much as a vacuum cleaner. The neck is cleared of preplatysmal fat in the submental and submandibular areas and along the sternocleidomastoid groove. If there is fatty thickness greater than 8 mm in the area below the undermining, I use a 2.4-mm single-hole cannula to feather this thickness out rapidly.

Careful evaluation of the preparotid area and along the sternocleidomastoid sulcus should be done. The 6-mm cannula quickly clears these areas of fat. If the skin flap is thin, care should be taken to avoid total denuding of the parotid fascia of fat.

Fig. 16-47. Excessive fat removal just lateral to the nasolabial fold noted by arrow.

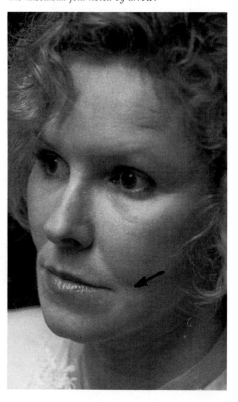

Suction Anterior to the Flap

Anterior to flap undermining, a 2.4-mm single-hole cannula is passed beneath the flap at the level of the lobule and through an alar stab incision. Pretunneling is very important. The pinch test is used first. If the jowl thickness is 10 or 12 mm, it is reduced by a few even strokes of suctioning to 6 to 8 mm. The reduction should not be overdone. The cannula is passed four to eight times in each tunnel. When a marionette deformity exists lateral to the oral commissure, a 1.5-mm cannula is useful. Skin undermining may need to be extended medially after suctioning is complete. It is impossible to suction this very medial area evenly after undermining has taken place. This is an area requiring finesse.

By tensing the flaps and by pinch and roll, the gradual removal is evaluated during extraction. It must be remembered that it is what is left behind that counts. Suctioning should not be done medial to the nasolabial fold or the pericommissural dimple because these are fixed points where muscle is attached to skin (Fig. 16-48).

Anterior Platysmoplasty

I split the intraplatysmal membrane vertically and elevate the platysmal flaps laterally along with the investing fascia. I remove subplatysmal fat as necessary. I elevate the platysma laterally and cut the medial bands for 2 to 2.5 cm at the level of the cricoid cartilage. The platysmal flaps are pulled toward the opposite side, and excess platysma is excised. There can be up to 2 cm of laxity on both sides. A midline repair is carried out with multiple 4–0 Mersilene (knitted Dacron polyester) to the advanced and slightly upwardly rotated platysmal flaps. If the investing fascia (the white membrane beneath the platysma) is not included, the repair will fail. Excess platysma below the last suture is trimmed toward the horizontal cut in the platysma. This anterior repair produces the best neck lines. Of course in a very thin neck, a plication technique such as that of Feldman is simpler and adequate.

Patient Studies

Closed Suction

Results of closed suction can be remarkable. A 35-year-old woman presented

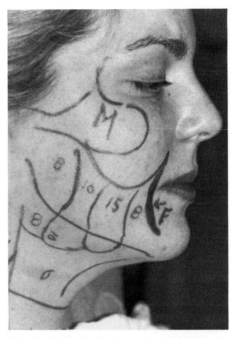

Fig. 16-48. The fixed pericommissural fold lateral to which there is fat and medial to which there is muscle. The fold is marked by the dark line with the arrow and the letter F. (From G.P. Hetter (Ed.). Lipoplasty. Boston: Little, Brown, 1990. Reproduced with permission.)

with chubby cheeks, no malar highlight, submental and submandibular fat, and no clear sternocleidomastoid definition. The eyelids showed fatty ptosis and lateral brow fat (Fig. 16-49A and C).

The postoperative views (Fig. 16-49B and D) show a woman appearing to have lost weight looking at least 10 years younger than in the preoperative views. The treatment consisted of upper lid blepharoplasty, lateral brow defatting, and suction through five ports, two alar, two sublobular, and one submental. No cheek or chin implant was used. The result was a fine malar highlight, clean mandibular line, and a fat cheek plane. There was no extension of the nasolabial line into the jowl segment after the operation. The patient did *not* lose weight postoperatively; the facial sculpturing only made it appear that way.

Face-Lift and Suction

The patient shown in Figure 16-50 requested a consultation for facial rejuvenation at the age of 67 years. The areas of her concern were a relaxed fatty neck,

jowling, wrinkling of the cheeks, and "a tired look." The areas of concern to me were brow ptosis with high hairline, ptosis of the malar soft tissues, fatty jowls, poor mandibular line, flaccid platysma with pre- and subplatysmal fat, and severe creping of neck skin. The upper and lower eyelids showed no fatty ptosis or clinically significant blepharochalasia. The chin was retrusive with geniomandibular groove atrophy (Fig. 16-50A, C, E, and G).

The patient underwent the following procedures directed at these findings: (1) an anterior hairline forehead lift with dissection and considerable resection of the procerus and corrugator muscles and attenuation of the frontalis muscle; (2) fat suction of the neck, jowls, and submandibular area through alar, submental, and sublobular ports; (3) a face-lift with anterior platysmoplasty and malarpexy and a long posterior hairline incision to fully advance the posterior cervical flap; and (4) extended chin-jowl implant of the Mittelman type.

The postoperative views reveal the following: Figure 16-50B frontal shows unhooding of the orbit, a fuller malar area, filling of the geniomandibular grooves, and a firm neck past the midneck crease. Figure 16-50D shows good malar highlight, improvement in contour of the alar-antral-zygomatic line, an improved mandibular line, mental prominence, and neck firming. (Note that the white linear scar on the left neck has not been raised because the vector of pull for the cervical flap is well below the mastoid.) Figure 16-50F shows unhooding of the lateral brow, filling of the geniomandibular groove combined with jowl fat removal resulting in tightening of the difficult "marionette" area, that the mandibular line ends in a prominent mentum, and a tight cervical envelope. Figure 16-50H demonstrates that the neck restoration remains tight in the flexed position.

Complications and Sequelae

The following complications may occur as in any face-lift: motor nerve damage, sensory nerve damage, skin necrosis, hair loss, infection, hematoma, and unpredictable scarring. Iatrogenic aesthetic sequelae seen too frequently are severe alterations of the hairline, loss of sideburn

Fig. 16-49A. Preoperative frontal view of a 35-year-old woman, 167 pounds, and 5 feet 9 inches. Note jowls, chubby cheeks, neck fullness, severe fatty ptosis of lids, and fatty excess of lateral brow. B. Postoperative frontal view at 4 months. Note defined mandibular line, impression of increased malar highlight, and opening up of orbital area. C. Preoperative lateral view. Note heavy jowl and neck, extension of nasolabial fullness onto and into jowl segment, and lateral brow fullness. D. Postoperative lateral view at 4 months. Note clean mandibular line, jowl and cheek reduction, malar definition, and lateral brow reduction with unhooding of eye.

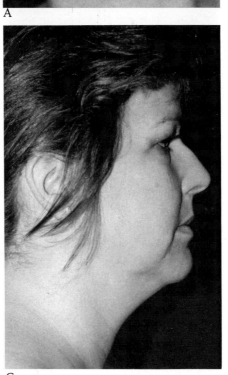
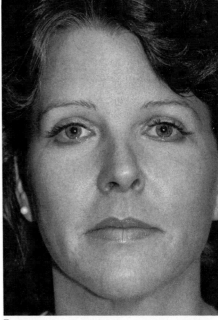
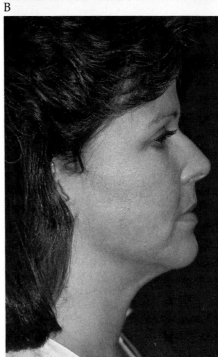

A

B

C

D

or temporal hair, elevation of neck creases onto the cheek or toward the lobule, descensus of the lobule or pixie ear, gathering about the ear, and failure to remove medial facial fat.

Deformities seen as a result of suction procedures are uneven resection, over-resection, step resection, adhesions, and dimples. Excessive injury to tissue conceivably could result in vascular embarrassment with resultant slough, which I have never seen. The dictum of the architect Mies van der Rohe, "Less is more," has validity in facial liposculpture also. Localized overresection is seen in Figure 16-47. Fat injection of iatrogenic defects can give improvement (Fig. 16-51). I usually wait for tissue softness to reappear—at least 4 but usually 6 months after the operation—before undertaking fat injections. More than one injection is usual.

Conclusion

The use of fine suction cannulas has allowed me to treat the fatty face and neck with greater success. Changes can be achieved in the areas of the cheek and jowl and the submental and submandibular areas, allowing the surgeon to achieve results approaching the Greco-Roman ideal. Suctioning allows a solution to the formerly difficult fatty problems of a face-lift. If the underlying fascia, platysma, and bone are not fully addressed, however, aesthetic shortcomings become evident.

The treatment of each of the four contour elements—skin laxity, fat excess, SMAS-platysmal defects, and bony contour deficiencies—is the key to good results. Fatty faces in particular can expect excellent improvement, but average faces benefit also. The next step in our quest for the finest in facial rejuvenation will be to find a skin peel treatment that restores the blush, quality, and texture associated with youthful skin.

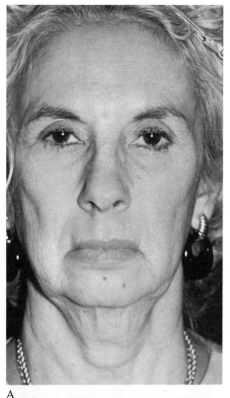

A

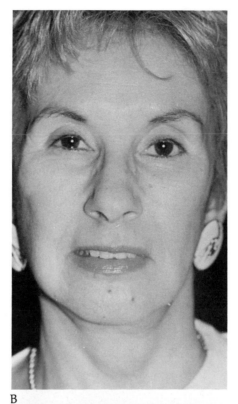

B

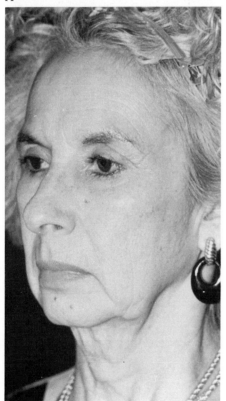

C

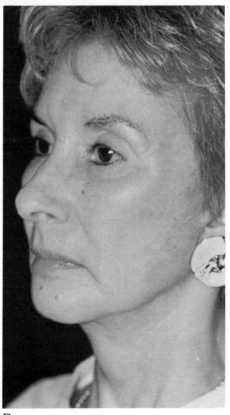

D

Fig. 16-50A. Preoperative view of 67-year-old woman. Frontal view shows severe relaxation of skin, fascia, and muscle and fatty depositions of jowl and neck. She has malar slumping, jowls, flaccid platysma, and brow ptosis. B. Postoperative frontal view at 6 months shows results of anterior hairline forehead-lift, face-lift with malarpexy, suction defatting of cheeks and neck, Mittleman chin-jowl implant, and anterior platysmoplasty. No blepharoplasty was performed. C. Preoperative left oblique view shows the severity of the problems in the lower third of the face: deficient bony prominence of chin, relaxed skin, fatty deposits, and flaccid fascia and platysma. D. Postoperative left oblique view shows the results of a lengthy postauricular incision where the vector allows complete restoration of the cervicomental angle without pulling neck creases toward the ear. Note correction of the pericommissural and nasolabial areas and the improved malar highlight and unhooding of the lateral orbit.

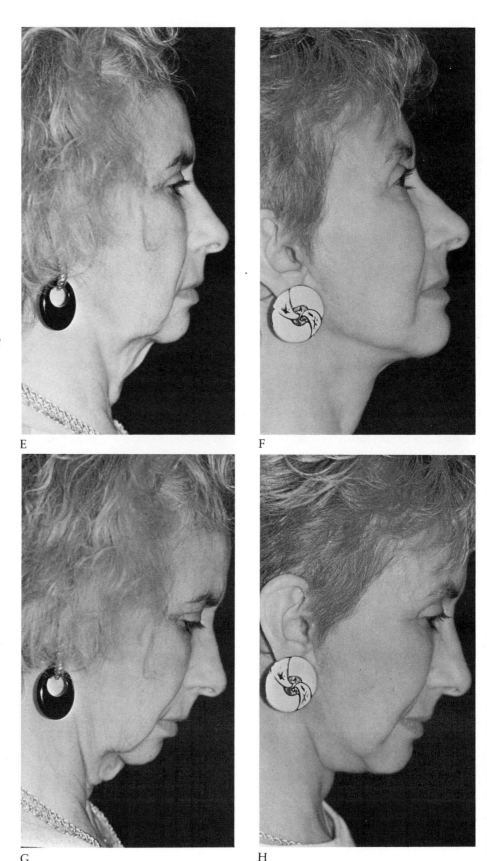

Fig. 16-50. (Continued). E. Preoperative right lateral view illustrates severe flaccidity and lack of mandibular line definition and dissociation of mentum from the mandibular line. Note continuation of nasolabial fold into the pericommissural fold and the jowl fold, which separates the chin eminence from the mandibular line. F. Postoperative right lateral view shows a cleaning of the mandibular line ending in the chin prominence, reestablishment of the cheek plane and malar highlight, and unhooding of the orbit. G. Right lateral "reading position" preoperative view shows the severe flaccidity of all neck layers. H. Right lateral "reading position" postoperative view shows that the tissues of the neck demonstrate tautness despite flexion of the head.

E

F

G

H

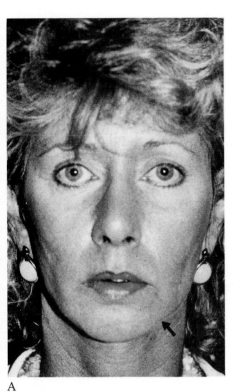 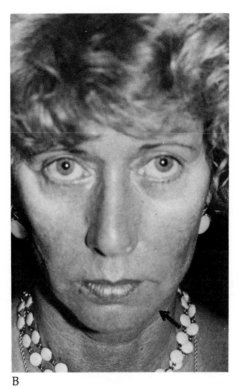

A   B

Fig. 16-51A. The arrow points to an area of overresection following suction of the anterior cheeks too close to the nasolabial line in a 50-year-old woman. B. After three fat injections in the course of 36 months, the area is improved. Whether the improvement will last for many years is unknown. The photograph was taken 5 years after the face-lift and 2 years after the last injection. The photograph was taken from above to show the geniomandibular area more clearly.

Suggested Reading

Clinics in Plastic Surgery: Body Contouring Surgery. Vol. 3. Philadelphia: Saunders, July 1984.

Clinics in Plastic Surgery: Lipoplasty. Vol. 16. Philadelphia: Saunders, April 1989.

Dermatologic Clinics: Liposuction. Vol. 8. Philadelphia: Saunders, July 1990.

Hetter, G.P. *Lipoplasty: The Theory and Practice of Blunt Suction Lipectomy* (2nd ed.). Boston: Little, Brown, 1990.

Illouz, Y.-G., and DeVillers, Y.T. *Body Sculpturing by Lipoplasty.* Edinburgh: Churchill Livingstone, 1988.

17

Lasers in Plastic Surgery

Lovic W. Hobby

History

In 1917 Albert Einstein proposed the quantum theory of radiation. The theory was that atoms are normally found in a state of energy called the resting state, in which the atom and its surrounding electrons are stable. Energy can be directed at the atom, causing a transition of an electron from its resting state to an excited state. This is an unstable condition, and the electron emits the energy previously absorbed and returns to its normal resting state. This emission of energy may be in the form of photons, which are the basic unit of electromagnetic radiation and light.

Einstein proposed that atoms, when subjected to a bombardment of energy, would enter this excited, unstable stage and release photons at an ever-increasing frequency, each electron stimulated by one photon, releasing two photons as it returned to its resting state.

It took scientists some time to advance these theories to a practical application. In 1954 Charles H. Towns put into operation the first microwave amplifier, or maser, at Columbia University. In 1958 he and Arthur L. Schawlow wrote a paper suggesting that the maser principle could be extended to include visible light. In 1960 Theodore H. Maiman from Stanford University was the first to observe stimulated emission of radiation with visible light using ruby crystals. He introduced the acronym laser for light amplification by stimulated emission of radiation. The ruby laser with its red light at 694.4 nm was the first laser to be used in medicine. Its light was absorbed by the pigmented tissue of the chorioretinal layer causing a chorioretinal scar. This was used as a welding mechanism in the reattachment of detached retinas. Reports of this work appeared in the scientific literature in 1963.

Within a year of the development of the ruby laser, four other types of lasers were available. The blue-green light of the argon laser at 488 to 514 nm was found to be well absorbed by hemoglobin and other pigmented tissues. It was clear that vascular tissue would be a selective target for this laser. This led to the treatment of diabetic retinopathies. Scientific documentation appeared in the literature in 1968. In 1971 Dr. Leon Goldman began to report his experience with lasers in the treatment of various skin diseases. In 1976 Dr. David Apfelberg began to focus specifically on the advantages of argon laser therapy for cutaneous vascular deformities.

Physics

The increasingly sophisticated laser machines of today follow the basic principles of the primitive laser used in 1960. The lasing medium is the ruby rod and the stimulated emission occurs in a cavity or lasing chamber. The energy is delivered to the lasing media electrically. This charge causes the necessary excitement of the atoms. As the atoms continue spontaneously to excite each other within the enclosure of the cavity, a state called population inversion is reached. At this point, there is massive excitation and increasing stimulation of photons of the same frequency traveling along the same axis. The lasing chamber is elongated with mirrors at each end. As the photons continue to collide, they eventually align themselves, moving back and forth along the long axis of the chamber reflecting off the mirrors. In the meantime the stimulated emission continues to increase, amplifying the process.

The mirror at one end has a small hole. Photons emerging through this hole make up the laser light. Theoretically this light can be in any wavelength within the electromagnetic spectrum. The spectrum ranges from very short wavelength gamma rays to long wavelength, low frequency radio waves. Wavelengths of surgical interest range from 10 to 400 nm in the ultraviolet, to 400 to 750 nm in the visible range, to 750 to 1,000,000 nm in the infrared spectrum.

Regardless of the wavelength, laser light has three unique characteristics. First, laser light is *monochromatic*. That is, it has a single color or a very narrow wavelength. This wavelength depends on the lasing medium. The specificity of laser light provides selective absorption of the energy by specific tissues in the body. Different substances absorb different wavelengths of light. These laser targets are known as *chromophores*. Common dermal chromophores include hemoglobin, oxyhemoglobin, collagen, and beta carotene. The only chromophore of clinical significance in the epidermis is melanin. The second characteristic of laser light is *coherence*. All the light waves in the laser beam are in step, and the crest of each light wave is aligned with the crest of every other wave. The third characteristic of rays is *collimation*, that is, they are all parallel. The combination of collimation and coherence produces a very low degree of divergence of the light. All the characteristics combine to produce intensely bright light, which is extremely pure and finely focused.

Not only does each laser system have its own particular type of light or wavelength, but also it has a specific manner of delivering this light. The most common way is with a continuous wave (CW). A continuous beam of laser light is emitted as long as the machine is on. The beam can be varied with shutters, which can be opened and closed at varying intervals. Some machines are capable of shutter openings as brief as 0.01 second, whereas more common shutter speeds are in the range of 0.1 to 0.2 second. These speeds are referred to as exposure times.

Much shorter exposures of laser light are provided by pulsed lasers. Such lasers build the energy up to a maximal point before it is released. After release, the energy must rebuild before it can be released again. Peak powers of pulsed lasers obtain much greater intensity than those of continuous-wave lasers. The end result is an exposure of target tissues to a much higher intensity of light over a much shorter period of time.

Superpulsed lasers are limited to the carbon dioxide systems and carry the principle of pulsed lasers even further. Pulses may be as short as 0.1 msec with pulse repetitions ranging as high as 1000 pulses per second. Here peak powers can be obtained in the range of several thousand watts per pulse. The end result is a beam that causes less thermal damage to tissues adjacent to target tissue.

Finally, Q-switched lasers accomplish the shortest pulse widths and the greatest frequency of pulses. These are in the range of 40 nsec and one million watts per square centimeter per pulse, achieved by a very fast electromagnetic or chemical switch.

Delivery of light energy from the laser system to the target is usually accomplished in one of two ways. Most frequencies are transmitted well through bundles of fiberoptic strands, thus enabling them to be used in endoscopy. This group includes the argon laser, the neodymium:yttrium-aluminum-garnet laser (Nd:YAG laser), and all the new-generation yellow-light lasers. The wavelength produced by the carbon dioxide laser, which is well into the infrared frequency, requires a system of articulating arms and right-angle mirrors, causing severe mechanical limitations.

Laser-Tissue Interaction

Once the laser energy is delivered to the target tissue, yet another new area of knowledge must be understood, that of the biophysics of laser-tissue interaction. Light energy can produce tissue reactions that are biologic, thermal, acoustic or photochemical. Medical interest at this time concentrates mainly on the thermal acoustic effects. In physics we know that when light strikes a target, it may be reflected, scattered, transmitted, or absorbed. For tissue to react to light, there must be absorption. This absorption almost always results in a transformation of light energy to heat energy. The site of absorption is determined by the location of the absorbing chromophore and by the wavelength. The longer the wavelength, the deeper is the tissue penetration. The degree of absorption is determined by the power density and duration of exposure.

Ideal laser therapy would involve delivering the laser light energy to the patient's tissues with totally selective destruction of the chromophore and no damage to the surrounding tissues. This could be achieved through absolute selectivity of the target tissue for the specific wavelength delivered. Power should be sufficient to destroy the target tissue, and exposure time should be short enough that no heat is dissipated to the surrounding tissues.

During the past 20 years, as the mechanics of lasers and the understanding of their effects on tissue have evolved, we have come closer and closer to the objective of ideal laser therapy. Specific characteristics of the individual laser systems and their clinical applications and safety requirements can best be addressed by discussing each of the lasers that have applications in plastic surgery.

Types of Lasers

Laser science has expanded in an explosive way in the past 20 years. There are now countless lasers in all walks of life. Lasers range from old dependable workhorses accepted and taken for granted to possibilities based on exotic and miraculous concepts still on the drawing board. They extend from the checkout counter laser in the local supermarket to lasers used in deep space weaponry, and their uses vary from medical science to military strategy. Relatively few of these lasers are used in medicine, and an even smaller group are applicable to plastic surgery.

Carbon Dioxide Laser

The carbon dioxide laser (CO_2 laser) has a wavelength of 10,600 nm, which is out of the visible light spectrum and into the far infrared spectrum. A lower powered helium-neon laser is usually piggybacked with the CO_2 laser to provide an aiming beam. The lasing medium is carbon diox-

Fig. 17-1. Keloid of earlobe excised with CO_2 laser fine focused to 0.2-mm spot size and 5 W power with 5-second exposure interval. Wound is packed open and allowed to heal secondarily. A. Preoperative appearance. B. Six months postoperatively.

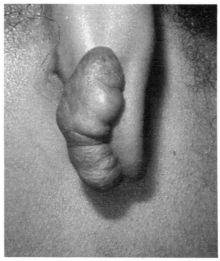

A

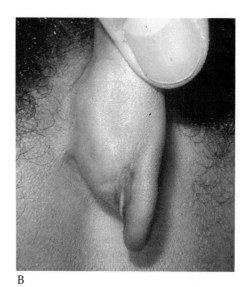

B

ide gas with nitrogen and helium gases added to improve energy transfer. The CO_2 laser is a nonspecific vaporizer of tissue with no selective color absorption. Its chromophore is any tissue with a water content.

As mentioned, a series of jointed, right-angle mirrors are required for delivery of the energy. The basic continuous wave can be altered by the usual methods of shuttering, but the laser also is specifically adapted to a superpulse mode to limit tissue destruction farther outside the path of the beam.

Clinically the CO_2 laser is extremely diverse. It can be used at a fixed focal length, which usually provides a cutting beam as small as 0.1 mm in diameter. Simply by moving away from the target, the surgeon can defocus the beam, thereby increasing the surface area treated and decreasing the power density on that surface. Rather than a cutting mode, this becomes a "painting" function. The painting technique can never be done by prescribed instrument settings. The surgeon needs to designate the proposed wattage and exposure duration and test on a tongue blade the actual degree of defocusing to be used. This test prevents initial errors involving the patient's tissues. The combination of cutting and painting offers the surgeon great versatility obtained simply by small hand motions. The two modes will be addressed separately.

Using the CO_2 laser as a cutting instrument should be limited to procedures in

which the laser is clearly better than a conventional scalpel. Use of the laser is clearly superior in some neurosurgical, gynecologic, otolaryngologic, and orthopedic procedures. Using it requires some judgment and restraint on the part of plastic surgeons, however. The CO_2 laser is reported to cause sealing of smaller vessels and lymphatics as it cuts, thereby providing some small-vessel hemostasis and a decrease in postoperative discomfort.

The CO_2 laser theoretically offers some advantage as a cutting tool in patients with bleeding disorders, low hemoglobin levels, or pacemakers or other electronic monitoring devices and in those who have contraindications to epinephrine injections. A theoretical advantage would be obtained in operating on highly vascular tissues or on infected surgical sites. Examples of such procedures include excision of decubitus ulcers, burn debridement, bone perforation for stimulation of granulation tissue, and excision of plantar warts. Excision of keloids is predictably successful only when earlobes are involved. Recurrence rates are high in other locations (Fig. 17-1).

The CO_2 laser cutting function has been the subject of many claims in the field of cosmetic surgery. It has been implied that this laser, along with the neodymium: yttrium-aluminum-garnet laser using contact sapphire tips, produces results superior to conventional cosmetic operations. The Nd:YAG laser is discussed later in the chapter.

Because of distortion in the news media, the public has developed a romance with lasers. Some people believe that the results of any procedure done with a laser are superior to the results accomplished with a conventional operation. The classic example is the new method of minimally invasive gallbladder operations. Patients call seeking *laser* gallbladder operations, unaware that the basis is fiberoptic not laser technology.

These misconceptions can be capitalized on in cosmetic surgery. A typical example is blepharoplasty. In the hands of a competent plastic surgeon, there is essentially no bleeding and no postoperative pain associated with the conventional operation. Unknowing patients, however, come seeking laser blepharoplasty, having heard of superior results with that technique. They are not aware that a laser operation involves increased expense, operating time, and risk. Furthermore, controlled studies have failed as yet to reveal any difference in the ultimate results. In fact there have been multiple instances of complications from unintentional laser beam exposure.

It should be noted that to provide the most acceptable scar, any skin incised with a laser requires scalpel reexcision of the edges before closure. In summary, we are still in an era in which lasers should be used only when they provide an advantage over conventional surgical procedures. Objectivity and restraint are required on the part of surgeons, because the mere mention of the use of lasers for

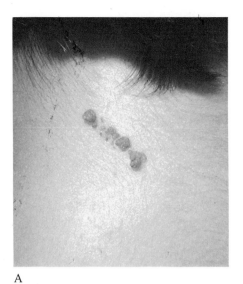

A

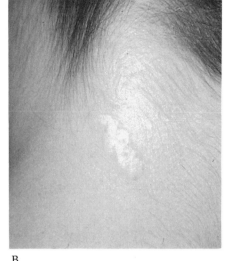

B

Fig. 17-2. Nevus sebaceus excised with CO_2 laser in the "painting" mode. Defocused to a spot size of approximately 3 mm. Lesion removed in layers under magnification until no visible pigment is seen. A. Preoperatively. B. One month postoperatively.

a procedure can be a means of practice enhancement.

Painting techniques provide a unique mode of treatment previously unavailable by conventional means. By appropriate defocusing, the surgeon can brush off layers of tissue only a few cells thick without bleeding. This technology can be applied to many conditions involving the skin.

Almost any type of wart can be treated either by excision in the cutting mode or by painting. Painting is usually done under magnification. The char is wiped away, and the area is repainted so that a progressive deepening of the excision occurs under controlled conditions. The method is especially effective for plantar warts, in which a conventional surgical procedure is usually associated with a considerable amount of postoperative pain and slow wound healing. Recurrent warts are also ideal for treatment by a CO_2 laser because a 1-cm margin around the wart can be painted to decrease the possibility of recurrence. The laser is effective in extensive condyloma acuminatum. Here countless lesions can be excised, leaving intact skin between the lesions to facilitate healing.

Many other epidermal lesions can be treated. Treatment of actinic cheilitis has certainly benefited from this mode. Treatment of other, deeper dermal processes has also shown excellent results. Xanthelasma can be treated by painting off the overlying epidermal layer and painting down through the fat structure until dermis is reached. This technique usually spares normal lid tissue and avoids the

threat of ectropion if multiple excisions are required over a period of years. Syringomas, trichoepitheliomas, and neurofibromas respond in a similar way. Linear epidermal nevi can be treated, again under magnification with whatever degree of defocusing to the appropriate spot size is indicated. Each nevus is treated with sparing of all the normal epithelium between nevi (Fig. 17-2). Dramatic results can be obtained with this method on even the largest of these nevi. A combination of cutting and painting can be used for dramatic improvement of rhinophyma in a relatively bloodless dermabrasion technique. Both of these modalities are being replaced by the new flash lamp pumped dye lasers.

The painting technique has been advocated for removal of tattoos, again a form of bloodless dermabrasion. I have found this application to be less controlled than similar treatment with the argon laser, which will be discussed later.

The CO_2 laser has been advocated also in the treatment of vascular lesions such as port-wine stains, telangiectasias, and hemangiomas; however, it is a completely nonselective modality. It seems ill advised to abandon lasers with specific photocoagulation chromophores when treating vascular lesions.

A wide variety of CO_2 laser models are available, ranging from low-powered mobile instruments to high-powered neurosurgical machines. Some lasers generate a maximum of as little as 5 watts of power, whereas others are in the 100-watt range. These devices can range in cost ap-

proximately from \$20,000 to \$100,000. Maintenance contracts are inexpensive, and repair bills are relatively small.

The CO_2 laser is the most dangerous of the lasers. Because its chromophore is anything with a water content, which is almost everything, it is always a potential hazard. The laser can readily set fire to drapes and scrub gowns. Its use in the vicinity of an endotracheal tube containing inflammable anesthetics or even oxygen requires special training, special equipment, and extreme caution. Catastrophic airway fires are a real danger. Protective eyewear can consist of anything without water content, which includes glass and plastic. Because the CO_2 laser wavelength is absorbed instantly by water with virtually no penetration, all of the immediate operative field other than the target should be protected by moist sponges or towels.

Neodymium : Yttrium-Aluminum-Garnet Laser

The Nd:YAG laser is a combination of lasing media that produces a wavelength of 1060 nm in the near infrared spectrum. The medium is composed of yttrium, aluminum, and garnet crystals that have been doped with neodymium ions. This laser has no specific chromophore. In fact, it is poorly absorbed by melanin, hemoglobin, water, and other normal chromophores, which results in a greater depth of penetration than other lasers. Its energy usually goes to 4 to 6 mm with a wide amount of diffuse tissue destruction. The light is delivered through a fiberoptic system in a continuous shuttered wave. Q-switched systems are now available.

The Nd:YAG laser is used most often on large vascular lesions. Treatment can be described as boring holes in the lesion. Flatter lesions require shorter exposure durations and lower power outputs. Bulkier lesions necessitate longer exposures and higher powers. Each hole is usually separated by a distance sufficient to prevent confluence of the coagulated areas. Multiple treatments may be required before maximal shrinkage is obtained. Scarring is always a factor to be considered because of the lack of specificity of the laser energy.

The Nd:YAG laser can be adapted to a cutting mode, but unlike the CO_2 laser, there is actual contact with the tissues. A quartz tip is attached to the end of the bundle of fiberoptic strands. This tip is heated by the laser light and cuts on contact. In the words of the industry, there is no longer an "air interface." This configuration provides hemostatic advantages that are especially helpful in the dissection of vascular tumors, such as strawberry hemangiomas of infancy. Larger vessels still need to be coagulated with electrocautery. Important advances in the management of large hemangiomas have been obtained by combining laser technology with preoperative selective embolization. Potentially life-threatening tumors now can be approached with considerably less fear than in the past.

Sapphire-tip contact laser technology has been expanded to involve procedures such as reduction mammaplasty and abdominoplasty. The method is touted as extremely advantageous because of the decreased blood loss. All but the smallest blood vessels still must be coagulated with conventional methods, however, and the procedure is extremely time consuming. Under normal conditions with competent surgeons, patients do not lose a large amount of blood in conventional procedures, and again the added risk, expense, and time of laser surgery make the advantage questionable. Claims have been made in the same areas of cosmetic surgery mentioned in the discussion of the CO_2 laser. Here too the only consistently demonstrable advantage is practice enhancement.

The Nd:YAG laser in the conventional format is inherently dangerous to patients because of its deep tissue penetration without simultaneous evidence of the depth on the surface. A great deal of clinical experience is required to prevent damage undetected at the time of the operation. Eye protection is necessary, but, unlike the CO_2 laser, the Nd:YAG wavelength does penetrate clear glass and plastic. Special filtered lenses are required.

Costs vary, but the Nd:YAG laser is not considered one of the more expensive lasers.

Excimer Lasers

Excimer lasers use halide gases that are stable only in their excited state. These are referred to as excimers, or excited dimers. Four of these halides can be used, providing four different ultraviolet wavelengths. Xenon fluoride (XeF) emits light at 351 nm. Xenon chloride (XeCl) emits light at 308 nm; krypton fluoride (KrF) at 248 nm; and argon fluoride (ArF) at 193 nm.

All these halides produce high-energy, short-duration pulses. The short wavelengths are all within the ultraviolet light spectrum, and their penetration into tissues is extremely shallow. Tissue can be cut precisely with little residual damage to adjacent tissue.

These lasers are well accepted in ophthalmology but have yet to become clinically feasible in plastic surgery. The halide gases are toxic and can be very dangerous if not contained. Also, the ultraviolet radiation has a cancer-producing potential in the tissue adjacent to the lased area.

Photocoagulation Lasers

The remaining lasers of interest to plastic surgeons all have wavelengths within the visible light spectrum.

Argon Laser

The lasing medium is argon gas. A blue-green light is produced in six different wavelengths, most of which are between 488 and 514 nm. The main chromophore is the color red. The energy can be delivered through a fiberoptic system. The

original mode is continuous wave, but the system also can be shuttered. Conventional handpieces provide spot sizes of 1, 2, and 5 mm. An area up to 1.3 cm in diameter, for example, can be treated by a robotic device such as a hexascan. The hexascan is a microprocessor handpiece that can be attached to the fiberoptic delivery system of several of the photocoagulation lasers. Multiple parameters can be designated by the operator, such as the size of the area to be treated and the length of pulses. The beam is scanned with a series of pulses of which the pattern covers a predetermined area. The pulses are delivered in such a sequence that no two pulses occur near each other either in time or in location. Thus small areas are treated over brief intervals of time, minimizing nonspecific tissue destruction. This device facilitates the treatment of large areas by a hexagonal pattern, which can be easily interfaced.

That the color red is the chromophore for the wavelengths of the argon laser was described by Bard Cosman as "a happy coincidence." When the light from an argon laser is beamed on any superficial vascular lesion, the light moves through the epidermis without effect. Technically, it goes through the wall of the abnormal vessel also with no effect; however, when the red of the blood inside the vessel absorbs the laser light, the light energy is transformed into heat energy. Thus a heat source originates from within the very vessels that the surgeon is seeking to destroy. This photocoagulation effect can be obtained in vessels of up to 0.5 mm in diameter. Vessels larger than that appear to have enough blood flow to cool the effect and prevent the coagulation. The laser is also limited in that it can penetrate tissues to a depth of only 1.0 to 1.5 mm.

Many models of argon lasers are available. These vary considerably in the amount of wattage produced and the degree of mobility. Some of the newer models are air-cooled and portable. Most, however, have special water and electrical requirements that make them entirely immobile. Their costs range from $30,000 to $75,000. Each laser should be studied for its specific safety precautions. The main danger from argon lasers is their ability to affect the retina. All operating room personnel and patients must have eye protection. A specific amber-colored lens different from any other photocoagulation laser protective device is required.

Port-Wine Stains. The argon laser was the first photocoagulation laser to gain popular use and was the workhorse of physicians treating superficial vascular lesions in the 1980s. The most prominent such lesion was the port-wine stain, or intradermal capillary hemangioma (some prefer the term *capillary malformation*). These lesions are among the most dramatic and devastating congenital anomalies. They originally were referred to as nevus flammeus because of the brilliant splash of color, usually appearing on the patient's face. In 1690 the Portuguese city of Oporto began to import wine into England, and the phrase *port wine* was introduced into the English language. The similarity in color between the red-purple wine and the nevus flammeus led to the coinage of the term *port-wine stain*, which became firmly entrenched in both the general and the medical literature by the 1800s.

The progressive nature of port-wine stains can be readily demonstrated histologically and clinically. The lesions are present at birth as pale, flat, pink lesions. Histologically only mild abnormalities can be demonstrated (Fig. 17-3). At puberty the lesions accelerate with darkening and a reduced tendency to blanch (Fig. 17-4). Thereafter, they become progressively darker, spongy, and protrusive. Individual bubbling or cobblestoning is often noted and is termed *lesional hypertrophy*. The darker the lesion originally, the more dramatically it is likely to deteriorate (Fig. 17-5).

In addition to the lesional hypertrophy, hemangiomas involving the full thickness of structures such as the nose, upper lip, or ear cause varying degrees of structural hypertrophy. By adulthood histologic analysis demonstrates masses of postcapillary venules representing a process of progressive ectasia. This stage results in a clinically significant entity that must be explained to patients to provide them with a comprehensive prognosis. The process is poorly understood by insurance companies, who frequently claim that treatment of port-wine stains is purely cosmetic (Fig. 17-6).

A dramatic response to argon laser therapy has been obtained in port-wine stains

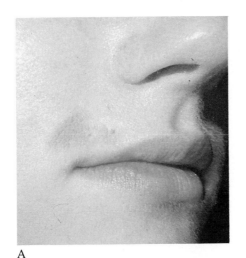
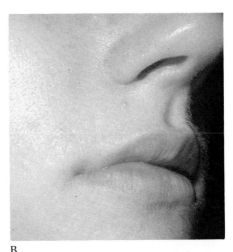

A   B

Fig. 17-3. Pale port-wine stain treated with argon laser, 1-mm spot size, 0.2-second exposure interval, and 0.8 W power. A. Preoperatively. B. Six months after one argon laser treatment.

Fig. 17-4. Port-wine stain in an adult showing dark coloration but no lesional or structural hypertrophy. Treated with the argon laser, 1-mm spot size, 0.2-second exposure interval, 0.8 W power. A. Preoperatively. B. Six months after one argon laser treatment.

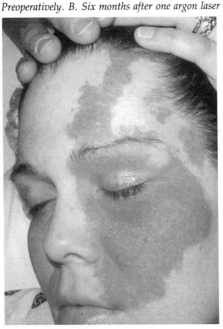
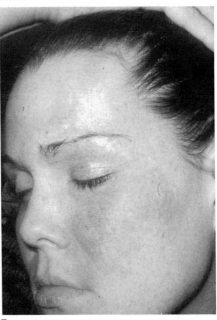

A   B

in the past few years. This treatment will continue to be appropriate as long as surgeons show restraint in patient selection. A four-point profile that defines the ideal candidate for argon laser treatment of port-wine stains should be used. This process will help surgeons to prevent pitfalls that involve scarring and that stem from the use of too much power on the wrong patients in the wrong locations. Of course other factors may cause complications, including abnormal wound healing and rare infections. To use the argon laser comfortably without test spots, the surgeon should require patients to satisfy these four criteria:

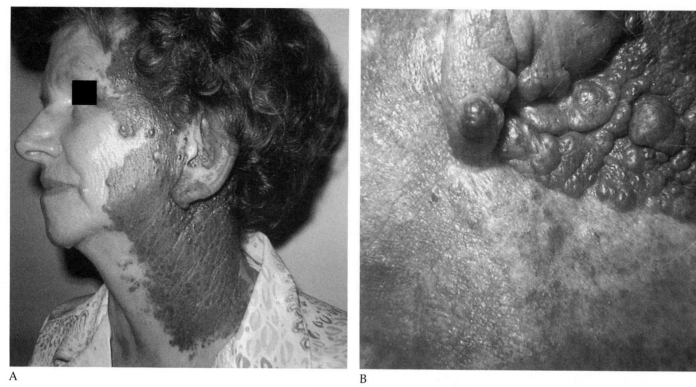

A

B

Fig. 17-5. *Port-wine stain with dark color and severe lesional hypertrophy. Treated with the argon laser, 1-mm spot size, 0.2-second exposure time, and 1.0 W power. A. Preoperatively. B. Six months after one treatment with argon laser. Postauricular area has not been treated.*

Fig. 17-6. *Port-wine stains demonstrating structural hypertrophy. A. Eyelid and upper lip. B. Left ear.*

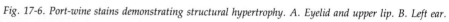

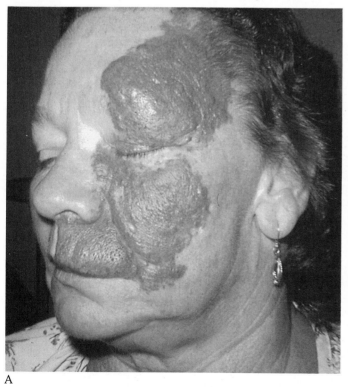

A

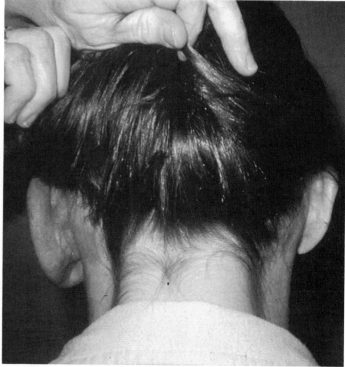

B

1. The patient should be at least one year past puberty.
2. The hemangioma should be on the head or neck.
3. The patient's complexion and the color of the lesion should have a satisfactory amount of color contrast.
4. The lesion should not blanch on pressure.

If the patient lacks any of these four points, it does not mean that the laser will not be effective, but it does mean that the results are not predictable. A test spot can assist the surgeon in making a decision regarding use of the laser in less-than-ideal candidates.

Once again, laser treatment should follow the principles of delivering the most effective dose of energy to the smallest amount of tissue over the shortest period of time to avoid nonspecific tissue damage. I prefer to use a 1.0-mm spot with a 0.2-second interval, and I begin at a strength that is known to be ineffective. The power can be increased in tenths of a watt until a minimal effective dose is obtained. Clinically this point is readily detectable by an instant gray-white spot after the pulse strikes the tissue. The therapy consists in treating the entire area in contiguous spots, firing the laser, observing the results, refiring if necessary, and moving to the next 1.0-mm area. The tediousness of this process could be relieved by using a robot scanning device such as a hexascan. I have found the more deliberate method, however, to be the most successful.

Except for very small lesions, argon laser therapy is done under general anesthesia. The heat produced in the tissue interaction with the laser light is extremely painful. On the other hand, the patient experiences little or no pain postoperatively. The vasodilative effect of general anesthetic agents enhances the color target and offers an additional benefit to the photocoagulation process. Additional target enhancement can be obtained by placing the treated part in a dependent position.

Because of the lack of complete specificity of tissue absorption of the argon laser energy, the treatment results in a superficial second-degree burn with demonstrable epithelial damage. The wound usually forms a fine scab on the fourth or fifth day, and the scab falls off within a week.

The treated area is red for several months, as would be expected with any similar burn. Sun protection is vital during this time. After 6 to 12 months, the area can be treated again if indicated.

Other Superficial Vascular Lesions. Many other superficial vascular lesions respond to photocoagulation therapy. Virtually any lesion that is red and superficial will respond, with the possible exception of an immature scar. I have found no advantage in treating such scars with the argon laser. On the other hand, the treatment of telangiectasias, spider angiomas, venous lakes, intraoral hemangiomas, acne rosacea, cherry hemangiomas, angiokeratomas, and angiofibromas can have quite remarkable results (Fig. 17-7). I have had some degree of success in approximately 50 percent of patients with familial hemorrhagic telangiectasias.

Argon laser therapy should never be used for superficial varicosities of the lower limbs. For the most part these vessels are too large and deep to be affected by laser energy. In addition, the skin overlying any treated area is imperceptibly thinned. The net result is usually a lesion more obvious than it was before treatment.

Strawberry Hemangiomas. Strawberry hemangiomas are the most common tumor of infancy. These tumors deserve particular attention because of their response to photocoagulation therapy. Only 30 percent of these tumors are present at birth. The others characteristically appear in the second week of life as small red dots and grow at a frightening rate for several months. Many of these occur in areas of the body in which function is not compromised, and many never show any clinically significant growth. These tumors may be left untreated.

On the other hand, there are hemangiomas that grow to alarming proportions and can cause serious problems. Any lesion in the areas of vital anatomy of the face, i.e., the tip of the nose, the filtrum, the eyelids, and ears, can cause permanent anatomic deformity even if the lesion eventually "resolves." Larger lesions can go on to cause high-output cardiac failure, airway obstruction, and Kasabach-Merritt syndrome. Tumors occurring on the upper eyelids can produce the surgical emergency of amblyopia. Histo-

logically this actively growing phase shows proliferating masses of endothelial cells, an abundance of mast cells, and only vaguely discernible vessel lumens.

Resolution can begin to occur any time after the end of the progressive stage, usually between the ages of 1 and 3 years. Clinically the first evidence is a central gray-white depressed area called a *herald spot*. Histologically vascular channels that have become more obvious now show thinning of their walls and a progressive deposition of fibrofatty tissue. This sclerosing of the blood vessels is seen as a mass of dense collagen and reticular tissue in islands of adipose tissue. Eventually the tumor may lose all its ability to carry blood, thereby losing most of its bulk and color.

Even at best, however, the skin overlying the original tumor site has a thin, shiny, slick texture. It has a tannish color and small vessels that are individually visible. This, added to the fact that underlying vital anatomic structures such as the nasal cartilages or the filtrum may be entirely destroyed, should make it readily apparent that these tumors should not be dismissed casually with the pronouncement, "Don't worry, they'll go away."

Developments in laser technology make it possible to construct guidelines for reasonable, selective intervention at all stages in the natural progression of hemangiomas.

The final decision, of course, must still be based on the surgeon's prediction of the residual deformity in the resolved hemangioma. During the proliferative stage, no one can anticipate precisely the extent of proliferation. The psychological trauma to the patient from living with such a deformity during the formative years must also be considered.

Patients with strawberry hemangiomas can be divided into four groups for consideration of therapy.

1. The *ideal patient* for treatment is only a few weeks old with a lesion only a few millimeters in diameter. At this point the lesion is always entirely capillary and superficial. Argon laser treatment can be administered in several seconds with no anesthesia. Healing is complete within a few days, and the problem is usually completely resolved with no clinically signif-

icant scarring. Occasionally an additional potential area of hemangioma may develop adjacent to the treated area; this requires retreatment (Fig. 17-8).

2. Patients with *active destructive* hemangiomas unfortunately are the ones most frequently seen by plastic surgeons. The lesion has already outgrown the predictions of the primary physician. The parents have panicked and have run out of patience, and the plastic surgeon is expected to provide the solution. The lesion has been allowed to progress beyond the early stage and may have developed a deep cavernous component in addition to the capillary component. This deep subcutaneous component does not respond to laser therapy because of the depth and size of the vessels. In some patients, however, growth of the lesion can be indirectly affected by treatment of the overlying capillary component. The purpose of treatment in these patients is to arrest growth, not to remove the tumor. Sometimes the added bonus of premature resolution results. All patients who still show clinical growth and who offer a superficial color target are candidates for treatment (Fig. 17-9).

3. Patients with lesions that have *stopped growing* may also be candidates for argon laser therapy if the lesion is causing functional problems. The most dramatic of these are upper eyelid lesions threatening to cause amblyopia. There can be airway obstruction involving the nostrils; hygienic dysfunction involving the perianal or vaginal regions; or lesions subject to chronic trauma, causing bleeding or ulceration. The unique nursing ulcer involving a hemangioma of the middle of the upper lip is an example. Rarely,

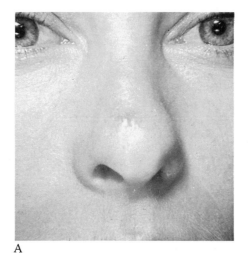
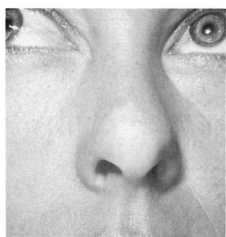

A

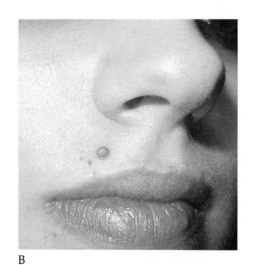
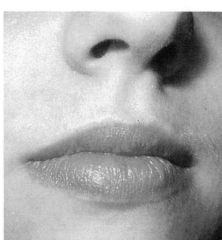

B

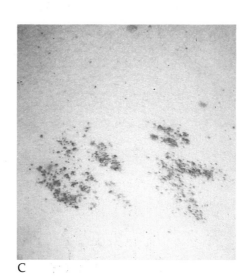

C

Fig. 17-7. *Superficial vascular lesions responding to argon laser therapy. All postoperative photographs demonstrate results 6 months after one argon laser treatment. A. Telangiectasia with raised central papule. B. Hemangioma of pregnancy. C. Nevus sebaceus. D. Intraoral hemangioma. E. Subconjunctival hemangioma.*

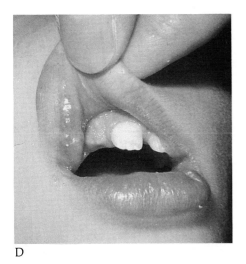

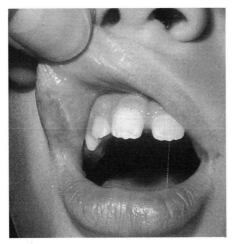

D

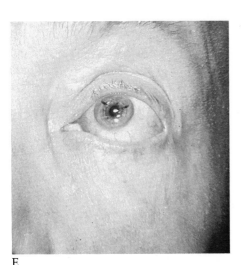

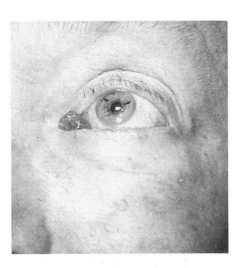

E

Fig. 17-7. (Continued)

Fig. 17-8. Early growing strawberry hemangioma. The patient was treated at the age of 2 months with the argon laser, 1-mm spot size, 0.2-second exposure interval, and 2.0 W power. A. Preoperatively. B. Six months after one argon laser treatment.

A

B

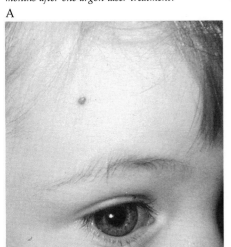

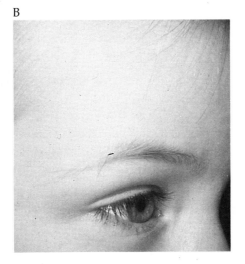

pathologic parental anxiety may justify laser treatment for the child. These lesions, as one might expect, show a greater tendency for refill and recurrence than lesions in the early (ideal) group, and treatment should be repeated until the lesion becomes stable (Fig. 17-10).

Larger lesions that produce the dramatic complications previously mentioned must be treated with the methods described in the section on the Nd:YAG laser.

Large doses of systemic prednisone or dexamethasone can provide useful adjunctive therapy for these lesions. The recommended dosage is usually 3 to 4 mg per kilogram. The drug is given over a 3-week period. If no response is noted, the medication should be discontinued. If a response is obvious, the drug can be continued for 3 more weeks and then tapered. Frequently a rebound phenomenon occurs on withdrawal of the drug. A second similar course can be instituted if this occurs. A third course is usually not recommended.

4. Some tumors have *stopped the process of resolution.* Patients with these tumors should not be treated until they are at least 6 years of age and have had no additional resolution for a year. At that point there is little hope for additional natural regression. If these lesions continue to present a color target, argon laser therapy is indicated for devascularization; it may also provide some reduction in size. If a conventional plastic surgical procedure is needed for additional debulking and sculpting, it is greatly facilitated by the previous laser devascularization (Fig. 17-11).

Fig. 17-9. *Actively growing strawberry hemangioma. The patient was treated at the age of 4 months with the argon laser, 1-mm spot size, 0.2-second exposure time, and 2.0 W power. A. Preoperatively. B. Six months postoperatively.*

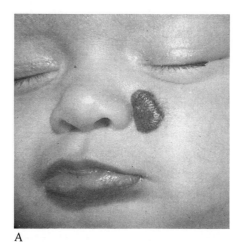

A

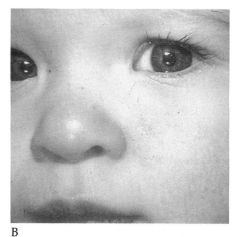

B

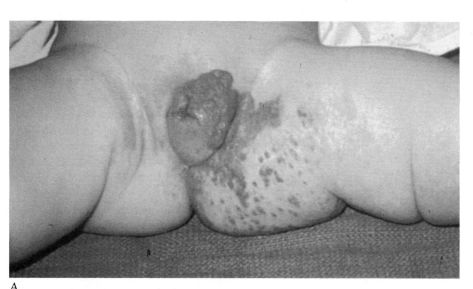

A

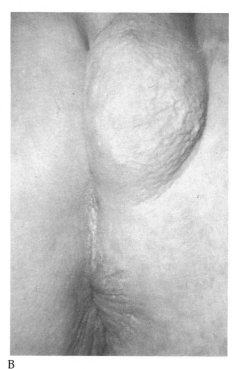

B

Fig. 17-10. *Massive strawberry hemangioma involving left labium majorum and left thigh causing hygiene problems, chronic ulceration, and hemorrhage. The patient was treated at the age of 8 months with the argon laser, 1-mm spot size, 0.2-second interval, and 2.0 W power. A. Preoperatively. B. Three months after second argon laser treatment.*

In summary, argon laser therapy is indicated for strawberry hemangiomas that are still growing, especially in areas of sensitive anatomy; causing functional problems; or still presenting a red color target after natural resolution is completed.

For decades plastic surgeons urged physicians not to treat strawberry hemangiomas because of their natural history of at least partial resolution. The theory was to let the hemangioma run its course and deal with the remaining reconstructive problems. We now have a prophylactic weapon to prevent these problems from occurring. Unless the lesion is already

large and widespread at birth, its growth usually can be interrupted in the first few weeks of life with a minimum of residual deformity and essentially no trauma to the patient.

If left to follow its natural course, a strawberry hemangioma produces an undue amount of anxiety during the proliferative stage in both the surgeon and the parents, to say nothing of the child in later years. No one can predict how large the lesion will become and how much tissue it will destroy. It lingers on and on, and has a less than satisfactory resolution. The daily concerns of peers, neighbors, and grandparents are also to be considered. All this

can be avoided by early prophylactic treatment; it is hoped that this will become the standard of care. In this enlightened age of medical knowledge, the plea of the informed plastic surgeon should no longer be "leave it alone"; it should be "lase it."

Yellow-Light Lasers

In the middle of the 1980s a new generation of lasers emerged, all using a wavelength range from 577 to 585 nm. These are commonly referred to as yellow-light lasers. One of these is a heavy metal vapor laser, and two derive their wavelength from dyes. This range of wavelengths is more specific for vascular le-

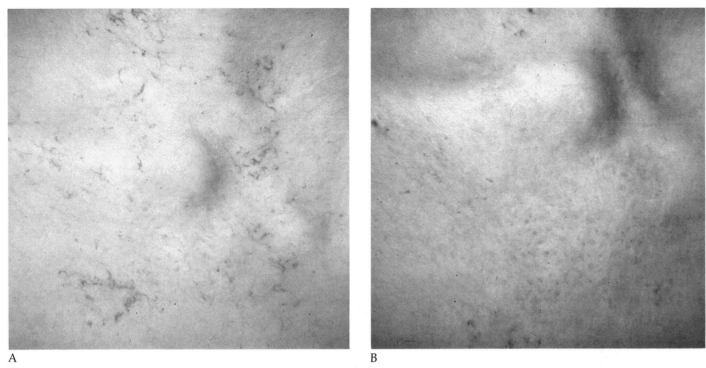

A   B

Fig. 17-11. Partially resolved strawberry hemangioma showing abnormal skin texture with some hyperpigmentation and individually visible vessels. Treated at the age of 12 years with argon laser therapy, 1-mm spot size, 0.2-second exposure time, and 2.0 W power. A. Preoperatively. B. Six months after one argon laser treatment.

Fig. 17-12. Absorption spectra of cutaneous oxyhemoglobin and melanin. Emission spectra of argon and yellow-light lasers.

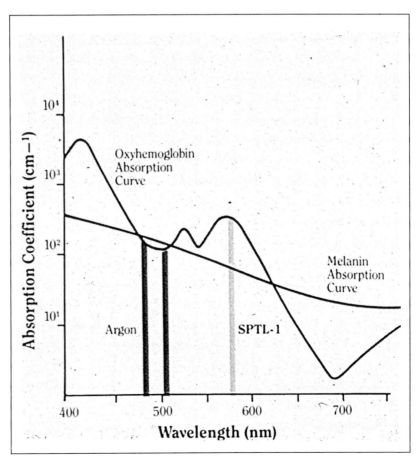

sions than is the range of the argon laser. Yellow-light lasers have the oxyhemoglobin of the red blood cell as their chromophore. In the high-500-nm range, much less light is absorbed by the melanin chromophore than by the oxyhemoglobin chromophore. It is clear that the absorption coefficients of oxyhemoglobin and melanin are much more widely separated in the 577- to 585-nm range than in the argon range (488 to 514 nm) (Fig. 17-12). The clinical significance is that the yellow-light lasers can be used with a greatly reduced risk of scarring.

Copper Vapor Laser

The lasing medium for this heavy metal laser is copper ore. It produces a wavelength of 578 nm (yellow) and a second wavelength of 510 nm (green). Gold ore may be substituted for the copper; the gold emits a wavelength of 628 nm (red). The desired ore is placed in the lasing cavity, and a high-powered electronic circuit is used to excite a gas discharge. The generated heat vaporizes the copper and produces metal vapor. The electrons from the gas form the lasing medium. This mechanism operates in pulse widths so small (25 nm) that clinically the light appears to be a continuous wave. It is claimed, however, that these pulses allow for some tissue cooling between deliveries of energy, thereby decreasing nonselective tissue destruction. Also, the beam can be shuttered to deliver exposure times of as little as 0.05 seconds up to a continuous beam.

The copper vapor laser also provides a new technology in the form of a variably sized handpiece, which can be adjusted to a diameter as small as 100 μ. This capability has fostered a discipline advocating individual vessel tracing techniques for the photocoagulation of superficial vascular lesions. This method is most advantageous in small lesions with individually visible vessels, such as spider angiomas. The procedure becomes prohibitively time consuming, however, in larger, more homogeneous lesions, such as port-wine stains. For the treatment of larger areas, this laser can be adapted to robot-like scanning devices such as the hexascan.

When the copper ore is replaced with gold ore, the laser produces a red light, which can be used in photodynamic therapy. This is a new tool with little clinical usefulness to date; it may be a great boon to medicine in the future. The technique involves the administration of a systemic photosensitizer, usually a hematoporphyrin derivative. Porphyrins can be selectively retained in tissues with predominately immature, fast-growing cells such as malignant tumors. The retained porphyrins photosensitize the malignant cells, which in turn become the chromophores of the 628-nm wavelength. Selective destruction of malignant cells results. Research in this field continues, and new developments are eagerly anticipated. The cost of the copper vapor laser is slightly more than $100,000, with an additional $25,000 for the robot device. The annual maintenance fees range from $9,000 to $11,000.

Continuous-Wave, Argon-Pumped, Tunable Dye Laser

This laser is one of two that use dye to produce its wavelengths. Organic fluorescent compounds dissolved in solvents such as alcohol are the active media. By selecting different dyes, different laser lights of virtually any wavelength within the visible spectrum can be produced.

Continuous-wave dye lasers are often pumped by another laser such as the argon laser. The argon laser acts as the energy source within the dye cavity. Either continuous or pulsed beams can be produced. Power output is usually limited because the wave-producing laser depends on the output of the pumping laser. The continuous-wave dye laser is versatile. It owes its popularity to its ability to produce the new-generation yellow light at 577 nm. It can be tuned through the range of the argon laser wavelengths up to the 639-nm length used for photodynamic therapy.

The continuous-wave dye laser also has the small-spot-size technology and the ability to adjust to a diameter as small as 50 μ. It can be shuttered to an exposure time as brief as 0.02 seconds. It is adaptable to the hexascan. The safety precautions and costs of this laser are similar to those of the copper vapor laser.

Flashlamp Pumped Dye Laser

The most recent addition to the new yellow-light generation of lasers is the flashlamp pumped dye laser. Its development is the product of technology sophisticated enough to produce a laser to meet a clinical need. The fact that argon laser therapy for port-wine stains was limited to postpubertal patients resulted in the denial of therapy to a vast population of infants and prepubertal children. Clinicians delayed treatment because of the probability of scarring but watched children suffer facial asymmetry from structural hypertrophy caused by growth of the tumor.

The flashlamp pumped dye laser does not cause scarring and can be used in all age groups. This improvement has been made possible through the combination of the new yellow-light wavelength and the use of a flashlamp pump as the energy source. Energy builds in the lasing cavity to a peak and is released at a very high power over an extremely small interval of time. This pulse width is less than the thermal relaxation time of typical port-wine stain tissue. The thermal relaxation time denotes the time during which a structure can contain heat from the laser within itself. The longer the target tissue receives laser light, the greater the ab-

sorption of laser energy and the greater the buildup of heat. As the structure (in this case cutaneous blood vessels) is heated, the thermal energy is at first retained. If the heating process continues, the structure can no longer contain the heat, resulting in a diffusion of the energy into surrounding tissues, which causes nonspecific damage. To achieve the best selective destruction of a port-wine stain, the laser pulse should be shorter than the thermal relaxation time of the tissue involved. Research demonstrated that the vessels making up port-wine stains have a thermal relaxation time of 1.0 to 10.0 msec. This laser has a pulse of 450 μsec. This difference in energy delivery is immediately apparent clinically. There is an almost instant blue-black bruise where the pulse strikes the skin. Close inspection reveals no epithelial damage. All continuous-wave photocoagulation delivery systems, despite the wavelength, cause some degree of epithelial damage.

Because no burn wound is produced, there is considerably less postoperative care, and essentially no scarring has been reported. This ability to keep the epidermis intact has removed the age limitations for laser therapy for port-wine stains. The recommended standard of care now calls for laser therapy to begin within the first or second month of life. This timetable provides several advantages clinically:

1. Considerable psychological trauma is avoided.
2. The area of hemangioma to be treated is much smaller.
3. The later asymmetry of facial features known as structural hypertrophy is greatly reduced.

There are some negative aspects, however. This laser was designed to work on pale, flat, childhood-type hemangiomas, and it is essentially limited to that kind of lesion. It is usually inadequate when used to treat three-dimensional or dark vascular lesions.

Because of its "gentleness," the flashlamp pumped dye laser requires multiple treatments (Fig. 17-13). The number of treatments for an individual patient cannot be predicted in advance. Adults frequently require 8 to 10 treatments before maximal improvement can be obtained. Very young children have the most dramatic and most rapid results, sometimes re-

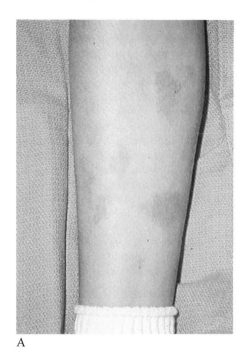

A

B

C

Fig. 17-13. Port-wine stain of lower limb in 11-year-old girl. A. Preoperatively. B. After one treatment with flashlamp pumped dye laser, 6.5 J/cm². C. After fourth treatment, same laser and strength.

Fig. 17-14. Port-wine stain near elbow in a 2-year-old. A. Preoperatively. B. After two treatments with flashlamp pumped dye laser, 6.0 J/cm².

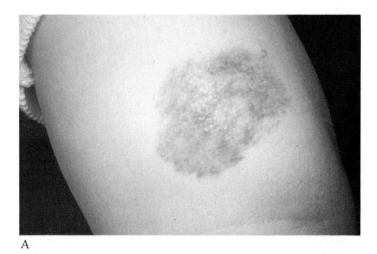

A

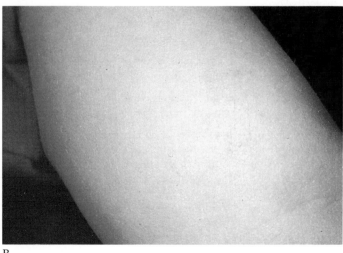

B

quiring no more than two or three treatments (Fig. 17-14).

Treatment with this laser is much less painful than with the argon laser but still has a clinically significant impact. General anesthesia is not used in patients younger than approximately one year of age. It is usually required in patients until the age of 8 or 9 years. Patients from about 8 to 13 years of age require an evaluation of motivation, maturity, and pain threshold. Anesthesia is rarely required after the age of 12 or 13 years.

This laser has applications for other pale, flat, vascular lesions, most commonly telangiectasias and spider angiomas. Like all photocoagulation lasers, this one has met with essentially no success in superficial varicosities of the lower limbs.

The flashlamp pumped pulsed dye laser is the most expensive of the frequently used lasers; it costs approximately $165,000. A yearly maintenance contract costs $25,000, and a considerable expense is involved in frequent replacement of the dyes. Other semiannual maintenance costs are also involved. These maintenance fees are disproportionately high compared with those of other photocoagulation lasers.

The high bolus of energy produced by the flashlamp pump demands specific safety considerations in several areas. Patients who require general anesthesia because of their age can often undergo the procedure without intubation because of the brief duration of treatment. The large 5-mm spot size enables even moderately large areas on children to be treated relatively quickly. Short procedures are usually done without intubation or an intravenous line. Hemangiomas located in the area of the mask can be treated by alternating access between the surgeon and the anesthesiologist. It is important to realize that no attempt should be made to insufflate a patient with a mask that is not tightly sealed to the face. If the laser is being used to treat tumors in the vicinity of the eyebrow and sufficient oxygen escapes from the mask, the bolus of energy from the laser can ignite the eyebrow. This produces a brush fire that rushes across the extent of the eyebrow. No epithelial damage is done and the eyebrow hairs grow back normally, but there is a considerable amount of inconvenience in the interim.

Eye protection is extremely important with this laser because of the bolus of energy released with each pulse. The risk of retinal damage is greater than with continuous wave lasers. The patient should wear opaque contact lenses whenever there is work to be done in the vicinity of the lids. At other times the lids should be taped shut. Patients who are awake for operative procedures away from the face should wear the same protective eyewear as the rest of the operating room personnel.

Pigmented Lesion Laser

The pigmented lesion laser is the newest to enter this highly competitive field. In many ways it is identical to the flashlamp pumped dye laser used for vascular lesions; it is referred to as a flashlamp excited pulse dye laser. It emits a wavelength of 510 nm, which is close to the green wavelength of the argon laser at 514 nm. It is identical to the 510-nm wavelength of the green portion of the copper vapor laser and can be exactly reproduced by the argon-pumped tunable dye laser.

It adds, however, the technology of the flashlamp excited pulse. This laser produces a pulse in the range of 300 nsec with a massive peak power of 3.5 milliwatts per pulse. It is claimed that the 300-nsec pulse width closely corresponds to the thermal relaxation time of the targeted organelles of melanin-containing cells. It is being held as the treatment of choice for any melanin-containing lesions with the exception, of course, of malignant melanomas. It is particularly recommended for solar lentigines, café au lait birthmarks, pigmented nevi, and freckles. Presumably its use would be contraindicated in lesions in which melanocytes descend into the deeper skin appendages such as hair follicles. Treatment would result in temporary depigmentation of the surface tissues followed by repigmentation as the melanocytes migrate back onto the surface from the appendages. It is assumed that giant hairy nevi are clearly beyond the scope of treatment with this device.

Of course, the greatest pitfall would be lack of restraint on the part of surgeons. The danger of treatment of countless potentially malignant lesions without the benefit of biopsy certainly looms as a frightening prospect.

The cost of this laser and its maintenance fees are essentially identical to those of the flashlamp pumped pulsed dye laser for vascular lesions. The safety requirements are also identical.

Many other lasers used to treat pigmented lesions are now emerging. These include several other continuous and Q-switched green light lasers and the Q-switched Nd:YAG laser, which offer wavelengths of 532 and 1064 nm.

Q-Switched Ruby Laser

Use of the ruby laser has changed from the treatment of relatively nonspecific chromophores to the extremely specific targets of some types of tattoos. With energy flows markedly reduced from those used in the 1960s, the Q-switched ruby laser can now achieve excellent results in the treatment of blue and black amateur decorative tattoos and blue and black traumatic tattoos. Again, the newer technologies of brief pulse widths and high boluses of energy are involved, thereby sparing the epidermis and specifically affecting the chromophores of the blue and black homemade dyes.

Most amateur and traumatic tattoos consist of several known pigments. These include india ink, pencil graphite, lampblack, boot polish, mascara, charred rubber, carbon particles, gunpowder, and paint. Professional tattoo pigments consist of cobalt to provide the blue color and black ferric oxides for the black color. Other pigments include chromium oxide for green; cadmium, ferric oxide, ochre, and sienna for yellow; mercuric sulfide for red; cobalt and magnesium for violet; and titanium dioxide for white. Clearly these present a multitude of chromophores, which would require a multitude of laser wavelengths, whereas the homemade and traumatic tattoos represent a much more homogeneous group.

Treatment is similar to treatment with the two previously described lasers in that multiple treatments are involved and no epidermal damage results. The end result can be the total removal of tattoo pigment with no scarring. There is no hypo- or hyperpigmentation and no destruction of hair follicles. This laser has the extremely high cost of the two previously discussed lasers and involves high maintenance fees. It, too, requires special eye protection for all those in the operating room.

Again, several other types of lasers are now available for tattoo removal. The Q-switched alexandrite laser, at 755 nm and 100 nsec, and the Q-switched Nd:YAG laser are playing important roles. The ruby laser is more effective for green light and the Nd:YAG laser for red light. The alexandrite laser appears to be better than others in overall color coverage, but it takes longer to achieve results.

This field is changing rapidly; knowledge of the subject is still in an immature state.

Safety

Because lasers are relatively new, the discipline of laser safety is also relatively new. Recommendations for precautions change as knowledge is acquired. The surgeon is the primarily responsible party in the operating room. His or her knowledge of laser physics and the potential of the laser being used must be applied not only to the surgeon and the patient but also to all operating room personnel. The Bureau of Radiation Hazards has defined most medical lasers as class IV, meaning that there is significant hazard to personnel exposed to laser effects. The American National Standards Institute (ANSI) is a group of professionals who meet to discuss such hazards. A guideline, ANSI Z 136.3, for the use of lasers in medical fields is available.

Perhaps of the greatest clinical significance in laser safety is the laser plume. All the cutting and puncturing type lasers, such as the CO_2 and the Nd:YAG, produce a copular plume. The photocoagulation lasers produce plumes whenever they are allowed to interact with the tissue sufficiently to cause carbonization. Plumes always result from interaction with hair and, frequently, with other melanin-pigmented lesions. For a number of years it was believed that the heat produced by the laser automatically sterilized the operative field. It is now known that the smoke in the plume can carry viable viral particles.

This knowledge resulted in the production of a new generation of suction machines known as smoke evacuators. Normal operating room wall suction rapidly becomes ineffective because of carbonization of its filter systems. These smoke evacuator machines have a wide-bore suction apparatus with a filter that should be in the range of 3.0 μ and should be changed between operations. The evacuator should vent to air outside the circulating area of the building. To provide the best current knowledge on this hazard, I include the report of the Ad Hoc Committee on Hazards of Laser Plume of the American Society of Laser Medicine and Surgery dated April 5, 1990:

The American Society of Laser Medicine and Surgery recommends the following guidelines in dealing with laser-generated plume. These guidelines are based on the assumption of the presence of a real hazard to those individuals who are exposed to the plume. The precise nature and extent of this hazard is currently unknown. For this reason, the extent of protection in practice that is necessary or possible is also not known. As such, these guidelines are presented as a means of providing suggested practice procedures to reduce potential risks until the hazard is better defined. Any organization or individual adopting these guidelines must frequently review them and update its information about the laser plume to assure that the guidelines will best meet the organization or individual's needs.

I. All laser personnel should consider the laser plume to be potentially hazardous both in terms of the particulate matter and infectivity.
II. Evacuator suction systems should be used at all times to collect the plume.
   a. The suction should have a high flow volume with frequent filter changes being made to optimize suction and filter capabilities.
   b. Filters should be chosen which allow for maximum filtering efficiency. Three microns is considered minimal for effective viral filtration.
   c. The suction tip must be placed as close to laser impact as possible.
   d. Evacuator suction tips should be cleaned (preferably sterilized) after each procedure.
III. Eye protection, masks, gloves, and gowns should be always worn during laser use by all laser personnel when laser plume is generated.
   a. Eye protection should be of a nature which would protect from splatter.
   b. Masks should have good effective filtration.
   c. Gloves should be preferably latex.

Hospital Organization and Establishing of Credentials

Wherever a laser is in use, all who are routinely involved should be united as a team. This is particularly true in the hospital operating room. These professionals should work according to a set of guidelines, preferably under the auspices of an organization within the hospital community. A committee should be convened to make decisions regarding lasers. A laser safety officer should be available to implement the decisions, and nurses should be specially trained. The committee should review requests for laser credentials. A physician applying should have a thorough knowledge of laser physics, safety, and applications, and should have clinical experience before being granted privileges.

Particular care must be exercised in granting these privileges. With all the attention focused on laser surgery, there is an incentive to become known as a laser surgeon. There is a temptation to present oneself as an accomplished specialist after a one-day laser course that grants an impressive-looking certificate. The American Society of Laser Medicine and Sur-

gery and the Laser Committee for the American Society of Plastic and Reconstructive Surgeons have developed guidelines for the standards of practice for the use of lasers in plastic and reconstructive surgery.

Conclusion

All plastic surgeons should at least be aware of what laser surgery has to offer. Many conditions requiring laser surgery also require conventional plastic surgery; an interdependence is necessary to obtain the best possible result. This principle can be demonstrated by treatment of partially resolved strawberry hemangiomas. These tumors can be devascularized with the laser but require a conventional operation to produce the best reconstruction. Port-wine stains also can be helped with lasers, but structural hypertrophy can be improved only by conventional plastic surgical debulking and sculpting methods (Fig. 17-15).

For the sake of the continuity of care of patients, plastic surgeons should renew their vital interest in laser surgery. They should reestablish themselves in this field by showing an increased participation with contributions in research and clinical applications. These actions will ensure that our patients have the benefit of expertise in this technology when indicated.

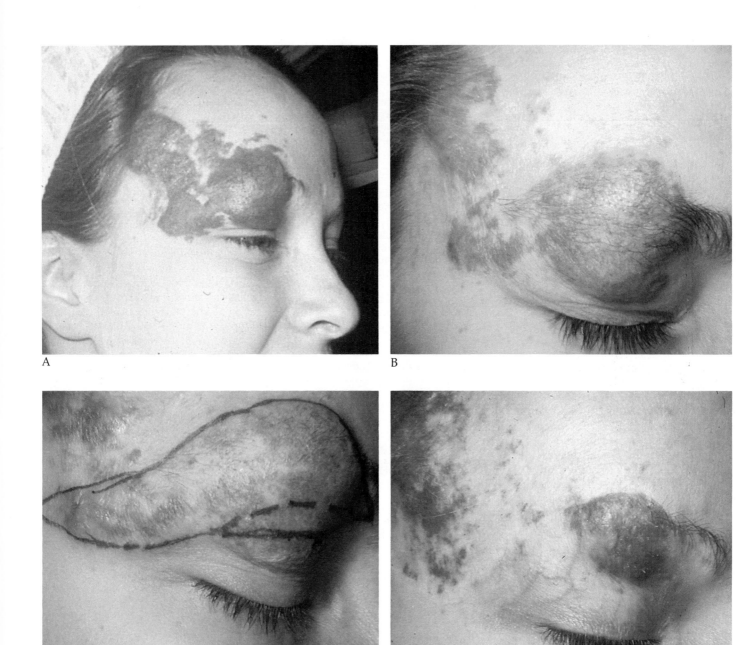

A

B

C

D

Fig. 17-15. Twenty-five-year-old woman with high-flow port-wine stain, forehead and brow, requiring a combination of laser therapy and conventional plastic surgery. A. Preoperatively. B. Hemangioma remaining after three argon laser treatments, 1-mm spot size, 0.2-second exposure time, and 2.0 W power. C. Lazy S *excision of portion of tumor. D. After excision. E. Tissue expander in place. F. Excision of temporal tumor and closure with the expanded tissue, excision of residual brow tumor, and closure with full-thickness skin graft.*

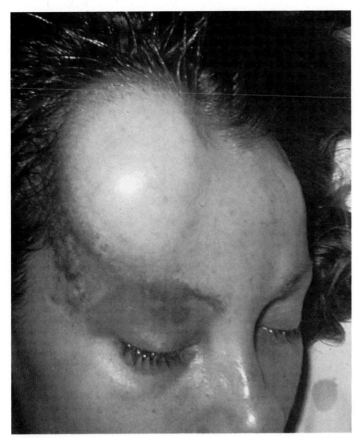

E

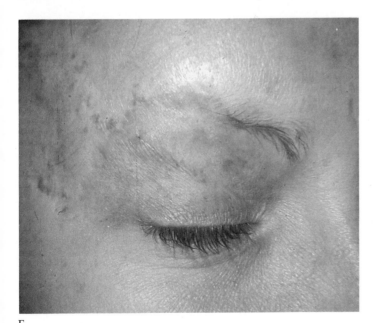

F

Suggested Reading

Apfelberg, D.B., Lane, B., and Marx, M.P. Combined (team) approach to hemangioma management: Arteriography with superselective embolization plus YAG laser/sapphire tip resection. *Plast. Reconstr. Surg.* 88:71, 1991.

Apfelberg, D.B., Maser, M.R., and Lash, H. Argon laser treatment of decorative tattoos. *Br. J. Plast. Surg.* 32:141, 1979.

Apfelberg, D.B., et al. Results of argon laser exposure to capillary hemangiomas of infancy: Preliminary report. *Plast. Reconstr. Surg.* 67: 188, 1981.

Barsky, S.H., et al. The nature and evolution of portwine stains: A computer-assisted study. *J. Invest. Dermatol.* 74:154, 1980.

Dover, J.S., et al. *Illustrated Cutaneous Laser Surgery: A Practitioner's Guide.* Norwalk: Appleton & Lange, 1990.

Garden, J.M. The dye laser. *Semin. Dermatol.* 6:264, 1987.

Hobby, L.W. Further evaluation of the potential of the argon laser in the treatment of strawberry hemangiomas. *Plast. Reconstr. Surg.* 71: 481, 1983.

Hobby, L.W. Argon laser treatment of superficial lesions in children. *Lasers Surg. Med.* 6:16, 1986.

Hobby, L.W. A practical guide to lasers in plastic surgery. *Perspect. Plast. Surg.* 1991.

McDaniel, D.H., and Mordon, S. Hexascan: A new robotized scanning laser handpiece. *Cutis* 45:300, 1990.

Mittelman, H., and Apfelberg, D.B. CO_2 laser blepharoplasty: Advantages and disadvantages. *Ann. Plast. Surg.* 24:1, 1990.

Nelson, J.S. Selective photothermolysis and removal of cutaneous vasculopathies and tattoos by pulsed laser. *Plast. Reconstr. Surg.* 88:723, 1991.

Noe, J.M., et al. Portwine stains and the response to argon laser therapy: Successful treatment and the predictive role of color, age and biopsy. *Plast. Reconstr. Surg.* 65:130, 1980.

Reid, W.H., et al. Experiences with the pulsed ruby laser treatment of tattoos (abstract). *Lasers Surg. Med.* (Suppl.) 2:50, 1990.

Soloman, H., et al. Histopathology of the laser treatment of portwine stains. *Invest. Dermatol.* 50:141, 1968.

18

Three-Dimensional Imaging: An Adjunct to Craniomaxillofacial Reconstruction

Bryant A. Toth   Bryan G. Forley

Advances in craniofacial surgical techniques have been paralleled by new developments in imaging technology. The advent of computed tomography (CT) facilitated a more informed approach to reconstructive procedures. The spatial relationship of the deformities, however, remained dependent on the mental integration of two-dimensional (2-D) images by the viewer. The evolution of three-dimensional (3-D) capabilities of CT enabled more precise, reproducible representation of the craniofacial problem with a variety of clinical applications for the surgeon.

The ability to produce a 3-D computed tomogram is a function of the digitalization of sequential 2-D CT slices, usually at 1.5-mm intervals. An image is generated by the assignment of a gray scale to the digital data based on the attenuation of a finely collimated x-ray beam by the volume of tissue (voxel) represented by each picture element (pixel). Soft tissue interference in the final imaging can be eliminated by selection of bone density digitalized data only. The image can be ro-

tated on a high-resolution video monitor through 360° in 5° increments. The source of image illumination also can be rotated through 360° to enhance surface details and depth perception. Sections can be removed from the image to allow viewing of the underlying structures (Fig. 18-1).

Preoperative planning is enhanced by the anatomic detail of 3-D CT imaging that may be impossible to reproduce at the time of an operation. This allows communication not only among members of the surgical team but also with the patient and family. Computed graphics techniques are being applied to the digitalized scan data for interactive surgical simulation as a planning and teaching tool. Various reconstructive approaches can be attempted on the computer monitor before the actual procedure, subsequently reducing operative time.

A milling machine has been linked in selected instances to 3-D CT to produce models of the deformity with a 1- to 3-mm level of accuracy (Fig. 18-2). The machine is driven by the position of surface points to generate a wax mold from which

a silicone or methyl methacrylate prosthesis can be derived. The model can be used as an alloplastic implant or as a template for autogenous bone. It enables a better understanding of the volume requirements necessary for reconstruction, thereby resulting in selection of the optimal donor site. The model also can be used to complement the medical record as documentation of what was done during the operation and for comparison after future growth and development.

Three-dimensional CT and model techniques should be applied selectively. The overlap of pixel values in the soft tissue range can present problems with thin bone. Minimally displaced fractures may result in misleading imaging because of volume averaging. This technology is too expensive to use unless clearly indicated.

Representative patients have been selected to show the range of potential applications of 3-D CT. These patients were gleaned from a series of 150 operations in which we used the CEMAX 1000 computer imaging system. This capability provided an exceptional opportunity to

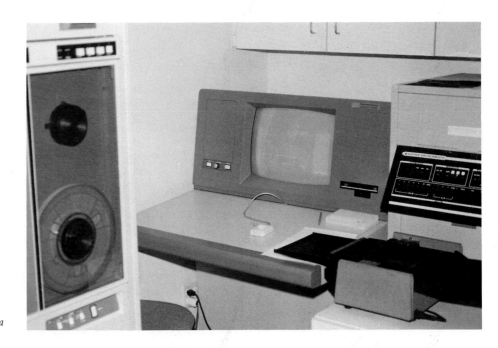

Fig. 18-1. Office-based CEMAX 1000 computer system for the imaging of 3-D CT scans.

Fig. 18-2. Milling machine linked to 3-D CT data to produce a prosthetic model or alloplastic implant.

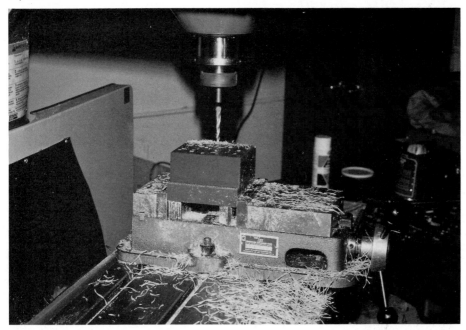

gain a greater understanding of the value of 3-D technology. Potential pitfalls and poor indications for use of the data also became apparent.

Applications

Congenital Deformities

Patient 1

A physical examination of a 1-month-old girl with Apert syndrome revealed marked shortening of the base of the skull

(Fig. 18-3). There was recession of the nasal bridge and supraorbital bar with shortening of the skull in an anteroposterior direction consistent with brachycephaly. The coronal suture appeared to be closed bilaterally.

Bilateral coronal suture synostosis was seen on 2-D and 3-D CT (Fig. 18-4). Shallow orbits and an abnormal nasofrontal region were seen on the 2-D scan. The spatial relations of these deformities are better visualized in the 3-D study. The patient underwent bilateral coronal suture release with a floating forehead frontocranial advancement at the age of $2\frac{1}{2}$ months (Fig. 18-5).

This patient's situation demonstrates the anatomic detail and reproducible imaging qualities of 3-D CT. The deformity is represented in an objective manner rather than subject to the mental integration required to interpret conventional 2-D CT scans. The presence of suture fusion and widely open metopic and sagittal sutures is clearly visualized. Shallow orbits with resultant orbital proptosis are also evident. The ability to represent the cranial base may allow for future development of surgical procedures to correct the synostosis of the cranial base inherent in conditions such as Apert syndrome.

The 3-D tomogram serves as a permanent record of the deformity, which can be used for comparison after future growth and development. Volumetric data can be

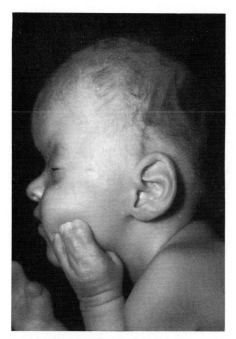

obtained from the 3-D scans and used in determining the adequacy of current and future surgical procedures. This capability is essential for the successful outcome of craniofacial procedures. The family can be informed of the specific nature of the child's deformity using the 3-D images. The surgical plan, however, was not altered by the additional imaging data for patient 1. Operations for bicoronal suture synostosis have been performed for many years without the benefit of 3-D CT.

Patient 2

A 5-year-old girl was referred for craniofacial consultation because of frontonasal dysplasia (Fig. 18-6). A physical examination showed her intercanthal distance to be 3.8 cm and her interpupillary distance to be 6 cm. There was a midline V-shaped depression in her skull based in the upper portion of the nose and open

superiorly. She also had a bifid uvula and a submucous cleft palate. The diagnosis was a Tessier O facial cleft.

Three-dimensional CT illustrated the absence of bone in the midline (Fig. 18-7). Midline hypoplastic structures also were clearly visualized. The patient underwent a transcranial exploration with repair of the hypertelorism. Cranial bone grafting of the orbital rims, orbital floor, and skull was required (Fig. 18-8).

This patient's situation illustrates the clarity of anatomic detail that can be achieved with 3-D CT. The actual bony detail of the defect itself is readily appreciated. A midline encephalocele or other associated midline defect could have been detected preoperatively. An experienced interpreter of a 2-D scan could have attained equivalent information but not in a readily transmissible visual format.

Fig. 18-3. One-month-old girl with Apert syndrome (patient 1). Recession of the nasal bridge and supraorbital bar is evident with shortening of the skull in an anteroposterior direction.

Fig. 18-4. Two-dimensional and 3-D tomograms of patient 1. A. The 2-D tomogram demonstrates shallow orbits and an abnormal nasofrontal region. B. The 3-D study enables better visualization of the spatial relations of these deformities.

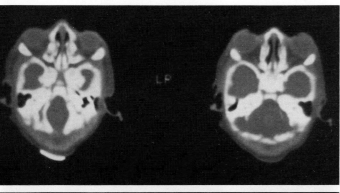

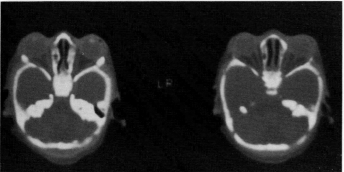

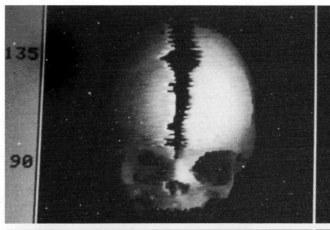

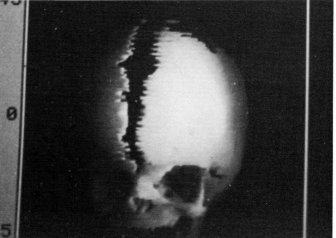

A

B

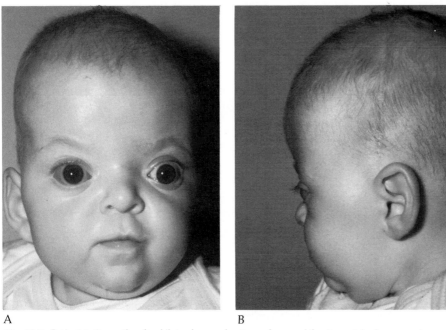

A   B

Fig. 18-5. Patient 1, 2 months after bilateral coronal suture release and frontocranial advancement.

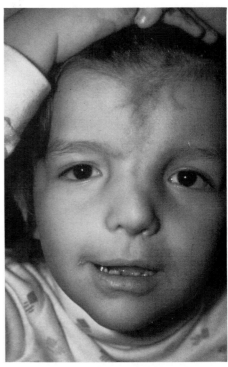

*Fig. 18-6. Five-year-old girl referred for frontonasal dysplasia (patient 2). She was found to have a nasally based **V**-shaped skull depression, a bifid uvula, and a submucous cleft palate.*

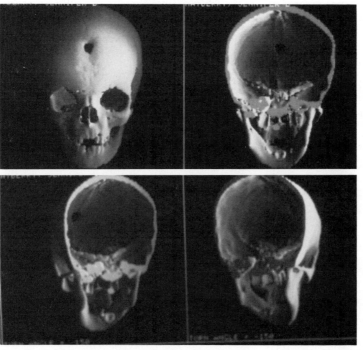

Fig. 18-7. Midline structural hypoplasia and absence of bone are clearly demonstrated in 3-D tomogram of patient 2.

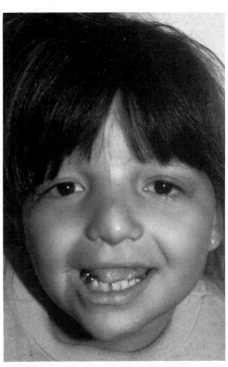

Fig. 18-8. Patient 2, 7 months after transcranial exploration and repair of hypertelorism.

Patient 3

A 6-month-old girl born with kleeblatt-schädel deformity underwent craniectomy soon after birth (Fig. 18-9). She subsequently experienced rapid, abnormal growth of the calvarium. A physical examination showed multiple areas of hypertrophic skull growth interspersed with soft areas.

Roentgenography of the skull (Fig. 18-10) and 2-D CT (Fig. 18-11) demonstrated large areas of nonossified calvarium. The 3-D reconstruction showed a moth-eaten appearance inconsistent with the physical findings (Fig. 18-12). Transcranial exploration was performed with a floating forehead advancement and craniectomy of abnormal bone. The skull was reconstructed with split cranial bone grafts (Fig. 18-13).

This patient's situation demonstrates the limitations of the current technology. The moth-eaten appearance is a result of the discrepancy between the extreme thinness of the skull and the thicker intervals between each of the scans, leading to a misrepresentation of the actual skull deformity.

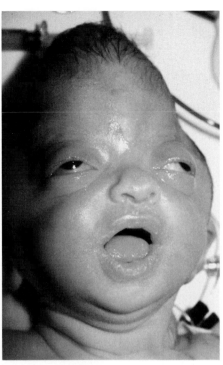

Fig. 18-9. Six-month-old girl (patient 3) with kleeblattschädel deformity who underwent rapid, abnormal calvarial growth following craniectomy at birth.

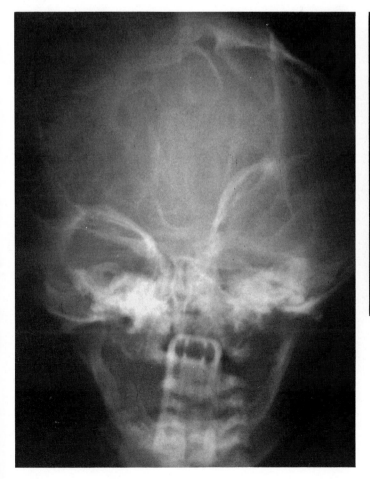

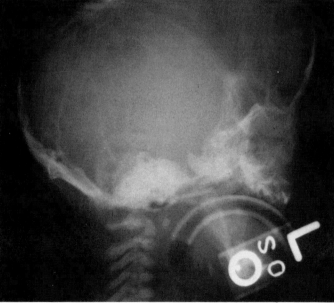

Fig. 18-10. Nonossified calvarium on plain roentgenogram of the skull (patient 3).

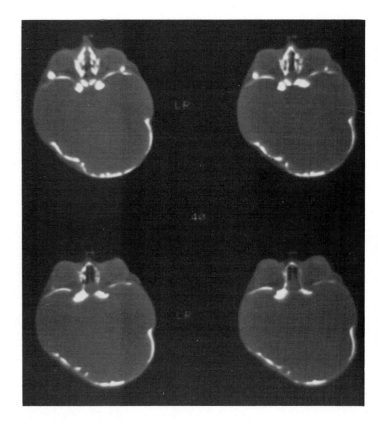

Fig. 18-11. *Large areas of nonossified calvarium on 2-D computed tomogram (patient 3).*

Fig. 18-12. *Moth-eaten appearance of calvarium in 3-D reconstruction is inconsistent with physical findings (patient 3).*

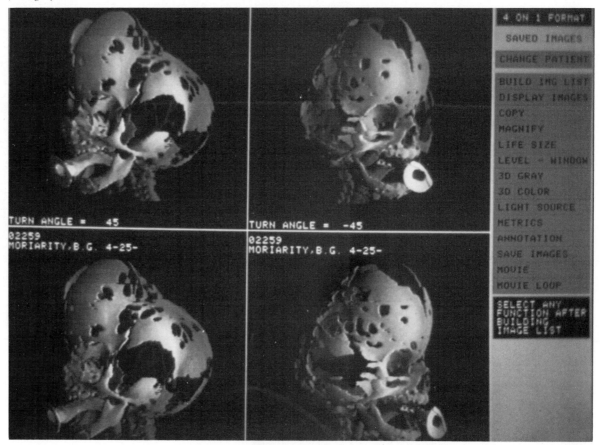

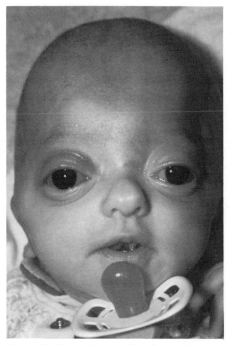

Fig. 18-13. Patient 3, 7 months after craniectomy of abnormal bone, floating forehead advancement, and split cranial bone graft reconstruction.

Patient 4

A 16-year-old boy with Treacher Collins syndrome had no prior surgical procedures. He sought evaluation for craniofacial reconstruction. The zygomatic hypoplasia characteristic of this syndrome was clearly demonstrated by 3-D CT (Fig. 18-14). This type of imaging allows improved preoperative planning by the surgical team. Counseling of the patient and family members is also enhanced with this technique.

Trauma

Patient 5

A 68-year-old man sustained a gunshot wound to the face one week before being transferred for surgical reconstruction. A physical examination revealed extensive soft tissue injury with gross distortion and fragmentation of the mandible.

Three-dimensional CT showed mandibular fracture lines near the mandibular mentum, at the right ramus, and at the right angle with absent bone (Fig. 18-15). The lateral and ventral aspects of the right maxillary sinus were also fractured. The patient underwent reconstruction with open reduction and internal fixation of all identified fractures using miniplates.

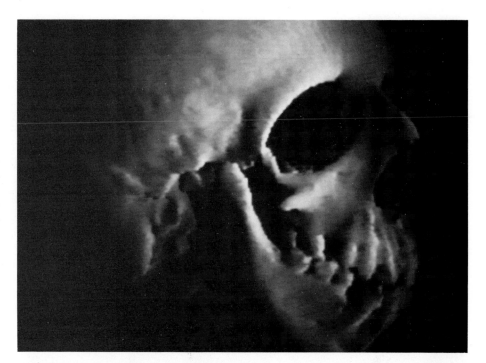

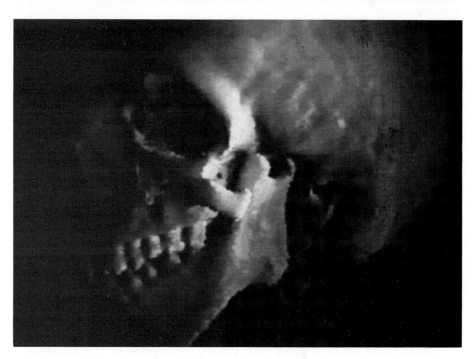

Fig. 18-14. Three-dimensional tomograms of 16-year-old boy with Treacher Collins syndrome (patient 4). The hypoplastic zygomatic deformity characteristic of this syndrome is clearly seen.

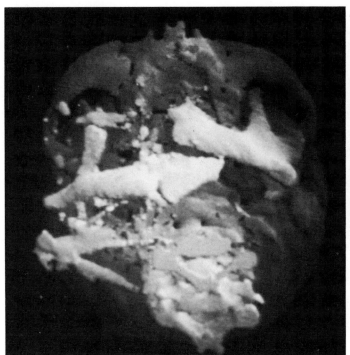

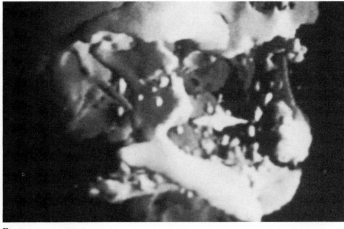

B

Fig. 18-15. Three-dimensional tomograms demonstrating multiple mandibular fractures at the mentum, the right ramus, and the right angle. The lateral and ventral aspects of the right maxillary sinus are fractured as well (patient 5).

A

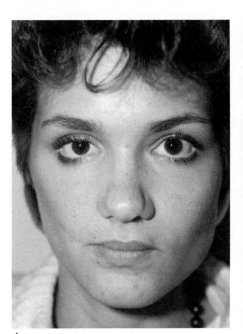

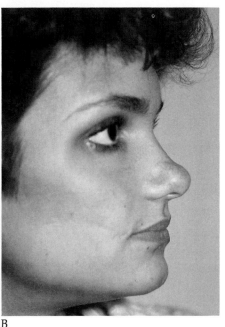

A   B

Fig. 18-16. Twenty-year-old woman (patient 6) with depressed right malar eminence following migration of a silicone implant used to reconstruct a traumatic fracture. (From B.A. Toth, D.S. Ellis, and W.B. Stewart. Computer designed prostheses for orbitocranial reconstruction. Plast. Reconstr. Surg. 81:315, 1988. Reproduced by permission.)

Its unpredictable nature makes complex facial trauma a clear indication for 3-D CT. Multiple, complex facial fractures are well-delineated. The location of bony fragments that cannot be visualized in two dimensions is readily apparent on inspection of 3-D computed tomograms. The spatial relations of the bony fragments in this patient would have been impossible to demonstrate without integration of the 2-D data into a 3-D format. Preoperative planning can be optimized by use of this imaging modality.

Patient 6

A 20-year-old woman was involved in a boating accident at the age of 16 years, which caused extensive comminuted fractures of the right zygoma, maxilla, zygomatic arch, coronoid process, and alveolar bone. The patient had several previous reconstructive procedures, including the use of two silicone implants. The implants migrated, depressing the right malar eminence (Fig. 18-16). Additional findings included right enophthalmos and dystopia caused by an untreated fracture of the orbital floor, a peripheral seventh nerve paresis with right lower eyelid ectropion, and reduced visual acuity from an injury to the optic nerve.

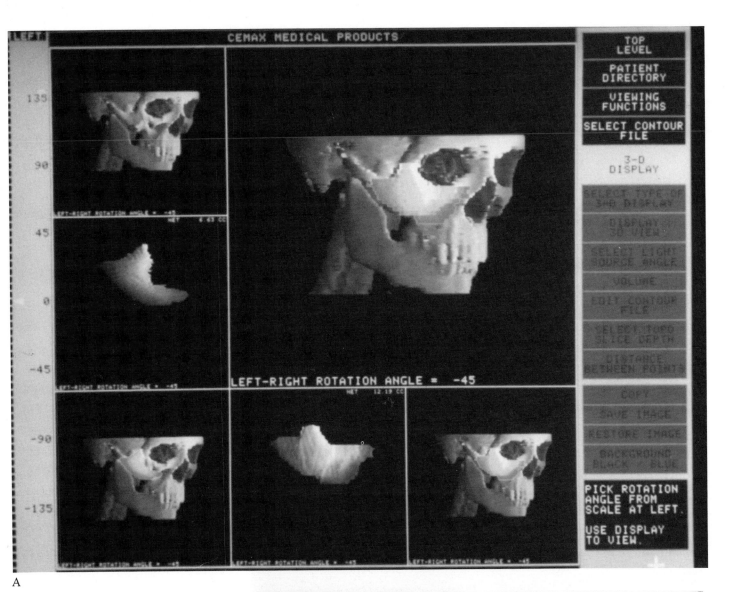

A

Fig. 18-17. Three-dimensional tomogram showing the zone of injury in the right malar eminence, zygomatic arch, and lateral orbital margin in patient 6. (From B.A. Toth, D.S. Ellis, and W.B. Stewart. Computer designed prostheses for orbitocranial reconstruction. Plast. Reconstr. Surg. 81:315, 1988. Reproduced by permission.)

Three-dimensional CT showed a complex deformity with marked posterior displacement of the right malar eminence and fractures of the zygomatic arch and lateral orbital margin at the level of the posterior globe (Fig. 18-17). The inferolateral portion of the right orbital margin was also displaced posteriorly along with the entire anterior wall of the right maxillary antrum. A hybrid resin model was manufactured from 3-D images generated preoperatively.

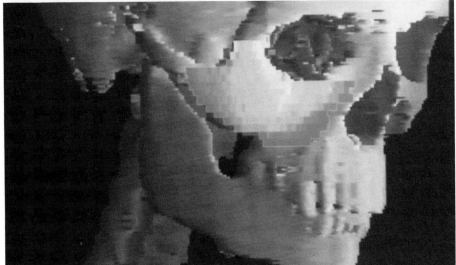

B

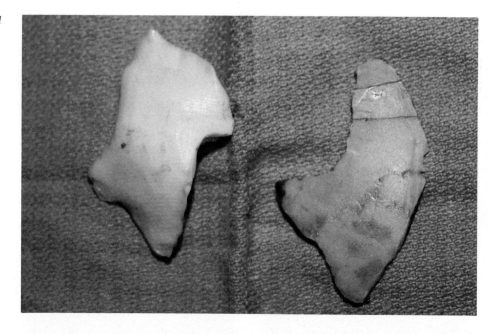

Fig. 18-18. The hybrid resin model (left) generated from the 3-D images and the cranial bone graft (right) used in patient 6. (From B.A. Toth, D.S. Ellis, and W.B. Stewart. Computer designed prostheses for orbitocranial reconstruction. Plast. Reconstr. Surg. 81:315, 1988. Reproduced by permission.)

A split cranial bone graft harvested from the right frontoparietal region was used to reconstruct the maxillary and zygomatic contour defects and repair the fracture of the orbital floor. The computer-generated model was used as a template to select the donor site by matching the contour of the cranial bone to that of the model (Fig. 18-18).

This patient's situation demonstrates the use of a computer-generated model as a template for delayed post-traumatic reconstruction. It was evident from analysis of the 3-D images that simply repositioning the existing alloplastic implant would not adequately correct the volume deficit. The template enabled us to make a bone graft in a more precise manner, matching the existing defect (Fig. 18-19).

Tumors

Patient 7

A 16-year-old girl was referred with the diagnosis of von Recklinghausen disease (Fig. 18-20). She had undergone multiple previous procedures for neurofibromatosis including a right orbital enucleation. A physical examination revealed orbital dystopia and soft tissue laxity of the right face. Three-dimensional CT revealed a large neurofibromatous lesion and absence of the posterior, inferior, and superior margins of the right orbit (Fig. 18-21). Parts of the right temporal and frontal lobes were seen to herniate into the orbit.

The patient underwent resection of the right orbital neurofibroma through a transconjunctival approach. The lesion was found to occupy nearly the entire right orbital cavity. Split skull cranial bone grafts were harvested by the bicoronal approach for use in orbital reconstruction. The facial laxity was corrected with a rhytidectomy and a fascial sling. A right lateral canthopexy also was performed.

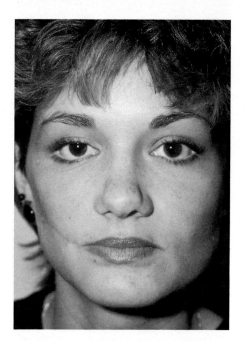
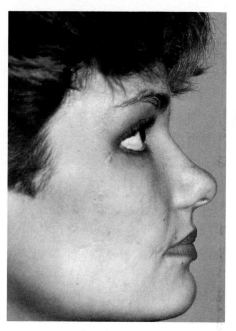

Fig. 18-19. Patient 6 after reconstruction of the maxillary and zygomatic contour defects and repair of the fracture of the orbital floor with cranial bone graft. (From B.A. Toth, D.S. Ellis, and W.B. Stewart. Computer designed prostheses for orbitocranial reconstruction. Plast. Reconstr. Surg. 81:315, 1988. Reproduced by permission.)

In this patient 3-D CT clearly demonstrated the extent of the bony deformity and the neurofibromatous mass. Preoperative planning of the volume requirements for graft harvesting was possible because the size of the cranial base defect was clearly demonstrated by 3-D CT.

Patient 8

A 3-year-old girl was noted to have left-sided facial swelling at the age of 2 years (Fig. 18-22). A physical examination showed that the girl had a markedly small oral aperture and facial asymmetry. Two-dimensional CT showed a huge mass in the left oropharynx extending and erod-

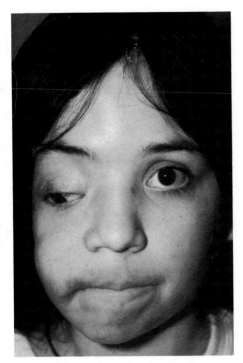

Fig. 18-20. Sixteen-year-old girl (patient 7) with orbital dystopia and right facial soft tissue laxity secondary to von Recklinghausen disease.

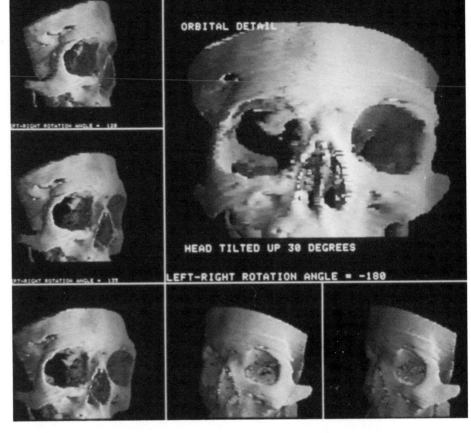

Fig. 18-21. Absence of posterior, inferior, and superior margins of right orbit in 3-D computed tomograms of patient 7.

ing through the bone into the middle cranial fossa (Fig. 18-23). Three-dimensional CT also was performed (Fig. 18-24).

The mass was found on biopsy to be consistent with fibrosarcoma, and the patient was treated with chemotherapy for one year because of the size and aggressive nature of the lesion. There was no clinically significant reduction in the size of the mass. The patient underwent exploration of the left infratemporal fossa with excision of its contents (Fig. 18-25).

This patient's situation exemplifies the ineffectiveness of 3-D CT in the evaluation of soft tissue. No useful information is added beyond that obtained by standard 2-D CT. Current technology limits the usefulness of 3-D CT in the head and neck to bony abnormalities. Magnetic resonance imaging (MRI), which is highly specific for soft tissue, is beginning to be used in the 3-D format.

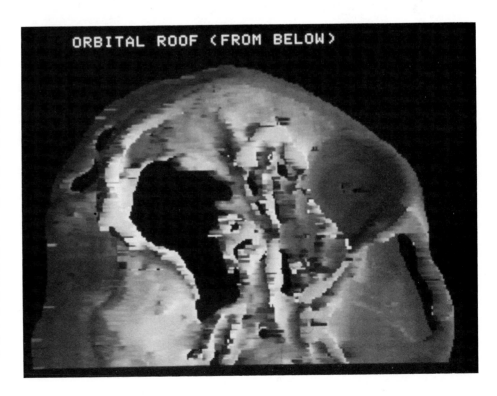

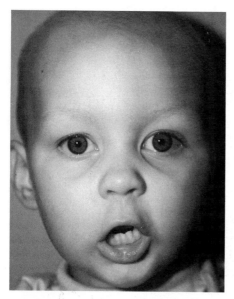

Fig. 18-22. Three-year-old girl (patient 8) with left-sided facial swelling found on biopsy to be consistent with fibrosarcoma.

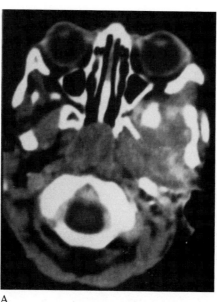

A

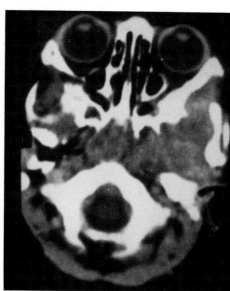

B

Fig. 18-23. Two-dimensional tomogram of patient 8 showing left oropharyngeal mass eroding through bone into the middle cranial fossa.

Fig. 18-24. Three-dimensional tomogram of left oropharyngeal mass in patient 8.

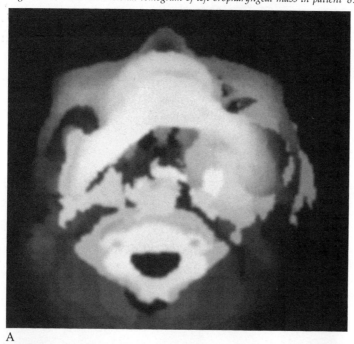

A

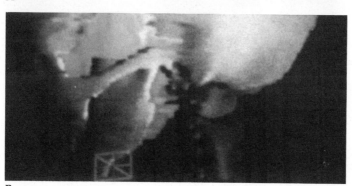

B

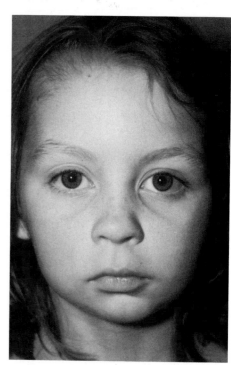

Fig. 18-25. Patient 8, 3 years after excision of the contents of the left infratemporal fossa.

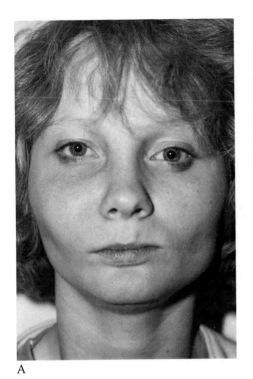

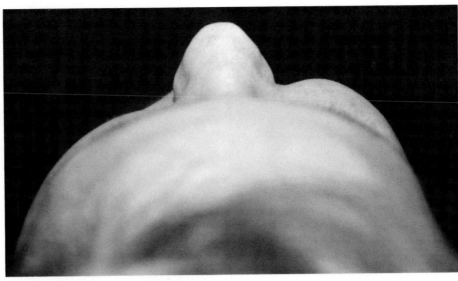

B

Fig. 18-26. Twenty-year-old woman (patient 9) with marked facial asymmetry caused by monostotic fibrous dysplasia of the right maxilla.

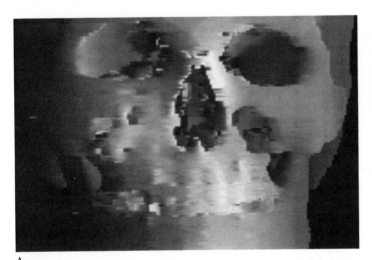

A

Fig. 18-27. Three-dimensional tomograms showing an expansile ossified lesion occupying the right maxillary antrum in patient 9.

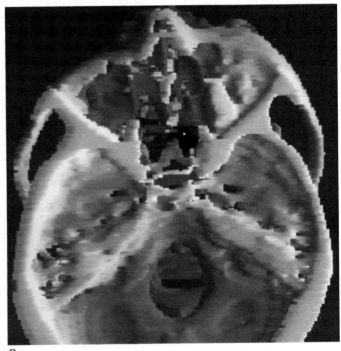

B

Patient 9

A 20-year-old woman was referred to us with a diagnosis of monostotic fibrous dysplasia of the maxilla. She had marked facial asymmetry (Fig. 18-26). Three-dimensional CT showed an expansile ossified lesion, which subsequently occupied the entire right maxillary antrum (Fig. 18-27). The soft tissues of the right cheek were displaced outwardly. An acrylic model was fabricated with the computer-controlled milling device by subtraction of the normal from the abnormal side on the basis of the data from 3-D CT (Fig. 18-28).

Bony osteotomy and contouring of the right maxilla to match the left were performed using the computer-generated template as an intraoperative guide during the surgical procedure. The volume of the fragments removed was compared with the volume of the template. This comparison allowed for a more precise understanding of the amount of bony subtraction needed (Fig. 18-29).

Fig. 18-28. Subtraction of the normal left maxilla from the abnormal right maxilla in patient 9 was used to generate an acrylic model that served as an intraoperative guide for bony recontouring.

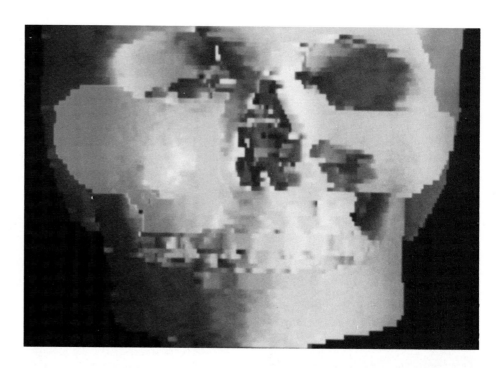

Fig. 18-29. Patient 9 after osteotomy and contouring of the right maxilla to match the left.

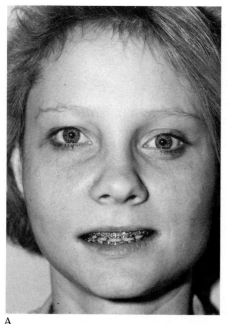

A

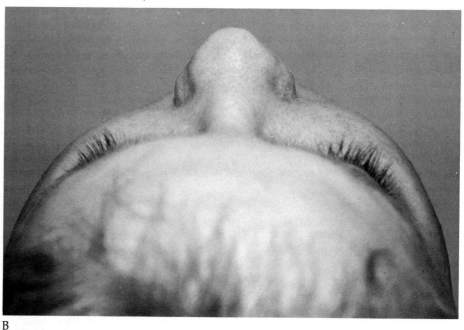

B

Patient 10

A 65-year-old woman underwent resection of a right frontal meningioma 10 years before being referred to us (Fig. 18-30). The margins of the tumor were positive, but the malignancy was low-grade. The patient had proptosis and a recurrent mass. The mass effect of the tumor had caused limitation of upgaze of the right eye. Resection and reconstruction were performed as staged procedures.

Two-dimensional CT done before resection of the tumor showed extensive soft tissue and bony involvement of the right orbitocranium, including the frontal bone, frontal sinus, and superior orbit. During the tumor resection, we removed a 10-by-10-cm section of the frontal bone, from the left frontal sinus to the right zygomatic arch, the right superior and lateral orbital rim, and the bony roof of the

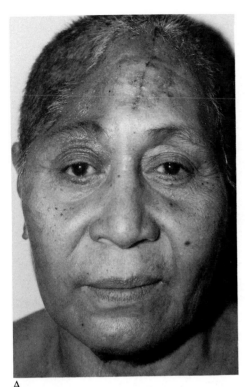

A

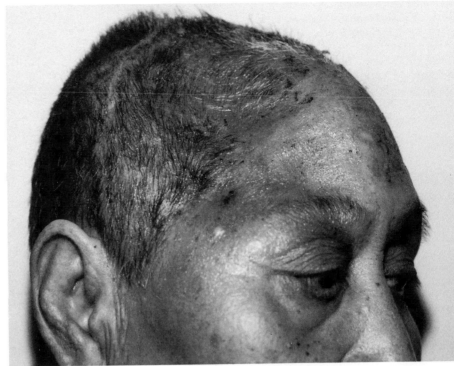

B

Fig. 18-30. Sixty-five-year-old woman (patient 10) 10 years after resection of a right frontal meningioma. She had a recurrent mass, proptosis, and considerable bony depression. (From B.A. Toth, D. DiLoretto, and W.B. Stewart. Multidisciplinary approach to the management of complex bony and soft tissue orbitocranial disorders. Ophthalmology 95:1013, 1988; and B.A. Toth, D.S. Ellis, and W.B. Stewart. Computer designed prostheses for orbitocranial reconstruction. Plast. Reconstr. Surg. 81:315, 1988. Reproduced by permission.)

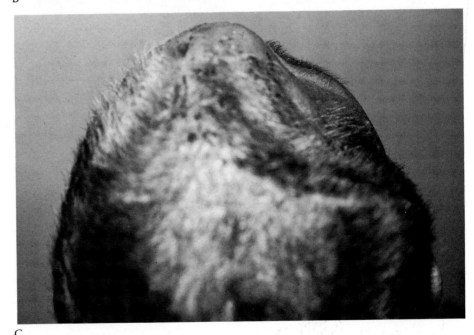

C

right orbit. The levator complex, extraocular muscles, lacrimal gland, and dura were left intact.

Reconstruction was undertaken 6 months after the resection. Three-dimensional images of the skull defect were obtained for use in preoperative planning (Fig. 18-31). There was no evidence of recurrent meningioma. A methyl methacrylate prosthesis for the skull and orbital defect was fabricated from a computer-generated model (Fig. 18-32). The surgical procedure consisted of a bicoronal approach with insertion of the methyl methacrylate prosthesis. Minimal intraoperative remodeling of the existing defect was required.

Manufacture of a prosthesis based on 3-D CT images enabled restoration of a symmetric forehead and orbit in this patient (Fig. 18-33). In addition, future need for resection of a recurrent lesion will be facilitated by the use of alloplastic rather than autogenous material.

Patient 11

A 41-year-old woman had a previous re-

section for a frontal meningioma (Fig. 18-34). This procedure was complicated by infection, which resulted in loss of the anterior bone flap. Two subsequent procedures were performed to reconstruct the defect with alloplastic material. After each operation, the prosthesis had to be removed because of infection. A physical examination revealed an 8-by-8-cm bony defect with gross deformity of the fore-

Fig. 18-31. Three-dimensional tomogram of patient 10, 6 months after recurrent tumor resection with removal of a portion of the right frontal bone 10 cm by 10 cm, the right superior and lateral orbital rim, and the roof of the right orbit. (From B.A. Toth, D. DiLoretto, and W.B. Stewart. Multidisciplinary approach to the management of bony and soft tissue orbitocranial disorders. Ophthalmology *95:1013, 1988. Reproduced by permission.)*

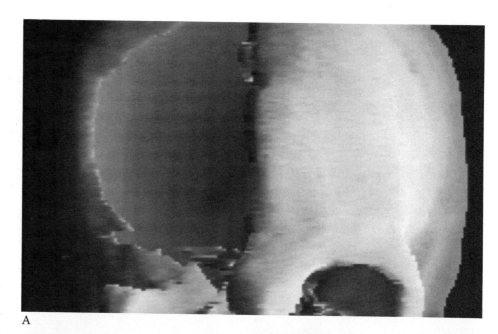

A

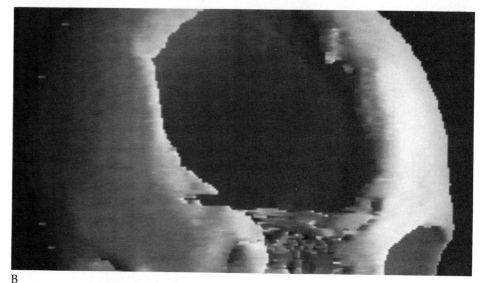

B

head and brow asymmetry. Three-dimensional CT demonstrated a large bilateral frontal bone defect (Fig. 18-35). An acrylic template of the bony defect was generated from the 3-D data.

The patient underwent reconstruction of the frontal bone defect using autogenous tissue. The template was used to locate an appropriate contour on the skull for use as a donor site. Three strips of split cranial bone were harvested from the occipitoparietal region and secured in position with wire using the template as a guide. The autogenous bone graft was placed into the frontal bone defect and fixed to adjacent bone (Fig. 18-36).

The size and contour of bone needed for reconstruction were precisely determined using the computer-generated template. This enabled the achievement of a more symmetric result than would otherwise have been possible (Fig. 18-37).

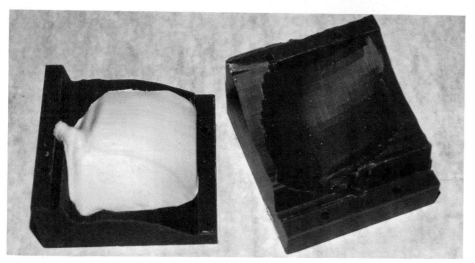

Fig. 18-32. Methyl methacrylate prosthesis fabricated from a computer-generated model for use in reconstructing the skull and orbital defect in patient 10. (From D. Ellis, B.A. Toth, and W.B. Stewart. Three-dimensional imaging and computer-designed prostheses in the evaluation and management of orbitocranial deformities. Plast. Reconstr. Surg. *81:315, 1988. Reproduced by permission.)*

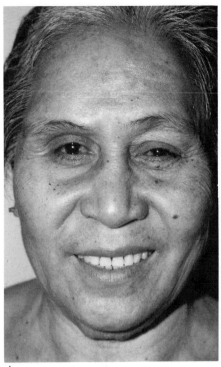

A

Fig. 18-33. Postoperative views of patient 10 after insertion of prosthesis. Good contour and symmetry were obtained. (From B.A. Toth, D. DiLoretto, and W.B. Stewart. Multidisciplinary approach to the management of complex bony and soft tissue orbitocranial disorders. Ophthalmology. 95:1013, 1988; and B.A. Toth, D.S. Ellis, and W.B. Stewart. Computer designed prostheses for orbitocranial reconstruction. Plast. Reconstr. Surg. 81:315, 1988. Reproduced with permission.)

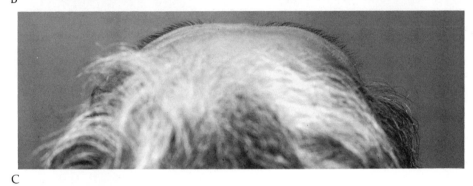

B

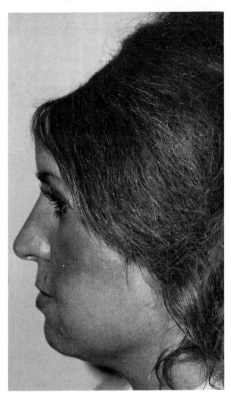

C

Fig. 18-34. Forty-one-year-old woman (patient 11) after resection of a frontal meningioma with bone flap and alloplastic prosthetic failure caused by infection. (From B.A. Toth, D. DiLoretto, and W.B. Stewart. Multidisciplinary approach to the management of complex bony and soft tissue orbitocranial disorders. Ophthalmology. 95: 1013, 1988. Reproduced with permission.)

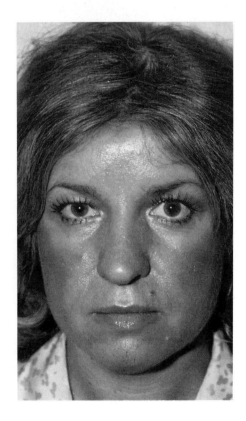

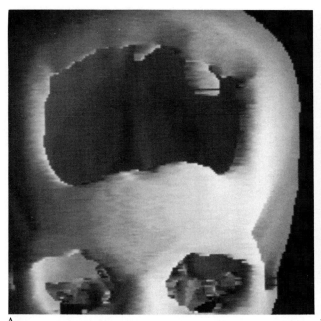

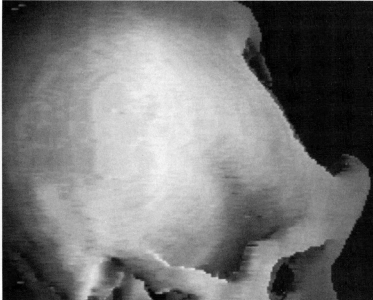

A

B

Fig. 18-35. *Three-dimensional tomograms demonstrate large bilateral defect of frontal bone in patient 11. (From B.A. Toth, D. DiLoretto, and W.B. Stewart. Multidisciplinary approach to the management of complex bony and soft tissue orbitocranial disorders. Ophthalmology 95:1013, 1988. Reproduced with permission.)*

Fig. 18-36. *Acrylic template adjacent to autogenous bone graft placed into frontal bone defect in patient 11. (From B.A. Toth, D. DiLoretto, and W.B. Stewart. Multidisciplinary approach to the management of complex bony and soft tissue orbitocranial disorders. Ophthalmology 95:1013, 1988. Reproduced with permission.)*

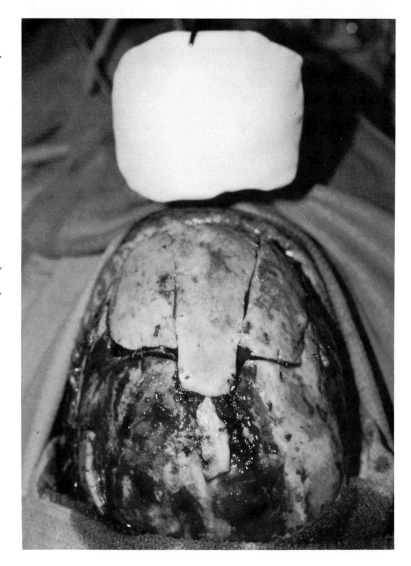

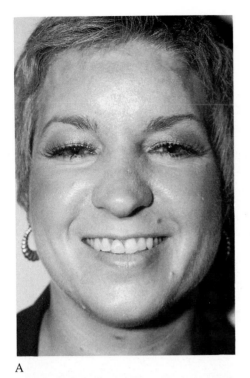

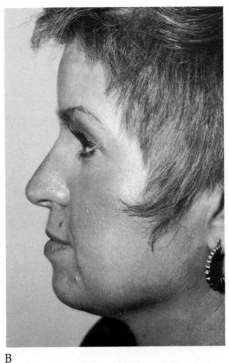

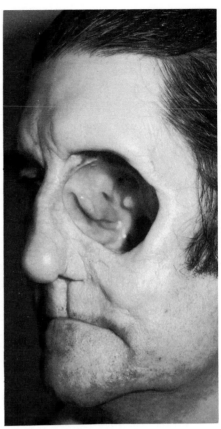

A

B

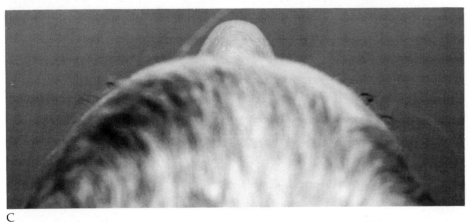

C

Fig. 18-37. Patient 11 after reconstruction of the frontal bone. (From B.A. Toth, D. DiLoretto, and W.B. Stewart. Multidisciplinary approach to the management of complex bony and soft tissue orbitocranial disorders. Ophthalmology 95:1013, 1988. Reproduced with permission.)

Fig. 18-38. Sixty-five-year-old man (patient 12) 9 years after left hemimaxillectomy and orbital exenteration for squamous cell carcinoma. (From W.B. Stewart and B.A. Toth. A multidisciplinary approach to orbital neoplasm. Clinics in Plastic Surgery 15:2, 1988. Reproduced with permission.)

Patient 12

A 65-year-old man had had a hemimaxillectomy and orbital exenteration for squamous cell carcinoma 9 years previously (Fig. 18-38). A split-thickness skin graft had been used to cover the posterior orbital area, and the patient was using a palatal obturator. He complained that food entered the orbital defect while he was eating. A physical examination showed a communication between the orbital cavity and the palate.

Three-dimensional CT was used to determine the total volume requirements of the defect (Fig. 18-39). The orbitofacial deformity was reconstructed using a free latissimus dorsi musculocutaneous flap with three discrete skin islands for use in the nasopharynx, palate, and orbit (Fig. 18-40).

Three-dimensional CT allowed precise selection of a suitable donor site for closing the defect (Fig. 18-41). The true volume requirements could not be obtained readily from 2-D CT.

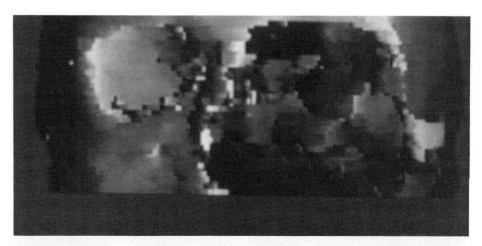

Fig. 18-39. The total volume requirements in patient 12 were determined using 3-D CT. (From W.B. Stewart and B.A. Toth. A multidisciplinary approach to orbital neoplasm. Clinics in Plastic Surgery *15:2, 1988. Reproduced with permission.)*

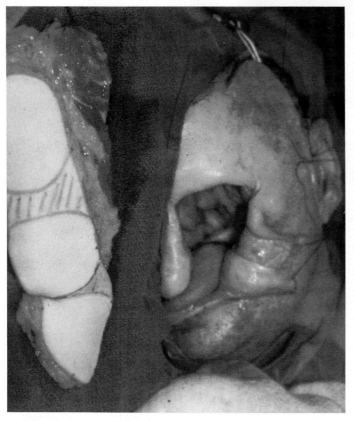

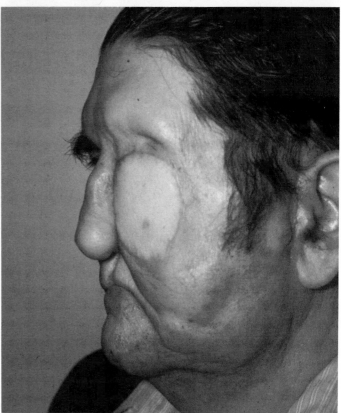

Fig. 18-40. Reconstruction (patient 12) using latissimus dorsi musculocutaneous flap with three discrete skin islands for use in the nasopharynx, palate, and orbit. (From W.B. Stewart and B.A. Toth. A multidisciplinary approach to orbital neoplasm. Clinics in Plastic Surgery *15:2, 1988. Reproduced with permission.)*

Fig. 18-41. Patient 12 after latissimus dorsi musculocutaneous flap reconstruction of the orbital defect. (From W.B. Stewart and B.A. Toth. A multidisciplinary approach to orbital neoplasm. Clinics in Plastic Surgery *15:2, 1988. Reproduced with permission.)*

Discussion

The anatomic relationships and reconstructive requirements of congenital, traumatic, and neoplastic disorders of the craniofacial skeleton are complex. Two-dimensional CT images are routinely used for preoperative analysis. Three-dimensional computer-generated images use the same database but allow a more precise contour and volume analysis in a format that is more easily interpreted.

The clear anatomic definition of the deformity serves as an objective foundation for preoperative planning among members of the surgical team (patients 1, 2, 4, and 7). Programs have been developed for interactive surgical simulation to preview surgical alternatives. The use of a computer-controlled milling device to produce a model of the bony defect has clearly been a useful adjunct to craniofacial operations for selected patients.

The model has been an excellent tool for improving the understanding of the deformity and of the planned operative procedure by the family. It functions as a permanent record for serial evaluation of growth, volume, and contour changes. These data can serve as an aid in monitoring both surgical and nonsurgical patients.

The fashioning of autogenous bone grafts (patients 6 and 11) has been enhanced by the contour and volumetric information provided by the model. The need for removal rather than repositioning of a displaced alloplastic implant may be evident from preoperative 3-D volumetric analysis (patient 6).

An alloplastic implant may be appropriate when the patient's age, disease process, and risks of infection and recurrence are considered (patient 10). The use of the model to generate a prosthesis decreases operative time by reducing the need for trimming and recontouring of the implant. The accuracy of standard intraoperative molding of a prosthesis is limited in the orbital region by the multiple contours present and the free margins at the orbital rim. Similarly, the dimensions required for musculocutaneous flap reconstruction of the orbit can be readily obtained from 3-D data (patient 12). The use of the model as a template for determining the amount of tissue excision necessary to achieve a symmetric result has also been valuable (patient 9). The model serves as a negative template for assessing the volume of bone that needs to be removed.

Limitations of 3-D CT technology include additional cost, increased scanning time, and exposure to radiation. The time and expense involved in preoperative planning, however, must be weighed against the decreased operative time and improved results. Furthermore, newer techniques are enabling a reduction in radiation exposure.

The use of 3-D imaging in lesions of soft tissue has been disappointing (patient 8). Current technology does not allow useful imaging of these lesions. The use of standard 2-D scans or MRI is recommended in these situations. In some patients (e.g., patient 3) the 3-D image is misleading because there is a discrepancy between the thinness of the bone and the intervals between the scans. The thin areas of bone are not recorded and the result is a moth-eaten appearance of the bone.

In conclusion, 3-D CT is an effective adjunct to craniomaxillofacial surgery. Its true value will be realized when it is used in appropriately chosen patients for extensive preoperative evaluation, planning, and management.

Suggested Reading

Gillespie, J.E., et al. Three-dimensional CT reformations in the assessment of congenital and traumatic cranio-facial deformities. *Br. J. Oral Maxillofac. Surg.* 25:171, 1987.

Gillespie, J.E., et al. Three-dimensional reformations of computed tomography in the assessment of facial trauma. *Clin. Radiol.* 38:523, 1987.

Guyuron, B., and Ross, R.J. Computer-generated model surgery: An exacting approach to complex craniomaxillofacial disharmonies. *J. Craniomaxillofac. Surg.* 17:101, 1989.

Jackson, I.T., and Bite, U. Three-dimensional computed tomographic scanning and major surgical reconstruction of the head and neck. *Mayo Clin. Proc.* 61:546, 1986.

Linney, A.D., et al. Three-dimensional visualization of computerized tomography and laser scan data for the simulation of maxillofacial surgery. *Med. Inf.* 14:109, 1989.

Marsh, J., and Vannier, M.W. The third dimension in craniofacial surgery. *Plast. Reconstr. Surg.* 71:759, 1983.

Toth, B.A., Ellis, D.S., and Stewart, W.B. Computer-designed prostheses for orbitocranial reconstruction. *Plast. Reconstr. Surg.* 81:315, 1988.

II
Skin and Adnexa

19

Benign Skin Tumors

Brian Cook   Susan D. Gass   Michael D. Lichter
Stephanie F. Marschall   Lawrence M. Solomon

Tumors of the Epidermis

Verrucae (Warts)

Verrucae are benign tumors of the skin and mucous membranes caused by human papillomavirus (HPV), a double-stranded DNA virus in the papovavirus group (Table 19-1). Warts are classified on the basis of their clinical appearance, their location, and the HPV type inducing the lesion (Figs. 19-1 to 19-5). HPV has not been cultured successfully, but typing through the use of DNA hybridization techniques is possible. To date, 55 HPV types have been identified. Warts occur most commonly in people who are between 12 and 16 years of age. Immunosuppressed hosts, especially those with impaired cell-mediated immunity, have an increased susceptibility to HPV. Patients with atopy, particularly atopic dermatitis, have functional T-cell depression of a relatively benign nature; however, these patients suffer from widespread common warts, which are relatively resistant to treatment. Highly immunosuppressed patients, such as those suffering from acquired immunodeficiency syndrome (AIDS), have an added increased

risk of malignant transformation of their lesions.

Epidermodysplasia verruciformis, a familial disorder, is characterized by the development of HPV-induced papules and macules that have malignant potential. These patients have depressed cell-mediated immunity.

Many methods are available for the treatment of warts, and we use them all, including physical, chemical, destructive, and chemotherapeutic agents. Salicylic acid and lactic acid, trichloroacetic acid, cantharidin, formaldehyde, and glutaraldehyde have been used for palmar and plantar warts. Podophyllin is the main treatment of anogenital warts, but it should not be used during pregnancy or on large bleeding surfaces because of its systemic absorption and possible neurotoxicity. Cryotherapy with liquid nitrogen is commonly used; disadvantages include pain and blister formation. Surgical methods such as excision, curettage, laser ablation, or blunt dissection are sometimes used. Topical 5-fluorouracil and intralesional bleomycin have been reported to be effective. Alpha-2-interferon is being investigated for treatment of warts.

Seborrheic Keratosis

Seborrheic keratoses are benign tumors in the epidermis that appear most commonly in the fourth and fifth decades of life (Fig. 19-6).

A variant of seborrheic keratosis is *dermatosis papulosa nigra,* which is characterized by small, deeply pigmented papules that usually occur on the face of deeply pigmented people (Fig. 19-7).

The *sign of Leser-Trélat* is the sudden appearance of or increase in the number or size of preexisting seborrheic keratoses. It is hypothesized to be a marker for an internal malignant tumor.

Methods used to remove seborrheic keratoses include curettage, shave excision, and cryotherapy, depending on the site being treated. Excision generally is not indicated; however, a lesion that becomes inflamed, crusted, eroded, or ulcerated or one that bleeds should be examined histologically.

Organoid Nevi

Epidermal nevi are hamartomas. They have been classified according to the predominant component: *nevus verrucosus* (keratinocytes), *nevus sebaceus* (sebaceous glands), and *nevus comedonicus* (hair follicles). *Epidermal nevus syndrome* refers to the association of epidermal nevi and extracutaneous abnormalities. Epidermal nevi are most often present at birth, but they may develop or first become visible to the naked eye during the first or second decade—rarely in the third decade—of life.

Table 19-1. Verrucae (warts)

Wart	Clinical characteristics	HPV type
Palmoplantar warts	Thick, hyperkeratotic surface with thrombosed capillaries	HPV 1
Common warts (verruca vulgaris)	Circumscribed, firm, rough keratotic papules singly or grouped; most common on dorsum of hands, periungual area, and knees	HPV 2 and 4
Flat warts (verruca plana)	Slightly elevated, smooth papules less than 5 mm in diameter; flesh colored to brown; most often on hands and face except in patients with epidermodysplasia verruciformis, in whom all the skin except the trunk can be involved	HPV 3 and 10
Epidermodysplasia verruciformis	Genetic predisposition to developing HPV-induced lesions, which are flat and wartlike, tinea versicolor–like, or psoriasiform; spares palms, scalp, and mucous membranes; can undergo malignant degeneration	HPV 5, 8, 9, 10, 12, 14, 17, 19–25, 36–38, 46, 47, 49, 50
Condyloma acuminatum (bowenoid papulosis)	Soft verrucous papules and cauliflower-like masses or small verrucous papules on the cervix, perineum, anogenital region, and penis; may undergo malignant degeneration	HPV 6, 11, 16, 18, 31, 32
Butcher hand warts	Rough keratotic papules on hands	HPV 7
Focal epithelial hyperplasia	Multiple discrete or confluent papules on labial, buccal, and gingival mucosa and tongue; occur most often in Native Americans	HPV 13

HPV = human papillomavirus.

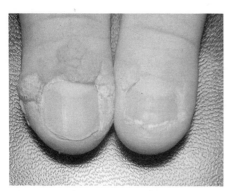

Fig. 19-1. Periungual verruca vulgaris.

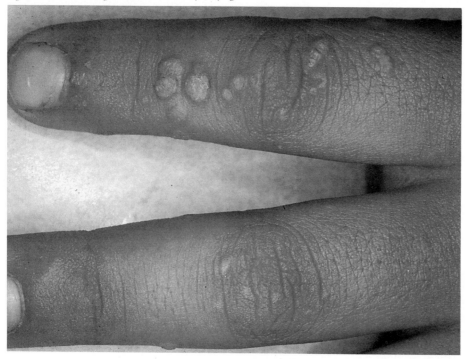

Fig. 19-2. Verruca vulgaris on the dorsum of the fingers.

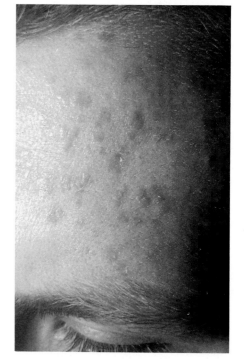

Fig. 19-3. Verruca plana of the forehead.

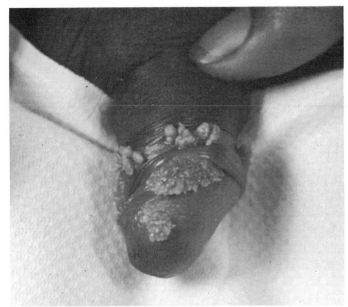

Fig. 19-4. Perianal condyloma acuminatam.

Fig. 19-5. Condyloma acuminatam of the penis.

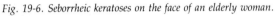

Fig. 19-6. Seborrheic keratoses on the face of an elderly woman.

Fig. 19-7. Dermatosis papulosa nigra primarily involving the malar area.

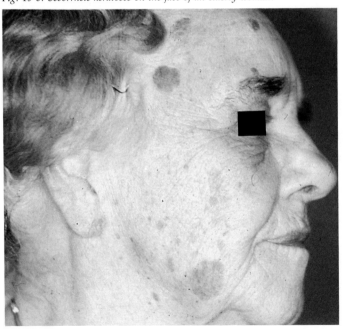

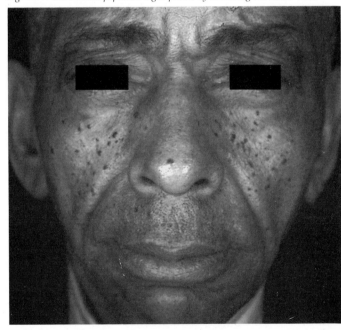

Nevus sebaceus of Jadassohn occurs in infancy as a smooth orange-yellow, slightly raised, hairless plaque on the scalp or face, often taking a linear distribution. During adolescence the lesions become darker, verrucous, and nodular, possibly because of hormonal stimulation, which may induce hyperplasia of the sebaceous and apocrine glands. The third stage, which occurs in approximately 5 percent of patients, is characterized by the development of benign and malignant skin tumors, most commonly syringocystadenoma papilliferum and basal cell carcinoma.

Nevus comedonicus is a hamartoma of the hair follicle. It appears as linearly grouped or zosteriform cystic dilatations with extensive keratotic plugging clinically presenting as open comedones. Sites of predilection are the face, neck, trunk, and upper limbs (Fig. 19-8).

Nevus unius lateris is a linear unilateral warty lesion that may extend from head to toe, may cross the midline, may occupy a single limb, or may limit itself to a digit. *Ichthyosis hystrix* produces a scaly, erythematous, or hyperpigmented whorled

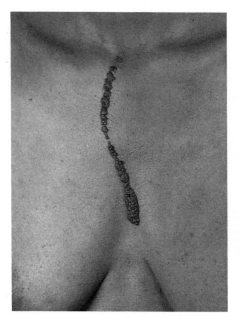

Fig. 19-8. Linear verrucous nevus of the chest.

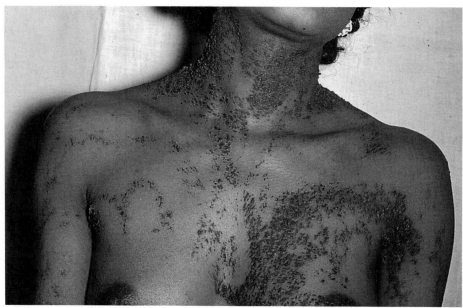

Fig. 19-9. Ichthyosis hystrix of the neck and trunk.

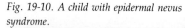

Fig. 19-10. A child with epidermal nevus syndrome.

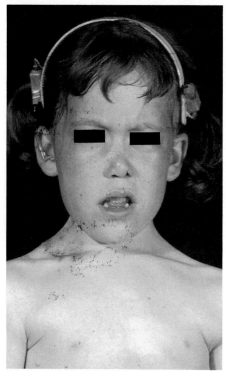

pattern on the trunk that stops abruptly at the midline; it has a distinctive histopathology (Fig. 19-9).

Patients with epidermal nevi should be screened for the *epidermal nevus syndrome*, which is the association of epidermal nevi with abnormalities in other organ systems, most often ocular, neurologic, or skeletal disorders. Central nervous system complications, most commonly seizures and mental retardation, are more common in epidermal nevi involving the head and neck. *Many cutaneous and systemic malignant tumors have been associated with epidermal nevus syndrome* (Fig. 19-10).

Patients with an epidermal nevus should be evaluated with a careful history and physical examination. Excision is the treatment of choice for small epidermal nevi. For larger lesions and facial lesions, topical treatments such as cryotherapy, topical or intralesional steroids, retinoic acid, and podophyllin ointment have been used with limited success. Laser ablation, dermabrasion, deep shave excision, and keratolytics also have been used. For nevus sebaceus, removal of the lesions before puberty is recommended because of its potential for malignant degeneration.

Keratoacanthoma

Keratoacanthoma is a rapidly growing tumor that originates from hair follicles and regresses spontaneously after a period of months (Fig. 19-11). Keratoacanthomas typically arise in elderly men and women on sun-exposed areas, specifically the face, the dorsa of hands, and the forearms. Men are affected three times as often as women. Sunlight is thought to be a factor in the production of keratoacanthomas, and lesions are more frequent in fair-skinned people. Patients exposed to tar derivatives and people who smoke have an increased incidence of these lesions, as do immunosuppressed patients.

A keratoacanthoma characteristically first appears as a dome-shaped, rapidly growing nodule with a central keratin plug; it attains a maximal size in 4 to 8 weeks. Generally the lesions are solitary, but multiple lesions may appear, especially in the familial variety, Ferguson-Smith. Fully developed lesions have a central, large, irregularly shaped crater filled with keratin. The lesion may be difficult to differentiate from squamous cell carcinoma. Keratoacanthomas often involute spontaneously, but we suggest treatment in the form of an excisional biopsy.

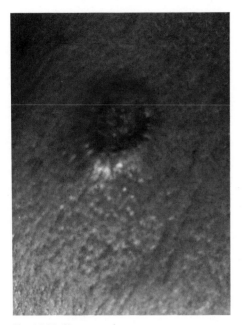

Fig. 19-11. Keratoacanthoma.

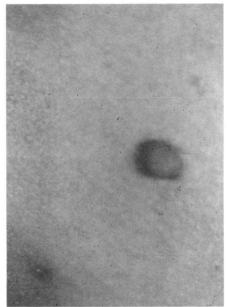

Fig. 19-12. Angiofibroma.

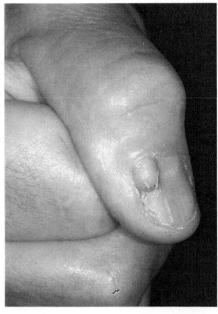

Fig. 19-13. Periungual fibroma, a lesion found in 50 percent of patients with tuberous sclerosis.

Tumors of Mesodermal Origin

Fibrous Tissue Tumors

Dermatofibromas are common dermal nodules located most frequently on the limbs. They are solitary or few in number with a diameter typically less than 1 cm. The epidermis is usually pigmented and may be slightly hyperkeratotic. Dermatofibromas generally arise in adult life and persist indefinitely without change. On physical examination, the lesions are usually flat and dimple on slight pinching of the surrounding skin. They are believed to arise from a connective tissue. In general a histologic examination reveals epidermal proliferation and newly formed collagen and fibroblasts between preexisting collagen fibers with a variable number of histiocytes. The treatment recommended is surgical excision with a histologic examination.

Soft fibromas, also called *acrochordons*, cutaneous tags, or fibroepithelial polyps, are soft, pedunculated tumors. The neck, axilla, flanks, and groin are the sites of predilection. Lesions are usually numerous and vary from 1 or 2 mm to 1 cm in diameter. Simple shave excision, cryosurgery, and electrodesiccation are the usual methods of removal. Strangulation with a thread is not recommended.

Facial *angiofibromas* are seen in tuberous sclerosis, an autosomal dominant disorder characterized by mental deficiency, seizures, and angiofibromas. They are small, red, smooth papules present in a symmetric distribution in the nasolabial folds, on the cheeks, and on the chin (Fig. 19-12).

Fibrous papules of the nose, a fairly common lesion, are dome-shaped, firm, small lesions on the lower portion of the nose. Treatment of these lesions is usually requested for cosmetic reasons and may be accomplished with a carbon dioxide laser or surgical excision.

Periungual fibromas, a type of fibrokeratoma, occur independently in 50 percent of patients with tuberous sclerosis (Fig. 19-13).

Connective tissue nevi are hamartomas that occur as slightly elevated, indurated nodules that may be grouped together in plaques or widely disseminated. The amount of collagen is increased, whereas the elastic tissue content varies. These lesions may occur as a strictly cutaneous defect sporadically without abnormalities in other organ systems or may be transmitted by autosomal dominant inheritance.

They may occur in the Buschke-Ollendorff syndrome with osteopoikilosis or as part of tuberous sclerosis, as the "shagreen patch."

A *giant cell tumor of the tendon sheath* is a common firm tumor attached to a tendon sheath. It is seen usually on the fingers, hands, wrists, or feet, and there is no tendency toward spontaneous resolution. The lesion may extend to skin or bone. Treatment consists of surgical excision (Fig. 19-14).

Giant cell epulis occurs in children, young adults, and pregnant women as a solitary gingival tumor. It is found in the area of the bicuspids and the anterior teeth. The lesion is a benign 1- to 2-cm firm, dark red tumor. Conservative surgical excision is considered the treatment of choice.

Desmoid tumors are benign fibroblastic proliferations. They are firm, tender masses that tend to invade muscle and are usually solitary. These lesions grow slowly but may attain a large size. Some authors believe that desmoid tumors are malignant soft tissue tumors because of their propensity for local invasion. Management of these tumors requires wide surgical excision.

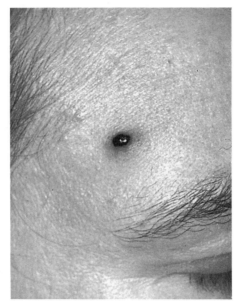

Fig. 19-15. Angiokeratoma.

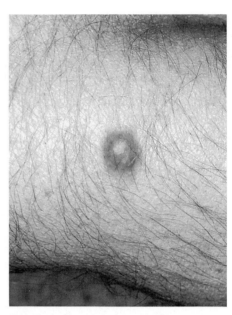

Fig. 19-16. Glomus tumor.

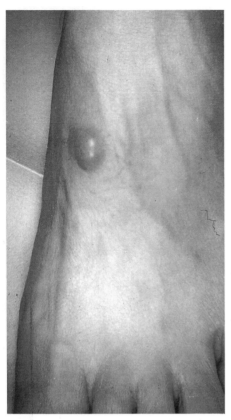

Fig. 19-14. Giant cell tumor of the tendon sheath.

Vascular Tumors

Senile hemangiomas (cherry hemangiomas) are common vascular tumors found on the trunk in adults. Lesions tend to be small and often are numerous. They contain a cluster of dilated capillaries in the upper dermis. Treatment is indicated only for cosmetic reasons.

Venous lakes are raised, violaceous lesions that occur on the exposed skin and lips of older people. Treatment, if cosmetically indicated, is vascular laser surgery.

Granuloma pyogenicum usually occurs as a solitary lesion that consists of a dark red, soft or firm pedunculated nodule. It grows rapidly and is most commonly found on the fingers or face. The oral cavity is a rather common site during pregnancy. Trauma may play a role in development. Granuloma pyogenicum responds well to laser treatment. The importance of this lesion lies in its resemblance to amelanotic malignant melanoma; therefore, laser ablation should take place only after a diagnostic biopsy has been done. Often the biopsy is curative.

Angiokeratoma is a term applied to several conditions that may or may not be associated with systemic disease (Fig. 19-15). *Angiokeratoma Mibelli* usually develops in childhood and is characterized by scattered hyperkeratotic red papules on the dorsum of the fingers and toes. *Angiokeratoma of the scrotum* consists of numerous hyperkeratotic red papules that arise in later life. *Papular angiokeratomata* are found in young adults as one to several papules on the lower limbs. These types of angiokeratomata are not associated with systemic disease. *Angiokeratoma circumscriptum,* sometimes present at birth, is characterized by reddish-blue papules or nodules that tend to cluster. These lesions usually have a deep hemangiomatous component and may be associated with several of the neurocutaneous diseases. The most important type of angiokeratoma occurs in association with Fabry disease and is called *angiokeratoma corporis diffusum.* This is an X-linked recessive disorder caused by a deficiency of the enzyme alpha-galactosidase A. In this condition, papular angiomas develop on the lower trunk and thighs in late childhood. In addition to the cutaneous findings, cardiovascular and renal disturbances develop.

Glomus tumors are tumors of vascular smooth muscle cells. They may occur alone or in small numbers. The solitary type is tender and is often found on the limbs, especially in the nail bed, although it does occur on other parts of the body (Fig. 19-16). It takes the form of a purple nodule composed of numerous vessels with surrounding sheets and strands of cuboidal glomus cells. Solitary lesions are treated by surgical excision. Laser ablation has been used for the multiple variety.

Tumors of Fat

Lipomas are solitary or multiple soft subcutaneous nodules that are freely mobile against the overlying skin. The back of the neck, the trunk, and the forearms are common locations. *Angiolipoma* is a variant that occurs as an encapsulated subcutaneous nodule, which is sometimes tender. These lesions can become evident at a young age. Multiple tender lipomas occur in Dercum disease (adiposis dolorosa). These lesions are indistinguishable from subcutaneous fat and may be removed surgically or by liposuction. If removed by liposuction, tissue should be sent for a pathologic examination to detect liposarcomas.

Nevus lipomatosus superficialis may be present at birth. It is composed of soft papules, nodules, or plaques usually seen on the thorax. Mature fat cells can be seen in the dermis on histologic examination (Fig. 19-17).

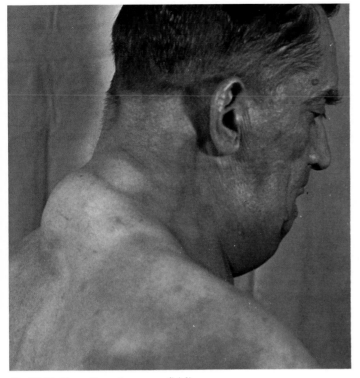

Fig. 19-17. *Nevus lipomatosus superficialis.*

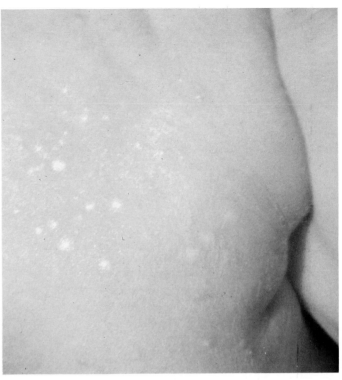

Fig. 19-18. *Milia, which may occur spontaneously, from trauma, or with bullous diseases.*

Tumors of Cutaneous Appendages

Tumors with Follicular Differentiation

Epidermal cysts are complex tumors that contain sebaceous material, keratin, and hair. For this reason, the old term *sebaceous cyst* is inappropriate. Epidermal cysts are slow-growing, elevated, firm round intracutaneous or intradermal tumors that vary from 1 to 5 cm in diameter. These nodules are found most commonly on the head, neck, and back. They cannot be distinguished clinically from pilar cysts. Excisional treatment is indicated for cosmetic reasons or if lesions become symptomatic.

Milia are keratinized cysts that may arise from the infundibulum of vellus hair follicles, sebaceous glands, or eccrine sweat ducts (Fig. 19-18). Clinically these tumors appear as solid, multiple, intraepidermal white papules 1 to 2 mm in diameter. Tumors may arise spontaneously or secondarily to trauma or subepidermal bullous disease. Simple extrusion of milial contents is the treatment of choice.

Dermoid cysts are thought to be the result of the sequestration of dysmorphic zones of skin along the lines of embryonic closure. The intracutaneous or subcutaneous tumors appear at birth as round, smooth-surfaced nodules, 1 to 5 cm in diameter. They are found most commonly on the face, often in a periocular location, particularly the lateral eyebrow.

Dermoid cysts are lined by epidermis to which are attached mature appended structures including hair follicles, sebaceous glands, eccrine glands, and sometimes apocrine glands. The need for excision of these lesions is dictated by their appearance.

Eruptive vellus hair cysts occur after occlusion of a vellus hair follicle at the level of the infundibulum as the result of a developmental abnormality. These tumors occur in children or young adults as an autosomal dominant trait with variable transmission. They are asymptomatic follicular papules 1 to 2 mm in diameter, arising most commonly on the chest and less commonly on the limbs and trunk. Clinically these tumors are difficult to distinguish from those of steatocystoma

multiplex, both occurring in similar anatomic locations. These lesions sometimes disappear spontaneously, but most often they persist indefinitely. Surgical excision of these tumors is impractical.

Pilar or *trichlemmal cysts* arise from the outer root sheath of the hair follicle and are clinically indistinguishable from epidermal cysts.

Pilomatricoma, or calcifying epithelioma of Malherbe, is an appended tumor with differentiation toward hair matrix, cortex, and inner root sheath cells. Most lesions arise in patients younger than the age of 20 years; there is a slight preponderance in females.

These tumors are usually solitary, firm, deep-seated blue nodules. They are most commonly located on the face and limbs and measure 0.5 to 3.0 cm in diameter. Pilomatricomas may be confused clinically with epidermal cysts, although the former are often much firmer on palpation. Treatment is by simple surgical excision.

Trichofolliculomas are common tumors with differentiation toward the inner and

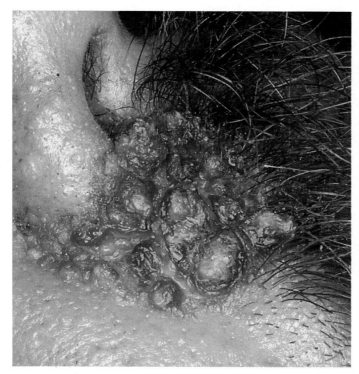

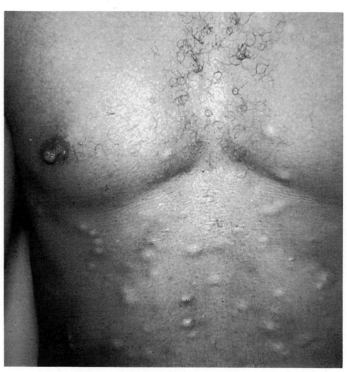

Fig. 19-19. *A close-up view of multiple tricholemmomas on the face associated with Cowden disease.*

Fig. 19-20. *Steatocystoma multiplex involving the chest.*

outer root sheaths of the hair. These tumors occur as solitary, small, skin-colored dome-shaped papules or nodules on the face and occasionally on the scalp or neck. Frequently a tuft of vellus hair is seen emerging from a central pore; when present such a tuft is highly suggestive of the diagnosis.

Trichofolliculomas are histologically well-differentiated tumors. The dermis contains an epidermally lined central large cystic space, often with extension to the surface.

Trichoepitheliomas are well-differentiated appended tumors with differentiation toward hair shaft cells. Lesions may be solitary or multiple. Solitary lesions are non-hereditary and develop in adults. Multiple trichoepitheliomas are transmitted as an autosomal dominant trait. Lesions initially appear during childhood and grow slowly in number thereafter. Multiple tumors are associated with the simultaneous appearance of cylindromas (turban tumor), and they may be difficult to distinguish clinically from angiofibromas found in patients with tuberous sclerosis.

Solitary lesions are skin-colored, smooth-surfaced papules or nodules, most commonly on the face.

Solitary trichoepitheliomas that do not show a high degree of differentiation toward hair follicles should be regarded as keratotic basal cell carcinomas and treated as such.

Tricholemmomas display epidermoid keratinization and occur fairly commonly as solitary and less commonly as multiple tumors. Individual lesions appear as nondescript skin-colored, dome-shaped papules most commonly on the face. Multiple tricholemmomas are markers for Cowden disease, an autosomal dominant condition characterized by the coexistence of multiple ectodermal, mesodermal, and endodermal hamartomas; punctate keratoderma of the palms; and lipomas. Cowden disease is associated with a high incidence of breast, thyroid, and gastrointestinal carcinoma (Fig. 19-19).

Tumors with Sebaceous Differentiation

Fordyce condition consists of ectopic sebaceous glands that appear as groups of small yellowish globoid deep-seated papules on the vermilion border of the lips and oral buccal mucosa. Lesions increase in number with age.

Sebaceous gland hyperplasia is a tumor of the sebaceous glands; two clinical forms exist. The first form occurs in newborn infants and represents increased sebaceous gland size and activity in response to maternal hormonal stimulation. These lesions resolve within the first few weeks post partum. Senile sebaceous gland hyperplasia occurs most commonly in patients older than 40 years.

Sebaceous gland hyperplasia appears as solitary or multiple, small, yellow-white, slightly umbilicated papules. The face, especially the cheeks and forehead, is primarily affected. The carbon dioxide laser is effective in the treatment of these lesions.

Steatocystoma multiplex is an autosomal dominant appendageal tumor. It usually first appears during adolescence as multiple, slow-growing, soft, freely movable cysts. Lesions are located on the upper anterior trunk, back, arms, thighs, and scrotum. They vary in size from 2 mm to several centimeters in diameter. Often

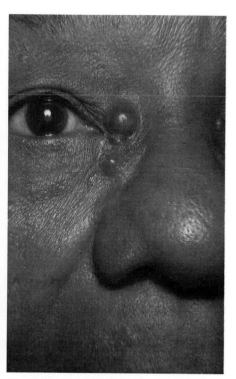

Fig. 19-21. Apocrine hidrocystoma (apocrine cystadenoma) of the face.

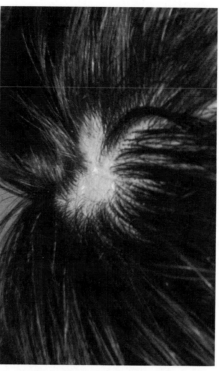

Fig. 19-22. Syringocystadenoma papilliferum of the scalp; one-third of lesions are associated with nevus sebaceus.

clinical distinction from epidermal cysts is difficult without a biopsy (Fig. 19-20).

The lesions may increase in both size and number with age. Surgical excision is generally unsatisfactory from the cosmetic point of view because of the large numbers of lesions.

Tumors with Apocrine Differentiation

Apocrine hidrocystoma (apocrine cystadenoma) appears as an asymptomatic, translucent, solitary, cystic blue nodule on the face. It results from a cystic proliferation of apocrine secretory cells (Fig. 19-21). Multiple tumors have been described as occurring on the ear, scalp, chest, and shoulders. These lesions are differentiated from blue nevi and melanomas by their cystic quality and lack of pigment. Treatment is surgical excision.

Bronchogenic cysts are common solitary nodules located in the midline on the anterior neck and chin, frequently at the sternal notch. They are apparent soon after birth. Clinically they are indistinguishable from thyroglossal cysts, and they must be differentiated from ectopic

thyroid by thyroid scan or ultrasonography. These cysts are lined with pseudostratified columnar epithelium; goblet cells, smooth muscle, and cartilage may occur in the cyst wall. Treatment is surgical excision.

Supernumerary nipples (polythelia) occur along a line from the anterior axillary fold to the medial thigh. They may be an isolated finding or may be associated with supernumerary breasts. Associated breast tissue may enlarge and become tender during puberty or pregnancy. Surgical excision is advisable because carcinoma of the breast has been found in these anomalies.

Syringocystadenoma papilliferum is a circumscribed hamartoma of the skin predominantly composed of apocrine glands. Clinically this lesion most commonly occurs as a plaque of grouped nodules on the neck, face, or scalp appearing at birth or during infancy. One-third of the lesions are associated with nevus sebaceus (Fig. 19-22). At puberty they enlarge, elevate, and become verrucous. Malignant transformation to basal cell carcinoma and, less frequently, squamous cell carcinoma has been reported;

hence surgical excision is recommended.

Hidradenoma papilliferum is a well-circumscribed, mobile, firm tumor of apocrine differentiation that occurs only in women, primarily on the vulva or in the perianal region. Histologically the tumor is composed of slender fronds of connective tissue with apocrine differentiation. It may be mistaken for an angioma, hemorrhoid, or epidermal cyst. A single instance of malignant transformation has been described. Treatment is surgical excision.

Cylindromas occur as multiple firm smooth nodules on the scalp that exhibit a distinctive mosaic-like structure. They appear in early adulthood and grow slowly; they may occur on the trunk and limbs. The differential diagnosis clinically includes tricholemmal cysts, which are mobile; trichoepithelioma; steatocystoma multiplex; and basal cell carcinoma. Malignant transformation has been described in solitary and multiple cylindromas. Surgical excision is the treatment of choice.

Tumors of Eccrine Differentiation

Eccrine hidrocystoma is a 1- to 3-mm translucent, cystic, solitary, often blue nodule, located most commonly on the eyelids and cheeks. It is more common on people who are exposed to extremes of heat such as cooks. Histologic analysis shows a single cystic cavity; serial sectioning may show an eccrine duct leading into the cyst, yet no connection with the epidermis is demonstrated. Treatment is excision or ablation.

Syringomas are common adenomatous tumors that present as 1- to 5-mm dermal papules on the eyelids, cheeks, neck, chest, or vulva. They occur after puberty and are usually multiple skin-colored papules in a bilaterally symmetric distribution. An eruptive variant occurs in which lesions arise in crops on the chest in young adults (Fig. 19-23). Most lesions we have seen treated by any method seem to have an unsatisfactory cosmetic result.

Eccrine poroma is an asymptomatic firm, solitary tumor primarily located on the ventral or lateral aspect of the foot, but it may be found on the hand, chest, or nose. A variant, eccrine poromatosis, with

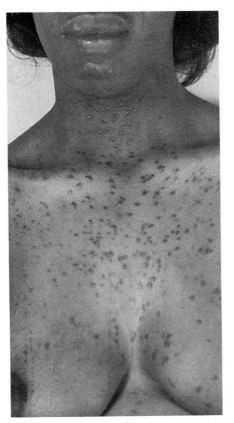

Fig. 19-23. Eruptive syringomas of the chest.

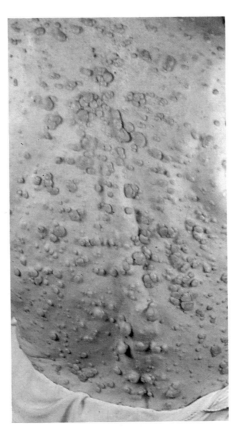

Fig. 19-24. Multiple neurofibromas in a patient with neurofibromatosis.

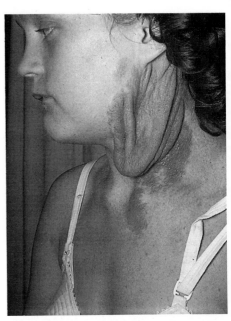

Fig. 19-25. Plexiform neurofibroma following the course of cervical nerves.

more than 100 nodules on the palms and soles, has been described. The structure is distinctive—broad anastomosing bands of uniform, small, cuboidal cells with intracellular bridges—and allows differentiation from verrucous carcinoma and verruca vulgaris. Malignant transformation has been described in poromas of long standing. A unique feature of this transformation is multiple cutaneous metastases. Treatment is early surgical excision.

Eccrine spiroadenoma is a benign tumor that occurs primarily as a solitary, firm, dark blue, tender nodule in early adulthood. The lesions may be multiple and zosteriform. Although they lack a characteristic location, most lesions are located on the chest and limbs. The diagnosis is made histologically. Malignant degeneration has occurred in long-standing solitary tumors, resulting in widespread metastases. Treatment is complete surgical excision.

Eccrine mixed tumor or chondroid syringoma is a 0.5- to 3-cm firm intradermal or subcutaneous nodule most commonly

found on the head and neck. Malignant chondroid syringomas have been reported; primarily they arise de novo, and widespread metastases have occurred. Treatment is surgical excision.

Tumors of Neural Crest Origin

Neural Tumors

A *neurofibroma* is an unencapsulated tumor that may occur anywhere on the body as a solitary, flesh-colored, soft pedunculated nodule. Single or multiple lesions can be associated with café au lait macules, axillary freckling, and pigmented iris hamartomas as a part of neurofibromatosis. Neurofibromatosis, or von Recklinghausen disease, has an autosomal dominant mode of inheritance; however, it frequently arises by spontaneous mutation (Fig. 19-24). Three particular forms of neurofibroma are to be noted. Mollusca fibrosa are soft dome-shaped nodules that may number in the hundreds; plexiform neurofibromas are

linear and follow the course of a nerve, most commonly the trigeminal or cervical nerves (Fig. 19-25). Finally, elephantiasis neurofibromatosa, which also follows nerves, is associated with an overgrowth of the subcutaneous tissue and skin with concomitant disfigurement. The condition requires aggressive surgical treatment, often with less than satisfactory results.

Neuroma represents a benign tumor of the peripheral nerves (Fig. 19-26). *Amputation*

Fig. 19-26. Neuroma involving a finger.

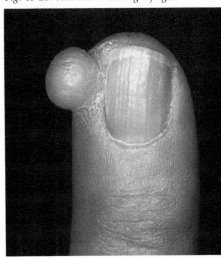

neuromas are sensitive to pressure, and *rudimentary supernumerary digits* are asymptomatic and located at the site of true supernumerary digits. Idiopathic cutaneous neuromas may be either single or multiple asymptomatic nodules that are located on the skin or oral mucosa; they have been associated with multiple endocrine neoplasia IIB. The lesions present as multiple small nodules on the lips, mucosa, tongue, nose, and eyelids. Recognition of this syndrome is critical because of associated intestinal ganglioneuromatosis, medullary thyroid carcinoma, and pheochromocytoma. In all patients the structure is distinctive, including large bundles of peripheral nerves. Treatment of individual lesions is surgical excision.

Granular cell tumor is a benign not infrequent tumor of Schwann cell origin found in the tongue (40%), skin, gastrointestinal tract, and skeletal muscle. The lesions may be solitary or multiple. Granular cell tumors of the skin are firm nodules that may be painful. The name is derived from the characteristic structure, large cells with pale cytoplasm filled with acidophilic granules, which distinguishes these from other tumors of the dermis. Pseudoepitheliomatous hyperplasia may occur in the overlying epidermis and should not be mistaken for squamous cell carcinoma. Malignant transformation to metastasizing granular cell myoblastoma has been reported. Treatment is complete surgical excision.

Cutaneous meningioma appears as cutaneous soft nodules with or without hair, possibly with a central depression, atrophy, or ulceration. Primary meningioma of intracranial origin extends into the skin directly or through a surgical defect. Primary cutaneous meningiomas occur on the scalp or forehead or paravertebrally. They may connect by a stalk to the central nervous system. They are benign and do not increase in size. Histologically secondary ectopic cutaneous meningiomas exhibit islands of cells with vesicular nuclei and pale-staining cytoplasm in a dense hyalinized stroma. Treatment is surgical.

Benign Pigment Cell Tumors

Four types of *lentigos* are recognized, including lentigo simplex, actinic lentigo, lentigo maligna (also called Hutchinson

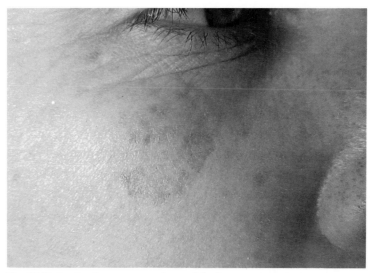
Fig. 19-27. Lentigo in a sun-exposed area of the face.

freckle), and ultraviolet A light (UVA)–induced lentigines (Fig. 19-27). Lesions of lentigo simplex develop in childhood; those of actinic lentigo develop after the fourth decade; and lentigo maligna develops in later life. Lentigines caused by ultraviolet A rays occur after multiple exposures to UVA or psoralen plus UVA (PUVA) in adolescence. Both lentigo simplex and actinic lentigo are benign lesions with no malignant potential. Lentigo maligna, on the other hand, may progress into invasive lentigo maligna melanoma in up to 30 percent of patients if left untreated.

Clinically lesions of lentigo simplex are evenly pigmented, well-demarcated macules without predilection for sun-exposed areas of the skin and measure 2 to 4 mm in diameter. In contrast, lesions of actinic lentigo occur most commonly on sun-exposed areas. Lentigo maligna begins as a fairly well-demarcated, unevenly pigmented macule, usually on the face or other sun-exposed area, and generally grows slowly to a size of 5 to 6 cm in diameter or larger. Ultraviolet A light (sunbed or tanning booth)–induced lentigines are sharply demarcated, irregularly shaped, darkly pigmented macules occurring on any exposed surface. Darkly pigmented, irregularly bordered lesions of lentigo simplex or UVA–induced lentigines should be subjected to biopsy or excised to differentiate them from malignant melanoma.

Surgical excision is the treatment of choice for lentigo maligna. Curettage and other destructive techniques are also acceptable for elderly people.

Becker melanosis, originally described as an organoid nevus with both epidermal melanocytic and dermal components, probably represents a localized area of androgen-hypersensitive cells. Lesions occur in all races with a male-female ratio of 5:1. Seventy-five percent of lesions occur before the age of 15 years, but lesions are not present at birth. In 25 percent of patients, a history of severe sunburn precedes the onset of the lesion.

Clinically lesions are island-shaped, well-demarcated, light brown to brown patches. They occur most frequently on the shoulder and chest but may appear on virtually any surface. Lesional hairiness is present more than 50 percent of the time. Once stable, lesions rarely fade, and malignant change does not occur. Associated developmental abnormalities include hypoplasia of the ipsilateral breast, areola, and nipple.

Lesions of Becker melanosis can be confused with those of giant congenital nevi and with the macule of Albright syndrome. Both are present at birth. Giant congenital nevi become elevated plaques. Becker melanosis is best left surgically ignored except perhaps for a small biopsy.

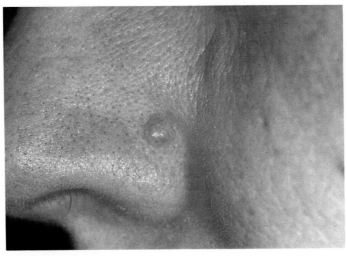

Fig. 19-28. Intadermal nevus on the nose.

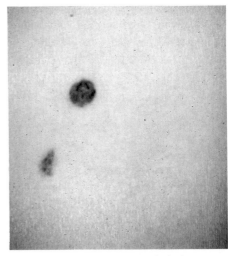

Fig. 19-29. Compound nevus on the back.

Café au lait macules are common cutaneous lesions that may be found at, or soon after, birth. They may be single inconsequential isolated lesions or they may be markers for several multisystem diseases. Lesions occur in all races and are found in 10 to 20 percent of the healthy population.

Clinically lesions are evenly pigmented light tan to light brown, well-demarcated macules with regular or irregular margins. Café au lait macules may be found on any cutaneous surface and have a tendency to disappear with old age.

Café au lait macules are markers for and are associated with many multisystem diseases. Most notably, lesions occur in patients with neurofibromatosis and Albright syndrome. Adults demonstrating six or more smooth-bordered café au lait macules measuring 1.5 cm or more in diameter have a greater than 95 percent chance of having neurofibromatosis. Café au lait macules in Albright syndrome are usually larger in size and fewer in number and have a characteristic ragged edge.

Acquired melanocytic nevi are composed of nests of nevus cells located in the epidermis (junctional nevi), dermis (intradermal nevi) (Fig. 19-28), or both (compound nevi) (Fig. 19-29). Nevus cells are dedifferentiated melanocytes and differ from melanocytes in their tendency to nest and in the absence of dendritic processes. Acquired nevi begin to appear at 6 to 12 months of age; most appear in ad-

olescence or early adulthood. Most lesions disappear late in life.

Acquired nevi can be found on any cutaneous surface, including the palms, soles, and nail beds, as well as the eye and oral mucosa. Junctional nevi are usually flat. Intradermal nevi are almost always papillomatous or dome-shaped. Compound nevi are usually slightly elevated or papillomatous with a flat pigmented ring at the periphery.

It is important to differentiate acquired nevi from congenital nevi, dysplastic nevi, and melanomas. Acquired nevi should be subjected to biopsy or completely excised if they change in size or color or become symptomatic.

Congenital nevi are melanocytic nevi that are present at birth and have an incidence of 1 percent. Congenital nevi range in size from less than 1 cm to garment sized or greater. Familial aggregations of both small and large congenital nevi occur frequently (Figs. 19-30 and 19-31).

Clinically congenital nevi appear the same as acquired nevi, except congenital nevi are usually larger. Various tumors and underlying bony abnormalities have been associated with giant congenital nevi. Giant, or garment-sized, congenital nevi also have an increased relative risk for the development of melanoma estimated to be at least 17-fold, with an estimated lifetime risk of at least 6.3 percent. Small congenital nevi (less than 3

cm) have an estimated relative risk for the development of melanoma of between threefold and 21-fold, and a risk of 0.8 percent to 4.9 percent by 60 years of age.

There is no unanimous opinion among dermatologists regarding the proper timing for surgical excision of congenital nevi. One treatment proposal suggests surgical excision of congenital nevi less than 1.5 cm in diameter after the age of 10 or 11 years if a given lesion is typical in appearance and stable in size. Giant congenital nevi (greater than 20 cm) unquestionably have an increased incidence of malignant change, even before the age of 5 years, and should be completely excised early in life, if possible. Appropriate surgical excision may require staged procedures or the use of tissue expanders. The limitations to surgical treatment are risk of anesthesia and lesser ability of an infant to withstand a serious operation.

A *halo nevus* is a melanocytic nevus surrounded by an area of depigmentation representing an area of tumor regression (Fig. 19-32). The overall prevalence of halo nevi is 0.9 percent; most nevi appear before the age of 20 years. Familial instances have been reported. Vitiligo, dysplastic nevi, and melanoma may occur more frequently in patients with halo nevi.

Halo nevi are typically pink or brown and are surrounded by a 0.5- to 5.0-mm halo of depigmentation. Halos can be seen sur-

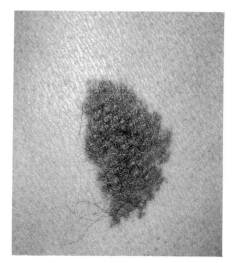

Fig. 19-30. Congenital nevus.

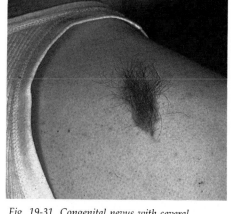

Fig. 19-31. Congenital nevus with several terminal hairs within the lesion.

Fig. 19-32. Halo nevus is a melanocytic nevus surrounded by an area of depigmentation.

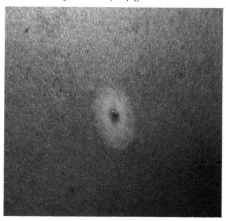

Fig. 19-33. Spitz nevus on the chest.

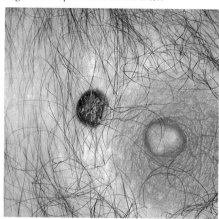

rounding acquired, congenital, and dysplastic nevi, as well as around melanomas. Multiple lesions have been reported frequently, and poliosis (white hair) may be seen in the depigmented areas.

It is important to differentiate benign halo nevi from tumor regression in dysplastic nevi and melanomas. Suspicious lesions should be excised completely.

Spitz nevi are benign melanocytic nevi sharing several histologic features with melanoma (Fig. 19-33). Lesions generally arise in children and young adults, with 25 percent of lesions occurring after the age of 30 years. Spitz nevi are usually hairless, pink-brown, solitary dome-shaped nodules measuring less than 6 mm in diameter. Histologically Spitz nevi can show clinically significant individual nevus cell atypia; however, an overall assessment of lesional architecture is usually sufficient to differentiate them from melanoma. Because it is often difficult to differentiate these lesions from melanoma clinically, suspicious lesions should be completely excised.

Blue nevi are acquired melanocytic nevi thought to represent ectopic collections of melanocytes in the dermis. The overall prevalence of blue nevi is 3.2 percent.

Treatment of typical-appearing blue nevi less than 1 cm in diameter is usually unnecessary. Existing lesions that change or lesions greater than 1 cm in diameter should be excised completely.

Dermal melanocytosis is thought to represent the failure of migration of dermal melanocytes to the epidermis during embryogenesis. Dermal melanocytosis can be classified as localized or generalized. Localized dermal melanocytosis of the sacrococcygeal region at birth is known as a Mongolian spot. These sacral lesions often disappear spontaneously. Localized dermal melanocytosis is most common in people of oriental descent; generalized dermal melanocytosis is rare.

There is no satisfactory treatment of persistent lesions of dermal melanocytosis.

Suggested Reading

Arons, M.S., and Hurwitz, S. Congenital nevocellular nevus: A review of the treatment controversy and a report of 46 cases. *Plast. Reconstr. Surg.* 72:355, 1983.

Bender, M. Concepts of wart regression. *Arch. Dermatol.* 122:644, 1986.

Brownstein, M.H., and Phelps, R.G. Papillary adenoma. *J. Am. Acad. Dermatol.* 12:707, 1985.

Cobb, M.W. Human papillomavirus infection. *J. Am. Acad. Dermatol.* 22:547, 1990.

Cook, B., and Solomon, L. Cylindromas. In *Birth Defects Encyclopedia.* Dover, MA: Center for Birth Defects, 1990. Pp. 1512–1513.

Fine, R.M., and Chernosky, M.E. Clinical recognition of clear-cell acanthoma (Degos'). *Arch. Dermatol.* 100:559, 1969.

Friedman, C.E., and Butler, D.F. Syringoma. *J. Am. Acad. Dermatol.* 16:310, 1987.

Knight, P.J., and Reiner, C.B. Superficial lumps in children: What, When, and Why. *Pediatrics* 72:147, 1983.

Kojima, T., Nagano, T., and Uchida, M. Periungual fibroma. *J. Hand Surg.* 12A:465, 1987.

Kullberg, B.J., and Nieuwenhuijzen Kruseman, A.C. Multiple endocrine neoplasia type 2b. *Arch. Intern. Med.* 147:1125, 1987.

Lanigan, S.W., and Robinson, T.W.E. Cryotherapy for dermatofibromas. *Clin. Exp. Dermatol.* 12:121, 1987.

Lee, S., Kim, J., and Kang, J.S. Eruptive vellus hair cysts. *Arch. Dermatol.* 120:1191, 1984.

Marschall, S.F., Ronan, S.G., and Massa, M.C. Pigmented Bowen's disease arising from pigmented seborrheic keratoses. *J. Am. Acad. Dermatol.* 23:440, 1990.

Paniago-Pereira, C., Maize, J.C., and Ackerman, A.B. Nevus of large spindle and/or epithelioid cells (Spitz's nevus). *Arch. Dermatol.* 114:1811, 1978.

Radentz, W.H., and Vogel, P. Congenital common blue nevus. *Arch. Dermatol.* 126:124, 1990.

Rhodes, A.R. Congenital nevi: Should they be excised? *J.A.M.A.* 262:1696, 1989.

Riccardi, V.M. Von Recklinghausen neurofibromatosis. *N. Engl. J. Med.* 305:1617, 1981.

Rodgers, M., McCrossin, I., and Commens, C. Epidermal nevus and the epidermal nevus syndrome. *J. Am. Acad. Dermatol.* 20:476, 1989.

Roth, D.E., Hodge, S.J., and Callen, J.P. Possible ultraviolet A–induced lentigines: A side effect of chronic tanning salon usage. *J. Am. Acad. Dermatol.* 20:950, 1989.

Smith, J., and Chernosky, M.E. Apocrine hydrocystoma. *Arch. Dermatol.* 109:700, 1974.

Solomon, L.M. The management of congenital melanocytic nevi. *Arch. Dermatol.* 116:1017, 1980.

Solomon, L.M., and Esterly, N.B. Epidermal and other congenital organic nevi. *Curr. Probl. Pediatr.* 6:3, 1975.

Sperling, L.C., and Sakas, E.L. Eccrine hidrocystoma. *J. Am. Acad. Dermatol.* 7:763, 1982.

20

Premalignant Skin Tumors, Basal Cell Carcinoma, and Squamous Cell Carcinoma

David T. Netscher   Maher Anous   Melvin Spira

We include here only the premalignant skin lesions that progress to basal cell carcinoma and squamous cell carcinoma and not those that are traditionally discussed with melanomas, that is, giant congenital nevi, dysplastic nevi, and lentigo maligna. For each of the premalignant lesions, we provide a clinical and histologic description and treatment options. Basal cell and squamous cell carcinomas are discussed separately, and reconstructive possibilities after tumor ablation are discussed by anatomic site involved and the special requirements of each region. We highlight, when appropriate, the natural history and treatment options unique to particular sites, including the hand, lip, eyelids, nasal vestibule, and external ear. We discuss the role of regional lymph node dissection in squamous carcinoma.

Premalignant Skin Tumors

Actinic Keratosis

Actinic keratoses are the most commonly occurring premalignant lesions of the skin. They are also called *senile keratoses* and *solar keratoses*. Most are caused by ex-

cessive exposure to sunlight and therefore occur on sun-exposed sites. They are rough and scaly, discrete epidermal lesions that are usually erythematous, but they range in color from yellow to dark brown (Fig. 20-1). They usually occur in genetically susceptible people, generally older men of Celtic origin. Marked hyperkeratosis may give rise to a cutaneous horn. Arsenical keratoses develop secondarily to exposure to inorganic arsenic compounds. They have a predilection for the palms and the soles, unlike actinic keratoses, which occur on the sun-exposed dorsum of the hand.

Actinic keratoses predominate on the nose, ears, cheeks, forehead, and dorsal surfaces of the hands and arms. They are frequently multiple and may be pruritic or painful. When the scales are removed, a bleeding surface remains. Lesions may coalesce, become superficially ulcerated, and bleed.

Histologic changes occur in both dermis and epidermis. In the epidermis there is a loss of the granular layer, disordered maturation and progression of the epidermal layers (dyskeratosis), and retention of nuclei in the keratin layer (parakeratosis). The keratotic layer is usually

thickened (hyperkeratosis). The basement membrane is thickened but intact. In the dermis there is frequently an inflammatory infiltration. The characteristic changes of elastosis are basophilic degeneration of connective tissue and fragmentation of elastic fibers.

Actinic keratoses frequently can be distinguished clinically; however, a firm diagnosis must be established by biopsy. Invasive squamous cell carcinoma is indicated by disruption of the basal membrane. In actinic keratoses, extension of abnormal epithelium along the processes of the skin adnexa may cause some confusion with squamous cell carcinoma.

Actinic keratoses can be considered to represent carcinoma in situ. Even though one study suggested that invasive squamous cell carcinoma develops in 20 percent of patients with actinic keratoses, the true incidence is probably much lower. Such carcinomas are less virulent than similar carcinomas arising in normal skin. Squamous cell carcinomas may arise de novo, but more commonly they arise from precursors. Thus actinic keratoses must be treated cautiously.

Treatment varies with anatomic location, the appearance of the lesion, and the age

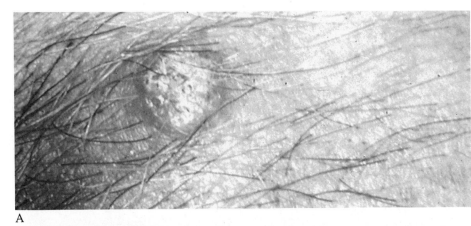

Fig. 20-1A. *Classic rough, scaly appearance of actinic keratosis. B. Diffuse facial actinic keratoses. C. Application of 5-fluorouracil initially causes marked erythema. D. Four weeks after last application of 5-fluorouracil. Actinic lesions have resolved.*

A

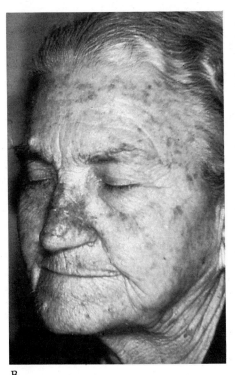

B

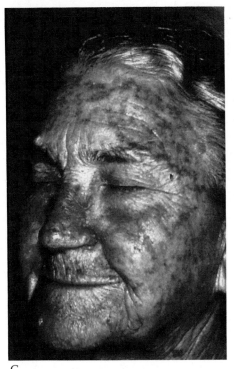

C

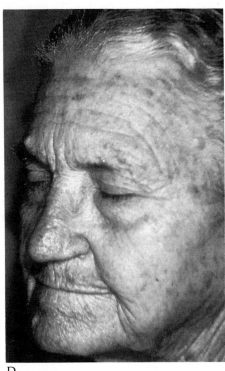

D

and general health of the patient. When appropriate, we prefer surgical excision of these premalignant lesions, particularly for larger, nodular lesions. Liquid nitrogen, superficial curettage, and light electrocautery are also acceptable modes of treatment. Topical application of 5-fluorouracil (5-FU) at least twice a day for 3 to 4 weeks is also commonly used. Such application is particularly useful for diffuse facial lesions when other forms of surgical therapy would be impractical (see Fig. 20-1). Lesions resistant to treatment with 5-FU may contain foci of squamous carcinoma. Systemic and topical retinoids also have been used to treat actinic keratoses.

Cutaneous Horns

Although cutaneous horns are not premalignant conditions, one should be aware of the lesions from which they arise. Cutaneous horns can occur in any lesion in which there is exaggerated hyperkeratotic growth that results in the compression of keratinous material into a conical mass. Thus cutaneous horns frequently arise from seborrheic keratoses, actinic keratoses, and infiltrating squamous cell carcinomas; extremely rarely they arise from basal cell carcinoma, keratoacanthoma, Kaposi sarcoma, and sebaceous adenoma. Up to 10 percent of patients have underlying squamous carcinoma.

These horns occur most commonly on sun-exposed parts of the skin—the face, the ears, and the dorsa of hands (Fig. 20-2). They seldom reach the remarkable proportions reported in the older literature, especially in areas in which access to health care is good; however, less dramatic, compacted growths are still common. Histologically the lesion consists of densely packed keratin, but the histologic structure of the underlying lesion is typical for the lesion involved.

Accurate determination of the underlying pathology requires excision of the lesion

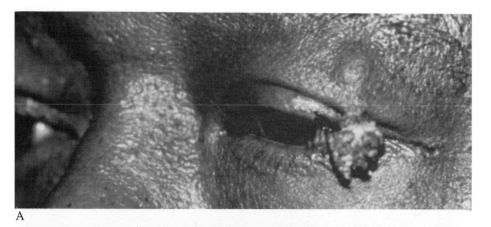

A

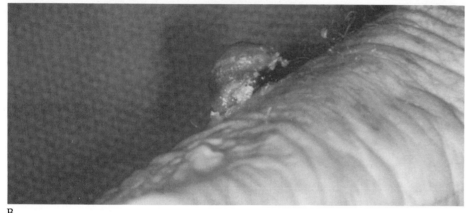

B

Fig. 20-2. Examples of cutaneous horns. A. On the eyelid. B. On the dorsum of the hand.

with a 1- to 2-mm margin of normal skin. Subsequent treatment depends on the nature of the underlying lesion.

Nevus Sebaceus of Jadassohn

Nevus sebaceus of Jadassohn is present at birth and gradually enlarges. The most common site is the scalp, but the face and neck, and more rarely the trunk and limbs, may be involved.

During childhood the lesion is quiescent; it is a circumscribed, slightly raised, yellow-brown plaque. At the time of puberty, it becomes much more noticeable, assuming a yellow, cobblestone appearance (Fig. 20-3).

The lesion is a hamartomatous conglomerate of large sebaceous glands associated with heterotopic apocrine glands and defective hair follicles. It is called an "organoid nevus" because it involves the entire skin organ and numerous skin adnexa.

In 10 to 20 percent of patients, nevus sebaceus evolves into a basal cell carcinoma. Complete excision before puberty is recommended.

Fig. 20-3A. Yellow-brown plaquelike lesion of nevus sebaceus. B. Nevus sebaceus in blacks may be darkly pigmented.

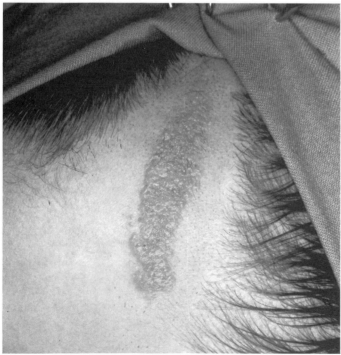

A

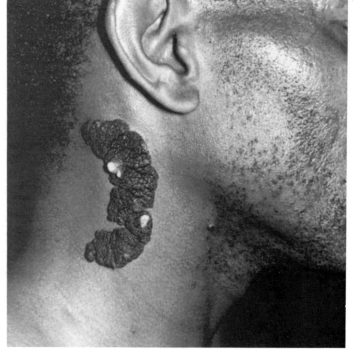

B

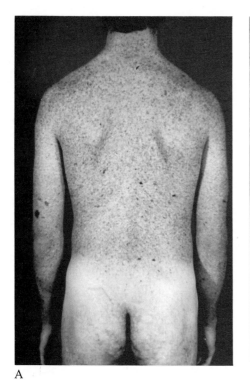 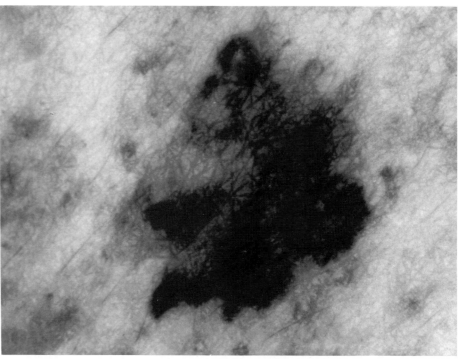

A   B

Fig. 20-4. Patient with xeroderma pigmentosum in whom malignant melanoma subsequently developed. (Courtesy of Don Gard, M.D.)

Xeroderma Pigmentosum

Xeroderma pigmentosum is a genodermatosis characterized by an autosomal recessive defect in which the DNA repair mechanism of ultraviolet light–induced damage is impaired. There is intolerance of the skin and eyes to ultraviolet light.

At birth, the skin appears normal. At the earliest exposure to sunlight, there is an exaggerated clinical sunburn reaction. With repeated exposure pigmentary changes occur, giving the appearance of intensely pigmented freckles (Fig. 20-4). Drying and thickening of the skin occur subsequently, with ultimate cutaneous and subcutaneous atrophy, particularly around the eyes, nose, and mouth. Early in the evolution of the syndrome, the eyes are painfully sensitive to light and they tear excessively. In more severe instances, there is progressive neurologic deterioration, leading to xerodermic idiocy. In many patients, multiple malignant epithelial tumors and melanomas appear in the first decade of life, and the patient dies in the second decade. The prognosis for these patients remains dismal. There is no specific treatment. Use of sun-protective clothing and topical sunscreens and an indoor life-style are the most effective preventive measures. The child must be monitored frequently to detect and treat the malignant cutaneous lesions.

Other Premalignant Skin Conditions

Epidermodysplasia Verruciformis
In this condition wartlike lesions occur on the face, neck, hands, feet, and trunk. The lesions have a viral cause (human papillomavirus, HPV-3, HPV-5) and degenerate into squamous cell carcinomas. T-cell function is defective.

Porokeratosis
A hereditary condition, porokeratosis is characterized by disseminated annular plaques with sharply raised horny borders. Approximately 13 percent of these lesions transform into basal and squamous cell carcinomas. The most common type is porokeratosis of Mibelli (Fig. 20-5).

Disseminated Superficial Actinic Porokeratosis
These lesions are smaller than those of porokeratosis of Mibelli, and the frequency of malignant transformation is not as high. Lesions occur primarily on sun-exposed parts of the body.

Rare Syndromes Associated with Skin Cancers
Basal Cell Nevus Syndrome

Basal cell nevus syndrome is also called Gorlin syndrome. The typical nevi are reddish brown in color, papular, and of various sizes. In most patients, the nevi appear after puberty. The lesions number from a few to many thousands in each patient. These lesions may become invasive basal cell carcinomas. The principal features of the syndrome are as follows (Fig. 20-6):

1. Multiple basal cell carcinomas scattered throughout the body

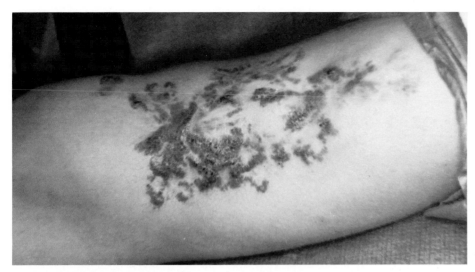

Fig. 20-5. *Porokeratosis of Mibelli. This lesion is on the anterior aspect of the thigh.*

Fig. 20-6. *Classic facial features of Gorlin syndrome with broad nasal root and hypertelorism. Multiple facial nevi have become invasive basal cell carcinomas. (Courtesy of Don Gard, M.D.)*

A   B

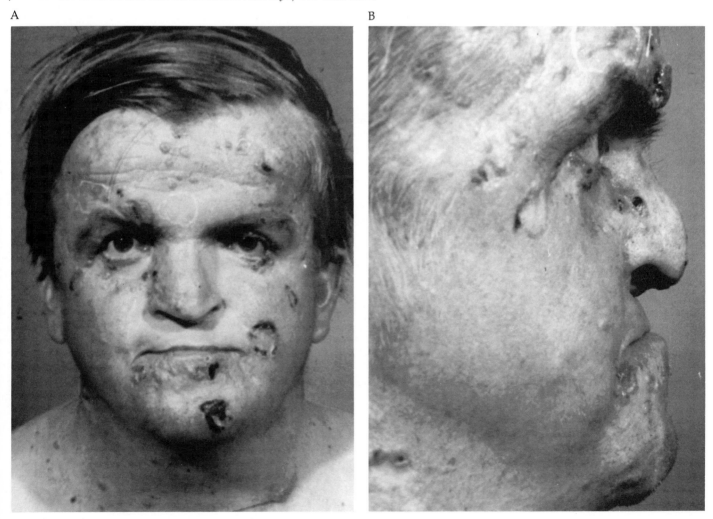

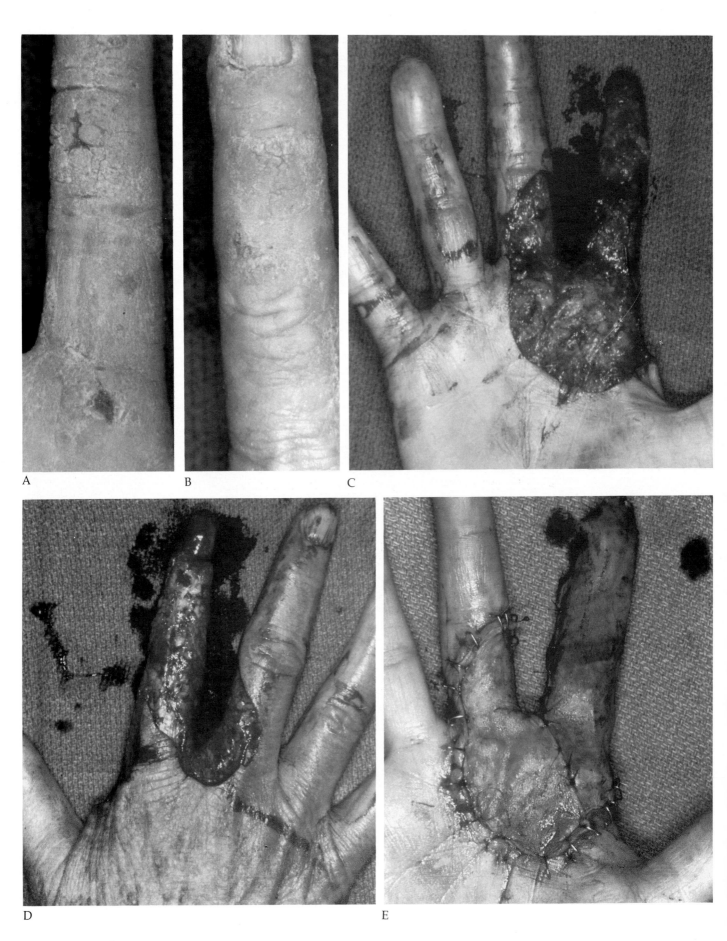

A

B

C

D

E

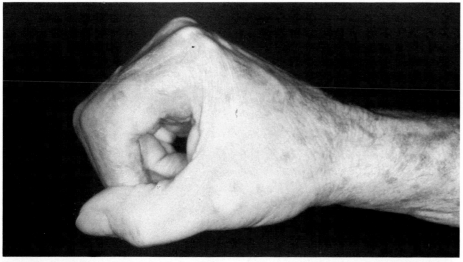

F

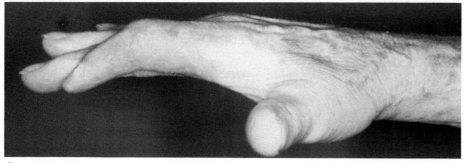

G

Fig. 20-7A, B. Bowen disease affecting the hand. This dry, crusting lesion was present for many years in this 70-year-old patient. She had numerous dermatologic treatments before a biopsy was finally performed. C, D. Surgical excision using the Mohs micrographic surgical technique. (Courtesy of Leonard Goldberg, M.D.) E, F, G. Immediate split-thickness skin grafting results in functional hand with normal sensation at index fingertip.

2. Jaw cysts
3. Skeletal abnormalities such as bifid ribs, scoliosis, brachymetacarpalism
4. Overdeveloped supraorbital ridges, broad nasal root, and hypertelorism
5. Palmar and plantar pits
6. Calcification of falx cerebri
7. Occasional neurologic abnormalities, including mental retardation and medulloblastomas

Bazex Syndrome

Bazex syndrome was first described in 1966 and is inherited as an X-linked dominant trait. It consists of follicular atrophoderma with multiple basal cell carcinomas, hypotrichosis, and hypohidrosis.

Other Syndromes

Other syndromes associated with skin cancers are Haber syndrome, dyskeratosis congenita, and Rothmund-Thomson syndrome. Haber syndrome is a variant of Bowen disease consisting of a familial rosacea-like eruption of the face and Bowen lesions on the covered areas of the body.

Carcinoma In Situ

Bowen disease is an intraepidermal squamous cell carcinoma (carcinoma in situ). It occurs predominantly in Caucasian males in sun-exposed sites. Grossly it presents as a brown verrucous plaque. Crusting with underlying serous oozing may be present (Fig. 20-7). When Bowen disease appears on the glans penis, it is called erythroplasia of Queyrat.

Although most carcinomas remain localized indefinitely, 10 percent of tumors become invasive after many years. When invasive carcinoma develops, it has a tendency to be more virulent than squamous carcinomas arising de novo; metastatic disease develops in at least one-third of patients. It has been reported that other skin and mucocutaneous lesions of premalignant or malignant nature develop in as many as one-half of these patients and that primary malignant extracutaneous tumors develop in 25 percent. The association with extracutaneous malignant tumors remains controversial, however.

Histologic features include hyperkeratosis, parakeratosis, acanthosis, and destruction of the normal progression of epidermal maturation. There is increased mitotic activity, and giant cells may be seen. The basement membrane remains intact. Histologically Bowen disease may resemble bowenoid variations of actinic keratosis and Paget disease. Immunohistologic techniques might distinguish among these conditions.

Surgical excision with a margin of normal tissue is the most effective treatment. Because of deep follicular involvement, curettage and topical application of 5-FU are frequently followed by recurrence.

Basal Cell Carcinoma

Basal cell carcinoma appears as an ulcer with raised, pearly edges and an erythematous base. Definitive diagnosis requires biopsy and histologic examination. If the lesion is small, excisional biopsy can be performed. For larger lesions, however, incisional biopsy or punch biopsy should be done and histologic confirmation obtained before a major ablative procedure is considered. Prior incisional biopsy of basal cell (or squamous cell) carcinoma does not adversely affect the prognosis or natural history of the tumor, provided the lesion is excised as soon as the histologic diagnosis is confirmed by permanent section.

Histology

Four clinical types of basal cell carcinoma are generally recognized (Fig. 20-8):

1. *Superficial basal cell carcinoma* is a scaly, erythematous lesion flush with the skin surface. It is frequently confused with eczema, actinic keratosis, or fungal infection.
2. *Nodular basal cell carcinoma*, also called adenoid-cystic basal cell carcinoma, is a flesh-colored nodular lesion with multiple telangiectatic vessels.
3. *Pigmented basal cell carcinoma* has a brown pigmentation, sometimes even blue-black, and may be confused with a melanoma or seborrheic keratosis.
4. *Morphea-like (sclerosing) basal cell carcinoma* presents as a firm plaque with surrounding "scar" tissue. There almost never is ulceration and there is little skin elevation.

Basal cell carcinomas are the most frequent form of skin cancer and occur predominantly on sun-exposed skin in direct proportion to the number of pilosebaceous units present. Fair-skinned, blue-eyed people engaged in outdoor occupations or activities have a high incidence of these tumors. Although metastases are extremely rare (less than 0.1%), these lesions can invade by direct extension and may result in death by invasion into vital structures or from superimposed infection.

Six histologic types have been described, which roughly parallel the clinical types—superficial, nodular, nodular-ulcerative, ulcerative, infiltrative, and morphea-like. Some authors believe the ulcerative, infiltrative, and morphea-like lesions behave more aggressively than the others. Such aggressive behavior remains unclear, however, except in the distinctive sclerosing lesions.

Histologically basal cell carcinomas arise from the basal layer of the epidermis and from the pilosebaceous adnexa. The characteristic cell has a large basophilic nucleus with minimal cytoplasm. Tumor cells at the periphery of any nest of cells are oriented with their long axes perpendicular to the nest giving a "picket fence" appearance. Mitotic figures are seen only occasionally. The presence of keratinocytic differentiation has resulted in the term *basosquamous carcinoma.* Such an entity may not exist, however; basal cell carcinomas that have squamous differentiation behave no differently from pure basal cell carcinomas. They are not an intermediate step toward squamous carcinoma. As already indicated, pigment may be seen in the tumor, and, in the morphea-like cancers, considerable dermal collagen compresses the tumor cells into cords.

Basal cell carcinomas were once thought to be multicentric. Often, however, these apparently disconnected lesions have been found on serial sections to be connected along rete ridges.

According to one study in the United States that investigated the anatomic distribution of basal cell carcinomas, 86 percent occur on the face and scalp, 7 percent on the neck, and 7 percent on the rest of the body. The most commonly occurring sites are the nose (25.5%), the cheek (16%), the periorbital region (14%), the

scalp (11%), and the ear and periauricular region (11%). A report from Australia showed a trend toward a greater proportion of lesions on the trunk and limbs.

Although basal cell carcinoma is the most commonly occurring skin cancer, it is relatively rare on some anatomic sites, such as the hand, penis, and lip. Squamous cell carcinomas are much more common than basal cell carcinomas at these sites. Although often affected by basal cell carcinoma, the external ear is more frequently affected by squamous cell carcinoma. Squamous cell carcinoma is the most common skin cancer on the external ear, accounting for 50 to 60 percent of the total number of tumors of that organ. Basal cell carcinoma accounts for 30 to 40 percent, and melanoma for the rest. All skin cancers are rare in the external auditory canal, but at this site also squamous cell carcinomas outnumber basal cell cancers.

Treatment

Radiation Therapy
Radiation therapy has an overall cure rate of 92 percent, but it requires specialized equipment. It is generally reserved for older patients because the resultant scar becomes worse with time and may later ulcerate. In selected sites radiation therapy may be the treatment of choice or it may serve as an adjunct to surgical excision, especially when the surgical margins are not clear in large, relatively inaccessible tumors. These lesions include invasive tumors at the medial canthus close to the lacrimal apparatus and invasive tumors at the pyriform aperture.

Electrodesiccation and Curettage
Electrodesiccation with curettage is one of the more common methods of treatment. Although it is a simple method of therapy, the procedure should be reserved for small lesions: The cure rate has been shown clearly to be inversely proportional to the size of the tumor. The cure rate was 100 percent for lesions less than 2 mm in diameter, but the recurrence rate was 50 percent for tumors larger than 3 cm in diameter.

Cryosurgical Therapy
Cryosurgical therapy has been reported to have an overall cure rate of greater than 97 percent. In that series, however, most

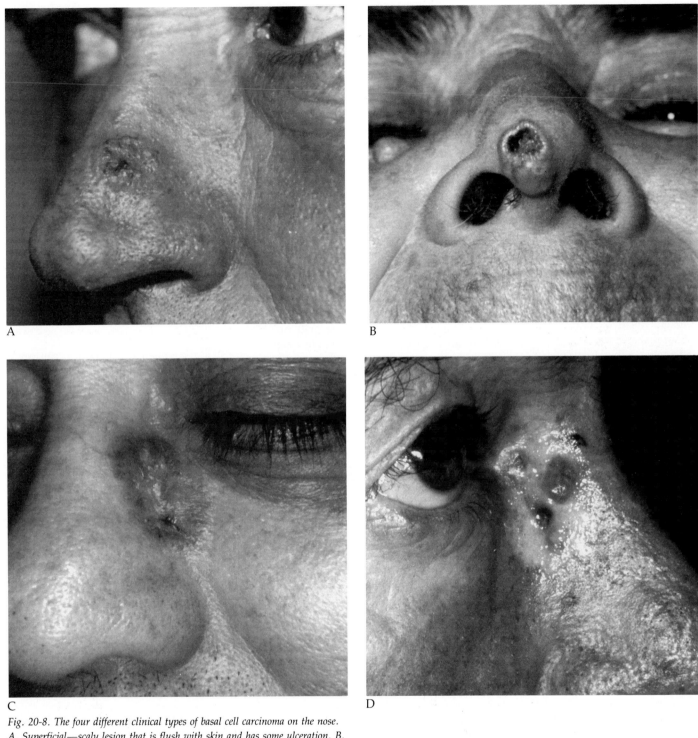

A

B

C

D

Fig. 20-8. The four different clinical types of basal cell carcinoma on the nose.
A. Superficial—scaly lesion that is flush with skin and has some ulceration. B.
Adenoid cystic—nodular lesion. C. Pigmented. D. Sclerosing—poorly defined
edges.

of the lesions were less than 2 cm in diameter. The morbidity is high and the cosmetic results unpredictable. The problems include a long period of edema (4 to 6 weeks), permanent loss of pigment, and atrophic or hypertrophic scars. Neuropathy from adjacent nerve injury may occur, particularly on digits or around the elbow. An inherent disadvantage is the lack of microscopic verification of complete eradication of the tumor.

The accepted indications for cryosurgical therapy are nodular or ulcerated carcinomas and tumors with well-oriented borders. Other indications might be for palliation in advanced tumors and the treatment of elderly patients and patients at poor surgical risk. Absolute contraindications to cryosurgical therapy are abnormal intolerance to cold, as in cryoglobulinemia, and morphea-like basal cell carcinoma. Relative contraindications are lesions that are recurrent, larger than 3 cm in diameter, adherent to bone or cartilage, directly over superficially located nerves (lateral borders of digits and ulnar groove of the elbow), or involving the vermilion border of the lip or the free margin of the eyelid (where a deforming cicatrix would be unacceptable).

Chemotherapy
Chemotherapy with topical 5-FU or with retinoids does not have acceptable cure rates for general use for basal cell carcinomas.

Surgical Therapy
Surgical excision gives an overall cure rate of greater than 90 percent. When excising a skin tumor, we prefer to use loupe magnification. This allows more accurate visual assessment of the tumor borders. The tumor border and margin of surgical excision should be marked before injection of the local anesthetic agent because injection causes tumor distortion and prevents accurate palpation of the tumor borders. Reconstruction of the surgical defect can generally be done by undermining of the edges and linear closure (Fig. 20-9).

The success rate depends primarily on the size of the lesion, the anatomic site, and the histologic type. In most instances, visual assessment of margins is accurate. A 2-mm surgical margin has been said to provide a 94 percent cure rate, except in morphea-like lesions. In many texts, however, margins up to 5 mm are rec-

ommended to achieve cure. Generally speaking, the larger the tumor, the wider is the surgical margin required to achieve cure. The confidence with which one can predict the adequacy of surgical excision depends not on the width of the surgical margin, but on the completeness with which the surgical margin is examined histologically.

The technique of micrographic surgery was developed by Frederick Mohs. At present fresh tissue modification does not involve using a fixative, as it originally did. Horizontal frozen sections of the entire undersurface of the excised tissue are made and examined microscopically. Cure rates by the Mohs micrographic technique are as high as 99 percent for primary lesions and 96 percent for recurrent basal cell carcinoma.

The use of frozen sections (with or without the Mohs micrographic technique) is expensive and so is not recommended for every patient. In a location where wide surgical margins can be taken safely and where repair does not involve rearrangement of local tissues (that is, repair requires direct suture closure only or the application of a skin graft), one can safely excise the lesion and await the pathologic interpretation of the permanent sections. In such a situation, if microscopic margins are involved, one can perform a reexcision without adversely affecting the probability of cure. We generally perform frozen sections in treating biopsy-proved recurrent lesions or in situations in which a more elaborate flap closure is planned for immediate reconstruction of the defect (even when one might believe a wide clinical tumor-free margin has been excised).

Some tumor types, especially morphea-like (sclerosing) lesions, have a propensity for large subclinical extension. As a result, it is hard to predict clinically the adequacy of surgical excision, and recourse is frequently made to frozen sections when excising these tumors.

Various anatomic sites show a higher than usual recurrence rate. Recurrent tumors are virtually unknown on the trunk, limbs, and cheeks. Recurrent tumors are distributed most frequently around the eyes, ears, and nose. One of the reasons for the high recurrence rates at these sites is the difficulty of achieving adequate margins during resection because of ad-

jacent vital structures or the desire to obtain a good cosmetic result.

In summary, basal cell carcinomas should be treated with an appropriate method according to their size, anatomic location, histologic characteristics, and whether they are primary or recurrent. Indications for the Mohs micrographic surgical technique include basal cell carcinomas with the following features:

1. Recurrence
2. Poorly delineated margins, either arising in scar tissue or morphea-like
3. Sites with relatively high rates of treatment failure—periorbital, periauricular, nasal, and perinasal
4. Critical location where maximal preservation of uninvolved tissue is desirable such as the eyelid
5. Large size—more than 3 cm in diameter

It is recommended that basal cell carcinoma with proved marginal involvement on initial treatment be reexcised once the wound is healed. This is because the generally accepted recurrence rate is 35 percent if nothing more is done, and one-third of recurrences are more extensive and more difficult to manage than the original tumor. One study found three histologic features to be predictive of recurrence: cellular palisading, ulceration, and lymphocytic infiltration. Irregularity in the peripheral palisade seems to have major prognostic significance with regard to tumor aggressiveness; thus management guidelines have been established to deal with tumors that have positive surgical margins. In one series no tumor with positive histologic margins and with minimal irregularity in the peripheral palisade layer (less than 25% of tumor cords) recurred in a 5-year follow-up study, demonstrating that these tumors can be safely observed. Tumors with an intermediate range of irregular palisading (25 to 75% of tumor cords) should be reexcised, however, if there is ulceration or sparse lymphocytic infiltration. All highly irregular lesions should be reexcised; the study found a 93 percent recurrence rate in these tumors when histologic margins were positive.

Recurrence

Recognition of recurrent basal cell carcinoma can be difficult. Clinical signs that

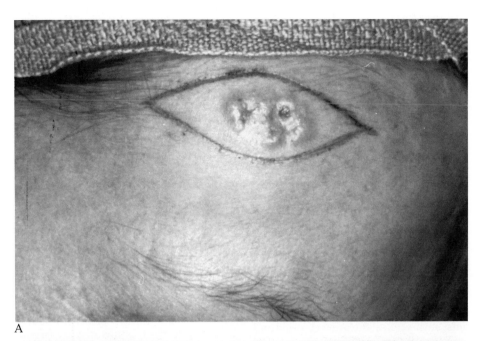

A

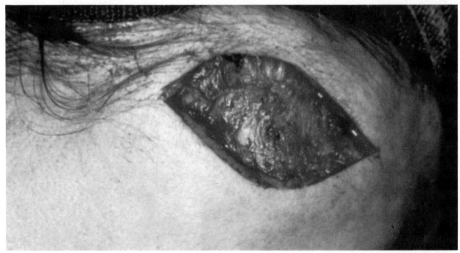

B

Fig. 20-9A. Margin of surgical excision of this basal cell carcinoma is marked out before infiltration of local anesthetic. B. The simplest, most practical method should be used to reconstruct the surgical defect, most frequently undermining and direct linear layered closure. C. Almost imperceptible scarring results after meticulous technique.

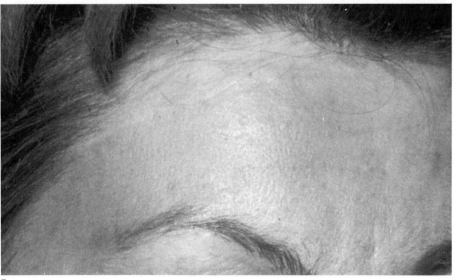

C

may alert the physician to a recurrence are as follows:

1. Scaling, erythema, crusting, or intermittent ulceration that developed within the previous scar
2. An enlarging scar with increased telangiectasis
3. Development of papules or nodules within the scar
4. Frank tissue destruction that might produce problems such as loss of eyelashes or progressive elevation of the nasal ala

Surgical margins considered adequate for excision of a primary tumor are not satisfactory in dealing with recurrent cancers because of distortion produced by scarring. The Mohs micrographic surgical technique proves invaluable for adequately tracing out tumor extensions beyond clinically detectable areas of disease.

Squamous Cell Carcinoma

Squamous cell skin cancers are only one-fourth as common as basal cell carcinomas. They tend to be more indurated, to grow more rapidly, to ulcerate sooner, and, seemingly, to have an even stronger actinic basis. Nearly all tumors arise in sun-exposed areas of the face, trunk, and limbs. They rarely arise in unaltered skin, and there is nearly always associated sun damage to surrounding skin, actinic keratosis, radiation keratosis, scar, or chronic ulceration.

Usually the lesions are ulcerated and crusted, but they may be raised, papillomatous, or verrucous. Verrucous carcinomas are well-differentiated squamous cell carcinomas capable of local invasion, but they rarely metastasize. Verrucous carcinomas occur most commonly on the palms and soles, where they are known as carcinoma cuniculatum. It may be difficult to distinguish verrucous carcinoma from pseudoepitheliomatous hyperplasia, which is a completely benign condition caused by chronic inflammation.

Squamous cell carcinomas arise from the prickle cell layer. The histologic findings are diagnostic. Surface epithelium is acanthotic and irregularly penetrating into the dermis. Variable parakeratosis and hyperkeratosis occur. Varying degrees of anaplasia and mitoses are found. Well-differentiated tumors contain numerous keratin pearl formations. Some highly anaplastic tumors are impossible to categorize by light microscopy. Immunoperoxidase stains distinguish desmoplastic melanoma and poorly differentiated squamous cell carcinoma from other spindle tumors. Epidermal cytokeratin antibody is specific for tumors of the squamous epithelium.

Prognosticators of tumor recurrence include the degree of differentiation, depth of invasion, and surface size. In one series the recurrence rate was 7 percent if the tumor was well differentiated, 23 percent if moderately differentiated, and 28 percent if poorly differentiated. Depth of tumor invasion to Clark IV or V levels (or below the reticular dermis) increases the risk of recurrence severalfold.

Perineural invasion is also related to poor prognosis; it occurs in 5 percent of all cu-taneous squamous cell carcinomas. Clinical signs include paresthesia and paralysis. In one study only one-third of patients with the histologic finding of perineural spread were free of disease at 5 years. When treated by micrographic surgical therapy, however, no tumor recurred in 17 patients with perineural invasion, but the follow-up period in this study was quite short (average of 16 months).

The incidence of regional node metastases for cutaneous squamous cell carcinoma is only 2 percent. In anatomic sites such as the scalp, nostril, ears, lower lip, and limbs, however, there is a greater propensity to metastases. Lesions with unusual causes such as Marjolin ulcer are also more prone to spread to lymph nodes (Fig. 20-10). For this reason treatment must be directed at the primary lesion and at regional nodes in selected patients. The place of node dissection is considered in the discussion of the individual anatomic sites. In a series from M. D. Anderson Hospital, burn scar carcinoma was shown to have a 35 percent incidence of regional metastases. A case can possibly be made for elective regional node dissection, particularly in Marjolin ulcer of the lower limb. Squamous carcinomas originating in decubitus ulcers, chronic sinuses, and radiation ulcers also behave aggressively.

A review of squamous cell tumors of the skin of the head and neck revealed that 14 percent had perineural invasion in one or more major nerve trunks. Regional lymph node metastases occurred more frequently in these patients. Whether the lesion is squamous cell carcinoma or basal cell carcinoma, perineural growth is considered to be a manifestation of aggressive tumor behavior. Recommended therapy for squamous carcinomas demonstrating perineural invasion is not only adequate resection of involved tissue and nerves but also regional lymphadenectomy followed by postoperative radiation therapy.

Treatment of the local lesion involves radiation therapy or surgical excision. Sometimes both may be required. The width of the surgical margin necessary to achieve cure is generally accepted to be considerably wider than for basal cell carcinoma. Thus the Mohs micrographic surgical technique should be considered for all large tumors (greater than 2 cm). Other indications for the Mohs micrographic excision include recurrent tumors, tumors with perineural invasion, and tumors in critical locations.

Cutaneous Malignant Tumors at Specific Anatomic Sites

Upper Limb

Basal cell carcinoma is rare on the hand; when present, it is usually located on the dorsum. When located near the nail bed, it can be mistaken for paronychial infection. If the nail matrix is involved because of proximity to periosteum, amputation at the distal interphalangeal joint may be required to reach normal tissue margins. Local excision of basal cell carcinoma on the dorsum of the hand is satisfactorily reconstructed with a skin graft (Fig. 20-11). On the dorsum of the arm, again, thin and pliable tissue must be used for reconstruction. Skin grafts remain useful. Local flaps, such as rotation advancement or bilobed flaps, may also be used. Incorporation of fascia in the cutaneous flap enhances its vascularity and reliability (Fig. 20-12).

Squamous cell carcinoma of the hand has a 10 percent 5-year mortality with a local recurrence rate of 22 percent and a lymph node metastasis rate of 28 percent. For lesions smaller than 2.5 cm in diameter, wide excision of a 2- to 3-cm clear margin is recommended. For larger lesions, however, because of the high rate of local recurrence, more radical excision is required; treatment may include ray or segmental amputation.

Lymph node metastases occur frequently (67% of the time) with recurrent squamous cell carcinomas of the hand. Lymphadenectomy is advised for recurrent tumors even if the lymph nodes are not clinically palpable. Routine prophylactic lymphadenectomy for primary tumors, however, is not beneficial. Awaiting the clinical presence of lymphatic metastases does not seem to worsen the 5-year survival rate. It is suggested that radiation therapy be added to lymphadenectomy if there is extracapsular nodal spread or if nodes are greater than 3 cm in diameter.

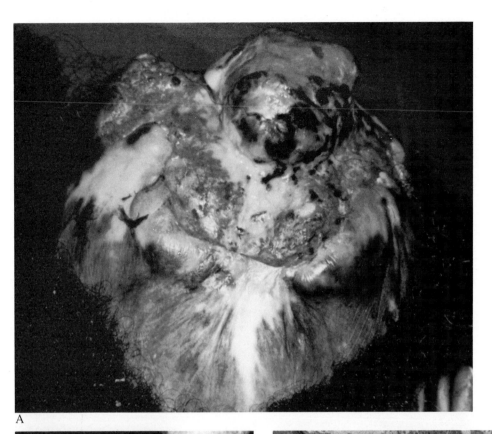

Fig. 20-10A. Obviously fungating squamous cell carcinoma on the scalp in an area of burn alopecia. B. A clinically less obvious squamous cell carcinoma in an unstable burn scar of the lower limb. C. Invasive carcinoma is seen on biopsy of this lesion.

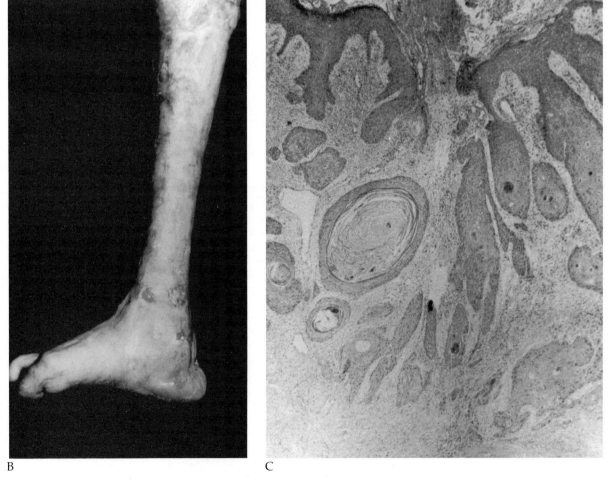

A

B

C

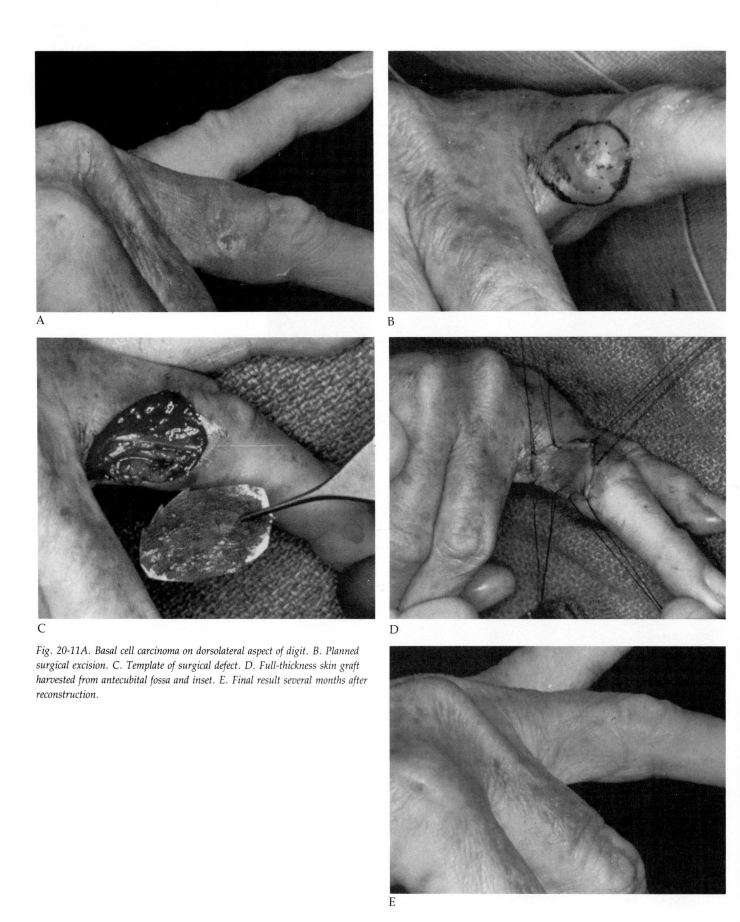

Fig. 20-11A. Basal cell carcinoma on dorsolateral aspect of digit. B. Planned surgical excision. C. Template of surgical defect. D. Full-thickness skin graft harvested from antecubital fossa and inset. E. Final result several months after reconstruction.

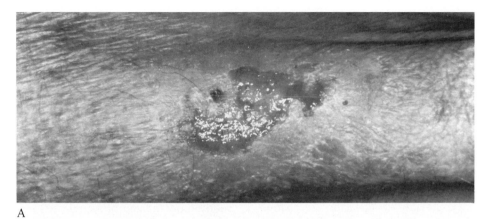

A

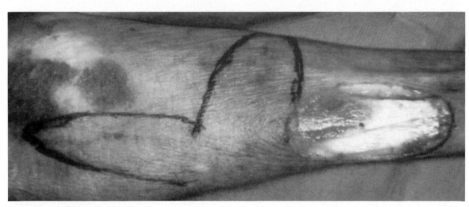

B

Fig. 20-12A. Forearm basal cell carcinoma in an elderly man who worked outdoors for many years. B, C. A bilobed fasciocutaneous flap was used to provide stable coverage of the exposed tendons. D. Final result.

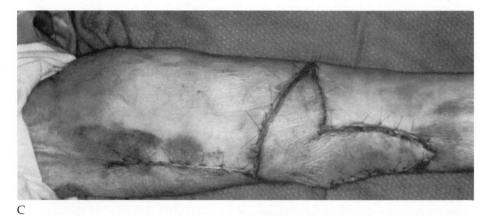

C

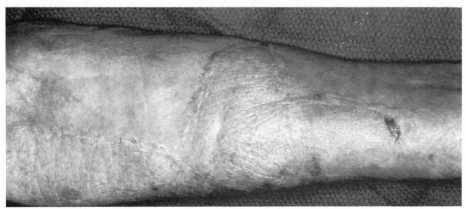

D

Squamous cell carcinoma involving the nail matrix and paronychium is often a difficult diagnostic problem. Distal phalangeal amputation provides a high cure rate. Tumor growth of these lesions is slow, and metastases are unusual. The Mohs micrographic surgical technique has a role, ensuring complete removal of disease with maximal preservation of normal tissue and digital function.

Nose

Excision of cancers from the nose follows the surgical principles already enunciated. Micrographic surgical technique is probably best used for tumors in the nasolabial region because of the propensity of these lesions to invade deeply toward the pyriform aperture and because of the higher rate of recurrence.

Squamous cell carcinoma of the nasal vestibule tends to behave differently. Aggressive local growth is indicated by a tumor that invades into the adjacent columella, floor of the nose, and upper lip and is associated with a high incidence of nodal metastases. Surgical and radiation therapy are equally effective for the primary lesion, but radiation therapy has the disadvantage of producing a local drying effect. Once the upper lip has been invaded, access is gained to the rich lymphatic system. Drainage may be homolateral or bilateral and includes the lower parotid nodes, buccinator nodes, and upper neck nodes. Because of the wide lymphatic drainage, one should await the clinical presence of lymph node metastases before performing a node dissection. Postoperative radiation therapy after the dissection should include the lymphatics between the neck and the primary tumor site.

Reconstruction of the nasal defect depends on the specific requirements of the anatomic site. One should try to resurface anatomic units. The contour and sebaceous nature of the tip and alae present special reconstructive challenges. Various local flaps can be used to cover small defects. A nasolabial flap pivoted proximally near the infraorbital margin enables cheek advancement to reconstruct the nasal-cheek angle and to prevent flattening of this angle, which might be caused by a nasolabial flap pivoted more inferiorly (Fig. 20-13). The nasolabial flap is also helpful in reconstructing the alae.

Local unilobar and bilobed flaps and the nasoglabellar sliding advancement flaps are also versatile reconstructive tools (Fig. 20-14). For larger defects involving more than one anatomic subunit, the forehead flap is our workhorse for reconstruction (Fig. 20-15). We have found that, before the pedicle of the forehead flap is separated, the flap can be safely thinned to achieve better contour. Only when satisfactory contour has been achieved is the pedicle finally divided. In the upper dorsum, where skin is thinner, a skin graft may provide a satisfactory reconstruction. Forehead tissue expansion has added an extra dimension to total nasal reconstruction.

Lip

Squamous cell carcinoma is much more common than basal cell carcinoma in the lip. The lower lip is far more frequently involved by cutaneous malignancy than is the upper lip. Malignant tumors of the upper lip are almost always basal cell carcinomas.

In contrast to squamous cell carcinomas of the oral cavity, squamous cancers of the lower lip do not have a tendency for regional node spread (less than a 10% chance). Early tumors are equally well treated by radiation or surgical therapy. Radiation treatment might be more appropriate for lesions at the commissure. Prophylactic lymph node dissection is not routinely indicated. Furthermore, in the presence of a palpable neck node, one should not proceed immediately to radical neck dissection, because up to 50 percent of patients have nodal enlargement on the basis of inflammatory changes only. This statistic contrasts with the situation of palpable neck nodes in the presence of oropharyngeal carcinoma, in which the nodes are histopathologically positive in 90 percent of patients.

In squamous cell carcinomas of the lower lip, three questions emerge: Which patients should have prophylactic neck dissection? How extensive should the neck dissection be? How is the opposite side of the neck to be treated? The risk of nodal metastasis increases to 60 percent if the tumor is poorly differentiated. Thus the indication for neck dissection in these patients is increased; however, only 2 percent of all lip cancers are poorly differentiated. In a reported series, neck me-

tastases occurred with 63 percent of T3 lesions (greater than 4 cm in diameter). Nodal metastases are also more common for lesions of the commissure. If the mental nerve is involved with the tumor, 80 percent of patients have positive nodes and the survival rate at 5 years is only 35 percent. Indications for neck dissection in the absence of clinically palpable nodes thus include (1) little likelihood that the patient will return for follow-up care; (2) primary lesion greater than 3 cm in diameter; (3) lesion at the commissure; (4) poorly differentiated or spindle cell carcinoma; and (5) mental nerve involvement. The initial procedure of choice is a bilateral suprahyoid dissection. If positive nodes are found on final pathologic examination, a modified radical neck dissection is completed on that side. Postoperative irradiation is reserved for patients with large primary lesions (T3) or mandibular invasion and for patients with extracapsular nodal spread.

Reconstruction of the lip defect depends on size. For the lower lip, full-thickness defects of up to 30 percent of the lip can be closed primarily, especially in older patients. Defects of 30 to 60 percent can be closed effectively by a unilateral or bilateral modified Bernard procedure or lip-switch pedicle from the upper lip. For large defects, it is important that reconstruction produce a competent oral sphincter. Gillies fan flaps or a Webster-Bernard approach may be used. One compromise may be to reconstruct with a Karapandzic technique, accept a microstomia temporarily, allow the tissues to stretch with time, and have the patient return for a lip-switch procedure to enlarge the oral opening (Fig. 20-16).

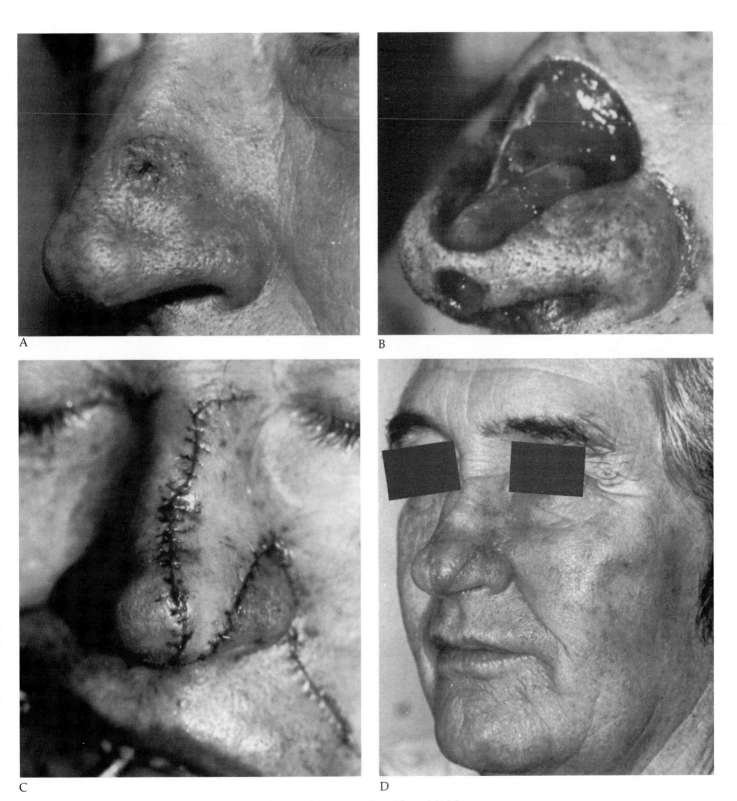

A

B

C

D

Fig. 20-13A, B. Excision of two basal cell carcinomas on the nose. C. Reconstruction with nasolabial flap pivoted at the infraorbital margin. D. Final result.

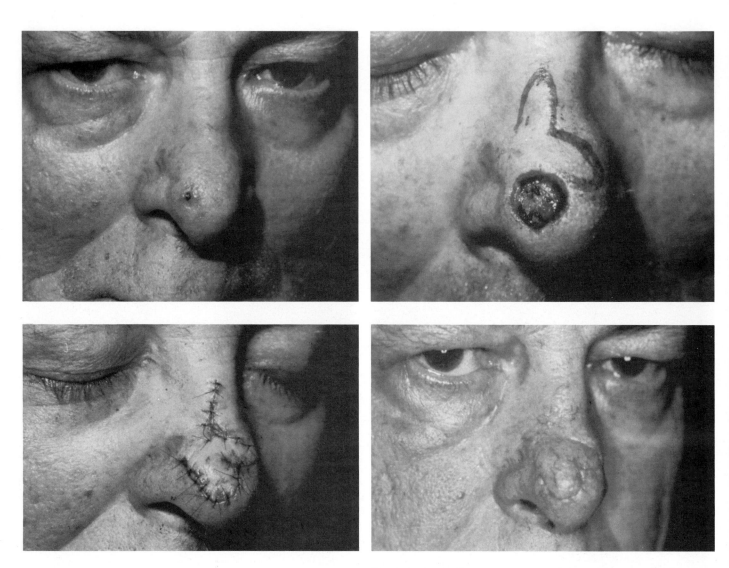

Fig. 20-14. *Basal cell carcinoma at the tip of the nose resected and reconstructed with bilobed flap.*

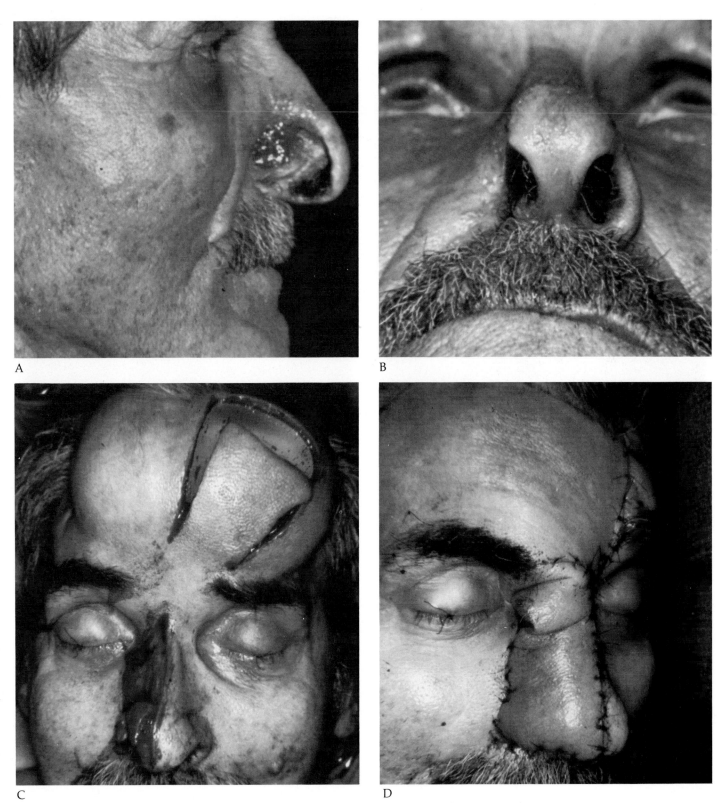

A

B

C

D

Fig. 20-15A, B. Nasal defect after tumor resection. C. Turn-in flaps for nasal lining and conchal cartilage to recreate contour of ala. Expanded forehead flap is used to reconstruct heminasal defect. D. Initial insetting of flap.

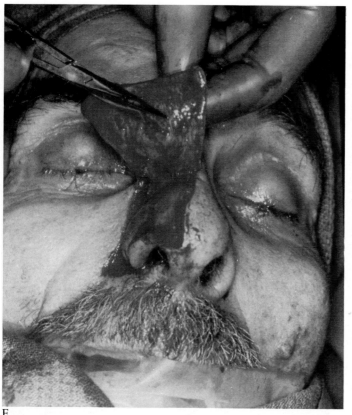

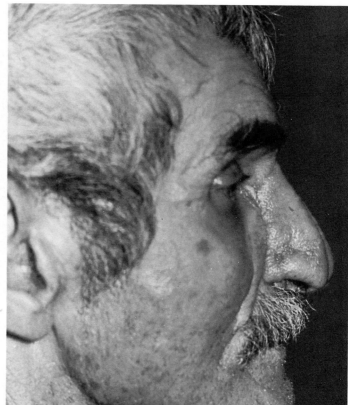

E

F

Fig. 20-15. (Continued) E. Flap thinned before division of pedicle. F, G. Final result.

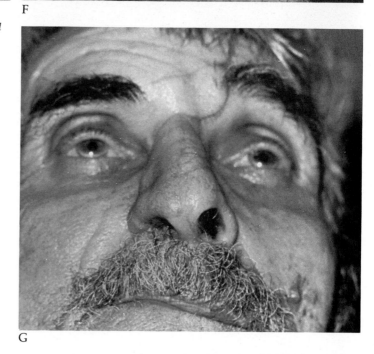

G

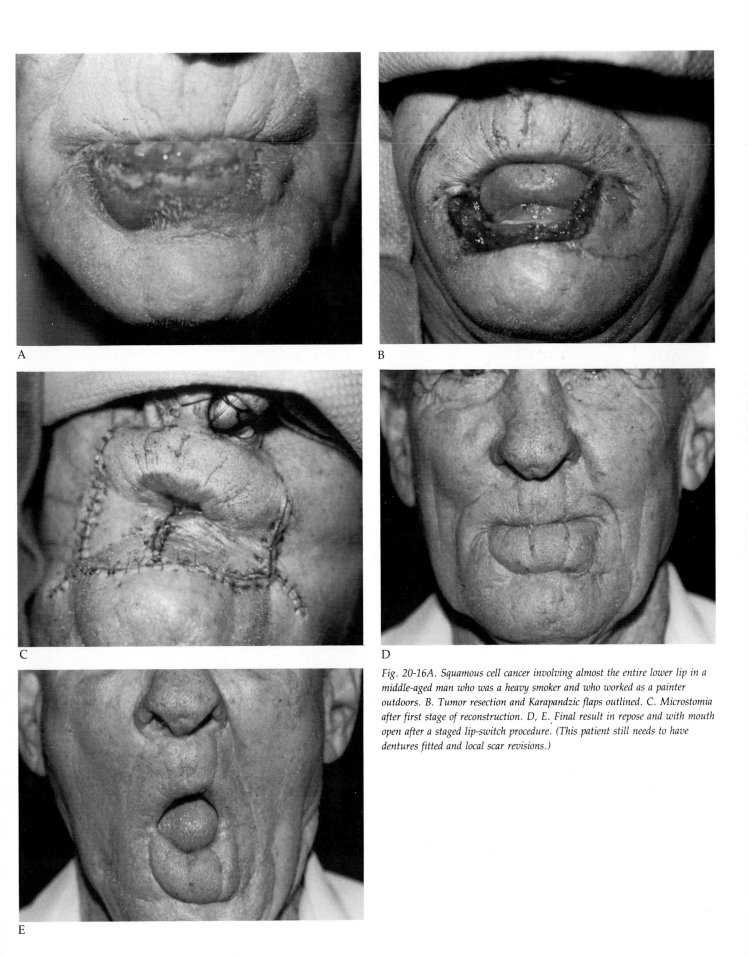

A

B

C

D

Fig. 20-16A. Squamous cell cancer involving almost the entire lower lip in a middle-aged man who was a heavy smoker and who worked as a painter outdoors. B. Tumor resection and Karapandzic flaps outlined. C. Microstomia after first stage of reconstruction. D, E. Final result in repose and with mouth open after a staged lip-switch procedure. (This patient still needs to have dentures fitted and local scar revisions.)

E

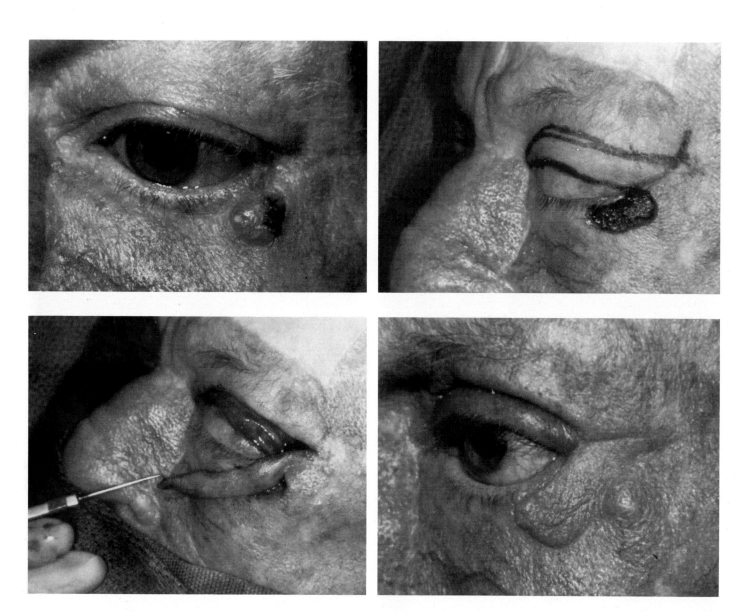

Fig. 20-17. Patient with lower lid basal cell carcinoma excised and reconstructed with skin-muscle Tripier flap from upper lid.

Eyelid

Basal cell carcinoma is the most common malignant tumor of the eyelid. Approximately 67 percent of the lesions occur on lower eyelids and 10 percent at the inner canthus. Squamous cell carcinoma is rare on the eyelids, representing about 2 percent of all eyelid lesions. The reported ratio of basal cell to squamous cell carcinoma is 30:1. Squamous lesions occur more commonly on the lower than the upper lid.

Some authors claim that radiation therapy is as effective as surgical intervention in the treatment of these lesions and is preferable because it avoids the problems of a complex surgical reconstruction. With proper shielding, intraocular complications are avoided. For medial canthal lesions, however, it is generally considered that the Mohs micrographic surgical technique offers the most reliable cure rate, because tumors at this site have a high recurrence rate and a propensity to invade the orbit. Use of the technique is supported by the finding of a recurrence rate of greater than 16 percent for medial canthal basal cell carcinomas following radiation therapy.

Reconstruction depends on the size of the defect and on whether or not the defect is full thickness. Smaller defects can be closed by direct suture after wedge excisions. We have found a Tripier skin-muscle flap from the upper lid to be ideally suited for resurfacing the lower lid (Fig. 20-17). Medial canthal defects are readily resurfaced with a thin skin graft; on occasion, when allowed to heal secondarily, the result is a surprisingly good cosmetic outcome. Tarsoconjunctival flaps are useful for large full-thickness defects of the lower lid. A lateral transposition tarsoconjunctival flap together with a lateral cantholysis and Tenzel flap may enable closure of defects of up to 60 percent of the lid width. For lateral defects of the lower lid, a Hewes upper-to-lower-lid transposition tarsoconjunctival flap may be used. If a medial canthal defect were to involve the lacrimal canaliculus, many surgeons would now teach that reconstruction ignore the canaliculus. In most

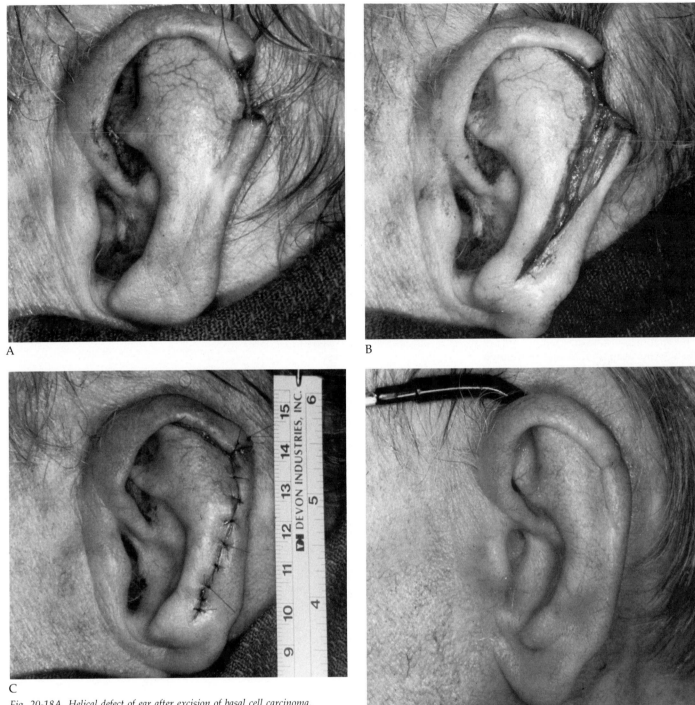

A

B

C

Fig. 20-18A. Helical defect of ear after excision of basal cell carcinoma.
B, C, D. Reconstruction of defect with Antia flap.

D

patients, epiphora is not a problem because most of the surface tear film (except for emotional tears) is lost by evaporation. If tearing becomes a problem, a Jones tube can be placed later between the conjunctival fornix and the adjacent nasal fossa. Placement of a tube later also has the advantage that the tube will be better positioned once cicatricial distortion has occurred. Finally, patients tolerate lower lid deficiencies if a good Bell phenomenon is present to protect the cornea.

External Ear

As already indicated, squamous cell carcinoma is the most common skin tumor of the pinna and of the external auditory canal. Most squamous and basal cell carcinomas along the helix cannot be differentiated from each other without a biopsy and are generally nonaggressive. As a rule, cartilage is excised with a conservative margin of tissue, and immediate reconstruction can be done such as with an Antia flap or a composite graft from

the opposite ear (Fig. 20-18). Larger helical defects may require staged reconstruction. Central defects of the concha are best skin grafted.

When it arises on the posterior auricle or central part of the ear, squamous carcinoma usually is not related to actinic damage, originates de novo, and behaves aggressively. The reported rate of lymph node involvement in such tumors is as high as 20 percent. In the presence of palpable lymph nodes, one must perform radical resection of the auricle, superficial parotidectomy, and radical neck dissection. Wound closure at the ear is best managed with a skin graft at this early stage. Postoperative radiation therapy may be required for the neck.

Excision of cancers at the external canal requires wide local-regional resection, frequently involving a temporal bone operation.

Summary and Conclusions

A variety of nonpigmented premalignant skin conditions have been discussed. Treatment should be directed not only at the specific lesion but also at prevention and early detection of malignant change. A final word of caution in treating suspected malignant skin tumors: A shave or punch biopsy should be performed to establish the diagnosis before a deforming surgical resection is undertaken.

Suggested Reading

Dellon, A.L., et al. Prediction of recurrence in incompletely excised basal cell carcinoma. *Plast. Reconstr. Surg.* 75:860, 1985.

Dillaha, C.J., et al. Selective cytotoxic effect of topical 5-fluorouracil. *Arch. Dermatol.* 119:774, 1983.

Dubin, N., and Kopf, A.W. Multivariate risk score for recurrence of cutaneous basal cell carcinomas. *Arch. Dermatol.* 119:373, 1983.

Goepfert, H., et al. Squamous cell carcinoma of nasal vestibule. *Arch. Otolaryngol.* 100:8, 1974.

Goodwin, W.J., and Jesse, R.H. Malignant neoplasms of the external auditory canal and temporal bone. *Arch. Otolaryngol.* 106:675, 1980.

Immerman, S.C., et al. Recurrent squamous cell carcinoma of the skin. *Cancer* 51:1537, 1983.

Jacobs, G.H., Rippey, J.J., and Altini, M. Prediction of aggressive behavior in basal cell carcinoma. *Cancer* 49:533, 1982.

Jones, E.W., and Heyl, T. Nevus sebaceous: A report of 140 cases with special regard to the development of secondary malignant tumors. *Br. J. Dermatol.* 82:99, 1970.

Kroll, S.S. Delayed pedicle separation in forehead flap nasal reconstruction. *Ann. Plast. Surg.* 23:4, 1989.

Loeffler, J.S., et al. Treatment of perineural metastasis from squamous carcinoma of the skin with aggressive combination chemotherapy and irradiation. *J. Surg. Oncol.* 29:181, 1985.

Luce, E.A. Carcinoma of the lower lip. *Surg. Clin. North Am.* 66:3, 1986.

Novick, M., et al. Burn scar carcinoma: A review and analysis of 46 cases. *J. Trauma* 17:809, 1977.

Plosila, M., Kiistala, R., and Niemi, K.M. The Bazex syndrome: Follicular atrophoderma with multiple basal cell carcinomas, hypotrichosis, and hypohidrosis. *Clin. Exp. Dermatol.* 6:31, 1981.

Rayner, C.R.W., Towers, J.F., and Wilson, J.S.P. What is Gorlin's syndrome? The diagnosis and management of the basal cell nevus syndrome, based on a study of thirty-seven patients. *Br. J. Plast. Surg.* 30:62, 1976.

Rodriguez-Sains, R.S., and Jakobiec, F.A. Eyelid and Conjunctival Neoplasms. In B.C. Smith et al. (Eds.), *Ophthalmic Plastic and Reconstructive Surgery.* St. Louis: Mosby, 1987. Pp. 759–770.

Schiavon, M., et al. Squamous cell carcinoma of the hand: Fifty-five case reports. *J. Hand Surg.* 13A:401, 1988.

Shanoff, L.B., Spira, M., and Hardy, S.B. Basal cell carcinoma: A statistical approach to rational management. *Plast. Reconstr. Surg.* 39:619, 1967.

Zacarian, S.A. Cryosurgery of cutaneous carcinomas: An 18-year study of 3,022 patients with 4,228 carcinomas. *J. Am. Acad. Dermatol.* 9:947, 1983.

21

Principles of Mohs Micrographic Surgery

June K. Robinson

Some malignant cutaneous tumors that spread contiguously are treated with great precision by Mohs micrographic surgery. Although initially called chemosurgery by Mohs in the late 1930s, the technique is now formally called Mohs micrographic surgery. This technique involves surgical excision with substantial modifications to obtain accurate histologic analysis of all margins. Unique frozen tissue sections and specimen mapping allow the surgeon to excise tumor and return to a specific area of the surgical wound to remove remaining tumor if still present. Thus a Mohs operation is performed as a series of excisions; a single physician serves as both the surgeon and the pathologist.

The goal is ablation of the malignant tumor with sacrifice of the least amount of normal tissue possible. The procedure usually can be completed on an outpatient basis over several hours using local anesthesia. The resulting defect can be repaired immediately or allowed to heal by secondary intention.

Indications
Histologic Characteristics

Skin cancer is the most common form of cancer; at least 500,000 patients are treated annually. Basal cell carcinoma is by far the most common lesion, its incidence estimated at 400,000 instances annually; the incidence of squamous cell carcinoma is 80,000 to 100,000 instances annually. For both of these tumor types, multiple treatment options are available, including Mohs micrographic surgery. Each patient must be evaluated for such characteristics as age; tumor histologic subtype, size, and location; previous therapy; and other medical problems to determine the optimal treatment plan.

Because it can detect only tumors that spread locally by contiguous cell extension into neighboring tissue, the Mohs technique is applicable only to tumors with these growth characteristics. Tumors that readily metastasize, by either hematogenous or lymphatic dissemination, cannot be treated solely with the Mohs procedure. For tumors with high metastatic potential, the Mohs procedure may be used to ensure removal of the primary tumor; however, elective node dis-

section may be necessary afterward. It must be emphasized that the technique provides a narrow margin of resection. Depending on the histologic description of the tumor and the depth of invasion, this margin varies from 1 to 4 mm. In aggressive squamous cell carcinoma, such a narrow margin is inappropriate and a surgeon skilled in Mohs surgery adjusts by taking a wider margin; this margin still does not normally exceed 1.0 cm.

Tumors amenable to excision with the Mohs surgical technique are basal cell and squamous cell carcinoma, Bowen disease and erythroplasia of Queyrat (both squamous cell carcinoma in situ), and dermatofibrosarcoma protuberans. Less common cutaneous tumors such as extramammary Paget disease, sebaceous carcinoma, microcytic adnexal carcinoma, and keratoacanthoma also can be treated by the Mohs technique, but the results for large series of patients have not yet been reported.

Mohs advocates the older, fixed-tissue micrographic surgical technique for melanoma. This technique involves the application of a fixative, zinc chloride paste, to a 1.0- to 2.0-cm zone surrounding the clinically evident melanoma. In excising the fixed tissue, another, wider margin (up to 2.0 cm) is excised around the area. During the 1970s and 1980s, Mohs used the fixed-tissue technique to excise margins of up to 3.0 cm. This was before narrower margins of surgical excision became acceptable. The cure rates reported by Mohs were similar to those reported by others performing excisions with margins up to 3 cm for the same types of tumors. Tumors of clinical stage I, thin melanomas of a Breslow thickness of less than 0.75 mm, have cure rates approaching 100 percent when treated with excision of 2- to 3-cm margins. I recommend that melanomas be treated with the standard surgical margins, with or without lymph node dissection, on the basis of the thickness of invasion and stage of the disease.

Other Indications

Tumors that recur after previous treatment are best treated by the Mohs procedure. When recurrent basal cell carcinomas are treated by surgical excision, radiation therapy, or curettage and electrodesiccation, the likelihood of another recurrence approaches 50 percent. In recurrent tumors, scar tissue from the previous procedure entraps malignant cells and acts as a barrier to the upward migration of the cells. The malignant growth continues at the depth of the initial wound and migrates horizontally before surfacing at the borders of the old scar. All the old scar tissue is removed with the Mohs technique. This is necessary to ensure that a second not yet clinically detectable area of noncontiguous cancer does not lurk within an area of scarring from the previous procedure.

Primary lesions in areas that demonstrate a high risk of recurrence when treated by other methods are suited to the Mohs method. Tumors with ill-defined clinical borders, because of either tumor type or occurrence in areas of extensive radiodermatitis, e.g., in patients who received x-ray therapy for acne or epilation of the face, also are well suited for Mohs micrographic surgery. In general, tumors larger than 2.0 cm in diameter are present for a longer time and have a greater likelihood of recurrence when treated by standard methods.

Some anatomic areas require maximal conservation of tissue to preserve func-

Table 21-1. Indications for Mohs micrographic surgical procedure

Recurrent tumors
Primary tumors
  In locations noted for frequent recurrence (periorbital region, nasal ala, nasolabial fold, periauricular region, temple, scalp)
  With indistinct clinical margins (morphea-like and metatypical basal cell carcinoma, tumor within area of extensive radiodermatitis)
  Larger than 2.0 cm in diameter
Tumors for which conservation of tissue is necessary
  Tumors of the eyelid
  Tumors of the fingers and toes
  Tumors of the penis
  Tumors of the nose

tion. For example, in squamous cell carcinoma of the hand the Mohs procedure may preserve tendons or prevent amputation of a digit (Fig. 21-1). In other instances, preservation of tissue may obviate exceedingly complex reconstructive procedures, which are less likely to yield a satisfying cosmetic result, such as loss of the nasal tip (Table 21-1).

Technique

Initially the patient has a biopsy of the tumor, which is processed by routine paraffin-embedded histologic methods. The biopsy allows accurate diagnosis of the type of the tumor. The Mohs technique is applied to the tumor remaining at the site of the biopsy to trace the extensions of the malignant growth in a series of layered excisions.

The clinically apparent border of the tumor is outlined with gentian violet and used to generate the surgical map with reference to regional anatomy. The affected area is prepared with a surgical antiseptic antimicrobial skin cleanser. The area is anesthetized by regional or local anesthesia or a nerve block, usually with 1% lidocaine with epinephrine 1:100,000. Unintentional nerve injury may be minimized by injection of additional local anesthetic or normal saline solution into the treatment site if the lesion overlies the course of a cutaneous nerve. This procedure causes the soft tissues to balloon

out, providing a safe distance between the level of excision and the deeper nerve structure. The operative field is covered with sterile towels or drapes.

The tumor is debulked by simple curettage. This process may help to reduce the number of excisional layers necessary to eradicate the tumor. The first micrographic specimen is obtained through excision of the base of the lesion in a saucer-like manner with a border of 2 to 3 mm of skin from the edge of the defect made by the curette. After the skin surface is superficially scored in a circle to indicate the area to be excised, a second set of score marks is made at the superior and inferior edges to preserve orientation of the specimen. These superficial incisions are made before the specimen is removed (Fig. 21-2A).

The piece of tissue is excised with the blade beveled slightly inward. The angle of the blade becomes more severely beveled as it cuts deep to the surface until the plane of the incision is horizontal to the skin surface (see Fig. 21-2B). This thin wafer of excised tissue has a thickness of 2 to 3 mm and is excised without any holes made in the specimen (see Fig. 21-2C). The tissue is held at only one edge with the forceps to preserve the proper orientation of the specimen. Once the specimen is removed, orientation is verified by aligning of the specimen in its original position using the scored incisions made previously. The specimen is placed with proper orientation on an anatomically marked transfer card.

Hemostasis of the wound is obtained with electrocautery with the aid of a forceps or hemostat. Larger transected blood vessels are ligated with sutures. If the operative field is large and there is considerable capillary bleeding, chemical cautery with aluminum chloride or ferric subsulfate solution or use of a hemostatic gauze may be helpful. If immediate repair is anticipated, however, chemical cautery is not used. A simple bulk dressing is placed on the surface, or a pressure dressing is applied when appropriate.

The specimen is subsequently prepared for frozen section. To ensure proper orientation of the specimen, a schematic drawing of the surgical defect is made with reference to regional anatomic landmarks. Aligning incisions are marked on the diagram (see Fig. 21-2C). The excised

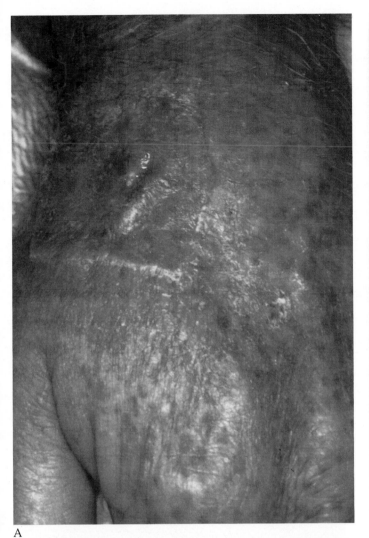

A

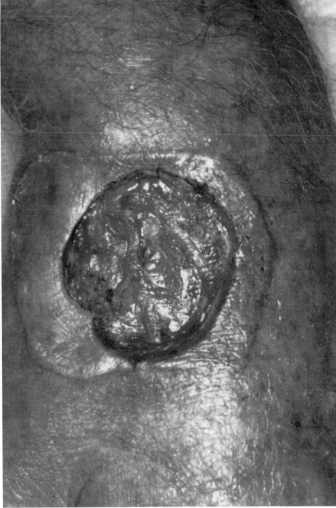

B

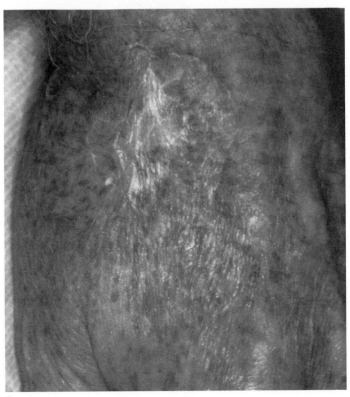

C

Fig. 21-1A. Squamous cell carcinoma, grade II, of the dorsum of the left hand recurred after standard surgical excision with repair using a full-thickness skin graft. B. Mohs micrographic surgical resection of the tumor spared the peritenon after this photograph was taken. A final phase of the procedure involved removal of the remaining graft, which showed no tumor involvement. The resulting defect was repaired with a split-thickness skin graft. C. At the 5-year follow-up examination, there was no tumor recurrence, and the hand was capable of full function.

Fig. 21-2. Mohs micrographic technique. A. After the tumor is debulked with a curette, the skin surface is scored in a circle 2 to 3 mm from the edge of the defect made by the curette. A second set of score marks indicates the superior and inferior edges of the specimen. B. The incision begins with the blade beveled at a 45° angle inward and is carried downward at an ever more acute angle until the blade is horizontal to the skin surface. C. The excised specimen has no holes, and orientation is verified by the scored incisions made previously. D. The specimen is divided into sections that fit onto the chuck of the cryostat. Indelible marking dyes are applied to the cut surfaces of the sections. E. A map is made of the excised specimen with reference to regional anatomy. Dyes are applied to the sections, and section numbers are recorded. (From J.K. Robinson. Mohs Chemosurgery. In A.R. Moossa, M.C. Robson, and S.C. Schimpff (Eds.), Comprehensive Textbook of Oncology *(2nd ed.). Baltimore: Williams & Wilkins, 1990. © 1990, the Williams & Wilkins Co., Baltimore.)*

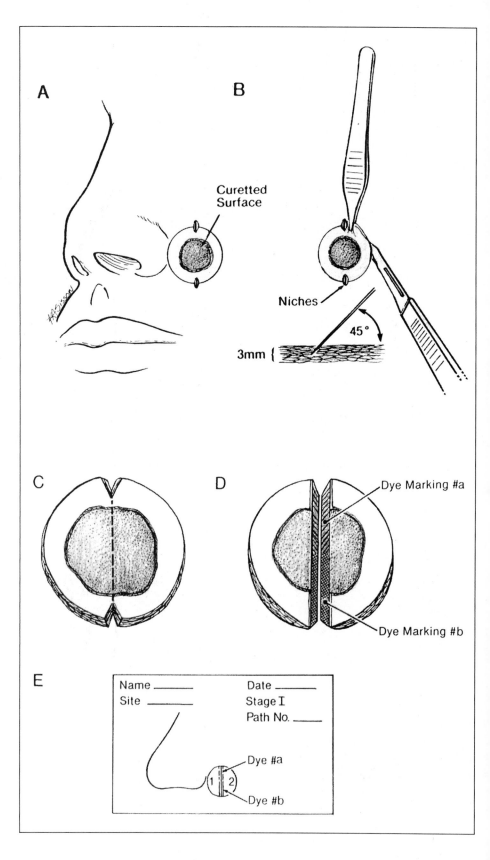

tissue is cut into pieces, each two square centimeters in size, which fit onto the freezing chuck of the cryostat (see Fig. 21-2D). Each of these blocks of tissue is given a number, which is known as the section number. Indelible marking dyes are applied to opposing cut surfaces of the sections (see Fig. 21-2E). The colored margins are recorded on the map. By convention, the broken lines on the map denote black dye (india ink) and the solid lines are red dye (merbromin). After dye is applied, the specimen is placed in a Petri dish on filter paper moistened with saline solution to await frozen section processing by the surgeon or a technician.

Frozen sections are cut sequentially from each section. The technician begins with the first section and continues with each consecutive section. Optimal cutting temperature medium is placed on the cryostat chuck, and the specimen is inverted and placed horizontally on the chuck so that

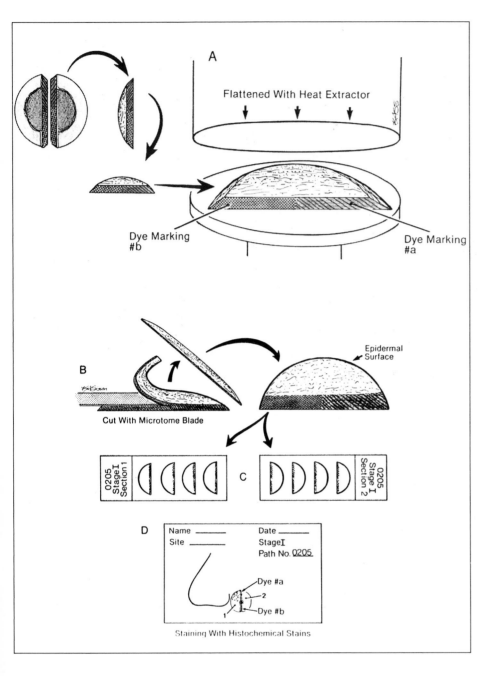

A

Flattened With Heat Extractor

Dye Marking
#b

Dye Marking
#a

B

Cut With Microtome Blade

Epidermal
Surface

0205
StageI
Section1

C

0205
Stage I
Section 2

D   Name _____   Date _____
     Site _____   StageI
                     Path No. 0205

                         Dye #a
                         2
                     1   Dye #b

Staining With Histochemical Stains

Fig. 21-3A. Mohs micrographic technique, continued. The specimen is inverted and placed horizontally on the chuck of the cryostat for sectioning. B. Serial sections are cut from the deepest margin. C. The sections are positioned on the slides and stained, and coverslips are placed. D. The surgeon reads the histopathologic characteristics of each section and pinpoints the location of residual tumor on the map. (From J.K. Robinson. Mohs Chemosurgery. In A.R. Moossa, M.C. Robson, and S.C. Schimpff (Eds.), Comprehensive Textbook of Oncology (2nd ed.). Baltimore: Williams & Wilkins, 1990. © 1990, the Williams & Wilkins Co., Baltimore.)

the deepest margin faces up (Fig. 21-3A). When the specimen is mounted, it is molded so that the skin margin is elevated until it is in the same plane as the rest of the specimen. The whole specimen is flattened with the heat extractor. The tissue is sectioned at a thickness of 4 to 8 μm (see Fig. 21-3B). The first sections processed represent the deepest and most lateral margins of that piece and are the most important. These sections are placed on a standard glass slide beginning at the end closest to the frosted portion. Deeper

sections into the block are actually closer to the epidermal surface and are placed on the slide in sequence, progressing away from the frosted end of the slide. Once all sections are positioned, the slide is dried on a slide warmer and stained with toluidine blue or hematoxylin-eosin (see Fig. 21-3C). Immunofluorescence or immunoperoxidase techniques combined with monoclonal antibodies to keratin distinguish basal cell and squamous cell carcinoma from normal tissue. Although they may be helpful in improving the his-

topathologic accuracy in a small number of tumors, these techniques are not sufficiently well developed or available for regular use.

After the sections are stained, a coverslip is applied and each slide is carefully examined microscopically. The surgeon pinpoints the exact position of residual tumor using the colors of the dyed margins and marks the position of the tumor on the map (see Fig. 21-3D). If residual tumor is present, the patient returns to the procedure room for removal of areas with persistent tumor. In this second stage of the surgical procedure, the excision is performed in a manner similar to that of the first stage. Each area of residual tumor is resected with a 1- to 2-mm area of clinically normal tissue surrounding it. The mapping, marking, and processing of specimens from the second and each subsequent stage of the procedure are carried out exactly as in the initial

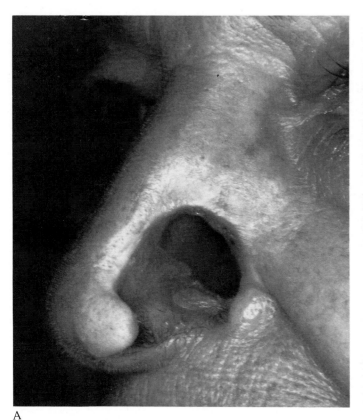
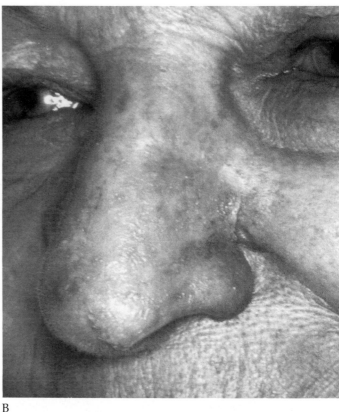

A

B

Fig. 21-4A. Resection of a recurrent basal cell carcinoma of the left ala by Mohs procedure resulted in full-thickness loss. Wound edges healed by secondary intention. B. The patient was fitted with a nasal prosthesis.

stage. These stages of the operation continue until the tumor is ablated, the last frozen sections showing no tumor. The final defect is measured and the size recorded.

This microscopic control allows the surgeon to formulate a three-dimensional view of the tumor extension, which is not always uniform in all directions and often extends considerable distances beyond the clinically apparent margins of the tumor. Once the tumor is resected, the resulting defect is evaluated to consider whether immediate repair should be undertaken or if the wound should be allowed to heal by secondary intention.

Reconstruction, Healing by Secondary Intention, or Prosthesis

The nature, location, and extent of the tumor influence the decision whether a wound should be repaired immediately or allowed to heal by secondary intention. Most tumors that have recurred after pre-

vious therapy have a slightly lower chance of cure with the Mohs technique than do primary tumors. When the risk of recurrence is too high and the process of healing by secondary intention is not likely to endanger an important function such as sight, hearing, or eating, the defect is allowed to heal by secondary intention. This method allows the surgeon to identify sites of subsequent recurrence earlier in the course of the disease. This procedure might be selected for aggressive primary tumors such as primary squamous cell carcinomas of the nasal vestibule or large metatypical basal cell carcinomas of the nose. In most such tumors, the recurrence occurs within 2 years of the resection. The surgical defect heals by secondary intention, and rehabilitation with a prosthesis is begun (Fig. 21-4). After 2 tumor-free years, reconstruction may be performed.

A period of 4 to 8 weeks is required for healing by secondary intention. Wound remodeling continues for an additional 6 to 8 months. The rate of healing depends on the site, size, and depth of the wound and the physical condition of the patient.

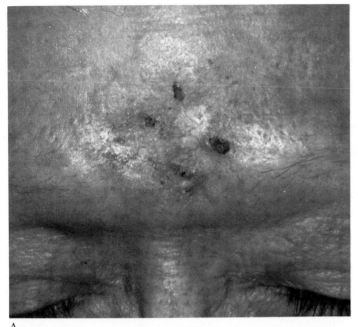

A

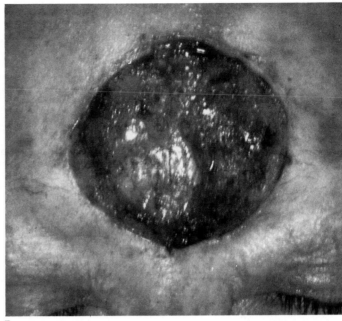

B

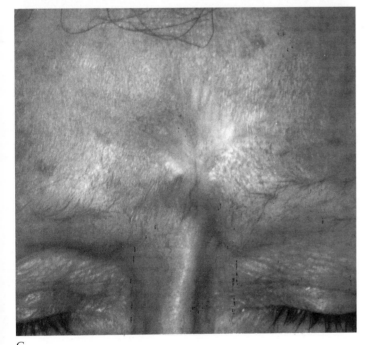

C

Fig. 21-5A. Recurrent basal cell carcinoma of central forehead before excision by Mohs technique. B. At the completion of the Mohs procedure, the defect includes resection of periosteum in the center of the wound. The area heals by secondary intention. C. The final result one year after the operation.

Limbs heal more slowly than the face, and large and deep wounds heal more slowly than small and superficial wounds. During this period, the patient cleanses the wound twice daily with hydrogen peroxide and applies an antibacterial ointment. Pain is uncommon after the operation. Postoperative discomfort is controlled with analgesics. If the defect is on a concave or flat surface of the face, the final cosmetic result from healing by sec-

ondary intention can be exceptional (Fig. 21-5). If healing by secondary intention does not yield acceptable results, consideration can be given to reconstructive surgery.

Resection of tumors on or near the margin of the lip, eyelid, and alar rim results in retraction of the free margin if healing is by secondary intention. Such retraction results not only in poor cosmetic appear-

ance but also in impairment of function, e.g., echlabion, ectropion, or malfunction of the nasal valve. In these instances, immediate reconstruction is indicated.

These reconstructions may involve liaison with surgeons in other specialties such as plastic surgery, oculoplastic surgery, hand surgery, neurosurgery, otolaryngology, and urology. Indeed, for deeply invasive carcinomas, the interspecialty consultation takes place before resection of the tumor begins. To determine whether or not a tumor is operable, extensive evaluation may be necessary. A complete physical examination, chest roentgenography, bone scanning, computed tomography, magnetic resonance imaging, ultrasonography, or other non-invasive radiographic examination may be necessary to evaluate the extension of the tumor and whether or not it has metastasized.

Suggested Reading

Mohs, F.E. Chemosurgery: Microscopically controlled methods of cancer excision. *Arch. Surg.* 42:279, 1941.

Mohs, F.E. The width and depth of the spread of malignant melanomas as observed by a chemosurgeon. *Am. J. Dermatopathol.* 6(Suppl. 1): 123, 1984.

Robins, P. Chemosurgery: My 15 years of experience. *J. Dermatol. Surg. Oncol.* 7:779, 1981.

Robins, P., Dzubow, L.M., and Rigel, D.S. Squamous cell carcinoma treated by Mohs surgery: An experience with 414 cases in a period of 15 years. *J. Dermatol. Surg. Oncol.* 7:800, 1981.

Robins, P., Pollack, S.V., and Robinson, J.K. Immediate repair of wounds following operations by Mohs fresh-tissue technique. *J. Dermatol. Surg. Oncol.* 5:329, 1979.

Robinson, J.K. Dermatofibrosarcoma protuberans resected by Mohs surgery (chemosurgery): A 5-year prospective study. *J. Am. Acad. Dermatol.* 12:1093, 1985.

Robinson, J.K. Expression of keratin proteins in deeply invasive basal and squamous cell carcinoma: An immunohistochemical study. *J. Dermatol. Surg. Oncol.* 3:283, 1987.

Robinson, J.K., and Gottschalk, R. Immunofluorescent and immunoperoxidase staining of antibodies to fibrous keratin. *Arch. Dermatol.* 120:199, 1984.

Swanson, N.A. Mohs surgery: Technique, identification, applications, and the future. *Arch. Dermatol.* 119:761, 1983.

Tromovitch, T.A., and Stegman, S.A. Microscopically controlled excision of cutaneous tumors: Chemosurgery, fresh tissue technique. *Cancer* 41:653, 1978.

22

Malignant Melanoma

Steven D. Macht   Joseph G. DeSantis

The malignant tumor resulting from the cancerous transformation of any cells capable of producing melanin is termed *melanoma*. Laennec in 1812 first used the term *melanoses* to describe the previously unknown disease. Lillian Norns, a general practitioner in Stourbridge, England, was the first to study melanoses in depth and made conclusions concerning its etiology and treatment that remain valid. Today the word *melanoma* is frequently prefixed by the term *malignant* to emphasize its aggressive character. The skin is by far the organ most frequently affected, although involvement of the eye is not rare, and primary tumors of the oral cavity, esophagus, rectum, gallbladder, vagina, adrenal glands, and leptomeninges have been reported.

Melanoma is not a common tumor, composing only 2 percent of all cancers. The incidence of the disease has increased markedly over the last several decades, however, and appears to be doubling every 8 to 10 years. Currently melanoma is second to lung cancer in frequency of cancers in women. More encouraging has been the decline in mortality from melanoma. Whether this is the result of a greater public awareness and subsequent

earlier presentation remains unclear. Surgical treatment has been less aggressive in the past 15 years. Still, melanoma claims the lives of approximately 25 percent of the patients who are affected by the disease. Despite a large body of research, many questions concerning melanoma remain unanswered, and many controversies regarding the appropriate treatment of the disease still exist.

Epidemiology

Melanoma is known primarily as a malignant tumor of Caucasians. Although any person may be afflicted with the disease, it is relatively rare in blacks and Asians. Only 1 percent of patients with melanoma are black, and in most black patients the least pigmented areas—the palms and the soles—are the sites of tumor occurrence. The typical patient may be described as having light skin, blue eyes, and light or red hair. He or she is more likely to burn than tan after sun exposure. The typical age of the patient is between 35 and 55 years, although an additional peak incidence occurs after the age of 65 years. Melanoma is rare in children. Although men and women are equally afflicted with the disease, women tend to

develop melanoma at an earlier age than men. Lesions on women occur with greater frequency on the legs, a more favorable site, whereas melanoma in men is more likely to occur on the trunk, a less favorable location.

The exact cause of melanoma is not known, although actinic exposure and heredity have clear roles in its development. Ninety percent of patients give a history of a severe sunburn at some point in their lives, and people with a history of episodic sun exposure are at greater risk than those with constant exposure. The incidence of melanoma among fair-skinned people corresponds with the proximity of these people to the equator. For example, there is a threefold greater incidence among people in the southern United States than among people in New England, and the highest incidence in the world is among the white population in Australia. Sun-exposed areas of the body are at greatest risk for melanoma, and the head and neck area has the highest incidence of the tumor.

First-degree relatives of patients with melanoma have a slightly increased risk for the disease. More dramatic examples of the influence of heredity in the devel-

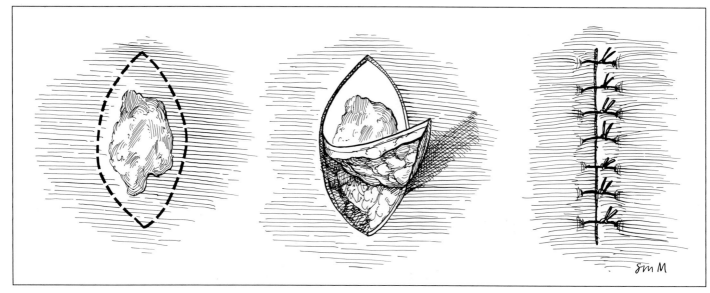

Fig. 22-1. Excisional biopsy (full thickness) is recommended for lesions less than 2 cm in diameter. Incisional biopsies should be reserved for larger tumors. Representative sections should include the most elevated portion, the most typical portion, and the transition from normal skin to tumor.

opment of melanoma are seen in xeroderma pigmentosum and the dysplastic nevus syndrome. Xeroderma pigmentosum is inherited as an autosomal recessive trait and results in a faulty DNA repair mechanism. People with this disease have a 3 percent incidence of melanoma. The dysplastic nevus syndrome is inherited as an autosomal dominant trait. The skin of patients with the disease demonstrates a large number of irregular nevi, and the incidence of melanoma among these people approaches 100 percent over a lifetime. Considering all patients with melanoma, however, less than 6 percent have a family history of the disease.

The relation of trauma to the occurrence of melanoma remains speculative. Anecdotal reports exist, but studies demonstrating a clear cause and effect relation are not available. A hormonal influence on the development of melanoma is suggested by an observed 5-year disease-free interval in pregnant patients with the diagnosis of melanoma. Attempts to use hormonal manipulation in the treatment of melanoma have not been successful thus far. Observations of a relation between previous petrochemical exposure and melanoma occurrence have been made, but studies demonstrating a clear correlation are lacking.

Diagnosis

Melanoma most often presents as a pigmented lesion greater than 6 mm in diameter with a history of change in appearance. The American Cancer Society has developed the ABCD system to help clinicians in identifying melanoma: A for asymmetry, B for border irregularity, C for color change, and D for diameter greater than 6 mm. Other characteristics that should alert the physician are bleeding, itching, ulceration, and an increase in size. In short, any skin lesion with a change in character should be viewed with suspicion, and a biopsy should be strongly considered.

In general, excisional biopsies are performed for lesions less than 2 cm in diameter (Fig. 22-1). The decision to perform an incisional biopsy rather than an excisional biopsy is also influenced by the site of the lesion and the relative difficulty of primary closure. An incisional biopsy must include the thickest area of the lesion, the most typical area of the lesion, and the zone of transition between the lesion and normal skin. The most important criteria in establishing the histologic diagnosis of melanoma are architectural rather than cytologic. Shave biopsies are

not acceptable. Punch biopsies and frozen section examinations are discouraged because of possible tissue distortion.

Histology

Clark categorized melanoma into four distinct groups based on gross and microscopic appearance: superficial spreading, nodular, lentigo maligna, and acral lentiginous (Fig. 22-2). Whether these distinctions represent discrete groups or points along a continuum remains debatable. More important is Clark's concept of horizontal versus vertical growth. Horizontal, or radial, growth represents the initial phase of melanoma development and is characterized by the proliferation of malignant melanocytes in the epidermis with no more than single-cell involvement of the dermis. Vertical growth refers to the proliferation of malignant melanocytes into the layers of the dermis and eventually into the subcutaneous fat. The earlier in the growth of the tumor the vertical phase occurs, the more aggressive is the course of the disease and the greater is the likelihood of systemic spread.

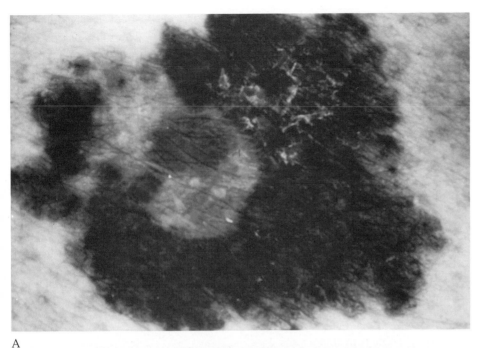

A

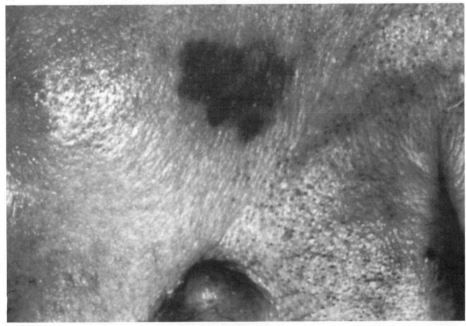

B

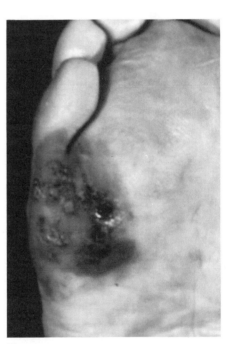

C

Fig. 22-2A. Superficial spreading melanoma.
B. Lentigo maligna. C. Acral lentiginous
melanoma. D. Nodular melanoma.

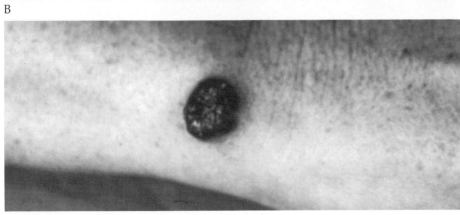

D

Superficial Spreading Melanoma

Superficial spreading melanoma has a relatively long radial growth phase lasting from 6 months to 7 years. The lesion is typically flat or slightly raised with an irregular contour and border. Initially the fine skin creases may be preserved within the lesion. The development of nodularity alerts the clinician to the transition to the vertical growth phase.

The superficial spreading lesion is the most common type of melanoma, representing 50 to 70 percent of instances. The most common locations of superficial spreading melanoma are the backs of men and the lower limbs of women. This type of melanoma has no gender predilection and can occur at any age. It is the type of melanoma most likely to arise in a preexisting nevus.

Lentigo Maligna

Lentigo maligna has a prolonged radial growth phase and may be confused with superficial spreading melanoma. In general, it is the least aggressive of the types of melanoma. It is preceded by the Hutchinson freckle, a flat, irregularly pigmented and progressively enlarging lesion always occurring on sun-exposed areas, typically the face or hands. This noninvasive form of the tumor may persist for 30 to 40 years. A change in color or shape and, in particular, the presence of nodularity suggest a malignant transformation.

Lentigo maligna melanoma represents 5 to 12 percent of all melanomas but 50 percent of tumors found on the head and neck. It is more common in women and most often afflicts people in their sixth, seventh, and eighth decades of life. The prognosis in patients with lentigo maligna melanoma is the most favorable among the types of melanoma.

Acral Lentiginous Melanoma

Like superficial spreading melanoma and lentigo maligna, acral lentiginous melanoma starts with a radial growth phase. The conversion to vertical growth, however, is earlier in the clinical course of acral lentiginous lesions, rendering them more aggressive and dangerous tumors.

Acral lentiginous melanoma accounts for 2 to 8 percent of tumors in Caucasians but 35 to 60 percent of melanomas in blacks and Asians. This type represents 35 to 60 percent of lesions in Hispanics also. These tumors are often large, not infrequently larger than 3 cm, and flat with irregular borders and heterogeneous coloring. They may resemble lentigo maligna melanoma. Unlike lentigo maligna, however, acral lentiginous melanoma occurs on unexposed areas such as the soles and palms, on the nail beds, and in mucosal areas. Typically elderly people are afflicted; the average age at the time of tumor occurrence is 60 years.

Nodular Melanoma

In contrast to the other types of melanoma, nodular melanoma has no horizontal growth phase. By definition, epidermal proliferation of tumor cells does not extend more than three retia from the area of dermal invasion. Predictably, this is the most aggressive type of melanoma. The polypoid subtype of nodular melanoma may be a more advanced form of the disease and has a particularly poor prognosis.

Nodular melanoma is second only to superficial spreading melanoma in frequency, representing 10 to 20 percent of tumors. It has never been found to develop from a preexisting nevus. The lesion typically presents as a darkly pigmented nodule or papule. Because there is no horizontal growth phase, there is a sharply demarcated transition between normal skin and the lesion. Nodular melanoma is found most frequently in middle-aged men.

Microscopic Classification

Depth of invasion is the single most valuable prognostic indicator of melanoma in the absence of metastatic disease. The separation of melanoma into the previously described types, although useful clinically, does not predict the aggressiveness of the disease independently of the depth of invasion. Two methods of evaluating tumor depth are widely used today, that of Wallace Clark and his associates and that of Alexander Breslow.

The Clark system was published in 1969 and classifies the level of tumor penetration based on the anatomy of the skin (Fig. 22-3). In level I, malignant cells are confined to the epidermis and there is no penetration of the basement membrane. Clark level I is identical to melanoma in situ. In level II, malignant cells have penetrated the basement membrane into the papillary dermis. Malignant cells reach but do not enter the reticular dermis in level III. In level IV tumor cells are present in the reticular dermis, and in level V malignant melanocytes have invaded the subcutaneous tissue. A clear relation between survival and level of penetration was demonstrated in Clark's original study and has been confirmed by many subsequent investigations. Survival rates were determined to be 98, 96, 94, 78, and 44 percent, respectively, for levels I, II, III, IV, and V in a recent study.

Breslow in 1970 developed a system of melanoma invasion based on tumor thickness. The tumor is measured from the top of the granular cell layer to the deepest portion or to the ulcer base if ulceration is present. Lesions are classified as low risk, less than 0.76 mm thick; intermediate risk, between 0.76 mm and 3.0 mm thick; and high risk, greater than 3.0 mm thick. Day and associates correlated tumor thickness with 5-year survival rate as follows: less than 0.85 mm, 99 percent; 0.85 mm to 1.69 mm, 94 percent; 1.70 mm to 3.60 mm, 78 percent; and greater than 3.65 mm, 42 percent.

The measurement of tumor thickness outlined by Breslow is more predictive of survival than the Clark system. The microscopic measurement of tumor thickness is currently considered the method of choice for characterizing melanoma.

Both the Clark and the Breslow classification systems have limitations. Neither system is of absolute value as a prognostic indicator of recurrent disease or the presence of lymphatic or systemic metastasis, but they are both valuable in predicting survival rate. The Clark classification lacks reproducibility in situations in which the papillary reticular dermal junction is poorly defined, as is typical of sun-damaged skin. Furthermore, difficulty arises in determining the exact number of malignant cells needed to upgrade a tumor to the next level. Potential errors in using the Breslow system occur in areas

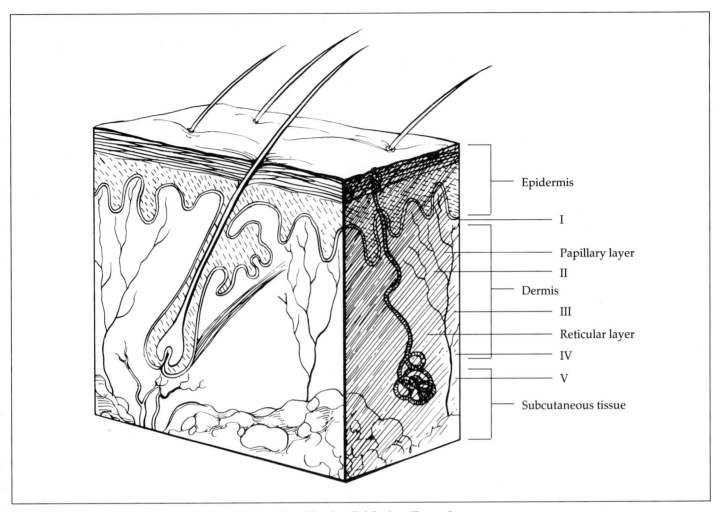

Fig. 22-3. Clark levels *are based on identification of tumor cells and the often ill-defined papillary and* reticular dermis. Breslow thickness *measures tumor thickness only and is unrelated to skin thickness.*

adjacent to hair follicles and sweat glands. Here, the invagination of the epidermal-dermal junction appears to carry tumor cells deeper into the dermis, leading to an overstaging of the lesion, the so-called adnexal drag (Fig. 22-4A). Severe beveling of the tissue, fixation artifacts, and tumor ulceration also can alter the microscopic measured thickness (see Fig. 22-4B). In addition, lymphatic infiltration may be mistaken for tumor, thus inflating the measured depth (see Fig. 22-4C). We believe it is optimal to obtain both a Clark and a Breslow histologic tumor stage for each melanoma.

Sometimes the depth of tumor invasion does not correlate well with prognosis even in the absence of recurrent or metastatic disease. These situations include amelanotic or nonpigmented lesions, desmoplastic lesions, and lesions demonstrating ulceration. All these situations

Table 22-1. Staging of malignant melanoma: American Joint Committee on Cancer staging system

Stage	Characteristic
Ia	Localized disease <7.6 mm thick or level II (T1, N0, M0)
Ib	Localized disease 7.6 to 1.5 mm thick or level III (T2, N0, M0)
IIa	Localized disease 1.51 to 4.0 mm thick or level IV (T3, N0, M0)
IIb	Localized disease >4.0 mm thick or level V or satellite lesions within 2 cm of primary lesion (T4, N0, M0)
III	Involvement of one regional lymph node station with movable nodes <5 cm in diameter or in-transit metastases >2 cm from primary (any T, N1, M0)
IV	Advanced local disease (any T, N2, M0) or systemic disease (any T, any N, M1 or M2)

From O.H. Beahrs and M.H. Myers. *Manual for Staging of Cancer.* American Joint Committee on Cancer. Philadelphia: Lippincott, 1992. Reproduced with permission.

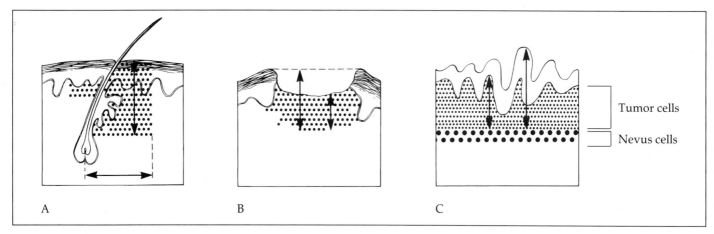

Fig. 22-4A. Adnexal drag. Infiltration of tumor down hair follicle should be measured laterally, not from skin surface. B. Ulceration. Measurement is made from ulcer base, not granular cell layer, and may underestimate virulence. C. Lymphocytic infiltration may be confused with tumor cells and should not be included in measurement.

may be associated with a lower survival rate than the depth of penetration would suggest.

Tumor regression previously was considered a sign of relatively poor prognosis in otherwise low-risk tumors. Tumor regression refers to areas within a tumor in which there is a marked reduction or absence of invading melanoma. Although this concept was initially supported, more recent investigators have not confirmed the importance of regression. Currently regression is not considered a sign of poor prognosis.

Melanomas arising on the back, arms, neck, and scalp, termed the *BANS* regions, had been correlated with a poorer prognosis. Larger studies have demonstrated no prognostic significance of the BANS regions independent of tumor thickness.

Recent advances in the histologic characterization of melanoma include the use of flow cytometry. Aneuploidy was found to be an independent predictor of recurrence in lesions less than 1.5 mm thick and in lesions greater than 3.0 mm thick. In addition, the use of melanoma monoclonal antibodies to detect nodal metastasis may prove to be of clinical value in the future.

Staging

Several systems for the staging of melanoma have been developed. The most comprehensive of these has been devised by the American Joint Committee on Cancer and consists of a four-stage system (Table 22-1). Lesions are assigned to stages I and II based on their Clark or Breslow thickness. A stage III melanoma has either involvement of one regional node group or fewer than five in-transit metastases. A stage IV lesion has advanced regional node disease such as large or fixed nodes, more than one regional node group involvement, or distant organ metastasis.

The original staging system, which is still in common use, consists of three stages (Table 22-2). The principal limitation of this system is that it does not take tumor thickness into account. The frequently used term *stage I melanoma* was derived from this older staging system and refers to a melanoma without regional or systemic metastases.

Table 22-2. Original staging system for malignant melanoma

Stage	Characteristic
I	Localized melanoma
II	Metastasis confined to regional lymph nodes
III	Disseminated melanoma

From G. McNeer and T. DasGupta. Prognosis in malignant melanoma. *Surgery* 56:512, 1964. Reproduced with permission.

Diagnostic Evaluation

The diagnostic evaluation of a patient in whom melanoma has been diagnosed starts with a total-body skin examination that includes the scalp. Synchronous tumors are not uncommon. A patient who has a single melanoma has a 600 to 900 times greater risk for a second primary lesion than does the general population. In patients with numerous irregular nevi, a "dysplastic nevi series" consisting of 32 total-body photographs should be performed. This procedure greatly facilitates follow-up examinations and allows an objective evaluation of changes in individual lesions. A physical examination also includes palpation of the cervical, axillary, and inguinal areas to detect adenopathy.

The minimal systemic evaluation of malignant melanoma includes a chest roentgenogram and liver function tests. Further testing could include computed tomography (CT) or magnetic resonance imaging (MRI) of the brain, chest, abdomen, and pelvis, and radionuclide bone scanning. The low yield of these additional studies among patients without symptoms has been documented by multiple investigators; the use of such tests should be based on the history, physical examination, and preliminary testing. Consideration of these methods is sometimes helpful if a major extirpative procedure is planned.

Surgical Treatment

The surgical treatment of primary melanoma is wide local excision. Controversy has arisen in determining precisely how wide an excision is needed to prevent local recurrence. The origin of wide excision for melanoma can be traced to William Simpson Handley. In 1907 Handley proposed a surgical treatment plan based on his impression of the centrifugal lymphatic spread of melanoma, which he noted in a single autopsy specimen. He recommended local excision of 1 inch cf skin and an additional 2 inches of subcutaneous tissue around the tumor. In accordance with this guideline, a 5-cm excision of normal tissue around a melanoma was considered standard management for many years.

Theoretically a wide buffer of normal tissue makes sense in terms of offering the patient the greatest likelihood of local cure. Olsen postulated that the primary melanoma can emit a virulent noxa capable of transforming normal cells for a distance around the tumor. This idea, together with the finding of "atypical melanocytes" within several centimeters of the primary tumor, suggests a benefit of wide excision. Clinical studies, however, have not supported the need for the 5-cm margin in early lesions. In 1977 Breslow and Macht suggested that melanomas less than 0.76 mm thick could be cured using 1-cm margins. Multiple retrospective studies that followed supported these impressions. A prospective, randomized study by Veronesi and associates was presented in 1988; it demonstrated the safety of a 1-cm margin in lesions less than 2 mm thick.

The optimal surgical treatment of lesions greater than 2 mm thick remains unclear. No prospective study is available that addresses the issue of margins, but retrospective investigations demonstrate no added advantage of margins greater than 3 cm in thicker melanomas. Our current practice is to excise lesions less than 2 mm thick with a 1-cm margin and to remove lesions greater than 2 mm thick with a 3-cm margin. Individualization is advised in areas adjacent to or involving critical structures such as the eye, nose, or ear. In these instances more limited resection can be considered in conjunction with appropriate discussion with the patient and close follow-up study.

The issue of whether or not to include underlying fascia with the melanoma resection has been controversial in the past. It is now well established that the resection of fascia does little to alter the course of the melanoma. In general, fascia is taken if it is close to a deep lesion or if removing it facilitates closure.

Reconstruction

Split-thickness skin grafting after excision of a melanoma previously was the standard method of reconstruction. It was believed that skin grafting as opposed to flap closure would allow earlier detection of local recurrence. Bagley and colleagues, however, showed no difference in survival rates in a comparison of primary closure with split-thickness skin grafting. No study has demonstrated a benefit of delayed closure over immediate reconstruction.

Currently the best reconstruction available is offered to the patient. A thin lesion excised with a 1-cm margin frequently can be closed primarily (Fig. 22-5). Facial lesions often require some ingenuity in the use of local flaps to close the defect without loss of function and with a minimal amount of distortion. Areas of resection on the limbs or trunk may be managed with local advancement or transposition flaps. Larger defects may require the use of a rhomboid, double rhomboid, or triple rhomboid closure or the double Z rhomboid closure described by Cuono. When a split-thickness skin graft is to be used, it is best to prepare the patient carefully with appropriate photographs to avoid unrealistic expectations.

Surgical Management of Regional Lymph Nodes

The incidence of metastasis to regional lymph nodes corresponds directly with the thickness of the primary melanoma. Lesions less than 0.75 mm thick are rarely associated with lymph node metastasis, whereas lesions greater than 3 mm thick spread to regional lymph nodes in 40 percent of patients. Clinically palpable lymph node metastases are treated by radical lymphadenectomy of the appropriate lymph node basin. Partial lymph node dissections are inadequate because metastatic disease often is present in grossly normal lymph nodes. Involvement of lymph nodes in the inguinal area requires a deep iliac node dissection in addition to the superficial lymphadenectomy to maximize survival (Fig. 22-6A). Axillary node metastases are treated with a level III axillary node dissection, which includes nodes medial to the pectoralis minor muscle (see Fig. 22-6B). Metastases to the cervical nodes should be treated with a modified or standard radical neck dissection (see Fig. 22-6C).

The role of prophylactic lymph node dissection in the treatment of melanoma remains unsettled. On an intuitive basis, it would appear that the removal of lymph nodes harboring microscopic metastases could favorably alter the course of the disease. The best indicator of the possibility of microscopic disease in the lymph nodes

Fig. 22-5. Wide excision and primary closure after appropriate undermining. This technique is used most often with thin melanomas.

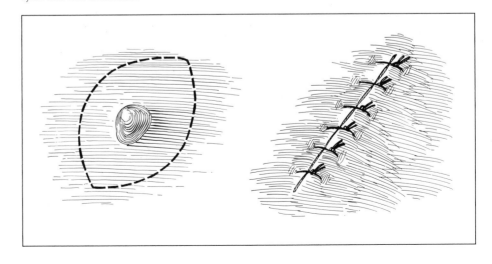

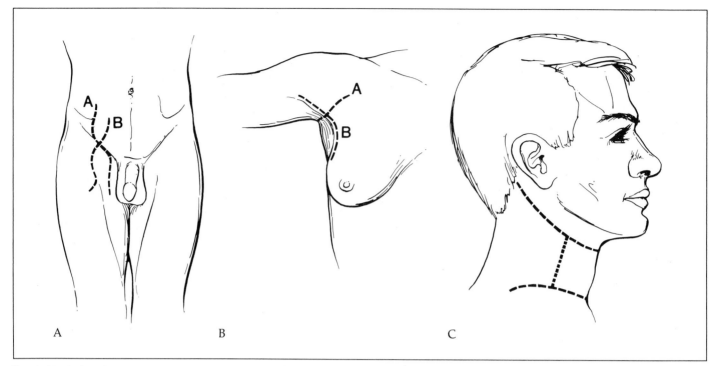

Fig. 22-6A. Options for incisions for superficial and deep inguinal lymph node dissection.
B. Recommended incisions for axillary dissection. C. Incision for modified radical neck dissection
(McPhee). Vertical component is used if greater exposure is needed.

is the thickness of the primary lesion. Several retrospective studies have demonstrated a beneficial effect of prophylactic lymph node dissection in lesions of intermediate thicknesses, that is, melanomas ranging in thickness from 1.5 mm to 3.0 to 4.0 mm.

Two prospective studies compared resection and resection plus prophylactic lymphadenectomy. Neither study demonstrated an increase in survival rate for the group who underwent lymph node dissection. These studies were criticized because of differences in the patient populations in the two groups, inconsistencies in clinical staging, and failure to identify a subset of patients who might benefit from lymph node dissection. Regarding the last point, a reanalysis of the data accounting for both tumor thickness and ulceration demonstrated a subgroup of patients with intermediate-risk lesions with a 22 percent improved 10-year survival rate. Two prospective, randomized studies currently are addressing the value of prophylactic lymph node dissection.

Until additional evidence is available, it is advisable to perform an elective lymph node dissection for lesions thicker than 1.5 mm when there is no evidence of systemic disease and when an identifiable lymph node basin is present. In areas where the lymph node basin is not clear, lymphoscintigraphy may be helpful in assisting mapping of the drainage pattern of the area in question. Some surgeons set an upper limit of tumor thickness of 3 or 4 mm for prophylactic lymph node dissection because very thick lesions have a high likelihood of systemic spread, thus negating the beneficial effects of lymphadenectomy. Our group does not set an upper limit of tumor thickness; we proceed with lymphadenectomy in thicker lesions if the evaluation for metastatic disease is negative.

Adjuvant Therapy
Radiation Therapy

Because melanoma is considered a radio-resistant tumor, the use of radiation therapy in the eradication of the disease is limited. Creajan and associates found no effect of radiation therapy on survival or disease-free interval in a prospective, randomized study. In special situations radiation therapy has been demonstrated to be effective in control of disease, in particular when a high dose per fraction technique is used, although this technique is associated with severe side effects. In general, standard radiation therapy is most useful in the palliation of advanced melanoma.

The successful treatment of melanoma by radiation therapy may lie in its use with other adjuvant modes, such as hyperthermia, chemotherapy, and immunotherapy. The use of chemical radiosensitizers such as 5-fluorouracil (5-FU) also may increase the usefulness of radiation therapy in the treatment of the disease. In addition, the use of fast neutrons in the local treatment of primary and recurrent melanomas has been encouraging.

Immunotherapy

Several clinical observations have suggested that the natural history of melanoma may be altered by the function of the immune system. For example, spontaneous regression of local and metastatic lesions has been noted. Also, it is well known that in 5 to 7 percent of patients with metastatic melanoma, no primary lesion is found, suggesting that the immune system may be capable of locally suppressing the tumor. In addition, the late recurrence of melanoma may be linked to a depressed immune system. A depressed immune system in patients with melanoma has been correlated with a poor prognosis.

Investigations into the use of immunologic stimulants to treat melanoma have used both specific and nonspecific agents. A large part of the research concerning nonspecific stimulants has involved bacille Calmette-Guérin (BCG), an attenuated strain of *Mycobacterium bovis*, now known to be a reticuloendothelial stimulant. Several studies have demonstrated a beneficial effect of BCG in the treatment of melanoma, but these investigations were not randomized and lacked adequate controls. Other investigators have not found a significant effect of BCG on the course of melanoma. Other nonspecific agents used in the treatment of melanoma have included *Corynebacterium parvum*, a gram-positive diphtheroid bacillus; levamisole, the levoisomer of the antihelminthic tetramisole; and transfer factor, an extract of lysed buffy-coat white blood cells. The results of these investigations have been inconclusive to date.

Interferon alpha has been known to decrease the proliferation of melanoma in vitro. Clinical trials using systemic interferon alpha demonstrated a 22 percent response rate, the response being transient in most instances. A greater response has been noted in intralesional therapy, but to date no increase in survival rate or disease-free interval secondary to the use of interferon has been documented.

The production of a vaccine specific to melanoma has been undertaken by various groups, again with inconsistent results. Investigations of randomized populations have not demonstrated a beneficial effect. An additional method of enhancing the immunogenicity of melanoma cells is to infect them with an oncolytic virus. This procedure has been undertaken by several investigators using viral oncolysate. Results are promising, although more trials are needed. In general the use of immunologic agents, both specific and nonspecific, in the treatment of melanoma remains in the realm of clinical protocols.

Chemotherapy

Despite a magnitude of clinical trials, few chemotherapeutic agents have been found to alter the course of metastatic melanoma. Dacarbazine (DTIC) has been the most widely studied and is thought to be the most effective single agent. Clinical response to DTIC is seen in 20 to 25 percent of patients, although a complete response is noted in only 4.5 percent of patients, and a long-term complete response is seen in only 1 to 2 percent. The other major monochemotherapeutic group of drugs is the nitrosoureas, which include carmustine (BCNU) and semustine (methyl CCNU). Partial response rates with these agents range from 10 to 20 percent. The high morbidity associated with these agents and their modest ability to influence survival time limit their usefulness in treating metastatic melanoma.

A search for a more effective, less toxic chemotherapeutic agent has led to the use of multiple agents. Most trials have included various combinations of DTIC, nitrosoureas, vincristine, bleomycin, and *cis*-platinum. Promising results have been claimed by some groups; the response rates range from 40 to 50 percent. Because other investigators have not demonstrated an improved remission rate, it remains unclear whether combination chemotherapy is superior to single-agent chemotherapy. A combination of chemotherapy and immunotherapy theoretically would be effective in the treatment of systemic melanoma. Most studies of chemoimmunotherapy have failed to demonstrate a benefit.

The use of chemotherapy in advanced melanoma must be individualized. It appears that chemotherapy may benefit a subset of patients, but the criteria by which this group may be identified have not yet been determined.

Isolated Limb Perfusion

The perfusion of high-dose chemotherapy into a vascularly isolated limb is a technique particularly suited to malignant melanoma for two reasons. First, a large percentage of melanomas occur on the limbs, and second, the systemic doses of chemotherapy needed to treat the tumor effectively are associated with a high morbidity. First described by Klopp and associates in 1950, isolated perfusion is not new. Work done by Creech and colleagues in 1958 led to the first use of isolated perfusion in the treatment of melanoma in humans using an extracorporeal oxygenator. Hyperthermia was shown to be effective in the killing of cancer cells in 1967, and the addition by Stehlin in 1969 of heat to the chemotherapy circuit increased the effectiveness of limb perfusion in the treatment of melanoma.

The method of isolated limb perfusion has been described in detail. The upper limb is perfused through the axillary vessels. Lesions of the foot are perfused through the popliteal vessels. The femoral vessels are used for melanoma of the lower leg and the lower thigh, and the external iliac vessels are used for lesions of the upper thigh. Perfusion of the regional lymph nodes is not consistently accomplished, and lymph node dissection should be performed when indicated. The vessels to be perfused are dissected, and the patient is systemically heparinized. Venous and arterial cannulas are placed. Isolation of the limb is accomplished by proximal tourniquet placement, ligation of smaller vessels, and proximal clamping of the perfused vessels. Venous blood is collected, pumped through an oxygenator, and warmed to 38° to 40°C (100.4° to 104°F). The chemotherapeutic agent is added to the perfusate, and the blood is returned through the arterial system. The most commonly used agents are L-phenylalanine mustard (L-PAM) and DTIC. The perfusion time ranges from 45 to 120 minutes. At the conclusion of the procedure, the limb is drained and flushed with crystalloid before the tourniquet is released.

As in the use of chemotherapy, the main issue regarding the use of isolated perfusion is identifying patients most likely to benefit from the procedure. The combination of surgical resection and isolated hyperthermic perfusion in patients with locally recurrent or in-transit disease may offer a better chance of survival. Isolated perfusion also has been demonstrated to offer effective palliation in patients with advanced local disease. The use of isolated perfusion in nonmetastatic and nonrecurrent disease has been controversial. Investigations using historical studies seem to indicate an improvement in survival rate. A prospective, randomized study of lesions thicker than 1.5 mm performed by Ghussen and associates demonstrated a longer disease-free survival time among patients who underwent surgical excision plus hyperthermic isolated perfusion than among patients who underwent excision without perfusion.

Isolated limb perfusion is a relatively safe procedure, provided the patients are well selected and carefully monitored intraoperatively for systemic leakage of the chemotherapeutic agent. Most complications are associated with technical problems, wrongly given systemic chemotherapy, and preexisting arteriosclerosis. Isolated perfusion is beneficial in patients with local recurrence, satellitosis, and intransit metastasis for palliation and possibly to increase survival time. It is also useful in selected patients with thick primary lesions in the absence of systemic disease.

Special Presentations of Melanoma and Its Precursors

Several clinical situations involving melanoma and lesions associated with melanoma deserve separate mention.

Compound Nevus

There is little question that giant congenital nevi carry a definite risk of conversion to melanoma. A giant nevus has been defined as a nevus present at or soon after birth whose area is greater than 144 square inches. Some authors consider congenital nevi to be giant if the lesion cannot be excised and the wound closed without deformity. The incidence of melanoma associated with giant nevi is unclear, but reported rates range from 2 to 31 percent. Sixty percent of these melanomas arise in the first decade of life, 10 percent in the second decade, and 30 percent throughout the remaining life span. It is recommended that excisions of giant congenital nevi be done early in life, usually when the patient is between 6 and 24 months of age.

The malignant potential of small congenital nevi is even clearer than that of giant nevi. The melanocytes of small and large nevi are likely to be similar; thus the malignant potential of the lesion is related to the number of cells at risk of conversion. The larger the lesion, the greater is the

risk, although all congenital nevi must be considered with suspicion. Thus even small congenital nevi should be excised at some point during childhood. In instances in which excision would leave a cosmetic or functional deformity, close observation is acceptable after the patient's parents are advised of the unknown risk that a malignant tumor will develop.

Familial Dysplastic Nevus Syndrome

The dysplastic nevus syndrome is inherited as an autosomal dominant trait. Patients with this syndrome have a risk for melanoma several hundred times that of the general population. The lifetime incidence of melanoma in these patients is close to 100 percent. Most affected patients have more than 100 nevi. A dysplastic nevus is usually larger than a typical mole and has more irregular borders, multiple colors, and indistinct margins. Most lesions have a pebbly surface, but the lesions may vary in their topography. Greene and associates described the lesions in detail.

Initial management consists of a representative biopsy of several lesions to establish the diagnosis and of excision or biopsy of any suspicious lesions. In general, multiple excisions of the nevi are not done, although excision of lesions in hidden areas such as the scalp has been advocated. Patients should be advised of the importance of self-examination and the avoidance of sunlight. Patients are followed by biannual complete skin examinations. A set of photographs known as a dysplastic nevus series is obtained at presentation and is used to detect changes in individual nevi.

Lymphatic Metastases with Unknown Primary Site

The clinical presentation of melanoma metastatic to lymph nodes without identification of a primary tumor is seen in approximately 5 percent of patients with melanoma. Most likely, this situation represents a complete regression of the primary tumor. Interestingly, these patients have a prognosis comparable to that of patients with lymph node metastasis and known primary melanoma. Treatment consists of lymphadenectomy of the ap-

propriate drainage basin. It is attractive to consider the use of isolated perfusion when a limb is involved to eradicate any undetected primary melanoma, but studies supporting the use of limb perfusion in this setting have not been done.

Locally Recurrent Melanoma

The development of a second melanoma within 5 cm of the excision scar of the primary lesion is considered a local recurrence and is presumed to be secondary to failure to eradicate all the malignant cells at the time of the original resection. Intransit metastasis and satellite metastasis represent lymphatic involvement and are typically found in the area between the primary lesion and the nearest lymph node basin. The overall incidence of local recurrence is approximately 3 percent but varies with the stage and thickness of the tumor. Most recurrences are seen within the first 3 to 5 years following initial treatment, but recurrences up to 23 years after excision have been documented.

The development of local metastatic disease is a poor prognostic sign. Ninety percent of patients were noted to have systemic metastases within 23 months of the development of local metastases. The median survival time after recurrence is approximately 27 months.

Despite the poor prognosis associated with local recurrence, all local recurrence is not invariably fatal. Management should be aggressive, and major resections should be considered for either restoration of local control or for palliation. As previously stated, radiation therapy has a role in local palliation, and isolated perfusion should be used in patients with local recurrence on a limb.

Regional and systemic metastases also should be treated aggressively in selected patients. Overett and Shiu demonstrated improved 5-year survival rates for metastatic lesions in lymph nodes, viscera, and bone that can be completely excised. There is no increased survival rate associated with incompletely excised metastatic tumors.

Follow-up Care

The goal of follow-up care of patients with melanoma is twofold: to monitor the patient for recurrence of the original tumor and to detect new melanomas. Treatment failures occur as local or nodal recurrences in two-thirds of patients and systemic recurrences in one-third of patients. Eighty percent of failures occur within 2 years of the diagnosis; thereafter, approximately 1 percent per year are distributed over the ensuing 20 years.

All patients need to be followed indefinitely. At minimum, patients are examined every 3 months for 2 years and yearly thereafter. Patients who may need to be followed more closely include those with thick or ulcerated lesions and those with lymph node metastases. Examination of the operative site and lymph node palpation are performed at each visit. A total-body skin examination is performed each year. Yearly chest roentgenograms and liver function tests are done as indicated by the history, physical examination, and baseline studies.

Conclusion

Malignant melanoma is a complex and difficult disease. The past several decades have seen an increased understanding of the surgical treatment of the disease. Currently most patients who have melanoma can be treated successfully. Future research will be directed at patients in whom surgical treatment alone is inadequate for cure. Although many methods are promising, indisputable consistent prolongation of survival time through their use has yet to be demonstrated in advanced melanoma. As a result, clinical trials are ongoing at many institutions, and it is exciting to realize that in the next several decades there will be a greater ability to treat this disease.

Suggested Reading

Balch, C.M. The role of lymph node dissection in melanoma: Rationale, results, controversies. *J. Clin. Oncol.* 6:163, 1988.

Balch, C.M., et al. A multifactorial analysis of melanoma: Prognostic histopathological features comparing Clark's and Breslow's staging methods. *Am. Surg.* 188:732, 1978.

Berman, C.G., et al. Lymphoscintigraphy in malignant melanoma. *Ann. Plast. Surg.* 28:29, 1992.

Breslow, A. Thickness, cross-sectional areas and depth of invasion in the prognosis of cutaneous melanoma. *Ann. Surg.* 172:902, 1970.

Breslow, A., and Macht, S.D. Optimal size of resection margins for thin cutaneous melanoma. *Surg. Gynecol. Obstet.* 145:691, 1977.

Clark, W.H., et al. The histogenesis and biological behavior of primary human malignant melanoma of the skin. *Cancer Res.* 29:705, 1969.

Creagan, E.T., et al. Adjuvant radiation therapy for regional nodal metastases from malignant melanoma: A randomized prospective study. *Cancer* 42:2206, 1978.

Cumberlin, R., et al. Isolation perfusion for malignant melanoma of the extremity: A review. *J. Clin. Oncol.* 3:1022, 1985.

Golomb, F.M., et al. Chemotherapy of melanoma. *Dermatol. Clin.* 3:335, 1985.

Harris, M.N., et al. Ilioinguinal lymph node dissection for melanoma. *Surg. Gynecol. Obstet.* 136:33, 1973.

Koh, H.K., et al. Adjuvant therapy of cutaneous malignant melanoma: A critical review. *Med. Pediatr. Oncol.* 13:244, 1985.

Macht, S.D. Current concepts in melanoma. *Otolaryngol. Clin. North Am.* 15:241, 1982.

Milton, G.W., et al. Prophylactic lymph node dissection in clinical stage 1 melanomas: Results of surgical treatment in 1319 patients. *Br. J. Surg.* 69:108, 1982.

Overett, T.K., and Shiu, M.H. Surgical treatment of distant metastatic melanoma: Indications and results. *Cancer* 56:1222, 1985.

Roses, D.F., Harris, M.N., and Ackerman, A.B. *Diagnosis and Management of Cutaneous Malignant Melanoma.* Philadelphia: Saunders, 1983.

Veronesi, U., et al. Thin stage 1 primary cutaneous malignant melanoma: Comparison of excision with margins of 1 or 3 cm. *N. Engl. J. Med.* 318:1159, 1988.

Wong, J.H., Cagle, L.A., and Morton, D.L. Surgical treatment of lymph nodes with metastatic melanoma from unknown primary site. *Arch. Surg.* 122:1380, 1987.

23

Vascular Malformations

Hugh G. Thomson   Patricia E. Burrows

Vascular lesions are the most common of the pediatric cutaneous anomalies. It is suggested that 2.6 percent of all newborn infants have some form of vascular malformation. Certainly by the age of one year, 10 percent of all Caucasian children are affected. Because this problem is common, patients are constantly being brought in by distraught parents for surgical opinions. The parents are anxious concerning the diagnosis, cause, and prognosis; their anxiety is compounded by the confusion caused by the multiple, conflicting opinions they have received.

After a careful history is taken and an examination of the patient performed, the parents must be counseled regarding what to expect of the deforming lesion on a short- and long-term basis. The use of serial slides or photographs of other patients with a similar lesion is a reasonable method of reassuring parents that a resolution or involution is anticipated. It is worthwhile to have the parents participate in the photographic analysis by standardizing photographs of their child every 6 months for comparison. An issue that has confused parents and referring doctors as well is nomenclature, which will probably never be uniform. Mulliken attempted to clarify this subject between

the years 1982 and 1990. Mulliken stated that "any classification of vascular anomalies based on descriptive terminology, e.g., strawberry hemangioma, is predisposed to inaccuracy because lesions that look similar may have quite different etiologies and behaviour." His major classification divides vascular anomalies into hemangiomas, which have a proliferative and involuting phase, and malformations, which are caused by inborn errors of vascular morphogenesis and have a normal endothelial cell turnover (Table 23-1).

Fortunately, the most common vascular lesions fall into the category of hemangioma and thus the prognosis is encouragingly predictable.

Hemangiomas

Types

Capillary, or Strawberry (Superficial Dermis Vascular Channels)

Capillary hemangiomas present at birth in 50 percent of patients as a small, pinhead, red lesion or a macular rash that grows rapidly in the next few weeks and becomes bright red and raised. The other

50 percent are not present at birth but appear within the following 2 weeks. Capillary hemangiomas occur more commonly in girls, with a ratio of 3:1, and are primarily singular, but they may be multiple (Fig. 23-1). Of clinical importance during the early rapid growth period is the increased number of mast cells, as described by Kessler, that surround the hemangiomatous vessels. These cells produce heparin, which has a suggested role in vasoproliferation. In a similar way Sasaki and Pang suggested the presence of hormone receptors that influence cellular proliferation. They demonstrated serum estradiol 17B levels in infants with proliferative hemangiomas to be four times higher than in controls. These factors relate to the natural regression of the lesions and to their response to hormone therapy.

The natural history of capillary and other hemangiomas is to involute with time. There is usually considerable evidence of involution by the time the child is 5 to 6 years of age. The final degree of improvement is achieved by the time the child is 8 years of age. Not all hemangiomas have the same percentage of involution. Almost 98 percent of the capillary has disappeared by the time the child is 8 years

Table 23-1. Clinical classification
of vascular birthmarks

Hemangiomas—proliferating and involuting
        phase
  Capillary
  Cavernous
  Capillary-cavernous
  Lobular capillary (pyogenic granuloma)
Malformations
  Capillary
    Nevus flammeus
      Parkes Weber syndrome
      Sturge-Weber syndrome
    Nevus araneus (spider)
    Nuchal nevus flammeus neonatorum
    Nevus flammeus
    Telangiectasias
      Cutis marmorata
      Rendu-Osler-Weber syndrome
  Capillary-lymphatic, capillary-lymphatic-
      venous
    Nevus flammeus with gigantism
    Verrucous
    Klippel-Trenaunay syndrome
    Parkes Weber syndrome
    Capillary-lymphangioma, lymphan-
      gioma-capillary
  Lymphatic
    Lymphangioma simplex and circum-
      scriptum
    Lymphangioma cavernosum
    Lymphangioma hygroma (cystoides)
  Venous
  Arteriovenous
    Aneurysms
    Truncal
    Nidal

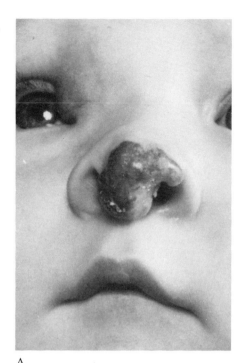

A

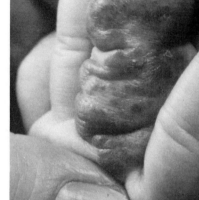

B

Fig. 23-1. Patient with three lesions involving tip of nose and medial canthus (A) and middle finger (B).

of age (Fig. 23-2). During the growth and the slow natural regression, or involution, there are definite stages of change. During the first 3 months rapid growth may take place with associated central ulceration and possible destruction of involved anatomic structures. At 9 months, however, a plateau is reached wherein the lesion continues to grow, but its growth rate parallels the growth of the child. When the child is one year of age, central gray zones or herald spots appear and coalesce. They are the first positive signs of ultimate regression and provide an excellent milestone to predict for the parent. Thereafter, growth parallels that of the child.

Cavernous (Deep Dermal and Subcutaneous Vascular Channels)

Cavernous lesions have an ill-defined margin and a bluish hue; they are usually nonlobulated (Fig. 23-3). These lesions lie in the deeper tissues and can distort the surrounding anatomic structures, including bony structures, because of their size. Cavernous lesions have a somewhat spongy feel on compression with no thrill. As with all vascular lesions, it is important to listen with the stethoscope to eliminate the possibility of a bruit, which indicates an arteriovenous (AV) shunting situation. The use of Doppler ultrasonography as described by Bingham might also be useful if a more complex situation is suspected. For lesions that are deeper with a less obvious bluish hue and no radiating venous channels, for example, in the frontal region, a differential diagnosis should include encephalocele, dermoid, ectopic glial tissue, and rhabdo- or fibrosarcoma.

The natural history is one of involution, but involution of a slower nature than seen with capillary hemangiomas, requiring the full 8 years before an estimate regarding the percentage of regression can be made. On average, 60 to 70 percent of these lesions regress with conservative management. Of course there also can be secondary bony deformities associated with pediatric vascular tumors. Secondary complications may require surgical in-

tervention before the child is 8 years of age.

Capillary-Cavernous

Capillary-cavernous lesions demonstrate a combination of both types of hemangioma and have a similar prognosis (Fig. 23-4). In general the lesions are larger and more disfiguring than capillary or cavernous lesions and have associated complications. Occasionally they demonstrate a high-flow situation that is not obvious on the initial physical examination, even if auscultation is performed. This type of additional involvement increases the potential for persistence and lack of resolution as well as for left ventricular strain or failure. At the same time, a rapidly enlarging, hot lesion without evidence of intrinsic bleeding is a diagnostic problem even with computed tomography (CT) and may require surgical resection.

Pyogenic Granuloma (Lobulated Capillary Hemangioma)

Unlike the preceding lesions, pyogenic granuloma is an acquired problem, the cause of which has not been definitely determined. Occasionally a parent states there was a scratch on the skin of the in-

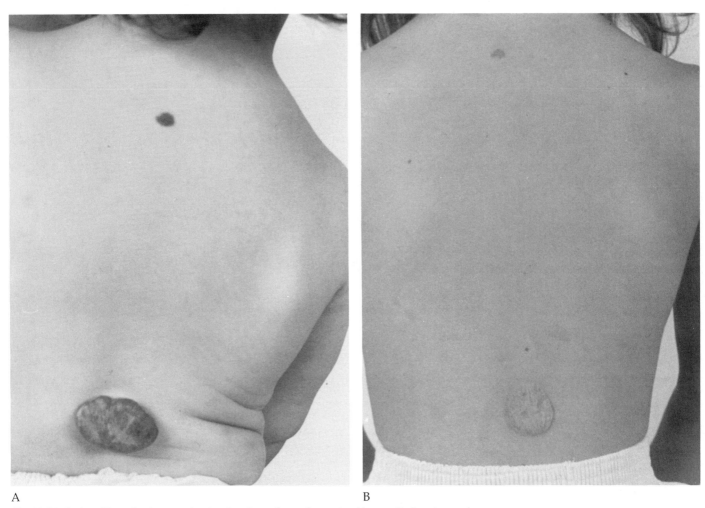

A   B

Fig. 23-2A. Lesion of lower lumbar area showing elevation and central, gray herald spots. B. Complete regression with slightly redundant skin.

Fig. 23-3A. Cavernous lesion involving tip of nose. B. Considerable spontaneous regression by the age of 6 years.

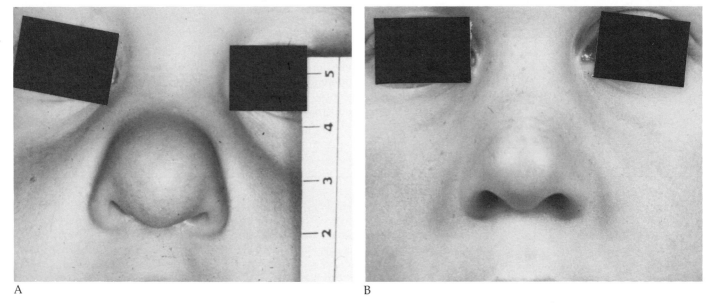

A   B

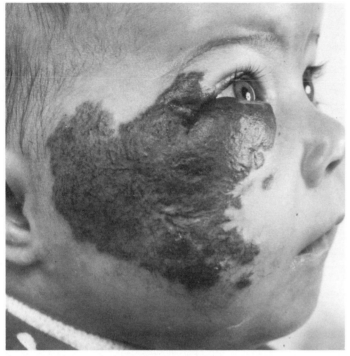
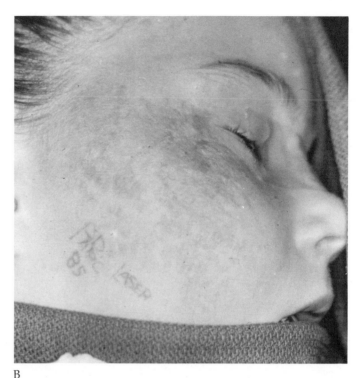

A

B

Fig. 23-4A. Diffuse capillary involvement of lateral V₂ with deep and surrounding cavernous hemangioma in preauricular, cheek, and mandibular regions. B. Almost complete regression of both lesions with residual telangiectasia appropriate for laser treatment.

volved area before the onset of a bright red spot. The lesion starts as a small, cherry-red zone 1 mm in diameter. It usually occurs on the face and grows rapidly into a pedunculated lesion that can measure 0.5 to 1 cm in diameter; there is a history of frequent arterial-like bleeds. Usually the patient is older than 2 years and the onset was 2 months before the first visit. These children are brought to the office or the emergency department with a bloody bandage covering the area. Conservative treatment with compression and silver nitrate sticks may temporize the acute bleed. Only shaving the lesion flush with the skin and electrocoagulation ensure a cure. This lesion rarely if ever requires repeated treatment (Fig. 23-5).

Indications for Early Treatment

The natural history of hemangiomas is one of spontaneous resolution by the time the child is 5 to 8 years of age. A few situations, however, require an active treatment approach because of the patient's needs or those of the parents.

Deprivation and Anisometropic Amblyopia

There is evidence to suggest that hemangiomatous closure of the eyelid during the first 6 months of infancy, even for a few weeks, can cause deprivation amblyopia. The use of intralesional injections of betamethasone (6 to 12 mg) and triamcinolone (40 mg) can be sight-saving. This treatment program may have to be repeated, however (Fig. 23-6). Similarly, if the upper lid is involved with a hemangioma of the cavernous type, the globe may be distorted, causing anisometropic amblyopia. This phenomenon can be simulated by a finger gently pressed medially from the lateral canthus. The degree of amblyopia can be monitored by ophthalmologic refraction. If the condition worsens, surgical excision has the potential to reverse the situation.

Kasabach-Merritt Syndrome

In Kasabach-Merritt syndrome thrombocytopenia and consumptive coagulopathy develop in a large hemangioma, usually in early infancy. The lesion usually demonstrates overlying cutaneous ulceration, rapid enlargement, and thus a congested

appearance. The secondary thrombocytopenia is believed to be caused by trapping of the platelets within the confines of the lesion. This situation requires urgent treatment in the form of systemic prednisone therapy (2 to 4 mg/kg/day) for a short term. This therapy should be given in consultation with an endocrinologist because of the potential for complications. A variety of other mechanical, cytolytic, and pharmacologic methods have been tried, including surgical removal, radiation therapy, embolization, and chemotherapy with cyclophosphamide, heparin, and drugs that inhibit platelets or fibrinolysis.

Most of the lesions associated with Kasabach-Merritt syndrome ultimately involute, and regression of the mass is associated with resolution of the bleeding disorder.

Microshunting Limb Lesions

The use of circumferential or other types of compression garments is helpful in hastening resolution if the lesion involves a limb. This is particularly true in a setting that includes excessive parental pressure, multiple small ulcerations, or left ventricular heart strain (Fig. 23-7).

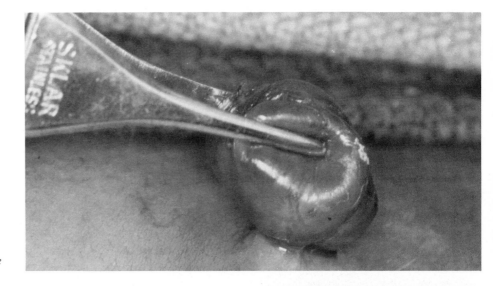

Fig. 23-5. Pedunculated pyogenic granuloma, ready to be shaved flush with skin margin and treated with electrocoagulation.

Fig. 23-6A. Hemangioma causing complete closure of the eyelid. B. Two weeks after cortisone injection. C. Appearance 3 years later demonstrating slight ptosis and telangiectasia.

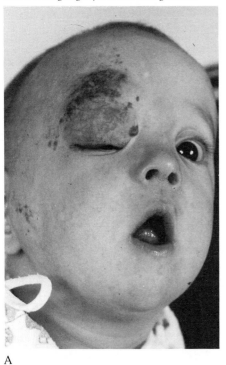

A

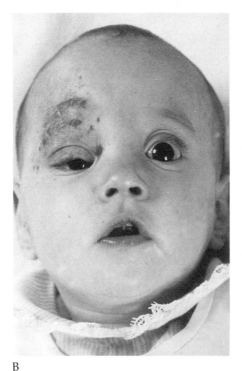

B

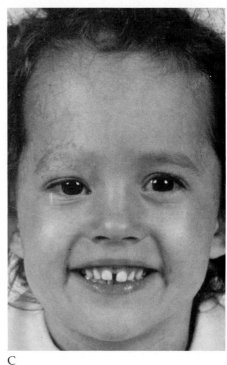

C

Obstructing Lesions

If the nasal vestibules are obtunded, respiratory distress might be anticipated, necessitating early treatment such as intralesional injection or compression (Fig. 23-8). Similarly, compression on the external auditory vestibule both externally and internally could cause hearing impairment early, but rarely is this bilateral and of clinical significance. Of more importance is a situation in which the larynx or trachea is compressed by a combined cutaneous-intracervical-thoracic lesion (Fig. 23-9). The patient may require systemic steroids with or without a tracheotomy.

Residual Problems

Partial Regression

For hemangiomatous lesions involving the upper or lower lips, there is always an element of regression but rarely total disappearance. In general, it is worthwhile to wait for as much resolution as possible—at least until peer pressure increases and body-image sensitivity develops, which is normally at 6 years of age. This course reduces the magnitude of tissue to be excised. The lesion may include baggy skin alone or excess skin plus a residual cicatricial hemangioma (Fig. 23-10). Occasionally the nose demonstrates a similar problem when an element of regression occurs, but a residual hemangioma results, necessitating surgical excision (Fig. 23-11).

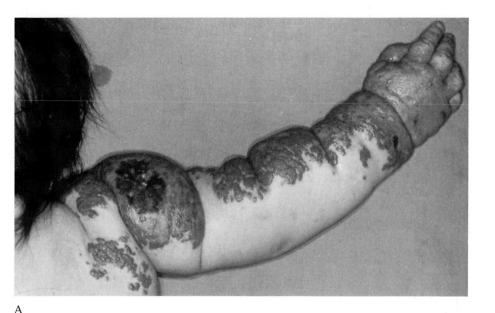

A

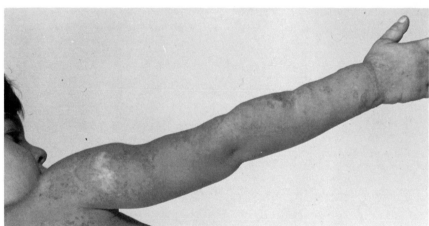

B

Fig. 23-7A. Microshunting hemangioma with additional cutaneous warmth and ulceration in deltoid region. B. Three years after use of compression garment. Note hypopigmented residual scar from healed ulceration in deltoid region.

Fig. 23-8A. Hemangioma obtunding right naris with compression. B. After cortisone injection and allowing 3 years for regression. C. Six weeks after surgical excision.

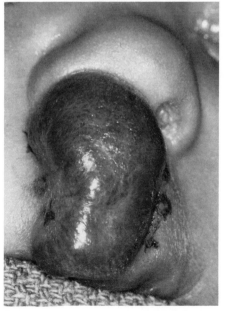

A

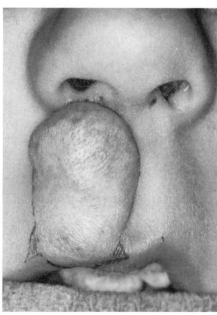

B

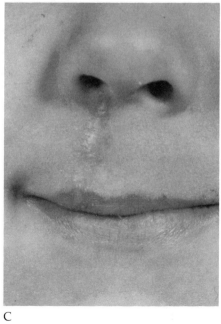

C

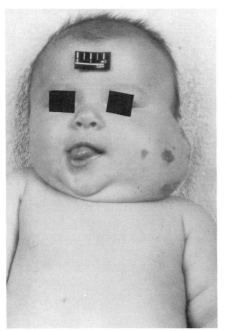
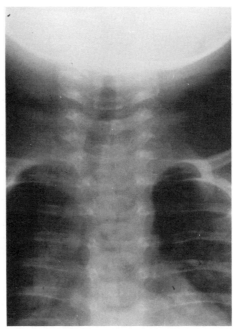

Fig. 23-9. Capillary-cavernous hemangioma of left cheek and neck with considerable unsuspected tracheal displacement.

Fig. 23-10A. Residual hemangioma of lower lip after 6 years of regression; it is an aesthetic problem. B. Soon after excision of lesion.

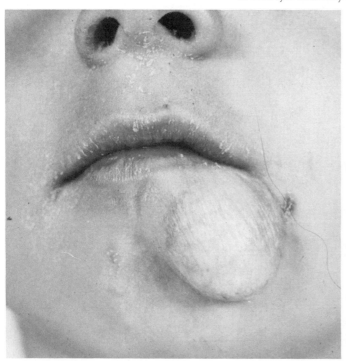
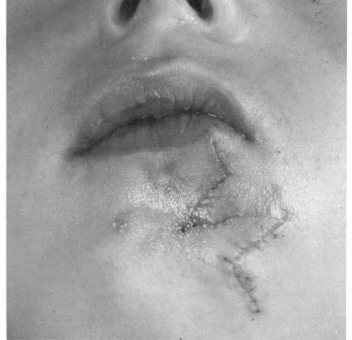

A

B

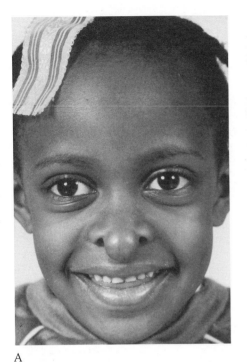
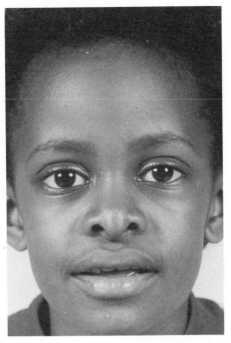

Overgrowth (Soft Tissue Gigantism)

Although almost total regression of the hemangioma may have occurred, there may be residual soft tissue excess that requires reduction (Fig. 23-12). This situation is more common in patients with capillary-cavernous hemangiomas, in which there is more deep tissue involvement than in other lesions.

Rebound Cortisone Injection

In an occasional patient who receives an injection of betamethasone and triamcinolone with an initial excellent response, the lesion reappears and is larger. This may be caused by macroshunting or formation of an AV fistula (Fig. 23-13). The anomaly may have been present initially but missed on the examination. One can become rather complacent about a routine-looking hemangioma; it is always necessary to auscultate.

A   B

Fig. 23-11A. Residual cavernous hemangioma of nasal tip and columella in 7-year-old girl. B. After midline excision.

Fig. 23-12A. Maximal regression of hemangioma with persistent gigantism. B. Step-wedge excision with Z-plasty. C. Eighteen months postoperatively.

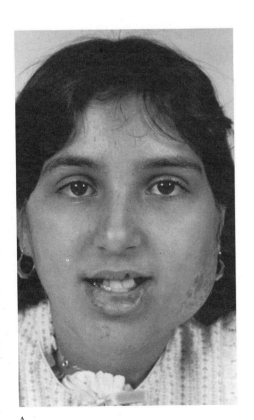
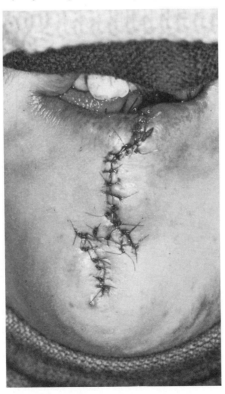
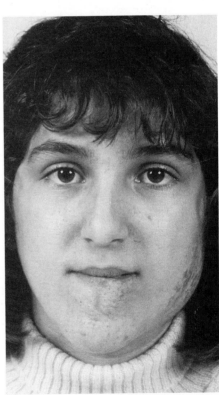

A   B   C

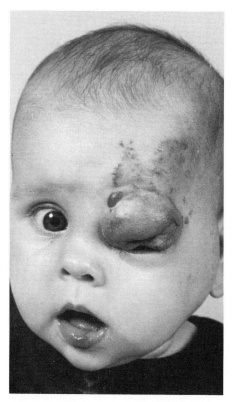

A

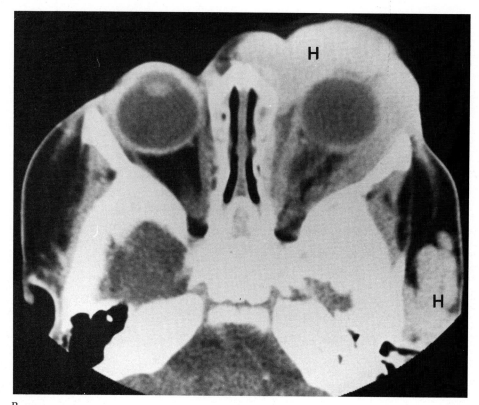

B

Fig. 23-13A. After cortisone injection for hemangioma with initial improvement and subsequent rebound closure. B. Contrast-enhanced transverse CT through orbits to show diffusely enhancing hemangioma (H). The lesion involves the eyelid and intraorbital structures with bony orbital enlargement; it is associated with inferior displacement of globe. Note additional preauricular hemangioma.

Malformations

Fortunately malformations are much rarer than hemangiomas. Usually present at birth, they can have a delayed clinical manifestation in adulthood after years of dormancy. As outlined by Mulliken in 1982, the Woolard concept of vascular maldevelopment has been a basis for various theories of the development of these malformations. Mulliken stated that during the stage of undifferentiation of the capillary network, disorganization in cell movement or segregation could cause a vascular abnormality. Like lymphatic anomalies, vascular malformations could be caused by dysmorphogenesis of the primitive jugular-subclavian and axillary sacs with a failure to reestablish venous connections. Permeating these theories is the concept of obstruction caused by hypo- or aplasia with sequestration of peripheral lymphatics. The clinical growth is usually parallel to that of the patient; however, bleeding or thrombophlebitis can cause acute enlargement, as can nonsuppurative lymphangitis. Various degrees of gigantism, or overgrowth, including that of bone, can occur.

The depth of involvement of vascular malformations is of clinical significance, and the predominant type of anomaly also is important. These two issues can be clarified by imaging techniques. There are basically two types of imaging: magnetic resonance imaging (MRI) and CT with enhancement (Fig. 23-14). Magnetic resonance imaging is superb for defining the extent of a lesion and its differentiation from normal tissues. It is also useful in demonstrating enlarged vessels in relation to a high-flow malformation. On the other hand, CT with enhancement can distinguish between capillary-venous lesions and lymphatic lesions; lymphatic lesions do not enhance. In addition, CT can outline bone and adjacent bony deformities. Arteriography and direct puncture angiography also play a diagnostic and therapeutic role.

Capillary Malformations

Nevus Flammeus (Port-Wine Stain)

Nevus flammeus, a flat red macular lesion, is present at birth, but it is not always vividly evident at delivery, becoming obvious during the neonatal period.

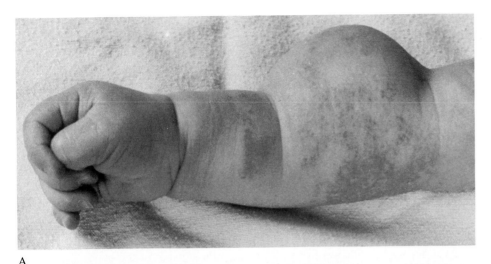

A

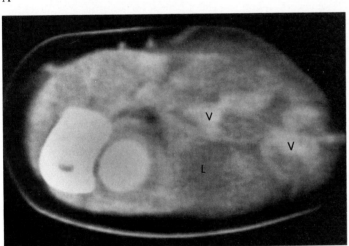

B

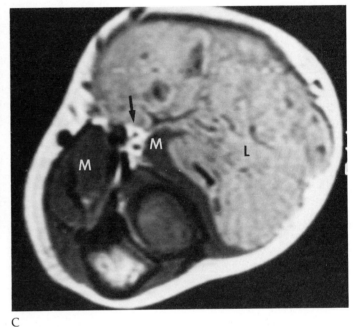

C

Fig. 23-14A. Combined lymphatic-capillary-venous malformation of the forearm. B. Contrast-enhanced transverse CT image of forearm shows mixed lesion containing low-density (lymphatic) (L) and contrast-enhancing (capillary-venous) (V) components. Angiographic confirmation was obtained. C. Transverse MRI through same forearm lesion shows more clearly the demarcation between lesion (L) and adjacent normal muscular (M) and neurovascular structures (arrow).

The lesion can be spotty or homogeneous with a mild-to-severe red hue. It can cross the midline with bilateral involvement but rarely does so when primarily unilateral (Fig. 23-15). It can be confused with nevus neonatorum, which is found in the glabellar-forehead region and regresses spontaneously by the age of 9 months. In contradistinction, nevus nuchae, also called stork bite or salmon patch, is found at the nape of the neck and persists in Caucasians throughout their lifetimes.

In general nevus flammeus most commonly involves the sensory distribution of the Vth cranial nerve and high cervical region. If the ipsilateral V_1 and V_2 areas are involved, glaucoma automatically is suspected. Intracranial involvement is possible in the form of Sturge-Weber syndrome, even in a patient without symptoms. Some investigators believe CT is imperative by the age of 5 years, particularly in children who are to play aggressive sports. If endoral mucosal involvement is present, there is commonly an element of gigantism of the involved facial soft tissues as well as bony overgrowth.

The methods of treating nevus flammeus are legion. It is only in recent years with

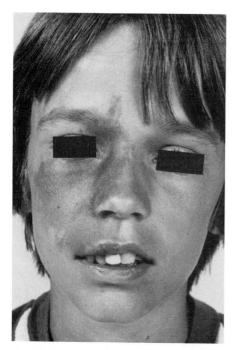

Fig. 23-15. *Nevus flammeus involving right V₂ with abrupt midline demarcation.*

the onset of laser therapy that true "cures" have been possible. We used an argon laser for 8 years with varied results. Throughout this time period, although the lesion disappeared, rarely if ever was the skin texture considered normal; we also found a 3 to 5 percent chance of varying degrees of hypertrophic burn scar formation, which caused us great concern. The relatively new flashlamp-pulsed tunable dye laser avoids this major problem and appears to be providing a higher percentage of cures. The original laser had an emission wavelength of 577 nm, raised recently to 585 nm. This wavelength provides selective absorption by the intravascular oxyhemoglobin and has a pulse duration of 450 μsec at 6 joules per square centimeter. This figure closely matches the thermal relaxation time for dermal blood vessels and precludes superficial skin necrosis and thus residual scarring. Unfortunately there is a drawback to this method of treatment: It requires a large number of treatments per area. Tan reported an average of 6.5 sessions per treated area. We are attempting to de-

crease the number of treatments using higher energy levels with more overlap and including larger areas with up to 1000 pulses. This procedure is usually done with general anesthesia; for small lesions either topical anesthesia or no anesthesia is used (Fig. 23-16).

Nevus Araneus (Spider Nevus)

Nevus araneus commonly occurs in girls 6 to 9 years of age on the anterior cheek; it can appear as an isolated lesion or as multiple lesions. There is a central arteriole with superficial vessels that radiate from the centrum. Other small, isolated lesions can be found elsewhere, usually on the dorsum of the hands and wrists. These blanch on compression. There is a natural tendency for spontaneous regression after puberty. If sensitivity is severe, the use of a pulse-dye tunable laser is worthwhile. These isolated lesions are to be differentiated from the autosomal dominant Rendu-Osler-Weber syndrome, which is also known as hereditary hemorrhagic telangiectasia.

Fig. 23-16. *Nevus flammeus treated with laser therapy. A. Lesion is gridded with skin-marking pen (light grid lines). B. After pulse-dye laser treatment is completed, lesion is much darker for 4 to 7 days.*

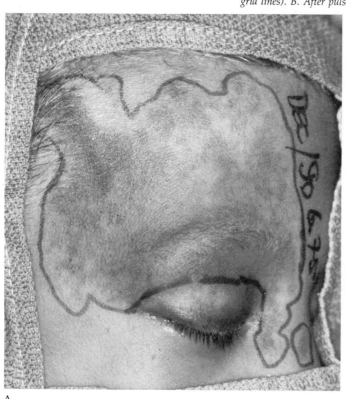

A

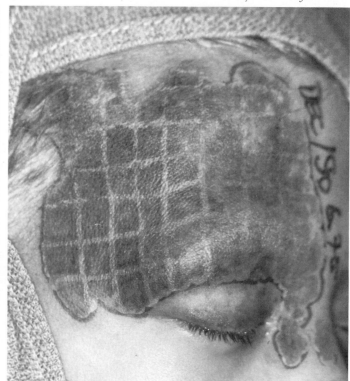

B

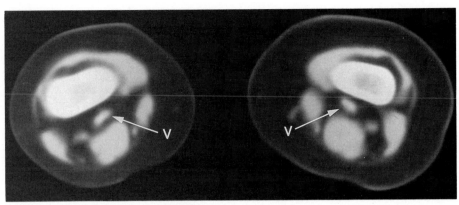

Fig. 23-17A. *Nevus flammeus and lymphatic gigantism with discoloration of left thigh and flank. B. Contrast-enhanced transverse CT image through lower thighs showing diffuse increased subcutaneous fat of left thigh with slight muscular enlargement. Vessels (V) appear normal.*

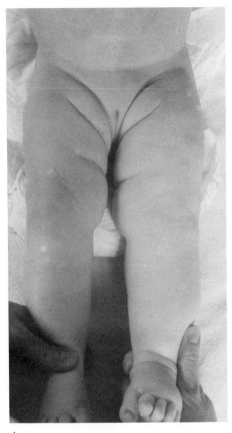

A

Nevus Flammeus Neonatorum

Nevus flammeus neonatorum is usually found in the glabellar and eyelid regions in newborn infants. The lesion usually disappears in 9 to 12 months. It is difficult to predict which lesions are of this type and will fade and which will persist, but the location in the central glabella and upper eyelids usually suggests nevus flammeus neonatorum rather than permanent nevus flammeus. If the lesion is elsewhere on the face, there is a greater likelihood that it will persist.

Nuchal Nevus (Salmon Patch, Stork Bite)

Nevus nuchae is a common finding in the posterior cervical hairline. It has a faint, homogeneous hue. The lesion usually has no clinical significance and persists into adulthood. Rarely if ever is any attempt made to treat this aesthetically insignificant lesion.

Cutis Marmorata Telangiectasia

Cutis marmorata telangiectasia is a congenital erythematous lesion with thinning of the skin and enlarged visible reticulated venous channels running throughout. It usually involves a limb and occasionally is associated with hypoplasia of the involved limb. There is a history of gradual improvement throughout infancy. It is reassuring to parents to be informed of the predicted improvement.

Capillary-Lymphatic and Capillary-Lymphatic-Venous Malformations

Capillary-lymphatic and capillary-lymphatic-venous malformations usually involve the lower and sometimes the upper limb with associated overgrowth, or gigantism. The flank and abdomen can be affected as well. Computed tomography or MRI is worthwhile to determine the extent of the lesion and extra- and intraperitoneal involvement (Fig. 23-17). The degree of enlargement is rarely excessive and can respond to a compression garment or segmental pumps. The capillary component can be treated, preferably early in the first year, with a pulse-dye tunable laser.

Verrucous Malformations (Keratotic Hemangioma)

Verrucous malformations are relatively rare lesions usually involving the limbs. They can be isolated or multiple and have raised, purple-red wartlike patches (Fig. 23-18). The lesions have a silvery scaly appearance with a history of intermittent, annoying venous bleeds. The lesions are usually deeper than anticipated and can penetrate through fascia into muscle.

Specific treatment should be primarily for bleeding but might occasionally be for aesthetic purposes.

The argon and tunable dye lasers can ameliorate the superficial bleeding problem, but only wide excision with or without a skin graft has curative potential. Late infiltration of the skin graft can occur even with this approach and after apparent total excision. These lesions are the most apparent components of the Klippel-Trenaunay syndrome (K-T).

Klippel-Trenaunay Syndrome

Klippel-Trenaunay syndrome is a combination of nevus flammeus and nevus avaneus with associated limb enlargement and anomalies of the major venous channels of the affected limb. It is usually unilateral and involves the lower limb, but the ipsilateral upper limb also may be involved and, rarely, a contralateral isolated limb as well. Cross-sectional imaging shows a spectrum of abnormalities, including increased subcutaneous fat, lymphedema, cystic lymphatic malformations, low-flow vascular masses, and ectopic or malformed vessels. Also, muscle enlargement or atrophy and increased or decreased length and thickness of bone may be demonstrated. If the major portion of the lower limb is involved, the abdomen, flank, and back are usually included (Fig. 23-19). In this situation, CT or MRI should be completed. Bladder involvement with associated hematuria occurs and can compound the problem. As-

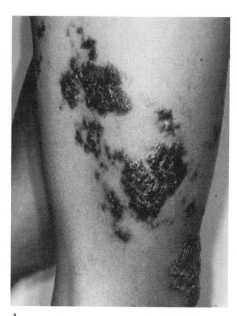

A

Fig. 23-18A. *Verrucous-venous malformation isolated to lateral thigh and knee. B. Another diffuse lesion extending from foot to groin.*

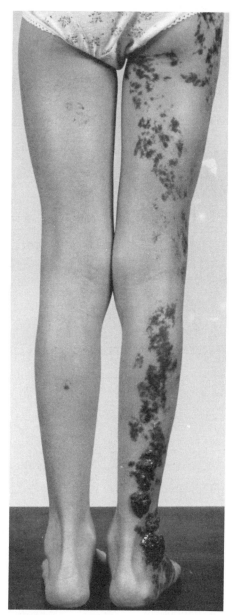

B

Fig. 23-19A. *Klippel-Trenaunay (K-T) diffuse involvement of right lower limb and flank. B. Contrast-enhanced transverse CT through midthigh demonstrating enlargement, subcutaneous stranding (S) of lymphangioma, large intramuscular lymphatic cysts (C), large anomalous vein (V), absent normal femoral vein, and small femoral shaft (F). The scan has been photographed light to emphasize the abnormal subcutaneous tissues.*

A

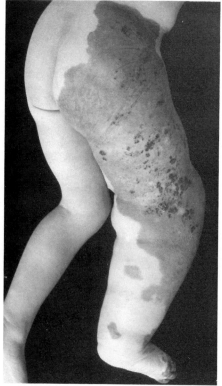

B

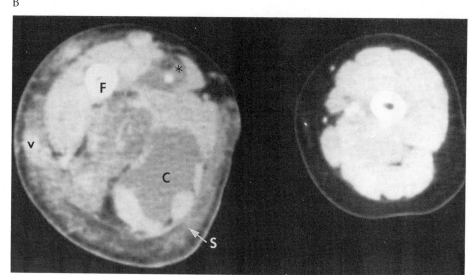

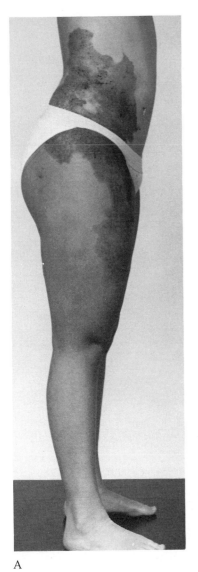
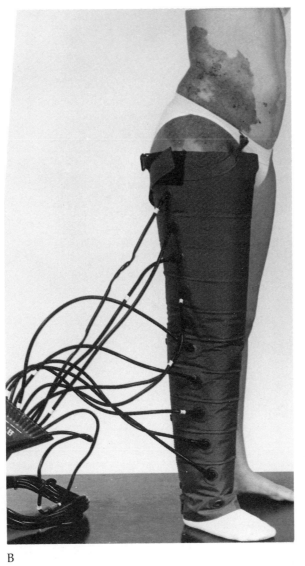
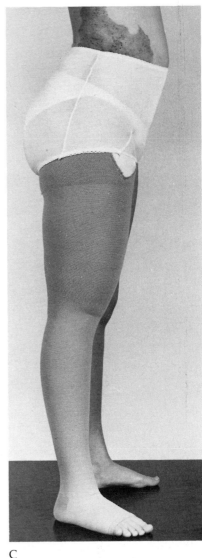

A   B   C

Fig. 23-20A. Klippel-Trenaunay syndrome involving right lower limb and flank. B. Segmental compartment pressurized unit in use. C. Support with elastic garment after removal of pressurized unit.

sociated with venous varices is lymphedema caused by lymphatic hypoplasia. The limb enlargement can be noted when compared with the opposite, normal side. Volumetric displacement is an excellent method of monitoring the progress of the lesion. In some situations, whether localized gigantism exists or enlargement is diffuse, amputation may be necessary for aesthetic and functional reasons. We have found the nighttime use of a segmental compression pump to be a worthwhile adjunct (Fig. 23-20). This treatment process can be monitored easily by volumetric displacement and should be used in conjunction with a daytime compression garment.

Parkes Weber Syndrome

Parkes Weber syndrome (PW), a rare condition, is similar to K-T, but there is, in addition, clinical evidence of an AV shunt. It is always worthwhile to examine patients with K-T carefully by palpation and by stethoscope to rule out the possibility of PW syndrome. Parkes Weber syndrome has the potential to cause left ventricular strain or failure. Angiography and embolization may be useful in these patients, especially in the presence of clinically significant cardiac volume overload or ischemic tissue complications.

Lymphangiohemangioma and Hemangiolymphangioma

This group of lesions comprises localized malformations that are primarily either blood vessel or lymphatic in composition. Mulliken prefers to describe these lesions as lymphaticovenous malformations. There is usually no tendency toward spontaneous regression in either of the basic components, and thus direct or specific treatment is necessary if some degree of improvement is to occur. Intervention frequently is not possible as in lesions involving the periorbital region or tongue (Fig. 23-21). There is often diffuse involvement that prohibits surgical intervention, but an embolization procedure may provide some short- or long-term improvement. Isolated lesions also can contain both lymphatic and blood vessel components. Contrast-enhanced CT is useful to demonstrate the different components of the lesion (Fig. 23-22). Subsequent treatment is often necessary because of persistent bleeding.

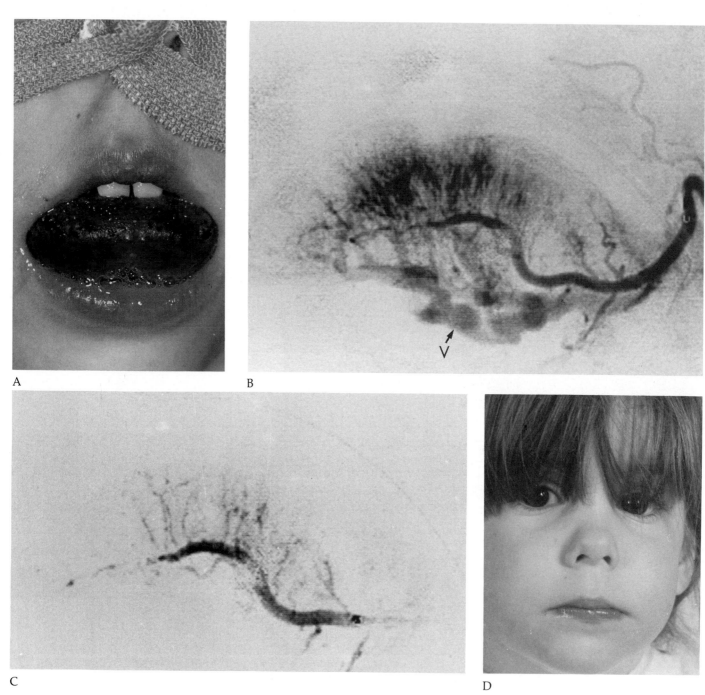

Fig. 23-21A. Tongue demonstrating hemangiolymphangioma just before selective arteriography. B. Lateral lingual arteriogram showing filling of small abnormal vascular spaces within the tongue and early filling of dilated veins (V). C. After selective embolization with polyvinyl alcohol sponge particles with decrease in flow and occlusion of many muscular branches. D. Twenty-four hours after embolization. The lesions did partially recur, however, 4 months after treatment.

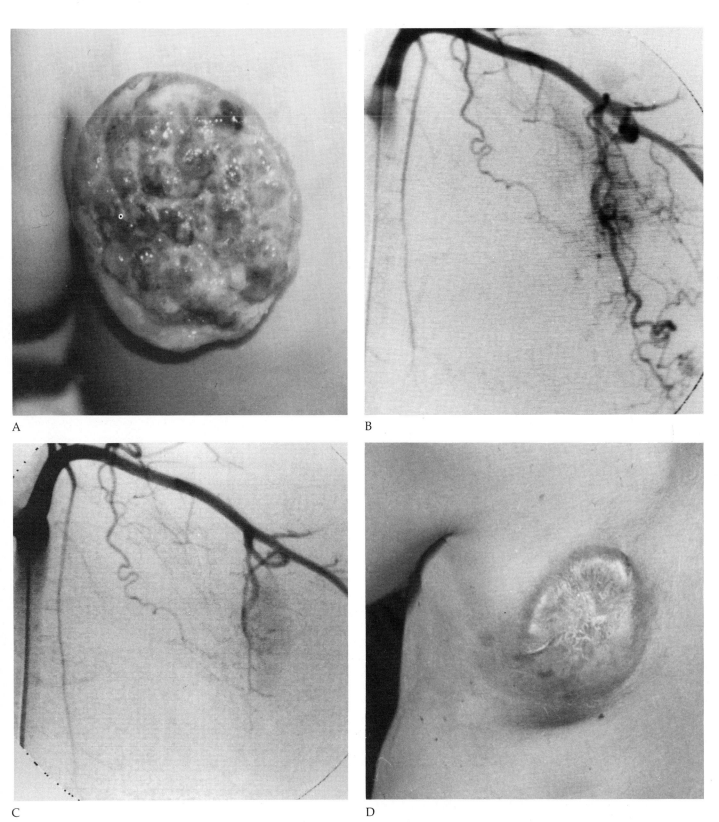

A

B

C

D

Fig. 23-22A. Lymphangiohemangioma of left back with fungating-exsanguinating lesion. B. Left subclavian arteriogram shows increased vascularity arising from lateral thoracic and subscapular arteries. C. After selective embolization with polyvinyl alcohol sponge particles. D. Clinical appearance 5 months after three embolization procedures. Three years later there was still no recurrence.

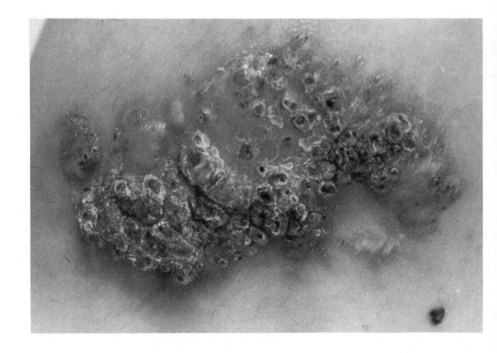

Fig. 23-23. Lymphangioma simplex and circumscriptum demonstrating raised blister-like lesions. These may be filled with venous blood from time to time.

Lymphatic Malformations

Lymphatic malformations (LM) can be localized in the superficial epidermal-dermal layers or diffuse in the deeper layers of the skin and soft tissues. They can cause distortion or obstruction of important structures such as the larynx and trachea. These ectopic lymphatic channels are lined with a thin layer of endothelium and filled with a proteinaceous clear yellow fluid. Occasional venous bleeding into the spaces can occur, giving rise to an acute increase in size, as can nonpurulent lymphangitis. The latter responds slowly to a 5-day course of antibiotics; penicillin is usually appropriate. It is worthwhile to forewarn parents of these two potential complications. For deep lesions MRI and CT, with and without enhancement, are helpful for diagnosis and determining anatomic location.

Lymphangioma Simplex and Circumscriptum

Lymphangioma simplex and circumscriptum appears within the skin itself, both superficially and deep. The lesions resemble small cauliflowers or warts filled with clear fluid. They may demonstrate intertriginous low-grade infection. Occasionally venous bleeds occur into these small vesicle-like lesions. Treatment can be attempted with electrocautery, the argon laser, or surgical excision. A split-thickness skin graft is usually required (Fig. 23-23).

Cavernous Lymphangioma

Cavernous lymphangioma is more extensive than the preceding types and has not only superficial and deep skin involvement but also subcutaneous and even fascial-muscular involvement. The extent of the lesion can be determined by imaging, which is imperative if wide surgical excision is to be considered. Some areas of the body present practical and philosophical limitations to this approach, namely the tongue and the breast (Fig. 23-24). There is evidence to support a conservative approach in a situation in which important structures would be sacrificed by an operation. Surgical excision is fraught with complications, primarily a risk of wound infection, peripheral nerve resection, and reappearance of residual lymphangioma.

Lymphangioma Hygroma (Cystoides)

Lymphangioma hygroma, lymph-filled endothelium-lined cysts, may be unilocular or multilocular. They are found primarily in the neck, but in 20 percent of patients they are located elsewhere, such as the axilla or the groin. The lesions tend not to encapsulate and thus have no true anatomic boundaries. Imaging is of great assistance in determining the extent of the lesion. Early surgical excision is necessary if respiratory tract obstruction occurs because of associated intrinsic in-

volvement or compression. There may be an opportunity to approach this problem in a more conservative way—by single or multiple aspirations and compression or injection of a sclerosant such as Ethibloc. This material was introduced recently, and the results, although encouraging, are not completely known. The injected material may form a hard lump that is slow to absorb and from time to time may erode through the skin surface (Fig. 23-25).

Venous Malformations

Venous malformations, a cutaneous group of lesions, can be confused with cavernous hemangiomas in that they are present at birth. They are clearly more superficial, however, and are filled with venous blood. They are compressible with no associated arterial component, such as a pulsatile phenomenon. These lesions are large dilated channels lined by endothelium and may show some evidence of smooth muscle too. Frequently there are phleboliths within the confines of the lesion. These are readily palpable and may even be tender when associated with thrombophlebitis.

If a venous malformation is suspected, it is worthwhile to image and localize the lesions with venous phase arteriography. The malformation may be treated by percutaneous injection of sclerosing agents

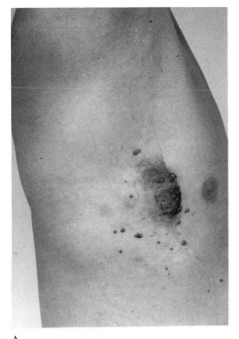

A

Fig. 23-24A. Cavernous lymphangioma involving
lateral chest wall. B. At time of excision, showing
smooth walled, multiseptate interior.

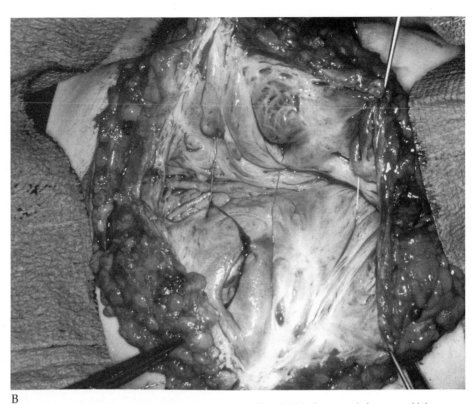

B

Fig. 23-25A. Large cystic hygroma of left
posterior triangle and trapezius region.
B. Enhanced transverse CT image through neck
shows intramuscular, nonenhancing, unilocular
cystic lesion (C). C. Several weeks after injection
with Ethibloc demonstrating small residual
fullness caused by firm Ethibloc mass. There was
no evidence of recurrence 6 months after
treatment.

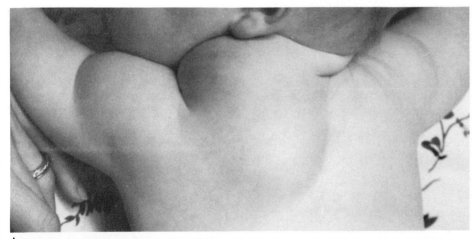

A

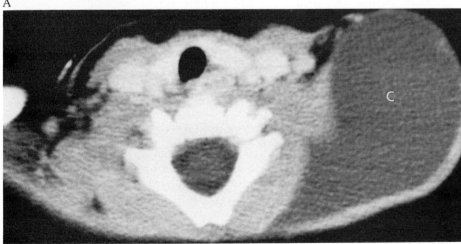

B

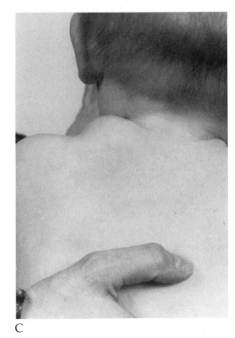

C

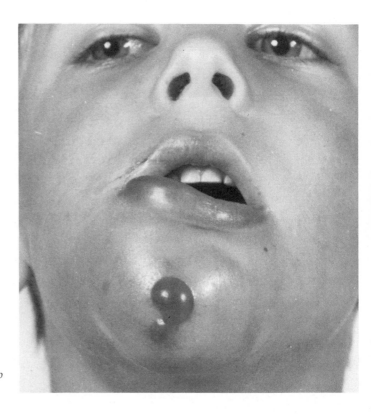

Fig. 23-26. Superficial skin blistering after percutaneous injection of 100% ethanol into venous malformation.

such as 100% ethanol or Ethibloc. The mass is cannulated percutaneously with a polytetrafluoroethylene (PTFE) sheath needle. Direct-puncture angiography is performed to confirm the intravascular positioning of the cannula. The contrast medium is then removed from the lesion and the radiopaque sclerosant is instilled under fluoroscopic control. The procedure results in initial thrombosis of the contents of the lesion with swelling, followed by regression of the swelling and the lesion in the course of 2 months. When ethanol is used most patients require three or four such procedures before regression is stable. This technique is generally safe, but skin necrosis can occur, especially with superficial lesions (Figs. 23-26 and 23-27). Another popular percutaneous sclerosant is recommended by Woods—sodium tetradecyl sulfate in aliquots of 0.05 to 0.1 ml at multiple sites with the total dose not to exceed 2.0 to 4.0 ml. Occasionally simple surgical resection can provide a worthwhile result (Fig. 23-28).

A different type of lesion, often clinically confused with a venous malformation, is the glomangioma. This lesion is painful and tender and of a considerably different basic pathology. It usually responds to wide excision and a skin graft.

Arteriovenous Malformations

The treatment of these rare congenital high-flow vascular malformations continues to frustrate therapists. Arteriovenous malformations can be truncal and large; or small and single, as a nidus; or multiple. Clinically they can remain hidden under other cutaneous vascular malformations, but they all have an increased temperature, which should cause suspicion, and they can be elicited by auscultation. This is not true, however, of the microshunting that can occur in some of the "hot," combined hemangiomas. Again, cross-sectional imaging and arteriography are primary requirements before therapy is considered.

Selective embolization remains the major method of palliation, presurgical size reduction, and even potential cure. Catheter delivery systems for embolization are now available in small and easily manipulated forms. In particular, the French No. 3 and No. 4 graduated-stiffness infusion catheters can reach tiny vessels with resultant superselection occlusion. A variety of embolic materials are available for temporary and permanent occlusion. Spring emboli (coils) in a wide range of diameters are used to occlude arterial

branches and fistulas. Detachable balloons have the advantage of being flow-directed and are also useful in occluding large vessels and arteriovenous fistulas. Liquid or particulate emboli are most frequently used to reach the nidus of an AV malformation. Polyvinyl alcohol foam is available in suspensions of differing particle sizes, ranging from 50 to 1000 μ. Liquids such as N-butyl-2-cyanoacrylate, ethanol, and Ethibloc are used to penetrate the capillary bed or to occlude the nidus of AV malformations. Both gelatin foam plugs and microfibular collagen are resorbable and thus are temporary occluding agents. Each of these materials has potential complications and should be used only by physicians with appropriate technical training and understanding of the vascular anatomy of the areas involved.

The decision to proceed with embolization is best made after discussion of the indications and treatment options for each patient. Embolization may be performed to improve symptoms or in combination with a surgical procedure, but it is not recommended in patients who do not have symptoms. The goal of embolization of AV malformations as primary treatment is to "cast" the nidus, preferably with a liquid embolic agent. Embo-

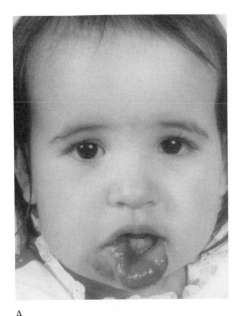

A

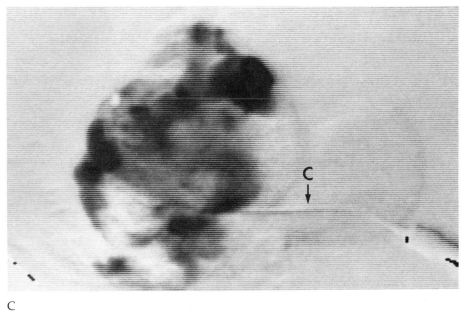

C

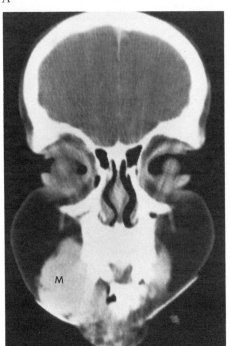

B

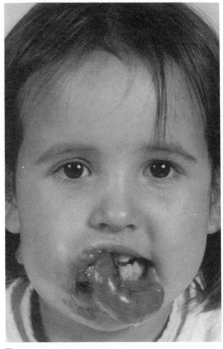

D

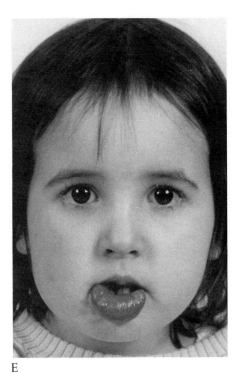

E

Fig. 23-27A. Venous malformation of lower lip. B. Coronal contrast-enhanced CT image through maxilla showing densely enhancing, well-defined right subcutaneous mass (M). C. Contrast-injection digital subtraction angiogram after percutaneous cannulation (C) of right facial mass. This lesion showed filling sinusoidal spaces before injection of the sclerosant. D. Intense lower lip swelling after injection, with zone of skin necrosis under right commissure. E. Considerable improvement is seen after eschar separation and healing.

lization should be distal, avoiding occlusion of the proximal trunks, because such occlusion is invariably followed by development of collaterals from less accessible areas, such as the basal intracranial arteries. Embolization can improve the symptoms of AV malformations, such as ischemic ulceration, bleeding, congestive heart failure, local pain, and mass effect, but it is usually not curative. Because embolization of recurrent lesions becomes progressively more difficult as the arterial access diminishes, techniques have been developed to treat the remaining nidus by percutaneous injection of liquid agents, such as cyanoacrylates and ethanol. The long-term results of repeated embolizations are not known, but some patients have done well. In particular, lesions involving the maxilla and mandible have been shown to heal after technically excellent embolizations. Embolization is not without associated complications, however.

Surgical intervention, with or without the adjunct of embolization, remains hazardous and frustrating regarding curing the macroshunt and aesthetic improvement. The proximal ligation of a truncal AV malformation simply encourages collaterals to open up and worsen the situation. If en bloc resection is deemed technically possible, however, preoperative embolization can be helpful to shrink the lesion and lessen blood loss (Fig. 23-29). This procedure can be augmented by the use of hypothermia, hypotensive anesthesia, and cardiopulmonary bypass.

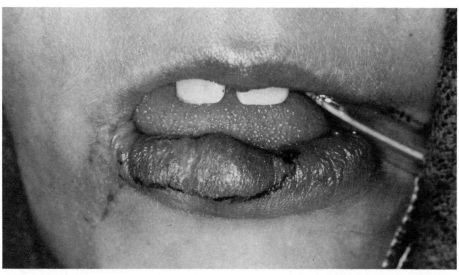

A

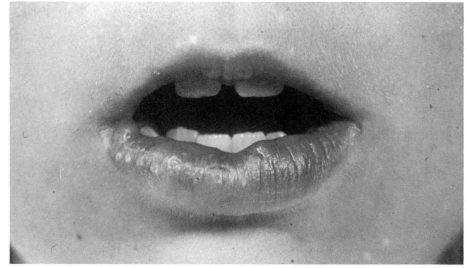

B

Fig. 23-28A. Venous malformation of leading edge of right lower lip. B. Four months after excision.

Suggested Reading

Apfelberg, D.B., Maser, M.R., and Lash H. Review of usage of argon and CO_2 lasers for pediatric hemangiomas. *Ann. Plast. Surg.* 12:353, 1984.

Azizkhan, R.G., et al. Mast cell heparin stimulates migration of capillary endothelial cells in vitro. *J. Exp. Med.* 152:931, 1990.

Burrows, P.E., Lasjaunias, P., and TerBrugge, K.G. A 4-F coaxial catheter system for pediatric vascular occlusion with detachable balloons. *Radiology* 170:1091, 1989.

Burrows, P.E., et al. Urgent and emergent embolization of lesions of the head and neck in children: Indications and results. *Pediatrics* 80:386, 1987.

Demuth, R.J., Miller, S.H., and Keller, F. Complications of embolization treatment for problem cavernous hemangiomas. *Ann. Plast. Surg.* 13:135, 1984.

Grabb, W.C., et al. Facial hamartomas in children: Neurofibroma, lymphangioma and hemangioma. *Plast. Reconstr. Surg.* 66:509, 1980.

Kushner, B.J. Intralesional corticosteroid injection for infantile adnexal hemangioma. *Am. J. Ophthalmol.* 93:496, 1982.

Lasjaunias, P., and Berinstein, A. *Surgical Neuroangiography.* Vol. 2. *Endovascular Treatment of Craniofacial Lesions.* Berlin: Springer, 1987.

Mulliken, J.B., and Young, A.E. *Vascular Birthmarks: Hemangioma and Malformations.* Philadelphia: Saunders, 1988.

Sasaki, G.H., Pang, C.Y., and Wittliff, J.L. Pathogenesis and treatment of infant skin strawberry hemangiomas: Clinical and in vitro studies of hormonal effects. *Plast. Reconstr. Surg.* 73:359, 1984.

Stevenson, R.F., Thomson, H.G., and Morin, J.D. Unrecognized ocular problems associated with port wine stains of the face in children. *Can. Med. Assoc. J.* 111:953, 1974.

Stringel, G., and Dastous, J.J. Klippel-Trenaunay syndrome and other cases of lower limb hypertrophy: Surgical implications. *J. Pediatr. Surg.* 22:645, 1987.

Tan, O.T., Sherwood, K., and Gilchrest, B.A. Treatment of children with port wine stains using the flashlamp-pulsed tunable dye laser. *N. Engl. J. Med.* 320:416, 1989.

Thomson, H.G. Cutaneous hemangiomas and lymphangiomas. *Clin. Plast. Surg.* 14:341, 1987.

Thomson, H.G., et al. Hemangiomas of the eyelids: Visual complications and prophylactic concepts. *Plast. Reconstr. Surg.* 63:641, 1979.

Woods, J.E. Extended use of sodium tetradecyl sulfate in treatment of hemangiomas and other related conditions. *Plast. Reconstr. Surg.* 79:542, 1987.

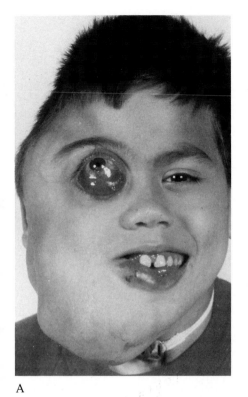

A

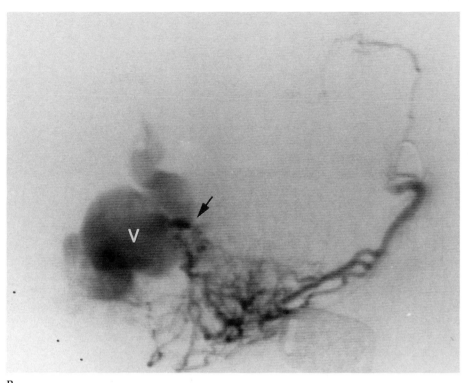

B

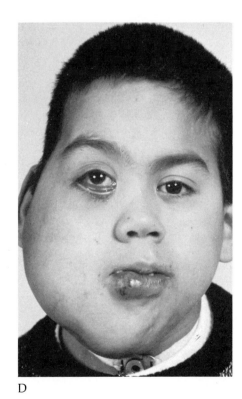

C

D

Fig. 23-29A. Patient with combined (AV) malformation with lymphatic component after ligation of right common carotid artery. B. Selective left facial arteriogram shows AV fistula (arrow) and venous pouch (V). C. After embolization with polyvinyl alcohol sponge particles, the venous pouch was injected percutaneously with N-butyl-2-cyanoacrylate to control acute oral bleeding. Repeat angiography 6 months later showed persistent occlusion of the fistula. D. After partial resection. (Courtesy of J. Posnick, H.S.C.)

24

Lymphedema

Bernard McC. O'Brien   P. A. Vinod Kumar

The treatment of lymphedema is a difficult and challenging problem. The condition is characterized by progressive swelling of a limb, induration, fibrosis, and repeated attacks of cellulitis. The protein-rich edematous fluid provokes an intense fibrous reaction, which further reduces the lymphatic transport. Treatment of lymphedema should be undertaken early, therefore, before irreparable damage to the lymphatics occurs.

Conservative, or nonoperative, treatment consists of hygienic measures to prevent or treat infection, manual lymphatic drainage to increase lymphatic transport, remedial exercise, and the retention of improvement, achieved by elastic support. Patient compliance is essential for the success of conservative therapy. Many patients find conservative treatment bothersome and the use of elastic support uncomfortable during the warm months.

Most surgeons advocate surgical intervention only for patients whose condition has not improved with conservative treatment. The surgical techniques used to treat lymphedema include drainage procedures, reduction procedures, and combined drainage and excisional proce-

dures. Reduction procedures are limited to excision of the excessive bulk of the limb. On the other hand, drainage procedures, such as lymphaticovenous anastomosis, aim at restoring the physiologic communication between the lymphatics and the veins. In lymphaticolymphatic anastomoses, used by some surgeons, lymphatic grafts bypass the obstruction in the lymphatics and reestablish lymphatic flow. These drainage techniques have greatly improved the results in the last decade. The results could be improved further with early referral, when there is little damage to the lymphatics.

Etiology

Primary Lymphedema

Primary lymphedema is the type found in 14 percent of instances of lower limb lymphedema (Microsurgery Research Centre statistics), but it is extremely rare in the upper limb. It may be caused by aplasia, hypoplasia, or varicosity of the subcutaneous lymphatics. It may present at birth (lymphedema), at puberty (lymphedema praecox), or in adult life (lymphedema tarda).

Secondary Lymphedema

Therapy for breast cancer is the cause of 90 percent of instances of upper limb lymphedema. Although either surgical or radiation therapy for carcinoma of the breast can cause lymphedema, it is the combination of these methods of treatment that causes most instances of lymphedema (Table 24-1). Seventy-five percent of all instances occur in the upper limb. The female-to-male ratio is 10:1.

Table 24-1. Cause of obstructive lymphedema in 134 patients treated by microlymphaticovenous operations

Cause	No. patients	Percentage
Breast carcinoma	92	69
Operation alone	12	
Radiation alone	1	
Operation and radiation	79	
Melanoma	13	10
Carcinoma of genital tract	8	6
Lymphoma	6	4
Trauma	4	3
Other	11	8

In contrast to these statistics, in China and other developing countries, filariasis or erysipelas causes lower limb lymphedema in more than 50 percent of patients.

Anatomy

Primary lymphatics arise in the interstitial tissue as capillaries that consist of an endothelial layer one cell thick. These lymphatic capillaries are valveless and enlarge to form secondary lymphatics. The secondary lymphatics have some valves, but it is only in the tertiary lymphatics that the valves become numerous and occur at regular intervals. Just proximal to each valve is an expanded sinus, which gives the characteristic beaded appearance on lymphangiography and as seen through an operating microscope. The tertiary lymphatic vessels branch and communicate with each other but do not increase in size as they ascend; they are about 0.5 mm in diameter.

The walls of the tertiary lymphatics consist of three layers—an outer adventitia, an intermediate muscular layer, and an inner endothelium. The muscular layer is responsible for rhythmic contractions of the lymphatics. The intrinsic lymphatic muscle contractions, together with the muscle pump action, the presence of valves, and the negative intrathoracic pressure, account for the unidirectional flow of lymph. The intralymphatic pressure is subatmospheric and becomes more so at the thoracic duct level. This descending gradient increases during deep inspiration and accounts for the flow of lymph in an anesthetized patient when the muscle pump action is absent. The main superficial lymphatic trunks accompany the main superficial veins, and the deep lymphatics accompany the deep artery and vein. There are only a few communications among the superficial and the deep lymphatics. The direction of flow is from the superficial to the deep lymphatics.

In the lower limb the superficial lymphatics accompany either the great saphenous vein or the small saphenous vein. The great saphenous system drains the posteromedial aspect of the leg into the inguinal lymph nodes. The small saphenous system drains the posterolateral aspect of the leg either by the popliteal node into the deep system or directly to the inguinal node.

The superficial lymphatics in the upper limb accompany either the basilic or the cephalic vein. Some lymph trunks in the basilic group drain into the epitrochlear lymph node at the elbow and into the deep system, but most drain directly into the axillary nodes. The lymphatics in the cephalic group also drain into the axillary nodes, but some of the more lateral ones in this group may bypass the axilla and drain into the supraclavicular nodes.

Pathophysiology

At the arterial end of the circulation, the hydrostatic pressure is higher than the osmotic pressure and drives protein-rich fluid into the interstitial tissue. Most of this fluid is returned to the circulation at the venous end, where the osmotic pressure is greater. The remaining high-molecular-weight proteins and their associated water are removed from the interstitial tissue by the lymphatics, but some are broken down into smaller particles by monocyte-derived macrophages before being absorbed into the veins.

Edema occurs only when the number of functioning lymphatics is reduced below a critical level or when there is an increased lymphatic load. Primary lymphedema may develop at birth (congenital lymphedema) or later (lymphedema praecox and lymphedema tarda). Secondary lymphedema can develop years after surgical or radiation therapy, initially there is an adequate number of functioning lymphatics, but the number is reduced gradually to below the critical level by scarring, infection, or the long-term effects of radiation. A decrease in the number of functioning lymphatics results in high-protein edema, which increases the tissue osmotic pressure and causes an additional shift of fluid into the interstitial tissue. This process provokes an inflammatory reaction resulting in perilymphatic scarring and obliteration of lymphatic trunks, reducing lymphatic transport even more.

The effect of lymphedema is seen mainly in the more expansile superficial tissue. There is increased thickness of the skin (primarily of the dermal elements) and scarring of the subcutaneous tissue. Extensive scarring in the subcutaneous tissue can result in venous obstruction, but this is a rare and a late phenomenon. Because the effect of lymphedema is superficial to the deep fascia, it was thought that the primary abnormality was in the superficial lymphatics and that the deep lymphatics were normal. This belief formed the basis of the buried dermal wick operation; however, experimental work demonstrated that it is the deep lymphatics that first show evidence of obstruction. The communications between the deep and the superficial lymphatics become incompetent, leading to dilatation of the superficial lymphatics in the more expansile subcutaneous tissue. Dilatation of the superficial lymphatics precedes the appearance of edema by months or years.

Lymphaticovenous communications can occur normally. These communications also are seen in abnormal circumstances but are not adequate to prevent edema. Researchers have attempted artificial lymphovenous anastomoses in an effort to drain the excess lymph in obstructive lymphedema. Mainly for technical reasons the initial emphasis was placed on anastomosis of a transected lymph node into the side of a vein. Although doubts exist whether these anastomoses continue to be patent, good clinical results have been reported. With microsurgical techniques, increased patency has been obtained by direct lymphaticovenous anastomosis and by lymphaticolymphatic anastomosis.

Diagnostic Tests

Investigations are carried out to establish the diagnosis when it is not clear from a careful history. It is essential to establish a diagnosis because in primary lymphedema the lymphatics are either hypoplastic or absent and are unsuitable for drainage procedures. Ten percent of our patients with secondary or obstructive lymphedema did not have lymphatics of a suitable size for microlymphaticovenous anastomoses, as we found at operation. It would be useful to know the condition of the lymphatics preoperatively thus avoiding an unnecessary exploration, but such a precise test is not available. In secondary lymphedema it is necessary also to exclude active malignant growth.

Lymphoangiography once was used to evaluate the suitability of lymphatics for an anastomosis. It provided good anatomic details of the lymphatics, but in one study 17 of 51 patients had an increase in edema after the procedure. It is therefore contraindicated.

Lymphoscintigraphy using ^{99m}Tc rhenium sulphide colloid or ^{99m}Tc pertechnetate stannous sulphur enables identification of the lymphatics and the draining nodes but does not enable direct visualization of the anastomosis; however, the rate of clearance of the radiotracer is good indirect evidence of lymphatic function. In addition, limb volume is measured at the wrist or ankle, elbow or knee, and arm or thigh. Linear measurements are made at the middle of the palm or foot and 15 cm above and below the elbow or knee. These measurements are repeated every 3 to 6 months. When the measurements are taken carefully, this is a satisfactory method of continued evaluation of the results of treatment.

Treatment

Aims

Lymphedema is not a curable condition, but it can be controlled. The aims of treatment are a permanent decrease in the size of the affected limb without the use of continued conservative measures; improvement of skin texture, softness, and consistency; and elimination of episodes of cellulitis. None of the current methods of treatment realizes these aims fully, but progress has been made in the last decade.

Conservative Treatment

Mild lymphedema can be managed effectively by nonsurgical measures. These modes are also essential preoperatively and postoperatively as an adjunct to various procedures.

The aims of conservative treatment are to reduce hydrostatic pressure, minimize valvular incompetence, decrease infection, and treat lymphangitis vigorously when it occurs. If excessive swelling is present, inpatient management is mandatory initially. Bed rest with the limb elevated and repeated elastic bandaging alternating with sequential compression pumping may be necessary to reduce the edema. Limb elevation reduces arterial hydrostatic pressure and thereby reduces the amount of fluid extravasated into the interstitial tissue. Intermittent use of an elastic or light rubber bandage increases tissue hydrostatic pressure and the return of edematous fluid through the lymphatics. A multichamber sequential pump is preferred to a single-chamber pump because the sequential compression starting distally in the limb propels the fluid proximally. The pressure in the chambers of this pump can be adjusted to the patient's comfort. When the pump is not in use, the elastic bandage is used. Massage by a physiotherapist is carried out intensively between weekly treatments, and this is sufficient to achieve a major reduction in volume. When the desired reduction is achieved, the limb is supported by a high-compression elastic garment worn during the day. Elastic bandages are applied at night. Subsequently the patient is taught to massage the limb and to inspect it for evidence of infection, which is treated vigorously with antibiotics. The patient returns to the hospital at a later date if additional reduction is necessary.

Drug Treatment

Benzopyrones (coumarin and 7 hydroxy-coumarin) have been used in the treatment of lymphedema. These drugs increase the proteinase activity, and the large protein levels are broken down into smaller groups. The resultant peptides and amino acids have a favorable osmotic balance and can diffuse readily into the local veins. This reduces protein concentration in the interstitial tissues and the associated edema. Drug treatment may have a place in the treatment of mild edema, although the benefit appears to be inconsistent and the drugs take a long time to act.

Surgical Treatment

Surgical treatment of lymphedema has hitherto been indicated when medical treatment has failed. With improved results of microlymphatic operations, however, surgical intervention now is indicated early, even in mild-to-moderate obstructive lymphedema, but it is always combined with conservative treatment. Operations for lymphedema are of two types: drainage procedures and reduction procedures.

Preoperative Management

The patients receive intensive conservative therapy for 5 to 7 days before the operation to decompress the leg as much as possible.

Drainage Procedures

Lymphatic Bridging Procedures. In lymphatic bridging, pedicled flaps and omental flaps are transposed across the lymphatic block. It was hoped that regeneration of lymphatics would establish communication between the blocked lymphatics and normal lymph trunks in the flap. Although regeneration of lymphatics can occur, it usually follows relatively minor incisions when the gap between the divided lymphatics is small. Delayed healing of the flap or infection reduces regeneration of the lymphatics, and with omental flaps intraabdominal complications from harvesting can occur. Because the incidence of complications is high and the results have been inconsistent, lymphatic bridging is not recommended.

Drainage into Deep Lymphatics. Drainage from the superficial into the deep lymphatics was attempted to establish an anastomosis between the superficial blocked lymphatics and the deep normal lymphatics. Because the primary abnormality may be in the deep lymphatics, however, it is unlikely that the dermal wick operation can drain the lymph from the superficial system to a blocked deep system. Sawhney, evaluating the procedure using radioactive serum albumin uptake (RISA), found no increase in lymph drainage, and the initial reduction in size was proportional to the excision of edematous tissue. This reduction was not maintained at follow-up examinations. These procedures are no longer recommended.

Lymph Node–Venous Anastomosis. Anastomosis of the transected lymph node to the vein was first carried out by Olszewski and Neilubowicz, who demonstrated patency of the anastomoses. Calnan and associates obtained 100 percent patency at one month, but all anastomoses were obstructed at 3 months. The technique is most useful in filarial lymphedema, and the results are better when more than one anastomoses are done.

Microlymphaticovenous Anastomosis.

Lymphaticovenous anastomosis (LVA) is preferred to lymph node–venous anastomosis (LNVA) because the latter is not possible when the draining regional nodes have been excised. In addition, better patency is obtained by LVA. The prime determining factor in the success of the anastomosis is the achievement of correct apposition of the cut edges of the vessels, which depends directly on the number and spacing of the sutures and on the tension applied when they are tied. Huang and colleagues observed that lymphatic pressure is higher than venous pressure normally, and it is even higher during muscular activity and in lymphedematous limbs. Because muscular activity increases lymphatic pressure without increasing venous pressure, lymph should drain through the anastomoses into the venous system. Huang's group also observed a fluctuation in lymphatic pressure correlated with rhythmic contraction of the lymphatics. The authors concluded that lymphatic flow depends principally on spontaneous intrinsic contraction of the lymphatics. Lymph flow is obvious under anesthesia: Within minutes of interdigital injection, patent blue dye is present in the lymphatics in the proximal part of the limb; it is present in the urine within 30 minutes. It has also been observed clinically that patients who have good results from surgical treatment do not have a relapse of lymphedema.

Surgical Technique for Drainage Procedures

After an intradermal test dose on the opposite limb, patent blue dye (1 to 2 ml) is injected subcutaneously in the interdigital webs of the hand or foot 20 to 30 minutes before the operation. A dermal flush of the dye indicates that the subcutaneous lymphatic trunks are sclerosed and that the dilated dermal and subdermal lymphatics are the main source of lymphatic drainage. It is a poor prognostic sign.

Exploration is performed under tourniquet but without exsanguination of the limb. This provides a bloodless field yet allows visualization of the veins and lymphatics. Dissection is carried out simultaneously in the medial upper arm or thigh and dorsum of the wrist or ankle. A transverse incision is made through the skin only, and the skin edges are sutured back to provide retraction. The subcutaneous tissue is gently teased apart under loupe magnification. Patent lymphatics are easily identified by their beaded appearance and their green color. All patent lymphatics and veins are marked with 5–0 silk loops and tagged with metal microvascular clips. When the lymphatics are sclerosed, it is difficult to differentiate them from a cutaneous nerve without the use of a microscope. Sometimes there is an abundance of lymphatics but only a few veins to match. It may be necessary to dissect the available veins distally to define additional tributaries suitable for anastomoses.

Lymphatics should have a diameter of more than 0.5 mm to be suitable for anastomosis. If suitable lymphatics are not found in the upper arm or thigh, exploration is made below the elbow or knee on the medial side. The tourniquet is released after completion of the exploration. The lymphatics are divided as proximally as possible in the wound and the veins are divided distally so that each can be transposed to facilitate anastomosis. The vein is irrigated with heparinized saline solution. The anastomosis is performed using 11–0 nylon with a swaged-on 70-μ needle. No clamps are used on the lymphatics, but a soft single clamp may be necessary on the vein. Because the lymphatic wall tends to collapse, a pair of No. 5 jeweler's forceps is inserted gently into the lumen of the lymphatics and spread slightly. The needle is passed through the lymphatic wall and through the vein (Fig. 24-1). Sometimes it is easier to pass the microsuture through the vein first (Fig. 24-2). The lymphatic vessel is pulled gently upward so that the lumen is visualized as a slit. The needle is inserted into the slit, ensuring that only a small segment of the lymphatic is penetrated by the needle.

Two guide sutures are inserted, and one or two sutures are made in the center of the vessels. The vessels are rotated, and one to three sutures are placed in the posterior wall. Four to six sutures may be used in the anastomosis. On completion of the anastomosis, the limb is massaged and the passage of dye across the anastomosis is verified. As many anastomoses as possible are performed. Occasionally, when venous tributaries are inadequate, an end-to-side anastomosis into a single vein is performed (Fig. 24-3).

In lymphedemas of the upper limb, a longitudinal elliptic wedge excision of skin and subcutaneous tissue from the posteromedial aspect of the upper arm is done, preferably at the primary operation. This excision is posterior to any lymphatic anastomoses in the upper arm. When adequate lymphatics are present only at the wrist, a segmental lipectomy on the medial aspect of the upper arm is performed. Even if liposuction of the medial forearm is done later, the lipectomy of the upper arm still allows any peripheral microlymphaticovenous connection to drain the lateral aspect of the limb. The subcutaneous tissue is sutured with 4–0 polyglycolic acid interrupted suture, and the skin with a subcuticular continuous polyglycolic acid suture. A simple noncircumferential dressing is applied.

When LVA was the only method of treatment, we reported that 42 percent of our patients had clinically significant improvement over a number of years (Table 24-2). When LVA is combined with a segmental reduction of the upper arm, this figure is raised to 60 percent (Table 24-3). The average reduction was 44 percent of the excess volume in both groups. Some of these patients showed a decrease in volume of more than 80 percent. It was observed that patients whose condition improved initially after microlymphaticovenous anastomosis continued to see improvement (Figs. 24-4 and 24-5). Huang and associates obtained good or excellent results in 79 percent of their patients, most of whom had lymphedema of the lower limb. Their results were better when the duration of edema was shorter and when the number of anastomoses performed was greater, but we could not find a similar correlation. Although long-standing obstruction does result in secondary sclerosis of the lymphatics that begins centrally, it is not clear how rapidly this sclerosis develops. The timing varies with individuals and is influenced by the frequency of cellulitis.

Lymphaticolymphatic Grafts

Baumeister developed and applied clinically lymphaticolymphatic grafts. In this method for upper limb lymphedema two to three lymphatic trunks with their afferent branches are harvested from the upper medial thigh. Three to five lymphatic tributaries are anastomosed distally to the proximal lymphatics in the

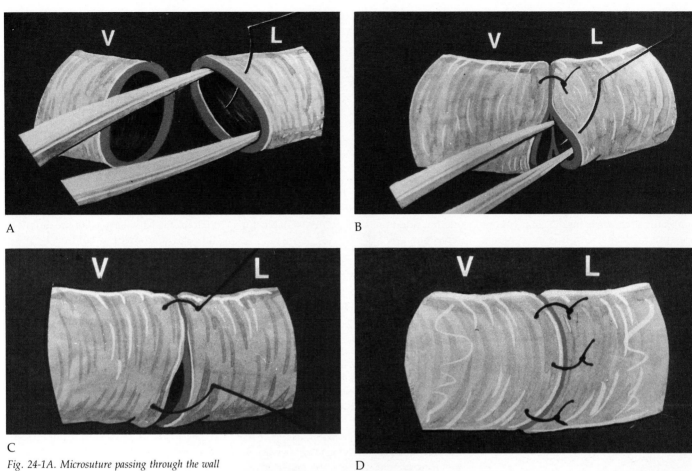

A

B

C

D

Fig. 24-1A. Microsuture passing through the wall of the lymphatic. A pair of jeweler's forceps gently opens the lumen of the lymphatic. B. The first suture has been tied and the second suture is being inserted through the lymphatic wall, again with the jeweler's forceps gently opening the lumen. C. Continuation of repair of the microlymphaticovenous anastomosis. D. Micro-lymphaticovenous anastomosis completed. E. Post-repair lymphaticovenous anastomosis in rabbit femoral lymphatic. Lymphatic shown to right (lymphatic side) of anastomosis, blood to the left (venous side). V = vein; L = lymphatic. (From B. McC. O'Brien, W.A. Morrison. Reconstructive Microsurgery. *Edinburgh: Churchill Livingstone, 1987. Reproduced with permission.)*

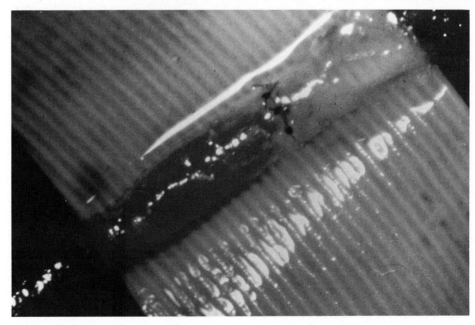

E

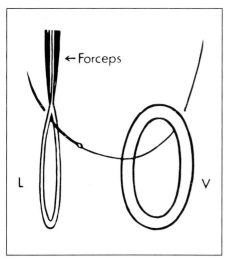

Fig. 24-2. A microsuture has been placed through the vein (V) first and then into the slitlike opening of the lymphatic (L). (From B. McC. O'Brien, W.A. Morrison. Reconstructive Microsurgery. Edinburgh: Churchill Livingstone, 1987. Reproduced with permission.)

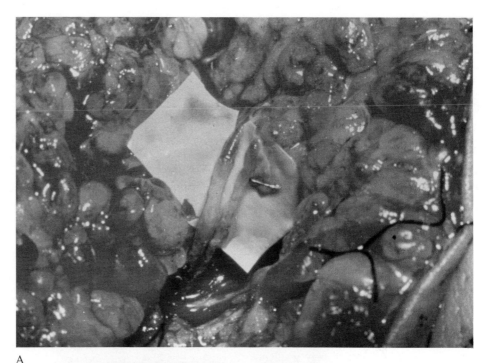

A

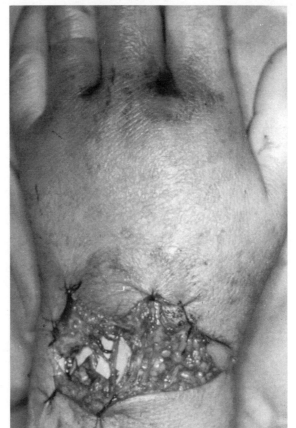

B

Fig. 24-3A. Two microlymphaticovenous anastomoses with the lymph stained with patent blue dye across the anastomoses in the upper forearm. B. Multiple microlymphaticovenous anastomoses on the dorsum of the wrist. Note patent blue injection site at the interdigital webs. (From B. McC. O'Brien, W.A. Morrison. Reconstructive Microsurgery. Edinburgh: Churchill Livingstone, 1987. Reproduced with permission.)

lymphedematous limb, and proximally the efferent trunks are anastomosed into a lymphatic trunk in the neck, thus bypassing the obstruction in the axilla. In lower limb lymphedema lymphatic trunks are harvested from the normal limb, but the afferent connection to the inguinal lymph nodes is retained. The connection is pedicled across the groin into the lymphedematous thigh, where it is anastomosed to lymph trunks. Baumeister demonstrated by lymphoscintigraphy a patency approaching 100 percent and an improved transport index. The transport index is determined from the scintigram by combining visual assessment of five criteria: temporal and spatial distribution of the radionuclide, appearance time of lymph nodes, and graded visualization of lymph nodes and vessels.

Baumeister reported the results of treating 36 patients with upper limb and 12 with lower limb lymphedema with lymphatic grafts. The mean follow-up period was 16 months. In the upper limb, 80 percent reduction in excess volume was achieved in patients followed for more than 3 years. The results improved progressively as the follow-up period lengthened. The main difficulty is determining the number of lymphatic grafts required to reduce the swelling adequately. The

Table 24-2. Objective results in 52 patients with unilateral obstructive lymphedema treated with microlymphatic anastomosis only

	Condition after treatment		
Factor analyzed	Improved	Unchanged*	Worsened
Number of patients	22(42%)	6(12%)	24(46%)
Mean volume change (%)	+44	−6	−29
Range of volume change (%)	+10 to +84	−2 to −9	−10 to −82
Number of anastomoses (mean)	5	6	6
Duration of edema (mean, years)	5	10	5
Mean follow-up period (years)	4.3	3.0	3.0

* Less than 10% volume change.

Table 24-3. Objective results in 38 patients with unilateral obstructive lymphedema treated with microlymphatic anastomosis and reduction

	Condition after treatment		
Factor analyzed	Improved	Unchanged*	Worsened
Number of patients	23(60%)	6(16%)	9(24%)
Mean volume change (%)	+44	+2	−35
Range of volume change (%)	+10 to +87	−5 to −9	−12 to −86
Number of anastomoses (mean)	4.1	4.2	4.3
Duration of edema (mean, years)	8	9	9
Mean follow-up period (years)	4.8	6.7	3.7

* Less than 10% volume change.

number of grafts used cannot be increased because doing so may result in lymphedema of the donor leg, although Baumeister states such lymphedema is minimal. It is not clear how lymphatic grafts can be used because patent lymphatics cannot be located in the upper arm in 25 percent of patients.

Reduction Procedures

Reduction procedures may be indicated in primary lymphedema and in secondary lymphedema when the lymphatic trunks are sclerosed and unsuitable for microlymphatic anastomoses or when conservative measures have failed or are not applicable. Posteromedial reduction of the upper arm is sometimes useful as an adjuvant in patients who have had microlymphaticovenous anastomoses, although it is preferable to perform the reduction at the primary operation.

Charles Procedure. Charles in 1912 reported excising the skin and edematous subcutaneous tissue circumferentially down to the deep fascia and applying a split skin graft. The cosmetic results of this procedure are unsatisfactory. The healing of the skin graft is often poor, resulting in unstable scars. Weeping of lymph from the graft surface is not uncommon. The results have been improved by using full-thickness grafts taken from the removed tissue. The Charles procedure has a limited application in severe elephantiasis. The method is never used in the upper limb.

Staged Excision. In the first stage the subcutaneous tissue and the excessive skin are excised from the posteromedial aspect of the limb. Two to three months later the procedure is repeated on the contralateral side of the leg. The results showed satisfactory reduction and improvement of limb function. The limb is supported with an elastic garment postoperatively.

Liposuction. Liposuction may have a place in the treatment of primary lymphedema and in secondary lymphedema when lymphaticovenous anastomoses are not possible or have failed or after inadequate reduction. After inadequate reduction liposuction should be done on the opposite aspect of the limb to the drainage area used for these anastomoses. The best results are achieved when skin elasticity is retained. An average reduction of excess volume of 23 percent was achieved in 10 of 11 patients. Liposuction can be combined with a drainage procedure.

Although reduction procedures achieve good reduction in limb volume, these results are maintained only if effective conservative therapy is continued indefinitely. The procedures do not cure the lymphedema, and the cosmetic result is sometimes unsatisfactory.

Postoperative Management

The postoperative management varies with the method of treatment. With reduction procedures the patient remains in the hospital in bed with the limb elevated for approximately 7 to 10 days, longer with the Charles procedure (average of 3 to 4 weeks). A compressive elastic dressing is applied. After the Charles procedure, the patient walks only when the graft has taken well and stabilized. The patients are measured and fitted with a custom-made elastic garment before mobilization.

After LVA the patient remains in the hospital for 3 to 5 days. A sequential compression pump is used alternating with massage, which is carried out reg-

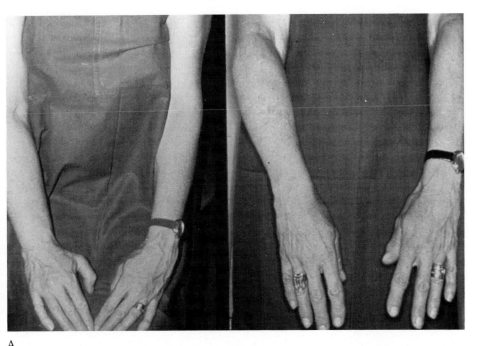

A

Fig. 24-4A. Left, obstructive lymphedema of right upper limb 6 years after radical mastectomy. Right, same patient after multiple microlymphaticovenous anastomoses in the medial aspect of the right upper arm 5 years postoperatively. Note the considerable reduction in volume of the upper limb. B. Percentage of reduction of excess volume over a 6-year period. Conservative measures were discontinued within 2 years and there was further improvement without such measures over the subsequent 4 years. The final reduction in excess volume was approximately 40 percent. C. Graph for same patient shows the change in circumference of the forearm over a 6-year period. The reduction is considerable, amounting to 7 cm with no conservative measures conducted during the last 4 years. (From B. McC. O'Brien, W.A. Morrison. Reconstructive Microsurgery. Edinburgh: Churchill Livingstone, 1987. Reproduced with permission.)

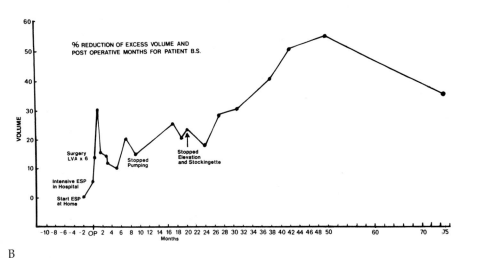

B

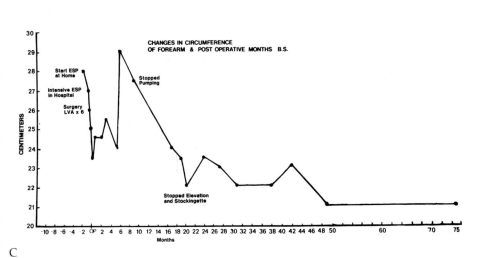

C

ularly by the physiotherapist and the patient up to the anastomosis to assist the flow of lymph and to keep the anastomosis patent. Antibiotics are used for the first week. Daily massage, wearing of a sequential elastic stocking, and bandaging are continued for about 3 months postoperatively; after that they usually can be discontinued. After lymphatic grafts Baumeister uses a similar regimen. He recommends wearing stockings for 6 months, however.

Conclusion

Currently there is no cure for lymphedema. Progress has been made by microlymphatic operations combined with conservative measures to relieve many of these patients of much of their swelling without resort to lifetime use of conservative measures. Additional work is required to increase understanding of the mechanism of lymphatic transport before a perfect solution can be found.

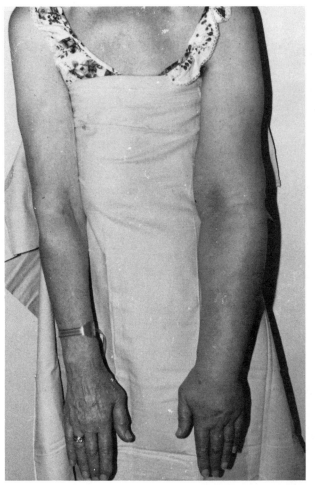

A

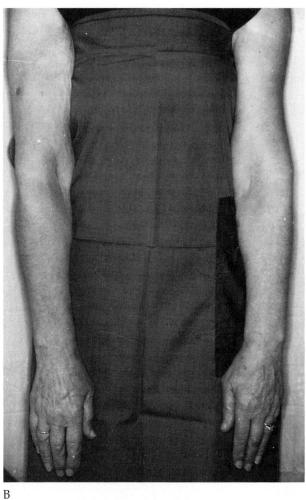

B

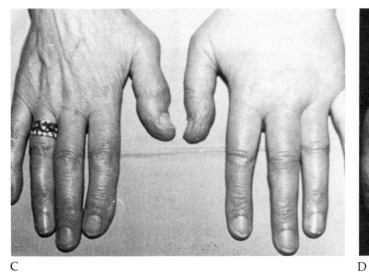

C

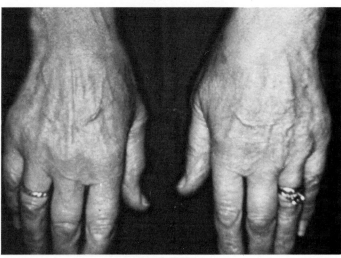

D

Fig. 24-5A. *Obstructive lymphedema of left upper limb of 2 years' duration. B. Same patient 12 months after multiple microlymphaticovenous anastomoses in the medial aspect of the left upper arm. C. Same patient with lymphedematous left hand preoperatively. D. Same patient 12 months after microlymphatic anastomoses with considerable reduction in volume. Note rings worn on left ring finger. (From B. McC. O'Brien, W.A. Morrison.* Reconstructive Microsurgery. *Edinburgh: Churchill Livingstone, 1987. Reproduced with permission.)*

Suggested Reading

Baumeister, R.G., and Siuda, S. Treatment of lymphedemas by microsurgical lymphatic grafting: What is proved? *Plast. Reconstr. Surg.* 85:64, 1990.

Charles, R.H. Elephantiasis Scroti. In A. Latham and T.C. English (Eds.), *A System of Treatment*, Vol. 3. London: Churchill, 1912.

Clodius, L., and Piller, N.B. Conservative therapy for postmastectomy lymphedema. *Chir. Plast.* 4:193, 1978.

Fox, U., Montorsi, M., and Ronafnoli, G. Lymphaticovenous shunt in the treatment of limb lymphedema. In Proceedings of the Sixth International Congress of the International Microsurgery Society, Sydney, Australia, 1981. P. 31.

Gilbert, A., et al. Lymphaticovenous anastomosis by microvascular technique. *Br. J. Plast. Surg.* 29:355, 1976.

Haung, G.K., et al. Microlymphaticovenous anastomosis in the treatment of lower limb obstructive lymphedema: Analysis of 91 cases. *Plast. Reconstr. Surg.* 76:671, 1985.

Knight, K.R., et al. Coumarin and 7-hydroxycoumarin treatment of canine obstructive lymphoedema. *Clin. Sci.* 77:69, 1989.

Neilubowicz, J., and Olszewski, W. Surgical lymphaticovenous shunts in patients with secondary lymphoedema. *Br. J. Surg.* 55:440, 1968.

O'Brien, B. McC., Chait, L.A., and Hurwitz, P.J. Microlymphatic surgery. *Orthop. Clin. North Am.* 8:405, 1977.

O'Brien, B. McC., and Franklin, J.D. Microlymphatic surgery. In Proceedings of the VIIth International Congress of Plastic Surgery, Brazil, 1979. Pp. 52–55.

O'Brien, B. McC., et al. Microlymphaticovenous anastomoses for obstructive lymphedema. *Plast. Reconstr. Surg.* 60:197, 1977.

O'Brien, B. McC., et al. Liposuction in the treatment of lymphoedema: A preliminary report. *Br. J. Plast. Surg.* 42:530, 1989.

O'Brien, B. McC., et al. Long term results after microlymphaticovenous anastomoses for the treatment of obstructive lymphedema. *Plast. Reconstr. Surg.* 85:562, 1990.

Pentecost, B.L., et al. A quantitative study of lymphovenous communications in the dog. *Br. J. Surg.* 53:630, 1966.

Rusznyak, I., Folldi, M., and Szabo, G. *Lymphatics and Lymph Circulation.* London: Pergamon, 1967.

Sawhney, C.P. Evaluation of Thompson's buried dermal flap operation for lymphedema of the limbs: A clinical radioisotopic study. *Br. J. Plast. Surg.* 27:278, 1974.

Yamada, Y. Studies on lymphatic venous anastomosis in lymphoedema. *Nagoya J. Med. Sci.* 32:1, 1969.

25

Hidradenitis Suppurativa

Norman Weinzweig

Hidradenitis suppurativa is a chronic, recurrent, inflammatory cicatricial disease of the apocrine sweat gland–bearing areas of the body, primarily the axillary and inguinal regions. It is a severely debilitating disease of unknown etiology. In the early stages, this condition may be treated conservatively by local wound care, good personal hygiene, and antibiotics. The chronic disease, however, is characterized by widespread involvement of the skin and subcutaneous tissues with scarring, multiple deep-seated abscesses, and draining sinus tracts; radical surgical resection is necessary.

Hidradenitis is a term derived from the Greek words *hydros* meaning sweat and *aden* meaning gland. More precisely, hidradenitis suppurativa is a disease of the apocrine rather than the eccrine sweat glands and might more appropriately be called *apocrinitis*, a term suggested by Harrison.

Eccrine and Apocrine Glands

Human skin contains two types of glands—sebaceous glands and sweat glands. Sweat glands are subdivided into two categories—eccrine glands and apocrine glands. These glands differ in histologic structure, location, and function.

Eccrine glands are small (20 μ), simple, tubular structures of cholinergic innervation. They are located superficially in the skin and open directly onto the skin surface. These glands produce odorless watery secretions that are "true" sweat. They are derived from the epidermis and distributed over the entire body; the highest concentration is in the palms, the soles, and the axillae. Eccrine glands function primarily in the regulation of body temperature.

Apocrine glands, on the other hand, have a limited distribution over the body surface. They are found predominantly in the axillae and groin but can also appear in the perineum and perianal regions, the pubis, the scrotum, the labia, the periumbilical area, the mammary areola (Montgomery areolar tubercles), the ear canal (ceruminal glands), and the eyelids (Moll glands). These compound, tubular glands of adrenergic innervation are larger (200 μ) than the eccrine glands and are located deeper in the dermis. They are derived from the hair follicle anlage and undergo decapitation secretion, in which a portion of the cytoplasm is "pinched off" and discharges its contents into the pilosebaceous apparatus. Apocrine glands produce thick milky secretions in response to pain, anger, and sexual arousal. In humans, they probably represent a vestigial structure; in other animals, however, they have mating and protective functions.

Epidemiology

The peak incidence of hidradenitis suppurativa occurs between the second and fourth decades of life. It is rare to see this disease develop before puberty. This age dependence is believed to be related to endocrine function because the apocrine glands are inactive until puberty and diminish in activity in advanced years. Hidradenitis suppurativa occurs in both sexes and equal frequency, although in women there is a greater tendency for axillary involvement, whereas in men there is a greater propensity for perineal involvement. The axilla is the most commonly affected region of the body with the perianal and genital areas second in frequency. The disease is found in all races, but there is an increased incidence among blacks, in whom apocrine glands are three times more prevalent than eccrine glands. Asian peoples are rarely afflicted. Because they are under adrenergic control, the apocrine glands respond to emotional stimuli, and menstrual and premenstrual exacerbations have been reported.

Etiopathogenesis

Numerous theories have been proposed for the precise etiology of hidradenitis suppurativa. The etiopathogenesis of this condition, however, is still unknown. Predisposing factors include excessive shaving, use of deodorant and depilatory creams, sweating with secondary maceration of tissue, plucking of axillary hair, and wearing of irritating, tight-fitting clothing. The involvement of these factors has not been entirely corroborated in the laboratory. Shelley and Cahn, in 1955, attempted to produce the disease experimentally in human volunteers by depilation and obstruction of the apocrine glands with keratinaceous material. They succeeded in only 3 of 12 patients, suggesting perhaps that this was an inappropriate model. Morgan retrospectively compared 40 patients with axillary and inguinal hidradenitis to age-matched controls and found no association of the disease with shaving or use of deodorants or chemical depilatories. Morgan also found no significant differences in the size and density of the apocrine glands of people with hidradenitis suppurativa compared with those of healthy persons studied. Despite sporadic reports in the literature linking hidradenitis suppurativa to increased levels of male sexual steroids in women with the disease and the proclivity of this disease to run in families, possibly with an autosomal dominant inheritance, no clear associations of hidradenitis suppurativa with endocrinologic or immunologic abnormalities or genetic transmission have been established.

A retrospective histopathologic study by Yu of diseased axillary skin suggested that hidradenitis suppurativa is a disease of follicular epithelium rather than of apocrine glands. This study seriously questions the original concept of hidradenitis as primarily a disease of apocrine glands. In 10 of 12 patients, squamous epithelium–lined structures in the form of cysts

or sinuses were identified in the dermis, and laminated keratin was present in all of these structures. Half of the cysts also contained hair shafts, suggesting that they are derived from hair follicles. Only 4 of 12 patients demonstrated inflammation of the apocrine glands, and in these patients inflammation was also seen around eccrine glands, hair follicles, and the epithelium-lined structures. In no patient was there gross dilatation of the apocrine glands. Squamous epithelium–lined structures, which probably represent abnormal hair follicles, appeared to be a more constant finding than inflammation of the apocrine glands, which seemed to be a secondary phenomenon.

Clinical Manifestations

The initial lesion in hidradenitis suppurativa is a superficial abscess that progresses to the characteristic indolent inflammatory disease. Apocrine gland occlusion is followed by ductal obstruction and dilatation with secondary infection by a variety of organisms including *Staphylococcus*, *Escherichia coli*, *Klebsiella*, and *Proteus* as well as anaerobes and coliforms in perineal disease. Infiltration of the apocrine glands with polymorphonuclear leukocytes and lymphocytes occurs in response to bacterial invasion.

The initial episode of hidradenitis suppurativa may resolve with local wound care, incision and drainage, good personal hygiene, and antibiotic therapy. If untreated, this indolent inflammatory process spreads to involve the adjacent eccrine glands and overlying skin, leading to multiple deep-seated abscess formation and extensive epithelium-lined sinus tracts. The disease progresses to the chronic condition with scar contractures, multiple areas of sinus tracking, and pseudoepitheliomatous hyperplasia beneath the dermis. Hidradenitis is usually confined to the skin and subcutaneous tissue and does not penetrate beyond the deep fascial barrier, even in the most advanced, neglected forms.

The pathologic features of hidradenitis suppurativa bear closest resemblance to those of acne. The epithelium-lined structures resembling comedones have a predilection for specific anatomic sites corresponding not only to the distribution of apocrine glands in the body but also to

the distribution of terminal hair follicles; their associated apocrine, eccrine, and sebaceous glands are secondarily involved.

The clinical course of hidradenitis is characterized by exacerbations and remissions. The average duration of the disease before definitive treatment is 3 to 6 years. Patients vary considerably in the extent of disease and areas of involvement. Although it most commonly occurs in the axillary and perineal and perianal regions, hidradenitis suppurativa has been reported in many other sites, including the breast and the beard-bearing portion of the neck (beard sicosis).

Treatment
Axillary Hidradenitis

Before treatment of axillary hidradenitis suppurativa can begin, the correct diagnosis must be established. Other diagnoses to consider include acne, cellulitis, simple furuncles and carbuncles, and infected epidermoid cysts.

In the early stages, I prefer to treat hidradenitis suppurativa of the axillary region by conservative measures, including warm compresses and good personal hygiene. Possible causative factors such as use of deodorant and depilatory creams and excessive shaving are strictly avoided. Incision and drainage of isolated abscesses is combined with culture-specific antibiotics. When cultures are sterile, broad-spectrum antibiotics are prescribed. Symptoms often resolve temporarily with this conservative management, but tend to recur with worsening severity within weeks or months.

After conservative measures fail, surgical excision becomes the mainstay of treatment. It is extremely difficult, if not impossible, to define specific indications for surgical management. This is a personal decision made by the patient with the surgeon's assistance. Considerations include duration and severity of symptoms, location and extent of disease, number of attempts at conservative management, and degree of interference with activities of daily living and employment. The patient may become incapacitated after several unsuccessful attempts at conservative treatment and strongly desire to undergo surgical treatment with a full understanding of expected results and req-

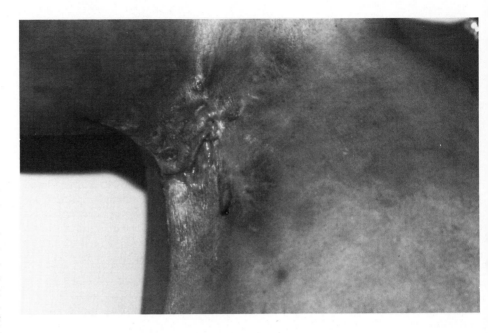

Fig. 25-1. Severe axillary contracture and multiple residual draining sinuses after several attempts at conservative management of axillary hidradenitis.

uisite compliance with postoperative care (Fig. 25-1).

The three chief goals of surgical management are (1) to completely excise all involved tissues; (2) to preserve function, avoiding or correcting axillary contractures; and (3) to obtain a satisfactory aesthetic result. It is critical to prevent recurrence that radical resection be performed of all involved and adjacent uninvolved apocrine gland–bearing tissue down to a clean, unscarred plane of subcutaneous tissue. The extent of the disease is delineated with a marking pen, and a small margin of adjacent healthy tissue is removed. The resected specimen is usually irregular in shape. Isolated areas of disease (satellitosis) are similarly excised and treated individually; no attempt is made to connect the defects and excise them as one large specimen. Wound closure after surgical resection can be accomplished in several ways depending on the size of the defect and the surgeon's preference. These include primary closure, skin grafting, and flap coverage. Any preexisting axillary contracture must also be released before closure. Whenever possible, wound closure is accomplished by well-concealed placement of incisions to minimize any cosmetic deformity.

My approach is to treat small axillary defects by primary closure in a manner similar to that described by Pollack in 1972. The patient is placed in the supine position with the affected arms brought out at an angle 80° to 90° from the body. The extent of involved skin and subcutaneous tissue is delineated with a marking pen. This irregular pattern is circumscribed with a small margin of unaffected tissue. No attempt is made to convert this irregular pattern into one that is more regular. Excision is performed, keeping the plane of dissection 0.5 to 1.0 cm deep to the diseased and scarred subcutaneous tissue to avoid injury to the underlying structures. This dissection is aided by steady upward retraction on the diseased tissue demar-

cating the plane between affected and unaffected tissues. After removal of the specimen, meticulous hemostasis is obtained with electrocautery. The wound is inspected for any residual disease, and the skin edges are minimally undermined and closed in layers. Large flat Jackson-Pratt drains are placed for suction. No. 1 nylon retention sutures are placed and left untied. They are followed by interrupted 000 polyglycolic acid subcuticular sutures and 4–0 nylon vertical mattress sutures. The retention sutures are tied over a gauze bolster dressing. The arm is placed in a properly fitted sling. Five to seven days after the operation, the dressing is taken down and mobilization by physical therapy is begun (Fig. 25-2).

This operation reduces the length of hospitalization, allows a large amount of tissue to be excised with a high rate of primary healing, allows both axillae to be operated on at the same setting without immobilization, and avoids skin grafting. Because axillary disease is bilateral in 75 percent of patients, simultaneous correction cuts hospitalization in half because the patient is neither immobilized nor dependent on the nursing staff for routine needs. The major disadvantage with this technique, however, is the inability to close wounds larger than approximately 15 cm by 8 cm. My experience with the Pollack technique has been highly successful. It is critical, however, that the

surgeon meticulously remove all diseased and scarred tissue and close the skin edges without great tension.

Watson, in a retrospective review of 72 patients, reported a 54 percent rate of reoperation for recurrences after excision and primary closure of axillary hidradenitis. The reoperation rate for excision and split-thickness skin grafting was 13 percent and for excision and local flap coverage, 19 percent. He advocated that axillary hidradenitis be treated surgically by wide excision of the affected skin and either split-thickness skin grafting or local flap coverage of the resultant defect.

Larger defects that cannot be closed primarily without tension may be treated by either split-thickness skin grafting or by flap coverage (Figs. 25-3 and 25-4). It is critical that the surgeon not compromise the excision to accomplish closure. Perhaps the high incidence of reoperation for recurrence after excision and primary closure in Watson's series is the direct result of closure of larger axillary defects under tension. As a rule, I avoid skin grafting this region. Major problems with skin grafting include axillary contracture, poor aesthetic appearance, hyperpigmentation, dryness, the need for prolonged immobilization, and a high incidence of partial skin graft loss with resultant contracture. I prefer flap closure, which allows a tension-free closure with incisions that

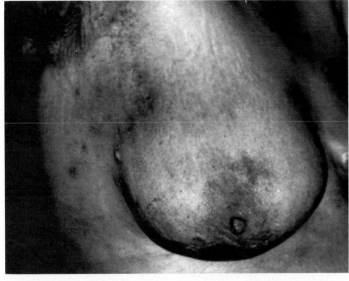

A

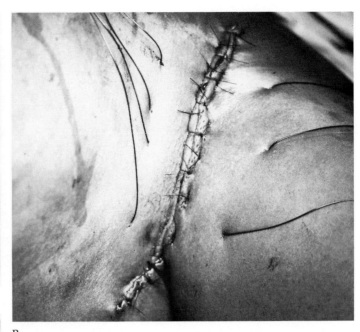

B

Fig. 25-2A. Axillary hidradenitis with multiple draining sinuses and a mild contracture. B. After wide excision of all involved tissue, the wound was closed primarily. Note the heavy nylon sutures placed before the application of a bolster dressing. C. Final result with primary healing and mobilization without restriction.

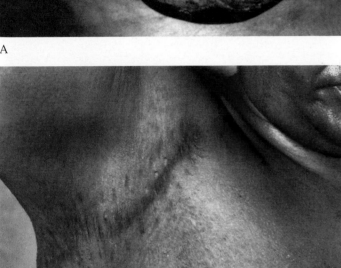

C

Fig. 25-3A. Residual axillary hidradenitis after previous limited resection. B. After wide excision of all involved tissue, the axillary wound was covered with a split-thickness skin graft. Stable coverage without restriction of arm movement 18 months postoperatively.

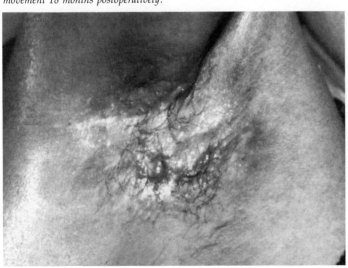

A

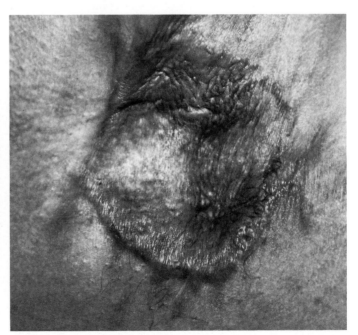

B

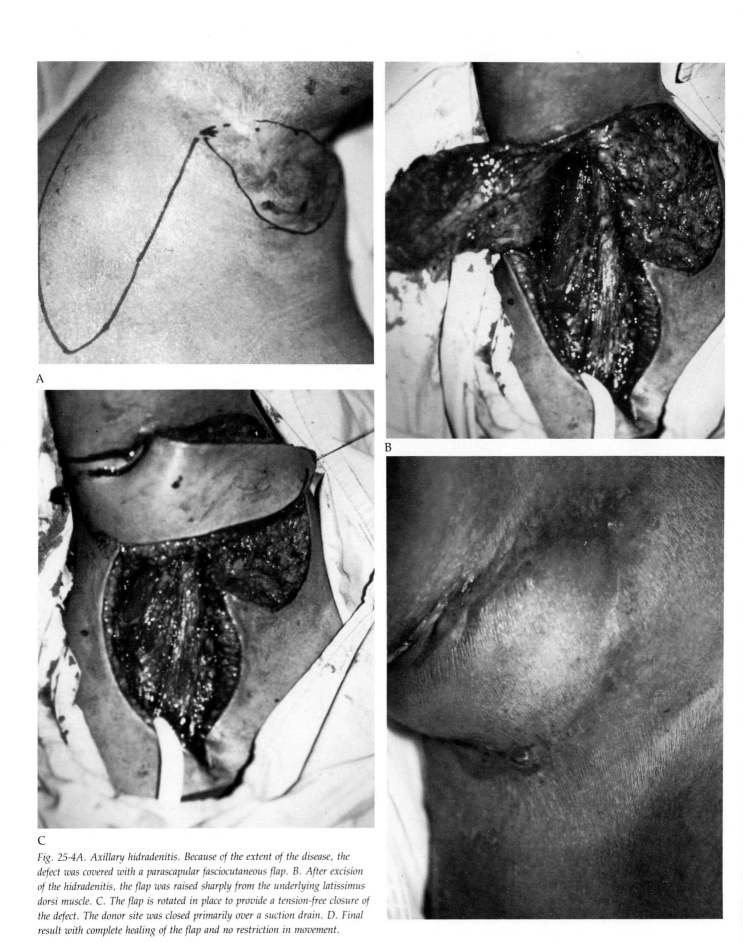

Fig. 25-4A. Axillary hidradenitis. Because of the extent of the disease, the
defect was covered with a parascapular fasciocutaneous flap. B. After excision
of the hidradenitis, the flap was raised sharply from the underlying latissimus
dorsi muscle. C. The flap is rotated in place to provide a tension-free closure of
the defect. The donor site was closed primarily over a suction drain. D. Final
result with complete healing of the flap and no restriction in movement.

are functionally and aesthetically acceptable. Proper flap design with a sufficient arc of rotation allows the suture line to be concealed in either the anterior or the posterior axillary folds in men or in the inframammary lines of the breasts in women. This method achieves the desirable cosmetic result yet facilitates early postoperative mobilization. In women an anteriorly based flap incorporating the anterior axillary fold is constructed. In men a posteriorly based flap incorporating the soft tissue overlying the latissimus dorsi or a scapular flap is preferred.

Before flap closure, a flat Jackson-Pratt suction drain is placed under the areas of dissection. The arm is placed in a properly fitted sling. When either of the foregoing techniques is used, both axillae may be operated on at the same time. One week after the operation, patients are allowed to abduct their arms to 90°. One month after the operation, they are allowed to progress to a full range of motion.

Hidradenitis Involving the Perineal Region, Groin, and Genitalia

Hidradenitis suppurativa involving the buttocks, perineum, groin, and pubic and genital areas is much less common than axillary hidradenitis. It is usually far more severe, however, with possible development of fistulous communications with the intestinal and urinary tracts, scar carcinomas, and iron deficiency anemia. Squamous cell carcinoma, developing in areas of chronic hidradenitis suppurativa, is extremely rare, usually occurring in patients who have had the disease for longer than 10 years, although one instance of carcinoma was reported in a patient who had hidradenitis for only 3 years. It is, therefore, the surgeon's responsibility to request careful microscopic evaluation of all specimens.

Hidradenitis of the buttocks and perineum is an extremely debilitating disease. It is characterized by malodorous drainage from multiple sinus tracts and deep-seated abscesses embedded within dense fibrous tissue, causing great pain, discomfort, and social isolation. Patients may become bedridden because of pain when their legs are in the characteristic abducted, semiflexed position. Reports in the literature describe eradication of the

disease by radical resection of the apocrine gland–containing tissues combined with subtotal vulvectomy or diverting colostomy; this therapy, however, increases patient risk, length of hospitalization, and cost. The need for a temporary colostomy is extremely limited with a well-planned preoperative and postoperative bowel regimen and should be considered only in the event of multiple fistulous communications.

The differential diagnosis for acute perineal hidradenitis includes acne, cellulitis, simple furuncles, infected epidermoid cysts, dermoid cysts, pilonidal cysts, and perirectal abscesses. In chronic disease lymphogranuloma venereum, Crohn disease, ulcerative colitis, tuberculosis, nocardial infection, actinomycoses, and anal fistulas must be considered.

Surgical Treatment

My approach to the treatment of perineal hidradenitis is to obtain a thorough history, including previous rectal problems, anal fistulas, or venereal disease. In severe instances, an extensive investigation must be performed to rule out any urinary or intestinal fistulas or other disease. After the definitive diagnosis is established, the patient is prepared for surgical treatment. Preoperatively the patient undergoes mechanical intestinal preparation and consumes a clear liquid diet. The patient's nutritional status is optimized. The patient is operated on under spinal or general endotracheal anesthesia in the supine lithotomy position with an indwelling urinary catheter in place (Fig. 25-5). This position provides excellent exposure for combined resections in the groin and perineal area. After the extent of diseased tissue including a small cuff of normal tissue is marked out, a knife or electrocautery is used to carry the resection down to the subcutaneous tissue 0.5 to 1.0 cm deep to the level of diseased tissue but not to the fascia. The resected specimen is often asymmetric and irregular in contour (Fig. 25-6). Great care is taken to avoid injuring the levator muscle, which lies very superficially. Injury to this structure can result in incontinence and stricture with tremendous morbidity. After meticulous hemostasis is obtained, the wounds are left open and packed with moist gauze.

Postoperatively the patient consumes a constipating diet for 5 to 7 days. Whirl-

pool baths are started immediately and saline dressings are applied to the wounds three times a day and maintained in place with fishnet-stocking gauze. Patients are encouraged to walk as tolerated after the operation and usually are discharged to go home 1 to 2 days after the operation. Wound healing by secondary intention and with no severe deformity occurs within 3 to 8 weeks of the operation depending on the size of the defect. During this healing period, patients are able to take care of themselves without problems, and some have returned to work.

Direct closure of extensive perineal excisional defects is not possible. I have obtained satisfactory and complete wound closure without severe deformity or contracture simply by allowing these defects to heal by the open method. After wide excision of all involved skin and apocrine tissues, the wound is allowed to granulate and epithelize spontaneously over several months. This simplified surgical approach to the management of hidradenitis suppurativa allows the patient easier postoperative care, early walking, no additional donor-site scarring, and early hospital discharge and return to work.

Silverberg reviewed the records of 20 patients with perineal hidradenitis who underwent an estimated average resection of 300 cm² and spontaneous healing by secondary intention without the interruption of normal bowel function. The average duration of the operations, even for severe disease, was less than one hour. Broad-spectrum antibiotics were given to control intraoperative bacteremia but discontinued in the postoperative period. The wounds were dressed four times daily with silver sulfadiazine. The patients were encouraged to walk as tolerated. By the third or fourth postoperative day, analgesic requirements were minimal. Patients were discharged after an average of 6 days. One year postoperatively, all patients had uncomplicated wound closure with unrestrictive, stable scars. There was minimal inconvenience or interruption of daily activities with minimal analgesic requirements. Complete healing took 2 to 5 months depending on the extent of resection. Ninety percent of the patients were satisfied. I have treated more than 25 patients in this man-

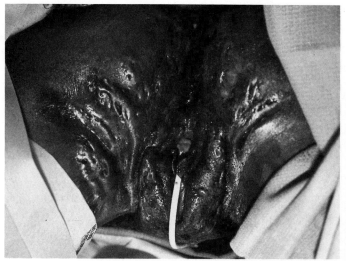

A

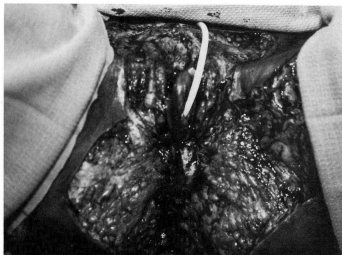

B

Fig. 25-5A. Severe hidradenitis involving the
genitalia, perineum, and buttocks. B. The
resection is done with the patient in the lithotomy
position. All wounds are left open to heal by
secondary intention. C. Three weeks
postoperatively. Clean contracted wounds with
near-total healing. D. Complete healing was
achieved by the sixth postoperative week. E. Final
result without limitation in motion and little
deformity despite the wide area of resection.

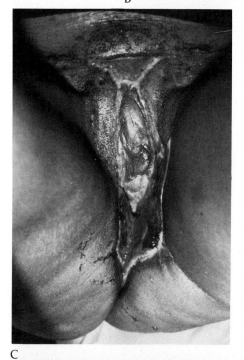

C

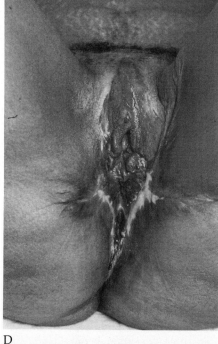

D

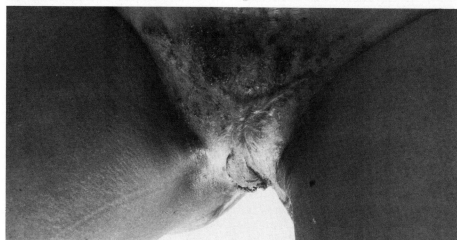

E

ner without any serious deformity, incontinence, infection, or other problem.

Harrison reviewed the records of 82 patients (118 excisions) who had been
treated by radical resection for intractable
hidradenitis suppurativa. Local recurrence rates varied with the disease site.
Recurrence rates were low after operations for perianal (0%) and axillary (3%)
hidradenitis and high after excisions for
inguinoperineal (37%) and submammary
(50%) disease. Recurrence was attributed
either to inadequate resection or to an unusually extensive distribution of apocrine
glands and, to a lesser degree, to physical
factors such as obesity, local pressure,
and skin maceration. One-fourth of the
patients had recurrent disease at a new
anatomic site.

Skin grafting of these extensive defects
has been advocated by some authors. Although skin grafting may facilitate rapid
healing with early wound closure, may
avoid the inconvenience of dressing

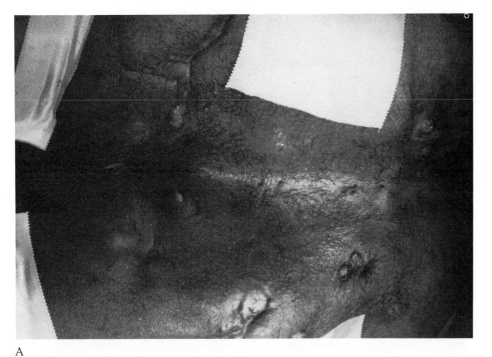

A

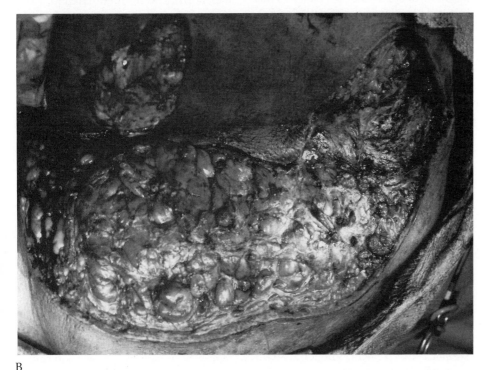

B

Fig. 25-6A Extensive hidradenitis of the perineum and buttocks. B. Superficial dissection of all involved areas was performed and meticulous hemostasis obtained. The dissection is carried only to the subcutaneous tissue. Thus rapid healing is achieved and the residual contour deformity is minimized. The dissection does not extend to the fascia, as is advocated by some authors.

changes, and may produce a less painful wound, there are several drawbacks. The major ones are prolonged operative time and donor site morbidity; the need for skin graft immobilization, which can be extremely difficult; and partial or complete skin graft loss, necessitating frequent dressing changes. If this approach is undertaken, skin grafting may be performed immediately after excision or after the wound is allowed to granulate. These grafts can be secured to the periphery and quilted centrally with either staples or sutures. The grafts are meshed and slightly expanded to allow drainage. Topical antibiotic ointment is applied. The patient can undertake unlimited walking and showering several days after the operation. Healing is complete 10 days to 2 weeks postoperatively.

Flap coverage may be performed after excision of perineal hidradenitis. Donor sites include the posterior thigh, the gluteus maximus muscle, and the lumbosacral area of the back, among others. Often these regions are involved with disease. These flaps may allow primary closure of the perineal defect with early return to activity. The main disadvantage, however, is that these perineal wounds are usually extensive defects that necessitate the use of multiple, large flaps with the concomitant problems of prolonged operative time, blood loss, and possibility of recurrence beneath the flaps. Nonetheless, this approach may be considered in specific situations. Large skin or musculocutaneous flaps are unnecessary for most patients. I do not use them except when vital structures such as nerves and vessels or bone are exposed after debridement.

Immunotherapy

Immunotherapy for hidradenitis suppurativa using staphylococcal bacterial antigen (Staphage Lysate) may offer a promising adjunctive approach to this disabling disease. This United States Food and Drug Administration–approved agent is specific for *Staphylococcus aureus*, one of the two predominant organisms found in cultures of patients with hidradenitis; the other is *Streptococcus viridans*. It has been postulated that the mechanism of action of the antigen is the induction-elicitation immune reaction. Induction of delayed hypersensitivity occurs in response to specific antigens. This phenomenon occurs in most healthy people from previous exposure to *S. aureus.* Elicitation of lymphokines and the activation of macrophages in response to antigens homologous with the pathogenic agent subsequently occurs. These "angry" macrophages are effective against *S. aureus* and various other intracellular pathogens indigenous to the patient with hidradenitis suppurativa.

Angel and colleagues, in a double-blind randomized trial, demonstrated a salutary effect of staphylococcal bacterial antigen in the treatment of recurrent hidradenitis suppurativa. Included in the study were patients with chronic recurrent hidradenitis suppurativa involving more than two sites that previously did not respond to antibiotics, conservative therapy, or local surgical treatment. Ten of twelve patients in the group that received antigen showed improvement—a decrease in the frequency of acute inflammatory lesions without surgical intervention. In the placebo group, 8 of 15 patients had new inflammatory nodules requiring surgical intervention, and only 2 patients showed improvement. Further study of immunotherapy for this disease is warranted.

Follicular Occlusion Tetrad

Hidradenitis suppurativa is one component of the follicular occlusion triad, which includes three extreme variants of postadolescent acne. The second component is dissecting cellulitis of the scalp, or *perifolliculitis capitis abscedens et suffodiens,* a severe form of acne involving the scalp. It is characterized by recurring bouts of inflammation and pustular nodularity, causing cicatricial fistulous tracts and scattered alopecia. The third component of the triad is acne conglobata, a widespread form of acne involving the back, buttocks, and chest. Brunsting in 1952 elucidated the histopathology and clinical similarities of these diseases. He described them as fulminant variants of acne vulgaris that share the following features: (1) glandular hyperplasia of the pilosebaceous apparatus; (2) follicular occlusion with double comedo formation; (3) bacterial invasion with suppuration; and (4) cicatrization. A fourth component, pilonidal sinus, has been added to form the follicular occlusion tetrad. Beard sicosis, a severe form of acne characterized by disease involvement of the hair-bearing beard area in men, is yet another manifestation of this process.

Dissecting Cellulitis of the Scalp

Dissecting cellulitis of the scalp is a rare, chronic, inflammatory disease of the scalp characterized by a confluence of painful, purulent nodules interconnected by deep sinus tracts, dense scarring, and cicatricial alopecia. The disease is localized to the vertex or occipital scalp and posterior neck. Postadolescent black men are affected predominantly. The etiology of this disease remains unknown, although it is probably similar to that of hidradenitis suppurativa, with follicular occlusion and secondary infection. The high incidence of sterile cultures indicates that bacterial infection is not of central importance but is rather a secondary event. Foreign body reaction and granuloma formation similar to tuberculous lesions occur, suggesting that this disease may represent an immunologic assault on the scalp in response to displaced follicular or hair antigens in the reticular layer. This explains the occasional success of steroid treatment.

The diagnosis of dissecting cellulitis of the scalp is made by physical examination confirmed by biopsy. On a microscopic level, the sebaceous glands are chiefly involved. Liquefaction necrosis occurs in the deep dermis and subcutaneous tissues, surrounded by an inflammatory infiltrate composed predominantly of neutrophils. The coalescence of multiple pustular nodules results in diffuse, rather than discrete, subcutaneous abscess formation usually centered over the vertex of the scalp. Convoluted ridges and atrophic scars remain. Alopecia occurs over these involved areas.

The differential diagnosis is limited to other scalp conditions, such as chronic lupus erythematosus, folliculitis decalvans, and dermatitis papillaris capillitii. None of these conditions, however, causes such deep inflammatory undermining of the scalp.

The clinical course of dissecting cellulitis is characterized by exacerbations and remissions. Patients do not usually show signs of systemic illness such as fever or leukocytosis. Laboratory values are normal. Cultures tend to be sterile. When cultures are positive, *S. aureus* and *Staphylococcus albus* are most commonly seen. Mycobacterial organisms have never been isolated.

Perifolliculitis capitis is refractory to conservative treatment with systemic antibiotics, hydrotherapy of the scalp to debride devitalized tissue, good personal hygiene, incision and drainage, and systemic administration of steroids. Nonetheless, initially these conservative measures should be taken. Culture-specific antibiotics are prescribed. When cultures are sterile, broad-spectrum antibiotics are administered. Alternate-day corticosteroid treatment has been more successful than antibiotics in controlling these symptoms, but the disease recurs as soon as the steroids are withdrawn. Low-dose radiation has been administered to the affected scalp with variable success. When conservative measures fail or when there is extensive involvement of the scalp, wide resection of all affected areas with immediate or delayed split-thickness skin grafting of the pericranium is the treatment of choice. Although this "scalping" procedure causes permanent alopecia, patients appear quite satisfied with the result and resume their normal activities. Recurrence is uncommon after this treatment. Alopecia may be corrected later by tissue expansion of the nonaffected hair-bearing areas of the scalp (Fig. 25-7).

Williams and associates reported on four patients with dissecting cellulitis of the scalp. These patients were all black men who had a long history of the disease (6 months to 17 years) with failure of previous treatment. They underwent wide resection of all affected areas, resulting in defects ranging in size from 100 to 250 cm^2. For all the patients, coverage was obtained with split-thickness skin grafts over the pericranium, three immediately and one 48 hours after the initial operations. All patients healed well. No skin graft loss was noted in any patient, and all patients were free of disease in follow-up periods ranging from 1 to 4 years postoperatively.

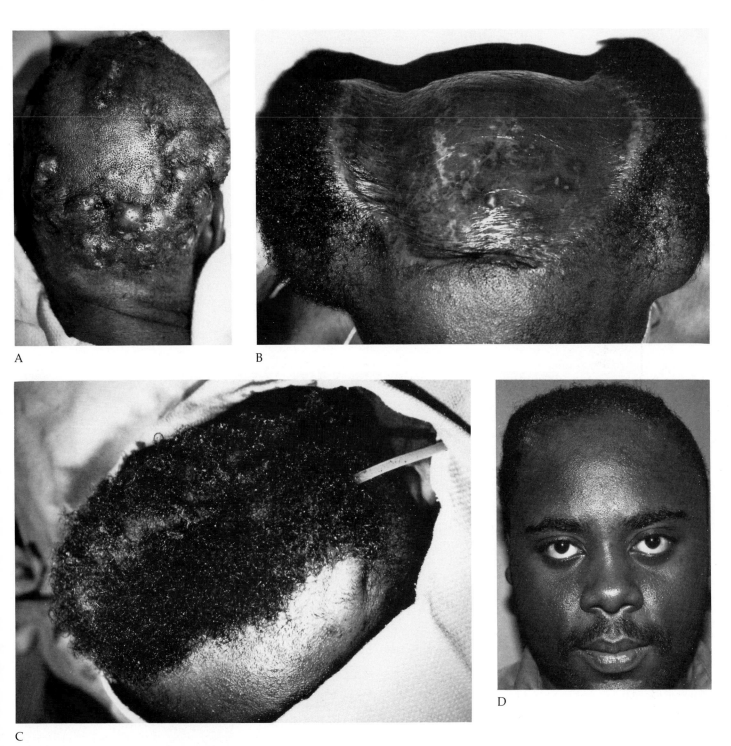

A

B

C

D

Fig. 25-7A. Extensive dissecting cellulitis of the scalp. All involved areas were resected to the level of the pericranium, and the residual wound was covered with a split-thickness skin graft. B. Six months after treatment. The anterior hairline was reconstructed with bilateral expanded temporoparietal flaps. C. Flaps are inset, and the anterior portion of the skin graft is removed. D. Final result with restored anterior hairline. A residual area of alopecia remains in the vertex of the scalp.

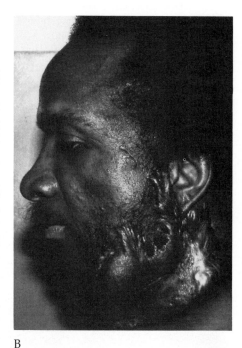

A

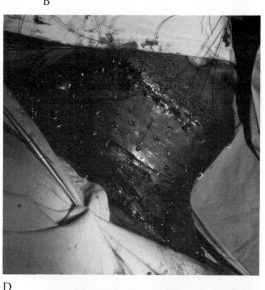

B

Fig. 25-8A, B. Sicosis with considerable involvement of the facial skin, draining sinuses, and scarring. C. All involved areas were resected down to healthy subcutaneous tissue. D. A split-thickness skin graft, applied directly to cover the defect, was immobilized with a stent. E. Final result with complete healing, no contour deformity, and no restriction in motion.

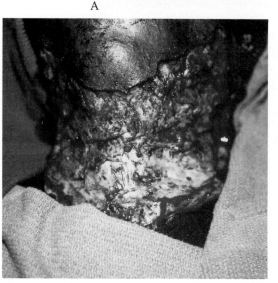

C

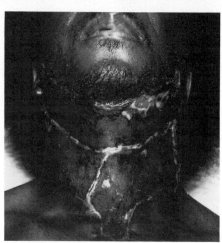

D

E

Beard Sicosis

Beard sicosis is a process similar to dissecting cellulitis of the scalp. It involves the hair-bearing area of the chin and neck. Patients have variable areas of involvement, draining sinuses, a history of superinfections, scarring, and keloid formation. This condition is treated by excision of all affected areas and coverage with split-thickness skin grafts to the subcutaneous tissue. In the postoperative period, compression garments are used to promote uniform healing without keloid formation.

Again, the key to the success of this procedure is meticulous dissection and excision of all involved areas. If this dissection is performed when gross infection is present, the skin grafting should be delayed for a few days, and the resected areas should be treated with moist dressings until permanent coverage is feasible (Fig. 25-8).

Acne Conglobata

Acne conglobata differs from hidradenitis suppurativa on a microscopic level in that the sebaceous glands in the pilosebaceous apparatus are involved. Moreover, all hair-bearing areas are susceptible, including the entire trunk, the buttocks, and the limbs, in addition to the areas usually associated with hidradenitis suppurativa. Florid acne conglobata does not occur until late in the second decade and in the third decade of life even though the sebaceous glands, which arise from the hair follicle, become active soon after birth. This condition has been attributed to a postadolescent sebaceous hyperplasia induced by hormonal influences and is almost exclusively limited to men. The pathophysiologic development of acne conglobata is similar to that of hidradenitis, with formation of multiple abscesses, phlegmon, fistulas, and sinuses.

Treatment of acne conglobata has been more difficult than that of hidradenitis suppurativa, primarily because of its more extensive distribution. Some satisfactory results with medical management have been reported using 13-*cis*-retinoic acid. This drug may have a direct inhibitory action on the sebaceous gland. Successful control with alternate-day corticosteroids also has been reported. When medical management fails and when there is extensive scarring, surgical excision is mandatory. Surgical management of acne conglobata is difficult and disappointing, usually producing less satisfactory results than the treatment of hidradenitis suppurativa. Dermabrasion has been used for permanent scarring with promising results. Nonetheless, acne conglobata appears most difficult to manage from both a medical and a surgical viewpoint.

Suggested Reading

Angel, M.F., et al. Beneficial effects of staphage lysate in the treatment of chronic recurrent hydradenitis suppurativa. *Surg. Forum* 38:111, 1987.

Ariyan, S., and Krizek, T.J. Hidradenitis suppurativa of the groin, treated by excision and spontaneous healing. *Plast. Reconstr. Surg.* 58:44, 1976.

Harrison, B.J. Recurrence after surgical treatment of hidradenitis suppurativa. *Br. Med. J.* 294:487, 1987.

Pollack, W.J., Virnelli, F.R., and Ryan, R.F. Axillary hidradenitis: A simple and effective surgical technique. *Plast. Reconstr. Surg.* 49:22, 1972.

Ramasastry, S.S., et al. Surgical management of massive perianal hidradenitis suppurativa. *Ann. Plast. Surg.* 15:218, 1985.

Silverberg, B., et al. Hidradenitis suppurativa: Patient satisfaction with wound healing by secondary intention. *Plast. Reconstr. Surg.* 79:555, 1987.

Thornton, J.P., and Abcarian, H. Surgical treatment of perianal and perineal hidradenitis suppurativa. *Dis. Colon Rectum* 21:573, 1978.

Watson, J.D. Hidradenitis suppurativa: A clinical review. *Br. J. Plast. Surg.* 38:567, 1985.

Williams, C.N., et al. Dissecting cellulitis. *Plast. Reconstr. Surg.* 77:378, 1986.

Yu, C.C.-W., and Cook, M.G. Hidradenitis suppurativa: A disease of follicular epithelium, rather than apocrine glands. *Br. J. Dermatol.* 122:763, 1990.

26

Thermal Burns: Resuscitation and Initial Management

John O. Kucan

Despite a proliferation in the number of burn prevention programs throughout the country, burn injuries continue to be an important cause of morbidity and mortality in all age groups. Burns have a multitude of causes, including scalding, chemicals, flame, electricity, and irradiation.

During the past 20 years, the care of the burned patient has greatly improved. These improvements are substantiated by a decreased mortality among people sustaining major thermal injuries. The commingling of a rapidly expanding body of knowledge pertaining to the basic pathophysiology of burn injury with the explosive growth in medical technology and surgical techniques and the adoption of the burn team concept has yielded salutary results.

A review of the objectives of burn care provides the outline for the management of the thermally injured patient. The first objective is to do no harm. Others include the prevention and treatment of shock, the control of bacterial growth, the conversion of an open wound to a closed wound, and the maintenance and preservation of body function and appearance while achieving healing within a minimal amount of time. In attaining these objectives, the preservation of the mental and emotional equilibrium of the patient must also be an important concern.

Management at the Scene

A primary goal in management at the scene of the accident is to stop the burning process. Smoldering clothing or clothing impregnated with chemicals may act as a continuing burning source unless promptly removed. In chemical injuries, copious irrigation of the affected area with water is the cornerstone of emergency management.

Once the burning process has been terminated and the clothes removed, the patient should be covered with clean, dry sheets. In high-voltage electrical injuries, the person first must be removed from the source of current, with great care exercised on the part of the rescuers so that they do not become victims.

All patients must be evaluated briefly but thoroughly to determine the patency of the airway and the status of breathing and circulation. In general, cooling of the burn should be avoided in burns of greater than 20 percent of the total body surface area (TBSA) or if the air temperature is below 10°C (50°F). Although cooling of the burn wound has been shown to decrease the depth of burning, the risk of hypothermia, especially in children, must be kept in mind. The patient should be wrapped in clean, dry dressings, but the application of topical antibacterial dressings should be avoided because these will only be removed when the patient arrives at a definitive care facility. The patient should be transported to the definitive care facility where triage can be accomplished and the determination of the patient's final disposition can be achieved.

Initial care of the burned patient begins with proper diagnosis. Evaluation of cardiopulmonary stability must be the initial priority in the management of this traumatic injury. Appropriate intervention to ensure continuance of these life-sustaining functions is mandatory. Care of the burn wound assumes a second-level priority; the burn wound should never take precedence over potentially life-threatening problems or complications.

BURN DIAGRAM, ESTIMATE

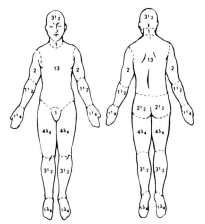

AGE: _____

SEX: _____

WEIGHT: _____

HEIGHT: _____

COLOR CODE

red - 3°
blue - 2°

Date of Burn _____

Date Revised _____

DOCTOR'S SIGNATURE

_____

Fig. 26-1. Burn diagram (estimate form) used to record location, depth, and extent of burn injury. (From J.O. Kucan. Comprehensive Care of the Burned Patient, *Vol. 3. St. Louis, Mosby–Year Book, 1990. Reproduced with permission.)*

A thorough and accurate accounting of the history of the accident along with the essential features of the patient's medical history must be obtained. The nature and circumstances of the injury should be elicited because they may provide pertinent information concerning the depth of the burn and the potential for life-threatening injuries or complications. A brief but thorough physical examination should be performed. As part of this examination, the location of the burn, the size of the burn wound, and the apparent depth of the injury should be recorded (Fig. 26-1). Any comorbid factors, such as advanced or young age, substance abuse, cardiopulmonary disorders, immunologic abnormalities, and inhalation injury, should be ascertained. On the basis of these findings, the burn may be classified according to the established American Burn Association criteria into one of three categories—minor, moderate, or major burn injury (Table 26-1). In obtaining the initial information, it is important to record both the time of injury and the patient's weight, because these are important factors in calculating the patient's initial fluid requirements.

The history of the injury may provide important clues to the depth of the injury. Flame or contact burns generally are deeper than scalds. Although the ability to differentiate definitively between deep partial- and full-thickness injuries continues to be elusive, the importance of such a distinction in the era of early excision and grafting has become less important. The involvement of special areas—the face, neck, hands, feet, and perineum—requires treatment in a specialized burn care facility. The aesthetic, functional, and wound care of these areas frequently exceeds the services available in a general hospital. One should never apologize for admitting a burned patient to the hospital. A conservative approach to the treatment of burn patients is preferable to the complications that may arise as the result of inappropriate or insufficient outpatient care.

AREA	Inf	1-4	5-9	10-14	15	Adult	2°	3°	Total	COMPLICATIONS LIST
Head	19	17	13	11	9	7				1.
Neck	2	2	2	2	2	2				2.
Ant. trunk	13	13	13	13	13	13				3.
Post. trunk	13	13	13	13	13	13				4.
R. buttock	2½	2½	2½	2½	2½	2½				5.
L. buttock	2½	2½	2½	2½	2½	2½				6.
Genitalia	1	1	1	1	1	1				7.
R. U. arm	4	4	4	4	4	4				8.
L. U. arm	4	4	4	4	4	4				9.
R. L. arm	3	3	3	3	3	3				10.
L. L. arm	3	3	3	3	3	3				11.
R. hand	2½	2½	2½	2½	2½	2½				
L. hand	2½	2½	2½	2½	2½	2½				
R. thigh	5½	6½	8	8½	9	9½				
L. thigh	5½	6½	8	8½	9	9½				
R. leg	5	5	5½	6	6½	7				
L. leg	5	5	5½	6	6½	7				
R. foot	3½	3½	3½	3½	3½	3½				
L. foot	3½	3½	3½	3½	3½	3½				
						Total				

Table 26-1. Categorization of burn injuries (American Burn Association)

Characteristics of burn	Major burn	Moderate burn	Minor burn
Partial thickness	>25% adults >20% children	15–25% adults 10–20% children	<15% adults <10% children
Full thickness	>10%	2–10%	<2%
Primary areas	Major burn if involved	Not involved	Not involved
Inhalation injury	Major burn if present or suspected	Not suspected	Not suspected
Associated injury	Major burn if present	Not present	Not present
Comorbid factors	Poor risk patients make burn major	Patient at relatively good risk	Not present
Miscellaneous factors	Electrical injuries		
Treatment environment	Usually specialized burn care facility	General hospital with designated team	Often managed on outpatient basis

Source: From J.O. Kucan. *Comprehensive Care of the Burned Patient*, Vol. 3. St. Louis: Mosby–Year Book, 1990. Reproduced with permission.

Inhalation Injury

The initial care of patients sustaining burns of the head and neck must concentrate on the issues of airway management and maintenance of adequate ventilation. Nearly 20 percent of patients admitted to burn centers have suffered various degrees of inhalation injury. At the present time, pulmonary complications associated with thermal injury constitute the primary cause of morbidity and mortality in burn patients. Furthermore, most burn victims who die at the scene die of the effects of acute asphyxia and inhalation injury rather than cutaneous burns.

Diagnosis

Patients who sustain inhalation injury may have a broad spectrum of symptoms, which range from minimal to severe. The diagnosis of inhalation injury is based on clinical evaluation, laboratory findings, and special diagnostic procedures. Despite a paucity of initial symptoms, severe life-threatening complications may develop; therefore, the identification of inhalation injury and the institution of prompt and directed treatment are essential.

The history of the injury provides important information regarding the potential for respiratory tract injury and its projected severity. A history of closed-space injury or extrication of an unconscious victim from a fire in an enclosed space strongly identifies a patient at risk. A thorough physical examination should be performed with specific emphasis on finding evidence of injury to the upper and lower respiratory tract. Deep partial- or full-thickness burns of the face; circumoral burns; and burns of the neck, singing of nasal hair, and injection or edema of the mouth and pharynx are all highly suggestive of inhalation injury. The presence of respiratory distress, progressive hoarseness, bronchorrhea, carbonaceous sputum, or conjunctivitis provides additional evidence of inhalation injury. Although initial chest roentgenograms may be normal, they do not preclude the presence of inhalation injury. An intraoral examination and indirect laryngoscopy may be helpful. Direct fiberoptic bronchoscopy, however, provides a definitive diagnosis because it positively identifies the airway changes consistent with inhalation injury. Three

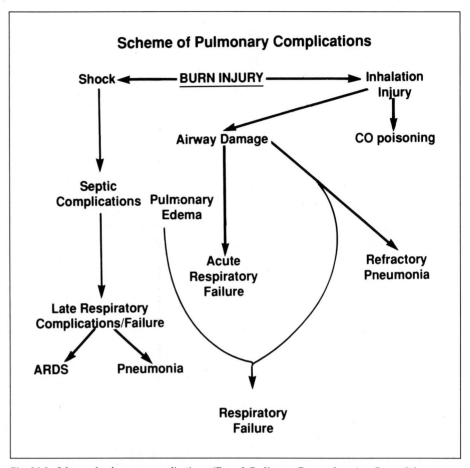

Fig. 26-2. *Scheme of pulmonary complications. (From J.O. Kucan.* Comprehensive Care of the Burned Patient, *Vol. 3. St. Louis, Mosby–Year Book, 1990. Reproduced with permission.)*

classic stages of inhalation injury have been described: (1) acute respiratory distress, occurring immediately after inhalation injury or arising within 12 hours of injury; (2) pulmonary edema, generally occurring from 18 to 36 hours after inhalation injury; and (3) bronchial pneumonia, developing 72 hours or longer after inhalation injury. The coexistence of inhalation injury and a cutaneous burn increases the mortality to nearly twice that seen with cutaneous thermal injury alone. Furthermore, the development of bronchial pneumonia after a thermal injury may carry a 60 to 70 percent mortality.

A number of pathologic processes may produce respiratory failure after thermal injury (Fig. 26-2). These include the direct toxic effects of smoke, the development of atelectasis and shunting, and numerous iatrogenic factors such as fluid overload, use of narcotic analgesics, patient

positioning, and controlled ventilation. Additional factors contributing to respiratory failure are aspiration, a generalized low-flow state, and trapping of neutrophils with liberation of superoxide radicals in the pulmonary microvasculature. The combined effect of multiple factors results in a profound, vicious circle, which may cause death. The effect of smoke on lung surfactant results in decreased pulmonary compliance, diminished oxygen exchange, atelectasis, and ventilatory failure. The presence of a circumferential chest burn may further restrict chest expansion and aggravate ventilatory problems.

The key laboratory studies necessary to make the diagnosis are determination of arterial blood gas and carbon monoxide levels. Pure carbon monoxide poisoning is seen occasionally and should be treated aggressively with 100% oxygen to displace carbon monoxide from the hemoglobin molecule. The role of hyperbaric oxygen therapy for this disease state has been well described. Carbon monoxide levels also may serve as a reliable indirect indicator of inhalation injury. The presence of hypoxemia, hypercarbia, and acidosis elucidated by arterial blood gas determinations provides additional important information regarding the presence and severity of inhalation injury.

Treatment

The treatment of inhalation injury and other pulmonary complications of thermal injuries is primarily supportive and expectant. Treatment should be implemented before the establishment of a definitive diagnosis. One hundred percent humidified oxygen is administered by a face mask or nasal cannula. The administration of intravenous bronchodilators may be helpful in relieving the early acute irritation of smoke on the tracheobronchial tree. Control of the upper airway must be achieved by prompt endotracheal intubation and ventilatory support. The absolute indications for endotracheal intubation include coma, respiratory depression, posterior pharyngeal wall swelling, progressive hoarseness, dyspnea, full-thickness circumoral burns, and circumferential burns of the neck (Table 26-2). It is important to note that not all patients with facial burns require endotracheal intubation; the procedure is not without inherent risks and dangers. Early tracheostomy should be avoided because of the associated two- to fourfold increase in pulmonary septic complications.

Fluid resuscitation must be carefully monitored and kept to a minimum to prevent or minimize pulmonary edema. Hypertonic fluid resuscitation should be considered in patients who have sustained inhalation injury to minimize free water loading. Invasive cardiopulmonary monitoring by Swan-Ganz catheters should be considered on an individual basis. In the presence of large cutaneous thermal burns, the correction of hypovolemia by exogenous colloid administration may be required. Diuretic therapy is frequently necessary to reduce the effects of pulmonary edema. The use of cardiac inotropic agents such as dopamine or dobutamine may be indicated. Sputum cultures and sputum for Gram stains are obtained when therapy is begun and daily thereafter. These results provide an ongoing monitor of the bacteriologic status of the tracheobronchial tree and enable the selection and institution of appropriate antibiotic therapy. Neither prophylactic antibiotics nor systemic steroids are indicated in the treatment of this disease state. Serial bronchoscopy may be of great value and should be used when clinically indicated. Despite maximal supportive therapy, the development of life-threatening complications in patients with inhalation injury is common. Nevertheless, the institution of proper therapy based on a high index of suspicion is lifesaving for a large number of patients with severe pulmonary injuries.

Fluid Resuscitation

Fluid resuscitation after thermal injury is an essential component of the initial care. It is generally accepted that patients with burn wounds of more than 15 to 20 percent TBSA require some type of intravenous fluid resuscitation. It must be remembered, however, that burn formulas serve only as guidelines for the initiation of resuscitation. Resuscitation should be individualized based on the patient's response. Successful resuscitation, therefore, requires continual monitoring of the patient with frequent corrections and adjustments in the rate of fluid administration. Resuscitation begins with a calculation of the patient's weight and percentage of body surface area that has been burned. A large-bore intravenous catheter is placed and fluid replacement is initiated. Current recommendations are for placement of peripheral intravenous catheters, avoiding central lines in resuscitating burned patients. In massive burn injuries, however, in which peripheral sites may be difficult to obtain, central lines should be placed, even through the burn wound. In patients who have sustained burns of more than 20 percent TBSA or in patients with facial burns, especially children, a nasogastric tube should be inserted. Placement of a Foley catheter is essential to assess urine output, an extremely important measurement for fluid resuscitation.

Numerous burn resuscitation formulas have been described, and all have been used successfully in resuscitating burned patients. The primary objective in initial fluid resuscitation is restoration and maintenance of tissue perfusion to avoid organ ischemia and to preserve the zone of stasis of the burn wound. The failure rate for initial fluid resuscitation is generally less than 5 percent in major burn centers. Nevertheless, inadequate fluid resuscitation after a major thermal injury is not an uncommon event when resuscitation is performed by personnel who do not have sufficient experience in this area. The problem of hypovolemia, which is now aggressively corrected, is not seen as frequently as generalized burn edema. The consequences of this fluid overload are decreased oxygen tension, additional ischemia to damaged cells, and pulmonary insufficiency, resulting in either chest wall or pulmonary edema. Overhydration may be as serious a problem as underhydration.

Fluid Monitoring

Successful burn resuscitation is based on appropriate monitoring. Arterial blood pressure, because of the initial catecholamine response, may not be a sensitive measurement of adequate fluid replacement. Pulse is generally more helpful. In older patients, however, the pulse may be unreliable because the heart is unable to increase its rate in response to volume deficits. Direct measurements of intracardiac filling pressures by pulmonary capillary wedge pressures may be misleading in patients who have sustained injuries of more than 20 to 30 percent TBSA. Because of the generalized capillary leak in these large burn injuries, it is not possible to replace fluids accurately on the basis of an attempt to increase filling pressures to an arbitrary level. Measurements of cardiac output may be helpful in these situations. It should be remembered that complications of central and Swan-Ganz

Table 26-2. Indications for endotracheal intubation

Supraglottic endema and inflammation on bronchoscopy

Progressive hoarseness or air hunger

Coma or respiratory depression

Acute respiratory distress

Full-thickness burns of face or perioral region

Circumferential neck burns

Source: Modified from J.O. Kucan. *Comprehensive Care of the Burned Patient*, Vol. 3. St. Louis: Mosby–Year Book, 1990.

lines are far greater in burned patients than in critically ill patients without burn wounds.

Urine output has consistently been found to be a useful guide because maintenance of renal blood flow reflects adequate perfusion to other organs as well. A urine output of 0.5 to 1.0 ml/kg body weight/ hour in an adult and of 1 ml/kg/hour in a child is considered sufficient. Acid-base balance is also a good measure of perfusion because a persistent base deficit is indicative of inadequate perfusion. In addition, serum lactate levels may provide important information regarding the adequacy of resuscitation. In inhalation injury, titration of fluid to the minimal amount required to maintain organ perfusion is vital.

Fluid Administration

In the presence of hemoglobinuria or myoglobinuria, an increase in fluid administration and the addition of an osmotic diuretic such as mannitol along with alkalizing agents such as bicarbonate in the intravenous fluids are necessary. In the initial stages, fluids containing salt but free of glucose are appropriate for resuscitation after a burn injury if given in sufficient amounts. The intravenous route is necessary in burns of more than 20 percent TBSA because a paralytic ileus usually accompanies burns of this size or greater. Lactated Ringer solution with a sodium concentration of 130 meq per liter is the most commonly used fluid. The presence of edema, which is a characteristic of thermal injury, results in the loss of effective intravascular volume and the translocation of proteins from the intravascular space into the tissues. The result is an osmotic gradient into the injured tissues. In burns of more than 25 to 30 percent TBSA, this capillary leak becomes generalized. Furthermore, alteration of the normal cell membrane potential results in the intracellular migration of sodium and a net increase of intracellular water, causing cellular edema. The result is edema formation within the interstitial space. Restoration of resting membrane potentials occurs approximately 24 to 36 hours after the thermal injury and depends on both the adequacy of volume resuscitation and the restoration of tissue perfusion.

Administration of colloid during the period of maximal edema helps increase the intravascular oncotic pressure, thereby drawing the edematous fluid from the interstitium back into the intravascular space. A complete restoration of intravascular volume during the acute phase is not possible despite adequate fluid resuscitation. Crystalloid resuscitation is based primarily on a calculated deficit in sodium ion, which has been lost from the extracellular space. This deficit has been estimated by Baxter to be 0.5 to 0.6 meq/ percent TBSA burned/kg body weight; therefore, fluid resuscitation approaching 4 ml/kg/percent TBSA burned is required during the first 24 hours. Half the required volume is given over the first 8 postburn hours and the other half during the succeeding 16 hours. It must be emphasized, however, that the rate of fluid infusion must be dictated by the patient's response according to the parameters used for monitoring (Tables 26-3, 26-4, and 26-5).

Because sodium is the major element in crystalloid resuscitation, with water serving as a solvent, a solution that would increase sodium concentration should have a theoretical advantage over isotonic or hypotonic solutions. The use of hypertonic solutions may decrease the net fluid flux into the burn wound. Hypertonic solutions have been reported to increase myocardial contractility, produce precapillary dilatation, and decrease vascular resistance. The theoretical advantages of

Table 26-3. Monitoring parameters

*Vital signs, sensorium, anxiety level
*Urine output
  Mean arterial pressure
*Cardiac output/index
  Pulmonary capillary wedge pressure
  Central venous pressure
  Peripheral vascular resistance
  Continuous tissue probes (pH, O_2, CO_2)
  Laser Doppler ultrasonography
  Laboratory tests
    *Hemoglobin/hematocrit
    *Serum electrolytes
      Serum and urine osmolality
      BUN, creatinine
    *Arterial blood gases
      Urinalysis

* Most important monitoring parameters.
BUN = blood urea nitrogen.

hypertonic fluid resuscitation include decreased edema formation and decreased incidence of paralytic ileus. Current indications for the use of hypertonic resuscitation include inhalation injury, burn wounds in excess of 40 percent TBSA, and hemodynamic instability in patients in whom fluid overloads would be poorly tolerated, such as elderly burn victims.

The disadvantages of this method are that it is somewhat complex and that careful monitoring is required. Complications may include hypernatremia, hyperosmolar coma, renal failure, and alkalosis with a left shift of the oxygen association curve. Serum sodium levels must be monitored closely in this group of patients, and the levels must not be allowed to exceed 160 meq per liter. If this degree of hypernatremia occurs, a slightly hypotonic solution such as lactated Ringer so-

Table 26-4. Parkland formula
for fluid resuscitation

Adults
  Lactated Ringer solution, 4 ml × wt (kg)
    × TBSA burned
    Half given over first 8 h
    Half given over next 16 h
Children
  Lactated Ringer solution, 3 ml × wt (kg)
    × TBSA burned
    Half given over first 8 h
    Half given over next 16 h
  Lactated Ringer solution maintenance
    every 24 h
    100 ml/kg for first 10 kg
    50 ml/kg for second 10 kg
    20 ml/kg for third 10 kg or portion
      thereof

TBSA = total body surface area.
Source: From J.O. Kucan. *Comprehensive Care of the Burned Patient*, Vol. 3. St. Louis: Mosby–Year Book, 1990. Reproduced with permission.

Table 26-5. Hypertonic formula
for fluid resuscitation

1 L lactated Ringer solution
(130 meq Na$^+$/L) + 100 meq Na$^+$ lactate = 230 meq Na$^+$/L
Infusion calculated as for Parkland formula

Source: From J.O. Kucan. *Comprehensive Care of the Burned Patient*, Vol. 3. St. Louis: Mosby–Year Book, 1990. Reproduced with permission.

lution is used until the condition is corrected.

Colloid infusions begin 16 to 24 hours after the burn and are given at a rate of 0.35 to 1.0 ml/kg/percent TBSA burned. The amount of colloid provided depends on the magnitude of the injury, the degree of hemodynamic instability, and the degree of concern over excess edema formation. The infusion is provided over a 6-hour period. Fresh frozen plasma is preferred because it contains protein fractions that have both oncotic and nononcotic properties. Fresh frozen plasma also contains clotting factors necessary to carry out early burn excision and fibronectin, an important opsonin for circulating microaggregates.

Specific concerns regarding the transmission of blood-borne diseases must be taken into account when considering fresh frozen plasma for colloid infusion. After the administration of crystalloid and colloid in the first 24 to 30 hours postburn, there occurs a gradual restoration of the altered cell membrane potential, a diminution of the capillary endothelial leak, and a gradual elimination of excess sodium ion. It is during this time that a second major source of fluid loss becomes readily apparent. Because the burned skin can no longer act as a barrier to water evaporation, evaporative losses from the burn surface begin to assume an ever-increasing importance. Initially the thick dry eschar of a full-thickness wound allows less net water loss than does the moist eschar of a partial-thickness burn wound. Nevertheless, these additional losses must be taken into consideration and replaced. An estimate of such losses can be obtained by a formula: Milliliters of evaporative loss equals 25 plus the percent TBSA burned multiplied by the surface area in square meters. Maintenance fluid in the form of dextrose and water should be initiated during this period. Dextrose is important because glucose stores are depleted during the initial catecholamine release and volume resuscitation. Additional potassium may be required. Serum sodium concentration is monitored every 4 to 6 hours, and free water is either provided or restricted on the basis of serum sodium concentrations. The need for a blood transfusion may become apparent, and blood replacement should be provided to maintain a hematocrit reading of 30 to 35 percent.

Assessment of the Burn Wound

During the period of initial resuscitation, careful assessment of circumferentially burned limbs and of the chest wall and neck is imperative. A restricting eschar overlying burn wounds in these regions may interfere with circulation or restrict chest wall movement. Patients with circumferential burns of the upper limb should be monitored carefully, therefore, for signs of impending compartmental syndrome. Clinical observation alone may be inaccurate, and the use of Doppler measurements may provide erroneous information. Direct measurement of muscle compartments provides the most reliable information on the status of these closed compartments.

The patient's ability to ventilate adequately in the presence of circumferential chest and neck burns must be carefully assessed. Escharotomy of the chest wall and neck may be necessary in patients who require continual augmentation of ventilator pressure to provide adequate ventilation. Surgical escharotomies should be carried out with attention to detail to achieve complete release with good hemostasis. An improperly performed escharotomy is of no benefit. Occasionally, most notably in the lower limb, escharotomy may be insufficient and fasciotomy may be necessary. High-voltage electrical injuries generally require fasciotomies and decompression of major neural structures in the known sites of compression neuropathy such as the carpal tunnel and the canal of Guyon. The morbidity associated with surgical escharotomy may be high. An alternative to surgical excharotomies is a medical escharotomy with sutilains ointment. Application of sutilains ointment to a fresh burn wound provides an effective means of decompressing circumferential burns of the limb and chest. This method is not useful, however, nor is it recommended for charred full-thickness burn wounds or when the time from injury to treatment has been prolonged.

Burn Wound Sepsis

The ultimate goal in the management of thermal injury is closure of the burn wound. Thus, after resuscitation, care of the burned patient is synonymous with care of the burn wound. During this time, every effort is made to prevent infection of the burn wound and to provide the appropriate conditions for either spontaneous or surgical closure of the burn wound. Before closure of the burn wound can be achieved, however, proper care must be delivered to the wound to enhance the healing of superficial partial-thickness wounds, to prevent the conversion of deeper partial-thickness wounds to full-thickness injury, and to prepare deep wounds for definitive surgical closure. Additional tissue damage must be avoided by the prevention of wound desiccation and infection.

The Nature of Sepsis

Infection and sepsis continue as the leading causes of morbidity and mortality in burned patients. Reasons for this increased infection rate include loss of the skin barrier to microbial invasion, immunosuppression as a result of thermal injury, and the presence of invasive tubes and catheters, which breach the normal anatomic barriers to infection. Therefore, the burn wound, along with the perineum, anus, and oral and pulmonary secretions, may serve as a major endogenous source of microorganisms. From these sites, the burn wound, lungs, and the various catheters and tubes serve as the major sites of bacterial lodgment.

Sepsis is a systemic response to actively invading and proliferating microorganisms. These organisms include bacteria, fungi, and viruses. The release of bacterial endotoxin produces an identical response. Sepsis must be differentiated from the postburn hypermetabolic state, which also may be characterized by fever, tachycardia, leukocytosis, increased cardiac output, and decreased peripheral vascular resistance along with an increased oxygen consumption. One can differentiate this state from sepsis by the presence or absence of impaired tissue oxygenation as evidenced by the presence or absence of lactic acidosis or hypotension. Two distinct septic states may be seen—the hyperdynamic state and the hypodynamic state. The hyperdynamic state, frequently indicative of gram-positive septicemia, is characterized by fever, tachycardia, warm and dry skin, mental changes, hyperglycemia, leukocytosis, and metabolic acidosis. The hypodynamic state is characterized by either fever or hypothermia, general coolness of the skin, tachycardia, hypotension, mental changes, and profound oliguria. Additional signs may be leukocytosis or leukopenia, hypoglycemia, metabolic acidosis, and hematologic changes, most notably thrombocytopenia and disseminated intravascular coagulation (DIC).

The physiologic changes associated with sepsis include decreased oxygen consumption, low arterial venous oxytension (AVO$_2$) difference, and diminished systemic vascular resistance. The status of the most common sites of infection in burned patients and the potential for the production of systemic sepsis in these sites must be carefully evaluated. Intravascular catheters carry a high risk of infection. It should be noted that in nearly 50 percent of patients, despite clinical evidence of sepsis, blood cultures remain negative. In addition, intra-abdominal sources of sepsis such as acalculous cholecystitis or pancreatitis must be considered. In patients with indwelling nasogastric or nasotracheal tubes, sinusitis may also be a source of sepsis.

Not all burn-related infections are attributable to bacteria alone. With the use of potent systemic antibiotics, and in the presence of an immunocompromised host, the incidence of fungal infections involving the burn wound, lungs, and intravenous catheters has increased. Continuous monitoring of potential sites of infection with special attention to the presence of fungi is imperative. Furthermore, *Candida albicans*, which was in the past the most common fungal isolate, is gradually being replaced by less common and perhaps more dangerous fungi such as *Aspergillus*, *Mucor*, and *Rhizopus*.

Effective management of septic complications is predicated on establishment of hemodynamic support, institution of appropriate systemic antibiotic therapy, and elimination of septic foci. Knowledge of the bacterial and fungal ecologic status of the burn treatment facility may be of great value in choosing appropriate systemic drugs. The maintenance of nutrition, aggressive management of the burn wound, and prompt and appropriate ventilatory and hemodynamic inotropic support are

essential elements in the care of these patients. It is also necessary to differentiate between sepsis emanating from the burn wound and that arising from other sources, such as septic thrombophlebitis, bacterial endocarditis, meningitis, urinary tract infections, sinusitis, acalculous cholecystitis, pneumonitis, and intra-abdominal abscess.

Treatment

Most infections in burn patients are endogenous. It has been clearly shown that burn wound sepsis is a quantitative disturbance in the resistance of the host and the resident bacteria. Early care of the burn wound, therefore, has been aimed primarily at preventing the increase of bacteria. After thermal injury, the resultant avascular burn wound provides an excellent culture medium for the bacteria that reside at the base of the hair follicles. Because of the avascular nature of the wound, systemic antibiotics are totally ineffective at controlling bacteria in the burn wound; therefore, topical antibacterial agents are necessary to control bac-

Table 26-6. Topical antibacterial agents

Characteristic	Silver sulfadiazine cream	Mafenide acetate cream	Silver nitrate soaks	Nitrofurazone ointment
Form of treatment	Occlusive dressing	Exposure	Occlusive dressings	Occlusive dressings
Concentration of active agent (%)	1.0	11.2	0.5	0.2
Advantages	Painless on application; wound readily visible when cream is applied without dressings; compatible with treatment of associated injuries; motion of involved joints is maintained	Penetrates eschar; wound not readily visible; compatible with treatment of associated injuries; no gram-negative resistance identified; motion of involved joints is maintained	No hypersensitivity; painless except at time of dressing change; no gram-negative resistance; reduces heat loss from wound; most compatible with hypertonic resuscitation regimen	Broad-spectrum activity, especially effective against silver sulfadiazine–resistant staphylococci, relatively nontoxic to epithelial cells
Limitations and side-effects	Poor penetration of eschar; bone marrow suppression with neutropenia; hypersensitivity (infrequent); resistance of many *Enterobacter cloacae* and of some *Pseudomonas*	Painful for 20–30 minutes after application to second-degree burns; accentuates postburn hyperventilation; hypersensitivity noted in 5% of patients; delays spontaneous eschar separation	No penetration of eschar; marked transeschar loss of Na+, K+, Ca^{2+}, and Cl−; methemoglobinemia (rare); dressings limit motion of involved joints; discolors unburned skin of patient, skin of attending personnel, and any environmental objects in contact ineffective in treating burn wound sepsis	No penetration; polyethylene glycol in base may produce renal impairment; increased BUN, anion gap, and metabolic acidosis

Source: Adapted from J.O. Kucan. *Comprehensive Care of the Burned Patient*, Vol. 3. St. Louis: Mosby–Year Book, 1990.

terial proliferation in the wound. There exists no ideal topical antibacterial agent. At present, a number of agents are used, each possessing beneficial characteristics and limitations (Table 26-6).

Silver sulfadiazine cream is the most widely used topical antibacterial agent in the United States. It is generally safe and effective in controlling bacterial proliferation, but it does not penetrate the burn eschar to any degree; therefore, its activity is primarily limited to the surface of the burn wound. It is painless and generally nontoxic and is well tolerated by most patients. Although it does not cause any metabolic disturbances, it may produce neutropenia. It also has been shown to delay wound healing.

Mafenide acetate, with an active ingredient concentration of 11.2%, was the first topical antibacterial agent shown to be effective against *Pseudomonas* burn wound sepsis. This agent has been relegated to second-line status because of the pain associated with its use on partial-thickness burn wounds and the induction of metabolic problems. It causes a metabolic acidosis and compensatory respiratory alkalosis because of carbonic anhydrase inhibition. It produces hyperventilation and may produce irreversible pulmonary edema in patients who have sustained inhalation injury. Because of its high osmolality, it is a strong desiccating agent. Nevertheless, mafenide acetate continues as the "gold standard" among topical antibacterials because of its ability to penetrate eschar, its broad spectrum of activity, and its great potency against both gram-positive and gram-negative organisms.

Silver nitrate, 0.5% solution, is not used frequently. It is generally ineffective in treating established burn wound sepsis because it does not penetrate eschar. In addition, evidence suggests that it may inhibit epithelization of partial-thickness wounds.

Nitrofurazone is effective in the treatment of staphylococci and is frequently substituted for silver sulfadiazine cream when the emergence of silver sulfadiazine–resistant staphylococci is noted in the burn wound. A number of experimental topical antibacterial agents continue to be evaluated and show great promise. It will be a number of years, however, before these

make their appearance on the market and enjoy widespread clinical use.

The effectiveness of burn wound topical therapy is assessed by quantitative bacteriologic analysis, histologic examination of burn wound biopsies, and the overall clinical status of the patient. The mere presence of bacteria is not the critical issue; it is the quantitative level of bacterial growth and the histologic presence or absence of bacterial invasion of unburned tissue subjacent or adjacent to the burn wound that provide the most useful information. Controversy continues regarding the reliability of swab techniques as opposed to biopsies in the longitudinal bacteriologic assessment of a burn wound.

Because all topical antibacterial agents have been shown to retard wound healing to some degree and to require frequent reapplication, small, clean, superficial burn wounds are perhaps best managed by the use of a nonadherent gauze dressing or the application of a biosynthetic skin substitute.

A burn wound that is to be treated with a topical antibacterial agent may be treated by either an open or a closed technique. There are advantages and disadvantages to both methods. With the open method, application of the topical antibacterial agent is easier, especially in areas where the application of dressings may be difficult. The disadvantages of this method include potential wound desiccation, increased patient discomfort, heat loss, and the risk of cross contamination. Situations that lend themselves to treatment by the open method include burns of the face, ears, and perineum, and superficial burns that have a low risk of infection or desiccation. Any deep burn, however, whether full thickness or partial thickness, may be treated by this method. Advantages of the closed technique include a decreased risk of wound desiccation, diminished heat losses, a decrease in the risk of cross contamination, and a potential debriding effect on the wound. In addition, an overlying dressing may provide a degree of comfort far greater than that achieved by the open technique. Disadvantages of this method include the expense of dressings and of additional nursing time and the potential risk of infection if the dressings are not changed frequently.

Metabolism and Metabolic Support

Major burn injury results in a hypermetabolic response directly proportional to the severity and degree of injury. The baseline energy expenditures and requirements may be increased as much as $2\frac{1}{2}$ times above normal in patients with wounds exceeding 30 percent TBSA. This increased energy expenditure is mediated by the neurohumoral axis in response to stress and represents a normal host response to major wounding. The consequence of this response to the patient is a markedly increased metabolism, and failure to replenish these energy sources may result in rapid weight loss and potentially fatal consequences. Nutritional support of burned patients should be initiated immediately after fluid resuscitation, preferably within 24 to 48 hours after the injury. Assessment of the nutritional needs of the patient and maintenance of these needs by appropriate intake coupled with continual monitoring is essential. Although numerous nutritional formulas are available for burned patients, indirect calorimetry at the bedside appears to be the most accurate method for monitoring the appropriateness of metabolic support. Certainly this is not required in patients with non-life-threatening injuries, but for critically injured patients attention to these details may make the difference between death and survival.

The enteral route is preferred to the intravenous route because the initiation and continuation of enteral feedings maintains the intestinal villi and augments production of immunoglobulin. The use of central venous lines and total parenteral nutrition in patients with thermal injuries should be avoided if at all possible; if these techniques are used, it should be with great trepidation. Septic complications are common; also, it was recently demonstrated that parenteral feeding fails to restore immunocompetence and may, in fact, unfavorably alter the prognosis in these patients. In patients who are at high risk for the development of septic complications and the resultant development of paralytic ileus, it may be useful at the time of initial surgical debridement to place a feeding jejunostomy tube, thereby allowing continuous feeding of an elemental diet in the face of absent gastrointestinal motility.

Monitoring of nutritional status and success of nutritional supplementation in burned patients are of major importance. Body weight provides a good indicator of the effectiveness of nutritional therapy. Although weight loss is common after major thermal injury, attempts should be made to prevent weight loss in excess of 10 percent of the patient's premorbid weight. Weight losses exceeding 10 percent of the preburned weight increase morbidity and mortality. Thus body weight should be recorded daily and under similar conditions each day. Furthermore, the maintenance of accurate records of intake and output and of caloric intake is essential. The provision of adequate nutritional support may require frequent readjustment and reevaluation.

Nutritional therapy can be evaluated with prognostic nutritional indices from the outset of the patient's care. Thus serum transferrin levels, hypersensitivity skin testing, anthropomorphic measurements, and total lymphocyte counts in conjunction with serum protein determinations and nitrogen balance studies are of great value. The goals of nutritional support are the maintenance of body weight, improved wound healing, and reduced morbidity and mortality. The inclusion of a dietitian as part of the burn team is essential in the attainment of these goals.

Immune Consequences

Because thermal injury results in a major alteration of the host immune system, the status of the immune system after a major thermal injury has become an object of focused attention.

There exist two major categories of phagocytic cells in humans: the circulating phagocytes of the blood, which include granulocytes and monocytes, and the fixed phagocytes, or macrophages of the tissue, which belong to the reticuloendothelial system. Neutrophils circulating cells are primarily involved in host defense against infectious agents. Present in high numbers, they possess greater phagocytic capabilities than do the other circulating leukocytes. Within minutes after tissue injury or microbial invasion, neutrophils begin to adhere to the endothe-

lium of blood vessels and migrate into the involved tissues. Once out of the confinement of the bloodstream, they are unable to return to the circulation. The extravasated neutrophils demonstrate chemotaxis in response to the various stimuli. Chemotactic factors include complement generating systems. The leukocytes themselves elaborate products that function as additional chemoattractants. Altered leukocyte chemotaxis and altered phagocytosis have been well demonstrated after thermal injury. In addition, a decrease in the complement components C3A and C5A also has been noted, suggesting that thermal injury nonspecifically activates the complement system. The resultant inflammatory response results in edema formation and a consumptive opsinopathy. As complement activity is suppressed, the response of chemotactic cells and phagocytosis is diminished. The complement system is a highly complex and integrated network of serum proteins that mediate both specific and nonspecific immunity. Defects in reticuloendothelial function occur after thermal injuries. These are caused by the disrupted interface between specific immune responses and phagocytosis.

The interaction of cell-mediated immunity (T-cell function), humoral immunity (B-cell function), and the complement system has a direct effect on opsonization. The decreased production of antibodies after thermal injury and the consumption of opsonins result in decreased phagocytosis. The reduction in macrophage phagocytosis results in decreased antigen processing and a decreased specific immune responsiveness. Furthermore, greater numbers of suppressor cells are generated. Fibronectin is also greatly decreased after thermal injuries, additionally reducing opsonic activity and, ultimately, reticuloendothelial function. Finally, antigen expression on the surface of the macrophage is markedly reduced, limiting lymphocytic activation and resulting in a decrease in both T-cell and B-cell immunity.

Cell-mediated immunity is a function of the T cell. T cells can differentiate into memory cells, which are capable of early and accelerated responses when restimulated by the original or cross-reactive antigenic factors. In addition, T lymphocytes can elaborate and secrete a variety of soluble mediators of the immune re-

sponse called *lymphokines*. These lymphokines are involved in the stimulatory and inhibitory capacity of T lymphocytes. Furthermore, T cells are composed of both helper and suppressor cells; a variety of T-cell responses and many B-cell responses depend intimately on the interaction with activated, regulator T cells. Adequate helper T cells are required for an antibody response when T cells are important regulators of these responses. Elevated suppressor cell activity is seen in burn injuries and has been associated with impaired host defense.

Humoral immunity is a function of B lymphocytes, which produce plasma cells. The plasma cell produces specific antibodies to invading microorganisms and their products. B-lymphocyte stimulation is through activation by T lymphocytes. When T-lymphocyte stimulation is inadequate, the production of antibody activity is markedly diminished. Antibodies serve multiple roles in host defense, including toxin neutralization, bacteriolysis in the presence of complement, and the opsonization of bacteria, which results in enhanced phagocytosis. Any defect in antibody production results in altered complement and altered white-cell function. This system interacts with cell-mediated immunity in that increased suppressor T-cell activity alters B-lymphocyte activation and thus greatly impairs immunoglobulin production.

Major thermal injuries produce a marked alteration in the immune response by directly affecting the complex interaction of the numerous components of the immune response. It is not clear at this time whether the alteration of immune function following thermal injury is a pure deficiency disease, is caused by circulating toxins, or is a combination of both elements. Nevertheless, the end result is an overstimulation of several immune system components, that is, suppressor T-cell stimulation and complement activation, and a depression of other components such as T-helper-cell and T-killer-cell activity and polymorphonuclear function.

Complications of Thermal Injury

As a result of improved resuscitation and a reduction in early mortality, the appearance of delayed systemic complications after thermal injuries has increased. The major risk factors influencing the incidence and severity of complications following burn injury include advanced or very young age, the presence of preexisting disease or associated injury, and the occurrence of the burn in a closed space.

Systemic complications following a burn injury may be caused by the burn injury itself or by inadequate treatment. Complications also may arise despite appropriate treatment. Although some complications are certainly avoidable and manageable, others occur as part of the continuum of the injury and may not be preventable or respond to effective treatment. In caring for burned patients, it is important to anticipate potential complications, minimize any iatrogenic factors, and identify developing complications at their onset. Because major organ system complications are potential threats to the survival of a thermally injured patient, a methodic review of each of the organ systems as part of the daily management of these severely injured patients is an essential component of care. This review aids in the early diagnosis and treatment of systemic complications.

Despite multiple causes and manifestations of systemic complications, treatment plans are guided by a few general rules. These include close monitoring, supportive care, and the timely institution of appropriate treatment. Frequently the therapies do not cure the complications (e.g., ventilator support in pulmonary failure), but serve to maintain homeostasis and support life until the organ system and ultimately the patient can recover. Frequent reevaluation and modification of the care plan may be necessary to address the everchanging findings in a critically ill patient. Prompt surgical treatment of some complications may be necessary to increase the potential for survival. Although the ideal therapy consists of total avoidance of complications, rarely is this goal possible. Keen awareness, vigilance, and an ability to react aggressively and appropriately constitute the basic requirements for effective management of systemic complications in burned patients (Table 26-7).

Cardiovascular Complications

Thermal injury may cause a number of cardiovascular complications, including acute myocardial infarction, hyperdynamic cardiac failure, acute hypertension, bacterial endocarditis, and septic thrombophlebitis and thromboembolism. Myocardial infarction may be seen soon after severe burn injury as a result of a massive reduction in cardiac output. Hyperdynamic cardiac failure is usually seen later in the course of burn injury as a result of sepsis. Acute hypertension after a burn injury is not uncommonly noted in children and may result in seizures and encephalopathy. Complications of endocarditis and septic thrombophlebitis are most often related to the use of central venous catheters, most notably pulmonary artery catheters. Recognition of the great risk associated with the use of these devices is imperative.

Respiratory Complications

The primary respiratory complications associated with thermal injury are inhalation injury, pneumonia, acute pulmonary edema, and acute respiratory distress syndrome (ARDS). Obstruction of endotracheal or tracheostomy tubes, laryngeal stenosis, tracheoesophageal fistula, and pulmonary embolism are other complications of note.

Renal Complications

Renal failure is the most common complication seen after a thermal injury. It is the result of inadequate resuscitation (hypovolemia), septic shock, or exposure to nephrotoxic substances. Metabolic acidosis is a renal complication that is often seen as the result of excessive bicarbonate loss from the kidney, most notably in conjunction with therapy with mafenide acetate.

Table 26-7. Complications of burn injuries

Organ system	Major complications
Respiratory	Inhalation injury, pulmonary edema, pneumonia, ARDS, embolism, sinusitis
Cardiovascular	Myocardial infarction, endocarditis, pericarditis, arrhythmias, hypertension, septic thrombophlebitis, embolism, thrombosis, ruptured vessel wall
Renal	Renal failure, hematuria, myoglobinuria
Gastrointestinal	Curling ulcer, hepatic dysfunction, paralytic ileus, acalculous cholecystitis, pancreatitis, mesenteric occlusion, superior mesenteric artery syndrome, peritonitis
Endocrine	Diabetes mellitus (insulin resistant), adrenal insufficiency, adrenal hemorrhage
Neurologic	Encephalopathy, CO poisoning
Musculoskeletal	Contractures, loss of limb
Hematologic	Anemia, coagulopathies
Immunologic	Sepsis, immunodeficiency
Metabolic-Nutritional	Prolonged catabolism, starvation

ARDS = adult respiratory distress syndrome; CO = carbon monoxide.

Gastrointestinal Complications

The commonly encountered gastrointestinal complications include gastroduodenal ulceration, hepatic dysfunction, pseudo-obstruction, prolonged paralytic ileus, superior mesenteric artery syndrome, pancreatitis, and acalculous cholecystitis. A high index of suspicion is essential in delineating gastrointestinal complications.

Endocrine Complications

Endocrine complications are not common after thermal injuries. Nevertheless, hormonal changes following burn injury are clinically significant and exert a profound effect on the host. These changes include disruption of the hypothalamic pituitary axis, changes in catecholamine and adrenal cortical hormone production, disruption of the normal insulin-glucagon interaction, and diminished production of thyroid hormone.

Metabolic and Nutritional Complications

The administration of incorrect amounts of protein, carbohydrate, fat, vitamins, and minerals may result in numerous problems, which range from poor wound healing to hyperosmotic coma and acute fatty liver. Improper management of gastric feeding tubes may set the stage for aspiration pneumonia and respiratory failure. The presence of nasogastric tubes may result in sinusitis or erosion of pharyngeal walls, nasal airway passages, or the nares. Perforation of the intestine also has been described. The complications associated with parenteral hyperalimentation (pneumothorax, hemothorax, sepsis, fatty liver, and hyperosmolar coma) must be considered when this route is to be used for nutritional support.

Musculoskeletal Complications

Loss of limbs after fourth-degree burn injuries or high-voltage electrical injuries is the most dramatic example of musculoskeletal complications. However, limb dysfunction secondary to scarring and disability secondary to prolonged ischemic changes, such as compartment syndrome, pressure necrosis, and infection, are also potential problems.

Hematologic Complications

Anemia and coagulopathy are the two key types of hematologic complications in burned patients. Initial hemolysis, altered red-cell half-life, exogenous blood losses, and diminished red-cell production are some of the more common factors causing anemia in burned patients. The disturbances in clotting mechanisms are seen within minutes of the burn injury as a result of the thermal injury itself. Later complications of clotting are generally caused by sepsis, massive blood transfusion, or a transfusion reaction.

Septic Complications

Sepsis, from whatever source, continues to be the most feared complication of a thermal injury. The sources of infection are not restricted to the burn wound itself, although the wound remains a major focus of attention. Furthermore, infection is not restricted to bacteria but may be caused by fungi or viruses.

Conclusion

Care of a burned patient is a complex undertaking that frequently continues long after the patient's discharge from the hospital. Numerous factors interact to determine the potential for survival and the quality of life after a thermal injury. It is incumbent on those who care for burned patients to minimize the controllable risk factors while maximizing the factors that bring about functional recovery. The care rendered to a burned patient in the initial postinjury hours and days may greatly influence the ultimate result. As leader of the burn team, a physician caring for burned patients should effectively use the expertise of the various members of the burn team. The physician must develop an organized and individualized plan of care for the burned patient and orchestrate its implementation from the time of the initial encounter, throughout the patient's hospitalization, and frequently beyond. Although the initial care of the burned patient represents a small part of the entire continuum of burn care, it represents a vital phase and frequently serves as a major determinant in the ultimate outcome.

Suggested Reading

Achauer, B.M., et al. Pulmonary complications of burns: The major threat to the burn patient. *Ann. Surg.* 177:311, 1973.

De Camara, D., Raine, T., and Robson, M. Ultrastructural aspects of cooled thermal injury. *J. Trauma* 21:911, 1981.

Hunt, J.L., Agee, R.N., and Pruitt, B.A. Fiberoptic endoscopy in acute inhalation injury. *J. Trauma* 15:641, 1975.

Metabolic and nutrition support for trauma and burn patients. Abstracts from Nutrition Symposium sponsored by Mead Johnson Nutritional Division, 1982.

Monafo, W.W. The treatment of burn shock by the intravenous and oral administration of hypertonic lactated saline solution. *J. Trauma* 10:575, 1970.

Munster, A.M. Immunologic Manipulation of the Injured Patient: Looking into the Future. In J.L. Ninnemann (Ed.), *Traumatic Injury: Infection and Other Immunologic Sequelae.* Baltimore: University Park Press, 1983.

Pruitt, B.A. Fluid and electrolyte replacement in the burned patient. *Surg. Clin. North Am.* 58: 1291, 1978.

Robson, M., Krizek, T., and Wray, R., Jr. Care of the Thermally Injured Patient. In G.D. Zuidema, R.B. Rutherford, and W.F. Ballinger (Eds.), *The Management of Trauma.* Philadelphia: Saunders, 1979.

Warden, G.D. *Immunology: Management of the Burned Patient.* Norwalk, Conn.: Appleton & Lange, 1987.

27

Burn Wounds: Excision and Grafting

Jeremy J. Burdge   Robert L. Ruberg

Burn wound management has changed considerably in the last 30 years. Increasingly effective topical antibiotics, improved critical care monitoring, readily available and "safe" blood products, improved anesthetic support, better understanding of the physiology of burn hypermetabolism, and increasingly aggressive nutritional support have dramatically improved burn care. Surgical treatment of the burn wound also has changed. Traditional wound management involved topical antibiotics and daily limited debridement of the burn eschar. Superficial and deep second-degree burns were allowed to heal spontaneously. Third-degree burns were often dressed and superficially debrided until separation of the burn eschar (usually at 2 to 4 weeks) and the appearance of healthy granulation tissue allowed skin grafting.

Within the last 20 years this conservative technique has been replaced with more aggressive and earlier surgical treatment of the burn wound. Now, excision of the burn wound and immediate coverage with autologous skin graft often can be accomplished within the first 72 hours after injury.

We cannot accept early excision of a burn wound as the standard of treatment for all burns, however, without critically examining several issues. When is the ideal time to perform excision and grafting of the burn? Does early excision of the burn improve survival or at least decrease hospital stay for patients surviving their burn? Which patients and what size burns are best suited to this treatment? Does earlier excision decrease the hypermetabolic demands or improve the immune competence of a burned patient? Does earlier excision improve the ultimate function of the structure burned or does it at least return the patient to employment sooner? Does earlier excision improve the final cosmetic result of the healed burn? All these questions need to be addressed before we can accept early excision of a burn as superior to conservative wound management. Finally, we must recognize the technical complexity of excision of a major burn and admit that not all surgeons or all hospitals have the resources to perform it successfully.

Timing of Burn Wound Excision

It is important to decide how early an excision is early enough. Initially when Jan-

zekovic described the technique, excision was performed as soon after the burn occurred as the patient's condition was hemodynamically stable, usually within the first 72 hours. This approach allows the surgeon to operate on a patient who is in a stable condition, after some edema has resolved and before the burn wound has become colonized. Although these advantages are important in relatively small, obviously third-degree burns (less than 20% of total body surface area, TBSA), this early an excision may not be practical in larger burns requiring repeated operations or in burns of indeterminate depth. Larger burns with obvious areas of deep second- or third-degree injury may require more than 72 hours for effective stabilization. For these burns we attempt to perform the first wound excision within 5 to 7 days.

At times it is difficult even for the most experienced observer to determine burn depth in the first 48 hours. Generally, superficial burns heal within 2 weeks with little functional or cosmetic deformity. Surgical excision may add little benefit in such instances. On the other hand, deeper dermal burns may not heal for up to 6 weeks, and complications of infection, hypertrophic scarring, and decreased function often develop. We operate on small, obviously, third-degree burns as soon as possible (24 to 72 hours after the injury). When we cannot initially distinguish between superficial and deep burns, i.e., in burns of indeterminate depth, we wait as long as 7 to 10 days for spontaneous healing and proceed with excision and grafting if necessary.

Effect of Early Excision on Mortality

It is difficult to show any statistically significant improvement in burn survival rate that can be attributed solely to early excision. Changes in burn mortality nationwide are not a reliable measure of the efficacy of early excision. There are too many unrelated variables in burn size, patient age, presence of inhalation injury, preexisting illnesses, and triage patterns. Comparisons between different burn units or comparisons with historical controls are equally unreliable.

Because early excision has become the standard of care in most burn centers, there are few well-controlled, randomized studies comparing excision with conservative separation of the eschar and grafting onto granulation tissue. In 1989 Herndon published the results of the only randomized comparison of early excision with conservative topical therapy and delayed grafting. His conclusion was that the type of treatment does not affect mortality in young children or the elderly, in patients with inhalation injury, or in burns involving less than 30 percent TBSA. This finding was probably based on a multiplicity of factors other than excision that affect mortality in these groups. Patients between the ages of 17 and 30 years with greater than 30 percent TBSA burns and no inhalation injury, however, had a statistically significant decrease in mortality (from 45% to 9%) when treated with early excision.

Despite the fact that there are few controlled studies of excisional therapy, there has been steady improvement in the size of burn that produces a 50 percent mortality (LA 50) in burned patients treated with early excision. In patients 40 to 65 years of age, the LA 50 has improved from a 38 percent to a 62 percent burn. Similarly, among patients older than 65

years, the LA 50 has increased from 23 percent to 33 percent. Herndon showed an LA 50 of a 90 percent TBSA burn in children from birth to 14 years of age using aggressive excision compared with an LA 50 of a 50 percent TBSA burn when using less aggressive therapy in historical controls. However, these improved survival rates are probably the result of multiple improvements in patient care, not of early excision alone.

McManus also reported improvement in survival rates among patients treated by early excision, but he warned that any advantages attributed to earlier surgical treatment may reflect patient selection only. Only patients healthy enough to tolerate an aggressive surgical procedure are considered for excision.

Although early excision and grafting cannot be rigorously proved to improve survival in all patients or in all sizes of burns, it is clear that the method does not increase mortality. Several studies, including one of our own, showed that even in patients older than 65 years excision of the burn with immediate grafting is safe and effective.

Whereas it is difficult to prove conclusively that earlier excision improves survival, many studies confirm that it has decreased hospital stay by as much as 50 percent for comparable burns when compared with conservative therapy. In a randomized, prospective study at the University of Washington, burns of indeterminate depth of less than 20 percent of the TBSA treated by early excision required a shorter hospitalization, lower hospital costs, and fewer reconstructive procedures than did burns treated by delayed healing. This seems to be true even in elderly patients. Slater noticed that patients older than 65 years spent 22 days in the hospital after early excision. Similarly elderly burned patients who had conservative treatment spent an average of 42 days in the hospital.

Effect of Excision on Burn Physiology

There has been some speculation that decreasing the burn size by early excision and grafting of the wound decreases septic complications, diminishes burn hypermetabolism, and improves immune

competence. It is unclear, however, whether improved immune function after early excision and grafting is caused by decreased necrotic debris in the wound or decreased circulating inhibiting factors because of the massive transfusions used during excision. Measured energy expenditure in burned patients would be expected to decrease as the patients' wounds close. If, however, energy expenditure (measured by indirect calorimetry) and protein degradation (measured by urine urea nitrogen level) are determined before and after wound excision, they do not decrease with progressive wound closure. This increased heat production, or "burn hypermetabolism," is caused by a combination of factors, including altered central thermoregulation and increased peripheral heat loss. Although early excision and grafting of the wound can decrease evaporative heat loss, it has little effect on the elevated metabolic rate seen in patients with burns.

The absence of physiologic improvement after partial burn excision is supported by Demling's research in a burned sheep model. He noted that there was a significant increase in oxygen consumption immediately after the burn. This increased oxygen consumption was not decreased by partial excision and closure of the burn wound. He concluded that early excision and grafting of the burn does not decrease the hypermetabolic state until the wound is *completely* covered. This conclusion agrees with our experience measuring nutritional indices in burned patients. Measurements of total protein, albumin, transferrin, and cell-mediated immunity (skin test anergy) rarely return to normal until the burn wound is completely closed, despite aggressive nutritional support.

A frequently cited reason for early excision of a burn wound is to decrease the septic complications. Once again, however, there is little statistical support for this conclusion. In a comparison of early excision and grafting with conservative therapy, Herndon could find no significant decrease in number of septic days at risk. Although McManus was able to show a decreased incidence of wound infections in patients treated with early excision, he was unable to tell whether this was caused by the surgical procedure or by improved topical bacterial control. Intuitively one would expect that the sooner a burn wound is closed, the fewer the septic complications. Certainly this factor must contribute to any improved survival time seen among patients treated by early excision. McManus has reported that burn wound sepsis is becoming a less frequent cause of death in patients with major burns.

Effect of Early Excision on Appearance and Use of Structure

Increased survival times and shortened hospital stays are not the only criteria for successful burn wound treatment. Does early excision improve the final functional or cosmetic result? One of the frequently cited criticisms of early excision is that the amount of tissue removed during aggressive early debridement is often greater than that removed with a more conservative approach. It is assumed that this factor produces an inferior cosmetic or functional result. In a review of 100 burns allowed to heal spontaneously, however, Deitch showed that those that healed in less than 14 days had less than a 14 percent incidence of hypertrophic scars. Burns healing in 14 to 21 days had a 33 percent incidence of scar hypertrophy, whereas those requiring greater than 3 weeks to heal had a 78 percent incidence of hypertrophic scars. In comparison, deep dermal burns treated by excision and grafting onto a remaining dermal base had a 15 percent incidence of hypertrophic scarring.

The question regarding final cosmetic result with early excision is difficult to answer because there are no randomized studies of similar wounds. Deitch's study, however, suggests that the cosmetic result from early skin grafting is comparable if not superior to that of delayed healing of the wound. In our own experience we frequently have had the opportunity to compare areas of healed deep second-degree burns with grafted areas on the same patient. We have repeatedly noted that the grafted areas are aesthetically superior.

It is equally difficult to compare functional results of different surgical and nonsurgical therapies. In 1979 Burke advocated earlier surgical treatment of burns of the dorsal hand. Burned hands treated by grafts seemed to regain functional motion earlier than those left to heal spontaneously. Salisbury found, however, that if comparable burn wounds were treated with aggressive physical therapy, there was no difference at one year in the final functional results between grafting and spontaneous healing. It has been our policy, therefore, to operate on isolated burns of the hand as soon as possible. In extensive burns, however, for which donor sites are limited, our primary goal is to maximize coverage as early as possible. Excision and grafting of the hand and of multiple digits is a time consuming operation. Because there is no long-term functional advantage to early skin grafting of hands, we do this at a later date, after larger areas are covered.

In addition to the therapeutic advantages of earlier excision and grafting of burn wounds, there are several advantages that affect patient comfort. When the hospital stay and the time required to achieve wound closure are shortened, the pain associated with prolonged, repetitive dressing changes decreases. In addition, earlier excision and grafting of the wound expedites return of the patient to the normal home and work environment. In one study, the patients who underwent excision and grafting returned to work twice as quickly as those who did not have operations. These factors are important to the patient and should be a consideration in determining the method of care.

Technique of Excision and Grafting

General Considerations

In 1972 Janzekovic noticed that excision of the necrotic debris of a burn immediately produced an acceptable wound for skin grafting. Excision eliminated the necessity for extensive dressing changes for debridement of the wound and allowed earlier closure of the burn. However, several factors prevented acceptance of this observation. (1) It was thought that excision removed excessive amounts of viable tissue; (2) donor sites were increased, requiring harvesting from difficult areas; (3) inexperience prevented many surgeons from accurately determining the appropriate depth of excision; and (4) excessive blood loss was thought to limit the extent of the operation. Fortunately, with experience many of these concerns lessened.

Effective topical antibiotics allow many deep partial-thickness burns to heal without conversion to full-thickness injuries. Although antibiotic therapy and spontaneous healing may decrease the extent of skin-grafted areas, the quality of the skin in these healed partial-thickness wounds is less than ideal. The epithelium is thin, friable, and prone to shear injury. In addition, many of these wounds produce hypertrophic scars, which contract, requiring additional surgical treatment. Often a well-healed skin graft gives a better final functional and cosmetic result than a spontaneously healed deeper wound.

Depth of Excision

It is often difficult to determine the appropriate level of excision. Tangential excision serially removes thin layers of necrotic debris until healthy unburned tissue is reached (Figs. 27-1 to 27-4). Although it is relatively easy to identify the punctate bleeding seen in healthy dermis, the exact level of excision in third-degree burns involving fat is more difficult to estimate. Healthy fat has a bright yellow color as opposed to the brown-yellow and hemorrhagic appearance of thermally injured fat. In addition, subcutaneous tissue that shows areas of venous thrombosis (see Fig. 27-3) should be considered necrotic and should be excised.

As opposed to tangential excision, excision to fascia removes all the burned skin and, possibly, viable subcutaneous tissue down to the fascia. Although it eliminates the necessity for deciding on the appropriate level of tangential excision, this procedure has several disadvantages. There are few data to support the idea that skin grafts take better on fascia than on healthy fat. In many patients, especially those with larger amounts of subcutaneous tissue, the contour and aesthetic deformity after fascial excision can be great. Finally, in a comparison of fascial and tangential excision, Jones noted that patients whose burns were excised tangentially to fat had better joint mobility and sensory function than patients

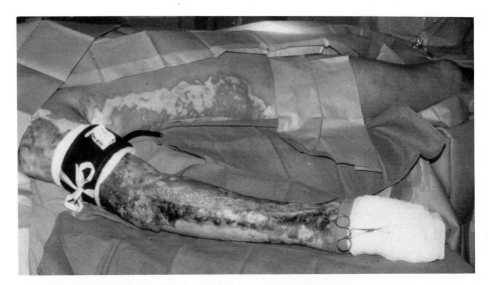

Fig. 27-1. Appearance before debridement. Note the tourniquet applied to reduce blood loss during the procedure.

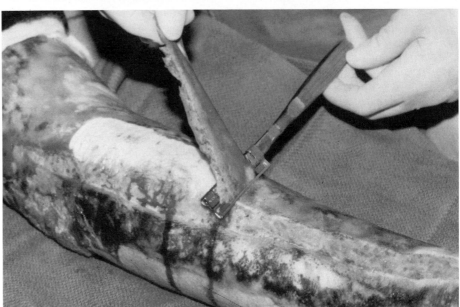

Fig. 27-2. Tangential excision of a thin layer of necrotic tissue with a dermatome.

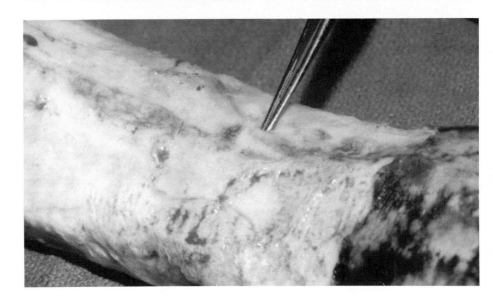

Fig. 27-3. Excision of a thrombosed vein during initial debridement.

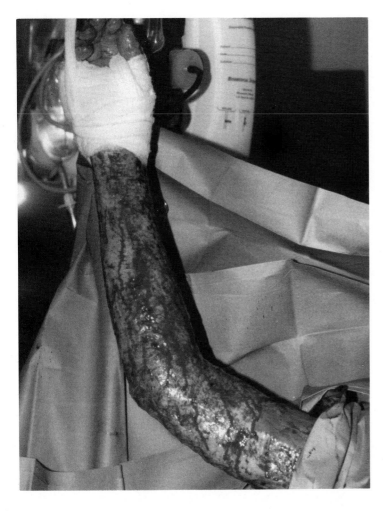

Fig. 27-4. Appearance after excision of all necrotic tissue.

whose burns were excised to fascia. The major advantages of excision to fascia are shortened operative time and reduced blood loss.

Under most circumstances, tangential excision, even to fat, seems to give better long-term function than does fascial excision. Therefore, we reserve fascial excision for patients with very deep burns (fourth degree); patients with extensive, life-threatening burns; or elderly patients who cannot tolerate a prolonged operation or massive blood loss.

Control of Hemorrhage

The major disadvantage of excision and grafting of a burn wound is the amount of blood lost during the procedure. In a retrospective study of blood loss during excisional therapy, Moran's patients lost nearly 200 ml of blood for each 1 percent of body surface excised and grafted. More standard methods of hemorrhage control,

such as electrocautery, are often ineffective in the face of innumerable punctate bleeding sites seen after tangential excision. We use several techniques to control excessive bleeding. Elevation of limbs during the operation decreases venous congestion and blood loss. Application of tourniquets (see Fig. 28-1) on the burned limb before excision is also helpful. Topical agents may be applied to the excised wound in an attempt to control hemorrhage. Epinephrine solution varying in concentration from 1:100,000 to 1:150,000 has been our most effective agent in this regard. Although there is some concern with epinephrine absorption, clinical complications are rare and usually are limited to tachycardia. We also have used topical thrombin but have not found it to be as effective as epinephrine for hemostasis. Vasopressin has long been recognized as a potent vasoconstrictor; it decreases blood flow to the skin without compromising cardiac output. By

infusing vasopressin (0.2 IU/kg/hour beginning one-half hour before and continuing for one hour after the operation), Achauer showed a 50 percent decrease in average blood loss per 1 percent TBSA debrided and a 50 percent decrease in the number of transfusions required.

Despite all these techniques to control intraoperative hemorrhage, burn excision continues to be a formidable procedure, and excision of more than 10 percent TBSA at one time may produce hemodynamic complications. In elderly patients or those in an unstable condition, fascial excision is preferable to tangential excision. When electrocautery is used at the fascial level, large areas of necrotic burn wound can be removed quickly with little blood loss.

Management of Donor Sites

Donor skin can be harvested from nearly any site on the body (Figs. 27-5 to 27-9); however, several techniques can help to decrease postoperative complications. The thickness of the donor skin is the primary determinant of how quickly the donor site heals and how often hypertrophic scarring develops. Except when functional or cosmetic considerations require thicker donor skin (i.e., burns of the face, hands, feet, and across joints), the donor skin should be no thicker than $^{12}/_{1000}$ inch. Donor sites harvested thicker than $^{12}/_{1000}$ inch or donor sites in elderly patients can be overgrafted with meshed thin split grafts to speed healing and to prevent hypertrophic scarring. Whenever possible, donor skin should not be harvested across flexion creases of the joints.

A variety of donor site dressings can decrease pain and minimize infection. Adhesive polyurethane sheets are particularly useful in decreasing postoperative pain in small donor sites; however, it is difficult to get these dressings to adhere to large wounds. Although synthetic skin substitute is effective at decreasing donor site pain, we have found it to be no more effective than other standard topical dressings in decreasing infection or speeding wound healing.

The scalp is a well-recognized but too infrequently used donor site. It has the advantage of being a frequently spared area in major burns. It provides an ideal color match for grafting facial burns. The donor site is hidden, making the scalp a preferred site in patients who have aesthetic concerns regarding donor-site scarring. The scalp heals more rapidly than some other donor areas, allowing for rapid reharvesting. Because the hair follicles arise in the subcutaneous tissue, transplantation of hair with a superficial scalp graft rarely occurs.

Harvesting the scalp does pose several technical problems. Since the galea is attached to the skull only by loose areolar tissue, which allows for motion of the scalp, harvesting of skin grafts may be difficult. In addition, the rich vascular supply to the scalp often produces a considerable amount of bleeding after harvesting. Both these problems can be di-

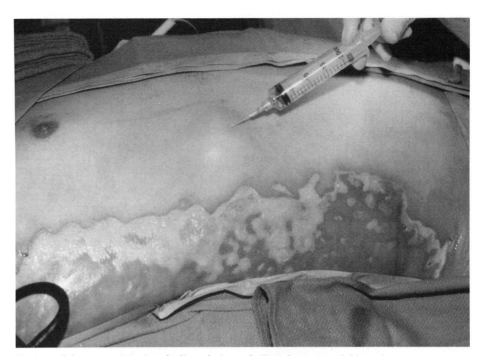

Fig. 27-5. Subcutaneous injection of saline solution to facilitate harvesting of skin grafts.

Fig. 27-6. Harvesting of long strips of split-thickness skin graft with a dermatome.

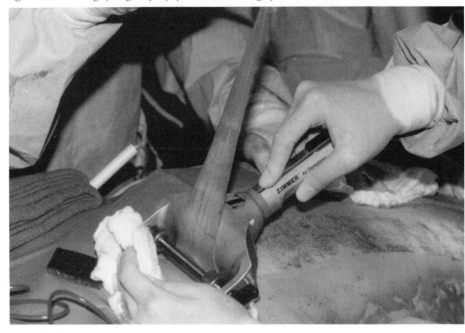

minished by injecting several hundred milliliters of saline solution into the subgaleal space. This maneuver improves the ease of harvesting by decreasing motion of the scalp, helps with tamponade the superficial vessels, and allows a smoother surface for harvesting. This injection technique also is useful in other irregular donor areas (see Fig. 27-5).

Although some authors report harvesting of up to 12 successive grafts from the scalp in children, our experience with this site in adults has not been without complication. Sparse hair growth, delayed wound healing, and patchy areas of alopecia are not uncommon after repeated harvesting of the scalp, especially in elderly people.

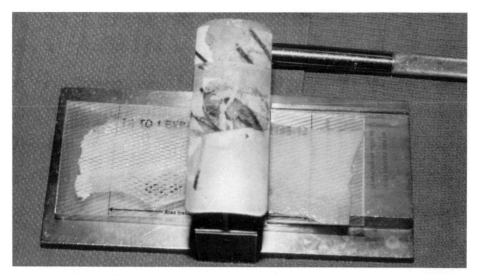

Fig. 27-7. Meshing of skin graft.

Grafting Techniques

Functionally and cosmetically important areas such as the face, neck, and hands are best treated with unmeshed skin grafts whenever there is adequate donor skin. This method decreases contraction of the grafts and avoids an unsightly "alligator skin" appearance. If meshed skin is used in these areas, care should be given to aligning the interstices of the mesh to parallel the normal skin creases and to avoiding overexpansion of the meshed skin. These steps ensure the best cosmetic appearance to the graft.

When large areas of burn need grafting, the sheet graft can be meshed (see Fig. 27-7) with an expansion ratio of 1.5:1.0 or 3:1. In patients with inadequate donor

Fig. 27-8. Application of skin graft to the debrided area.

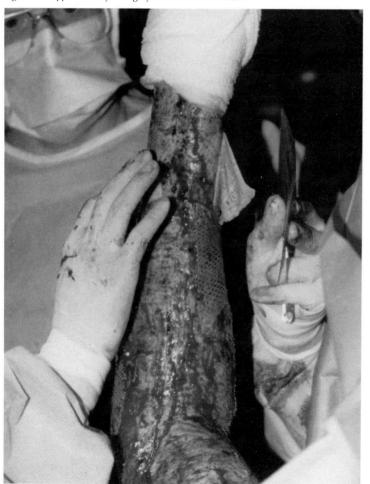

Fig. 27-9. Stabilization of the skin graft with staples.

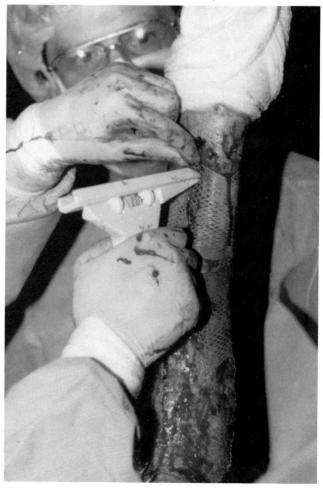

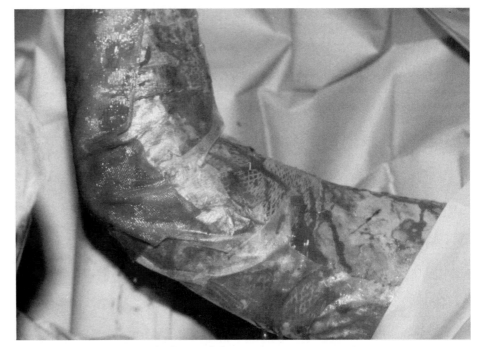

Fig. 27-10. *Inner layer of gauze has been applied.*

skin, Alexander described widely expanded split grafts covered with allograft as a useful technique for early closure of large burns. Fang described a similar technique of microskin grafting that involves transplantation of minced pieces of autologous skin using sheets of allograft as a carrier. Both these techniques have the advantage of allowing an expansion ratio of more than 10:1 while achieving early closure of the wound with allograft. These techniques have the disadvantages inherent in all thin skin grafts—increased contracture across flexion creases and poorer cosmetic results.

Use of Dermatomes

A wide variety of dermatomes are available to burn surgeons. The traditional hand-powered dermatome has been almost universally replaced by electric and pressurized air-driven dermatomes. However, the "drum style" (Padgett or Reese) dermatome continues to be useful for selected patients. These dermatomes easily harvest uniform thicknesses of skin from difficult rounded areas of the body, such as the hips, buttocks, and anterior abdomen. The uniformly high quality of skin harvested with these dermatomes makes them ideal for coverage of the hand or face. Unfortunately, these dermatomes are not suited for harvesting large, flat areas when extensive grafts are required.

The older-style Brown dermatome also has been replaced with dermatomes that allow better control of donor skin thickness. The electric motor–driven (Padgett) dermatome harvests skin of uniform,

well-controlled thickness. It has the disadvantage, however, of requiring gas sterilization after each use and is therefore not available for multiple patients on the same day. Our dermatome of choice for most burns is the air-pressure-driven dermatome made by Zimmer (see Fig. 27-6). It has all the advantages of the Padgett electric dermatome and is easily sterilized between operations.

Treatment of Difficult Burn Areas

Burns of the back and buttocks have been difficult to graft because of the pressure and shear force placed on the grafts by a bedridden patient. Postoperative use of low-pressure beds has diminished the extent of skin graft lost.

Facial burns are best treated by excision and grafting of entire aesthetic units, even when this requires excision of small areas of unburned skin. Burns of the eyelid often produce ectropion and exposure of the cornea, leading to ulceration and even extrusion of the lens. Permanent tarsorrhaphies are to be avoided if possible because they often pull apart and produce more destruction of the lid margin. Our best treatment is early release of the

burned eyelid and grafting with full-thickness or thick split-thickness skin. Even with aggressive surgical therapy, ectropion commonly recurs, requiring repeat release and grafting.

Microstomia secondary to deep burns of the lips is best treated with early dynamic splinting of the commissures. Early grafting of the infraclavicular areas in extensive burns provides a relatively clean area for subclavian venous access.

Dressings and Postoperative Care

Most of the skin grafts we apply are held in place by skin staples (see Fig. 27-9). However, skin grafts over irregularly contoured areas such as the face and hands are often sewn in place with absorbable chromic catgut sutures. The initial dressing is applied in the operating room by the burn team, including, whenever possible, the nurses (Figs. 27-10 and 27-11). This dressing comprises an inner layer of fine nylon gauze followed by a layer of petrolatum gauze impregnated with antibiotic ointment (either povidone-iodine or polymyxin-bacitracin) and covered with an outer layer of gauze burn packs. The nylon gauze allows serous drainage

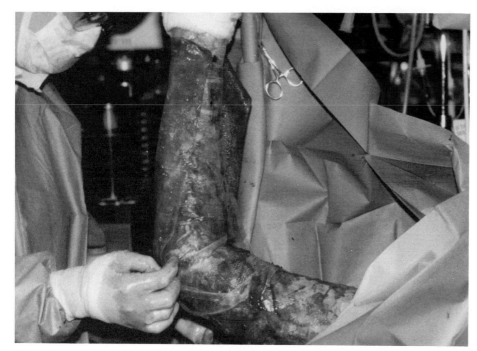

Fig. 27-11. Outer layer of gauze impregnated with antibiotic ointment is applied.

to escape the wound. At the same time it prevents adherence of the graft to the overlying dressing and accidental removal with subsequent dressing changes. Skin grafts across joints are immobilized with splints fashioned in the operating room. This dressing is left in place for 48 hours, at which time the petrolatum gauze and overlying burn packs are changed by the physicians. The skin staples and nylon mesh are removed 72 hours after application. Physical and occupational therapy is resumed 5 days after the operation. Patients with lower limb grafts begin walking at this time with elastic wrap supports.

Conclusion

Small burns (less than 20% TBSA, full-thickness or deep partial-thickness injuries) are best treated by early excision and grafting. This decreases hospital stay, cost, pain, and time away from work or family. Larger burns appear to have a decreased mortality, a decreased rate of infectious complications, and fewer wound complications when treated by early excision and skin grafting. In addition, the earlier the wound is permanently closed

with skin, the sooner patients have the advantages of reduced hypermetabolism and improved immune function. Patients treated by earlier, more aggressive operations require fewer late reconstructive procedures and have an earlier return to normal function. Therefore, excision and grafting must be considered an essential part of the modern care of burns.

Suggested Reading

Achauer, B.M., Hernandez, J., and Parker, A. Burn excision with intraoperative vasopressin. *J. Burn Care Rehabil.* 10:375, 1989.

Alexander, J.W., et al. Treatment of severe burns with widely meshed skin autograft and meshed skin allograft overlay. *J. Trauma* 21:433, 1981.

Burdge, J.J., et al. Surgical treatment of burns in elderly patients. *J. Trauma* 28:214, 1988.

Deitch, E.I. Prospective study of the effect of the recipient bed on skin graft survival after thermal injury. *J. Trauma* 25:118, 1985.

Demling, R.H., and Lalonde, C. The effect of partial burn excision and closure on postburn oxygen consumption. *Surgery* 104:846, 1988.

Demling, R.H., and Lalonde, C. Oxygen consumption is increased in the postanesthesia period after burn excision. *J. Burn Care Rehabil.* 10: 381, 1989.

Engrav, L.H., et al. Excision of burns of the face. *Plast. Reconstr. Surg.* 77:744, 1986.

Fang, C.H., et al. A preliminary report on transplantation of microskin autografts overlaid with sheet allograft in the treatment of large burns. *J. Burn Care Rehabil.* 9:629, 1988.

Heimbach, D., et al. Early excision of thermal burns: An international round-table discussion. *J. Burn Care Rehabil.* 9:549, 1988.

Herndon, D.H., et al. A comparison of burn wound excision on measured energy expenditure and urinary nitrogen excretion. *J. Trauma* 10:1103, 1970.

Janzekovic, Z. A new concept in the early excision and immediate grafting of burns. *J. Trauma* 10:1103, 1970.

Jones, T., McDonald, S., and Deitch, E.A. Effect of graft bed on long term functional results of extremity skin grafts. *J. Burn Care Rehabil.* 9: 72, 1988.

McManus, W.F., Mason, A.D., and Pruitt, B.A. Excision of the burn wounds in patients with large burns. *Arch. Surg.* 124:718, 1989.

Moran, K.T., et al. A new algorithm for calculation of blood loss in excisional burn surgery. *Am. Surg.* 54:207, 1988.

Salisbury, R.E., and Wright, P. Evaluation of early excision of dorsal burns of the hand. *Plast. Reconstr. Surg.* 69:670, 1982.

Snelling, C.F.T., and Shaw, K. The effect of topical epinephrine hydrochloride in saline on blood loss following tangential excision of burn wounds. *Plast. Reconstr. Surg.* 72:830, 1983.

Zingaro, E.A., Capozzi, A., and Pennisi, V.R. The scalp as a donor site in burns. *Arch. Surg.* 123:652, 1988.

28

Reconstruction of Burn Deformities of the Head and Neck

Bruce M. Achauer

Efforts to minimize the potentially disabling deformities of burns of the head and neck should be initiated during the acute period. Priorities include functional goals, such as preserving sight and oral competence, minimizing tissue loss, and preventing deforming chondritis and neck contracture. To minimize later problems, sheet grafts are used if possible for initial coverage. Open techniques are preferred because a sterile wound does not exist and bacterial proliferation may occur under a tie-over dressing.

If possible, potential flap sites are not used as skin graft donor sites. As soon as wound coverage is obtained, an initial discussion with the patient and family outlines the events to follow. The psychological help of support groups and psychologists is a priority during this period. It is difficult for patients to appreciate the magnitude and time span of the coming hypertrophic scar phase. Motivation to wear the splints and pressure garments must be continuously reinforced. The whole burn team—doctors, nurses, therapists, psychologists, and previous burn patients—is needed to sustain a patient through this period.

Ideally, reconstructive efforts for improved appearance are delayed until a mature scar is present. The length of time is highly variable (6 months to 2 years) and can vary even in the same patient from one anatomic area to another. When the red, thick, immobile scar tissue has passed from red to purple to brown in color and becomes supple, definitive reconstruction can be done without fear of unexpected changes. An additional reason for waiting out this period is that many times surgical procedures can be avoided by effective pressure treatment of the scars. Functional problems should be dealt with as early as necessary to prevent complications. Reconstructive procedures done during the early stage include full-thickness grafts on eyelids to prevent corneal exposure; operations on the oral commissure to allow oral competence, access for dental care, and adequate nutrition; and neck releases for future inductions of anesthesia, head movement, and mandibular function. The major problem with early surgical intervention is that additional procedures may be required after the scar has matured.

Even though reconstructive surgical therapy is not planned for several months, it is worthwhile for the reconstructive surgeon to be involved during the acute phase. The patient can see that something will be done, and the physician can develop a concept of what is needed and what the patient's priorities and expectations are. Together patient and surgeon can formulate a treatment plan.

General Principles
Aesthetic Units

The face is composed of regions that are seen as units (Fig. 28-1). Seams should be made to lie on the edges of these units, not course through them. Often unburned skin is sacrificed to preserve the unit during resurfacing procedures. Procedures done without attention to this concept leave aesthetically inferior patches.

Timing

Even though scar maturation has not occurred, an early start may be necessary to give the patient a psychological boost with some demonstrable progress. In the interest of time, several procedures should be done simultaneously. Procedures on noncontiguous areas of the face and on other areas of the body should be

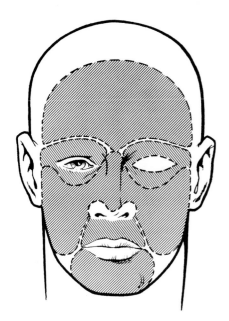

Fig. 28-1. Aesthetic units of the face. (Adapted with permission from M. Gonzalez-Ulloa. Restoration of the face covering by means of selected skin in regional aesthetic units. Br. J. Plast. Surg. 9:212, 1956, and from B.M. Achauer (Ed.). Burn Reconstruction. New York: Thieme, 1990.)

planned to minimize the number of hospitalizations and exposures to anesthesia. Scar revisions and releases should be continued until the patient realizes the diminishing returns. Many patients cannot accept that "nothing more can be done." Something more can always be done, but it may not be worth the time and trouble. Patients soon realize this without the abrupt withdrawal of support.

Priorities

Functional considerations are the first priority. After that, the overall problem must be assessed to determine the most important feature to be restored. Severely burned faces have no distinguishing features; therefore, a total nose reconstruction might be a priority to make a dramatic change and provide a face with individuality. A temporal artery island flap for mustache or eyebrow reconstruction might be a patient's priority.

Materials

For large areas, thick split-thickness skin grafts are used. Theoretically, skin as close to the face as possible should be used as a donor site because of color match. The availability of such skin is not predictable, however; donor site deformities, such as hypertrophic scarring, can render skin in the neck and upper chest unacceptable if other areas are available. Smaller areas, such as the lip, lid, or nose, may be resurfaced with full-thickness grafts. These grafts provide a superior color match, but there are a limited number of donor sites. The order of preference is postauricular, supraclavicular, inguinal, and brachial. In children, large sheets of full-thickness skin are available from the abdomen. Flaps are reserved for reconstruction of special features—nose,

eyebrows, and ears. Flaps tend to obscure facial angles and fine movements and their use is therefore controversial for cheek or neck reconstruction.

Scar Excision

Scar excision should be done when possible for facial burn scars. Large scars can be eliminated by repeated excisions. The scars must be surrounded by normal skin for this technique to be applicable. Nasolabial scars and scalp burns are especially appropriate. Successive excision was an extremely popular technique in the 1940s and 1950s and was the first line of treatment for extensive burn scars. Multiple partial excisions with either a rotation or advancement skin flap from the neck or postauricular region are simple, first-line techniques. These techniques are still useful and should not be discarded.

Tissue Expansion

Tissue expanders have added another dimension and also should be considered. Tissue expansion is an extension of the aforedescribed principles and has many applications to burn reconstruction. New normal tissue forms adjacent to the deformity, and there is no donor site. Tissue expansion is useful for scalp, cheek, and neck deformities (Fig. 28-2).

Fig. 28-2A. The tissue expander in the neck and cheek region is noted to be fully expanded intraoperatively. B. After removal of expander with excision and advancement flap.

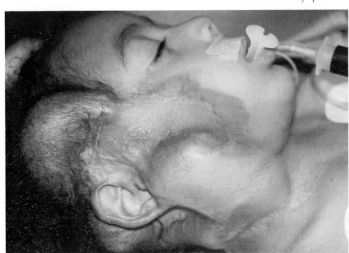

A

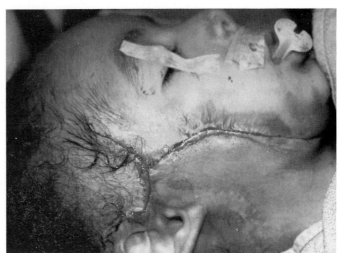

B

Burns of the Scalp

Deep burns of the scalp are more common in children than in adults—25 percent of children will have alopecia compared with only 7 percent of adults. The initial surgical treatment is split skin grafting if a suitable graft bed is available.

Classification

Minor
Burns of up to 15 percent of the scalp can be treated by early skin grafting. Reconstruction is usually done by staged excision if the defect is not too extensive in any direction.

Moderate
Defects of 15 to 40 percent of the scalp are not suitable for staged excision. Tissue expansion is ideal for these defects because of the lack of a donor defect and the advantage of replacing like tissue. Early care should be directed toward preparing for this type of reconstruction. If the skin graft can be placed expeditiously, this is the best early treatment. As soon as a wound has healed, tissue expanders can be placed beneath adjacent normal scalp. Tissue expanders can even be considered for placement at the time of injury, but insertion at this time is much more risky than insertion later.

Extensive Injuries Without Brain Involvement
Some injuries are too large or too deep to be reconstructed by tissue expansion. In these more complex injuries, early closure is crucial. Skin grafting is done if possible. Multiple scalp flaps as described by Orticochea and Jurkiewicz and Hill also should be considered. Distant flaps, especially free flaps, should be considered.

Extensive Injuries with Involvement of the Full Thickness of the Skull or Deeper
In these difficult injuries, coverage is required as a lifesaving measure. Immediate reconstruction with free tissue transfers is required; the most common tissue used is the omentum.

Treatment

Hair transplants (punch grafts) can be transferred successfully into a burn scar, but the results have not been rewarding and the method is not recommended as a primary mode of treatment. Tissue expanders are helpful in scalp defects and should be considered first (Fig. 28-3). No donor site defects occur, the procedures are not complex, and large areas can be reconstructed. It is possible with repeated expansion to use 30 to 40 percent of the scalp to cover the remaining 60 to 70 percent.

Electrical burns of the scalp are often deep and may involve one or both tables of the calvarium. Traditionally these burns have been treated by drilling bur holes in the outer table, waiting for granulation tissue to develop, and applying a skin graft to the defect. This is a slow process with questionable long-term results. Because it is nonviable bone, the outer table becomes a sequestrum and delays healing. It is more logical to remove the entire outer cortex, but the skin grafts are often unstable. Flap coverage is greatly preferred. For larger defects, free flaps are ideal. The omentum and the latissimus dorsi muscle are the most commonly used flaps.

Burns of the Forehead

It is unusual for the forehead to require flap reconstruction; usually a good quality sheet split-thickness skin graft serves well. It is quite acceptable to use a thin, patchwork graft during the acute period to obtain a sterile, closed wound. Later, the entire forehead unit can be replaced with a transversely oriented, medium thickness, split skin graft. Some surgeons prefer a mesh graft that is not expanded. Oriented transversely, the lines in the graft are said to mimic normal forehead lines.

Deeper wounds are usually caused by electrical injuries. If the periosteum is devitalized, flap coverage is required. First consideration should be given to fascial flaps. These thin, well-vascularized flaps are surfaced with a good quality split-thickness skin graft. The temporoparietal flap can be positioned to cover the forehead with the use of interpositional vein grafts. About one-third of the forehead can be covered with this flap. Other potential fascial flaps are the radial artery forearm and the scapular fascial flaps. For extensive forehead defects, the scapular flap is the right size but too thick. With subsequent thinning, however, excellent reconstruction is possible (Fig. 28-4). A final possibility is a pedicled scalp flap. A defect can be readily covered without microvascular technology. The hair-bearing upper layers can be removed later and replaced with a skin graft. Millard called this the crane principle.

Burns of the Ear

Ninety percent of patients with facial burns have burns of the ear. In addition to loss of the auricle from direct thermal injury, a suppurative chondritis occurs 2 to 3 weeks after injury in 20 to 30 percent of facially burned patients. Purdue and Hunt reported successful treatment with mafenide, local debridement, and early grafting. Grant has recommended early (24 to 48 hours postburn) excision of the burned auricular skin by dermabrasion followed by application of thin skin grafts. A fascial flap from the temporoparietal area has been described for total ear reconstruction, and its use has been reported for immediate vascularized coverage of the burned ear.

Many surgeons do not consider ear reconstruction after burn injuries to be worthwhile. Many disfiguring defects can be improved dramatically with relatively simple procedures; in severe injuries, one must consider the initial decision to undertake reconstruction. If no auricle remains and there is only burned skin in the area, reconstructive time and effort may be better used in other anatomic areas. Some patients cannot accept a prosthetic ear and insist on reconstruction. Patients must understand that many procedures may be required for reconstruction and that the result may not be as realistic as they hoped.

Classification

Mild
The helix and the upper part of the auricle are lost without extensive scarring.

Moderate
The concha is nearly normal, although it may adhere to the side of the head. The upper half of the ear is missing. The antihelix and its anterior and posterior crura are missing.

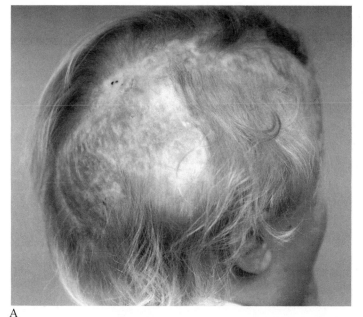

A

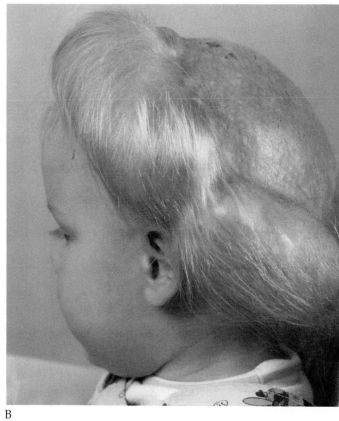

B

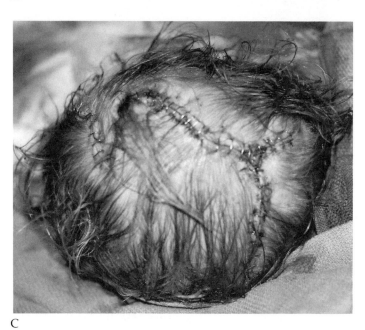

C

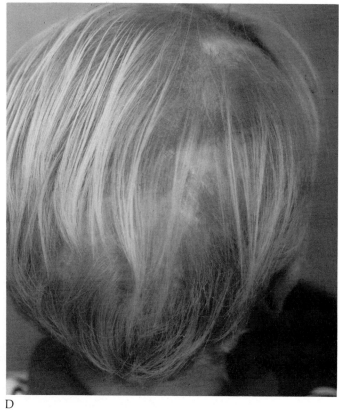

D

Fig. 28-3A. Burn alopecia. B. Two tissue expanders are in place and appropriately expanded. C. Expanders have been removed and advancement flaps accomplished. D. Postoperative result.

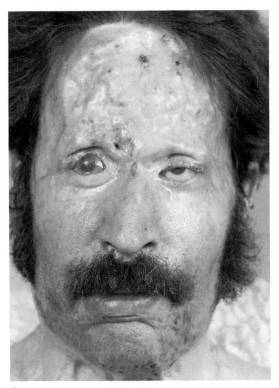

A

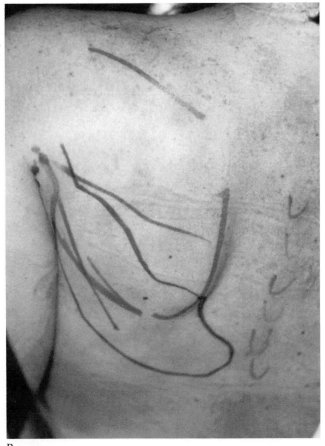

B

Fig. 28-4A. Severe forehead injury resulting from electrical burn. B. Mapping of scapular flap. C. Postoperative result. The flap has been defatted once.

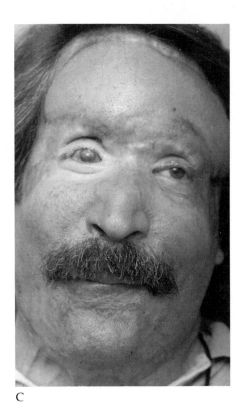

C

Severe

A remnant of concha is left; the external ear orifice is normal or stenosed, and the local soft tissues are scarred.

Treatment

There have been many advances in total ear reconstruction. Realistic ears are possible for patients with microtia. These refinements can be transferred to burn patients. Although scarred tissue in the area complicates ear reconstruction, there are several advantages in burned patients compared with patients with congenital anomalies. A concha is always available, the ear location is never in doubt, and the burns are often symmetric. Skin coverage is a greater problem in burned patients and must be addressed before cartilage grafts are inserted. Polymeric silicone frameworks do not have a place in reconstruction of a burned ear. (There is a 70% rate of silicone framework exposure in burned patients.) The temporoparietal flap mentioned earlier can be used for a vascularized cover.

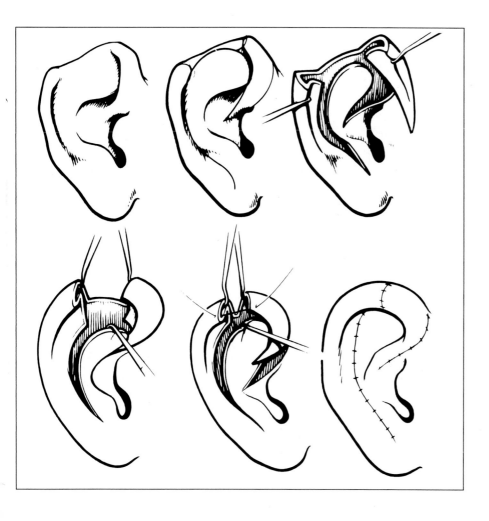

Fig. 28-5. Antia procedure. (Redrawn with permission from N.H. Antia and V.I. Buch. Chondrocutaneous advancement flap for the marginal defect of the ear. Plast. Reconstr. Surg. 39:472, 1967, and from B.M. Achauer (Ed.). Burn Reconstruction. New York: Thieme, 1990.)

Helical defects can be classified as either partial or complete. Partial defects can be corrected by the use of remaining ear tissue. An example is the Antia flap (Fig. 28-5), which produces a well-shaped but smaller ear (Fig. 28-6). Alternatively, the conchal cutaneous flap described by Davis is useful for defects of the upper third of the ear (Fig. 28-7). If the entire helix is missing, a tubed skin flap may be required (Fig. 28-8). Such a flap can be made from pre- or postauricular skin if that skin is unburned.

The classic method of cervical or supraclavicular tubed skin flaps are still useful for an extensively burned ear. In other types of ear deformities, the donor-site scar from skin tubes is too great, but in a severely burned patient a few more scars are not important, whereas a restored structure is precious. The fascial flap should be mentioned again; Dufourmentel recommended it for helical rim reconstruction by forming a roll and covering it with a skin graft.

Fig. 28-6A. Burn injury involving entire helical rim. B. Postoperative view following a combination of the Antia procedure and reconstruction with postauricular flaps.

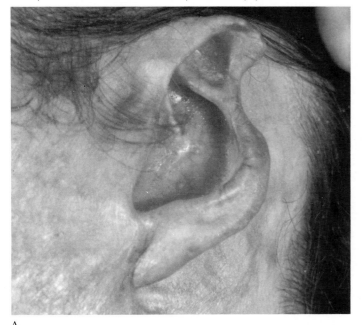
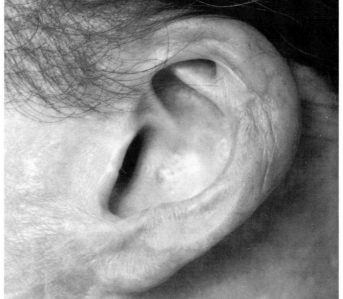

A   B

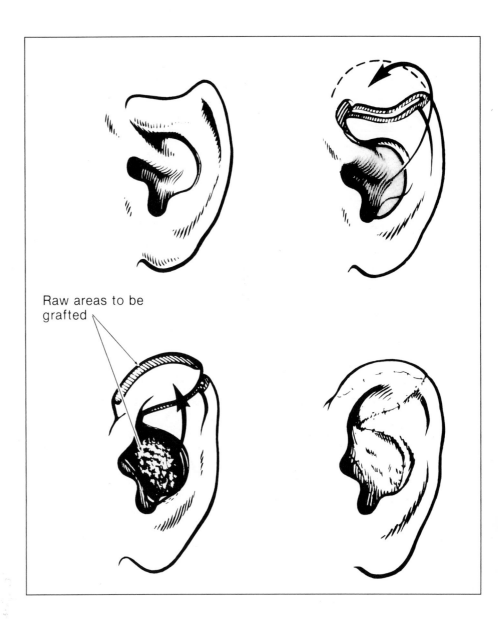

Raw areas to be grafted

Fig. 28-7. Conchal transposition flap. (Redrawn with permission from M.B. Donelan. Conchal transposition flap for postburn ear deformities. Plast. Reconstr. Surg. 83:641, 1989, and from B.M. Achauer (Ed.). Burn Reconstruction. New York: Thieme, 1990.)

Cartilage grafts are needed for many subtotal reconstructions. The ipsilateral concha should be considered first. Many burned patients have bilateral deformities, so contralateral cartilage may not be available. If conchal cartilage is not available, costal cartilage can be used.

Earlobe deformities are common in burn injuries and are rewarding to reconstruct. Most often the earlobes have adhered to the adjacent neck skin. Simple division with careful closure with a Z-plasty or local flap is all that is needed. Several local flaps have been described for earlobe reconstruction in absent earlobes.

The external auditory meatus may become stenotic because of scar contracture. If the stenosis is diagnosed early, a splint

may be manufactured to control the scar contracture and forestall surgical correction. If surgical release is required, local flaps should be considered. Usually skin grafts are required. After the grafts take, the patient must wear a conformer in the canal for several months to prevent a recurrence. If flaps can be interdigitated among the grafts, recurring stenosis may be prevented.

Burns of the Eyebrows

Eyebrows are frequently destroyed in facial burn injuries. Reconstruction is virtually always possible but is not necessarily desirable. For women, "reconstruction" may be done with an eyebrow

pencil. In some patients with partial eyebrow loss, reconstruction may call more attention to the scarring than the original defect might have. However, for severely burned patients who have few features to give visual relief from a sea of scar, dramatic eyebrows are a great asset.

The simplest method of eyebrow reconstruction involves a composite free graft from the scalp. A single strip the approximate size of the remaining eyebrow is used. Mustardé suggested narrow strips with a later excision of the intervening scar. Brent added the concept of medial accentuation by using a short strip to mimic the normal medial curve. Cronin advocated punch grafts for fill-in defects. When cutting the scalp, one must take

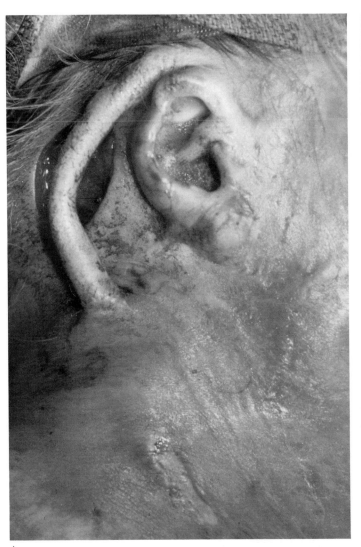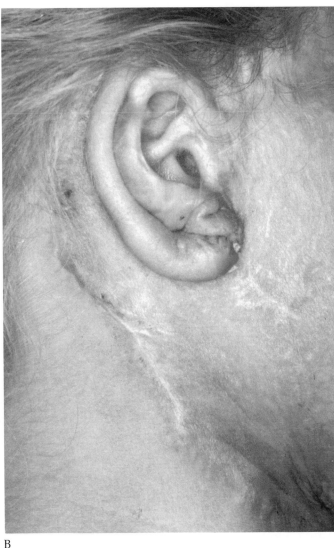

A   B

Fig. 28-8A. Near-total loss of ear. Staged reconstruction with tubed pedicle flap. B. Postoperative result.

care to make the incisions parallel to hair follicles to avoid damaging the roots. Temporal or occipital sites are preferred to mimic normal hair direction. Graft take can be unpredictable because the graft area is placed in a scar. If the free grafting technique has failed, or a prominent eyebrow is desired, the island flap technique is indicated.

An island of hair-bearing scalp is located over a branch of the superficial temporal artery of sufficient length to reach the eyebrow area. A Doppler flow probe is used to trace the vessel and aid in dissection during the operation. A commodious tunnel should be made to avoid kinking. Hair often falls out postoperatively and returns in 2 to 3 months. This

is a reliable technique with rewarding results if done in properly selected patients. Pensler found the complication rate with island flaps much greater than with composite grafts. The island flap is reserved for male patients with unilateral alopecia and heavy hair density in the remaining eyebrow.

Burns of the Eyelid

Initially great care must be taken in treating eyelid burns to avoid corneal damage and to preserve eyelid motion and integrity. Immediate care involves copious irrigation and ophthalmologic consultation. Within a few hours, edema of the

lids prevents easy inspection and access. After the edema recedes, exposure can be a problem, especially if a Bell phenomenon is lacking. During this period ophthalmic ointments (antibiotics and methyl cellulose) should be applied copiously. In severe burns, a scleral lens is required until grafts are applied. Tarsorrhaphies have been greatly overused. They are almost never required, are frequently ineffective, and greatly distort lid anatomy. In addition, an adequate release and skin grafting are made more difficult because the recommended overcorrection is much more difficult. As soon as a full-thickness burn of an eyelid is diagnosed and necrotic material is debrided, definitive repair should be done. Full-thickness grafts from the retroauricular or supraclavicular area are preferred. If full-thickness grafts are not available, thick split grafts are used. Preputial skin has been used, but objectionable pigmentation has been seen; therefore, it should be used only when other tissue is not available.

Eyelid burns (partial and full thickness) often require careful pressure therapy for several months. Custom-fabricated splints are made to be inserted inside the patient's face mask. A great deal of patience and expertise on the part of the therapist are required, as is a great deal of cooperation by the patient. With persistence, most late ectropions can be avoided.

Late ectropion may occur even in ideal circumstances. Ectropion repair has been a common reconstructive procedure; in fact, the first use of full-thickness skin grafts was for repair of eyelid burn ectropion. In the presence of an adequate Bell phenomenon, it may be acceptable to await scar maturation for definitive correction. Lubrication may be required at night during this period. It should also be understood that the tears of a burned patient may lack lipid material because the meibomian glands have been destroyed. Tears evaporate more rapidly, therefore producing a dry eye and conjunctivitis. Additionally, the lacrimal apparatus may be disturbed by blockage of the ducts or pulling away of the punctum from the globe. Lower lid ectropion is much more common than upper lid ectropion.

There are several important technical details in correcting eyelid ectropion. If a complete release and overcorrection are not done initially, a reoperation may be required. Only upper or lower lids on each side should be done at the same time. If both upper and lower lids on the same side are released at the same time, overcorrection is much more difficult. The release should be carried beyond the medial and lateral canthal areas to ensure a complete release. It has been stated that portions of the levator muscle frequently must be incised transversely if these areas inhibit full mobilization of the lid. The muscle regains full attachment through the scar bed under the graft. Adequate immobilization of the lid and graft is obtained with a tie-over dressing.

In severe, acute burns with loss of all the lash-bearing lid margins, the "masquer-ade" procedure may be indicated. In this procedure, the conjunctival margins are sutured together and a single graft is placed over both upper and lower lids. Several weeks later, the lids are separated.

Burns of the Nose

Almost all facial burns involve the nose because of its central location and projection. For a severely burned patient, successful nasal reconstruction is crucial for restoring self-esteem. Most problems are not complex and may be handled by routine plastic surgical techniques.

Classification

Burn Scar Deformity Without Major Tissue Loss
These problems are the most frequently encountered. The deformities consist of hypertrophic scars, scar bands, discoloration, hyper- and hypopigmentation, and asymmetry. The major corrections required are scar revision and resurfacing skin grafts. Aesthetic units are the major reconstructive guidelines.

Nasal Ectropion
Nasal ectropion is the classic nasal burn deformity resulting from a loss of alar rim substance. As the scar heals and matures, a scar contracture pulls the tip of the nose up, everting the nostrils. The lower lateral cartilages rotate externally. Local flap reconstruction and skin grafts are used for correction.

Subtotal Tissue Loss
In a subtotal nose deformity, more than the tip is involved but not the entire nose. More tissue is imported and flaps are usually required, but total reconstruction is not required. Local scar flaps are useful in this situation.

Extensive Tissue Loss
In a number of instances virtually all the soft tissue of the nose is destroyed or deformed. In these patients a total nose reconstruction is the best choice. Because the borderline between "subtotal" and "extensive" is not well defined, each reconstructive surgeon has to make his or her own determination. A more precise way to make this judgment is needed.

Nostril Stenosis
This unusual deformity is quite distinct from all others. If there is minimal tissue loss and scar contracture, the nostrils can close almost totally.

Treatment
Scar deformities are the most common problem and also the most straightforward to correct. Linear scars may be excised or reoriented with Z-plasties, W-plasties, and local flaps. Larger deformities are treated by total or, occasionally, partial resurfacing of the nose with a full-thickness skin graft. Supraclavicular or postauricular donor sites are selected if possible for the best color match. Aesthetic units are used. Resurfacing the nose is a worthwhile procedure that uniformly produces satisfying results. The procedures presented by Brown and McDowell more than 30 years ago are as applicable today as they were then.

The alae are contracted or missing to some extent in almost all nasal burns. The deformity ranges from barely noticeable to totally missing alae. Individual strategies are required for each patient. Not only is rim substance lost, but the force of the contracting scar pulls the end of the nose up, causing the nostrils to become everted. The lower lateral cartilages rotate externally and turn outward with exposure of the vestibular lining. The nasal covering is thin, shiny, and irregular; the scar epithelium is frequently unstable and easily traumatized. The term used to describe this deformity is *nasal ectropion*. Procedures to correct these problems include composite grafts from the ear and local flaps with or without skin grafts. Most problems can be improved sufficiently with these techniques. The columella usually is involved also and is too prominent. Often the columella can be deemphasized by shortening the caudal septum. Composite grafts may be used to form a columella if necessary. If the alae and columella are severely distorted, flap reconstruction of the entire nasal surface should be considered.

In severe injuries, particularly when a number of facial features have lost all individuality because of extensive scarring, flap reconstruction of the entire nasal surface is often the cornerstone of facial reconstruction and, eventually, of the patient's successful rehabilitation. It is best

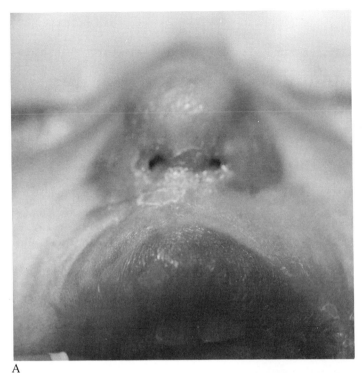

A

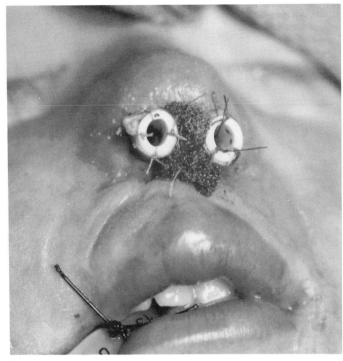

B

to anticipate this eventuality during the acute phase of the burn injury and save an appropriate donor site for this critical reconstruction. These situations are most often encountered in severely burned patients, and traditional sites for nasal reconstruction (forehead, deltopectoral area) may be unavailable. Several delay procedures may be necessary because random pattern flaps are required. Creativity may be necessary in immobilizing the patient during the transfer. Free flap techniques also should be considered. With the patient in unconventional positions, early division of the flap is desirable. Quantitative fluorescin injection studies with the base of the flap clamped indicate the earliest safe time to divide the flap.

The typical burn deformity results in enlarged nostrils; however, nostril stenosis develops in some patients. This is an unusual and most disturbing situation for the patient and one that is difficult to correct. The patient needs to be fully committed to a successful outcome because splints must be worn in the nostrils for at least 6 months postoperatively (Fig. 28-9).

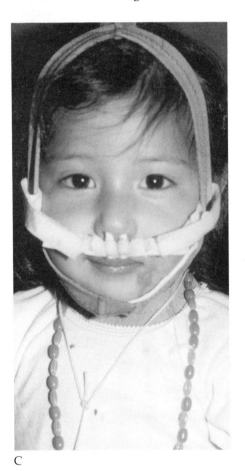

C

Fig. 28-9A. Severe stenosis of the nostrils. B. Skin grafts are sutured around splints, which are sutured into place. C. Headgear must be worn continuously for several months. D. Long-term postoperative result.

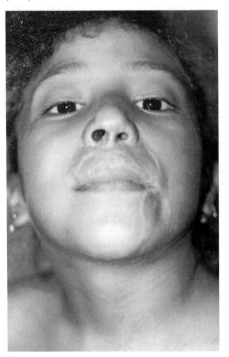

D

Burns of the Mouth

Classification

Minor
Less than one-third of the upper or lower lip or of the commissure or less than one-sixth of both lips with the commissure is injured.

Major
More than one-third of the upper or lower lip or of the commissure or more than one-sixth of each lip with the commissure is injured.

Severe
The same dimensions as for moderate burns are injured, considerable epithelium and muscle are lost, and the buccal sulcus is involved.

Electrical Burns

Oral burns are common injuries in toddlers (74% of patients are between 6 and 36 months of age). Curious children of this age place everything they encounter into their mouths. Unfortunately, this includes extension cords (usually empty receptacles of multiple-plug extension cords or the live ends of unused cords). Saliva completes the electrical circuit and an electric arc forms. The resulting burn usually results from the intense heat produced (3000°C). Involvement of an oral commissure is most common and produces the most noticeable deformity.

Most authors recommend allowing the wound to heal and the scar to mature, correcting the deformity several months after the burn. Even proponents of early surgical intervention state that the type of primary care is not an important influence on the necessity for additional surgical treatment. Ortiz-Monasterio performs a repair 2 weeks after the injury in moderate and severe deformities.

Burn scar contracture has been shown to be influenced by splinting if the splinting is done promptly and adequately. This concept was applied to burns of the oral commissure by Colcleugh and Ryan. An orthodontic appliance was made for each patient with prongs extending beyond each oral commissure. The appliance could be removed for eating and cleaning. This type of treatment should be attempted when possible. It is also useful in postsurgical reconstruction to prevent recurrence of contractures.

Microstomia

Severe facial burns are prone to produce microstomia. This can be a disabling condition that interferes with eating, oral hygiene, and the administration of general anesthesia. Surgical release is often necessary early in the postburn period because of these functional problems. Early splinting has been advocated by Hartford. A device is commercially available in adult and pediatric sizes and can be adjusted for each patient and as the treatment progresses. It should be applied as early as possible (the second or third week postburn) but can also help reverse contractures that are several weeks old.

Burns of the Lip

Upper Lip

Most scar contractures of the upper lip can be resolved with standard pressure therapy. If releases are required, full-thickness grafts are preferred, but they are not as crucial as they are for burns of the lower lip, in which recurrence of contracture is more common. If the central upper lip anatomy has been lost, it can be restored by a composite graft from the ear (Fig. 28-10). Some patients prefer to wear a mustache. In this case, an island flap based on the superficial temporal artery and vein works well.

Lower Lip

Applying skin grafts to the lips is technically difficult. It is virtually impossible to immobilize the lips or eliminate contamination with saliva and food. Feeding through a small, soft nasogastric tube is recommended for 5 to 7 days postoperatively. A foam rubber sponge is sutured over the graft to provide pressure and immobilization. For reconstructive procedures, full-thickness grafts are much preferred. It is important to follow aesthetic units in this area. After good quality skin coverage has been obtained and the vermilion margin is in a normal position, attention is directed to forming a good lip-chin sulcus and thinning the lower lip. Direct excision of orbicularis and scar tissue is effective in thinning the lower lip. A chin implant is helpful in obtaining a satisfactory relation between lip and chin.

Burns of the Neck

Great progress has been made in the prevention of neck contractures. Before current methods of splinting were developed, most patients with full-thickness burns of the neck had contractures. Bunchman found that 84 percent of patients with full-thickness burns treated before 1968 had neck contractures, whereas only 51 percent of patients treated after 1968 had them. The severity of contractures seen also was reduced in the latter series. The change in treatment is the use of a full-contact orthoplast neck conformer early in the treatment (as soon as edema subsides). Cronin described a similar pressure treatment for grafts applied after release of neck contractures. A number of measures can be instituted to keep the neck extended until splints can be applied. A short mattress can be used so the patient can extend his or her head over the edge of the bed. Early grafting and the use of a thick sheet graft are helpful in preventing contractures. As soon as wound healing has occurred, a splint or pressure garment must be worn 24 hours a day for at least 6 months. Close follow-up care with required adjustments and continued therapy also are essential.

Classification

Despite the most conscientious care, neck contractures still develop. Neck contractures are classified as follows.

Mild
The scar band involves less than one-third of the anterior surface of the neck. This type of burn usually can be treated surgically by local flaps or Z-plasties. If the contracture involves more than 20 percent of the anterior surface of the neck, tissue expanders might produce a more aesthetically pleasing result and should be considered.

Moderate
More than one-third but less than two-thirds of the anterior surface of the neck is involved in the burn. Local flaps are generally inadequate. Tissue expansion should be the first consideration, followed by skin grafts and distant flaps. A combination of local flaps and split-thickness skin grafts often works well.

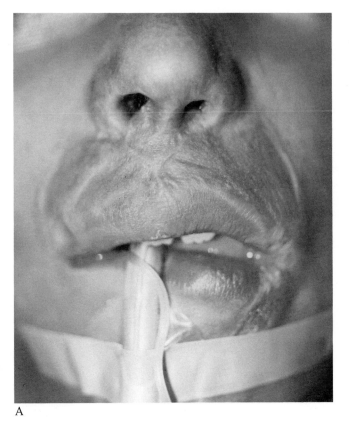

A

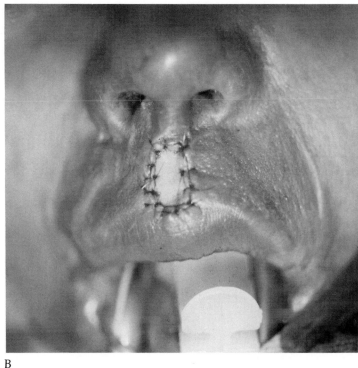

B

Fig. 28-10A. Preoperative view showing absence of filtrum. B. Immediately postoperatively, graft is shown sutured into place. C. Final result.

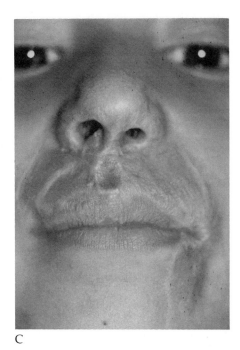

C

Severe

More than two-thirds of the anterior surface of the neck is involved in the burn. Local flaps are not adequate; tissue must be imported in the form of a skin graft or flap.

Extensive (Mentosternal Adhesion)

This extreme deformity is usually seen in neglected burns, particularly when appropriate medical care is unavailable. The defect left by surgical release is extensive. A skin graft is usually required.

Treatment

Any skin grafting to the neck requires a full-contact splint for several months to prevent a recurrence. An orthopedic four-poster neck brace has proved useful for the immediately postoperative period until graft take occurs.

Administering anesthesia to patients with severe neck contractures is probably the most hazardous procedure in reconstructive burn surgery. Intubation ranges from difficult to impossible. Mask ventilation also may be compromised. The surgeon should be prepared to do an immediate scar release to allow intubation. If the scar transection fails to allow intubation, a tracheostomy may be necessary. Intubation over a flexible bronchoscope can prevent most of these difficult situations.

If scar bands involve only a portion of the neck surface, local flaps and Z-plasties should be sufficient. When most of the neck is involved, a skin graft is required. The standard procedure is to transect the scar bands (dissection usually involves the platysma muscle and superficial cervical fascia) until a complete relaxation of the neck is obtained. The resulting defect is covered precisely with a medium-to-thick sheet of skin graft secured with a tie-over dressing. The neck needs to be immobilized for 5 days to allow for graft take.

Neck contractures have been corrected with flaps for many years. Although some spectacular results have been reported, the result is often disappointing because the flap obscures the normal neck angles. These procedures also involve

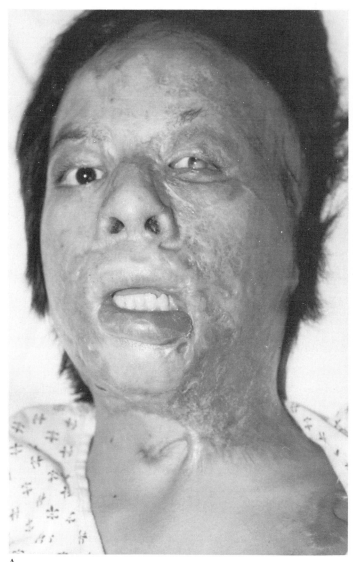

A

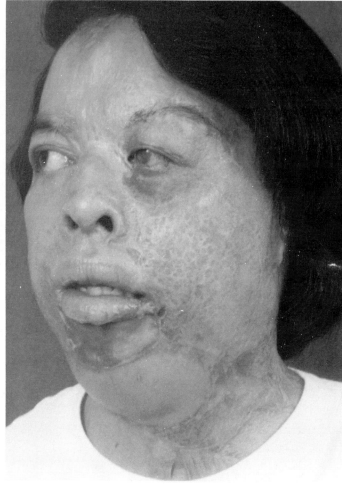

B

Fig. 28-11A. Severe neck contracture. B. After scapular flap reconstruction and after several defatting procedures.

several operations, large donor defects, and skin that is often not available in severely burned patients. The scapula free flap can be used (Fig. 28-11), but it usually requires several defatting procedures.

Suggested Reading

Achauer, B.M. *Burn Reconstruction.* New York: Thieme, 1990.

Achauer, B.M., Salibian, A.H., and Furnas, D.W. Free flaps to the head and neck. *Head Neck Surg.* 4:315, 1982.

Brent, B. Earlobe construction with auriculo-mastoid flap. *Plast. Reconstr. Surg.* 57:389, 1976.

Brent, B. The correction of microtia with au-togenous cartilage grafts. I. The classic deformity. *Plast. Reconstr. Surg.* 66:1, 1980.

Falvey, M.P., and Brody, G.S. Secondary correction of the burned eyelid deformity. *Plast. Reconstr. Surg.* 63:564, 1979.

Furnas, D.W., Achauer, B.M., and Bartlett, R.H. Reconstruction of the burned nose. *J. Trauma* 20:25, 1980.

Furnas, D.W., et al. A pair of five-day flaps: Early division of pedicles after serial cross-clamping and observation with oximetry and fluorometry. *Ann. Plast. Surg.* 15:262, 1985.

Gonzalez-Ulloa, M. Restoration of the face covering by means of selected skin in regional aesthetic units. *Br. J. Plast. Surg.* 9:212, 1956.

Gottlieb, L.J., Parsons, R.W., and Krizek, T.J. The use of tissue expansion techniques in burn reconstruction. *J. Burn Care Rehabil.* 7:234, 1986.

Grant, D.A. Minimizing Deformities in the Burned Ear. In J.B. Lynch and S.R. Lewis (Eds.), *Symposium of the Treatment of Burns,* Vol. 5. St. Louis: Mosby, 1973.

Hoopes, J.E. Multiple Excision of the Face. In I. Feller and W.C. Grabb (Eds.), *Reconstruction and Rehabilitation of the Burned Patient.* Ann Arbor, Mich.: National Institute for Burn Medicine, 1979.

Orticochea, M. New three-flap scalp reconstruction technique. *Br. J. Plast. Surg.* 24:184, 1971.

Purdue, G.F., and Hunt, J.L. Chondritis of the burned ear: A preventable complication. *Am. J. Surg.* 152:257, 1986.

Salisbury, R.E., and Bevin, A.G. The Eyebrow: Total and Partial Loss. In R.E. Salisbury and A.G. Bevin (Eds.), *Atlas of Reconstructive Burn Surgery.* Philadelphia: Saunders, 1980.

29

Reconstruction of Burn Deformities of the Extremities and Trunk

Warren L. Garner   David J. Smith, Jr.

Reconstructive strategies for thermally injured patients should not be postponed until the late phases of recovery, but should begin at the moment of initial treatment. Optimal recovery and the best possible functional and aesthetic results are most likely to be achieved when the reconstructive potential of each injury is considered with the initiation of treatment.

The initial treatment of the burn injury can improve the final result of the reconstruction in several ways:

1. Appropriate fluid resuscitation and invasive monitoring maximize tissue perfusion and result in increased tissue survival. Thus the area of tissue damage is decreased as is the subsequent area of reconstruction.
2. Early excision and grafting aid the reconstructive process by closing wounds earlier and decreasing the amount of hypertrophic scarring.
3. Healed wounds are less painful, and patients are more likely to participate actively in physical therapy.
4. Active participation of a burn team early in the recovery process has been shown clearly to maximize the rehabilitation of burned patients physically, psychologically, and socially.

The goals of any burn reconstruction are first to restore function, and second to restore appearance. After initial wound closure, we usually intervene surgically when the patient's progress has plateaued, before the anticipated level of recovery is achieved. Because most problems after a burn injury are the result of limitation of motion, we emphasize mobilization therapy with active and passive range-of-motion exercises, dynamic splinting, continuous passive motion, and nighttime static splints to achieve and maintain the best results. This type of program gives patients the opportunity to participate actively in the therapy and thus increases motivation to recover.

Limitation of motion is the result of two processes—hypertrophic scarring (HTS) with contraction and joint contracture. The causes of HTS remain unknown. It is likely, however, that scar development is related to the cell stimulation that results from the body's response to traumatic injury. The inflammatory process leads to the release of polypeptide growth factors at the site of the injury. These factors, as a group, lead to collagen and matrix protein deposition in the areas of injury and inflammation. When the injury is extensive or chronic, there is a greater degree of inflammation. The resulting increase in cytokine release may induce an intense and ongoing cellular response, resulting in a hypertrophic scar. The local fibroblast response to the massive cytokine release may be a long-standing up-regulation of collagen synthesis, clinically seen as fibrosis. An alternative hypothesis is that the early fibrotic response that develops after the initial cytokine response establishes a local wound environment devoid of oxygen. The wound environment exerts selective pressure for cells that tolerate hypoxia. Hypoxia and its sequela, lactic acidosis, are inducers of collagen synthesis, leading to perpetuation of the fibrotic process.

As wounds remodel during the later phases of healing, the additional problem of wound contraction develops. The activity of fibroblasts during this period causes the reorganization and contraction of collagen fibers, as demonstrated by Ehrlich. This process continues until an opposing force is encountered, when the contracted, redundant collagen is degraded. Practically, this process leads to

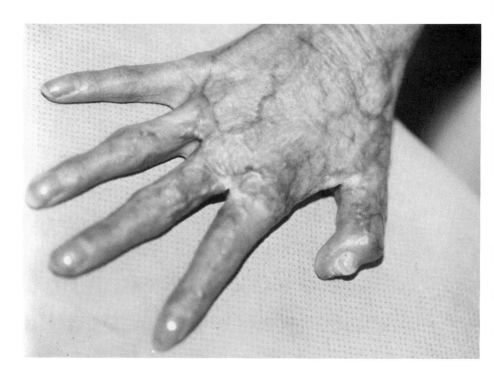

Fig. 29-1. A severe burn injury 6 months after coverage. The thumb–index finger web space has contracted, resulting in a flattened hand with decreased opposition. This patient did not participate in therapy with pressure garments or web spacers or in physical therapy.

the contraction of tissue until the limits of motion are reached. For example, the thumb and index finger contract together until the first web space is lost (Fig. 29-1), the arm contracts against the chest wall, and the axillary skin fold disappears. Active and passive motion, splinting, and external pressure are used during the remodeling phase of wound healing to help resist the contractile forces and maintain tissue length.

When tissues around a joint contract, inflammation of the overlying skin and subcutaneous tissue causes a generalized remodeling response. The ligamentous structures of the joint are included in the remodeling process. When the surrounding skin limits joint motion, the joint structures remodel and contract to the limits of motion. This phenomenon can cause ligaments and joint structures to shorten permanently. Splinting, again, is essential during this period to maintain capsule and ligament length.

Principles of Reconstruction

Hypertrophic scar, scar contraction, and established scar contracture are important problems in postburn reconstruction. The

unifying circumstance in all these problems is a lack of normal tissue. Wound contracture during scar remodeling effectively removes tissue from the site of injury, producing a functional tissue deficit that limits mobility and distorts the remaining tissues. Correction of this problem requires the transfer of additional normal tissue into the region. The transfer can be achieved by skin grafting, flap transfer, or Z-plasty. Each technique has advantages in specific situations, and the choice must be individualized.

In general, we perform most reconstructions using flaps or Z-plasties. These techniques add healthy tissue to the deficient areas, interpose normal tissue between regions of scar, and allow early mobilization of the parts operated on. Most problems with the distal extremities can be solved by Z-plasty. Problems at the elbow or knee are treated with either Z-plasties or flaps, depending on the size of the defect and the quality of the surrounding tissue. Axillary contractures usually require the addition of tissue provided by flap transfer. We reserve skin grafting for unusual circumstances—when Z-plasties are not possible, when local flaps are not available, and when the defect is small enough that it does not require coverage with a free flap. Although skin grafting is the simplest method of

adding tissue, there are several disadvantages: (1) Skin grafts require stabilization during the initial healing period, preventing immediate active mobilization and necessitating continued splinting; (2) grafts always contract, a process contrary to the desired result of release and lengthening; and (3) in addition, reharvesting donor sites can increase the risk of additional HTS. For these reasons, we seldom use skin grafts for reconstruction of contractions and contractures.

Aesthetic considerations become important when functional problems have been solved. The best reconstruction involves initiating treatment of the burn injury with the final aesthetic result in mind. General considerations include the use of sheet, rather than meshed, grafts at the time of initial wound closure. Different locations have a tendency toward better or worse cosmetic results. Knowing the differences can influence the choices for wound closure. For example, because grafts on the palmar surface of the hand always become hyperpigmented, and this area usually heals without clinically significant contraction, we seldom graft palmar burns. Burns of the dorsal hand usually heal with less hypertrophy and a better color match; because the dorsum of the hand is frequently an area of deep burns, early skin grafting is an excellent solution. All treatments of the anterior chest tend to hypertrophy, making successful reconstruction difficult. The reasons for these differences are unknown, but they may be related to a combination of factors, such as skin tension, motion, and regional vascularity.

Complete control of the hypertrophic scar remains beyond the means of the reconstructive surgeon. It is possible, however, to decrease HTS by several techniques. Wounds covered within 3 weeks of an injury are much less likely to hypertrophy. This supports the concept of early excision and grafting. After the burns have healed, wounds either developing or at high risk for the formation of a hypertrophic scar should be treated by pressure garments. Application of 30 mmHg of pressure through tight-fitting garments appears both to limit the degree of hypertrophy and to decrease the time to scar resolution. Other modes also have been reported to be successful. Ahn reported the use of silicone gel to decrease the development of HTS. We have found silicone gel extremely useful in the treatment of localized areas of HTS.

Z-Plasty

Z-plasty and its variations are an important tool in postburn reconstruction. The technique uses paired transposition flaps to lengthen linear scars and to reorient the contractile forces, which helps prevent recurrent contractures. A Z-plasty also can be used to interpose normal skin between sections of scar, improving the biomechanical performance of the region. Construction of the standard single Z-plasty requires placement of extensions at 60° from the scar. The skin and subcutaneous tissue are elevated as flaps and rotated into place. Theoretically, when the limbs are equal in length to the scar and the angle between them is 60°, the gain in tissue length is about 75 percent. However, the exact increase in length of any particular scar is difficult to predict because scars are three-dimensional not two-dimensional, and both scarred tissue and normal adjacent tissue contract and expand unpredictably. When the Z-plasty is constructed at the edge of a region of HTS, the normal skin flap advances easily

into place, whereas the hypertrophic limb advances little. For this reason, we incise one limb first, verifying the axis of rotation and the length of release into which the second limb is inset. Sometimes dense scar rotates little, and a single flap is rotated within the incised scar, producing what is functionally a half Z.

Several common variations of the Z-plasty should be reviewed. The four-flap Z-plasty achieves maximal gain in length when there is normal tissue on either side of a scar band. Double opposing Z-plasties usually use smaller limbs to achieve lengthening and are most useful when longer limbs are anatomically impossible. A modification we use frequently in our clinical practice for the release of thumb–index finger web space contractures is the five-flap ''jumping-man'' technique. This technique uses opposing Z-plasties and a central advancement flap.

Specific Injuries
The Hand

Early wound closure is the best method for preventing contractures of the hand and to maintain function. After successful

grafting, both pain and edema are reduced, improving the ability of the patient to participate in active hand therapy. When the patient is not using the injured hand, splints are extremely helpful in preventing contractures. We use the position of advantage applied to the burned hand by Krizek and associates (Fig. 29-2). This position maintains maximal collateral ligament length by placing the hand in metacarpophalangeal (MP) flexion and interphalangeal (IP) joint extension. We usually splint the hand to maintain this position using low-temperature thermoplastic splinting material. In some injuries, particularly in deep or recently grafted burns, we use longitudinal Kirschner wires to maintain position (Fig. 29-3). The thumb is placed in radiopalmar abduction to prevent contraction of the thumb–index finger web space. After the grafts have taken, pressure garments are usually used to limit the development of HTS. Custom-fabricated silicone elastomer inserts also can be used to apply pressure directly to the interdigital web spaces to prevent the development of postburn syndactyly (Fig. 29-4).

Fig. 29-2. Low-temperature thermoplastic screening material can be molded to form individualized splints. These splints are used to maintain position when the part is not in use or at night.

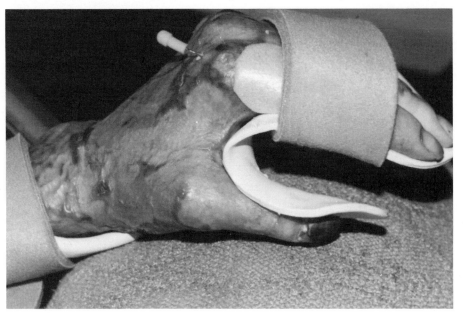

Fig. 29-3. This patient underwent excision of deep wounds of the dorsum of the hand. The digits were stabilized by Kirschner wires and grafts.

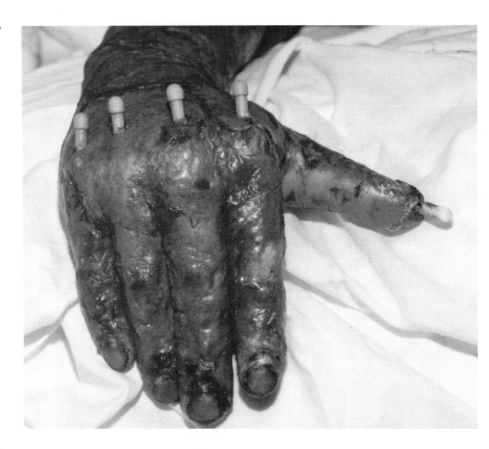

Fig. 29-4. Dorsal webbing at interphalangeal spaces often can be treated with elastomer inserts. These are held in place by a pressure garment and need adjustment as the scar tissue matures.

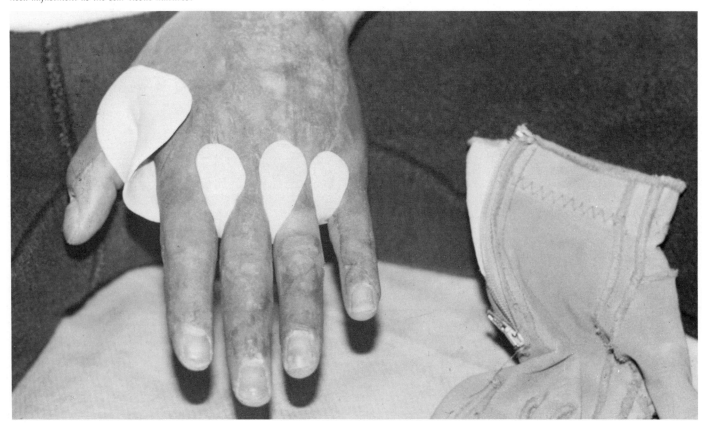

Fig. 29-5A. Dorsal web contractures often occur at the junction between the dorsal skin graft and the skin of the unburned web space. These contractures can be treated by a variety of Z-plasties. A five-flap "jumping man" is drawn on the thumb–index finger web. A five-flap V-M is drawn on the index finger–long finger contracture band. B. Released web space contracture showing healed Z-plasty. C. Resolved interphalangeal web space contracture.

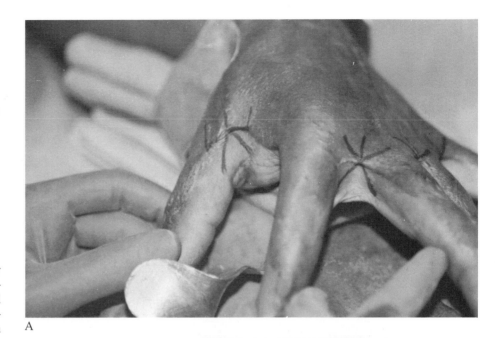

A

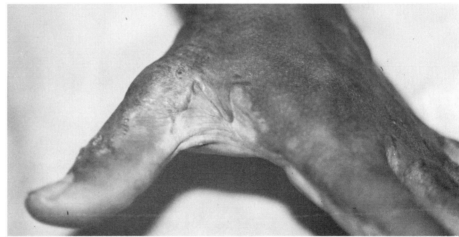

B

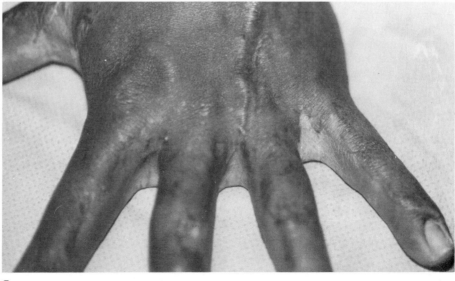

C

Despite these measures, burn syndactyly occurs in some patients. Surgical intervention is necessary to correct established contractures. All three methods of reconstruction—Z-plasty, local flaps, and skin grafting—can be used. We most often use double Z-plasties to correct interphalangeal contractions. The five-flap jumping-man repair is used for thumb–index finger contractures (Fig. 29-5). Severe syndactyly may require flap repair with or without additional skin grafting. The amount of tissue needed to reconstruct the thumb–index finger web space can be substantial. Local flaps may not provide adequate tissue for this purpose, necessitating skin grafting.

Nail-bed contractures may result from the contraction of the dorsal skin of the distal phalanx. The resulting lack of tissue distorts the eponychial fold and causes abnormal nail growth. This process is best controlled by prevention, which can be achieved with early excision and grafting using unmeshed thick partial-thickness or full-thickness grafts as suggested by Heimbach. When the problem is established, proximally based lateral digital flaps as recommended by Achauer provide an easy and effective treatment (Fig. 29-6).

Patients with severe burns of the digits, or who lose grafts to infection, are at risk for loss of extensor tendons with secondary joint exposure and infections. Percutaneous Kirschner wire pinning of the IP joints in extension and the MP joints in flexion stabilizes the joints. Fingers with this degree of injury can be stabilized and skin grafted; however, there is usually so much scarring that the functional result is poor.

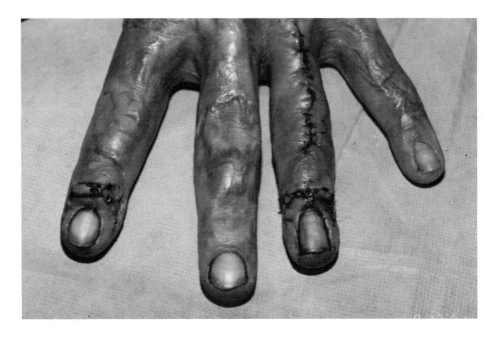

Fig. 29-6. Early postoperative result after nail-fold release with proximally based lateral digital flaps to the index and ring fingers. Excision and closure of a dorsal band on the ring finger also was performed.

Some patients sustain deep third-degree burns of their hands, exposing the deeper structures. Electrical burns are particularly likely to cause these injuries. For these burns, transfer of vascularized tissue is necessary. We have used a variety of flaps to achieve wound closure. Donor site availability is often the single most important determinant of flap choice. We have used groin flaps, chest and abdominal wall flaps, and free radial forearm flaps for this purpose (Fig. 29-7). Other options include a lateral arm flap or a temporoparietal fascial flap. Free flaps are technically more demanding, but they provide thin, pliable skin to the reconstructed hand and allow earlier mobilization than do pedicled flaps.

The Wrist and Elbow

Skin contractures in the upper extremity occur when a single linear band of scar forms that limits excursion of the adjacent joints. Flexion contractures across the wrist and elbow are the most common; they occur because flexion is stronger than extension across these joints. The Z-plasty techniques are useful in treating these problems both to alter the shape of the scar and to increase its length. For a relatively long contracture, a series of Z's

is usually the most successful in restoring length and limiting flap tip necrosis.

The Axilla

Axillary contractures are usually associated with burns of the trunk and the upper extremity. When the burn involves only one of these areas, contraction pulls normal tissue from the unburned region into the axilla. Scar contracture and tissue remodeling can remove the skin of the axillary fold, resulting in a general lack of tissue, rather than a linear band of scar. For this reason, transposition flaps are used in this area more often than in contractions of the arm and hand. When linear bands exist, however, Z-plasties retain their effectiveness. The hair-bearing skin of the central axilla is usually spared from burn injury. This tissue should not be transposed to other locations, however, because the hair and the apocrine glands are likely to cause considerable residual problems. Local rhombic and other random flaps from the chest skin can be used to release lesser contractures as long as they are designed on unburned skin. Fasciocutaneous flaps, on the other hand, can be designed on burned skin. Local fasciocutaneous flaps on the upper arm can be based on perforators from the brachial or collateral arteries and rotated to

release contractures of both the anterior and the posterior axillary areas (Fig. 29-8). Parascapular flaps also can be used for axillary coverage.

The Trunk

Few postburn functional problems require reconstruction in the chest, abdomen, or back. The aesthetic deformities, however, are a source of great concern. There is a tendency toward HTS that should be managed early. Pressure garments are helpful in preventing maximal scar development and reducing the incidence of HTS. When unsightly scars occur, the best reconstructive technique is excision and grafting with non-mesh split-thickness grafts. This procedure should be delayed until the scars have matured fully to reduce the possibility of HTS.

The Breast

Burns of the anterior chest can cause considerable distortion of the breast in children and adolescents. Direct thermal injury can lead to loss of the breast bud and subsequent lack of breast development. The area around the nipples should be debrided conservatively and only after non-

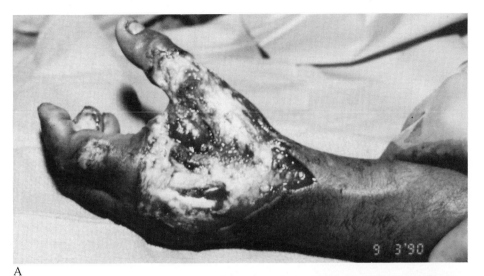

A

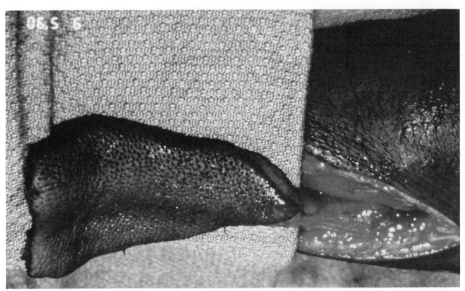

B

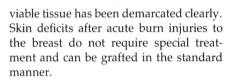

Fig. 29-7A. This patient sustained a high-voltage electrical injury to the radial-dorsal aspect of the right hand. After debridement, both extensor tendons were exposed and the metacarpophalangeal joint was exposed and left open. B. A radial forearm flap was used for immediate wound coverage. C. Successful wound coverage was achieved. A thumb–index finger web space Z-plasty was necessary to fully restore web space length.

C

viable tissue has been demarcated clearly. Skin deficits after acute burn injuries to the breast do not require special treatment and can be grafted in the standard manner.

Abnormal breast development can result from regional scar formation, distorting the skin position and leading to an abnormal breast contour and location. Furthermore, complete coverage of the breast by hypertrophic scar tissue can prevent expansion of the developing breast mound by direct pressure.

The surgical treatment of the contracted breast has been well described by Neale. The breast mound should be fully released and allowed to develop before nipple-areolar reconstruction is begun. An inframammary incision in most instances sufficiently releases contraction, but superior and lateral incisions may be necessary depending on the location of the contracture. The release should extend to the fascia of the pectoralis and rectus muscles if needed. Usually the subcutaneous fat separates from the breast tissue, allowing the surgeon to sculpt the breast. A contralateral unburned breast provides a useful model. After complete release of the skin envelope, the skin defect is covered with moderate-thickness skin grafts (Fig. 29-9).

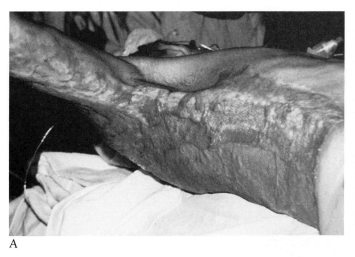

A

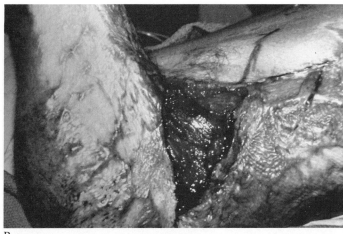

B

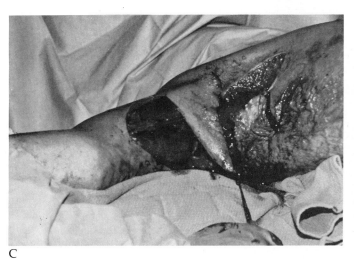

C

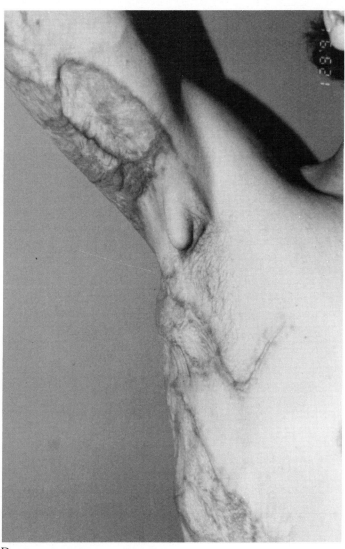

Fig. 29-8A. Severe axillary contracture after a burn injury. B. After release of the axillary contracture, the tissue deficit becomes apparent. A Z-plasty marked on the lateral unburned chest also is shown. C. Rotation of an antebrachial fasciocutaneous flap into the axillary defect. The donor site was skin grafted. Additional Z-plasties were performed on the chest wall. D. The final result 6 months after the reconstruction. Complete release of the axillary contracture was achieved with good motion of the shoulder joint.

D

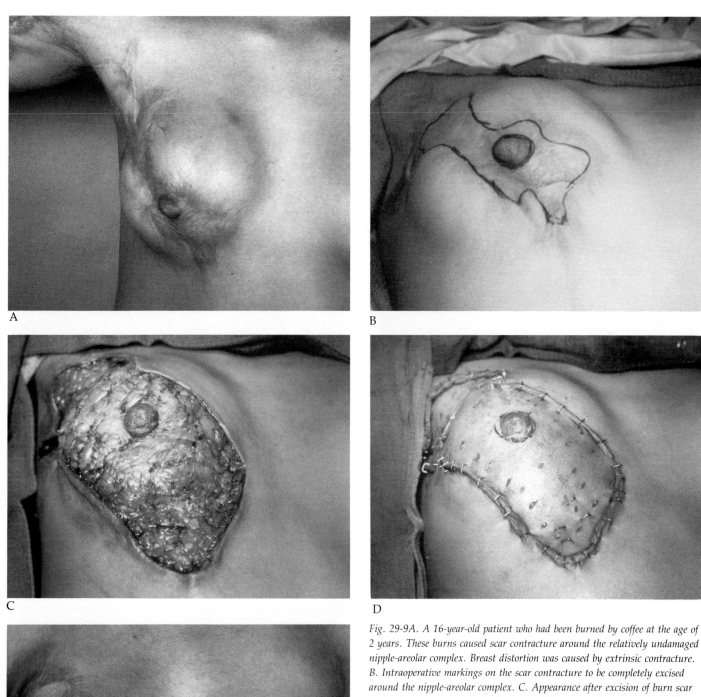

A

B

C

D

Fig. 29-9A. A 16-year-old patient who had been burned by coffee at the age of 2 years. These burns caused scar contracture around the relatively undamaged nipple-areolar complex. Breast distortion was caused by extrinsic contracture. B. Intraoperative markings on the scar contracture to be completely excised around the nipple-areolar complex. C. Appearance after excision of burn scar contracture. The breast instantly regained its normal size and contour. D. Split-thickness skin graft (0.02 inch) applied to cover the defect. E. Appearance 2 years after treatment with symmetry of the inframammary creases and full development of the breast. (Courtesy of Henry W. Neale, M.D.)

E

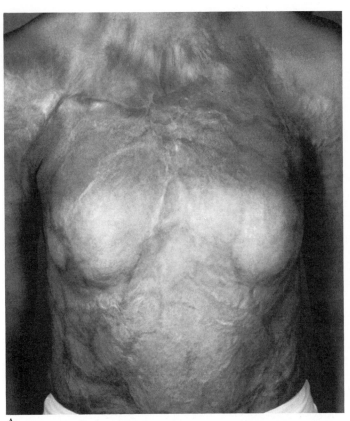

A

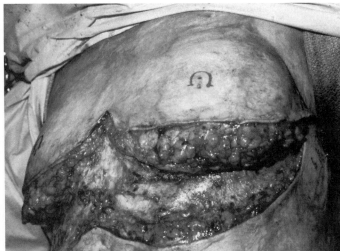

B

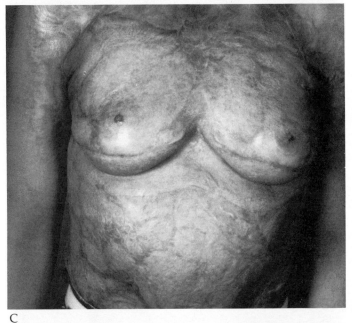

C

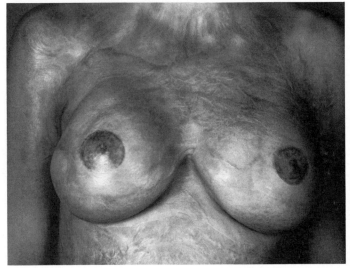

D

Fig. 29-10A. Sixteen-year-old patient after flame burns to the anterior trunk. Breast mound development is progressing, but scar contracture inhibits lower breast development causing blunting of the inframammary creases. B. Surgical release of contractures down to chest wall fascia and inframammary crease. C. Appearance one year after nipple and areolar reconstruction and split-thickness skin graft. Normal inframammary creases and symmetric breast contouring. D. Appearance 4 years after photograph in C was taken. Nipple and areolar tattooing and bilateral augmentation with a permanent expander-prosthesis for patient's desired breast augmentation. (Courtesy of Henry W. Neale, M.D.)

Fig. 29-11A. Contracture and deformity of the dorsum of the foot and toes of a 14-year-old girl several years after burn, which was not treated. B. Preoperative radiograph demonstrating that despite the skeletal deformity, the joint spaces remain intact. C. The contracture of the dorsum of the foot has been released and transosseous pins have been used to maintain the toes in position. The skin defect was covered with a split-thickness skin graft.

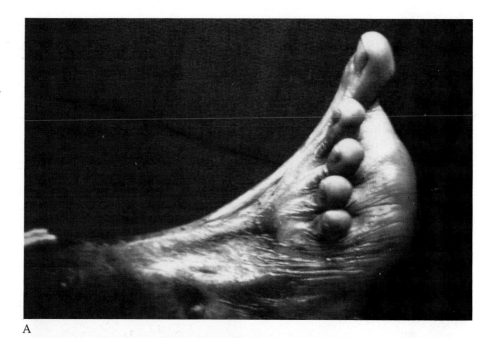

A

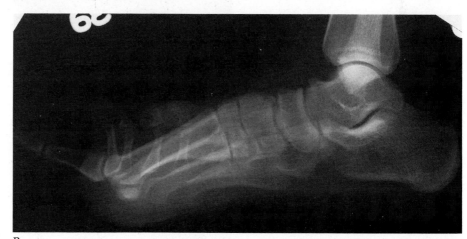

B

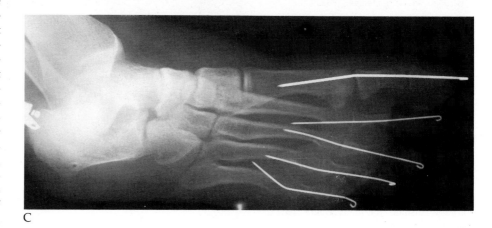

C

A hypoplastic breast mound can occur after long-standing contractures, previous debridement, or deep burns. Breast reconstruction techniques should be used to form an appropriate breast mound. If tissue expanders or implants are used, care must be taken to fully cover the implant with muscle to minimize erosion through stiff hypertrophic or thin grafted skin. Nipple reconstruction is usually delayed and performed several months after reconstruction of the breast mound (Fig. 29-10).

The Lower Extremity

Reconstructive problems are less obvious in the lower extremity, although healing is slower and HTS is more common. The problems may be less urgent because the patient's expectations are lesser and because there is less need for fine motor function in the feet than in the hands. Flexion forces across the joints of the lower extremity have contractive tendencies, but gravity and walking help splint and stretch tissues into the proper position. Patients who do not walk, particularly those who are critically ill, benefit from positioning and splinting. Of particular note is the fact that patients in air-fluid beds tend to sustain straight hip flexion contractures. When isolated scar bands develop, the best solution is usually a Z-plasty. Contractions of the thin dorsal skin of the foot can become a problem in young children. The tendency to form hypertrophic scars and the lack of toe flexion with walking may result in dorsal deviation of the toes. Inserts combined with pressure garments help some patients. In others excision of the hypertrophic scar and Kirschner wire pinning of the phalanges is necessary (Fig. 29-11).

Chronic ulceration of the distal lower limb is frequently seen after severe burn injuries. Hypertrophic or thinned skin is less able to resist the wear and tear of daily living. Patients with underlying circulatory problems, atherosclerosis, and diabetes are particularly at risk. These ulcers usually occur in the distal third of the lower extremity, an area where few surgical options are available. Free tissue transfers are usually the best solution (Fig. 29-12). Fasciocutaneous flaps such as the radial forearm or lateral arm flap work well, although we find that the donor site is most often chosen on the basis of availability of areas of unburned skin.

Suggested Reading

Achauer, B.M. *Burn Reconstruction*. New York: Thieme, 1991.

Achauer, B.M., and Welk, R.A. One stage reconstruction of the postburn nail-fold contracture. *Plast. Reconstr. Surg.* 85:937, 1990.

Alexander, J.W., MacMillan, B.G., and Martel, L. Correction of postburn syndactyly: An analysis of children with introduction of the V-M plasty and postoperative pressure inserts. *Plast. Reconstr. Surg.* 70:345, 1982.

Budo, J., Finucan, T., and Clarke, J. The inner arm fasciocutaneous flap. *Plast. Reconstr. Surg.* 73:629, 1984.

Cormack, G.C., and Lamberty, M.A. Fasciocutaneous vessels in the upper arm: Application to the design of new fasciocutaneous flaps. *Plast. Reconstr. Surg.* 74:244, 1984.

Hunter, J.H., et al. (Eds.). *Rehabilitation of the Hand* (2nd ed.). St. Louis: Mosby, 1984.

Krizek, T.J. Management of burn syndactyly. *J. Trauma* 14:590, 1974.

Maruyama, Y. Ascending scapular flap and its use for the treatment of axillary burn scar contracture. *Br. J. Plast. Surg.* 44:97, 1991.

Ostrowski, D.M., Feagin, C.A., and Gould, J.S. A three-flap web-plasty for release of short congenital syndactyly and dorsal adduction contracture. *J. Hand Surg.* 16A:634, 1991.

Peterson, S.L., et al. Postburn heterotopic ossification: Insights for management decision making. *J. Trauma* 29:365, 1989.

Salisbury, R.E., and Dingeldein, G.P. The Burned Hand and Upper Extremity. In D.P. Green (Ed.), *Operative Hand Surgery* (2nd ed.). New York: Churchill Livingstone, 1988. Vol. 3, P. 2135.

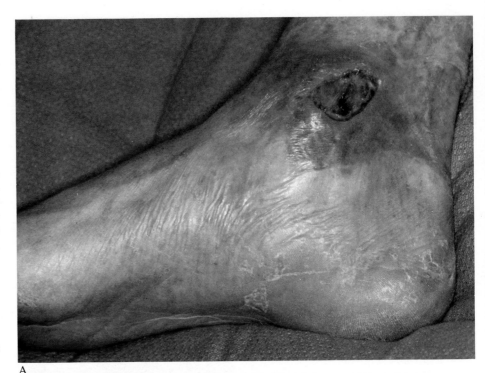

A

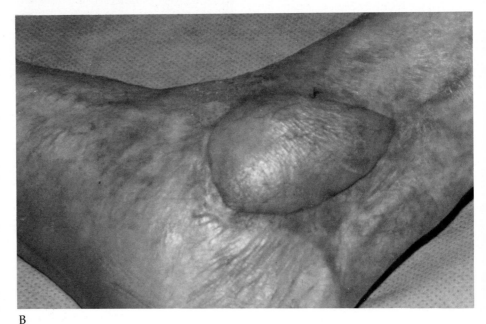

B

Fig. 29-12A. Chronic unstable scar and ulceration of the medial malleolus several years after a burn. Note the fibrotic burned skin around the ulcer. B. Appearance after debridement and coverage with radial forearm flap.

30

Electrical and Chemical Injuries

Martin C. Robson   Peter G. Hayward

Although they are in some ways similar to thermal burns, electrical and chemical injuries are distinct in many ways. To arrive at a rational approach to management, it is paramount to understand their pathophysiology and clinical presentation.

Electrical Injuries

An electrical injury is a unique and thoroughly devastating form of trauma. Electrical injuries are arbitrarily divided into high-tension and low-tension injuries determined by the voltage responsible for the damage. The dividing line is 1000 volts. This classification has important clinical implications. Low-voltage injuries mimic thermal burns and have zones of injury from the surface extending into the deeper tissue. High-voltage injuries consist of varying degrees of cutaneous burns combined with "hidden" destruction of the deeper tissues. A high-voltage injury results in progressive tissue necrosis, somewhat resembling the injury of crush trauma, and is extremely difficult to manage. These injuries often require repeated operations. Major amputations are common for these wounds, which frequently

produce severe cosmetic and functional disability.

Pathophysiology

Much progress has been made in unifying theories of electrical injury. This new theoretical base concerns the surgeon because it shapes rational surgical planning. The surgeon's greatest problems are the unpredictable, patchy distribution of necrosis and the progressive nature of the disease. The distribution of tissue injury after a high-tension injury is variable, often involving periosseous tissues and sparing overlying soft tissue. Furthermore, the injury progresses clinically, with tissues that were apparently viable at initial debridement undergoing late necrosis.

Recent advances suggest that these clinical features are the result of an initial cellular injury caused by joule heating or membrane disruption depending on whether the tissues through which the current passes are arranged in a series or are parallel to each other. When the tissues are in a series, the initial tissue destruction caused by contact with high-voltage electricity is basically a thermal injury. Passage of electric current through

a solid conductor results in conversion of electric energy into heat. The parameters dictating the amount of energy or current delivered to a victim are found in Ohm's law:

$$\text{Current} = \text{voltage/tissue resistance}$$

The amount of heat produced is described as joule heating:

$$\text{Heat (joules)} = \text{current}^2 \times \text{tissue resistance} \times \text{duration of contact}$$

These equations are of more than passing interest to surgeons because they summarize all the factors involved in electrical injuries and help explain why the clinical features are so variable.

Several theories have been postulated to explain the pathologic changes seen after joule heating. In a specific patient, the explanation of tissue damage depends on the direction of the injuring current. Tissue resistance increases progressively from nerves to blood vessels to muscle to skin to fat, and finally to bone. Current traveling *across* the axis of a limb passes through these tissues in a serial manner, generating the most heat at the bone ac-

Fig. 30-1. Model system to demonstrate temperature distribution when tissues are arranged in series (A) and when they are parallel to each other (B). Current traversing the cross section of a limb travels through tissues arranged in series. Each of the tissues in the series has a different conductivity, and the temperature increases as a result of joule heating as the current passes through the limb. (From R.C. Lee and M.S. Kolodney. Electrical injury mechanisms: Dynamics of the thermal response. Plast. Reconstr. Surg. 80:663, 1987. Reproduced with permission.)

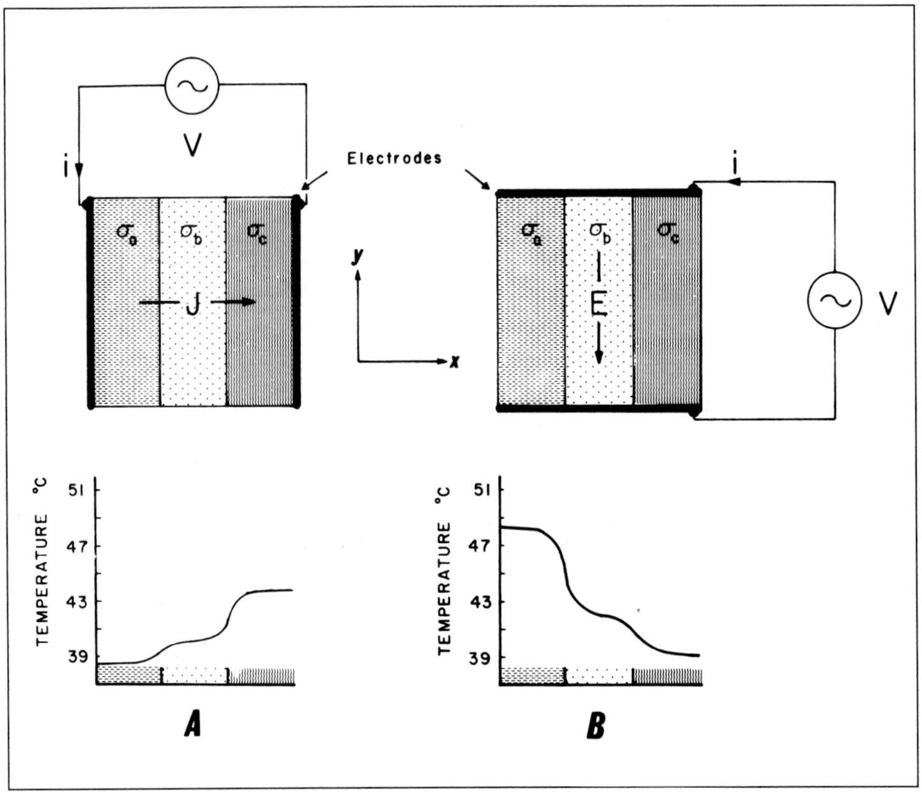

Fig. 30-2. When electrical contact occurs as depicted here, the current passes through tissues that are parallel to each other. The heat generated by the joule effect is not sufficient to account for the observed clinical injury. (From R.C. Lee and M.S. Kolodney. Electrical injury mechanisms: Dynamics of the thermal response. Plast. Reconstr. Surg. 80:663, 1987. Reproduced with permission.)

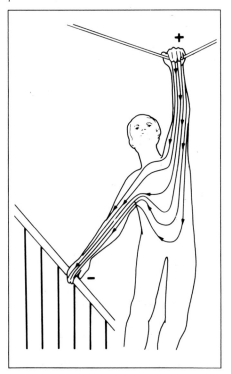

cording to the joule effect (Fig. 30-1). This explains the greater necrosis in the deep periosseous tissues. Current traveling *along* the axis of a limb passes through tissues that are parallel to each other, and the limb acts as a volume conductor with a uniform resistance (Fig. 30-2). As a result, current, flow, amperage, and temperature rise uniformly throughout the limb. By the time the current arcs, the temperatures of both muscle and bone are equal. Bone, however, takes longer to dissipate the heat. This prolonged elevation in temperature accounts for the periosseous core of necrotic muscle seen clinically. Current traversing the long axis of the limb reaches a very high density around joints where low-resistance muscle is replaced by highly resistant bone and tendon. As a result, severe tissue damage may be seen at the elbow, for example, although the forearm is relatively unaffected. Occasionally tissues arranged parallel to each other do not generate large amounts of heat. Cell membranes are still disrupted, however.

At a cellular level, initial microscopic studies of questionably viable muscle confirm the patchy nature of electrical in-

juries (Fig. 30-3). Normal muscle cells are immediately adjacent to necrotic cells with pyknotic nuclei, and normal patent vessels exist adjacent to thrombosed vessels, similar to the zone of stasis in a thermal burn. Recent electron microscopic studies have shown extensive membrane damage to muscle cells exposed to large current loads. This damage includes formation of defects (pores) in the cell membrane that lead to rhabdomyolysis. Such damage also triggers the production of elevated levels of arachidonic acid metabolites (Fig. 30-4). The prolonged elevation in the level of thromboxane, a potent vasoconstrictor, plays a key role in the progressive microvascular ischemia in electrically injured tissues, leading to progressive necrosis.

Clinical Evaluation

The history is critical in evaluating patients with electrical injuries. Because patients often have amnesia or partial amnesia about the electrical insult, relatives or fellow workers have to be closely questioned. The physical setting of the injury often indicates the voltage involved. Home injuries, for instance, usually in-

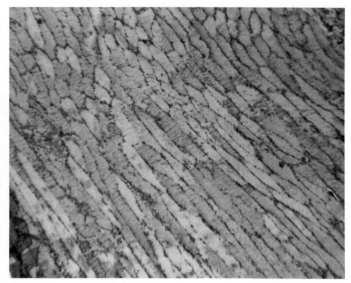

Fig. 30-3. Histologic section of muscle 24 hours after an electrical injury. Note the patchy necrosis and nonuniform appearance of cells.

Fig. 30-4. Eicosanoid production by metabolism of arachidonic acid. Pathway can be triggered by disruption of cell membrane by electric current. (From J.P. Heggers and M.C. Robson. Prostaglandins and thromboxane. Crit. Care Clin. 1:59, 1985. Reproduced with permission.)

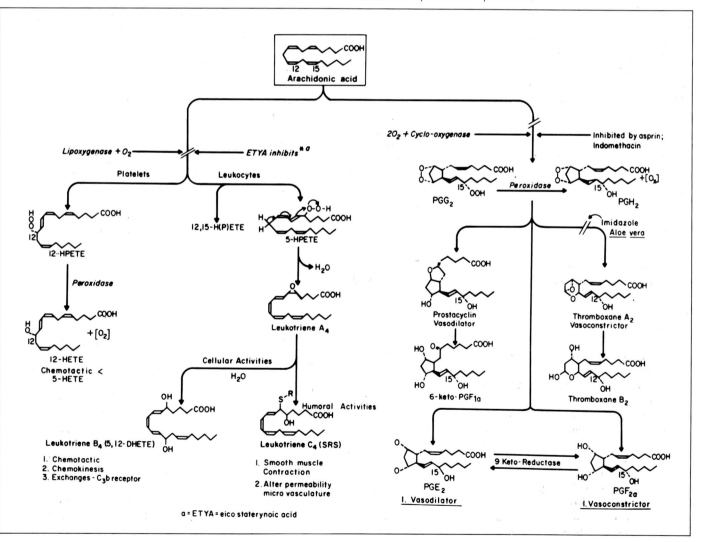

volve contact with 110 to 220 volts, whereas industrial or power-line injuries are usually high tension (>1000 volts). Baseline data are required to monitor the cardiac and neurologic state of the patient. It is essential to know if a cardiac arrest occurred at the injury scene.

Severe trauma is commonly associated with electrical injury. Victims may be thrown a distance or may fall from a height after contacting the electrical source. Historical evidence should alert the physician to the need for a thorough examination to diagnose related trauma.

The physical examination begins with the establishment of airway patency. The chest is examined for symmetric expansion, percussion, and bilaterality of breath sounds. Pneumothorax is not uncommon in high-tension injuries. Cardiac rate and rhythm are examined and electrocardiographic monitoring instituted. The peripheral circulation is examined and the need for urgent escharotomy or fasciotomy determined. Although evaluation of muscle compartmental pressures may be an adjunct in making this determination, clinical judgment should take precedence. When there is doubt about peripheral blood flow, a serial examination should be performed by an experienced surgeon. There should be a high index of suspicion regarding compartmental pressures, because underlying, deep muscle may be injured despite a lack of injury in the overlying skin.

In the evaluation of mental and neurologic status, level of consciousness and orientation to person, place, and time are important. A rapid neurologic examination should check for focal motor and sensory deficits. Respiratory paralysis and limb paralysis are not uncommon. Although these disturbances may subside spontaneously, permanent residual disability has been reported. Hemiplegia, aphasia, cerebellar dysfunction, and epilepsy all have been reported after electrical injuries, even when the contact does not involve the cranium. Indeed, physiologic spinal cord transection occurs in up to 25 percent of patients with high-voltage electrical injuries. It is essential to document neurologic findings at the time of admission to the hospital to differentiate these from postelectrocution neurologic syndromes, which can develop during the initial admission or months to years later.

After the initial triage, a detailed system review should be carried out. Multiple systems can be involved in electrical injuries. The surgeon should look specifically for the presence of shock, bony injuries, and occult abdominal trauma.

Electrical injuries often have an associated thermal burn. However, fluid loss may exceed that predicted by the size of the thermal burn. In severe electrical injuries, necrosis of large volumes of muscle contributes to extremely large fluid losses. Blood loss may occur as a consequence of vascular injury, from associated fractures, or from chest or abdominal trauma. Shock should never be attributed to an uncomplicated electrical injury. The possibility of associated hemorrhage or perforation of an intra-abdominal viscus always must be considered.

Bony injuries are evaluated for both associated fractures and direct injury to the bone caused by electrical conduction. As noted before, physical trauma is often associated with electrocution, especially with power-line workers. In fact, bony fractures have been reported in 10 percent of all instances of electrocution. The violent tetanic muscular contraction that results from contact, particularly with alternating current, may result in a variety of fractures and dislocations. Fractures contribute not only to blood loss but also to delayed rehabilitation if not diagnosed in an unconscious patient. Direct electrical damage results in extensive destruction of bone, common in very high-voltage electrical injuries. Grossly, the bone is avascular and may be exposed and appear whitened. Even nonexposed bone may be damaged. Up to 15 percent of patients have bone sequestra after very high-voltage injuries, and direct bony damage and exposure caused by electrical contact is never trivial. Excellent results have been achieved using early flap repair to cover such bony injuries, but the repair must be performed before sequestration (Fig. 30-5). This possibility should be kept in mind when formulating a management plan for such a patient.

Nausea, vomiting, and prolonged paralytic ileus are common after electrical injuries. The surgeon should be careful to differentiate these abdominal signs from those secondary to a perforated viscus or transmural injury to the colon (Fig. 30-6). The latter injuries may occur without direct electrical injury to the abdominal wall. In any case, peritoneal irritation indicates the need for an exploratory laparotomy.

Once these preliminary examinations are complete, attention is turned to the wounds. Three types of skin damage may result from electrical injury: (1) contact burns at points of current entry and exit from the body, (2) arc burns caused by current exiting and reentering adjacent parts or body parts in proximity, and (3) thermal burns from ignition of clothing because of the degree of heat generated by the flux of current. The total body surface area (TBSA) burned should be recorded. One must realize, however, that the injury may be underestimated because deep muscle necrosis can be hidden beneath apparently uninjured skin. An attempt should be made to locate the contact wounds. The scalp and the soles of the feet should not be overlooked. One must bear in mind that wounds may appear trivial at the body surface.

Laboratory tests complete the clinical evaluation. Hemoglobinemia may be observed as a result of lysis of red cells. Similarly, myoglobin is released from damaged muscle. The presence of both hemoglobin and myoglobin in the urine must be detected, and "dipstick" techniques are not universally reliable. In electrical injuries, discolored urine should be treated as myoglobinuria as a matter of urgency. If not cleared from the renal tubules, these pigments precipitate and cause secondary renal failure. Prophylactic treatment is in order; one should not wait for laboratory confirmation of myoglobinuria.

Blood abnormalities can occur after massive destruction of tissue, especially of muscle. Concentrations of creatinine, creatine phosphokinase (CPK), serum glutamic oxaloacetic transaminase (SGOT), and lactate dehydrogenase (LDH) may be elevated. To differentiate these conditions from cardiac damage may require isoenzyme assays. A standard 12-lead electrocardiogram (ECG) is essential in evaluating cardiac damage caused by electrocution or prolonged ischemia after cardiac arrest at the time of injury. If the ECG is normal on admission and there is no history of cardiac arrest or cardiopul-

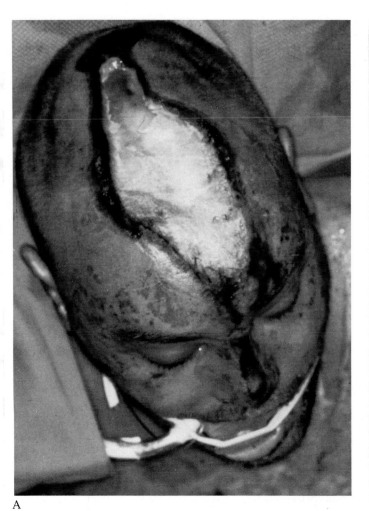

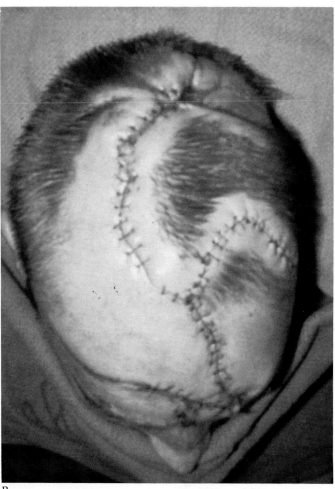

A   B

Fig. 30-5. Exposed nonviable bone (A) can be covered successfully with viable flaps (B) without the need for radical debridement.

Fig. 30-6. Hidden injuries to viscera are not rare after electrical trauma. This patient required a laparotomy and exteriorization of an injured colon.

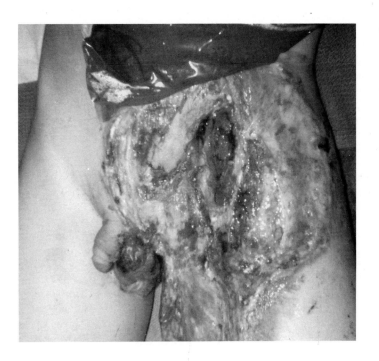

monary resuscitation, cardiac complications of electrocution are unlikely. Conversely, an abnormal ECG or enzyme studies or a cardiac arrest at the scene calls for continuous cardiac monitoring.

Any site of electrical injury should be subject to a roentgenographic examination. A chest roentgenogram may reveal a pneumothorax, a hemothorax, or a transected aortic root. Because of the possibility of coexisting trauma, roentgenograms of the cervical, thoracic, and lumbar areas of the spine are usually indicated in high-voltage injuries or if a fall has occurred.

Roentgenograms of the skull are obtained if indicated. When a perforated viscus is suspected, a barium or meglumine diatrizoate (Gastrografin) contrast study is useful.

The use of technetium-99m pyrophosphate muscle scans has been advocated to determine how much muscle is not being perfused. "Cold" areas on the skin may suggest irreversibly necrotic, non-salvageable tissue, whereas "hot" areas indicate that 20 to 28 percent of the muscle fiber is necrotic. We have not found this technique to add to clinical management. More accurate imaging technology such as nuclear magnetic resonance spectroscopy may soon add to the preoperative determination of the extent of muscle necrosis. For clinicians, the benefits of this advanced technology are to be weighed against its availability and the logistic considerations of moving a critically injured patient to a scanning facility.

Nonoperative Management

If the initial ECG is abnormal, continued cardiac monitoring is necessary with pharmacologic treatment of any arrhythmia. Prolonged respiratory support may be required because a coma occasionally occurs. In severe electrical injuries, fluid loss exceeds that predicted by the area of the thermal burn. Large volumes of necrotic muscle lead to extremely large fluid losses. These losses are compounded by associated vascular injuries, fractures, and chest or abdominal trauma. Resuscitation with lactated Ringer solution may be begun with the Baxter or Parkland Hospital formula using 4 ml/kg/percent TBSA burned. A brisk urine flow should be promoted because of the threat of myoglobinuria. Established myoglobinuria should be treated by starting a urine flow of at least 70 to 100 ml/hour using 10% mannitol diuresis if necessary. Addition of bicarbonate to the resuscitation fluid results in alkalinization of the blood and improves solubility of chromogens such as hemoglobin and myoglobin in the urine.

As in thermal injuries, nasogastric suction may be required for 24 to 48 hours. If there is no persistent ileus, enteral nutrition should begin as soon as is practical.

Avoidance of wound sepsis is critical in view of the large amount of necrotic tissue present. In one study of electrical injuries,

7 percent of deaths were caused by sepsis. Topical antimicrobials with maximal penetrating ability are preferred. Mafenide acetate is particularly well suited for these wounds. It can penetrate to the deep levels of injury, and it is the antibacterial of choice for *Clostridium*, which thrives in the necrotic muscle caused by electrical injuries.

Careful monitoring of affected limbs is essential. Ischemic compression and nerve compression are possible because unseen injury may have occurred in deep muscular compartments. Intracompartmental swelling may be marked. Careful observation of limbs that have already been surgically released should be continued because of the risk of late thrombosis of injured vessels. Serial palpation of limbs for tenseness, evaluation of capillary refill, and Doppler measurement, and intracompartmental measurement, all help to determine the need for vascular decompression.

Because paresthesia and numbness can result from electrocution itself, these symptoms do not necessarily indicate compression. This makes the diagnosis of nerve compression more difficult; however, changes over time do indicate a need for decompression.

The role of enzymatic agents like sutilains ointment (Travase) has not been defined in electrical injury. Compression in electrical injuries arises from the deep tissue compartments and the surface eschar; therefore, enzymatic or "medical" escharotomy may not be sufficient. Nonoperative enzymatic digestion of necrotic tissue has not been adequately studied in electrical injuries and cannot be recommended at this time.

Operative Management

Operative management of electrical injuries is virtually always necessary. We believe that electrical injury results in progressive tissue injury. As a result, only life-threatening and limb-threatening problems should be operated on acutely. Definitive wound closure should be delayed until the injury is fully demarcated. This approach maximizes the chance for definitive, one-stage reconstruction. It also minimizes the risk of premature closure over partially necrotic tissue.

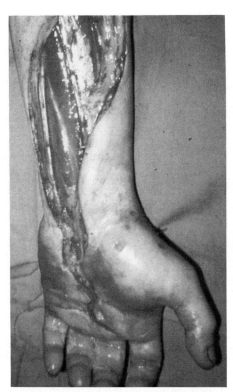

Fig. 30-7. *Escharotomy does not usually suffice in electrical injuries. Fasciotomy as demonstrated here is usually required to release the muscular compartment.*

In a high-voltage injury, the periosseous necrosis generates massive edema beneath what may appear to be uninjured skin. Therefore, escharotomy and fasciotomy are necessary soon after the patient is admitted to the hospital (Fig. 30-7). There should be a high index of suspicion regarding the possibility of compartmental syndromes. As noted, the need for such releases can be determined by physical examination, using compartmental pressure measurements as an adjunct. Major nerves are particularly susceptible to increased pressure in closed compartments, however, and escharotomy or fasciotomy alone or in combination may not be sufficient to decompress major nerve trunks. This is particularly true of the upper limb. We recommend decompression of the median and ulnar nerves as an emergency procedure in high-voltage injuries to the hands. In the lower limb a complete four-compartment fasciotomy is required.

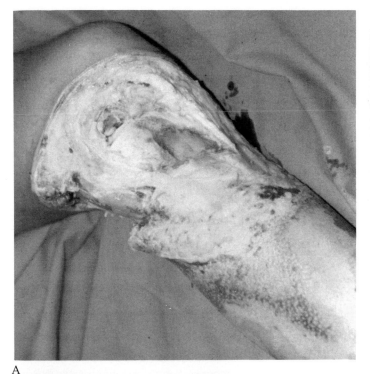

A

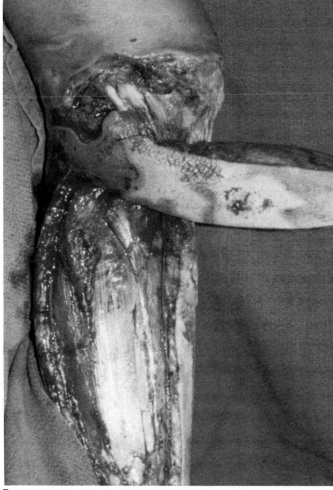

B

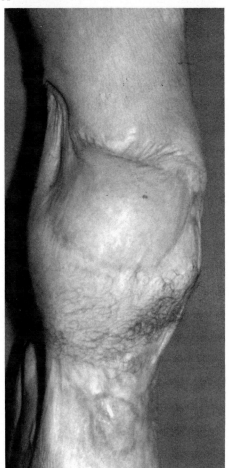

C

Fig. 30-8. An exposed knee joint (A) can be closed with a musculocutaneous flap (B) to give a satisfactory result (C).

Debridement of obviously necrotic tissue should be performed as early as feasible. This debridement should be combined with any escharotomies, fasciotomies, and nerve decompressions required. Because the lesion is progressive, wounds should not be closed definitively at the time of initial debridement. Like thermal burns, low-voltage injuries can be debrided using a layered or sequential tangential technique. Debridement in a high-voltage injury is much more demanding. Necrotic tissue may extend beneath what appears to be normal, uninjured skin and as far as 25 cm from the point of entry and exit of the current. Therefore, a careful survey should be made of all muscle compartments. Viability can be checked by frozen section, but from a practical point of view the most reliable test is the ability of the muscle to bleed and contract.

Once it is established, the definitive wound should be closed. Although skin grafts almost always suffice as closure for thermal burn wounds, flaps are frequently necessary for closure of electrical burn wounds. Flap coverage is required not only to cover injured bone but also to produce a stable, well-vascularized site for secondary reconstruction (Fig. 30-8). An increasing number of early wound closures using free tissue transfers are being reported. Because large neuromuscular units are frequently destroyed by high-tension injuries, the possibility of functional free muscle transfers should be considered early, particularly for the upper limb.

High-tension injuries often necessitate amputations. When possible amputation should be delayed until the limb threat-

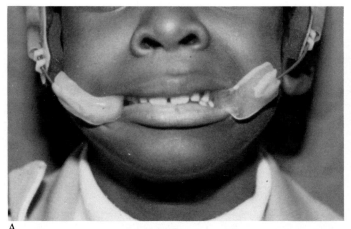

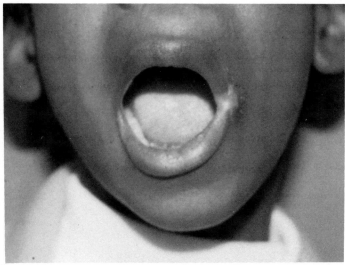

Fig. 30-9. *Conservative treatment of the oral commissure by dynamic splints (A) yields satisfactory results (B).*

A

B

ens to cause overwhelming sepsis. Even exposed, charred, and superficially infected bone can be salvaged with coverage by a vascularized flap. If they are required, amputations should be done in an open circular method and closed at a later date.

Intraperitoneal injuries are not rare among major electrical injuries. The principles of progressive disease apply to the torso as well as to the limbs. When such injuries are suspected, a laparotomy is required, and exteriorization or resection may be indicated. A second-look operation may be considered depending on the appearance of the organs at the initial laparotomy.

Electrical injury to the oral commissure is common, particularly among infants. Four treatment plans have been promulgated over the years, including (1) immediate excision within 12 hours of injury, (2) delayed primary excision and reconstruction 4 to 7 days after injury, (3) delayed reconstruction after complete healing by secondary intention, and (4) immediate and prolonged postburn splinting in an attempt to allow healing without deformity. We have had good results with the last, conservative approach with essentially no need for late reconstruction (Fig. 30-9). This approach requires patience and an excellent rapport with the child's parents, whose support is essential to compliance with splinting. Secondary hemorrhage from the labial ar-

teries is rare but needs to be discussed with the parents. When the conservative approach is untenable because of logistics or lack of compliance, we opt for conservative excision and closure with secondary reconstruction of the commissure.

Complications

Despite expert management, patients with electrical injuries frequently have complications. Acute complications, such as myocardial damage, arterial mural necrosis, rupture, and occult injuries to the abdominal viscera have already been discussed. Many late complications are caused by the complex, incompletely understood pathophysiology of the injury. This group includes lesions of the cardiac system, the central and peripheral nervous systems, and the eyes.

Cardiac dysrhythmia or ECG changes are present initially in 10 to 30 percent of patients. However, right bundle branch block, supraventricular tachycardia, and focal ectopic arrhythmia may present months after the injury and may persist.

Cerebral complications can be devastating; cortical encephalopathy, hemiplegia with or without aphasia, striatal syndrome, and brain-stem dysfunction all have been reported. These problems may occur 6 to 9 months after the injury. Secondary epilepsy also can appear late. Spinal cord syndromes similar to progressive muscular atrophy, amyotrophic

lateral sclerosis, or transverse myelitis may occur after a latent period of days to months. Peripheral nerve lesions can appear up to 3 years after the injury. Histopathologic changes of affected neural tissue have shown perivascular hemorrhage, demyelination with vacuolization, reactive gliosis, and neuronal death. These facts suggest that high-tension electrical injury institutes chronic, progressive cellular damage. It is disturbing that this cellular injury may be occult at the time of the initial diagnosis of the electrical injury.

The progressive onset of cataracts also is associated with severe electrical injuries. The cataracts can be delayed for several years, although the onset of blurred vision usually begins about 6 months after the injury. Some lens opacification develops in up to 30 percent of people receiving an electrical burn with contact above the clavicles; thus all patients should have an ophthalmologic assessment and be warned of this complication.

Chemical Injuries

Although chemical burns account for only 3 percent of all burns, they account for more than 30 percent of burn deaths. This statistic reflects the distinct nature of chemical burns both locally and systemically compared with other thermal injuries. Locally chemical burns cause continued destruction after the agent is removed. In addition, many chemical injuries cause systemic complications because of percutaneous or transpulmonary absorption. The surgeon should be mindful of both local and systemic toxicity during treatment.

Pathophysiology

Chemical agents cause injury by one of five mechanisms: (1) oxidation, (2) reduction, (3) corrosion, (4) protoplasmic poisoning, or (5) the ischemic concomitant of vesicant activity. *Oxidizing agents* become oxidized on contact with body tissue. Continued absorption by-products from this reaction account for further toxicity. Commonly encountered oxidizing agents are chromic acid, sodium hypochlorite (household bleach), and potassium permanganate. *Reducing agents* produce protein denaturation by binding free electrons in tissue proteins. Such reducing agents include alkyl mercuric agents, hydrochloric acid, and nitric acid. *Corrosive agents* denature tissue protein in a variety of ways. Their net effect is eschar formation and a shallow, indolent ulcer. Corrosive agents include phenols and cresols, white phosphorus, dichromate salts, sodium metals, and lyes. *Protoplasmic poisons* form salts with proteins or bind and inhibit calcium and other inorganic ions necessary for tissue viability and function. Protoplasmic poisons include "alkaloidal" acids, acetic acid, formic acid, and metabolic competitors or inhibitors, including oxalic and hydrofluoric acids. *Vesicant agents* produce ischemia with anoxic necrosis at the site of contact. Examples are cantharides (Spanish fly), dimethyl sulfoxide (DMSO), mustard gas, and lewisite. Agents that are desiccants produce their deleterious effects by causing dehydration damage, by producing excessive heat in the tissue, or by both reactions. Examples of this group are sulfuric acid and muriatic acid.

Clinical Evaluation

The overriding need is to identify the agent involved. With this knowledge both local and systemic toxicity can be gauged. To estimate the severity of a chemical injury, the physician needs to know (1) its strength, (2) the quantity of the agent, (3) the manner and duration of skin contact and progression, (4) the depth of penetration, and (5) the mechanism of action. During the clinical evaluation, two associated facts must be remembered. First, in the process of removing saturated clothing and irrigating the injury, the treating physician may become a secondary victim. Emergency department personnel should be appropriately clothed and wear gloves. Second, as the initial assessment is occurring, copious irrigation must begin without delay.

The initial evaluation should include an adequate history and physical examination, determining the confines of the chemical injury and ruling out associated injuries. Additional laboratory tests are dictated by the specific agent involved. A chest roentgenogram is indicated whenever a patient may have inhaled toxic vapors. Although the same TBSA nomograms are used as with thermal burns, the need for repeated assessment is greater. Commonly the initial estimate of the extent of injury changes after irrigation. Once the agent has been removed or neutralized, these wounds can be treated like any other burn on the basis of depth. However, depth assessment is not always easy, and initial appearances are frequently deceiving. Chemical agents frequently produce a discolored eschar. For example, a phenol burn may prove superficial despite a bronzed or dry, white eschar, whereas other agents such as nitric acid may progress to total obliteration of the surface anatomy.

Management

As a rule, all patients with chemical burns need to be admitted to the hospital because the extent of the injury cannot be appreciated fully at the time of initial evaluation.

Management of a chemical injury must include an assessment of possible systemic manifestations and of the localized wound. When the chemical agent is absorbed, appropriate corrective or neutralizing therapy needs to be instituted. For example, hypocalcemia can result with absorption of oxalic and hydrofluoric acid. Methemoglobinemia and hemolysis occur with absorption of cresol. Systemic toxicity may result from inhalation of vapors or transcutaneous absorption. An ingestion injury should suggest an associated inhalation injury. Organ-specific toxicity, such as hepatic necrosis and nephrotoxicity, may require intensive care. These complications can be seen with absorption of tannic acid and, to a lesser extent, of chromic, formic, and picric acids, and of metallic phosphorus.

Whatever the chemical agent, first aid consists of removing saturated clothing and irrigating with massive amounts of water. No superior agent has been described. Early and continued lavage has been associated with lessened tissue damage and shorter hospital stays. The volume of water dissipates the heat generated by dilution of the agent. In addition, copious irrigation or hydrotherapy effectively cleanses the wound of active surface chemicals, dilutes the chemical already in contact with the tissue, and may restore tissue water lost to the hydroscopic effect of some agents. Water constitutes immediate first aid and should continue at the scene for 20 to 30 minutes and thereafter for a period of time between 2 and 12 hours. Up to 48 hours of continuous irrigation may be necessary for burns involving the eye. Irrigation should be continued for up to 6 hours for acids and for longer periods for alkalis. The extended period of irrigation for alkalis is necessitated by the bonding of alkalis to tissue proteins. A general rule is that irrigation should be continued until the patient notices a decrease in pain, burning, or stinging. Measurement of skin surface pH is also often helpful. It should be noted that although it has been found to be therapeutic, prolonged irrigation may not be as helpful if not instituted within the first hour after the injury.

In contrast to water, specific neutralizing agents evoke an exothermic reaction that produces heat that increases tissue damage. In general such agents should be avoided. The one exception is hydrofluoric acid burns. This acid and several other chemicals elicit typical injuries and cause specific complications.

Hydrofluoric acid is the strongest of the inorganic acids. Its highly ionized acid moiety promotes penetration and binding of the fluoride ion. Within the soft tissues, the fluoride becomes insoluble only as calcium or magnesium fluoride. In short, it penetrates until it is neutralized by combining with calcium and magnesium from either serum or bone (Fig. 30-10). Treatment, therefore, is aimed at precipitating insoluble salts of the fluoride ion using calcium, magnesium, and occasionally ammonium. Immediate treatment, as with all burns, includes massive copious

Fig. 30-10. Hydrofluoric acid burns of digits of both hands.

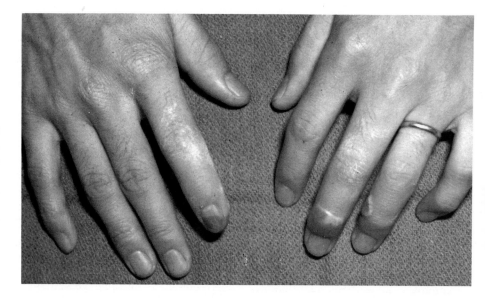

irrigation at the scene with water for 20 to 30 minutes. Some industrial hygienists have found it helpful to use dilute bicarbonate from vats that are constantly available at sites of potential hydrofluoric acid accidents. Following this immediate period of irrigation, flushing the surface with aqueous benzalkonium (a quaternary ammonium compound) helps precipitate any residual fluoride and seems to reduce the stinging pain of the burn. If available, a topical salve incorporating magnesium hydroxide and magnesium sulfate in a water-soluble base may be applied for the period of time required to transfer the victim to professional care.

For burns involving less than 20 percent TBSA, a solution of 10% calcium gluconate is injected directly into the burn and its immediate periphery at a dose of approximately 0.5 ml per square centimeter. An alternative delivery of calcium is by the use of moist compresses for 24 hours consisting of a 50:50 dilution of calcium gluconate and DMSO (Fig. 30-11). Extensive hydrofluoric acid burns may produce total body calcium changes, which may result in life-threatening arrhythmias. Continuous cardiac monitoring is essential in these patients. Individual reports have shown that calcium replacement in these patients requires careful and repeated monitoring of serum calcium concentration to avoid overdose or secondary relapse.

Contact with gasoline may produce a trivial-appearing, second-degree exfoliation, as occurs when someone is trapped in a motor vehicle. Gasoline burns can cause devastating systemic consequences. Continuous exposure or immersion can lead to absorption of gasoline through the skin, which can lead to multiple organ failure and death. The odor of gasoline on the breath following cutaneous absorption of the hydrocarbon is an ominous physical finding. Cerebral dysfunction ranging from disorientation to coma may be seen. Systemic toxicity may progress with upper airway obstruction within 6 hours. By 24 hours, hepatic enzyme levels

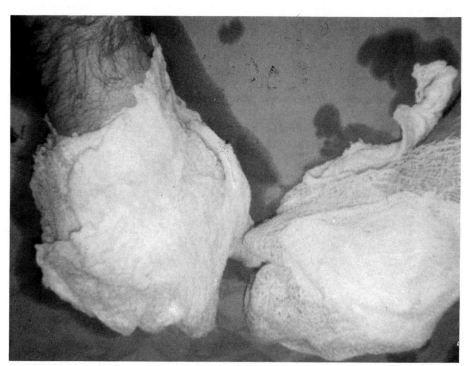

Fig. 30-11. Treatment of hydrofluoric acid burns can be effected by immersing hands in dimethyl sulfoxide (DMSO) and calcium gluconate or applying soaks of a 50:50 solution to the injured parts.

can be elevated and urine output drops. Nephrotoxicity becomes progressive. Gasoline is excreted by the lungs, and absorption of the hydrocarbon not only destroys the surfactant of the respiratory tract but also poisons all membranes. Segmental atelectasis and pulmonary infiltrates are seen. In the wake of pulmonary,

hepatic, and renal failure come gastrointestinal (GI) disturbances, neurologic changes, and cardiomyopathy. Death usually ensues within a week. Although hemodialysis has been suggested as a means of eliminating the absorbed hydrocarbon, reports of successful treatment are few.

Leaded gasoline carries the added toxicity of tetraethyl lead. There have been sporadic reports of lead toxicity following gasoline immersion. Serum measurements are unreliable because lead is heavily organically bound. Acutely, the presence of lead toxicity must be followed in the urine. Levels greater than 150 μg of lead in a 24-hour urine collection suggest severe toxicity. Treatment should include either dimercaprol (BAL) or ethylenediaminetetraacetic acid (EDTA) for 5 days followed by a 10- to 14-day course of penicillamine.

Phenols act as local anesthetics and can produce considerable damage before pain is felt. A gray discoloration of the skin precedes frank necrosis. The agent has strong penetrating abilities particularly if solubilized in water. For this reason polyethylene glycol (PEG) as a 50% dilution is the agent of choice for irrigation. Phenols are highly soluble in PEG, although methylated spirits or vegetable oils can be used. It is critical to remove as much phenol as possible to avoid systemic poisoning. Convulsions, cerebral depression, hemolysis, and renal and liver failure all have been reported.

Molten tar or asphalt produces a scald burn without secondary toxicity. Emergency treatment should consist in cooling the molten material with cold water (Fig. 30-12). Efforts to remove the hardened tar with vigorous cleansing can induce more damage by avulsing the interface between heat-damaged cells, thus deepening the burn. Tar itself is relatively sterile, and no vigor need be exerted to remove the substance. Rather, the wound should be gently cleansed with soap and water and dressed with a petrolatum-based ointment. Dressings can be changed at intervals with gradual separation of the tar and often spontaneous healing of the burn. Once all the tar is removed, the burn can be reassessed with regard to the need for surgical treatment.

A similar approach can be taken to the management of injuries from molten metal and molten sulfur. Industrial sulfur is transported in the molten state, and exposure yields a hard cast not unlike that of tar or asphalt. The element itself has no local toxicity and can be allowed to separate by conservative means as with a tar burn. Although petrolatum does not dissolve the mineral, it forms an interface

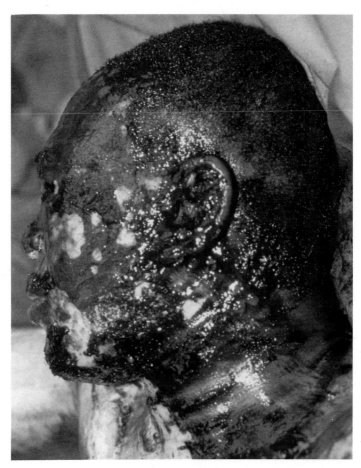

Fig. 30-12. Tar burns can be dramatic but often have little underlying damage. Cooling is a more important treatment than is removal of the tar.

between the cast and the skin that allows atraumatic separation over time. Burns from molten sulfur must be differentiated from burns caused by ignition of sulfur. In the latter injury, the flame burn is compounded by inhalation injury caused by hydrogen sulfide gas.

The depth of injury from chemicals may not be immediately evident. Once demarcated, partial-thickness injuries can be managed by standard conservative means; spontaneous healing is the rule. Blisters should be debrided to remove any absorbed and dissolved chemical within the blister fluid. Full-thickness injuries can be treated with standard topical antimicrobial therapy and allowed to demarcate. Debridement and closure can then be carried out by the standard grafting techniques used for other full-thickness injuries.

Suggested Reading

Luterman, A., and Curreri, P.W. Chemical Burn Injury. In J.A. Boswick (Ed.), *The Art and Science of Burn Care*. Rockville, Md.: Aspen, 1987, Pp. 233–239.

Monafo, W.W., and Freedman, B.M. Electrical and Lightning Injury. In J.A. Boswick (Ed.), *The Art and Science of Burn Care*. Rockville, Md.: Aspen, 1987, Pp. 241–253.

Robson, M.C., Hayward, P.G., and Heggers, J.P. The Role of Arachidonic Acid Metabolism in Electrical Injury. In R.C. Lee (Ed.), *Electrical Trauma: Pathophysiology and Clinical Management*. London: Cambridge University Press, 1991.

Robson, M.C., and Smith, D.J. Burned Hand. In M.J. Jurkiewicz et al. (Eds.), *Plastic Surgery: Principles and Practice*. St. Louis: Mosby, 1990, Pp. 781–802.

Robson, M.C., Smith, D.J., Jr., and Heggers, J.P. Innovations in Burn Wound Management. In M.B. Habal et al. (Eds.), *Advances in Plastic Surgery*. Chicago: Year Book, 1987, Vol. 4, Pp. 149–176.

Zachary, L.S., et al. Treatment of experimental hydrofluoric acid burns. *J. Burn Care Rehabil.* 7: 35, 1986.

31

Radiation Injuries

Ross Rudolph

Clinical Findings

Patients with radiation skin injury continue to be seen by plastic surgeons in spite of improved techniques in radiation therapy. The overall incidence may be diminishing as radiation therapists become more sophisticated in ways to avoid skin injury. Because of a long lag time between exposure to radiation and skin ulceration, however, there exists a substantial population of patients who either have or will have radiation skin injury.

Typically visible skin damage develops 5 to 20 years after the radiation therapy, which was generally but not always given for a malignant tumor. Older techniques of radiation therapy, which delivered more radiation to the skin, appear to be more likely to cause such injury. Typically the acute injury to the skin at the time of treatment caused redness, skin blistering, and pain. This reaction resolved and was replaced later with fibrosis, telangiectasia, and hyperpigmentation. The radiation injury may produce a visible outline of the radiation therapy port. If it remains unchanged, this fibrotic skin reaction requires no treatment other than protection and lubrication. Unfortunately, however,

such radiation skin damage may be painful or can proceed to frank ulceration (Fig. 31-1).

Radiation skin ulcers have a deep punched-out appearance. Lined with shaggy and infected necrotic tissue, they are surrounded by a rim of inflamed and tender skin. Such ulcers are often quite painful. Underlying bone or cartilage may be exposed, particularly on the anterior chest. Hallmarks of such ulcers are their inability to heal spontaneously regardless of topical treatment and their tendency to worsen with time. Radiation injury to the skin requires surgical treatment when it becomes either painful or ulcerated, and the presence of severe and increasing pain demands a comprehensive approach.

Another postradiation concern for the surgeon is the inability of elective surgical incisions to heal. This is rarely a problem if the irradiated skin looks and feels normal. If the skin is thin, densely fibrotic, and telangiectatic, however, surgical incisions may dehisce, *especially if there is tension on the wound*. Operations on such visibly damaged skin should be avoided, if possible, but may be essential as for treatment of a tumor recurrence. If sur-

gical treatment is essential, wound closure tension must be avoided. Muscle or musculocutaneous flaps may be necessary for wound closure if tension is otherwise unavoidable.

The cause of chronic radiation skin damage has never been clearly delineated. Traditionally, radiation skin injury, skin ulceration, and inability to heal after an operation has been ascribed to a decreased blood supply. However, recent clinical studies demonstrating fluorescin perfusion of radiation ulcers and ongoing transcutaneous oxygen partial pressure measurement in irradiated patients suggest that a decreased blood supply may not be the only cause of radiation injury. Laboratory studies involving tissue culture, surgical delay of flaps within irradiated tissue, and electron microscopy of both human and experimental irradiated tissues have added weight to this hypothesis. Just as radiation therapy is designed to damage cancer cells permanently, so there may be injury to fibroblasts and endothelial cells and the stem cells for both lines. Such injury would reduce the ability of tissue to repair minor skin trauma. Fibroblast and endothelial stem cell injury may be at least as impor-

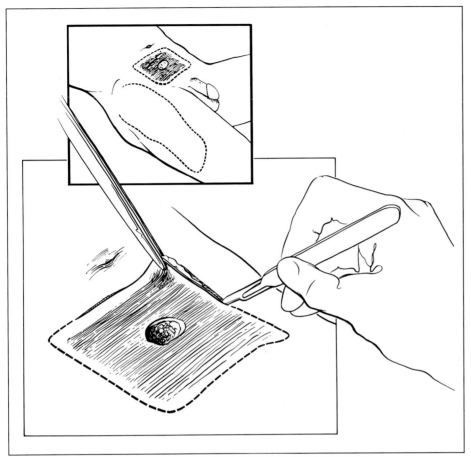

Fig. 31-1. Wide surgical excision of radiation ulcer and surrounding radiation-damaged tissue. Excision should extend beyond the visible radiation change and go into well-vascularized healthy bleeding tissue whenever possible. Immediate reconstruction should be planned.

tant as the reputed decreased blood supply in radiation injury.

The concept that irradiated skin is not hypoxic but rather contains damaged cells and their progenitors has allowed a modification of surgical strategy for dealing with irradiated skin. If such skin were uniformly hypoxic, *any* elective reconstructive technique would be avoided, especially those involving flaps and grafts. Yet it is possible to reconstruct a missing nipple and areola after partial mastectomy and irradiation, for example, using local flaps and full-thickness skin grafts with complete survival of these flaps and grafts. These procedures have succeeded when the irradiated breast tissue has a completely normal texture and appearance and should probably be avoided if the skin has visible radiation damage. The key to success of such procedures appears

to be the avoidance of wound closure tension. The irradiated but normal-appearing skin apparently is able to sustain local flaps and skin grafts (that is, it is not hypoxic) as long as tension is avoided. Radiation-damaged fibroblasts and their stem cells may not be able to repair wounds when tension exists that could be overcome in a nonirradiated wound with cells capable of normal repair.

Preoperative Management Techniques

Minimal management of a radiation injury falls into three main categories: (1) local treatment to prevent ulceration, (2) limited debridement of necrotic tissue to

reduce infection, and (3) hyperbaric oxygen treatment.

Local treatment of the radiation injury can be used when the skin is fibrotic and prone to minor breakdowns following trauma yet is not painful or progressively ulcerating. Preventive measures include appropriate padding and lubrication of the skin, because the lubricating sebaceous glands may not be functional in heavily irradiated skin. Small traumatic injuries to irradiated skin can be treated with topical cleansing and antibacterial ointments and may not progress to major wound breakdown.

If frank ulceration occurs, such ulcers often are filled with infected necrotic tissue. Limited local debridement of the necrotic tissue *without debriding into bleeding viable tissue* is appropriate to reduce the infection level. After debridement, topical agents such as half-strength Dakin solution (0.25%) or silver sulfadiazine applied twice a day reduce the bacterial count and the odor caused by infection of necrotic tissue. These measures are particularly appropriate in a dying patient with a radiation ulcer who is not a candidate for major surgical excision and reconstruction. Wide excision of the irradiated tissue into bleeding tissue should not be done without plans for *immediate* appropriate closure.

Hyperbaric oxygen has been championed by Marx, particularly for treatment of osteoradionecrosis of the mandible. Marx has shown improved healing in a large series of patients with osteoradionecrosis using hyperbaric oxygen treatments before and after surgical reconstruction. Although it is not always necessary, particularly if a skin and subcutaneous ulcer can be excised completely and covered promptly, hyperbaric oxygen has proved to be a valuable adjunct when underlying bone has undergone osteoradionecrosis. The hyperbaric oxygen appears to promote both local healing and the ability to accept reconstructive tissue such as grafted bone.

Definitive Surgical Treatment

For a patient with progressive painful ulceration following radiation therapy, surgical treatment is the only method of cure.

Excision

The first part of such treatment is complete surgical excision of the irradiated tissues. Not only the ulceration but also all visible tissue altered by radiation should be removed deep enough to uncover well-vascularized and bleeding tissue. The only exception to complete debridement occurs when the undersurface of the irradiated wound is composed of important structures such as the bladder, intestines, or major blood vessels, in which case complete excision cannot be done. Under these circumstances, the principle of "biologic scavenging" may be of benefit: Healthy tissue is placed on top of the wound still containing some radiation-damaged tissue.

In most instances, however, the surgeon should plan to remove the entire visibly irradiated area. When the radiation damage has been sufficient to cause ulceration, it usually is obvious where the extent of the radiation port was (see Fig. 31-1). When the radiation port is not apparent, experimental studies suggest that tissue culture comparing growth rate of fibroblasts from irradiated tissue with those of control tissue may be of help in determining the margin of irradiated tissue. In general, sufficient tissue for repair should be available so that a wide excision can be done. Infusion of fluorescin has *not* proved useful in delineating where the radiation injury stops, because the dye typically perfuses the entire irradiated ulcer.

Reconstruction

Reconstruction involves immediate coverage of the irradiated wound excision. Temporary wound dressings such as cadaveric allograft can be used, but they are not ideal; typically an excised irradiated wound continues to undergo necrosis unless immediately covered with live autogenous tissue.

Most irradiated wound problems occur on the anterior trunk or in the lower jaw and upper neck region. The musculocutaneous flap has become a mainstay of treatment, especially on the trunk. These flaps transfer a large volume of healthy nonirradiated tissue into the excised defect. Flaps should be selected that do not produce a large functional defect at the donor site.

Radiation injuries caused by breast irradiation on the upper anterior chest are repaired after excision with either a latissimus dorsi or a transversus abdominis musculocutaneous (TRAM) flap. When chest wall ulceration is present with exposure of bone or cartilage, many surgeons prefer the latissimus dorsi flap because it transfers a large muscle segment. In the lower jaw and upper neck region, pectoralis major musculocutaneous flaps have proved exceptionally safe and useful.

When musculocutaneous flaps are not available, free flaps involving microvascular anastomoses have proved useful. Particularly in the head and neck, such free flaps can include a vascularized bone graft when taken from areas such as the lateral lower leg, including the fibula, or from the iliac crest or scapular spine area. If a musculocutaneous flap is readily available, it may be selected because of its ease and safety. However, when microvascular free flaps are done frequently and bone is required, a free flap represents an excellent approach. A free flap has the additional potential advantage of being less bulky than a pectoralis major musculocutaneous flap, depending on the donor location.

Another potential flap, particularly for a chest or upper abdominal defect in a patient who has not had a previous abdominal operation, is made from omentum. This well-vascularized tissue can be brought out over synthetic mesh and covered with a split-thickness skin graft.

A third common area for radiation ulcers, besides the breast and head and neck areas, is the lower abdomen or groin after pelvic irradiation. The tensor fasciae latae flap is particularly useful for this location. The flap transfers a large area of healthy tissue with almost no functional loss.

The tensor fasciae latae muscle is a thin, small flat muscle on the lateral thigh. As noted by Mathes and Nahai, this muscle allows transfer of an unusually large cutaneous area in relation to its size. The muscle originates from the outer iliac crest and is supplied by the transverse branch of the lateral circumflex femoral artery. The blood supply is a dominant single pedicle 8 to 10 cm below the anterior superior iliac spine.

Figures 31-2 and 31-3 demonstrate the use of a tensor fasciae latae flap for reconstruction of a lower anterior abdominal radiation ulcer. The ulcer and surrounding radiation port are completely removed (see Fig. 32-1), and hemostasis is obtained. The tensor fasciae latae musculocutaneous flap is elevated from distal to proximal on its proximal vascular pedicle (see Fig. 32-2). The skin is incised distally and the fascia lata identified. Dissection of the fascia lata and skin as a unit proceeds proximally. The rotation point is approximately 10 cm below the anterior superior iliac spine, and the feeding vessel into the muscle must be preserved. It is not necessary to dissect as far proximally as the vessel pedicle if the flap rotates easily with less proximal dissection.

Adequate flap length *must* be planned to reach the entire excision site *without tension*. The elevated flap, composed of tensor fasciae latae muscle, fascia lata, and overlying subcutaneous tissue and skin is rotated anteriorly 90° into the defect. Although not shown in Figure 31-2, which involves rotation of the entire flap, an island pedicle can be used to avoid a prominent proximal dog-ear if an excellent blood supply is ensured. The donor site may be closed primarily in some patients, but the patient in Figures 31-2 and 31-3 required a split-thickness skin graft.

In planning a musculocutaneous flap repair of a radiation ulcer, tension on the closure site must be prevented. Adequate flap length and mobility are essential to allow the flap to sit comfortably into the defect. The pull of gravity on an edematous flap can cause it to separate from the residual irradiated wound bed. Hence flaps should be designed to avoid the traction of gravity. For example, a pectoralis musculocutaneous flap to the lower jaw should be an island flap, with the muscle pedicle supported by a local skin bridge, rather than being totally external and hanging from the recipient site.

Local skin flaps, whether delayed or not, and skin grafts should be avoided in reconstructing radiation ulcers. Such local flaps and grafts have a high failure rate, although they are successful in reconstructing irradiated tissues that appear normal. This failure of grafts and local flaps is probably caused by tension on flaps and the parasitic nature of skin grafts on the irradiated wound bed. Even

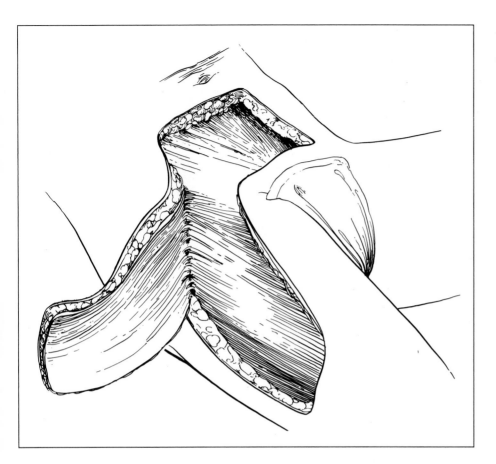

Fig. 31-2. Elevation of a tensor fascia lata musculocutaneous flap to be transferred into the defect made by excision of a radiation ulcer.

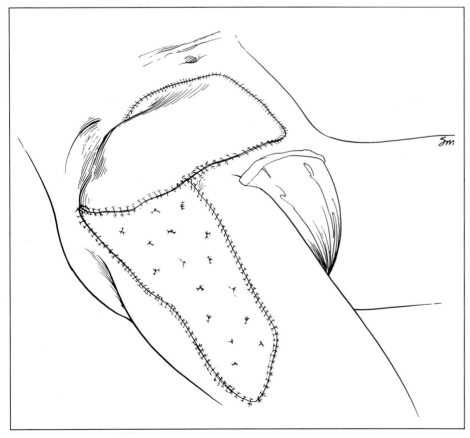

Fig. 31-3. Completed transfer of tensor fasciae latae musculocutaneous flap. Donor site has split-thickness skin grafts harvested from the contralateral thigh and buttock.

musculocutaneous or free flaps should be designed to be nonparasitic; that is, they should bring and maintain a permanent blood supply rather than having to be divided later.

Postoperative Care

Because cellular dysfunction is probably an important cause of radiation ulceration and poor wound healing, provision of cellular nutrition is also important. In the repair of a radiation ulcer, a high-protein, high-calorie diet is advisable. Patients with radiation ulcers are often debilitated and malnourished. In addition to protein and carbohydrate supplementation, administration of vitamins B and C and of zinc may improve healing. Rather than testing for low levels of vitamins and zinc, it is usually advisable to provide such supplementation empirically with the expectation that levels of these nutrients will be low (or low normal). Finally, avoidance of smoking by the patient and the administration of nasal oxygen, 3 to 4 liters per minute at normal atmospheric pressure, may be helpful. These measures increase the oxygen partial pressure and its effect on collagen synthesis in the newly repaired wound, as shown conclusively by Hunt. Broad-spectrum antibiotics should be used because radiation ulcers are invariably reported to be infected when excised.

Conclusion

Older techniques of radiation therapy for malignant tumors often produce radiation skin damage. Initially the only problems may be dense fibrosis, pigment changes, and telangiectasia, but these conditions may proceed to painful and progressive ulceration. Management may include gentle debridement of necrotic tissue and administration of hyperbaric oxygen. In most instances, definitive wide excision of the entire irradiated field and area of ulceration is required with coverage using musculocutaneous or free flaps with an excellent blood supply that can provide nonirradiated tissue for healing. Attention to nutrition and oxygenation is an important ancillary measure.

Suggested Reading

Marino, H. Biologic excision: Its value in the treatment of radionecrotic lesions. *Plast. Reconstr. Surg.* 40:180, 1967.

Marx, R.E., and Johnson, R.P. Studies in the radiobiology of osteoradionecrosis and their clinical significance. *Oral Surg.* 64:379, 1987.

Mathes, S.J., and Nahai, F. *Clinical Atlas of Muscle and Musculocutaneous Flaps.* St. Louis: Mosby, 1979. Pp. 63–85.

Rudolph, R. Complications of surgery for radiotherapy skin damage. *Plast. Reconstr. Surg.* 70:179, 1982.

Rudolph, R. Radiation Ulcers. In R. Rudolph and J.M. Noe (Eds.), *Chronic Problem Wounds.* Boston: Little, Brown, 1983. Pp. 87–94.

Rudolph, R., and Hunt, T.K. Healing in Compromised Tissues. In R. Rudolph (Ed.), *Problems in Aesthetic Surgery*: Biological Causes and Clinical Solutions. St. Louis: Mosby, 1986. Pp. 65–98.

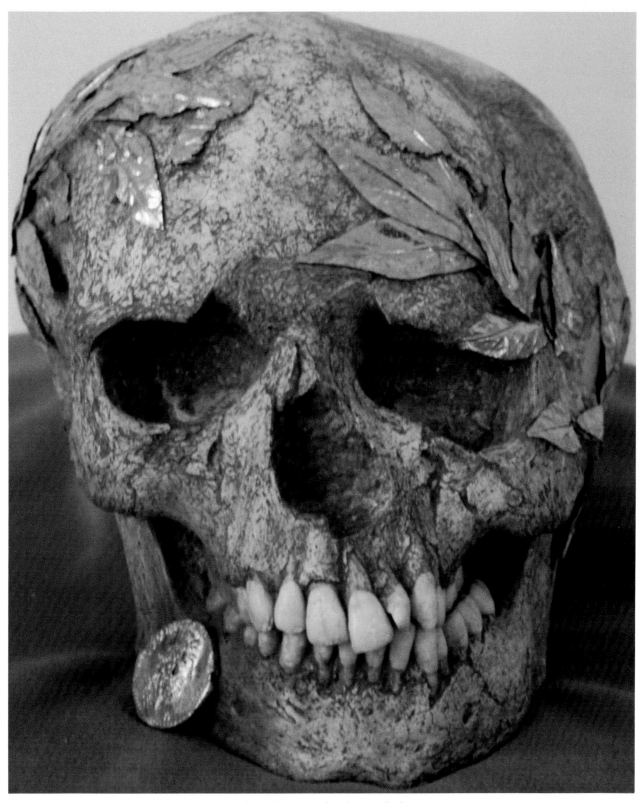

Skull of an athlete crowned with a wreath of golden olive branches. A silver coin has been placed in the mouth as the fare for the trip to the underworld, circa 37 A.D. Aghios Nicolaos Archaeologic Museum. Aghios, Nicolaos, Crete, Greece. Reprinted with permission.

III

Head and Neck

Congenital Anomalies

32

Craniofacial Embryology

Robert M. Greene   Wayde M. Weston

It is of course impossible in the space of one short (or even long) chapter to discuss the many facets of normal embryology of the head and neck. Such a treatise would include a description of the embryogenesis of the bony cranium, the pharyngeal arches, the teeth, the ear, the eye, and the central nervous system. Several discussions of these topics exist; the reader is referred to Sadler [67] and Moore [55], who provide excellent overviews of craniofacial embryogenesis.

The purpose of this chapter is, first, briefly present the normal embryogenesis of the human midfacial region with emphasis on the development of the primary and secondary palates and, second, to provide readers unfamiliar with cellular and molecular aspects of the developing orofacial region an up-to-date construct of what we currently understand to be the facts in the field as they relate to normal and abnormal craniofacial development.

Origins and Early Migrations of Facial Tissues

During the third week of human development, the embryo consists of two epithelial sheets of cells, or germ layers—the hypoblast (endoderm) atop of which lies the epiblast (ectoderm). A third germ layer is formed by mass migration of epiblast cells toward and into a midline groove, the primitive streak (Fig. 32-1). These cells migrate between the epiblast and hypoblast and form the mesoderm. Cells that migrate anteriorly give rise to the notochord, whereas cells located adjacent to the notochord proliferate and give rise to the paraxial mesoderm. In the head, these cells form most of the skeleton and connective tissue of the brain and skull. More laterally, the mesodermal layer is called lateral plate mesoderm and is represented in the developing face as the cells forming the pharyngeal arches.

Under the inductive influence of the notochord, the ectoderm overlying the notochord thickens to form the neural plate (Fig. 32-2). By the end of the third week of development, the lateral edges of the neural plate elevate as the neural folds (Fig. 32-3), which approach one another and fuse in the region of the future neck. This fusion proceeds in a cephalic and caudal direction, thereby forming the neural tube (Fig. 32-4). As the neural folds fuse, a population of cells, the neural crest, leaves the lateral border of the neurectoderm, undergoes extensive migrations throughout the embryo, and gives rise to an extensive array of tissues [43].

In the development of the head and neck, paraxial mesoderm gives rise to the cranial base, all voluntary muscle of the craniofacial region, and most of the meninges. Lateral plate mesoderm forms the laryngeal cartilages (arytenoid and cricoid) and associated connective tissue. Cranial neural crest cells migrate into the pharyngeal arches and into the facial region (Fig. 32-5), where they form the mandible and skeleton of the midface and all the cartilage, bone, sensory neurons, glandular stroma, dermis, and dentin in this region. A unique feature of embryonic facial development is that one of the functions performed by mesoderm in other parts of the body, the formation of the skeleton and connective tissue, is performed by the neural crest cells.

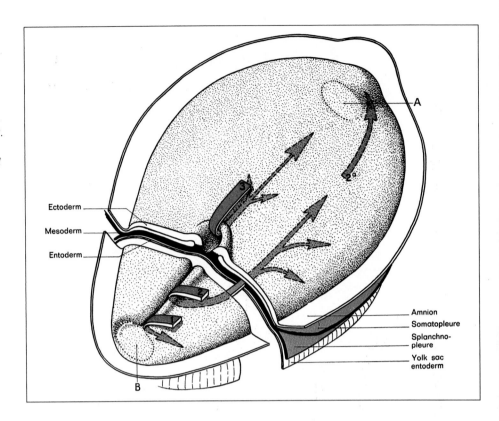

Fig. 32-1. Schematic representation of a dorsal view of a human embryo during the fifteenth to sixteenth day of development depicting cell migration at the time of gastrulation. Arrows indicate the direction of ectodermal cell movements. A and B indicate the regions of the future pharyngeal (A) and cloacal (B) membranes. (From H. Tuchmann-Duplessis, G. David, and P. Haegel. Illustrated Human Embryology. Vol. 1. Heidelberg: Springer, 1972. P. 21. Reproduced with permission.)

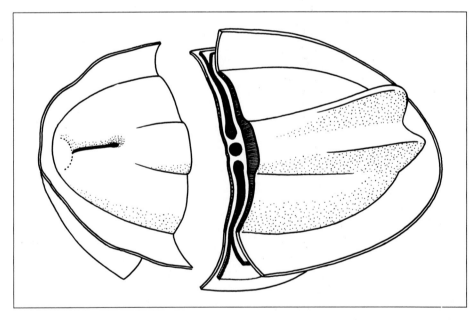

Fig. 32-2. Schematic representation of a dorsal view of a human embryo during the eighteenth day of development depicting the thickened ectodermal neural plate in the midline. (From H. Tuchmann-Duplessis, G. David, and P. Haegel. Illustrated Human Embryology. Vol. 1. Heidelberg: Springer, 1972. P. 30. Reproduced with permission.)

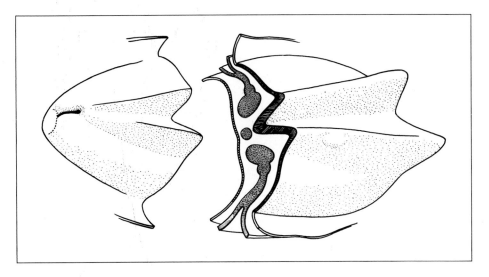

Fig. 32-3. Schematic representation of a dorsal view of a human embryo during the twentieth day of development depicting the elevation of the lateral edges of the neural plate as neural folds. (From H. Tuchmann-Duplessis, G. David, and P. Haegel. Illustrated Human Embryology. *Vol. 1. Heidelberg: Springer, 1972. P. 30. Reproduced with permission.*)

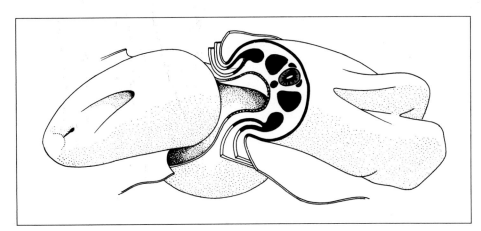

Fig. 32-4. Schematic representation of a dorsal view of a human embryo during approximately the twenty-second day of development depicting closure of the neural axis in the middle portion of the embryo to form a neural tube. The anterior and posterior ends of the neuraxis remain open as the anterior and posterior neuropores, respectively. (From H. Tuchmann-Duplessis, G. David, and P. Haegel. Illustrated Human Embryology. *Vol. 1. Heidelberg: Springer, 1972. P. 32. Reproduced with permission.*)

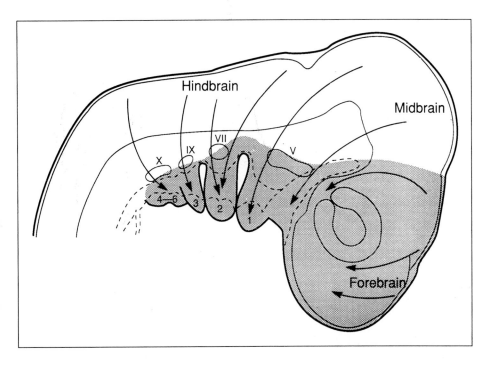

Fig. 32-5. Schematic representation of the migration pathways (arrows) of neural crest cells from fore-, mid-, and hindbrain regions into their final locations (shaded areas) in the pharyngeal arches and face. (Reproduced with permission from Langman's Medical Embryology (6th ed.). Baltimore: Williams & Wilkins, 1990. P. 298. © 1990, the Williams & Wilkins Co., Baltimore.)

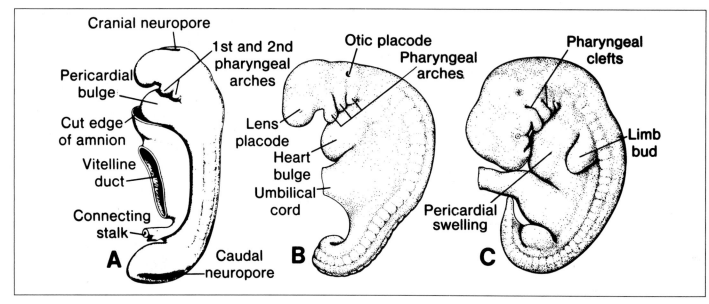

Fig. 32-6. Schematic representation of a series of human embryos depicting development of the pharyngeal arches. A. Approximately 25 days. B. 28 days. C. 5 weeks. (Reproduced with permission from Langman's Medical Embryology (6th ed.). Baltimore: Williams & Wilkins, 1990. P. 299. © 1990, the Williams & Wilkins Co., Baltimore.)

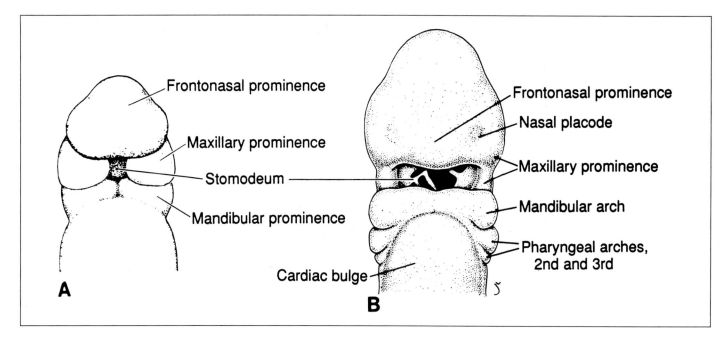

Fig. 32-7A. Schematic representation of a frontal view of an embryo of approximately 24 days. The stomodeum is surrounded by the frontonasal, maxillary, and mandibular prominences. B. A slightly older embryo. (Reproduced with permission from Langman's Medical Embryology (6th ed.). Baltimore: Williams & Wilkins, 1990. P. 301. © 1990, the Williams & Wilkins Co., Baltimore.)

Pharyngeal Arches

During the fourth and fifth weeks of embryonic development, a series of ridges (pharyngeal arches) separated by grooves (pharyngeal clefts) appears on the ventrolateral surface of the head region (Fig. 32-6). In humans, five branchial arches, separated by four grooves, develop in sequence. Each arch contains a cartilaginous core, an aortic arch, and a specific cranial nerve destined to supply the structures derived from the arch. At the same position as the ectodermal invagination of each pharyngeal cleft, the endoderm of the pharynx exhibits laterally directed evaginations called pharyngeal pouches, which normally do not establish continuous lumina with corresponding clefts.

The pharyngeal arches make major contributions to the embryonic development of both the head and the neck. The midfacial region, which develops mainly be-

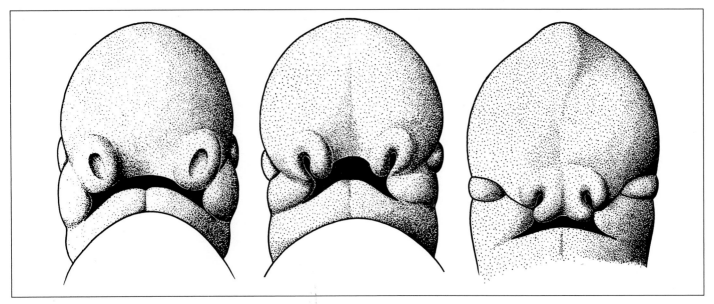

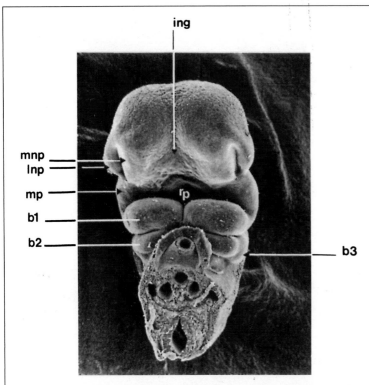

Fig. 32-8. Schematic representation of a frontal view of the developing embryonic orofacial region during the fourth to fifth week of gestation when the nasal placodes have appeared (left), the fifth to sixth week of gestation when the nasal pits form (middle), and the sixth to seventh week of gestation when the nasal cavities form (right). (From H. Tuchmann-Duplessis, G. David, and P. Haegel. Illustrated Human Embryology. Vol. 2. Heidelberg: Springer, 1972. P. 13. Reproduced with permission.)

Fig. 32-9. Scanning electron micrograph of a rat embryo 11.9 days postconception. Nasal placodes have been transformed into nasal grooves by the medial nasal (mnp), lateral nasal (lnp), and maxillary processes (mp). b = branchial arch 1–3; rp = Rathke pouch; ing = internasal groove. (From C. Vermeij-Keers. Craniofacial Embryology and Morphogenesis: Normal and Abnormal. In M. Stricker et al. (Eds.), Craniofacial Malformations. Edinburgh: Churchill Livingstone, 1990. P. 32. Reproduced with permission.)

tween the fourth and eighth weeks of gestation, arises largely from the first pharyngeal arch, which contains cells derived from the lateral plate mesoderm and mesenchymal cells derived from the cranial neural crest. For an excellent discussion of the specific nervous, muscular, and skeletal derivatives of each pharyngeal arch and of the epithelial derivatives of the pharyngeal clefts, the reader is referred to Sadler [67]. With regard to the face proper, the first pharyngeal arch bi-furcates into maxillary and mandibular processes, which flank the stomodeum, or future oral cavity (Fig. 32-7). By the end of the fourth week of development, an anterior view of the developing face presents a midline frontonasal prominence and paired maxillary and mandibular prominences (Fig. 32-7). The nasal placodes arise as bilateral thickenings of the surface ectoderm of the frontonasal prominence. During the fifth week of development, nasal pits bounded by the me-dial and lateral nasal processes develop (Figs. 32-8 and 32-9). During the fifth and sixth weeks of development, the maxillary processes enlarge; grow medially, compressing the medial nasal processes toward the midline; and fuse with these processes (Figs. 32-8 and 32-10). Thus the upper lip is formed by the two maxillary and two medial nasal processes. The two merged medial nasal processes form not only a portion of the upper lip but also, within the oral cavity, the portion of the

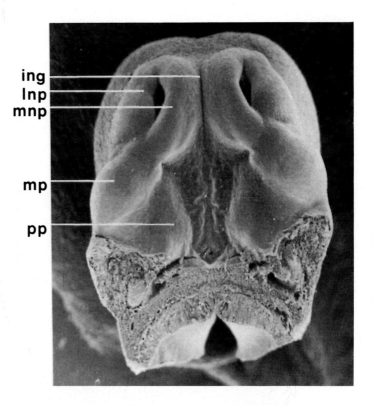

Fig. 32-10. Scanning electron micrograph of a rat embryo 13 days postconception. Inferior view of the roof of the oral cavity (tongue and mandible removed). pp = palatine process; ing = internasal groove; lnp = lateral nasal process; mnp = medial nasal process; mp = maxillary process. (From C. Vermeij-Keers. Craniofacial Embryology and Morphogenesis: Normal and Abnormal. In M. Stricker et al. (Eds.), Craniofacial Malformations. Edinburgh: Churchill Livingstone, 1990. P. 39. Reproduced with permission.)

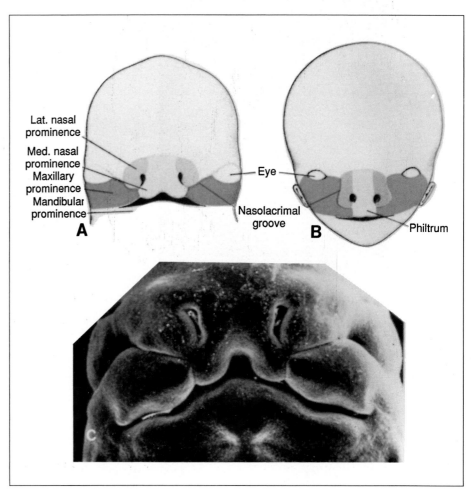

Fig. 32-11. Frontal aspect of the face. A. Seven-week embryo. The maxillary prominences have fused with the medial nasal prominences. B. Ten-week embryo. C. Scanning electron micrograph of a mouse embryo at a similar stage to A. (Reproduced with permission from Langman's Medical Embryology (6th ed.). Baltimore: Williams & Wilkins, 1990. P. 316. © 1990, the Williams & Wilkins Co., Baltimore.)

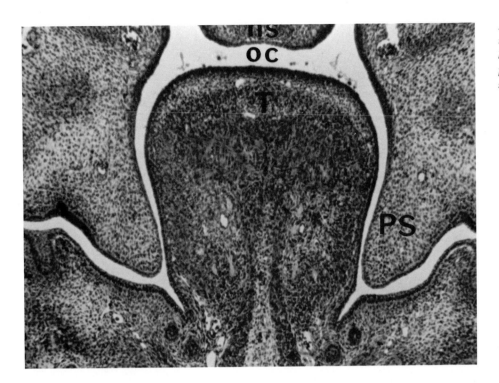

Fig. 32-12. Photomicrograph of a coronal section through a fixed, Paraplast-embedded, fetal mouse head demonstrating the relation of the vertical palatal shelves (PS) to the tongue (T) and nasal septum (NS). OC = oral cavity. (×20.)

maxilla containing the four incisor teeth and the primary palate (Fig. 32-11).

The lateral nasal processes initially are separated from the maxillary processes by the nasolacrimal groove (see Fig. 32-11), which in adults forms the nasolacrimal duct connecting the medial corner of the eye with the inferior meatus in the nasal cavity. The lateral nasal processes ultimately form the sides of the nose. The lower lip and mandible are formed by the mandibular prominence of the first pharyngeal arch during the fourth week of gestation. Subsequent to these events, mesenchyme from the second branchial arch invades the maxillary and mandibular arches and differentiates into the muscles of facial expression, which are innervated by the facial nerve (CN VII), the nerve of the second arch.

During the seventh week of gestation in humans, the secondary palate originates as bilateral extensions from the oral aspect of each maxillary process. These extensions, termed *palatal processes*, first grow vertically on either side of the tongue (Fig. 32-12) then undergo a series of movements that result in their fusion with one another, with the primary palate anteriorly, and with the nasal septum superiorly (Figs. 32-13 and 32-14). Although

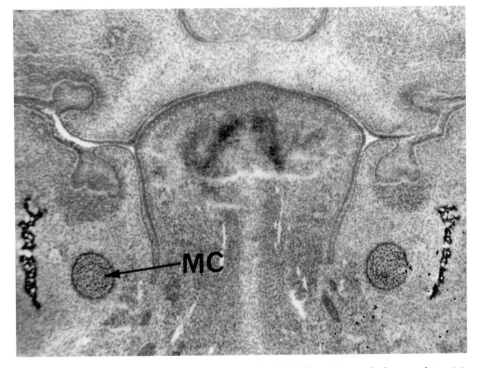

Fig. 32-13. Photomicrograph of a coronal cryostat section through an unfixed frozen fetal mouse head demonstrating homologous palatal shelves above the tongue and in contact with one another and the nasal septum. MC = Meckel cartilage. (×12.5.)

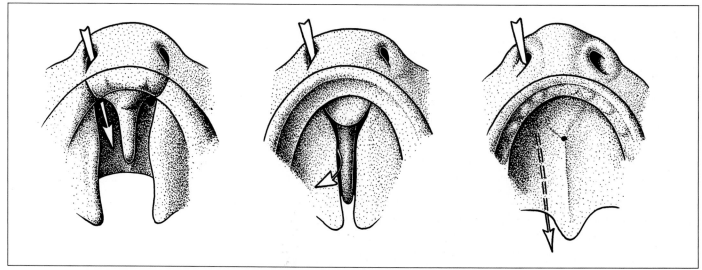

Fig. 32-14. Schematic representation of a ventral view of the developing human oronasal cavity with the tongue and mandible removed. The palatal shelves are depicted as lateral to the intervening tongue (left) and perpendicular to the plane of the page; superior to the tongue (middle) and parallel to the plane of the page; and fused with each other and the primary palate to give rise to the definitive adult palate (right). (From H. Tuchmann-Duplessis, G. David, and P. Haegel. Illustrated Human Embryology. Vol. 2. Heidelberg: Springer, 1972. P. 17. Reproduced with permission.)

the precise mechanisms responsible for movement of the palatal processes are not known, current thinking focuses on a functional role for extracellular matrix components or intracellular contractile elements, or both.

Palatal ontogeny also depends on differential, temporal, and spatial patterns of cell proliferation. The importance of proper quantitative and spatiotemporal growth in the craniofacial region is illustrated by the fact that inhibition of palatal mesenchymal cell proliferation or of normal craniofacial growth can result in a cleft palate [28]. For an excellent review of growth during craniofacial development, the reader is referred to Stricker et al. [76].

Cells of the medial edge epithelium (MEE) of the approximating palatal shelves undergo a precise sequence of changes, including cessation of DNA synthesis, synthesis of cell surface adhesive glycoconjugates, autolytic degeneration of some of these cells [29], and transformation of others into mesenchyme [21], allowing confluence of the mesenchyme from adjacent palatal processes. The future hard palate becomes ossified by intramembranous bone formation followed by bony invasion from the maxilla. This sequence of events gives rise to the secondary palate, or roof of the oral cavity.

Molecular Determinants of Craniofacial Development

As mentioned, the embryology of the craniofacial region has been amply described. However, in part because of the complexity of facial morphogenesis, a satisfactory understanding of the molecular determinants governing facial development has yet to be achieved. The powerful force of reductionism in biology results from the need to understand biologic phenomena at a more basic level. Past morphologic and biochemical analyses have provided fascinating insights regarding control of cellular growth and differentiation of embryonic orofacial tissue. The conceptual chasm between the gene and metazoan embryogenesis is rapidly narrowing as advances in molecular analysis of gene function in the embryo provide a greater understanding of the molecular aspects of normal and abnormal craniofacial ontogeny [72, 73].

Regulatory Signaling Molecules

Cyclic Adenosine Monophosphate
A substantial body of data has developed suggesting that normal growth and dif-

ferentiation of embryonic palatal tissue depend on the presence and interaction of various hormones and growth factors regulating intracellular levels of cyclic adenosine monophosphate (cAMP). Additionally, a positive correlation has been demonstrated between teratogenic agents and mutant genes known to adversely affect palatal development and alterations in palatal cAMP levels [26, 32, 58].

The singular role of intracellular cAMP is to activate cAMP-dependent protein kinases (cAMP-dPK) (EC 2.7.1.37) that act to mediate the biologic activities of cAMP by catalyzing the phosphorylation of specific cellular proteins. Despite the similarities among tissue cAMP-dPKs, the physiologic actions of cAMP are diverse. Changing levels or the cellular and subcellular distribution of cAMP-dPKs may account for the multiplicity of cellular responses to cAMP. Indeed, analysis of cAMP-dPK isozyme ratios during the period of palatal ontogeny reveals striking temporal alterations [46] that reflect alterations in steady-state levels of mRNAs for individual cAMP-dPK subunits [27] and alterations in cellular localization of the enzymes [47]. The complex regulatory ability of this family of enzymes was highlighted by studies involving cDNA cloning and sequencing, which indicate the existence of four different regulatory subunits, RIα [45, 68], RIβ, RIIα [69], and RIIβ [39], and three different catalytic subunits, Cα, Cβ, and Cγ [8, 14, 78]. Thus the particular combination of subunits expressed and available for cAMP binding and subsequent protein phosphorylation may be critical in defining a specific cellular response.

The additional specificity of cAMP action is thought to reside in the specific endogenous substrate proteins phosphorylated by cAMP-dPK inasmuch as they represent the final effectors for some of the cAMP-mediated actions in embryonic craniofacial tissue. For example, the means by which cellular regulatory signals affect gene expression has been clarified by the identification of sequence-specific DNA-binding proteins that associate with specific cis-acting elements and mediate a transcriptional response to signaling molecules such as cAMP. In mammalian cells, a conserved cis-acting cAMP-response element (CRE) with enhancer characteristics has been identified in the promoter of several cAMP-regulated genes. The linkage among cAMP, cAMP-dPK, and the activation of specific genes in mammalian cells is mediated by one or more trans-acting DNA-binding proteins that recognize this CRE [52]. This CRE-binding transcription factor (CREBP) is a substrate for cAMP-dPK [25], such that phosphorylation of CREBP increases transcription of cAMP-regulated genes [42, 52]. Thus, depending on flanking sequences, the CRE is likely to be the target sequence for a diversity of binding proteins, suggesting that the CRE motif could serve multiple regulatory functions.

Protein Kinase C

Receptor-mediated hydrolysis of inositol phospholipids is a common means for the transduction of extracellular signals into the cell. Hydrolysis of phosphatidylinositol 4,5-bisphosphate (PIP_2) results in the intracellular release of two second messengers, inositol triphosphate and diacylglycerol (DAG). Inositol triphosphate mediates Ca^{2+} mobilization from intracellular stores [10, 11], whereas DAG activates protein kinase C [56]. Both have a transient existence and are rapidly degraded but not before eliciting dramatic effects on cellular metabolism. Cellular responses may be immediate, such as secretion of cellular constituents, or long-term, such as alterations in gene expression and cell proliferation. The multiplicity of these responses was reviewed by Nishizuka [57].

Hydrolysis of inositol phospholipids also may be a metabolic process that is critical for ensuring proper growth and differentiation of embryonic orofacial tissue. Support for such a hypothesis comes from evidence that phosphatidylinositol metabolism in embryonic palatal mesenchymal cells can be modulated by corticoids [30] and that some prostaglandins, important factors in palatal tissue differentiation, also stimulate phosphatidylinositol turnover [49].

The cells of most tissues transduce information across the plasma membrane either by the generation of cAMP or the induction of a rapid turnover of inositol phospholipids. Although protein kinase C and cAMP-dependent protein kinase transmit information along different intracellular signal pathways, similar cellular responses are often evoked [10]. Moreover, these two enzymes often phosphorylate the same proteins [40]. An intriguing possibility is that these two pathways, both operative in cells of the embryonic palate, cooperate positively to amplify cellular responses or developmental processes during orofacial ontogeny.

Growth Factors

Much of organogenesis is thought to involve the actions of locally derived factors that regulate cell proliferation and differentiation. Among the classic growth factors, only epidermal growth factor (EGF) has been investigated extensively as a possible regulatory molecule in palatal ontogenesis. Current evidence supporting the hypothesis that EGF or a related peptide—transforming growth factor-alpha (TGF-α)—modulates development of the secondary palate has been reviewed [62]. More recent studies have demonstrated the presence of several other growth factors and their messenger RNAs (mRNAs) in the tissues of developing craniofacial structures [7, 22, 34, 44, 60, 61, 77].

Normal growth of the entire craniofacial region is critical for proper development of the palate in both humans and laboratory animals. Normal development of the mammalian secondary palate depends particularly on differential patterns of cell proliferation, which vary both temporally and spatially within the palatal processes. The action of transforming growth factors–beta-1 and –beta-2 (TGF-β1, TGF-β2), which are present in developing orofacial tissue [60, 61], is in part characterized by changes in the expression of growth regulatory genes. Transforming growth factor–beta either stimulates or inhibits proliferation depending on the cell type and the presence of other growth factors. These polypeptide signaling molecules, together with fibroblast growth factor [63], therefore may represent local regulators of embryonic craniofacial cellular proliferation.

Both the temporal and the spatial distribution of extracellular matrix components are known to play a critical role in the normal ontogeny of the mammalian palate. Glycosaminoglycans (GAGs), primarily hyaluronic acid and chondroitin sulfate, and collagen, tenascin, and fibronectin are distributed throughout the mesenchymal core of the palate [33, 38, 70]. Transforming growth factor–beta-1 (TGF-β1) has been shown to increase expression of genes encoding collagen [37], GAGs [6], fibronectin [18], and tenascin [59]. Indeed, TGF-β was able to stimulate GAG production synergistically in murine embryonic palatal mesenchymal cells [16]. Thus TGF-β may also act to regulate extracellular matrix metabolism by neural crest cells as they migrate into the branchial arches.

Localization of TGF-β isoforms and their mRNAs appears to change temporally throughout development in a manner consistent with a role for the protein in mediating epithelial-mesenchymal interactions [1, 22, 34, 51, 61]. The importance of these interactions has been established in the developing palate: In a series of recombination studies, mesenchyme exhibited a regional control on the overlying epithelium [19]. The tissue-specific localization of both TGF-β protein and mRNA suggests a role for these molecules in morphogenesis and tissue differentiation. Although the pattern of localization for the TGF-βs in organs and tissues undergoing epithelial-mesenchymal interactions suggests paracrine regulation, the precise way in which TGF-β exerts its effects remains to be determined. These observations, combined with the demonstration that TGF-β can regulate various aspects of mandibular development [74], suggest a critical role for this paracrine-autocrine factor in craniofacial ontogeny.

Epithelial-Mesenchymal Interactions

It is well documented that the epithelia of many developing organs depend on tissue interactions with adjacent mesenchyme. The reciprocity of this interaction is well illustrated in developing palatal tissue. Viability [66], proliferation [4], and chondrogenic and osteogenic differentiation [31, 79] of mesenchymal components in the developing facial region require reciprocal interaction with epithelia. Using homologous, heterologous, heterochronic, and isochronic combinations of embryonic mandibular and palatal tissue, Ferguson and Honig [19] demonstrated that palatal MEE differentiation is specified by the underlying mesenchyme and that signaling of MEE differentiation occurs in a species-specific manner.

Although the nature of putative signaling molecules in the embryonic craniofacial region is not known definitively, available evidence allows consideration of several candidates. Embryonic palatal tissue grown in organ culture exhibits epithelial differentiation identical to that seen in vitro [71, 75] and embryonic mouse first branchial arch tissues differentiate into cartilage, bone, and tooth in vitro in serumless, chemically defined medium [74], indicating that locally derived autocrine or paracrine factors or both are involved in the induction of tissue differentiation. Epidermal growth factor has been shown to influence mouse palatal MEE differentiation by action on the underlying mesenchyme [81]. Studies have demonstrated the presence of several additional locally derived growth factors in the tissues of developing craniofacial structures [7, 22, 34, 44, 60, 61, 77]. One of these, TGF-β, can stimulate the synthesis of the molecules of the extracellular matrix, fibronectin, type IV collagen, and hyaluronic acid by palatal mesenchymal cells [16, 70]. In other systems, it can stimulate epithelial cells to synthesize receptors for some of these molecules. Thus interaction between epithelium and mesenchyme in the embryonic palate may be under the control of TGF-β by modulation of the extracellular matrix and other growth factors.

Homeobox-Containing Genes

Several genes thought to be important in orchestrating embryonic development have been isolated on the basis of their homology to motifs within *Drosophila* control genes or human transcription factor genes. One such example is the homeobox (Hox) gene family, members of which are expressed with spatial and temporal specificity during development. Several transcription factors are encoded by homeobox genes, suggesting that a general function of homeodomain proteins is to regulate transcription. A homeobox is a 183 bp region that encodes a DNA-binding domain present in three major classes (maternal effect, segmentation, and homeotic) of developmental control genes in *Drosophila* [24]. The cloning and characterization of one maternal effect gene in *Drosophila*, the gene *bicoid (bcd)*, has occasioned much excitement inasmuch as its product, the *bicoid*-encoded homeodomain protein, may play a key role in embryonic development of the head. Maternal effect genes specify the anteroposterior polarity of the multicellular zygote. Several *bcd*-activated homeobox genes, specifying patterned domains in the embryonic head, have been identified, and it is thought that these genes control development of the head [15, 20].

Little is known regarding the function of vertebrate homeogenes, although studies involving microinjection of specific mRNAs and gene transfer experiments using transgenic mouse technology promise to offer insights into molecular regulatory mechanisms operative during embryogenesis. Indeed, some studies already have offered fascinating glimpses into the molecular control of craniofacial development. Ectopic overexpression of Xhox-3 in the anterior region of frog embryos, achieved by microinjection of Xhox-3 mRNA, resulted in abnormal development of the anterior embryonic structures [64]; ectopic expression of the Hox 1.1 gene in anterior structures of transgenic mice also resulted in craniofacial malformations [5]. In the latter study a combination of craniofacial anomalies similar to retinoic acid–induced embryopathy was noted. Moreover, retinoic acid, a human craniofacial teratogen, induces the expression of many homeobox-containing genes, including Hox 1.1 [50]. These data therefore collectively suggest

that induced expression of these homeogenes in cranial regions, where they are not normally expressed, interferes with normal embryogenesis of cranial structures and that retinoic acid–induced craniofacial embryopathy may involve ectopic expression of homeobox-containing genes.

Neural crest cells, as already discussed, play a critical role in normal craniofacial ontogeny. The generation of transgenic mice bearing random integrations of transgenes in their genomes has provided direct experimental evidence for a possible functional role of neural crest cells in craniofacial development. The abnormalities seen in the Hox-1.1 gain-of-function transgenic mutant described earlier [5] are thought to be caused by the disruption of cranial neural crest migration into, or function within, the first branchial arch. This implicates cranial neural crest cells as potential targets for Hox gene function. The generation of transgenic mice, in which overexpression of the Hox-1.4 gene provided a gain-of-function mutant exhibiting megacolon [80], thought to be caused by a lack of neural crest–derived enteric ganglia, additionally supports this notion. The expression of a new mouse Hox locus, Hox-7, in the mesenchyme of embryonic mandibular and hyoid arches and in cephalic neural crest cells [9, 35] will no doubt accelerate the search for a functional role of Hox genes and neural crest cells. Whether homeobox-containing genes do indeed play a role in anteroposterior positional specification in the cranial region [36] or have other equally important regulatory functions is a fascinating question only now being explored.

Molecular Genetic Approaches

The frequency of cleft lip with or without cleft palate is approximately 1 in 800. Genetic factors are thought to play an important role in the etiology of this defect because the risk of recurrence of cleft lip and palate (CL/P) is nearly 40-fold greater in siblings of people with CL/P than in the general population. Several reports describe cleft palate as X-linked [12, 13, 48, 65]. Additional evidence for this mode of inheritance of cleft palate comes from the use of restriction fragment length polymorphisms (RFLPs) for linkage studies.

In one such study, cleft palate and ankyloglossia (CP/A) was mapped to the q13 to q21 region of the X chromosome [53], and of late CP/A has been even more precisely mapped on the X chromosome [54]. An association has been found between two RFLPs at the TGF-α gene locus and the occurrence of clefting in patients with nonsyndromic CL/P [3]. This finding suggests that either the TGF-α gene or the adjoining DNA sequences also contribute to CL/P in humans.

Reverse genetics has become a powerful molecular tool with which to investigate inherited single-gene disorders in humans. This approach involves mapping a gene to a particular chromosome, cloning the DNA sequence related to the gene, and finally using the DNA sequence data to identify the protein encoded by that gene. Thus one can acquire knowledge of the protein that may be altered in a particular disease state. The gene for Duchenne muscular dystrophy has been mapped [17] and sequenced [41] and the protein product identified [2] by these reverse genetic techniques. Identification of the chromosomal localization of genes associated with specific craniofacial malformations such as CP/A [53] and Stickler syndrome [23] provides the first step toward isolation of the gene and related protein products responsible for these disorders. Such studies afford exciting new opportunities to understand the pathogenesis of various craniofacial dysmorphologies.

References

1. Akhurst, R., et al. TGF-beta in murine morphogenetic processes: The early embryo and cardiogenesis. *Development* 108:645, 1990.
2. Arahata, K., et al. Immunostaining of skeletal and cardiac muscle surface membrane with antibody against the Duchenne muscular dystrophy peptide. *Nature* 333:861, 1988.
3. Ardinger, H., et al. Association of genetic variation of the transforming growth factor-alpha gene with cleft lip and palate. *Am. J. Hum. Genet.* 45:348, 1989.
4. Bailey, L., Minkoff, R., and Koch, W. Relative growth rates of maxillary mesenchyme in the chick embryo. *J. Craniofac. Genet. Dev. Biol.* 8:167, 1988.
5. Balling, R., et al. Craniofacial anomalies induced by ectopic expression of the homeobox gene Hox-1.1 in transgenic mice. *Cell* 58:337, 1989.

6. Bassols, A., and Massague, J. Transforming growth factor β regulates the expression and structure of extracellular matrix chondroitin/dermatan sulfate proteolgycans. *J. Biol. Chem.* 263:3039, 1988.
7. Beck, F., et al. Histochemical localization of IGF-I and -II mRNA in the developing rat embryo. *Development* 101:184, 1987.
8. Beebe, S., et al. Molecular cloning of a tissue-specific protein kinase (C$_\gamma$) from human testis representing a third isoform for the catalytic subunit of cAMP-dependent protein kinase. *Mol. Endocrinol.* 4:465, 1990.
9. Benoit, R., et al. Hox-7, a mouse homeobox gene with a novel pattern of expression during embryogenesis. *EMBO J* 8:91, 1989.
10. Berridge, M. Inositol triphosphate and diacylglycerol: Two interacting second messengers. *Ann. Rev. Biochem.* 56:159, 1987.
11. Berridge, M., and Irvine, R. Inositol triphosphate: A novel second messenger in cellular signal transduction. *Nature* 312:315, 1984.
12. Bixler, D. X-linked cleft palate. *Am. J. Med. Genet.* 28:503, 1987.
13. Björnssen, Å., Árnason, A., and Tippet, P. X-linked cleft palate and ankyloglossia in an Icelandic family. *Cleft Palate J.* 26:3, 1989.
14. Chrivia, J., Uhler, M., and McKnight, G. Characterization of genomic clones coding for the Cα and Cβ subunits of mouse cAMP-dependent protein kinase. *J. Biol. Chem.* 263:5739, 1988.
15. Cohen, S., and Jürgens, G. Mediation of *Drosophila* head development by gap-like segmentation genes. *Nature* 346:482, 1990.
16. D'Angelo, M., and Greene, R. Transforming growth factor–β modulation of glycosaminoglycan production by mesenchymal cells of the developing murine secondary palate. *Dev. Biol.* Submitted for publication, 1991.
17. Davies, K. E., Parson, P.L., Harper, P.S., et al. Linkage analysis of two cloned DNA sequences flanking the Duchenne muscular dystrophy locus on the short arm of the human X chromosome. *Nucleic Acids Res.* 11:2303, 1983.
18. Dean, D., Newby, R., and Bourgeois, S. Regulation of fibronectin biosynthesis by dexamethasone, TGFβ, and cAMP in human cell lines. *J. Cell Biol.* 106:2159, 1988.
19. Ferguson, M., and Honig, L. Epithelial-Mesenchymal Interactions During Vertebrate Palatogenesis. In E. Zimmerman (Ed.), *Current Topics in Developmental Biology.* New York: Academic, 1984. Pp. 137–164.
20. Finkelstein, R., and Perrimon, N. The orthodenticle gene is regulated by bicoid and torso and specifies *Drosophila* head development. *Nature* 346:485, 1990.
21. Fitchett, J., and Hay, E. Medial edge epithelium (MEE) transforms to mesenchyme

after embryonic shelves fuse. *Dev. Biol.* 131:455, 1987.
22. Fitzpatrick, D., et al. Differential expression of TGF beta isoforms in murine palatogenesis. *Development* 109:585, 1990.
23. Francomano, C., et al. The Stickler syndrome: Evidence for close linkage to the structural gene for type II collagen. *Genomics* 1:293, 1987.
24. Gehring, W. Homeo boxes in the study of development. *Science* 236:1245, 1987.
25. Gonzalez, G., et al. A cluster of phosphorylation sites on the cyclic AMP–regulated nuclear factor CREB predicted by its sequence. *Nature* 337:749, 1989.
26. Greene, R., and Garbarino, M. Role of Cyclic AMP, Prostaglandins, and Catecholamines During Normal Palate Development. In E. F. Zimmerman (Ed.), *Current Topics in Developmental Biology.* New York: Academic, 1984. P. 65.
27. Greene, R., et al. Transmembrane and intracellular signal transduction during palatal ontogeny. *J. Craniofac. Genet. Dev. Biol.* 11:262, 1991.
28. Greene, R., and Pisano, M. Analysis of Cell Proliferation in Developing Orofacial Tissue. In G. L. Kimmel and D. M. Kochhar (Eds.), *In Vitro Techniques in Developmental Toxicology: Use in Defining Mechanisms and Risk Parameters.* Boca Raton: CRC Press, 1989. Pp. 91–101.
29. Greene, R., and Pratt, R. Developmental aspects of secondary palate formation. *J. Embryol. Exp. Morphol.* 36:225, 1976.
30. Grove, R., Willis, W., and Pratt, R. Studies on phosphatidylinositol metabolism and dexamethasone inhibition of proliferation of human palatal mesenchyme cells. *J. Craniofac. Genet. Dev. Biol.* 2:285, 1986.
31. Hall, B. The induction of neural crest derived cartilage and bone by embryonic epithelia: An analysis of the mode of action of an epithelial-mesenchymal interaction. *J. Embryol. Exp. Morphol.* 64:305, 1981.
32. Harper, K., Burns, R., and Erickson, R. Genetic aspects of the effects of methylmercury in mice: The incidence of cleft palate and concentrations of adenosine 3′:5′ cyclic monophosphate in tongue and palatal shelf. *Teratology* 23:397, 1981.
33. Hassell, J., and Orkin, R. Synthesis and distribution of collagen in the rat palate during shelf elevation. *Dev. Biol.* 49:80, 1976.
34. Heine, U., et al. Role of transforming growth factor-β in the development of the mouse embryo. *J. Cell Biol.* 105:2861, 1987.
35. Hill, R.E., Jones, P.F., Rees, A.R., et al. A new family of mouse homeobox-containing genes: Molecular structure, chromosomal location, and developmental expression of Hox-7.1. *Genes and Dev.* 3:26, 1989.
36. Holland, P. Homeobox genes and the vertebrate head. *Development* [Suppl.] 103:17, 1988.

37. Ignotz, R., Endo, T., and Massagué, J. Regulation of fibronectin and type I collagen mRNA levels by transforming growth factor-β. *J. Biol. Chem.* 262:6443, 1987.

38. Jahnsen, T., et al. Molecular cloning, cDNA structure, and regulation of the regulatory subunit of type II cAMP-dependent protein kinase from rat ovarian granulosa cells. *J. Biol. Chem.* 261:12352, 1986.

39. Kishimoto, A., et al. Studies on the phosphorylation of myelin basic protein by protein kinase C and adenosine-3',5'-monophosphate–dependent protein kinase. *J. Biol. Chem.* 260:12492, 1985.

40. Koenig, M., Monaco, A., and Kunkel, L. The complete sequence of dystrophin predicts a rod-shaped cytoskeletal protein. *Cell* 53:219, 1988.

41. Kurisu, K., et al. Immunohistochemical demonstration of simultaneous synthesis of types I, III, and V collagen and fibronectin in mouse embryonic palatal mesenchymal cells in vitro. *Collagen Rel. Res.* 7: 333, 1987.

42. Lamph, W., et al. Negative and positive regulation by transcription factor cAMP response element-binding protein is modulated by phosphorylation. *Proc. Natl. Acad. Sci. U.S.A.* 87:4320, 1990.

43. Le Douarin, N. *The Neural Crest.* Cambridge: Cambridge University Press, 1982.

44. Lehnert, S., and Akhurst, R. Embryonic expression pattern of TGF beta type-1 RNA suggests both paracrine and autocrine mechanisms of action. *Development* 104:263, 1988.

45. Lee, D., et al. Isolation of a cDNA clone for the type I regulatory subunit of bovine cAMP-dependent protein kinase. *Proc. Natl. Acad. Sci. U.S.A.* 80:3608, 1983.

46. Linask, K., and Greene, R. Ontogenetic analysis of embryonic palatal type I and type II cAMP-dependent protein kinase isozymes. *Cell Differ. Dev.* 28:189, 1989.

47. Linask, K., and Greene, R. Subcellular compartmentalization of cAMP-dependent protein kinase regulatory subunits during palate ontogeny. *Life Sci.* 45:1863, 1989.

48. Lowry, R. Sex-linked cleft palate in a British Columbia Indian family. *Pediatrics* 46:123, 1970.

49. Macphee, C., et al. Prostaglandin F$_2$ stimulates phosphatidylinositol turnover and increases the cellular content of 1,2-diacylglycerol in confluent resting Swiss 3T3 cells. *J. Cell. Physiol.* 119:35, 1984.

50. Mavilio, F., et al. Activation of four homeobox gene clusters in human embryonal carcinoma cells induced to differentiate by retinoic acid. *Differentiation* 37:73, 1988.

51. Miller, D. A., Lee, A., Pelton, R.W., et al. Murine transforming growth factor β2 cDNA sequence and expression in adult tissues and embryos. *Mol. Endocrinol.* 3:1108, 1989.

52. Montminy, M., and Bilezikjan, L. Binding of a nuclear protein to the cyclic-AMP response element of the somatostatin gene. *Nature* 328:175, 1987.

53. Moore, G., et al. Linkage of an X-chromosome cleft palate gene. *Nature* 326:91, 1987.

54. Moore, G., et al. X chromosome genes involved in the regulation of facial clefting and spina bifida. *Cleft Palate J.* 27:131, 1990.

55. Moore, K. *The Developing Human* (4th ed). Philadelphia: Saunders, 1988. Pp. 170–205, 402–420.

56. Nishizuka, Y. Turnover of inositol phospholipids and signal transduction. *Science* 225:1365, 1984.

57. Nishizuka, Y. Studies and perspectives of protein kinase C. *Science* 233:305, 1986.

58. Olson, F., and Massaro, E. Developmental pattern of cAMP, adenyl cyclase, and cAMP phosphodiesterase in the palate, lung, and liver of the fetal mouse: Alterations resulting from exposure to methylmercury at levels inhibiting palate closure. *Teratology* 22:155, 1980.

59. Pearson, C., et al. Tenascin: cDNA cloning and induction by TGF-β. *EMBO J* 7:2977, 1988.

60. Pelton, R., et al. Differential expression of genes encoding TGF's β1, β2, and β3 during murine palate formation. *Dev. Biol.* 141: 456, 1990.

61. Pelton, R., et al. Expression of TGFβ2 RNA during murine embryogenesis. *Development* 106:759, 1989.

62. Pratt, R. Role of Epidermal Growth Factor in Embryonic Development. In A. Moscona and A. Monroy (Eds.), *Current Topics in Developmental Biology.* New York: Academic, 1987. Pp. 175–193.

63. Richman, J., and Crosby, Z. Differential growth of facial primordia in chick embryos: Responses of facial mesenchyme to basic fibroblast growth factor (bFGF) and serum in micromass culture. *Development* 109:341, 1990.

64. Ruiz i Altaba, A., and Melton, D. Involvement of the Xenopus homeobox gene Xhox3 in pattern formation along the anterior-posterior axis. *Cell* 57:317, 1989.

65. Rushton, R. Sex-linked inheritance of cleft palate. *Hum. Genet.* 48:179, 1979.

66. Saber, G., Parker, S., and Minkoff, R. Influence of epithelial-mesenchymal interaction on the viability of facial mesenchyme in vitro. *Anat. Rec.* 225:56, 1989.

67. Sadler, T. *Langman's Medical Embryology* (6th ed). Baltimore: Williams & Wilkins, 1990. Pp. 297–346.

68. Sandberg, M., Skalhegg, B., and Jahnsen, T. The two mRNA forms for the type Iα regulatory subunit of cAMP-dependent protein kinase from human testis are due to the use of different polyadenylation site signals. *Biochem. Biophys. Res. Commun.* 167: 323, 1990.

69. Scott, J., et al. The molecular cloning of a type II regulatory subunit of the cAMP-dependent protein kinase from rat skeletal muscle and mouse brain. *Proc. Natl. Acad. Sci. U.S.A.* 84:5192, 1987.

70. Sharpe, P., and Ferguson, M. Mesenchymal influences on epithelial differentiation in developing systems. *J. Cell Sci.* [Suppl.] 10:195, 1988.

71. Shiota, K., et al. Development of the fetal mouse palate in suspension organ culture. *Acta Anat.* 137:59, 1990.

72. Slavkin, H. Gene regulation in the development of oral tissues. *J. Dent. Res.* 67:1142, 1988.

73. Slavkin, H. Cellular and Molecular Determinants During Craniofacial Development. In M. Stricker et al. (Eds.), *Craniofacial Malformations.* New York: Churchill Livingstone, 1990. Pp. 15–26.

74. Slavkin, H., et al. Early embryonic mouse mandibular morphogenesis and cytodifferentiation in serumless, chemically defined medium: A model for studies of autocrine and/or paracrine regulatory factors. *J. Craniofac. Genet. Dev. Biol.* 9:185, 1989.

75. Smiley, G., and Koch, W. An in vitro and in vivo study of single palatal processes. *Anat. Rec.* 173:405, 1972.

76. Stricker, M., et al. Craniofacial Development and Growth. In M. Stricker et al. (Eds.), *Craniofacial Malformations.* New York: Churchill Livingstone, 1990. Pp. 61–90.

77. Stylianopoulou, F., et al. Pattern of the insulin-like growth factor II gene expression during rat embryogenesis. *Development* 103: 497, 1988.

78. Uhler, M., et al. Isolation of cDNA clones coding for the catalytic subunit of mouse cAMP-dependent protein kinase. *Proc. Natl. Acad. Sci. U.S.A.* 83:1300, 1986.

79. Wedden, S. Epithelial-mesenchymal interactions in the development of the chick facial primordia and the target of retinoid action. *Development* 99:341, 1987.

80. Wohlgemuth, D., et al. Transgenic mice overexpressing the mouse homeobox-containing gene Hox-1.4 exhibit abnormal gut development. *Nature* 337:464, 1989.

81. Yoneda, T., and Pratt, R. Mesenchymal cells from the human embryonic palate are highly responsive to epidermal growth factor. *Science* 213:563, 1981.

33

The Cleft Palate–Craniofacial Team

Howard Aduss

The craniofacial team provides an effective alternative form of health care designed to solve the problems caused by specialization and fragmentation in the usual medical setting. The purpose of the team is to meet the multiple needs of patients with craniofacial anomalies and the needs of their families. As an interdisciplinary clinical unit, the craniofacial team provides coordinated care in a cost-effective manner with careful attention to priorities. As medicine and the associated health sciences have become increasingly specialized and the information within each specialty has become more focused, problem solving requires greater interaction with and reliance on the expertise of peers. The interdisciplinary team is the logical response to the complex needs of the "whole patient" and his or her family.

The purpose of this chapter is to examine the development of craniofacial teams and the dynamics of team interaction and to identify the factors that contribute to effective team care.

The Development of Craniofacial Teams

Historically it was the responsibility of the surgeon to provide a child with a cleft lip and palate with optimal aesthetic and functional results. Ironically it was the surgeon's lack of success in meeting this responsibility that led to the development of the cleft palate team. In contrast, because of the success of the cleft palate team, the more expanded craniofacial team has been readily accepted as a natural progression to meet the greater needs of patients with more complex craniofacial malformations.

The earliest cleft palate teams—interactions between surgeons and associated health professionals—arose soon after the turn of the twentieth century. Anesthetic techniques were developed that allowed sufficient operative time for the talented pioneers of plastic and reconstructive surgery to perform surgical procedures that met the needs of patients with cleft lip and palate. Veau, Gillies, Kilner, von Langenbeck, and Wardill, to mention a few, perfected techniques that form the basis of today's operations for the treatment of cleft lip and palate. When

surgical intervention failed to achieve the desired goals of aesthetics and function, however, the patient was referred to a prosthodontist for palatal obturation and to a speech and language pathologist.

The climate was ripe for the development of more elaborate cleft palate teams in the 1930s. The 1930 White House Conference emphasized the concept of the whole child. The development of roentgencephalometry provided a method for the analysis of craniofacial growth and development and for the evaluation, in part, of velopharyngeal function. During this same period, it was recognized that highly compartmentalized medical specialty training was inadequate to solve complex problems and that a team of clinicians was required. Passage of the Social Security Act, in 1935, established the Crippled Children's Program, and through the efforts of Dr. Herbert Cooper, the care of children with cleft lip and palate was ultimately included within this program. In 1938 Cooper established the first cleft palate clinic in Lancaster, Pennsylvania.

Seminal activities related to the development of cleft palate teams took place also in another part of Pennsylvania during the 1930s. The distinguished speech and language pathologist and psychologist, Dr. Herbert Koepp-Baker, while serving as director of the speech clinic at Pennsylvania State University, began collaborating with Dr. Cloyd Harkins. Harkins, a dentist, was making prostheses for patients with clefts. Several years later, the relationship between Koepp-Baker and Harkins fostered the formation of the American Association of Cleft Palate Rehabilitation, the forerunner of the American Cleft Palate Association and the present American Cleft Palate–Craniofacial Association.

During the 1940s, there was increased collaboration among specialists involved in the treatment of cleft lip and palate, and the first federally funded research and training program was established at the University of Illinois at Chicago. At some point during the subsequent 40 years, the name of the center was changed to the Center for Craniofacial Anomalies. The name change reflected the expanded role of the center's team to include all craniofacial malformations, but it did not change the center's original mandates: to provide a training program for specialists interested in craniofacial malformations with additional training in their field; to promote knowledge of all dimensions of the malformation process; and to foster research supportive of the overall program of education within the academic and clinical communities.

Advances in the treatment of cleft lip and palate and other craniofacial malformations have come about through the efforts of those involved in team care. As noted earlier, patients whose condition did not improve with surgical treatment were referred to prosthodontists and speech and language pathologists for rehabilitation. The goal of this referral was to provide an adequate speech mechanism. If the patient could communicate, at least part of the overall goal of treatment was achieved.

In 1975 a conference was held at the University of Iowa to examine the objectives of management of cleft lip and palate. The goal of the treatment of cleft lip and palate, as defined by this interdisciplinary group of specialists, was the "rehabilitation" of "an individual who for reasons which relate to the cleft defect does not differ significantly from his peers in

health, education, and the ability to interact socially." In a few short years, the goal progressed from "rehabilitation" to "habilitation" and from the single aim of communication to the expanded objective of "treating the whole patient." This growth could not have taken place without the interaction of a team of specialists who recognized that a patient with a cleft lip and palate is a growing and changing person and that the needs of a patient vary over time. Additionally, the team of specialists came to recognize that no member of the team is omniscient, but that there are periods in the course of habilitation when the expertise of one colleague takes precedence over that of the others. This is not a small task since most specialist training emphasizes individuality.

Members of the Team

At this point it is appropriate to identify the individual specialists who compose a craniofacial team and to list the responsibilities of each member. With this information, anyone wishing to start a team would know which specialists to consider for membership, and individual members would know what was expected of them. Theoretically, all would proceed smoothly; unfortunately, this tidy package has the highest likelihood of failure because it does not recognize that the needs of a population and the availability of specialists in one geographic area are entirely different from those of another. For example, the logistics of a large rural area are entirely different from those of a tertiary care medical center in an urban setting. To overcome these differences and to function effectively at a variety of levels, teams should be organized in response to the following questions: (1) What are the needs of our patients? and (2) how can we best meet those needs? In short, the team should not be specialist-oriented; it should be patient-oriented. The orientation should be based on developmental thresholds and the needs of the family. For example, the immediate need of a newborn infant with a craniofacial malformation is physiologic stability, whereas the immediate needs of the family are psychosocial support and edu-

cation. The pediatrician and psychologist can meet these needs, but the surgeon responsible for repair of the lip should make every effort to visit the mother and counsel both parents before the baby leaves the hospital.

There are specialists who traditionally compose a craniofacial team, and the American Cleft Palate–Craniofacial Association is developing guidelines for team composition. At this time, three levels of teams are being considered: the cleft palate team, the orofacial team, and the craniofacial team. On each team the pediatrician is the patient's physician, and until the pediatrician establishes physiologic stability, the patient is not eligible for diagnostic evaluation, treatment planning, or specialized treatment. The psychologist or social worker provides support for the family and addresses the needs of the "whole" patient. Once the patient's condition is stable, and after integrating the information provided by his or her colleagues on the team, the surgeon may elect to operate. The dental specialist, most often an orthodontist, provides information regarding craniofacial growth. The otologist and audiologist monitor and maintain the status of the hearing mechanism, an essential part of intellectual development. The speech and language pathologist bears the primary responsibility for communication. All members of the team need to keep in mind that the purpose of the team is to meet the needs of the whole patient and the family. Participation on a team requires not only individual expertise but also a willingness to interact with other specialists to understand their needs and the goals of their treatments. This objective can be accomplished only with face-to-face meetings of the specialists on the team, careful record-keeping within the team, and regular redefinition of the patient's and the family's short- and long-term needs.

Team Dynamics

Craniofacial teams represent one of several types of programs that fall into the category of "human service teams." Brill defined such teams as a group of people, each of whom possesses particular expertise, each of whom is responsible for making individual decisions, who together hold a common purpose, who meet together to communicate, collaborate, and consolidate knowledge from which plans are made, actions determined, and future decisions influenced.

In short, teams are interactive groups comprising professionals from a number of disciplines. Unless a group of clinicians meets these criteria, the individuals cannot call themselves a team. Tuckman and Jensen have suggested that teams go through a series of stages in the course of their development.

Stage 1:
Testing and Dependency

At this stage of development, dependency needs are high and members rely on a leader to provide structure and direction for their activities. Trust in other members is low, and members are cautious in their interactions. Although they are working together, members do not feel responsible for the group as a whole. The leader is encouraged to make all the decisions.

Stage 2:
Conflict

The conflict takes the form of a battle for position in the pecking order within one's own discipline or between disciplines. Eventually, the conflict may become polarized between those who support and those who oppose the leader. It is during this stage that alliances are formed. Reticent members may rely on a spokesperson, and members may focus on those less competent and isolate them. Among other characteristics of this stage, emotions run high. Despite the difficulties of this stage of development, the team gains in cohesion and becomes less dependent on the leader.

Stage 3:
Cohesion and Consensus

As members develop trust in each other, confidence in their ability to meet the demands of the task, and the courage to speak out about their dissatisfactions, they develop a team structure. Through open discussion, they reach a consensus on issues related to team interactions. At this point in development, the team becomes "our team." At this point too, new members are more easily accepted onto the team. The dependency on the leader is further reduced and is replaced, in part, by a coalition of members of which the leader is a part; decision making within the group is done by consensus or by the member with the relevant expertise.

Stage 4:
Functional Role-Relatedness

At this point, the team has developed its own character and structure. Individuals have established their special areas of competence, and there is recognition that some members have competence in peripheral areas as well. Different members take on leadership roles as their competence becomes relevant. Members are at ease with one another and responsibilities are easily distributed. Dissatisfactions are aired as they arise and are resolved by negotiation and compromise and on the basis of the goals and values that were established by the team.

Effective Team Care

Readers who are members of teams have already identified their team's stage of development. Unaffiliated readers are now aware that effective teams go through an extended period of growth and adjustment. In addition to an understanding of team dynamics, a necessary first step for effective participation on a team is that members have a cognitive awareness and understanding of behaviors, attitudes, and values relevant to interpersonal relationships, the team environment, team leadership, and team process. Brill suggested that younger and older professionals often are well-suited for teamwork and that middle-aged participants may have the most difficulty on a team. These are people who have established themselves, who are anxious about maintaining their positions, and who may therefore be less flexible, creative, and accepting of differences.

Coupled with an awareness of team dynamics is a recognition of how the com-petitive, individualistic education and training specialists receive can affect their performance. Each team member is an expert in his or her own field. Others come to them for definitive judgments. To be placed in a problem-solving environment with other experts, in which no one person knows all the answers and in which decision making may have to be modified by the more immediate needs of others or depend on the judgments of others, is contrary to the education and training most specialists have received. Yet team care is highly successful because those who are willing to learn, to grow, and to gain the respect of their fellow professionals have developed a health care delivery system that works: The interdisciplinary team not only meets the complex needs of the patient and the family but also provides an intellectual challenge to its members.

In several areas of the United States, more than one team may serve the same geographic area. The Illinois Association of Craniofacial Teams is an excellent example of a federation of teams, from within Illinois and the surrounding states, who have joined together to foster communication among member teams and to develop an awareness of team care within the public and private sectors. The Illinois Association of Craniofacial Teams has developed an excellent relationship with the state agencies that support the care of children who require the care of an interdisciplinary team and has been the source of information on team care for hospitals throughout the state. The Illinois experience has demonstrated that effective team care can have a global effect when all the teams in an area share their experience.

Conclusion

The craniofacial team is an effective form of health care delivery designed to meet the multiple and complex needs of patients with craniofacial malformations and the needs of the family. Teams provide interactive face-to-face encounters of professionals from a number of disciplines. They meet together to communicate, collaborate, and consolidate knowledge; from these meetings plans are made, actions determined, and future decisions influenced.

Suggested Reading

Brill, N.I. *Teamwork: Working Together in Human Services.* Philadelphia: Lippincott, 1976.

Farrell, M.P., Heinemann, G.D., and Schmitt, M.M. Informal roles, rituals, and styles of humor in interdisciplinary health care teams: Their relationship to stages of group development. In Proceedings of the 7th Annual Conference on Interdisciplinary Health Team Care, 1985. Pp. 37–55.

Kobes, H.R., and Pruzansky, S. The cleft palate team: A historical review. *Am. J. Public Health* 50:200, 1960.

Koepp-Baker, H. The Cleft Palate Team. In W.C. Grabb, S.W. Rosenstein, and K.R. Bzoch (Eds.), *Cleft Lip and Palate.* Boston: Little, Brown, 1971.

Parameters for evaluation and treatment of patients with cleft lip/palate or other craniofacial anomalies. (Suppl. 2) *Cleft Palate–Cranifac. J.* 30: March, 1993.

Pruzansky, S. The foundations of the Cleft Palate Center and Training Program at the University of Illinois. *Angle Orthod.* 27:69, 1957.

Slater, P.E. Microcosm: *Structural, Psychological, and Religious Evolution in Groups.* New York: Wiley, 1966.

Tuckman, B.W. Developmental sequences in small groups. *Psychol. Bull.* 63:384, 1965.

Tuckman, B.W., and Jensen, M.A.C. Stages of small group development revisited. *Group Organization Studies* 2:419, 1977.

Wallace, A.F. A history of the repair of cleft lip and palate in Britain before World War II. *Ann. Plast. Surg.* 19:266, 1987.

Will, L., et al. The team approach to treating cleft lip/palate and other craniofacial anomalies in Illinois. *Ill. Dent. J.* 58:112, 1989.

34

The Clinical Use of Cephalometrics

R. Bruce Ross

Cephalometrics refers simply to head measurement, although the term has become synonymous with the tracing and measuring of cephalometric roentgenograms. There are only two reasons for measuring and evaluating faces—to identify the morphologic characteristics of a population and to identify the morphologic characteristics of an individual.

Population characteristics are determined with cephalometrics by establishing the mean values and other statistics for a variety of facial measurements of a group of people. Groups can then be compared, such as patients with prognathism with people with normal jaws; Asians with Caucasians; those who received one treatment with those who received another treatment or those who received no treatment at all. In this kind of clinical research, the aim is to define and quantify every conceivable morphologic detail. This chapter is not concerned with the methods used for research cephalometrics.

A clinician using cephalometrics does not use the same methods of analysis as a research scientist does. A clinician has entirely different requirements. The reasons for evaluating a patient, each requiring a different cephalometric approach, are as follows:

1. *To evaluate changes in a patient's facial morphology over a period of time.* The cephalometrics are simple for monitoring growth changes or treatment-induced changes. Structures of interest are traced from a lateral cephalometric roentgenogram, and a reference line is located that is stable (and has not been affected by treatment), such as the cranial base line nasion to basion. Two or more tracings are superimposed on the nasion-basion line and observed (Fig. 34-1). The tracings can be superimposed on any other area of interest, and simple measurements of differences can be made with a millimeter rule. This provides greater accuracy and understanding of the changes than does the acquisition of a mass of somewhat abstract numbers. Why create complicated artificial configurations when the real thing is available?

2. *To identify any dysmorphology,* that is, to identify precisely how the patient deviates from "normal." For a dysmorphologist this information may be of considerable importance, providing clues to the embryogenesis and cause of the condition and to the identification of syndromes. The cephalometrics used must be complex, similar to those used in the population research previously mentioned. The surgeon does not need this kind of information, but it is natural to wish to know the general morphologic characteristics of a patient. For a person with an odd-looking face and cranium whose problem is difficult to visualize, a series of age- and sex-related templates can be placed over the cephalometric roentgenogram (or a tracing of it) to compare different areas and structures and the overall configuration (Fig. 34-2). This method gives a good "feel" for the patient's condition without requiring specific measurements.

3. *To identify a dysmorphology or deviation from the normal that is important to a patient* in that it constitutes a problem that requires treatment. It cannot be overemphasized that a dysmorphology per se is of no consequence unless it causes a problem. If there is no problem, the identification of a deviation from the average, however obvious, is merely of academic interest. There are two situations, however, in which dysmorphia does constitute a problem—when it interferes with function or when it causes psychosocial difficulty.

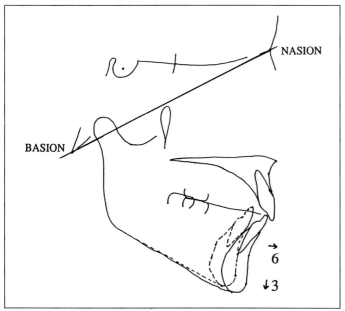

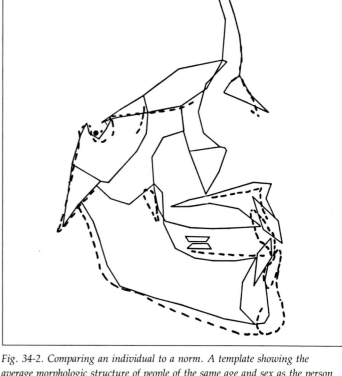

Fig. 34-1. Comparing changes over time or with treatment. A simple tracing of a cephalometric roentgenogram can be superimposed on a second roentgenogram or tracing to accurately identify and measure the changes that have occurred. In this example the morphologic changes following a mandibular advancement are determined by superimposing tracings on the unchanged areas. The soft tissues could also have been traced to show changes. Additional follow-up tracings can be added to complete the long-term picture. A collection of traditional cephalometric measurements would have almost no additional value.

Fig. 34-2. Comparing an individual to a norm. A template showing the average morphologic structure of people of the same age and sex as the person being analyzed provides an enormous amount of information without the necessity for actual measurements. Age per se is not dependable. It is better to use a template close to the same overall size. Different areas can be evaluated by moving the template around. Solid line = template; interrupted line = patient tracing.

An example of a dysmorphology that interferes with function is hemifacial microsomia (Fig. 34-3), in which the dysmorphology of the middle ear interferes with hearing. There are no functional problems related to the mandible in this instance, however, because the absence of a condyle does not cause a functional problem except in the strictest definition of the term. The mandible supports the essential functions of chewing, breathing, and speaking, and there are no long-term problems with these functions related to the complete absence of the left temporomandibular joint. If something works, it does not require fixing, even if it looks odd on a roentgenogram. Functional problems are never identified by cephalometric measurements. In fact, a functional problem rarely results from dysmorphology of the skeletal structures; it is dysmorphology of the soft tissues and organs that is invariably the cause.

The second situation in which dysmorphology is clinically significant is when it causes a psychosocial problem (either real

or imagined) because of the concept of acceptable facial aesthetics held by the person and by the society in which he or she functions. A severe morphologic deviation might induce low self-esteem, might incur a career or economic disadvantage, might interfere with personal relationships and social activities, and might even precipitate a direct verbal, physical, or psychological attack. The standards for facial aesthetics are somewhat vague, as they are in the case of function, and are generally not correlated with cephalometric measurements.

The focus of diagnosis and treatment planning, especially by orthodontists—but also by craniofacial, plastic, and oromaxillofacial surgeons—has been on the skeletal elements, which (with few exceptions) have little or no functional or aesthetic significance by themselves. The skeletal elements of functional importance are the teeth and, to a limited degree, the jaws. Most jaw dysmorphology, even that routinely treated surgically, has a minor influence on function. If we admit

this, treatment planning becomes simple. If we insist, however, that there is some master plan for the arrangement of all the bones of the craniofacial complex that is intrinsically normal and must be attained, if possible, treatment planning remains exceedingly complex.

Methods of Cephalometry

1. Radiography. Routine head films are a source of a great deal of diagnostic information for people with craniofacial malformations or diseases, but they should not be used for accurate measurement. Cephalometric roentgenograms are discussed in detail in this chapter. Computed tomography (CT) and computerized reconstructions are improving rapidly and are preferable for all but profile analysis.
2. Dental Models. A great deal of information is available from the analysis of a set of dental models. Much of this infor-

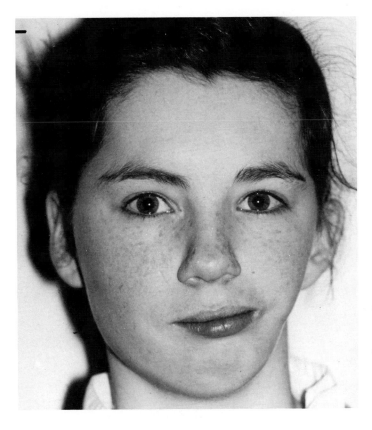

Fig. 34-3. Dysmorphology interfering with function and aesthetics. A child with hemifacial microsomia illustrates the gross dysmorphology that often accompanies this condition. The functional interference, however, is not with the mandible, because the jaw functions well in spite of the absence of a condyle. An aesthetic problem exists because of the mandibular dysmorphology. It is important to make this distinction.

mation is available only from this source.
3. Direct Measurements. Anthropometric data are valuable in local areas such as the eye, ear, and nose for reconstruction, but for the face in general they are not dependable, and the measurements produced are rarely of much use.
4. Photogrametrics. Photographs, although perhaps the most used planning aid, are not always reliable for measurements. Minor changes in head position can alter most of the measurements considered useful.
5. Direct Observation. Artistic and diagnostic sense is a marvelous tool that has fallen into disrepute to some extent. The discriminating judgment of a clinician viewing a patient is probably the most important component of good diagnosis and treatment planning.

Cephalometric Roentgenograms

In spite of the limitations of this representation of the head, cephalometric roentgenograms remain the most useful, practical, and effective clinical tool for treatment planning for both orthodontics and orthognathic surgery. Because cephalometric roentgenograms have a standardized orientation and size, measurements can be made on them to compare, with great precision, one group with another or an individual with a standard, to determine changes with time, to determine the effects of treatment, or to obtain other quantitative data.

Although measurements can be linear, such measurements are not recommended in the evaluation of a patient, because it is relative size rather than absolute size that is important to facial balance (a larger than average mandible should be present in a larger than average head). Proportions can be calculated from linear measurements, and this is an improvement, but there is no way of knowing with certainty which element of the several used for the proportion is abnormal and in what direction it is skewed. Constructed lines and points derived from anatomic references are often essential, but their use is abused in current practice, and meaningless relationships often are derived. Angular measurements eliminate the size variability and are probably the most popular form of cephalometric measurement. Again, however, there is a tendency to interpret the resulting angle in terms of the one landmark of greatest interest and to forget that there are two other landmarks that also are capable of great variation.

I become agitated when clinicians attempt to describe a functional or aesthetic problem and plan treatment on the basis of constructs depending on the Frankfort horizontal plane, head position, cranial base structures, or some other almost totally irrelevant evaluation. An obsession with numbers and needlessly complex systems has rendered analysis almost unintelligible. The disturbing specter of computer-generated plans has appeared, and these plans are, unfortunately, becoming popular. Orthodontists are responsible for this bizarre state of affairs; they have carried their enthusiasm for the total diagnosis of morphologic variation into a totally inappropriate area. My experience has led me to the startling conclusion that all formal cephalometric analyses are of academic interest only and are unnecessary. The measurements that are helpful for treatment planning are limited in number and are generally simple to acquire.

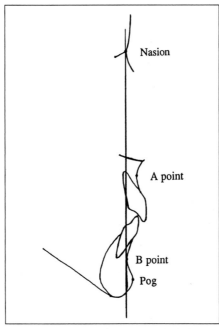

Fig. 34-4. Normal jaw relations. A simple but satisfactory evaluation of the jaw relations can be made by dropping a line from the nasion through point B and noting the position of point A. If point A is approximately 0 to 5 mm in front of point B, jaw relations are satisfactory and the teeth can be aligned by orthodontic treatment. If point A is behind point B, the face is straight with either mandibular protrusion or maxillary retrusion or both. If point A is more than 5 mm in front of point B, the face is convex with either mandibular retrusion or maxillary protrusion or both. The range is entirely arbitrary but helps to determine the indications for an orthognathic operation.

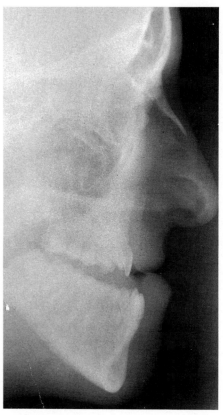

Fig. 34-5. Soft tissue cephalogram. A cephalometric roentgenogram taken to show the soft tissues as well as the underlying skeletal profile is extremely valuable for treatment planning.

Functional Measurements

Functional alterations to the facial skeleton are not usually required, other than for severe hypertelorism in which binocular vision is affected, when there is interference with respiration, or when one or both jaws need to be moved to establish reasonable jaw relations. Jaw relations and dental occlusion have been the focus of cephalometrics, but considering only function, the value of cephalometric roentgenograms is limited indeed. Dropping a line from nasion to point B and seeing whether point A falls a few millimeters in front of it (the usual in well-balanced jaw relations) is about all that is required for determining anteroposterior relations of the jaws (Fig. 34-4).

Once the dental compensations that can or should be accomplished are determined, the amount of jaw movement required to achieve balance is clear. Which jaw should be moved? It is unlikely to matter for function, especially if the movement is 5 mm or less. The determining functional factors include the soft tissue adjustment necessary after movement (tongue size and posture, soft palate function) and the stability of the surgical movement related to muscle stretching, muscle tone, and factors such as scar tissue. The skeletal and soft tissue measurements available from a cephalometric roentgenogram provide little assistance in making these decisions.

Vertical dysmorphologies producing an anterior dental open bite or deep bite generally require alteration of the planes of the maxilla or mandible. Again, vertical cephalometric measurements of the skeleton contribute little to the evaluation. Transverse (width) deficiencies of the maxilla inducing dental crossbites or reduction in the nasal airway are better determined clinically than by any cephalometric measurement.

Aesthetic Measurements

Aesthetic data must be gathered from the soft tissues, not from the skeleton. It is true that to establish satisfactory facial aesthetics in virtually every instance of extensive dysmorphology it is necessary to establish a good underlying skeletal base, with or without additional soft tissue operations. It makes good sense, however, to establish the soft tissue contours that would be most attractive and to try to alter the skeletal pattern to achieve them.

Patients must always be observed and photographed in three-quarter views as well as full frontal and profile views. The patient must be observed while animated (smiling, talking, eating, and pursuing

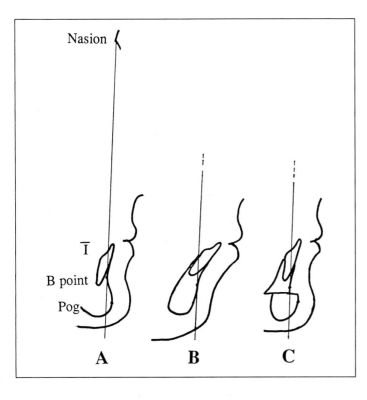

Fig. 34-6. Skeletal and dental effect on lower face aesthetics. A. An excellent relation of lower incisor edge and chin point (pogonion, Pog) to the nasion–point B line. The incisor (I) is a few millimeters in front, and Pog is the same or slightly farther in front. B. A poor relation. The incisor is protrusive, and Pog is behind the line. This situation is frequently encountered with mandibular micrognathia. Correction requires retraction of the incisor, preferably by orthodontics, and advancement of the Pog by genioplasty, as in C.

ordinary activities) and at rest. The soft tissue profile must be evaluated in both the horizontal and vertical planes for harmonious contours and pleasing proportions. It is a mistake to alter the facial skeleton on the basis of some cephalometric standard and assume this will produce better facial aesthetics. The norms provided are population averages and have no relevance to individuals. A sella-nasion-A point (SNA) angle 5° less than the mean for the population provides little information regarding whether or not a person has a jaw imbalance or what the soft tissues of the face look like.

The middle face (nose, cheeks, upper lip, nasolabial groove, maxillary incisors) is evaluated as a unit. One must not be preoccupied with the silhouette, however; it is only one aspect of the side view. The most important relationships in most instances are such features as height and depth of the cheeks relative to the inferior orbital margins (it is almost impossible for cheeks to be too high and prominent), position of the alar bases, and nose depth and protrusion from the cheeks. One common decision is whether or not to advance or retract the lower maxilla. This decision should be based first on the mid-

face evaluation without reference to the lower face. One should use a hand or a screen to block out the lower face and, looking at the rest of the face, try to determine whether the midface appears flat or is satisfactory and whether the nose is prominent or set back.

The maxillary incisors are the key to planning treatment of the midface, so one must be particularly astute in determining (1) whether the incisors are protrusive or retrusive and their angulation and (2) the amount of tooth showing. The desirable amount of tooth showing when the lip is at rest is about 2 to 3 mm, perhaps slightly more during conversation. A full smile or hearty laugh should expose almost all of the central incisors but little or no midline gingiva.

The lower face, which includes the lower lip, mental sulcus, chin point, submandibular soft tissue, and neck, is evaluated. The shape of the lower face is greatly influenced by the underlying skeleton and teeth, and it is simple to evaluate these relations on a cephalometric roentgenogram (Fig. 34-5). Using the same nasion–to–point B line as in Figure 34-4, it can be seen in Figure 34-6 that in a well-defined and attractive chin both the pogonion and

the tip of the lower incisor should lie about 3 to 5 mm ahead of the line. If they are farther ahead than that, the mental sulcus may become too deep; if they are less than 3 mm ahead, the mental sulcus may be too flat or absent. If either pogonion or the incisor is behind the line, the external appearance will almost certainly be affected. Obviously much depends on the overlying soft tissues, which can alter the requirements. For example, a thick soft tissue "button" over the pogonion is a common finding. Orthodontic treatment can either advance or retract the tip of the incisor, and a genioplasty can advance or retract the chin point. The lower lip is usually normal and unfurls or relaxes if placed in a proper relation to the upper teeth and upper lip.

The anterior midface should be blocked out so the surgeon can concentrate on the chin and lower contours of the mandible from all angles. There may be a true prognathism or retrognathism; there may be an illusion produced by an abnormal maxilla, or there may be an excess of height and width that gives a "heavy" chin and the illusion of a prognathism. The protrusion or retrusion of the lower face is evaluated superiorly relative to the

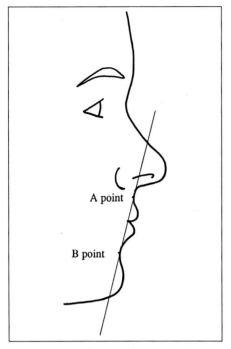

Fig. 34-7. The aesthetic profile. One simple method of evaluating or planning the profile is illustrated. A line passing through the soft tissue points A and B should cut off the lower half to third of the nose. This is an extraordinarily constant finding in well-balanced faces.

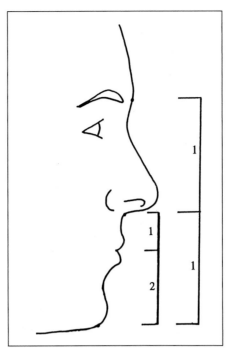

Fig. 34-8. Vertical proportions of the face. The 1:1 and 1:2 ratios are good guidelines.

maxilla and inferiorly relative to the neck. Aesthetically the midface relations are more important, but the relation of chin to neck sometimes dictates treatment.

After the characteristics of each element are established, they are put together. As a starting point, a simple reference plane can be used to establish a concept of a harmonious profile. A line passing through the deepest concavity of the lower lip and the deepest concavity of the upper lip should pass through the middle to lower third of the nose (Fig. 34-7). This concept is embarrassingly simple at first glance, but it is amazingly constant in balanced faces.

Vertical proportions are relatively easy to determine from a profile photograph (a frontal photograph never should be used for vertical measurements), provided the photograph properly captures resting lip relations in contact. As shown in Figure 34-8, the middle face (eyebrows to subnasale) should be almost exactly the same height as the lower face (subnasale to menton). The distance from subnasale to lip contact should be about one-half the distance from lip contact to menton.

Dysmorphologies that are apparent when a patient is viewed from the front are combinations in all three planes of space. Anteroposterior and vertical disproportions are best analyzed from the profile view, the frontal view being used to confirm or add details. Asymmetries occur in all three planes of space, and are corrected for aesthetic, not functional, reasons. Midline (eyes, nose, and chin) and vertical plane (orbit and lip) asymmetries are usually far more obvious and unaesthetic. Anteroposterior and facial-width asymmetries are rarely noticed. Cephalometric measurements are complicated by the fact that in such instances the ears often are displaced, so the head is rotated by the head holder and appears more asymmetric than it really is. It is better to trust the clinical diagnosis and location of the problem and transfer that information to the frontal cephalogram.

One effective clinical procedure for evaluating asymmetries requires a transparency with etched horizontal and vertical lines at approximately 2-cm intervals. This transparency is easy to make from a sheet of clear plastic. The examiner should sit directly in front of the patient, eyes at the level of the patient's, and hold the transparency close to the patient's face. The patient's head should not be tilted down or up. The reference lines are established; the eyes (orbits) provide the horizontal plane, unless an orbital operation is planned. The desired midline of the face is a line dropped from between the eyes perpendicular to the eye plane. This requires a judgment in many instances because the orbits are often asymmetric as well. In hemifacial microsomia, the orbit on the affected side is often lower than the other one. In that case, a reference horizontal that is not level with the orbits is established, some residual facial asymmetry must be accepted, or the affected orbit must be surgically altered (Fig. 34-9). Noting the relation of the maxillary dental midline to the facial midline is important; it is easy to determine and can be used to verify both the posteroanterior (PA) cephalometric roentgenogram and the model set-up on the articulator.

Vertical deviations of key landmarks must be established. I place a tongue depressor on the tip of one maxillary cuspid and parallel to the eye plane and measure the vertical distance to the tip of the other cuspid. This measurement is used to verify

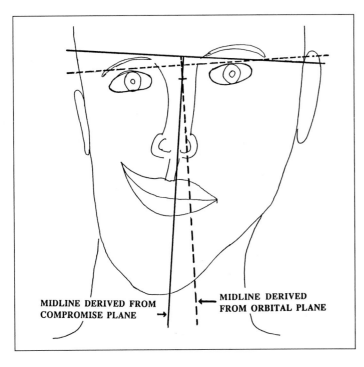

MIDLINE DERIVED FROM
COMPROMISE PLANE →   ← MIDLINE DERIVED
                             FROM ORBITAL PLANE

Fig. 34-9. Facial asymmetries. The reference line for evaluating asymmetries must be established, usually a perpendicular line dropped from the orbital plane (interrupted lines). For the patient in this sketch, one would not wish to use the orbital plane; the right orbit is lower, and the midline plane derived from it would be unrealistic. The choice is to compromise by taking a more representative midface line (clinical judgment, the solid line in the diagram) or surgically altering the position of the orbit. Once established, distances of various structures from the midline are noted.

the orientation of the roentgenogram and the accuracy with which the dental models have been mounted. The roentgenogram and model set-up can be used to plan the leveling of all the facial planes (maxillary, maxillary incisal, lip, occlusal, and mandibular) and midline corrections.

Treatment Planning

I plan in the following order—face, jaws, teeth. The changes to the face are planned first to achieve the best aesthetics and any specific functional requirements. Function almost always is well served by the changes necessary to achieve a well-balanced face. Correcting the face and thereby achieving facial balance should result in the correction of abnormal jaw relations.

The skeletal movements necessary to accomplish the desired facial changes are determined. Compromising the facial plan should be considered only if the changes required are not surgically feasible or make the operation unnecessarily complicated. Additional fine-tuning of jaw relations will be necessary, but they should not affect the facial plan. The jaw relations should not be changed for tooth position. The correction of the teeth should be routine. An orthodontist can

cope with minor variations in jaw relations by compensations in the placement of the teeth.

The most common major flaw in planning in the literature and in presentations by noted clinicians is that the jaws are not adequately corrected. This undercorrection is invariably caused by the placement of the dental arches in an ideal relation. It is far better to correct the face and jaws and to let the orthodontist achieve an ideal occlusion.

This chapter concludes with a description of my approach to cephalometric techniques for a variety of problems. I use a horizontal viewbox inset into a worktable and have close at hand all planning aids, including a detailed clinical assessment and the general surgical goals. Up to this point I have not traced or measured the facial skeleton and have used the roentgenograms as visual references for diagnosis, but without any measurements on them. The measurements I have are the few made in the clinic on the patient. I work directly with the soft tissue cephalogram (see Fig. 34-5) for planning and have the regular cephalometric and orthopantomograms, photographs, and models for reference. I begin by drawing two registration crosses on the cephalo-

gram for ease of later superimposition. I do not trace the cephalogram for analysis, only for the finished treatment plan.

Mandibular Advancement or Setback

For the sake of argument accept that in Figure 34-10A the midface is excellent, with or without some incisor changes or other subtleties, and only mandibular correction is necessary. The first and most important question is where to put the soft tissue chin. One could draw a chin point (soft tissue pogonion) as a small arc on a piece of tracing paper and move it around horizontally and vertically on top of the cephalogram until it was in a spot where it looked right. Regardless of any cephalometric measurement, a satisfactory chin position probably would be determined. This position could be overcorrected to allow for relapse.

Rather than guess, however, I establish a range. I place a sheet of tracing paper on the roentgenogram (I do not tape it down; I move it around as planning proceeds). I then trace the crosses I drew on the cephalogram. I plan a straight face for a retrognathic patient and a convex face for a prognathic patient to allow for some relapse. To establish the maximal corrected

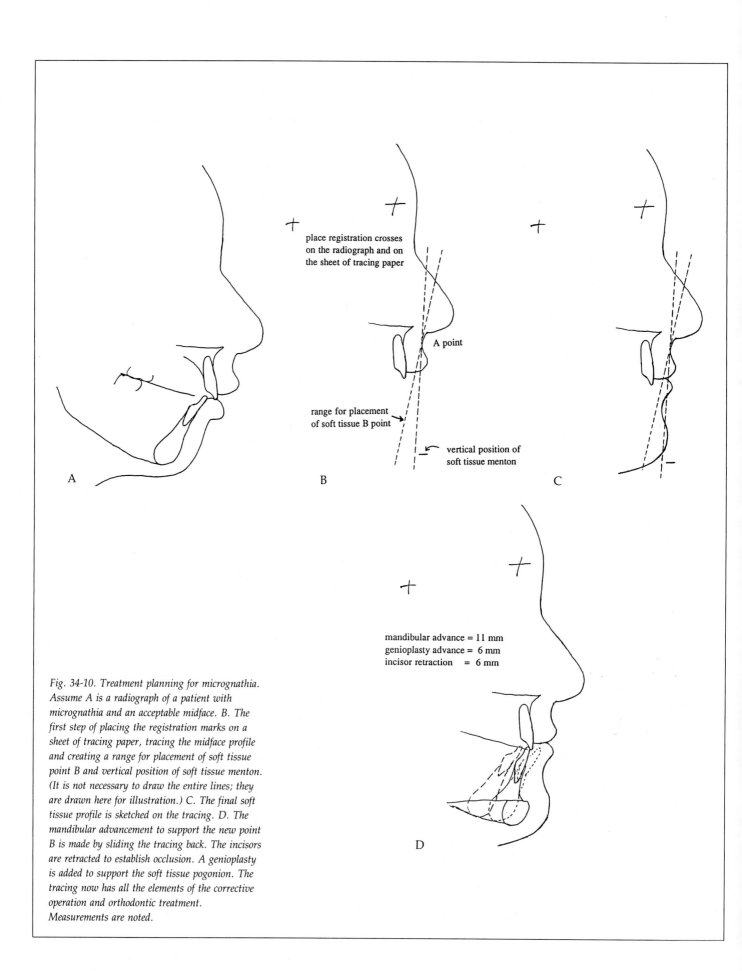

place registration crosses
on the radiograph and on
the sheet of tracing paper

A point

range for placement
of soft tissue B point

vertical position of
soft tissue menton

B

C

mandibular advance = 11 mm
genioplasty advance = 6 mm
incisor retraction   = 6 mm

A

D

Fig. 34-10. Treatment planning for micrognathia.
Assume A is a radiograph of a patient with
micrognathia and an acceptable midface. B. The
first step of placing the registration marks on a
sheet of tracing paper, tracing the midface profile
and creating a range for placement of soft tissue
point B and vertical position of soft tissue menton.
(It is not necessary to draw the entire lines; they
are drawn here for illustration.) C. The final soft
tissue profile is sketched on the tracing. D. The
mandibular advancement to support the new point
B is made by sliding the tracing back. The incisors
are retracted to establish occlusion. A genioplasty
is added to support the soft tissue pogonion. The
tracing now has all the elements of the corrective
operation and orthodontic treatment.
Measurements are noted.

forward position of a retrognathic chin, I draw a line that crosses the upper third of the nose and passes through the concavity of the upper lip (soft tissue point A) (see Fig. 34-10B). I draw a second line that crosses the middle of the nose and goes through the concavity of the upper lip. This produces an overcorrected maximal and minimal position for the soft tissue point B for a patient with severe or moderately severe retrognathia. For a prognathic mandible, the origin of the line for the maximal position is the middle of the nose and for the minimal position it is the lower third of the nose. The many other less important factors noted determine where the final point B should be.

I place the chin point (soft tissue pogonion) about 4 to 5 mm in front of the soft tissue point B. This makes for the best chin-lip contour. I establish the vertical position of the chin from the guidelines previously noted (see Fig. 34-8). I trace in the "givens" (forehead, nose) and the new soft tissue chin and add the lower lip and mental groove, completing the aesthetic facial plan (see Fig. 34-10C).

I add the skeletal changes to the tracing (see Fig. 34-10D). In general, I advance the mandible until the skeletal point B is correct with the new soft tissue point B; I slide the tracing back to the position where the soft tissue thickness between the skeletal point B and the new soft tissue point B is correct. I have previously decided whether or not the inclination of the lower incisor is the desired one for a satisfactory relation to the skeletal chin and point B. In retrognathic patients the incisors are usually proclined, and in prognathic patients they are usually retroclined; corrections are usually required for the best facial aesthetics. If incisor changes are indicated, I can easily place them on the tracing. I trace in the symphysis and teeth. Additional chin advancement, if required, is accomplished by an advancement genioplasty. Mandibular height is reduced by a vertical reduction genioplasty.

I now move the tracing back (and down, if there is to be a vertical reduction genioplasty) until the bony chin is in the proper position relative to the new soft tissue chin (the thickness of the soft tissue should remain the same) and trace the lower symphysis contour. If there is a discrepancy between the new bony chin and the symphysis at point B, a genioplasty is required, and the distances can now be measured. I superimpose the tracing on the crosses again, lightly trace the original symphysis with a dotted line, and measure the distance from the original to the new position of the bony chin and point B.

Cephalometric tracings provide plans that are an approximation and that must be transferred to the model set-up for the actual measurements the surgeon will use. The plan *must* be rechecked on the patient in the clinic.

Maxillary Advancement

I arrive at the tracing table with a good idea from the clinical examination of how much advancement of the maxilla is required to achieve a good midface aesthetic result. I place crosses on the soft tissue cephalogram. On a sheet of tracing paper I trace the maxilla. I incorporate any change in incisor position by rotating the tracing with the fulcrum just below the apex of the central incisor. I move the tracing until the maxilla is in the desired advanced position and check this position with the mandible. If the maxilla now assumes a good relation with the mandible, no mandibular operation is required. If so, the profile can be checked with the nose–upper lip–lower lip line. With a Le Fort I procedure the upper lip point A moves only about half as much as the maxillary advancement, and the tip of the nose moves even less.

If the new maxillary position is not in good relation to the mandible, there are three choices: (1) Move the mandible as well; (2) leave the mandible and let the orthodontist achieve a good occlusion by dental compensations; or (3) alter the maxillary position to achieve a good relation to the mandible. I dislike compromising the predetermined best maxillary position, but that is preferable if it means only a slight compromise and a mandibular operation can thereby be avoided. There is a range of maxillary advancement within which aesthetics are subjective and almost too subtle to detect. One sees patients, however, for whom a 10- to 15-mm advancement was indicated and a totally inadequate 5- to 6-mm advancement was performed because the teeth seemed to fit well. An orthodontist can rearrange the teeth a surprising amount, but it must be taken into consideration that with extreme movement some relapse can be expected.

When I am satisfied with the position of the maxilla, I trace on the crosses. I trace the new soft tissue profile of the midface and forehead. I complete the tracing by adding the mandible. If the mandible is to be operated on as well, I follow the procedure described for mandibular advancement. Thus, in two-jaw operations the maxillary portion is planned first and the mandibular portion planned to harmonize with it.

Problems of Vertical Dimension

A typical patient with a problem of vertical dimension has a long face, open bite, and excessive "show" of the maxillary incisors. The first decision to make is whether the vertical height of the maxilla should be altered by impaction. This is definitely a clinical decision based on appearance and function, not on cephalometry. Altering the height of the anterior maxilla is determined by how much of the maxillary incisor is visible at rest, during conversation, and especially in smiling and laughing. With almost any length of upper lip, one should try for 2 to 4 mm of exposed incisor at rest and conversation, almost all of the incisors showing in maximal smile, but no gingival tissue visible above the teeth in the midline.

The second decision concerns the vertical change in the posterior maxilla to maintain the occlusal plane or to tip the maxilla to close an open bite. The third decision is whether or not the maxilla should be advanced. Again this is a clinical, not a cephalometric, decision. Once I make these decisions, I transfer them to the tracing as for maxillary advancement. I trace the maxilla on a sheet of tracing paper and move it to the desired vertical and anteroposterior position with the amount of tipping estimated (Fig. 34-11A and B).

The next step is critical: locating the presumed center of rotation of the mandible. (I use a point just below the center of the head of the condyle; the exact position is not important at this stage of planning unless the patient has a very unusual closure path.) I put the pencil on this rotation point and rotate the tracing paper (and

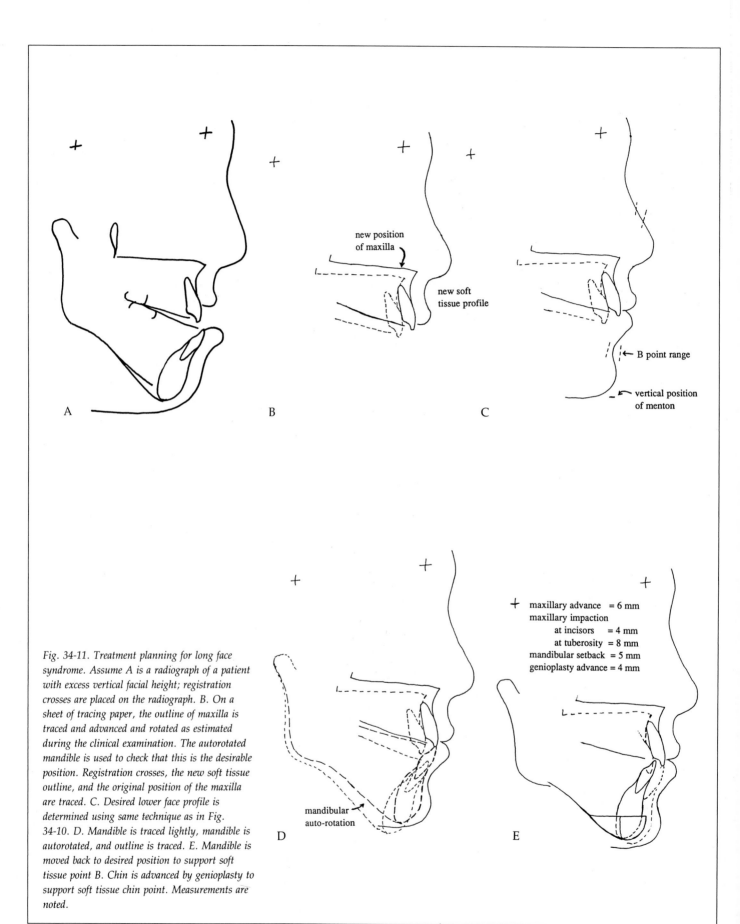

new position
of maxilla

new soft
tissue profile

← B point range

← vertical position
of menton

A

B

C

maxillary advance = 6 mm
maxillary impaction
at incisors = 4 mm
at tuberosity = 8 mm
mandibular setback = 5 mm
genioplasty advance = 4 mm

mandibular
auto-rotation

D

E

Fig. 34-11. Treatment planning for long face
syndrome. Assume A is a radiograph of a patient
with excess vertical facial height; registration
crosses are placed on the radiograph. B. On a
sheet of tracing paper, the outline of maxilla is
traced and advanced and rotated as estimated
during the clinical examination. The autorotated
mandible is used to check that this is the desirable
position. Registration crosses, the new soft tissue
outline, and the original position of the maxilla
are traced. C. Desired lower face profile is
determined using same technique as in Fig.
34-10. D. Mandible is traced lightly, mandible is
autorotated, and outline is traced. E. Mandible is
moved back to desired position to support soft
tissue point B. Chin is advanced by genioplasty to
support soft tissue chin point. Measurements are
noted.

thus the maxilla) down until the maxillary and mandibular teeth contact. I note whether the maxillary and mandibular occlusal planes meet and whether the maxillary rotation and anteroposterior relation of maxilla to mandible are slightly overcorrected. If the anteroposterior relations are close to ideal, I might increase or decrease the maxillary advancement to avoid the necessity of operating on the mandible. When such slight adjustments are made, rotate the tracing paper with the traced maxilla back up to the desired vertical position and transfer the registration crosses to the tracing paper. Next the soft tissue response to the maxillary movement can be added to the tracing (see Fig. 34-11B).

The tracing proceeds as described for mandibular advancement. I determine the desired profile using the nose-lip-line and locate the new soft tissue point B (see Fig. 34-11C). I establish vertical proportions as before. If the two vertical proportions (1:1 upper to lower face, 1:2 upper lip to lower lip and chin) give conflicting indications of where the menton should be, I strongly favor the second of the two proportions, but I almost always compromise a little. If the upper lip is excessively long or short, I do not try to lengthen or shorten the lower face height to achieve the ideal proportions.

I trace the mandible lightly using an interrupted line, rotate it into contact, and trace it with a dotted or interrupted line. The difference between the two lines clearly indicates the amount of autorotation and the autorotated position of the mandible (see Fig. 34-11D). The mandible must be advanced or set back (by sliding the tracing forward or backward) to achieve a corresponding skeletal point B, which I indicate on the tracing. I can then directly measure the amount of mandibular movement as the distance between the solid and the dotted mandibles. The position of the new soft tissue pogonion determines where the skeletal pogonion must be, and this invariably requires a genioplasty, particularly a vertical reduction genioplasty and often an advancement as well (see Fig. 34-11E).

The treatment plan tracing is now complete, ready to be used for planning orthodontic treatment before surgical correction. When this tracing is done just before the operation to finalize the surgical

movements, the measurements are available to transfer to the mounted dental casts. When a discrepancy occurs, it is the measurement from the mounted casts that are to be used (the amount of maxillary posterior impaction and the amount of mandibular advancement are more accurately determined on the model). Transverse (width) alterations to the maxilla or rotations for asymmetry are done on the model.

Asymmetries

I mark two registration crosses on the posteroanterior cephalometric roentgenograms. I place a sheet of tracing paper on which I have drawn a T over the cephalogram so that the horizontal arm lies on the orbital plane (if that has been established clinically as an appropriate plane from which to establish the asymmetry of the face) and the perpendicular arm is in the midline (crista galli or the midpoint between the orbits). The perpendicular line indicates the midline of the face. I check that this line passes through the incisor teeth as it was found to do during the clinical examination. I draw a line through one maxillary cuspid tip parallel to the orbital plane and check that the opposite cuspid is higher or lower by the amount that was determined on the patient in the clinic. The usability of the cephalogram is thus verified.

I work on the maxilla first. With a ruler, I draw on the maxillary, mandibular, and occlusal planes, and the incisal plane if it is different. I determine the vertical differential between sides. I decide on the basis of the vertical height requirements (incisor show anteriorly is the major determinant, as is the posterior occlusion) whether to raise one side, to lower the other, or to do a bit of both. This leveling of the planes alters the midline, so the maxilla must be adjusted to the right or left by rotation or bodily movement. The fine details are best left to the mounted models, which provide much more three-dimensional information. I usually do not bother to trace the maxilla and mandible, but simply transfer the measurements to the model.

I determine whether the mandible can be rotated keeping the same occlusion with the maxilla or if more or less mandibular rotation is required to center the midline of the symphysis on the midline of the

face. I check the vertical levels of the gonia. Detailed movements are easier to envision with the mounted models and the disarticulated mandibular model. It is even more important than usual in these instances to *take the plan back to the clinic and check it on the patient.*

There are no cephalometric measurements of any meaning for the transverse dimensions. Differential maxillary width corrections are best left to the model, on which arch asymmetry can be evaluated and related to the clinical findings.

Conclusion

Facial analysis and treatment planning require only a few measurements. Clinical judgment, templates, and direct comparisons are of greater value. A clinician using cephalometrics should not try to use an analysis designed for growth research. Many of the common skeletal cephalometric standards are population averages and are of little relevance to an individual patient's treatment.

Suggested Reading

Bell, W., Proffit, W., and White, R. *Surgical Correction of Dentofacial Deformities.* Philadelphia: Saunders, 1980.

Epker, B.N., and Fish, L.C. *Dentofacial Deformities.* St. Louis: Mosby, 1986.

Jacobson, A., and Canfield, P. *Introduction to Radiographic Cephalometry.* Philadelphia: Lea & Febiger, 1985.

35

The Classification and Management of Facial Clefts

J. C. van der Meulen

Through the ages, the fate of children with facial clefting has been an unhappy one. They were either worshipped as deities or rejected as diabolical quirks of nature. Integration in society was made possible only recently by the pioneering work of Tessier, who revolutionized surgery of the craniofacial skeleton. This chapter focuses on the soft tissue problems that continue to remain a challenge.

Identification of Clefts

Normal facial growth depends on a harmonious integration and interaction of the parts. A study of the developing face of an embryo shows that dramatic changes occur in an extraordinarily brief period of time (the period between 17 and 27 mm crown-rump length, CRL). In a 17-mm CRL embryo the facial processes have fused, marking the end of the transformation phase. Morphogenesis of the craniofacial skeleton begins with the formation of the sphenoid body and its extensions. It continues with the formation of the middle and anterior fossae and a reduction of the interorbital distance. Ev-

olution proceeds with the union of the two nasal halves and the development of the nasomaxillary complex, which expands forward, downward, and laterally. In a 27-mm CRL embryo the skeleton is completed with a lengthening of the mandibular ramus, which adapts itself to the formation of the nasomaxillary complex.

Malformations may have their origin at different stages and different sites of development. Identification of a malformation on a *chronologic basis* allows distinction between primary, or true, and secondary, or false, clefts. Primary, or true, clefts can be produced only at an early stage of facial development (the transformation phase) and only in four locations. These locations are the junctions between the lateronasal process and the maxillary process, between the medionasal process and the maxillary processes, between the maxillary processes where the palate is formed, and between the maxillary and mandibular processes. Arising at an early stage (before 17 mm CRL), the clefts automatically become associated with bony deficiencies. Secondary, or false, clefts have their origin at a later stage of development when the facial processes have fused and the differentiation phase has

begun. They are caused by abnormal ossification within or between the ossification centers.

Identification of a craniofacial cleft on a *topographic basis* allows distinction between the ossification centers from which the parts of the skeleton are formed and the parts themselves. Identification of a craniofacial cleft on a chronologic and topographic basis shows that all malformations can be graded and related to the form at a certain stage of embryonic life. The earlier the developmental arrest, the more severe is the malformation. When the insult strikes early, the final relations among the skeletal parts have not yet been achieved, and the position of these parts is therefore still subject to the changes induced by the constant interactions between normal growth on the one hand and absence of growth on the other.

An early failure of differentiation involving the internasal and nasal areas prevents normal approximation of the facial halves and causes teleorbitism. A late failure is restricted to bifidity of the nasal tip. An early failure of differentiation involving the nasomaxillary and maxillary areas causes separation of the central and lat-

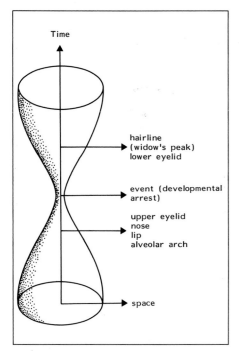

Fig. 35-1. Hourglass deformity. Space-time diagram illustrating evolution of skeletal and soft tissue malformation.

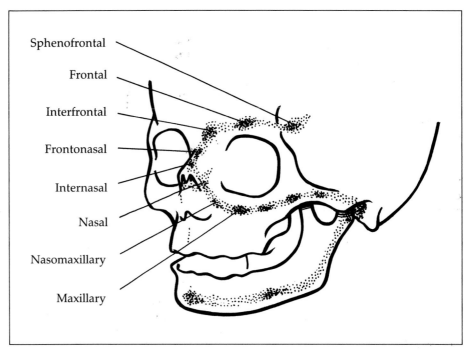

Fig. 35-2. Helix of craniofacial dysplasias (D).

eral parts of the skeleton and cranial drift of the nose. A late failure has no such effect.

In the years preceding the era of craniofacial surgery, it was customary to regard these clefts as a two-dimensional problem. Tessier was the first to emphasize the intimate relation between soft tissues and skeleton when he presented his classification of clefts around the orbit. He stated that "a fissure of the soft tissues corresponds as a general rule with a cleft of the bony structures." The anomaly therefore presents a three-dimensional problem in the sense that the bony tissues also are involved and that the severity of the skeletal defects is reflected in that of the soft tissues.

The appearance of these pseudoclefts can be understood when one visualizes what may happen when development is arrested in one skeletal area while it continues in the normal adjacent tissues. An hourglass deformity may be produced with the transition in the middle as the original site of the evolutionary disturbance. This part, behaving as a scar, prevents the surrounding tissues from expanding normally. As a result, a series of opposed V-shaped anomalies develops, affecting the hairline, nose, maxilla, lips, and eyelids. The character of these anomalies varies with the area of skeletal involvement and the nature of the adjacent tissues. The direction of these pseudoclefts, colobomas, and peaks is predominantly craniocaudal. The evolution of these clefts is in fact a four-dimensional problem. The illustration of this process resembles the space-time diagram found in *A Brief History of Time* by S. Hawking (Fig. 35-1).

Classification of Clefts

The production of bone in the ossification centers is a key element in craniofacial morphogenesis. Deficiencies in bone formation therefore reflect the topography of these centers. The architectural design of the skeleton can in fact be compared with a helix, the symbol of life in some cultures, and in Figure 35-2 is symbolized by the letter **S**.

The ossification centers in the upper section of the helix form the anterior wall of the brain, and those in the middle section delineate the nasal aperture, the orbital cavity, and the auditory meatus. The skeletal primordia in the lower section provide a floor for the oral cavity. The spectrum of facial dysostoses is dominated by the clefts, which have their origin in the middle section of the helix formed by the internasal, nasal, nasomaxillary, maxillary, and malar structures. The facial clefts in these areas are named after the site of the developmental arrest and are the subject of this chapter.

Surgical Principles

The ultimate goal of reconstructive surgery is to achieve an optimal result in a minimum of time with a minimum of scarring and morbidity. In the general euphoria following Tessier's presentation of his pioneering work, it was sometimes overlooked that the best results were obtained with adult patients. At that time pediatric craniofacial surgery was still in its infancy. This situation has changed, and craniofacial surgeons who are now studying the results of early surgical in-

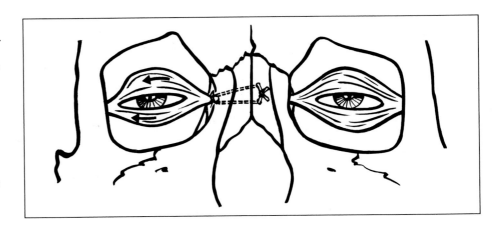

Fig. 35-3. Technique of canthopexy. A hole is bored at the site of insertion of the canthal tendon. The diameter is sufficiently wide to allow the tendon to enter it as deeply as possible. After it is identified, the tendon is secured with a monofilament nonabsorbable 000 suture, leaving both ends long. Parallel to and just below the bridge of the nose, two holes are burred on the contralateral side. The direction of the canals is such that the tip of the bur becomes visible in the hole that was previously made. Through these canals two hollow needles are passed, which serve as guides for the ends of the sutures. The needles are withdrawn, and the procedure is concluded with the tying of a firm knot.

tervention have begun to realize that optimal results can be considered optimal only when they are also stable.

Reestablishment of facial integrity in patients with median or paramedian clefts involves all disrupted structures—the skeleton, muscles, and skin. It is therefore based on the following principles:

1. *Reconstruction of the skeleton by the removal of abnormal elements, the transposition of skeletal parts,* and *the apposition of bone grafts.*
2. *Reinsertion of the muscles by transposition and fixation of dystopic remnants.* An intact muscular layer serves to establish and maintain form, to animate the face, and to stimulate growth.
3. *Restoration of the skin by transposition and apposition of flaps.* The cutaneous layer provides protection for the underlying structures and preserves facial contour by its fixation to the skeleton at strategic points.

Application of these principles is usually rewarded with good results, but failures are still observed at each level of reconstruction. Failures at the first level of reconstruction may be caused by inadequate mobilization and fixation of skeletal parts, lack of cartilaginous or bony growth, and loss of bone by resorption.

Failures at the second level causing canthal drift may be related to the loss of tensile strength in the fixed tissues after the canthopexy (Fig. 35-3). This loss is gradual, and during the period of weakness alterations in the structure of tissues are caused by external factors. This remod-

eling capability is a characteristic of young patients. A devascularized, fragile orbital wall undergoing creeping substitution is particularly vulnerable in the presence of not one but several laterally directed forces that exert traction on one point: the medial canthus. These forces are (1) the extensive subcutaneous scar contractions that occur in the first 2 months postoperatively; (2) the contraction of the orbicularis oculi muscles by the canthal ligaments; and (3) those generated by inadequate periosteal release of the tissues overlying the orbital frame, inadequate fixation of the bony structures in the midline, and inadequate exenteration of the tissues inside the interorbital space. In addition, the apposition of new bone by the periosteum in the weeks after its release and reattachment and the formation of an abundance of scar tissue in the medial canthal area must be considered.

Failures at the third level of reconstruction may be explained by the eternal conflict between surgical correction and scar formation, which is the reason that much of the initial benefit of the operation can be erased with growth. A discrepancy in growth between the scarred area and the adjacent normal tissues is a natural phenomenon, which should be expected.

Mastery of surgery implies that surgeons are, first of all, aware of the limits of surgery. Only then will their results become predictable and reproducible. Unfortunately, there is a fine line between doing too much and doing too little. A surgeon who does too much may ruin the face of a child. A surgeon who does too little may ruin the soul. In trying to define the limits

of craniofacial surgery today, it seems that surgeons have almost reached their limits at the first and second levels of reconstruction.

A growing, rebuilt nose has not yet been reported, and a canthus that remains fixed under all circumstances is also somewhat illusory. Room for improvement seems to exist only at the third level, at which a surgeon makes incisions and, consequently, scars. It is therefore to this aspect that the energy of the surgeon must be devoted. The detrimental effect of scarring, however, can be minimized or avoided by accurate timing of the correction, meticulous planning of the incisions, and secure anchoring of the tissues.

Timing of the Correction

The desire to correct a malformation soon after birth is understandable from several points of view; however, extensive rearrangement of skin should be avoided in a growing child. Local expansion of the surface followed by local rearrangement of skin and necessary stabilization of the result by the insertion of a bone graft or a temporary implant may help to improve the appearance and to avoid unnecessary scarring. Repetition of this procedure at desired intervals until growth of the facial skeleton is complete may enable the surgeon to achieve the envisaged result and minimize scarring.

Planning of the Incision

If possible, incisions should be made away from the midline of conspicuous areas, such as the forehead, nasal dor-

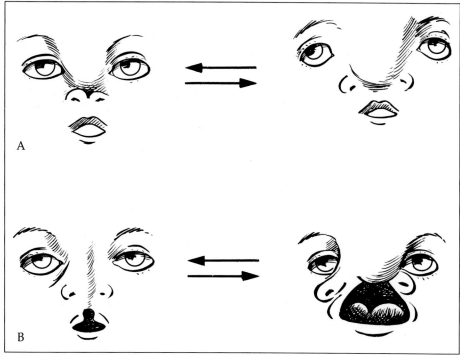

Fig. 35-4. Spectrum of malformations caused by internasal dysplasia.
A. Without cleft lip. B. With cleft lip.

sum, or philtrum; hidden in creases or folds; and parallel to the lines of minimal tension.

Anchoring of the Tissues

Even when parallel to the lines of minimal tension, a scar may be subject to tangential or shearing forces. The effect of these forces is particularly harmful in the early postoperative period, when scar tissue is still young. Fixation of the skin to the skeleton at strategic points, such as the medial and lateral canthal area, and careful re- and appositioning of muscles when required help improve scar formation.

Internasal Dysplasia

The term *internasal dysplasia* refers to a developmental arrest in the groove separating the two nasal halves before union has occurred. The anomaly is also known as the Tessier no. 0 cleft. Depending on the time of the developmental arrest, a wide spectrum of abnormalities can be observed (Fig. 35-4). In less severe instances, the anomaly is characterized by bifidity of the columella, of the nasal tip, of the dorsum, and of the distal part of

the cartilaginous septum. Occasionally a median cleft of the lip, a median notch in the cupid's bow, or a duplication of the labial frenulum is found. In more severe instances the nasal halves are widely separated and teleorbitism is present. The premaxilla is never absent, but it can be retarded in development and bifid. The maxilla may show a keel-shaped deformity, in which the incisors are rotated upward in each half of the alveolar process. Sometimes a medial cleft of the palate also is found, and this may extend upward to the cribriform plate as an inverted V.

The distance between the palate and the cranial base is short, and the remaining internasal space is occupied by a partially duplicated cartilaginous mass. In extreme instances the two nasal halves may be separated by a lipoma or meningoencephalocele. The wider the cleft is, the greater is the interorbital distance, the shorter is the nose, and the more arched is the maxillary vault.

Surgical Treatment

The Nose
Reconstruction of a bifid nose may require the following steps:

1. *Resection of anomalous and excessive cartilage.*
2. *Restoration of a nasal framework using a costal, calvarial, or iliac bone graft.* It should be borne in mind that this framework will not grow and that some degree of resorption is bound to occur. To minimize this problem, the graft must be rigidly fixed and covered with well-vascularized tissue.
3. *Elongation of the mucosal lining of the roof of each nasal half when retrusion exists.*
4. *Approximation of the alar cartilages over the new skeleton whenever possible.*
5. *Reconstruction of the nasal dorsum by one of various methods.*

In instances of less severity, excision of the depressed area followed by linear closure may be sufficient. In more severe instances advancement of the contracted skin toward the tip of the nose in a V-Y manner has frequently been advocated. This technique carries the risk of conspicuous scarring, is inadequate, and therefore is outdated. Skin expansion before a more definitive repair may allow resurfacing of the nasal tip and columella and positioning of the scars in less con-

Fig. 35-5. Patient with severe internasal dysplasia corrected by expansion and local transposition of skin. A. Frontal view over bone implant (preoperative). B. Expansion of nasal skin. C. Redistribution of nasal skin. D. Frontal view (postoperative).

A

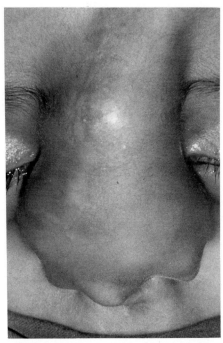

B

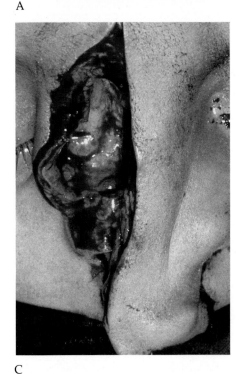

C

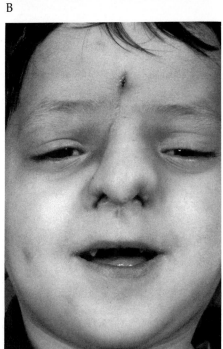

D

spicuous areas (Fig. 35-5). In some patients who have a surplus of skin in the internasal area, there is no need for expansion. Reconstruction of the nasal tip is achieved by rotation and advancement of the dorsal skin over the inferior cartilaginous domes after release of the flap in the glabellar area (Figs. 35-6 and 35-7). Rotation of a forehead flap is rarely indicated (Fig. 35-8).

The Skeleton

In more severe anomalies, the type of correction is dictated by the degree of orbital hypertelorism and maxillary involve-

ment. When the maxillary deformity is of little importance, reduction of the interorbital distance by movement of the orbits medially can be considered. Medial movement of orbit and maxilla by means of a medial faciotomy, however, is indicated for patients with a more pronounced maxillary deformation. The concept of the split face, or facial bipartition,

was originated when the association of teleorbitism and maxillary malformations was observed and the possibility of correcting these skeletal anomalies in one procedure was considered. The technique allows a rotatory movement in each facial half, reducing the interorbital distance, tilting the alveolar arches, and lowering the height of the palate (Fig. 35-9).

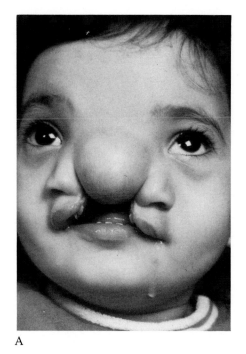

A

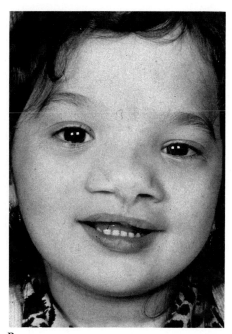

B

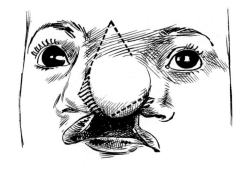

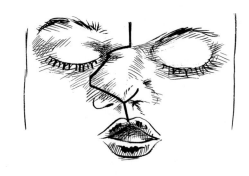

Fig. 35-6. Patient with severe internasal dysplasia corrected by split-face procedure and local transposition of skin over bone implant. A. Frontal view (preoperative). B. Frontal view (postoperative). C. Technique of skin transposition.

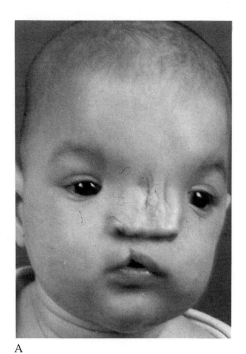

A

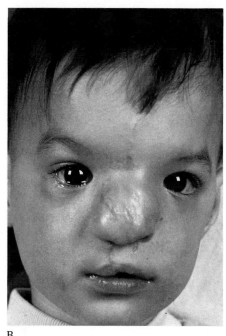

B

Fig. 35-7. Patient with severe internasal dysplasia corrected by split-face procedure and local transposition of skin over bone implant. A. Frontal view (preoperative). The unilateral cleft lip was repaired elsewhere. B. Frontal view (postoperative).

Fig. 35-8. Internasal dysplasia corrected by medial fasciotomy procedure and transposition of forehead flap. A. Frontal view (preoperative). B. Lateral view (preoperative). C. Same patient, frontal view (postoperative). D. Lateral view (postoperative).

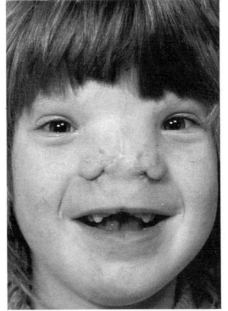

A

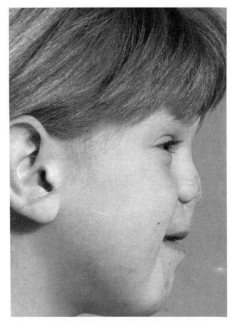

B

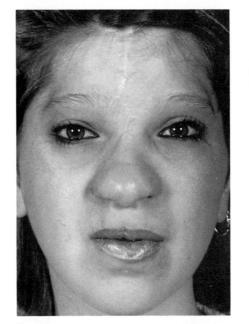

C

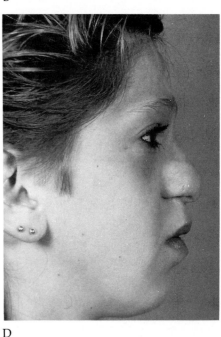

D

Nasoschizis

The term *nasoschizis* relates to clefts of the lateral part of the nose. The spectrum of these anomalies ranges from a small notch in the alar rim to a wide defect involving one or both nasal halves (Fig. 35-10). Direct access to the pyriform aperture and to the floor of the anterior cranial fossa is thus provided. Clefting of the alveolar arch between the central and lateral incisor is commonly associated. Notching of the nasal bone or at the junction of the nasal bone and frontal process of the maxilla in combination with teleorbitism is seen in more severe instances. In the literature these clefts are commonly referred to as Tessier no. 1 or 2 clefts, although Tessier himself is not convinced that there is such a "distinct" entity as the no. 2 cleft. Nor is it possible to differentiate between these clefts on an embryologic basis.

Surgical Treatment

The Nose

Reconstruction of the nose is done by one or more of the following steps:

1. *Restoration of a nasal framework.* This procedure is required only in severe instances of teleorbitism. In patients with lesser defects of the nose, the septum is normal.

2. *Closure of the disrupted mucosal lining by mobilization and approximation of the edges.* The passage thus made is normally sufficient. In selected patients it may be necessary to lengthen the roof of the nasal cavity by transposition of flaps.

3. *Reconstruction of the nasal surface by rearrangement of the skin.* In minor degrees of nasoschizis, this can be achieved by transposition of V-shaped flaps in a Z configuration. In major degrees of the anomaly, the available surplus of skin in the nasal

dorsum is rotated. In the early days of craniofacial surgery a laterally pedicled flap was used, resulting in scarring of the nasal dorsum (Fig. 35-11). Nowadays coverage is achieved with a medially pedicled flap. Rotation is facilitated by a backward cut in the glabellar area (Fig. 35-12). This approach makes it possible to position the final scars on the lateral aspect of the nose and in the alar rim, where they are least visible (Fig. 35-13).

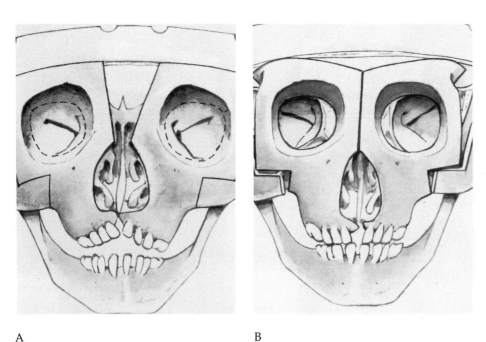

A   B

Fig. 35-9. Medial fasciotomy, split-face, or facial bipartition, procedure.

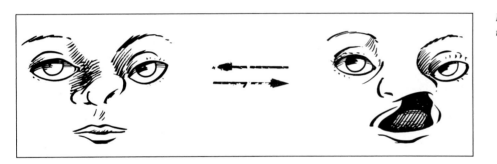

Fig. 35-10. Spectrum of malformations caused by nasal dysplasia (nasoschizis).

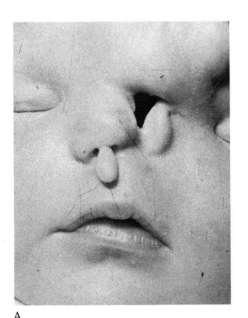
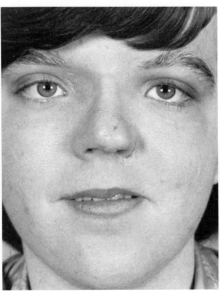

Fig. 35-11. Patient with severe unilateral clefting of the nose (nasoschizis). A. Frontal view, soon after birth. B. Frontal view, soon after final correction by redistribution of skin over nasal dorsum. The resulting scars cross the nasal surface and are less than optimal.

A   B

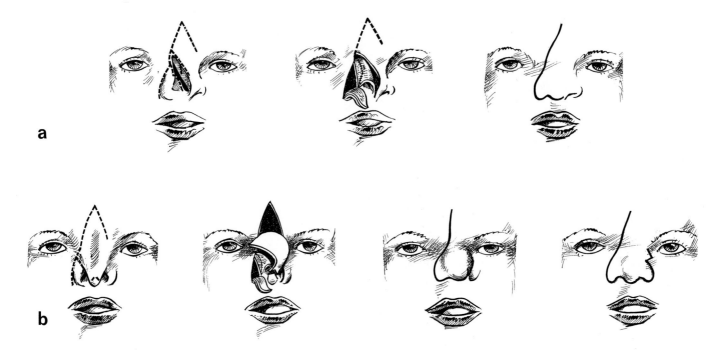

Fig. 35-12. Technique of skin transposition used for nasoschizis. A. In unilateral anomaly.
B. In bilateral anomalies.

The Skeleton

In patients with teleorbitism, reduction of the interorbital distance is indicated. This goal can be achieved by medial movement of the orbit in toto or by a facial bipartition procedure, depending on the absence or presence of alveolar clefting.

Nasomaxillary Dysplasia

Nasomaxillary dysplasia requires a distinction between incomplete and complete clefting (Fig. 35-14). An incomplete, or naso-ocular, cleft results when the disturbance in fusion is restricted to the lateronasal and maxillary processes. The cleft runs from the alar base, which is drawn upward, to the inferiorly dislocated medial canthus. In these patients, the lip develops normally.

A complete, or oronaso-ocular, cleft occurs when fusion between the medial nasal and maxillary processes also is disturbed. This cleft starts in the upper lip as an ordinary cleft and passes through the nasal aperture, skirting the foot of the distorted and superiorly dislocated ala nasi. The cleft continues to the inner canthus, which is always drawn inferiorly.

Upward rotation of the premaxilla is common. There is a retrusion of the maxilla medial to the infraorbital foramen, and its frontal process is deficient or even absent. Teleorbitism is commonly seen. The nasolacrimal apparatus is anomalous in most instances.

The appearance of an incomplete or a complete cleft depends on the period in which the arrest occurs. If the arrest occurs before the different processes have merged at the 17 mm CRL stage, the lacrimal canal does not form and a so-called primary, or transformation, defect forms. If the disturbance takes place after closure of the ectoderm of the face has been completed and a canal has been produced, a secondary, or differentiation, defect results.

Maxillary Dysplasia (Medial)

Maxillary dysplasia is caused by a developmental failure involving the medial part of the maxillary ossification center. The resulting secondary cleft extends from the lip, midway between the philtrum and the oral commissure, and proceeds laterally from the intact but superiorly dislocated nasal aperture to a lower lid coloboma. The maxilla, medial to the infraorbital foramen, is always hypoplastic, causing severe retrusion of the rim of the pyriform aperture and a funnel-shaped concavity (infundibulum) in the medial or anterior part of the orbital floor. There may be a cleft in the alveolus between the lateral incisor and the canine tooth, and the premaxilla may be rotated upward. Not surprisingly clefting of the palate, complete or partial, also has been reported, and malformations of the nasolacrimal apparatus have been observed in most patients. A wide spectrum of anomalies may be observed (Fig. 35-15).

Surgical Treatment

From a surgical point of view, the treatment of nasomaxillary dysplasia has much in common with the treatment of maxillary dysplasia. Cranial drift of the nose and premaxilla is always associated with considerable shortening of the distance between the lower eyelid or medial canthus and the alar base. In both malformations, there also may be a cleft of the upper lip. The eyeballs are usually unprotected, and the anomaly must, therefore, be treated as an emergency.

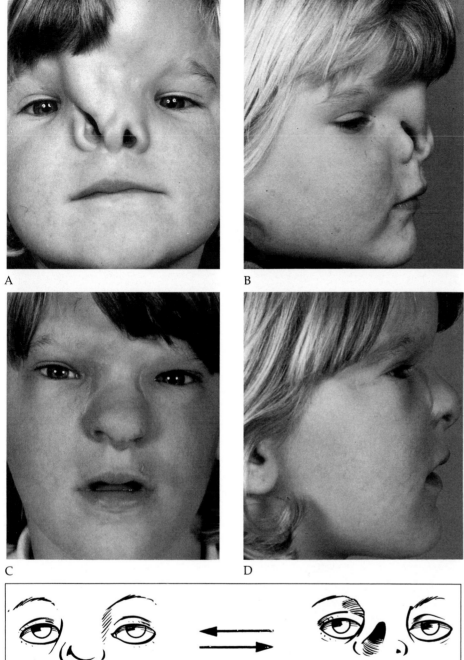

A

B

C

D

Fig. 35-13. Patient with severe bilateral clefting of the nose (nasoschizis). A. Frontal view (preoperative). B. Lateral view (preoperative). C. Frontal view (postoperative). D. Lateral view (postoperative).

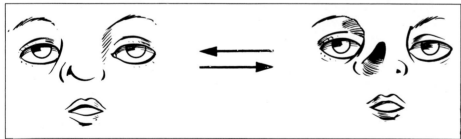

Fig. 35-14. Malformations caused by nasomaxillary dysplasia. Left. incomplete. Right, complete.

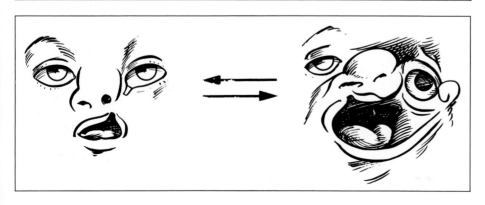

Fig. 35-15. Spectrum of malformations caused by maxillary dysplasia (medial).

Fig. 35-16. Patient with severe unilateral maxillary dysplasia. A. Before correction with median forehead flap. B. After correction, many years later. The lower eyelid on the affected side needs to be raised in combination with onlay grafting of the hypoplastic maxilla.

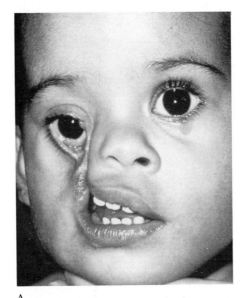

A

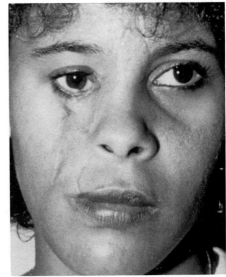

B

Fig. 35-17. Patient with severe unilateral incomplete nasomaxillary dysplasia. A. Before correction. B. Planning of the incision, which allows for movement caudally of the distorted nostril. C. After correction, frontal view. D. After correction, caudal view.

The Soft Tissues

In the past, the soft tissue defects in these anomalies were usually closed by the transposition of skin raised in one or more of the available donor areas: the forehead (Fig. 35-16), the upper eyelid, the glabella, and the cheek. All too frequently these corrections have been marred by an undesirable patchwork of flaps characterized by differences in color and texture and separated by scars crossing the nasal dorsum, the cheek, and the lip in various directions. Although it reflects the magnitude of the problem, this patchwork is no longer acceptable; it is avoidable by application of the following principles:

1. *Dissection of the medial and lateral edges of the cleft.* The periosteum is mobilized exposing the anterior wall of the maxilla, the alveolar arch, the orbital floor, and the infraorbital foramen and nerve. The orbicularis oculi and oris muscles are freed from their distorted positions. If necessary, the lateral canthus is released and a subciliary incision of the lower eyelid is made to allow for additional mobilization of the skin of the cheek.

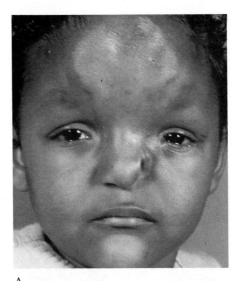

A

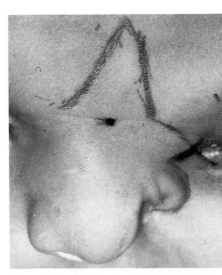

B

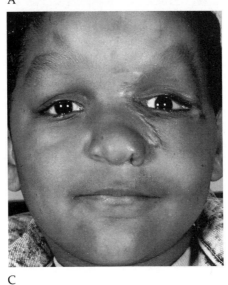

C

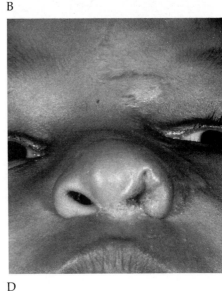

D

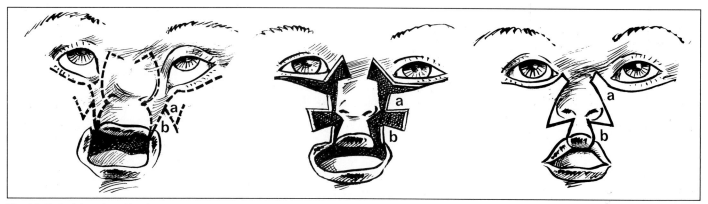

Fig. 35-18. *Incisions that allow for optimal redistribution of skin from nose and cheek. Left, preoperative. Center, intraoperative. Right, postoperative.*

Fig. 35-19. *Patient with severe bilateral maxillary dysplasia. A. Preoperative view. B. Postoperative view (3 months). The scars have not yet softened. Further improvement by medial movement of the paranasal scars will be required in the future. The final position of the scars should resemble the pattern of the Weber-Fergusson incision.*

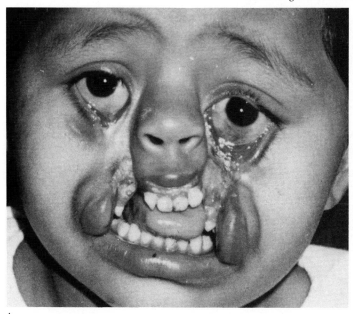

A

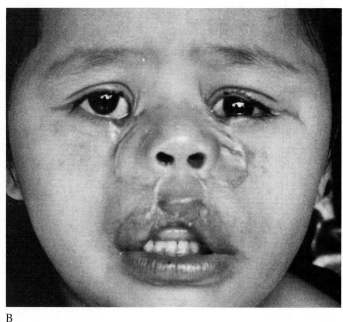

B

2. *Approximation and fixation of the periosteal muscular and mucosal elements.* The defect in the alveolar arch is bridged by transposition of periosteum and mucosa. The muscular layer in the lateral part of the lip is attached medially, its upper part anchored to the septal base. The muscular layer in the lower eyelid is attached to the medial canthus. The conjunctival defect is closed by apposition of its edges, if necessary by insertion of a mucosal graft.

3. *Elongation and integration of the cutaneous edges of the cleft.* Lengthening on the lateral aspect is achieved by two incisions: One is oblique and directed inferiorly; the other is parallel to the edge, directed superiorly. The flap thus formed can be rotated over 90°, transporting skin to the medial canthal area, where it is most needed. Lengthening of the medial aspect of the edge is obtained by incision in the lip immediately below the distorted alar base and in the nose high up in the glabellar region. In incomplete nasomaxillary dysplasia, the dissection on the medial aspect is limited to the nose (Fig. 35-17).

Rotation and approximation of the designed flaps (Fig. 35-18) allow closure of the skin defect. The main advantage of this procedure is that a maximal result is obtained with a minimum of scarring (Fig. 35-19). Medial movement of the skin of the cheek in a second stage allows serial excision of the skin on the nasal aspect of the scar and makes it possible to complete treatment with a scar similar to that of a Weber-Fergusson incision. Such a scar is less visible because of its optimal position.

The Skeleton

Management of skeletal anomalies is first determined by the condition of the hypoplastic maxilla. Movement of the roof of the maxillary sinus caudally, retrusion of the anterior wall of this cavity, and movement of its medial wall laterally are commonly observed. Correction of the first and second of these abnormalities can be achieved by application of bone grafts. Obliteration of a defect in the alveolar arch with bone grafts is never indicated. This procedure would interfere with the repositioning of the dislocated nasal structures, which is achieved by the contraction of scar tissue and by the restoration of muscular activity after closure of the soft tissue defects. The management of skeletal anomalies also depends on the presence of teleorbitism and orbital dystopia, which occasionally are seen in combination with nasomaxillary dysplasia. A patient with complete nasomaxillary clefting is a candidate for a hemifacial bipartition procedure because the position of the displaced orbitomaxillary unit in relation to the remaining part of the face can be improved. The hypoplastic dimensions of the maxilla are not altered by this technique, however; additional surgical intervention at a later stage is required.

Suggested Reading

Ortiz-Monasterio, F. Reconstruction of major nasal defects. *Clin. Plast. Surg.* 8:565, 1981.

Rieger, R.A. A local flap for repair of the nasal tip. *Plast. Reconstr. Surg.* 40:147, 1967.

Stricker, M., et al. *Craniofacial Malformations.* New York: Churchill Livingstone, 1990.

Tessier, P. Anatomical classification of facial, craniofacial and laterofacial clefts. *J. Maxillofac. Surg.* 4:69, 1976.

Tessier, P. Fentes orbito-faciales verticales et obliques (colobomas) completes et frustes. *Ann. Chir. Plast.* 14:391, 1969.

Tessier, P. Colobomas: Vertical and oblique complete facial clefts. *Panminerva Med.* 11:95, 1969.

Van der Meulen, J.C., et al. A morphogenetic classification of craniofacial malformations. *Plast. Reconstr. Surg.* 71:560, 1983.

Van der Meulen, J.C. The pursuit of symmetry in craniofacial surgery. *Br. J. Plast. Surg.* 29:85, 1976.

Van der Meulen, J.C. Medial faciotomy. *Br. J. Plast. Surg.* 32:339, 1979.

Van der Meulen, J.C., et al. Pathology and treatment of nasoschizis. *Ann. Plast. Surg.* 8:474, 1982.

Van der Meulen, J.C., and Vaandrager, J.M. Surgery related to the correction of hypertelorism. *Plast. Reconstr. Surg.* 71:6, 1983.

Van der Meulen, J.C. Oblique facial clefts: Pathology, etiology and reconstruction. *Plast. Surg.* 76:212, 1985.

36

Craniosynostosis and Craniofacial Dysostosis

Daniel Marchac   Dominique Renier

History

In the field of craniofacial surgery, my main contribution has been a group of techniques for primary correction of craniosynostosis. They were developed mainly from 1973 to 1977 and were detailed in a textbook published in 1982. It is time to reassess these techniques and the usefulness of the basic concept by observing the long-term results.

A brief history of the treatment of craniosynostosis may be useful. Skull deformities linked to premature fusion of cranial sutures were recognized and described by Virchow and others. Since the end of the nineteenth century the surgical decompression that seemed necessary in many instances was performed by strip craniectomies along the fused sutures or elevation of bone flaps or both. Despite interposition of various materials to slow down reossification, recurrences were frequent and repeated operations were routine, to the point that the Polish neurosurgeon Powiertowski proposed in 1965 to perform a total craniectomy followed by protection and remodeling with a headcap. This technique was well accepted for a time and was performed in many neurosurgical centers. It was aban-

doned because of the large number of poor reossifications and defective head shapes. Nevertheless, the method is advocated periodically by neurosurgeons who find it simpler to perform than a correction by craniofacial techniques. In fact, it was when I was presented with patients with deformed skulls as sequelae of total craniectomies that I introduced the concept of frontocranial remodeling for craniosynostosis.

Paul Tessier, whose work I observed from 1962 to 1970, developed the concept of the advancement of the supraorbital bar, or bandeau. It was used to correct the recessed forehead of adults with Crouzon and Apert syndromes who had a simultaneous Le Fort III facial advancement.

In 1973 I described the correction of a forehead that was obliquely recessed as the sequela of craniectomy or caused by oxycephaly by an advancement and rocking of the supraorbital bar and exchange and rearrangement of free bony pieces of the cranial vault. A bony Z-plasty in the temporal fossa allowed an easy and stable fixation.

In 1976 I began working in the large pediatric neurosurgical division of the Hôpital des Enfants-Malades and was

challenged by the primary treatment of craniosynostosis in infants. Pediatric anesthesiology improved greatly during these years, allowing the safe performance of sophisticated operations. A few years earlier neurosurgeons had been asked to minimize operations on children and to operate on infants as quickly as possible.

In addition to classic neurosurgical techniques, such as craniectomies and bone flaps, bone mobilization was proposed. The procedures included mobilization of the calvarial bones without mobilization of the supraorbital bar, partial mobilization with limited reconstruction, and partial mobilization with temporal muscle attachment restraining mobilization.

In 1976 my neurosurgical colleague Dominique Renier and I developed a procedure for the correction of the principal types of craniosynostosis. The operation was based on the concept of the forehead comprising two main components—the supraorbital bar and the upper forehead (Fig. 36-1). The main goal was the reconstruction of the anatomy as closely as possible to normal. It did not take into account the tremendous growing force of the infant's brain.

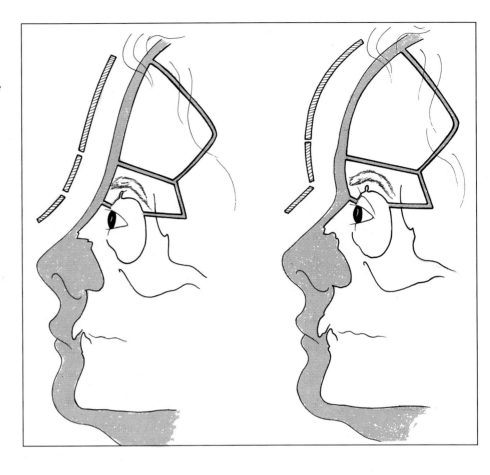

Fig. 36-1. The two components of the bony forehead. The supraorbital bar is responsible for the frontonasal angle and the projection of the eyebrows. The upper forehead, made of one piece of bone, has a gentle convexity up to the top of the cranium. A. Before advancement. B. After advancement. (From D. Marchac and D. Renier. Craniofacial Surgery for Craniosynostosis. Boston: Little, Brown, 1982. Reproduced with permission.)

To use the procedure for the recessed forehead of brachycephaly, we developed in 1977 the concept of the *floating forehead* (Fig. 36-2). The corrected and advanced forehead is fixed only to the root of the nose and to the orbital wall without connection to the cranial vault. The brain can therefore push anteriorly. We hoped initially that it would also push the midface of craniofacial dysostosis forward.

We have now operated on well over 900 patients with craniosynostosis. Since 1977 we have introduced only minor modifications, and limited variations have been reported by other authors. Our multidisciplinary craniofacial team has examined and followed these patients, and it is time to evaluate the functional and aesthetic results to see if the techniques should be modified (Table 36-1).

Simple Craniosynostosis

Craniosynostosis is quite frequent—1 per 1000 to 1500 births. Various factors have been postulated to be the cause during pregnancy (viral diseases, fetal malposition), and there is a high incidence (39% in our series) of a family history of the condition.

Classification

According to the sutures involved, the conditions observed *at birth* are as follows:

Trigonocephaly—metopic suture, triangular shape of the forehead, hypotelorism
Scaphocephaly—longitudinal suture, anteroposterior elongation, depressed middle portion of vault
Plagiocephaly—unilateral coronal synostosis, deformed vault with unilaterally recessed forehead, recessed and elevated orbit, deviated root of the nose
Brachycephaly—bilateral coronal synostosis, recessed vertical forehead with transverse enlargement, bulging temporal fossae

During the first years of life, a child may have oxycephaly with progressive upper coronal and longitudinal suture involvement. The features are a pointed head and an obliquely recessed forehead.

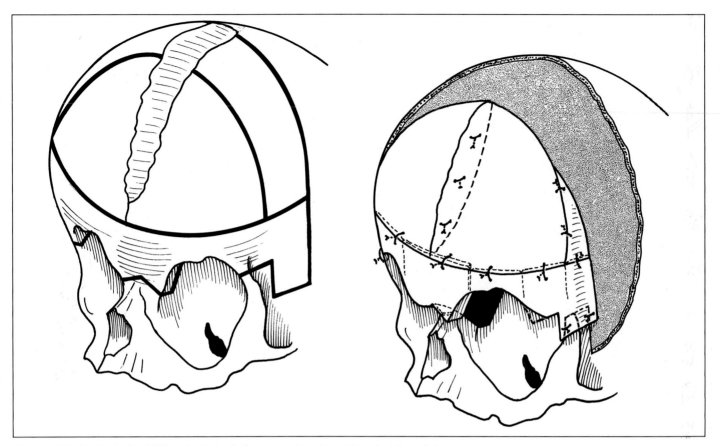

Fig. 36-2. The floating forehead. When the forehead advancement is performed in early infancy (before 6 months), the rapidly expanding brain pushes the forehead forward. The advanced forehead (2 cm) therefore is attached only to the face (root of the nose, lateral wall of the orbits) and not to the posterior cranium.

Table 36-1. Operations for craniosynostosis, 1976–1993

Condition	Number of patients examined	Number of patients operated on	Percentage operated on
Trigonocephaly	124	104	84
Scaphocephaly	482	321	67
Plagiocephaly	181	177	98
Brachycephaly	79	72	91
Oxycephaly	120	80	67
Lambdoid suture synostosis	10	7	70
Rare forms of craniosynostosis	80	70	88
Associated syndromes	51	44	86
Crouzon syndrome	60	54	90
Apert syndrome	62	54	87
	1247	983	

Trigonocephaly

Trigonocephaly is caused by a premature fusion of the midline metopic suture. Aggression during pregnancy seems a predominant factor in this synostosis. We treated a homozygous twin whose sibling was not involved (Fig. 36-3). The triangular shape of the forehead with a midline crest, recessed lateral orbital walls, and hypotelorism makes trigonocephaly easily recognizable. The hypotelorism is clear on roentgenograms even though it is not always visible clinically.

The principle of correction is simple—straightening the supraorbital bar and reconstructing a proper upper forehead—and can be done in several ways (Fig. 36-4). We usually readjust the two hemiforeheads or reverse the forehead—the new anterior part is the former posterior part. Several technical points are important:

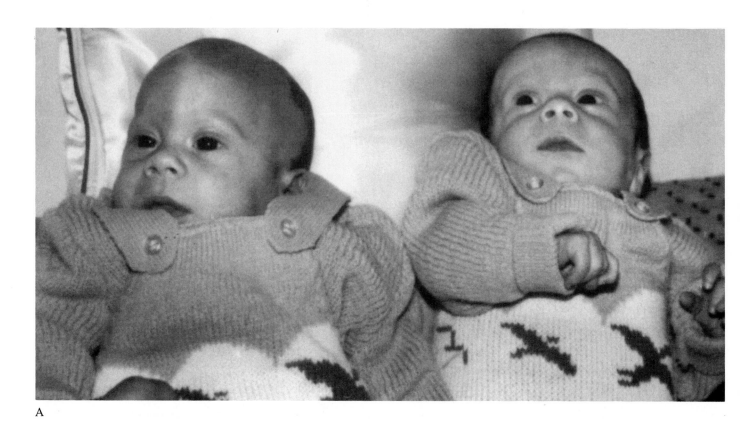

A

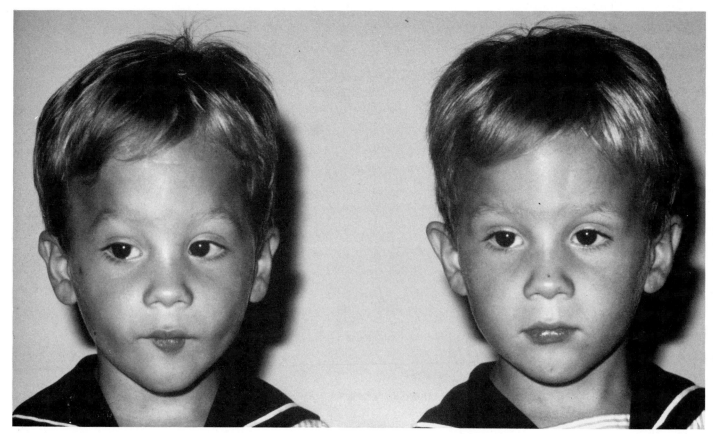

B

Fig. 36-3A. One of two homozygous twins presented with severe trigonocephaly; the other was normal.
B. The two brothers at 3 years of age after frontal remodeling on the affected one at 6 months of age.

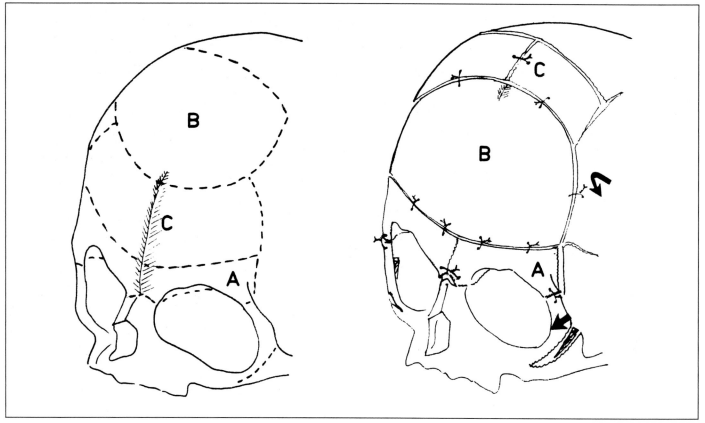

Fig. 36-4. Correction of trigonocephaly. The supraorbital bar (A) will be straightened after deposition. The upper forehead will be repaired in different ways, but use of the superior part (B) is common. The two hemiforeheads (C) are readjusted. The lateral wall of the orbit is advanced, and the temporal bone is moved outward with greenstick fractures. (From D. Marchac and D. Renier. Craniofacial Surgery for Craniosynostosis. *Boston: Little, Brown, 1982. Reproduced with permission.)*

1. It is not necessary to correct the hypotelorism by splitting the nasal bones and wedging a bone graft in between. We performed this step on five patients at the beginning of our experience and noticed no difference between these patients and those in whom the nose was left intact. We therefore discontinued this maneuver, which carries the risk of opening the nasal fossae.

2. The lateral orbital walls are always set backward. We move them forward by doing a vertical osteotomy through the lateral wall of the orbit, 1 cm from the orbital rim, down to the sphenomaxillary fissure and orbital floor. A greenstick fracture allows the forward advancement of the lateral wall as necessary, usually 7 to 8 mm. A triangular bone graft is wedged in the defect and maintains the advancement. This maneuver not only corrects the recession of the lateral wall of the orbits but also allows it to be fixed to the lateral part of the straightened supraor-

bital bar, giving stability and continuity.

3. For several years, we fixed the supraorbital bar only to the midline, to the root of the nose, but we observed one instance of frontal asymmetry, and now we prefer better stabilization.

4. The temporal region is usually narrow so we enlarge it with a few greenstick fractures, cutting several parallel slits and elevating the bone with strong bone crushers (Fig. 36-5).

Scaphocephaly

Premature fusion of the longitudinal suture, starting at the level of the coronal suture, is the most frequent synostosis in our series. The degree of malformation is variable and different techniques are required to correct it. From simplest to most complex these techniques are as follows:

1. A mild form of scaphocephaly seen early can be corrected before the infant is 6 months of age by a wide strip craniectomy of the sagittal suture or two para-

median craniectomies if one does not want to injure the sagittal sinus.

2. In more pronounced deformities of the vault, or those seen later, parietal flaps are used. These flaps are elevated; the adjacent lateral temporoparietal bone is moved outward by greenstick fractures; and the flaps are fixed in an outward position with bony struts.

3. In many patients not only is there a saddle depression of the cranial vault with temporoparietal narrowing, but the frontal area bulges forward and the occipital area bulges backward. To correct the forehead, it is rarely necessary to mobilize the supraorbital bar. It is sufficient to cut horizontally just above it and to rock the upper forehead backward. The occipital area is also pushed forward after complete cuts are made laterally and a greenstick fracture is made in the midline. Utmost care must be taken with the lateral venous sinuses, which are fragile and difficult to repair.

Fig. 36-5A. Typical trigonocephaly with hypotelorism, shown just before frontocranial remodeling. B. At 10 years of age, with a normal appearance.

All the intermediate parts of the skull are elevated in several pieces and cut transversely, as the segments of a barrel. These segments can be manipulated to change their curvature with rib benders and with the help of incomplete cuts. They are rearranged to reproduce a satisfactory shape. Usually the most anterior fragment comes behind while the preoccipital piece fits well behind the forehead (Figs. 36-6 and 36-7). Laterally these segments should be cut rather low, but it may be useful to open the remaining bone further, close to the base of the skull, by outward greenstick fractures. The anteroposterior dimension should be reduced and the cranial width increased.

In infants it is not necessary to fix all the bony pieces by wiring, apart from the frontal bone. Fixation with absorbable sutures or even gluing of the bony segments to the dura with fibrin glue is sufficient. Sometimes, a large polyglactin net is used to maintain the bony pieces in the desired position while the scalp flaps are brought over it. It is important to have the baby lie on the back of his or her head in the postoperative period. The occipital correction, the most dangerous part of the operation, can be avoided if the deformity is not too prominent. One should not hesitate, however, to correct the bulging forehead by rocking it backward and enlarging the temporal fossae.

Plagiocephaly

Unilateral coronal synostosis produces an asymmetry that should be corrected. Because the deformity is unilateral, most authors advocate a unilateral correction. We believe, however, that a bilateral correction is more satisfactory in infants for the following reasons:

1. The apparently normal side often presents compensatory bulging and should be corrected.
2. Symmetry is easier to achieve by bilateral remodeling. The upper forehead selected as one piece has the proper double curvature, and its rigidity helps maintain the reconstructed supraorbital bar. When fixing the corrected supraorbital bar into place, one finds there is often a slight advancement on the midline. This is helpful

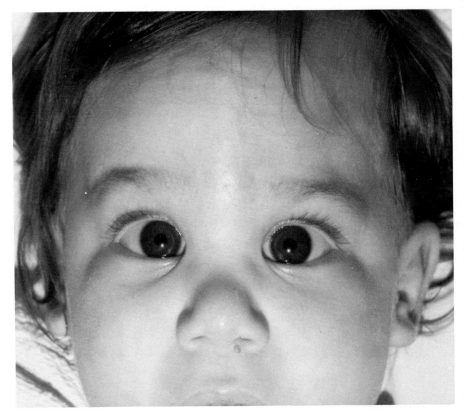

A

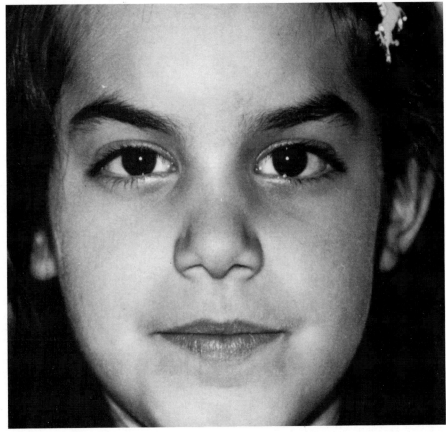

B

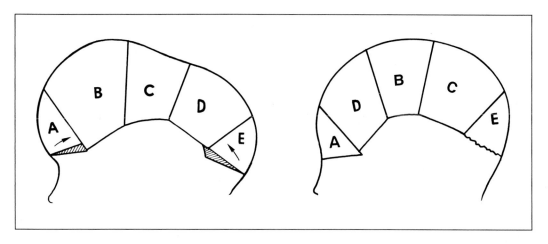

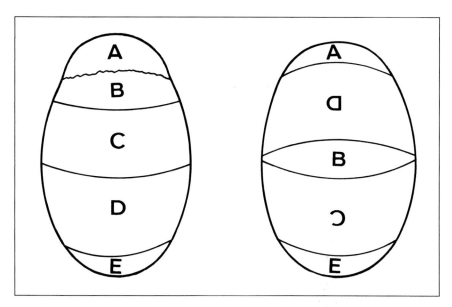

Fig. 36-6. Correction of scaphocephaly. In severe forms, one performs a total vault remodeling: The forehead is pushed backward; the occipital area is brought forward; and the intermediate bony pieces of the cranial vault are elevated like parts of a barrel, remodeled, and exchanged to produce a normal curvature transversely and longitudinally. (From D. Marchac and D. Renier. Craniofacial Surgery for Craniosynostosis. Boston: Little, Brown, 1982. Reproduced with permission.)

Fig. 36-7. Pre- and postoperative roentgenograms illustrating the remodeling technique for scaphocephaly.

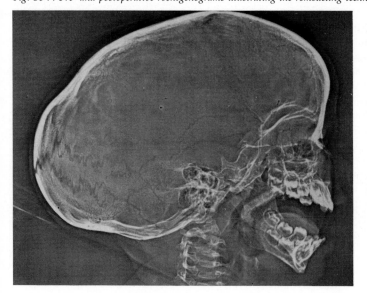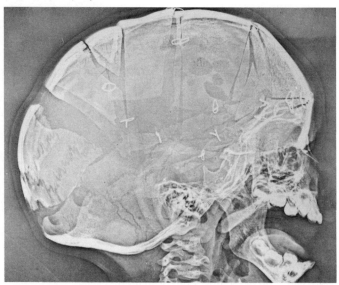

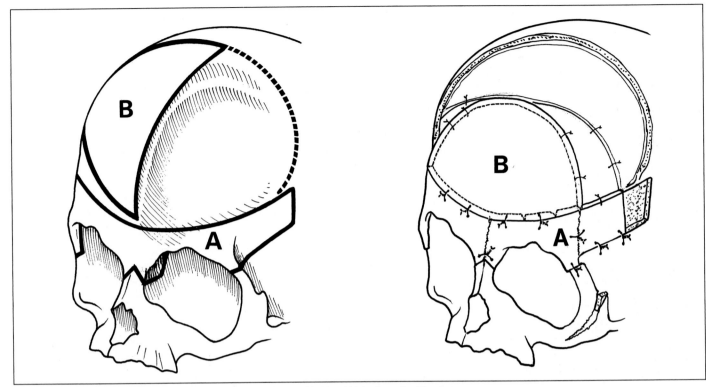

Fig. 36-8. Bilateral correction of plagiocephaly. The distorted supraorbital bar (A) is elevated with a long, wide temporal tenon. It is straightened and put back in an advanced position. The lateral wall of the orbit is advanced considerably. The upper forehead (B) is reconstructed with a single piece of bone of the proper shape on the vault. Defects are closed. (Part A from D. Marchac and D. Renier. Craniofacial Surgery for Craniosynostosis. Boston: Little, Brown, 1982. Reproduced with permission.)

to obtain a smooth curve and therefore to avoid a possible midline depression.

3. Complete transection of the anterior cranial base, from one temporal fossa to the other, seems to provide a better release from the restricting forces of the premature synostosis.

To begin the operation one draws a horizontal line 1 cm above the orbits. This line often is deviated, going higher on the affected side. A resection is made on the lateral orbital margin to allow the supraorbital bar to be put back horizontally. The supraorbital bar is short on the "normal" side and has a long temporal tenon on the affected side (Fig. 36-8).

A suitable upper forehead is selected with the help of forehead templates (Fig. 36-9). We try as much as possible to find this upper forehead in the anterior part of the cranium to limit the dissection. The forehead template helps to determine where the future upper forehead will be adjusted and to cut the remaining skull so it will fit precisely.

After elevation of the upper forehead and

of the bar, the orbital roof on the affected side is corrected. It is usually angulated upward because it is very thick at the summit of the angle. This piece is removed with a bone cutter, and the two remaining parts of the orbital roof—medial and lateral—are brought down by making greenstick fractures with a strong forceps.

The lateral orbital wall is moved forward. After elevation of the periosteum of the orbit down to the sphenomaxillary fissure and elevation of the temporal muscle, the lateral wall is cut down to the fissure. A curved osteotome allows greenstick fractures to bring the lateral wall forward. A triangular graft, usually taken from the resected orbital roof, is wedged in the gap and maintains the anterior projection. The asymmetry of the supraorbital bar is corrected by making incomplete posterior cuts and greenstick fractures of the malformed portion to give it a normal curvature.

Often there is double angulation, the lateral part of the recessed side also having rotated horizontally and the lower part lo-

cated too far anteriorly. One can try to correct this problem without breaking the supraorbital bar. If the bar breaks a wire is necessary to restore continuity. The supraorbital bar is wired back, with care taken to advance it sufficiently on the recessed side. The tenon allows maintenance of the desired projection.

The upper forehead is adjusted. All temporal defects are carefully repaired with the remaining bone from the forehead. After irregularities are burred out and the temporal muscle is reattached, the skin is put back. If it still looks asymmetric, the forehead must immediately be advanced additionally.

We have found that overcorrection is rare, whereas undercorrection is frequent. The bony correction must seem slightly exaggerated to be satisfactory. Although the nose and orbit improve with time (Fig. 36-10), the forehead remains constant—if it is undercorrected it will remain so (Fig. 36-11).

Fig. 36-10. Self-correction of nasal deviation. A. At 6 months of age, this unilateral coronal synostosis shows a nasal bone deviation toward the left (affected) side. B. Five years after the bilateral frontocranial remodeling illustrated in Fig. 36-8, the nasal skeleton, untouched during the operation, has straightened itself spontaneously. Note advancement of left orbital wall. C. The infant at 6 months of age. D. The same child at 11 years of age. ▶

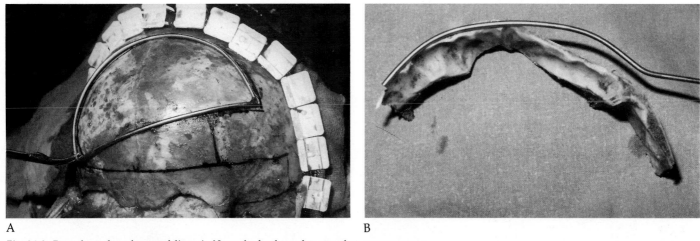

A

B

Fig. 36-9. Frontal templates for remodeling. A. Upper forehead templates to select a proper upper forehead. B. Supraorbital bar templates to control the curvature.

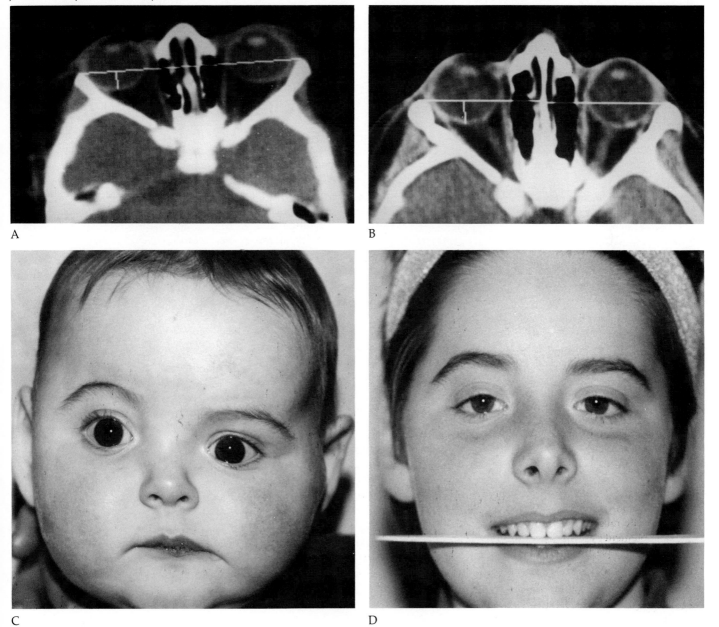

A

B

C

D

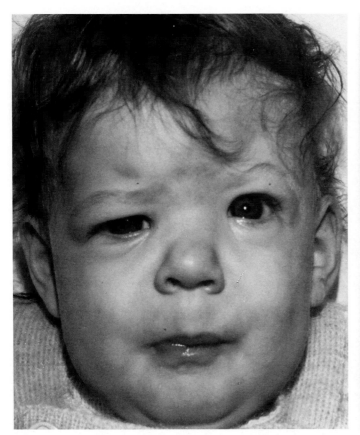
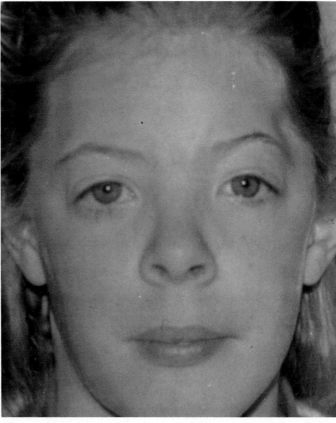

A   B

Fig. 36-11A. Severely distorted face in a 6-month-old infant affected with left unilateral coronal synostosis, just before frontocranial remodeling. B. At 12 years of age the symmetry of the face is good, but there is a small depression of the left temporal area.

If the cranial vault is severely asymmetric behind the coronal sutures, we often elevate parietal flaps and correct the asymmetry, mostly by rotating and exchanging the bony pieces. Usually we do not correct the posterior parietooccipital asymmetry, which is often observed in unilateral coronal synostosis. It seems to be related to a compensatory push from the brain, because it is rare to find a stenosed lambdoid suture. Correction involves risk at the level of the venous sinuses and extensive dissection. This posterior asymmetry usually diminishes with time after the frontal correction.

Brachycephaly

Bilateral coronal synostosis is responsible for a vertically recessed forehead. Transverse enlargement or turricephaly is often associated, because the brain seeks sufficient space in other directions.

When examining a patient with brachycephaly, one wonders always if the mid-

face is involved or not. The coronal suture continues medially to the cranial base and the sphenoidal region, and evaluation of possible cranial base involvement is difficult roentgenographically. Clinically, one examines the relation between mandible and maxilla; often there exists an end-to-end relation, or even a moderate maxillary retrusion. When brachycephaly is associated with faciocraniosynostosis, as in Crouzon and Apert syndromes, there is usually some degree of immediate facial retrusion. The floating forehead advancement is intended to remodel and advance the restricted forehead without limiting the anterior push of the brain; this push is supposed to be transmitted to the midface (see Fig. 36-2).

After the scalp and the periosteum are elevated separately to give more elasticity, the supraorbital bar is marked with two long temporal tenous. The superior forehead is selected. The midline fontanelle is often open, and it may be nec-

essary to select an upper forehead made of two pieces to be readjusted together.

The temporal fossa usually bulges outward. The convex bone is deposited in one piece and put back after it has been turned 180°, producing a concavity.

The supraorbital bar is remodeled. The desired shape, with angles at the level of the lateral orbital wall, is obtained by incomplete posterior cuts. A bone graft is fixed on the midline for transverse reinforcement. This remodeled supraorbital bar is fixed in an advanced position (usually 2 cm) to the root of the nose and the lateral sides of the orbits. A horizontal graft is placed between the root of the nose and the supraorbital bar. Laterally the fixation is sometimes difficult if the junction between the malar bone and the frontal bone is not stable. We fix the bones to the lateral wall of the orbit by two wires, sometimes with a bone graft as reinforcement to bridge the junction of the bar and the lateral orbital wall. It is fundamental to stabilize this advanced bar because the pressure of the forehead skin tends to rock it upward.

We have tried to improve fixation by the use of miniplates with a T shape, the vertical branch being located along the lateral orbital wall and the horizontal branch on the supraorbital bar. Although the fixation is stable, we have stopped using it in infants because, after some years, miniplates were found lying intracranially on the dura, the screws leaving holes in the dura when removed. One can, of course, remove these miniplates after a few months. It is not worthwhile to have children undergo another operation for removal of the miniplates, even if minor, if it can be avoided. When absorbable miniplates become available, we will use them, but for now we use wires only and sometimes additional bone grafts.

A fundamental measure to avoid displacement of the supraorbital bar consists in avoiding any dressing on the forehead. Only the coronal incision is covered by a light dressing. Once the supraorbital bar is solidly secured, the upper forehead is constructed, usually with the previous forehead remodeled.

We also carefully reconstruct the temporal areas lateral to the upper forehead. A wide gap is left behind the advanced forehead and the remaining cranium. If exaggerated tension occurs at scalp closure, a wide posterior undermining of the scalp is performed.

Initially the advancement of the forehead seems exaggerated, with a steplike appearance above the nose (Fig. 36-12). After a few months the appearance is quite normal. We have never regretted the magnitude advanced of a brachycephalic forehead (Fig. 36-13).

This advancement produces an important space between the advanced forehead and the frontal dura. The dead space is obliterated in about 2 to 3 weeks by the distention and advancement of the dura. It is not necessary therefore to incise the dura and to suture a patch, as has been proposed.

Evaluation of Treatment

The results of frontocranial remodeling for craniosynostosis must be evaluated both functionally and aesthetically. The

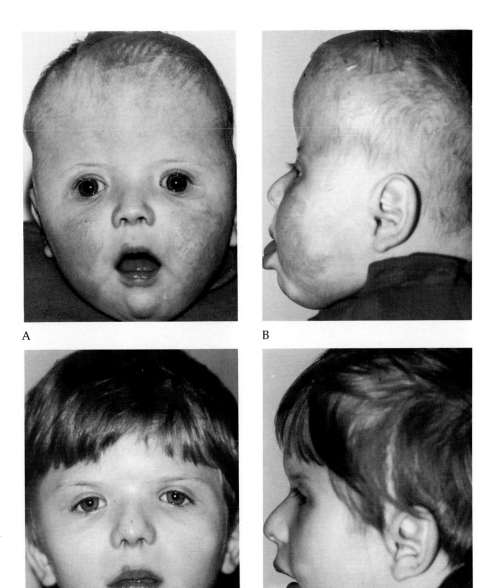

Fig. 36-12. Surgically treated brachycephaly. A, B. An infant with severe brachycephaly before frontal advancement. C, D. At 5 years of age, with a good forehead contour and projection of the supraorbital bar.

functional results are assessed on the basis of absence of neurologic problems such as seizures or headaches, the quality of vision, and the intelligence level. It is difficult to assess intelligence quotient (IQ) in infants, but a series of usable tests has been developed by our psychologists, and all our patients are evaluated. Our results show that the IQ is higher when the children are operated on in infancy than when the operation is delayed. It is also better than in children who are not

operated on. The prognosis is usually worse when there is an associated anomaly. Reoperations are rare. Classic neurosurgical techniques, on the other hand, frequently require reoperations.

The morphologic results are evaluated as we evaluate all our aesthetic results of cosmetic or reconstructive operations. The patient should be examined from a distance of 50 cm—normal conversational distance—in average daylight and, if pos-

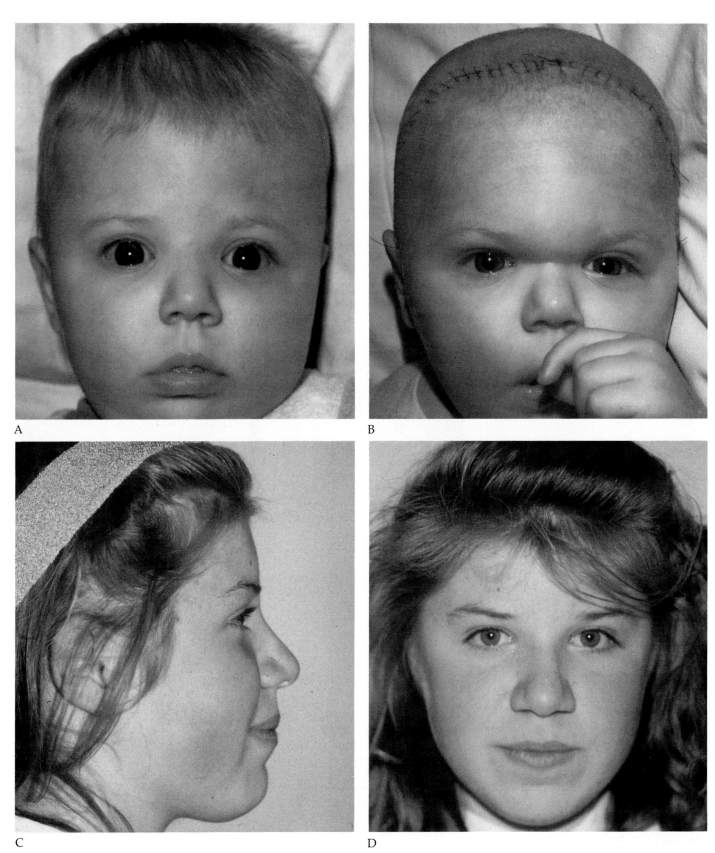

Fig. 36-13. *Brachycephaly. A, B. Before and just after the frontal advancement. C, D. At 12 years of age after floating forehead advancement in infancy.*

sible, by a person other than the surgeon who does not know about the previous condition. The rating is given on a scale of 1 to 4. A rating of 1 is excellent. Nothing abnormal can be detected. There is no deformity and no scarring. A rating of 2 is good. There is an existing deformity or scar, but it is minimal. Revision can be considered for improvement but is not mandatory. A rating of 3 is mediocre. A deformity or scar is visible and presents a problem. If revision is possible, it should be undertaken. A rating of 4 is poor. A serious deformity is obvious, and a reoperation must be considered.

Although the evaluation is done by someone other than the surgical team, we have compared our own evaluations with those of the uninitiated observers. We found that the ratings of the surgical team were more severe, probably because we were more aware of minor imperfections.

We based our evaluations on the treated area without taking into account untreated areas. For example, in patients with Crouzon or Apert syndrome who underwent frontal remodeling, we rated the appearance of the forehead, not the appearance of the midface, which was not treated. The overall results of frontocranial remodeling for craniosynostosis have been satisfactory (Table 36-2).

We found on the whole that the principles of frontal remodeling have not changed and that the correction of the different types of craniosynostoses has not changed a great deal since the period from 1973 to 1977. Nevertheless, the following features are different:

1. The fixation is more stable, especially for trigonocephaly and brachycephaly.
2. The procedure involves the area in front of the coronal sutures as much as possible.
3. The shape of the temporal area is carefully reconstructed: A bone graft is always placed at the sides of the upper forehead.
4. The distorted skull behind the osteotomy lines is straightened by greenstick fractures, and incisions are made perpendicular to the edge of the skull remodeling.
5. The remaining cranial defects are closed by splitting calvarium or using strips of bone dust mixed with fibrin glue.

Indications for Treatment

When a deformity is obvious or there is risk of brain compression, the question of whether or not to operate has not been raised. Frontocranial remodeling is the operation of choice. Its results are superior to those of the classic craniectomies. When a deformity is less severe and the functional risks are not obvious, the following studies can be performed to determine whether the operation should be performed on a functional basis.

1. Roentgenography may show fingerprinting.
2. Visual problems may be observed on an examination of the fundus.
3. Intracranial pressure recording seems to be the most reliable way to determine whether there is increased intracranial pressure. We prefer the transdural measurement. A small scalp incision allows a bur hole to be made, and the recording chamber can be plugged into the bur hole and connected to a recording apparatus. Variations in intracranial pressure are recorded for 12 hours. An EEG is performed at the same time.

4. Intracranial volume can be measured by calculating the surface areas of additional horizontal slices from a cranial computed tomogram.

We reiterate that the intracranial pressure test is at present the most important examination. If the pressure is increased, the operation should be performed. If the pressure is normal, there is no functional problem and it is up to the parents to decide whether or not they want the child to have the operation. The parents must be told that if it is performed later in the child's life, the operation will be more difficult and the final results may not be as good as those of an operation performed when the child is an infant.

One would hope that the roentgenographic measurement of intracranial pressure would give information similar to that provided by intracranial pressure measurement. However, many comparative studies must be made before roentgenography can replace intracranial pressure recording in doubtful situations.

For brachycephaly we recommend a floating forehead advancement when the infant is 2 to 3 months of age or weighs 5 kg. For all other craniosynostoses, the frontocranial remodeling advancement is performed ideally when the child is 6 to 8 months of age, but definitely before he or she is 12 months of age.

Rare and Complex Forms of Craniosynostosis
Oxycephaly

Mostly found in North Africa, oxycephaly is the only late-appearing craniosynostosis. When the child is about 2 or 3 years of age, coronal and metopic sutures fuse and the anterior part of the skull recedes. A bulge often occurs at the midline, at the bregma, and the child appears to have a pointed head. Brain compression is frequent, and this form of craniosynostosis is often discovered because the child has visual problems, headaches, and vomiting. Decompression is therefore urgent and is obtained by rocking the supraorbital bar to reconstruct a frontonasal angle and by exchanging bony pieces of the cranial vault.

Sometimes, there is little distortion and the shape is practically normal, but the

Table 36-2. Evaluation of late morphologic results of frontocranial remodeling for craniosynostosis

Condition	No. patients	Results (no. patients)			
		Excellent	Good	Mediocre	Poor
Trigonocephaly	6	4	2	0	0
Plagiocephaly	17	9	8	0	0
Brachycephaly	12	6	5	1	0
Total	35	19	15	1	0

Note: The 35 patients available for study were operated on when they were younger than 18 months; had nonsyndromic craniosynostosis; underwent mobilization of the supraorbital bar and forehead; and participated in the follow-up study for 10 years.

skull is just too small anteriorly and has fingerprinting. This is a harmonious oxycephaly. The same principle of correction is used as for the usual oxycephaly, but one should be careful to keep a good balance of the forehead while advancing it.

Cloverleaf Skull

A trilobed skull is a severe condition usually associated with facial retrusion. The synostosis between the temporal and parietal bones produces a deep groove that is also found in the dura after bony elevation. We have performed several Z-plasties of the dura to release this dural band.

Synostosis of the Lambdoid Suture

Synostosis of the lambdoid suture can occur alone but it is usually associated with brachycephaly or plagiocephaly. It can be treated by a posterior displacement similar to a frontal advancement, but with two lateral tenous. A strong fixation is necessary because it is difficult to avoid having the baby rest on his or her back.

Associated Forms of Craniosynostosis

Different types of associated *craniosynostoses* were observed in 9 percent of the patients in my series. The prognosis for these associated forms is not as good as that for the isolated forms.

Malformations Associated with Craniosynostosis

One must always look for other malformations. Skeletal anomalies, especially of hands and feet, must be sought. Renal and cardiac problems can also be associated with craniosynostosis. Besides causing operative and postoperative problems, the associated anomalies usually carry a poorer functional and aesthetic prognosis.

Hydrocephalus, the most frequent of these anomalies, represents a problem because the brain should be able to expand to fill the newly remodeled skull. But the brain should not exert too much pressure if the hydrocephalus has not been treated.

If a shunt has been installed, it could be too effective and prevent the brain from filling the dead space. If the neurosurgeon decides to place a shunt before the frontocranial remodeling is done, it is advisable to interrupt the shunt while the craniosynostosis is being treated.

Craniofacial Dysostosis

Dysostosis involves the midface, essentially at its junction with the cranial base. The sphenoid bone seems to play a key role in the development of the midface. The most well-known craniofacial dysostoses are Crouzon and Apert diseases, but many syndromes, such as Pfeiffer and Carpenter syndromes, also can present a facial retrusion, which is the major feature of craniofacial dysostosis. Facial retrusion is associated with various types of cranial vault deformities, the most frequent one being brachycephaly.

To treat craniofacial dysostosis, one usually has to advance the frontal bone and the midface for both functional and aesthetic reasons. Several possibilities are offered:

1. *Staged advancement.* The forehead is advanced first and the face later.
2. *Monobloc advancement.* The forehead and face are advanced simultaneously, and the whole orbits are mobilized with the midface, as described by Ortiz-Monasterio.
3. *Simultaneous advancement* of the frontal bone and of the midface by Le Fort III osteotomy.

The simultaneous or monobloc advancement seems a logical solution when both the frontal bone and the midface are recessed. These procedures carry a higher risk of complications, however, because there is a communication between the anterior cranial base and the nasal fossae. It has been advocated that this opening of the nasal fossae be avoided by dissecting in front of them, but experience shows that an opening is difficult to avoid when the advancement is great. The frontal dead space may also be avoided by lowering the top of the head to force the brain to move forward.

Another possibility, proposed by Anderl, is to leave the cranial base intact and to advance the frontal bone in front of the

supraorbital bar at the same time as a Le Fort III osteotomy is performed. This procedure is more applicable to older children and adults.

Craniofacial Dysostosis in Infants

When a newborn infant has a craniofacial dysostosis, one can choose to perform isolated frontal remodeling or a monobloc frontofacial advancement. An early monobloc procedure is vigorously advocated by Muhlbauer, from Munich. A careful dissection is performed in front of the nasal capsule, which is left in place. Dysjunction is obtained by gentle spreading and a series of tractions. Fixation is made by long miniplates adjusted on the malar bone in front and the temporal cranial vault in back. These miniplates are removed after 3 months.

This operation allows immediate dramatic correction of exorbitism and reestablishes a normal relation of face and cranium (Fig. 36-14). For two reasons my group is nevertheless reluctant to perform this operation when there is not major exorbitism and the eyes do not require protection:

1. This is an extensive operation for an infant and it involves a copious loss of blood. A communication between the cranial base and the nasal cavities is difficult to avoid and carries a risk of meningitis and osteitis.
2. An early midfacial advancement made through the pterygomaxillary junction may further deteriorate the limited growth potential of the midface.

We therefore reserve the monobloc operation for severe exorbitism. Otherwise we perform a frontal advancement and a later facial advancement. The frontal advancement is a floating forehead in infants 6 months of age and younger and a frontal advancement with temporal tendon in older infants, because the push of the brain diminishes considerably after 6 months of age. The facial advancement is performed when the child and the parents believe it to be necessary. Ideally, one would prefer to wait until the eruption of the permanent teeth is complete, at about the age of 12 years. Orthodontic preparation would allow a perfect occlusion after the facial advancement and per-

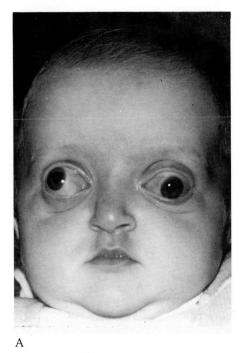

A

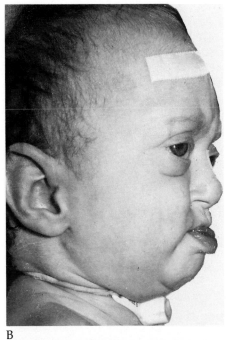

B

Fig. 36-14. Monobloc frontofacial advancement.
A, B. A 3-month-old infant with
faciocraniosynostosis (Crouzon disease). C, D.
After the monobloc frontofacial advancement.

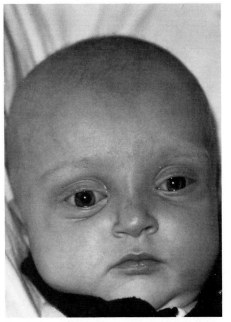

C

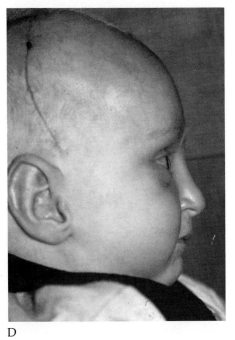

D

manent results. This is the treatment given when the retrusion is moderate and well tolerated.

In most instances of craniofacial dysostosis, the facial retrusion accentuated by the early frontal advancement is obvious and causes social problems at school age. We, therefore, usually perform the Le Fort III facial advancement when the child is 4 to 6 years of age. The occlusion is

rarely satisfactory, and we try to correct the orbital retrusion and shortened nose, advancing the maxilla as much as possible and fixing it with miniplates.

The family is warned that a second facial advancement will usually be necessary after completion of dental growth. In most instances a lower osteotomy—Le Fort I—is sufficient, the orbital area and root of the nose remaining satisfactory.

Special mention must be made of the root of the nose. For too long massive bone grafts have been used between the area of the glabella and the advanced nose. An enlargement of the upper part of the nose and a poor definition of the frontonasal angle were the results.

It is important to obtain a thin nose. Sometimes it is useful to narrow the advanced root of the nose by removing lateral or paramedian bony pieces. The bone graft should be well adjusted. We usually use a cranial graft, on which greenstick fractures are made to produce the shape of a roof in continuity with the nose. Careful fixation is obtained with wires or miniplates or both. Laterally we usually perform an interlocking procedure at the superolateral angle of the orbit and add bone grafts to improve the orbital contour.

Fig. 36-15. Advancement and bipartition for Apert syndrome. A, B. A 7-year-old patient who had a floating forehead advancement in infancy. A severe maxillary retrusion is developing. C, D. After facial advancement associated with bipartition to correct the teleorbitism.

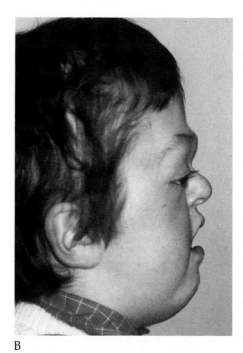

A

B

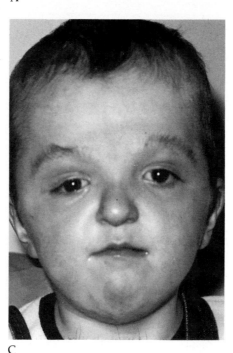

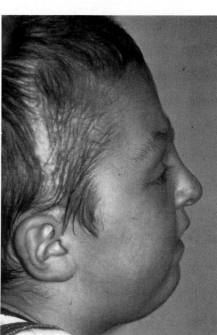

C

D

Apert Syndrome and Bipartition

The Apert syndrome represents a special challenge because of the associated facial retrusion with a short nose; teleorbitism; and narrow upper dental arch with inverted V shape of the teeth. The bipartition associated with the facial advancement is of special interest in Apert syndrome. The principle is that of a midline splitting of the facial mass, with a V resection at the level of the root of the nose. This medial resection allows the orbits to be brought together, correcting the teleorbitism, and the maxilla to be expanded simultaneously.

In patients who have not been operated on before, a total bipartition can be performed, mobilizing all the orbits and allowing the forehead to be corrected. In patients who have had their forehead corrected previously, a Le Fort III procedure with midline splitting through nose and palate is performed, leaving the forehead intact (Fig. 36-15).

Conclusion

The treatment of craniosynostosis, and even more so of craniofacial dysostosis, is a team effort that requires the close cooperation of all the members of the craniofacial team. Evaluation of the patient requires, besides the care of a plastic surgeon and a neurosurgeon, the collaboration of a radiologist, psychologist, geneticist, otorhinolaryngologist, and an ophthalmologist. The role of the anesthesiologist is of course fundamental. Most of what we achieve is possible only because of impressive progress in pediatric anesthesiology and intensive care.

Suggested Reading

Anderl, H., et al. Fronto-facial advancement with bony separation in craniofacial dysostosis. *Plast. Reconstr. Surg.* 71:303, 1983.

Bartlett, S., Whitaker, L., and Marchac, D. The operative treatment of isolated craniofacial dysostosis (plagiocephaly): A comparison of the unilateral and bilateral techniques. *Plast. Reconstr. Surg.* 85:677, 1990.

Benattar, A. La craniectomie extensive dans le traitement des craniostenoses. (Etude de 37 cas.) Thèse Méd. Paris, 1977.

Gault, D., et al. The calculation of intra-cranial volume using CT scans. *Childs Nerv. Syst.* 4: 271, 1988.

Hoffman, H.J. Early Craniectomy and Stripping in Craniofacial Synostosis. In J.M. Converse, J. McCarthy, and D. Woodsmith (Eds.), *Symposium on Diagnosis and Treatment of Craniofacial Anomalies.* St. Louis: Mosby, 1979. P. 287.

Le Merrer, M., et al. Conseil génétique dans les craniosténoses. *J. Genet. Hum.* 36:295, 1988.

Marchac, D. Radical forehead remodeling for craniostenosis. *Plast. Reconstr. Surg.* 61:823, 1978.

Marchac, D., et al. A propos des ostéotomies d'avancement du crâne et de la face. *Ann. Chir. Plast.* 19:311, 1974.

Marchac, D., and Renier, D. *Craniofacial Surgery for Craniosynostosis.* Boston: Little, Brown, 1982.

Marchac, D., and Renier, D. Craniosynostosis. *World J. Surg.* 13:358, 1989.

Muhlbauer, W., Anderl, H., and Marchac, D. Complete fronto-facial advancement in infants with craniofacial dysostosis. In Transactions of the 8th International Congress of Plastic Surgery. Montreal, June 26, July 1, 1983.

Ortiz-Monasterio, F., Fuente El Campo, A., and Carillo, A. Advancement of the orbits and the face in one piece combined with frontal repositioning for the correction of Crouzon's deformities. *Plast. Reconstr. Surg.* 61:507, 1978.

Powiertowski, H., and Matlosz, Z. The treatment of craniostenosis by a method of extensive resection of the vault of the skull. In Proceedings of the 3rd International Congress on Neurosurgery. *Surg. Excepta Med. Int. Cong. Series* 110:834, 1965.

Renier, D., et al. Intracranial pressure in craniostenosis. *J. Neurosurg.* 53:370, 1982.

Rougerie, J., Derome, P., and Anquez, L. Craniosténoses et dysmorphies cranio-faciales. Principes d'une nouvelle technique de traitement et ses résultats. *Neurochirurgie* 18:429, 1972.

Tessier, P. Recent improvement in the treatment of facial and cranial deformities in Crouzon's disease and Apert's syndrome. In *Symposium on Plastic Surgery of the Orbital Region.* St. Louis: Mosby, 1976. P. 271.

Virchow, R. Uber den Cretinismus, nametlich in Franken, und uber pathologische Schadelforamen. *Ver Phys. Med. Cesselsch. (Wurzburg)* 2:230, 1981.

37

Frontoethmoidal Meningoencephalocele

David J. David   Richard H. C. Harries

A *cephalocele* is a congenital herniation of intracranial contents through a cranial defect. When the herniation contains brain and meninges, it is termed a *meningoencephalocele*. Spring in 1854 wrote what was probably the first extensive monograph on the subject. He stated that Le Dran introduced the term *hernia cerebri* in 1740; however, Le Dran's patient probably had a cephalhematoma. Spring himself tried to distinguish between meningocele and cerebral hernia, the latter being divided into encephalocele and hydroencephalocele when hydrocephalus was present. The term *meningoencephalocele* seems appropriate because it describes the contents of the hernia. This chapter discusses frontoethmoidal meningoencephaloceles, which, by definition, present on the front of the skull and are seen externally. Modern methods and investigation offered by a multidisciplinary craniofacial unit enable these lesions to be studied more thoroughly and treated more effectively than in the past.

Etiology

In western Europe, North America, Japan, and Australia, these lesions are relatively rare; occipital cephaloceles are much more prevalent. In Southeast Asia frontoethmoidal meningoencephaloceles are by far the most common type of cephalocele, and this appears to be the case in parts of the Indian subcontinent and in southern Russia. For frontoethmoidal meningoencephaloceles, siblings and offspring do not show any increased incidence of anencephaly or myelodysplasia, and even in high-risk areas it is unusual to find more than one frontoethmoidal meningoencephalocele in the same family. Parents can be reassured accordingly. Recent work by the Australian Cranio-Facial Unit with Southeast Asian patients revealed that frontoethmoidal meningoencephalocele may have a genetic basis. It was found that advanced parental age was frequent in instances of this defect, suggesting that an autosomal dominant mutation may be involved, and this, if confirmed, would have important implications in genetic counseling. However, the lack of familial instances and geographic distribution of meningoencephalocele argues strongly against dominant mutation as a cause.

Classification

Meningoencephaloceles may be subdivided into occipital, parietal, basal, and sincipital types. The last group was further classified by Suwanwela and Suwanwela in 1972, based on a paper by Meyer published in 1890, into the following categories:

Frontoethmoidal
  Nasofrontal
  Nasoethmoidal
  Naso-orbital
Interfrontal
Craniofacial clefts

The bony defects associated with sincipital meningoencephaloceles have been included in many attempts to classify craniofacial clefts. Two of the most recent and important endeavors are Tessier's anatomic classification and Mazzola's morphologic classification based on embryologic considerations. However, it is important to note that there is a fundamental difference between the etiology and pathology of frontoethmoidal meningoencephaloceles and of meningoencephaloceles associated with facial clefts.

Pathology

To appropriately treat patients with frontoethmoidal meningoencephalocele, it is vital that the underlying pathology be clearly understood.

The term *frontoethmoidal meningoencephalocele* describes the site of the cranial end of the bony defect, which is always in the position of the foramen cecum at the junction of the frontal and ethmoidal bones. The posterior margin of the defect is formed by the crista galli. This margin is often distorted, and the cribriform plate is usually tilted downward as a deep central trough, the anterior end of which is well below the planum sphenoidale. The cribriform plate forms an angle of 45° to 50° with the orbitomeatal plane.

The cranial exit holes vary in size and shape. All nasofrontal defects appear round and central, whereas naso-orbital defects are usually bilobed. Nasoethmoidal meningoencephaloceles are particularly variable in the shape of the bony defect. The morphology of the defects of the facial bone shows even more variation.

In the nasofrontal type, the exit holes are at the junction of the frontal and nasal bones, the nasal bones being attached to the inferior margin of the defect (Fig. 37-1). In the nasoethmoidal type, the facial defects lie between the nasal bones and the nasal cartilage, the nasal bones being above and the nasal cartilages below. The nasal bones are deformed and often broadened with distorted margins. The nasal septal cartilage is pushed downward and backward. The frontonasal angle is obliterated, producing an overhanging ledge (Fig. 37-2). When the facial defect is confined to the nasal pyramid, the exit hole is small and oval and the medial walls of the orbit are not involved. If, however, the meningoencephalocele is larger, the facial defect extends more laterally and the anterior margins of the medial orbital walls are eroded and become crescent shaped. It is as though the meningoencephalocele had blown out onto the face through the weakened junction of the frontal and ethmoidal bones, displacing the otherwise normal orbits and nasal capsule, widening the orbits, and lengthening the face. In contrast, midfacial clefts appear to have a deficiency of tissue at their margins.

Naso-orbital meningoencephaloceles present onto the face through exit holes in the medial orbital wall, in the frontal process of the maxilla and lacrimal bones (Fig. 37-3). The bony tract is usually long and shaped like an inverted Y. The inverted Y is sometimes asymmetric. These meningoencephaloceles come through the frontal process of the maxilla onto the face, leaving the nasal bones intact anteriorly and the lacrimal bones and the lateral plate of the ethmoid bone intact posteriorly. A bony tunnel is thus formed through the substance of the ethmoid bone. The developing orbits may be grossly expanded by the meningoencephaloceles (Fig. 37-4).

Viable neural tissue is often seen at the neck of the meningoencephalocele, but tissue distal to the exit hole consists mostly of glial tissue infiltrated with fibrous trabeculae (Fig. 37-5). When the soft tissue mass of the meningoencephalocele extends into the orbits, it often fuses with periosteum, making excision of the orbital component of the mass extremely difficult.

A

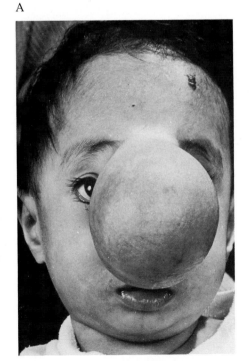

B

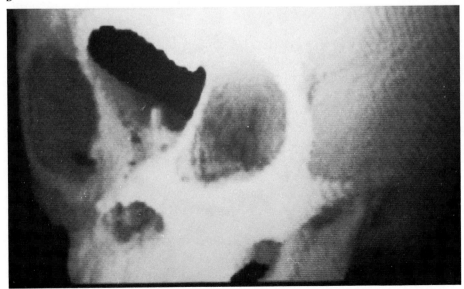

Fig. 37-1A. A large nasofrontal type of frontoethmoidal meningoencephalocele. B. Three-dimensional computed tomogram demonstrates the downward tilted cribriform plate with the crista galli forming the posterior margin of the cranial defect and the nasal bone forming the inferior margin of the facial defect. (From D. David et al. Meningoencephaloceles: Classification, pathology, and management. Adv. Plast. Reconstr. Surg. 5:85, 1989. Reproduced with permission.)

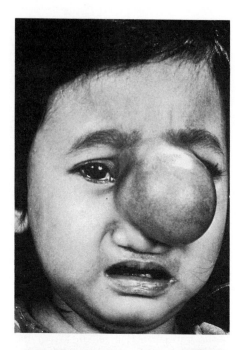

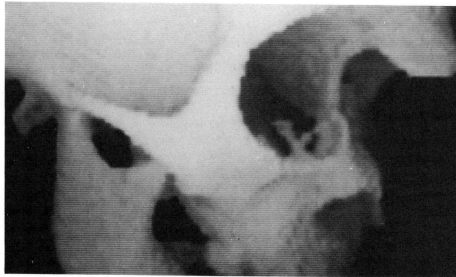

Fig. 37-2. A nasoethmoidal frontoethmoidal meningoencephalocele. Note the deformed nasal structures secondary to the facial exit holes. The frontonasal angle is obliterated.

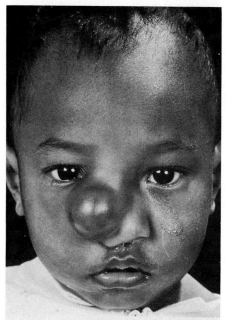

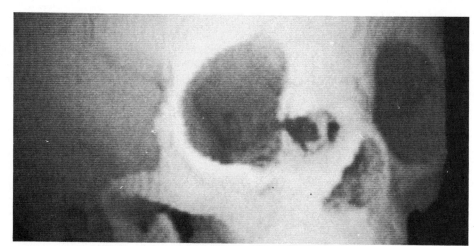

Fig. 37-3. A naso-orbital frontoethmoidal encephalocele. A bony tunnel through the ethmoid bone exits onto the face through the frontal process of the maxilla, leaving the nasal bones intact anteriorly. (From D. David et al. Meningoencephaloceles: Classification, pathology, and management. Adv. Plast. Reconstr. Surg. 5:85, 1989. Reproduced with permission.)

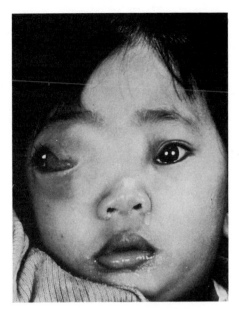

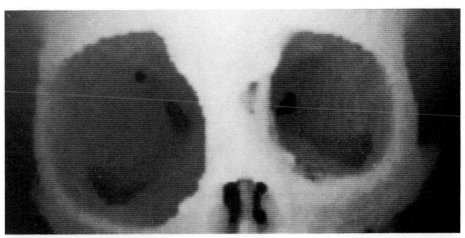

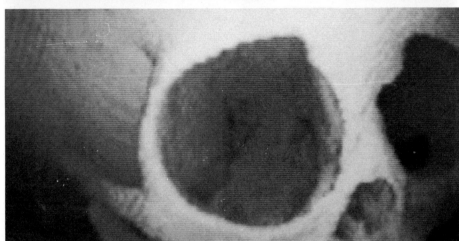

Fig. 37-4. A naso-orbital frontoethmoidal encephalocele. The massive orbital expansion is well demonstrated. (From D. David, et al. Frontoethmoidal meningoencephaloceles. Clin. Plast. Surg. 14:83, 1987. Reproduced with permission.)

Fig. 37-5. Viable neural tissue is often seen at the neck of the meningoencephalocele, but tissue distal to that is largely glial tissue with fibrous trabeculae.▼

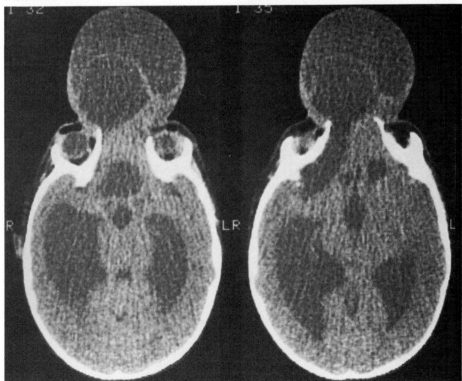

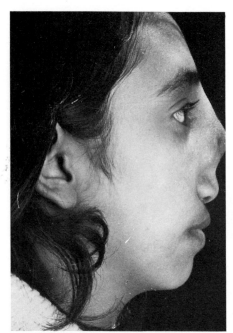

Fig. 37-6. *A typical long face of an adult patient with a frontoethmoidal meningoencephalocele. (From D. David, et al. Frontoethmoidal meningoencephaloceles: Morphology and treatment. Br. J. Plast. Surg. 37:271, 1984. Reproduced with permission.)*

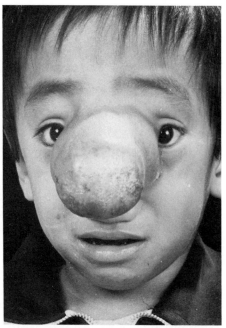

Fig. 37-7. *The skin overlying a frontoethmoidal meningoencephalocele, if involved, is full-thickness but dysplastic. (From D. David, et al. Meningoencephaloceles: Classification, pathology, and management. Adv. Plast. Reconstr. Surg. 5:85, 1989. Reproduced with permission.)*

Clinical Features

Frontoethmoidal meningoencephaloceles are usually grotesque deformities associated with gross facial disfigurement. The face appears to be longer than normal (Fig. 37-6), although this is hard to measure with ordinary cephalometric techniques, because some of the bony landmarks, particularly in the glabellar region, are obliterated. The pyriform aperture and nasal cartilages are misshapen, the aperture being shorter and broader than usual and displaced inferiorly. The Australian Cranio-Facial Unit has not seen a bifid nose or a midline nasal cleft in any of its patients. Telecanthus is an invariable feature; medial canthal dystopia is less common. Hypertelorism is a frequent finding (see Fig. 37-16A), but it is less severe than that seen with midline facial clefts. Some patients have dental malocclusion, which may be related to the attachment of the vertical plate of the ethmoid bone to the titled cribriform plate. The cribriform plate is retrodisplaced, presumably inducing secondary maxillary hypoplasia. Whenever it is involved, the nasal skeleton is distorted; the over-

lying skin is of full thickness but often discolored or ulcerated (Fig. 37-7).

Ocular problems are not uncommon. Micro-ophthalmia can occur, resulting from massive extrusion of the hernia into the orbit. Decreased visual activity is common if the globe is displaced, causing traumatic corneal ulceration. The most common ophthalmologic finding is lacrimal drainage dysfunction (see Fig. 37-16A). The function of the elongated and often tortuous drainage system is rarely corrected after the operation. Orbital expansion or dystopia (see Fig. 37-4) is present in all patients with naso-orbital meningoencephaloceles. Developmental retardation, hydrocephalus, and epilepsy are less frequently seen, and, perhaps surprisingly, anosmia is unusual.

Diagnostic Testing

Patients with frontoethmoidal meningoencephaloceles are best investigated using the team approach so successfully adopted by craniofacial units. The plastic surgeon, neurosurgeon, otorhinolaryn-

gologic surgeon, ophthalmologist, radiologist, dentist, psychologist, and social worker are all involved before the operation. A full neurologic examination is of utmost importance. Delineating developmental and intellectual parameters as well as visual acuity and sense of smell is an important facet of the preoperative evaluation. Radiographic assessment of both the skeletal lesions and the cerebral anatomy using plain roentgenograms and computed tomography (CT), including three-dimensional CT is vital when investigating these patients. Antenatal diagnosis by B-mode ultrasonography is now possible. Alpha-fetoprotein assay is not useful because the meningoencephalocele is fully epithelized with normal or dysplastic skin.

Operative Treatment

Operative treatment has three main aims: (1) to conserve cerebral function, (2) to prevent infection, and (3) to make facial appearance acceptable. The first aim is less easily achieved than one would wish because the herniated cerebral tissue within the cephalocele is usually too adherent to be extricated, and distal to the dural constriction it is likely to be gliotic and dysplastic. The second aim, prevention of cerebral infection by occluding the congenital craniofacial fistula, is relatively easy. The third aim can be difficult to realize, especially when there is marked teleorbitism and orbitofacial deformity.

The basis of surgical planning is the radiographic assessment, which consists above all of CT with reconstruction in three dimensions. This is particularly important because the nature of deformity in frontoethmoidal meningoencephalocele is so variable that each operation must be specifically tailored to the deformity. There is *no* standard operation for frontoethmoidal meningoencephalocele. After radiographic analysis the deformity can be assessed and the correction planned with a combination of osteotomies, bone grafts, and soft tissue operations.

There are two key principles of surgical treatment:

1. The operation should be performed by the transcranial approach so that the defect can be isolated intracranially and pos-

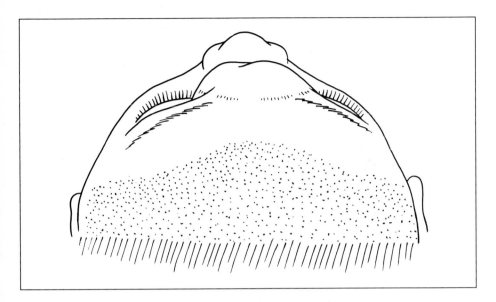

Fig. 37-8. The operation begins with shaving of the patient's scalp in preparation for raising the bicoronal scalp flap. Patient has already undergone orotracheal intubation and insertion of central and arterial lines.

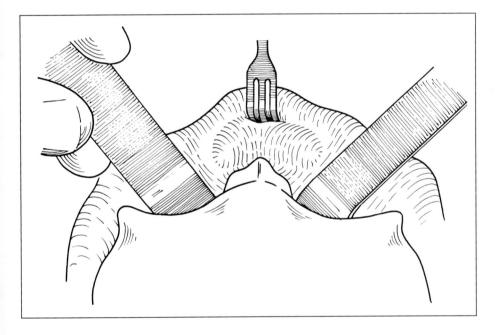

Fig. 37-9. Subperiosteal dissection reveals the neck of the frontoethmoidal meningoencephalocele emerging from its facial exit hole.

sibly intradurally with careful repair of the dura.

2. Complete bony reconstruction of the orbits and, if necessary, translocation of the orbits should be performed when required. The surgeon should, if possible, repair the bony and soft tissue deformities at the same time.

The patient is prepared for the operation by orotracheal intubation and insertion of central and arterial lines (Fig. 37-8). Access is gained by a bicoronal scalp flap. When there is a large soft tissue mass on

the face, or when there is previous facial scarring, an additional nasal incision is made to allow removal of the facial mass and trimming of the facial skin. The first step is wide subperiosteal exposure to outline the facial exit holes of the meningoencephalocele (Fig. 37-9). Planned osteotomies are marked out on the skull. In many instances the subcranial aspects of the bony reconstruction are made at this stage (Fig. 37-10), possibly involving osteotomies or bone grafts. The neurosurgeon performs a small bifrontal craniotomy, exposing both frontal lobes, and

the frontal bone is temporarily removed as a free graft (Fig. 37-11). If the bone removed is thick enough, it is split and the inner table is used for grafting; otherwise, two or even three ribs are harvested, one with a small cap of costal cartilage for use as a bone graft for the nose.

Before the bony orbital part of the operation is undertaken, the neurosurgical dissection of the anterior fossa is performed. The roofs of the orbits and the dural neck of the meningoencephalocele are exposed extradurally as far as the cra-

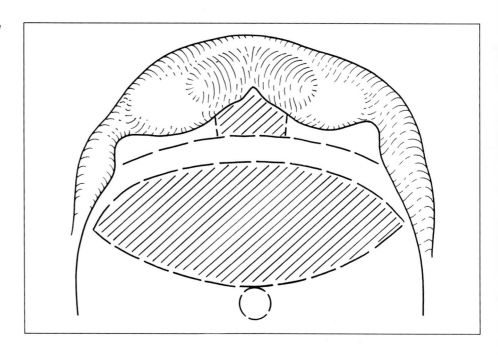

Fig. 37-10. The proposed osteotomies. Operatively these orbital and frontal osteotomies are marked out. The central nasal segment is removed, and not replaced, if hypertelorism is to be corrected.

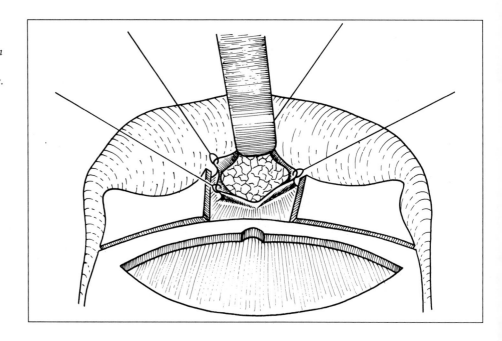

Fig. 37-11. Dura overlying neck of meningoencephalocele is opened and the contents are dissected out. Free frontal bone graft has been removed to assist with cutting or orbital osteotomies and removal of meningoencephalocele.

nial bone defect. Additional exposure is often obtained by excising a rectangle of bone from the glabellar region; this is replaced if there is no hypertelorism to correct. The dural sac of the meningoencephalocele is opened on both sides (see Fig. 37-11); cerebral herniation is inspected and, as much as possible, is conserved. The neck of the encephalocele is transected and the dural defect repaired, usually with a piece of temporalis fascia (Fig. 37-12). The remaining orbital oste-

otomies are made. In the nasoethmoidal type of meningoencephalocele, the medial orbital walls often are found to be defective and the angle of the cribriform plate is so steep that the translocated orbits come to overlie the cribriform plate. In some naso-orbital lesions, one or both orbits may be grossly expanded by the increased soft tissue volume. Osteotomies need to be designed to decrease the orbital size and may need to be supplemented by bone grafting of the or-

roofs, floor, and medial and lateral walls. When there is clinically significant teleorbitism affecting both orbits, the orbits are translocated medially to move the eyes (Fig. 37-13). Less severe deformities may require movement of one orbit only or osteotomy of only the medial orbital walls. Canthopexy and bone grafting of the nasal defect are final procedures.

Before external dissection of the soft tissue mass, it is our custom to cannulate

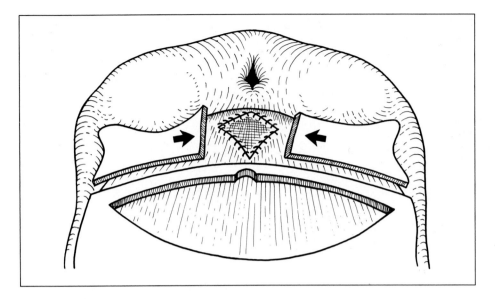

Fig. 37-12. *Meningoencephalocele has been removed and the dural defect repaired using temporal fascia. Orbits sectioned with the osteotome are moved medially as required. Nasal skin defect is closed in layers.*

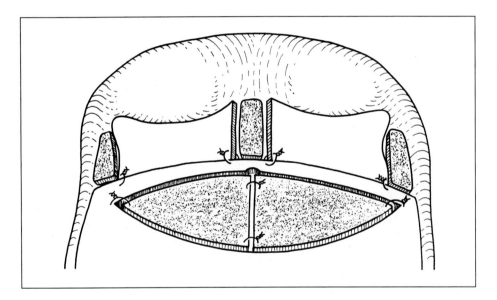

Fig. 37-13. *Hypertelorism has been corrected. Osteotomies are fixed with interosseous wires. The remaining bony defects of the nose are bone grafted if required using split calvarium and rib. Bicoronal scalp flap is replaced and closed in layers.*

intracranial pressure is high, there should be no delay in performing a shunt. We prefer ventriculoperitoneal drainage.

In older patients, particularly those with meningoencephaloceles of the nasoethmoidal variety with longer faces, we have not found it necessary to use the more complex face-shortening operations described by Jackson and associates. The operative program we use was devised for established deformities presenting later in childhood. We have limited experience with operations undertaken in patients in their infancy (1 to 3 months), but we believe that this is the ideal time to intervene, both to promote parental acceptance and ultimate psychological well-being and in the hope, as expressed by Naim-Ur-Rahman, that facial deformity will be avoided. The rationale for this hope is the concept that the skeletal deformities relate to the space-occupying effect of the hernia of extruded brain and not to some intrinsic deformity in the facial structures. If this view is correct, early complete surgical intervention should allow the developing brain and eyes to mold the orbital skeleton and the forces

the inferior lower lid canaliculus and inject dye into the nasolacrimal drainage apparatus. The soft tissue mass is often very vascular, and careful dissection is required to separate it from the overlying skin; the canaliculi and nasolacrimal apparatus often are stretched and distorted. Care must be taken not to remove excessive skin from the midline over the nose, because the soft tissue in this area has the capacity to "take up" in the first few months postoperatively.

Frontoethmoidal meningoencephaloceles often are associated with hydrocephalus. If this is severe and progressive, a ventriculoperitoneal or ventriculoatrial shunt

may be required. However, we usually defer this operation until the completion of the one-stage transcranial operation for the cephalocele, controlling intracranial pressure intraoperatively by draining the dilated ventricles through a separate burhole incision. This strategy allows regulation of intracranial pressure during the operation and for 2 or 3 days thereafter, avoiding the occasional complications (postoperative extradural hemorrhage, infections) sometimes associated with an internal shunt. The hydrocephalus associated with cephaloceles sometimes arrests spontaneously, even when quite severe. However, if the hydrocephalus is clearly progressive and the postoperative

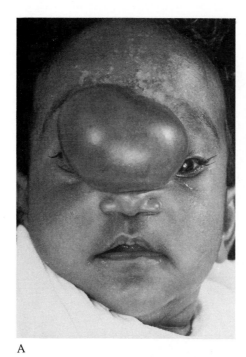
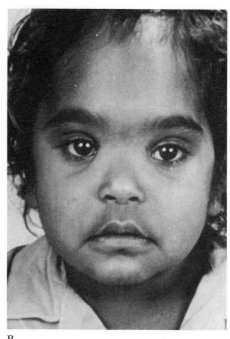

A   B

Fig. 37-14. Facial growth can approach normality after early removal of frontoethmoidal meningoencephaloceles. Child preoperatively at 4 months of age (A) and postoperatively at 3 years of age (B). (From D. David, et al. Meningoencephaloceles: Classification, pathology, and management. Adv. Plast. Reconstr. Surg. 5:85, 1989. Reproduced with permission.)

Fig. 37-15. Preoperative (A) and postoperative (B) views of patient whose left orbit only was moved after removal of meningoencephalocele. (From D. David, et al. Frontoethmoidal meningoencephaloceles: Morphology and treatment. Br. J. Plast. Surg. 37:271, 1984. Reproduced with permission.)

generated by the nasal airway, speech, and mastication to remodel the facial deformity. In operations on infants, it is necessary only to translocate and reconstruct the medial orbital walls with canthopexy and insertion of a nasal bone graft in addition to removing the contents of the meningoencephalocele. However, long-term studies are needed to validate this belief.

Operative Complications

All patients undergoing transcranial correction of frontoethmoidal meningoencephaloceles by the Australian Cranio-Facial Unit so far have survived the operation. The operation is usually accomplished in 2 to 4 hours. Complications have included two instances of acute postoperative hydrocephalus; three instances of rhinorrhea, which cleared spontaneously; and one secondary encephalocele in the frontal region as a result of raised intracranial pressure and inadequate reconstruction of the frontal bone, which necessitated a secondary operation. The same patient also had an infection of the left medial canthal region, which settled with antibiotics. Several patients squinted postoperatively, but in all but two of these patients the squinting resolved spontaneously. In these two patients the squinting was of sufficient severity to warrant further surgical correction. The most serious long-term problem

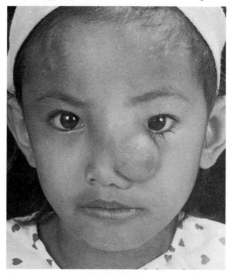

A   B

is epiphora resulting from malfunction of the nasolacrimal apparatus. Even in patients in whom the nasolacrimal apparatus has been demonstrated to be intact, it is often so deformed that the tortuous

ducts fail to function. Postoperative follow-up study over many years has shown that in almost all instances the condition settles down eventually. The explanation for this is obscure.

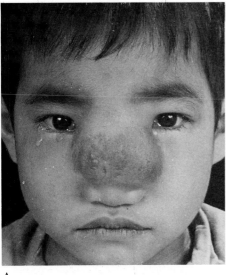
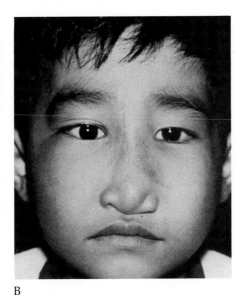

A   B

Fig. 37-16. Preoperative (A) and postoperative (B) views of a child in whom both orbits were translocated after transcranial removal of the meningoencephalocele. Note the resolution of epiphora. (From D. David, et al. Frontoethmoidal meningoencephaloceles: Morphology and treatment. Br. J. Plast. Surg. 37:271, 1984. Reproduced with permission.)

Fig. 37-17. Preoperative (A) and postoperative (B) views of a child in whom medial wall osteotomies, transnasal canthopexies, and nasal bone grafts were performed after removal of the meningoencephalocele. (From D. David, et al. Frontoethmoidal meningoencephaloceles: Morphology and treatment. Br. J. Plast. Surg. 37:271, 1984. Reproduced with permission.)

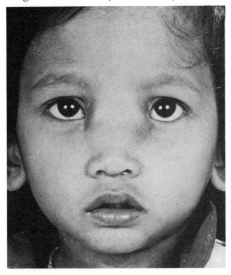
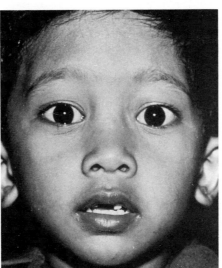

A   B

A number of patients have required the removal of their transnasal canthopexy wire and minor secondary bone grafting to the nose and cheeks. As far as facial growth is concerned, the results in patients who underwent the operation in infancy appear to confirm the proposition that the facial skeleton readjusts itself to the normal growth forces after removal of the displaced dysplastic brain (Fig. 37-14). However, we have not yet validated this impression with long-term craniometric data. It should be realized that cosmetically suboptimal results are often unavoidable when the meningoencephalocele is large and has dysplastic overlying skin. Various results are demonstrated in Figures 37-15 to 37-17.

Conclusion

Until recently, frontoethmoidal meningoencephaloceles were initially treated by neurosurgeons; plastic surgeons were, as a rule, consulted secondarily to deal with established deformities. The advent of craniofacial surgery allows definitive correction of the deformity in a single stage. Division of the neck of the encephalocele is not enough to wither the distal component of the extruded tissue or to prevent distortion of the developing skeleton. Craniofacial surgery is recommended with removal of the extruded brain, repair of the dura and anterior cranial fossa, and the appropriate osteotomies and bone grafts, preferably in the first 3 months of life; the hope is that the soft tissues will establish normal growth forces of the craniofacial skeleton and allow the face to assume more normal proportions. The simplest operation, namely moving the medial orbital walls with bone grafting and canthopexies, is the operation of choice in the early years of life. In older patients, however, the displaced orbits can be reconstructed in three dimensions if necessary.

We have not attempted to describe the details of each operation because in these days of the well-established craniofacial unit, it is now an accepted principle that the details of each operation be designed to fit the specific deformities present. The advent of CT techniques that give accurate three-dimensional images has allowed the surgical team the opportunity to plan surgical maneuvers, tailoring each operation to each deformity. It is important to realize that careful selection of patients should be practiced so that only those sufficiently able to benefit from the operation undergo it.

Suggested Reading

Aung, T., and Hta, K. Epidemiology of fronto-ethmoidal encephalomeningocele in Burma. *J. Epidemiol. Community Health* 38:89, 1984.

David, D.J., et al. Fronto-ethmoidal meningoencephaloceles: Morphology and treatment. *Br. J. Plast. Surg.* 37:271, 1984.

David, D.J., Simpson, D.A., and Cooter, R.D. Meningoencephaloceles: Classification, Pathology, and Management. *Adv. Plast. Reconstr. Surg.* 5:85, 1989.

Hemmy, D.C., and David, D.J. Skeletal morphology of anterior encephaloceles defined through the use of three dimensional reconstruction of computerised tomography. *Paediatr. Neurosci.* 12:18, 1986.

Jackson, I.T., Tanner, N.S., and Hide, T.A. Frontonasal encephalocele: "Long nose hyperteleorism." *Ann. Plast. Surg.* 11:490, 1983.

Le Dran, H.F. *Observations in Surgery.* London: James Hodges, 1740.

Mazzola, R.A. Congenital malformations in the fronto-nasal area: Their pathogenesis and classification. *Clin. Plast. Surg.* 3:573, 1976.

McLaurin, R.L. Cranium Bifidum and Cranial Cephaloceles. In P.J. Vinken and G.W. Bruyn (Eds.), *Handbook of Clinical Neurology: Part I. Congenital Malformations of the Brain and Skull.* Amsterdam: North Holland Publishing, 1977. Vol. 30, Pp. 209–218.

Naim-Ur-Rahman, N. Nasal encephalocele: Treatment by transcranial operation. *J. Neurol. Sci.* 42:73, 1979.

Simpson, D.A., David, D.J., and White, J. Cephaloceles: Treatment, outcome, and antenatal diagnosis. *Neurosurgery* 15:14, 1984.

Spring, A. Monographic de la hernie de cerveau et do quelques lesions voisines. Memoires de L'Academie Royale de Medicene de Belgiques, 1854.

Suwanwela, C. Geographic distribution of fronto-ethmoidal encephalomeningocele. *Br. J. Prev. Soc. Med.* 26:193, 1972.

Suwanwela, C., and Suwanwela, N. A morphological classification of sincipital encephalomeningocele. *J. Neurosurg.* 36:201, 1972.

Tessier, P. Anatomical classification of facial, craniofacial, and laterofacial clefts. *J. Maxillofac. Surg.* 4:69, 1976.

von Meyers, E. Uber Eine Basale Hirnhernie In Der Gregend Der Lamina Cribrosa. *Virchows Arch. [Pathol. Anat.]* 120:309, 1890.

38

Mandibulofacial Dysostosis

H. F. Sailer   Klaus W. Grätz   Michael C. Locher

Mandibulofacial dysostosis (Treacher Collins syndrome, Franceschetti-Zwahlen-Klein syndrome) is a rare autosomal dominant craniofacial malformation. Nevertheless, it often occurs as a sporadic mutation in a family previously unaffected. The phenotypic expression of the syndrome affects primarily the first and second branchial arches bilaterally and causes several facial disfigurements. The syndrome is caused by a fetal vascular anomaly that deprives the first branchial arch of its blood supply, which originates mainly from the stapedial artery between the third and fifth weeks of gestation. Poswillo produced a phenotypic copy of this syndrome in mice using teratogenic doses of vitamin A.

Since the early descriptions of the syndrome by Thompson in 1846, Barry in 1889, and Treacher Collins in 1900, many reports have described its facial characteristics—an antimongoloid obliquity of the palpebral fissure, notched lower eyelids, coloboma, ovoid orbital apertures, microphthalmia, hypoplasia of the malar and mandibular bones, a large mouth with irregular teeth and malocclusion, and a deformed external and sometimes middle and inner ear. Associated with these characteristics may be deafness, preauricular sinuses, dwarfism, cardiac and skeletal defects, and abnormalities of the upper airway. Obstructive sleep apnea in Treacher Collins syndrome also has been related to mandibular hypoplasia.

Treatment of this disease is regional reconstructive surgery. In 1982 a radical procedure was developed by Tessier and Tulasne. In its severe expression, this syndrome still represents one of the most challenging reconstructive problems for the craniomaxillofacial surgeon.

Principles of Treatment

The philosophy of treatment of craniofacial deformities and malformations depends on the length of experience of the particular surgeon and the analysis of the achieved results. The Department of Maxillofacial Surgery of the University Hospital in Zurich, Switzerland, has a tradition of almost 40 years of treatment of facial deformities. The Treacher Collins syndrome was one of the first malformations in which the sagittal splitting method and the sliding chin advancement technique were performed in a highly effective and elegant way. Over the years and with the development of craniofacial surgery, the following treatment principles were established in Zurich. Some of them are relevant to the treatment of the Treacher Collins syndrome.

1. Visible scars are considered a defeat in maxillofacial plastic surgery. The incisions routinely used nowadays are the bicoronal and the buccal sulcus incisions. Supraorbital, infraorbital, and submandibular skin incisions have been abandoned. The transconjunctival approach is still accepted and used for exposure and microplating of the infraorbital rim.
2. Autologous bone and cartilage grafts are not used because the donor site morbidity includes pain, infection, and other complications; because these grafts leave visible scars on the thorax, iliac crest, and elsewhere; because hospitalization may be prolonged; and because free autologous onlay bone grafts undergo some degree of absorption regardless of the origin of the graft, whether it be the iliac crest, the ribs, or the calvarium.

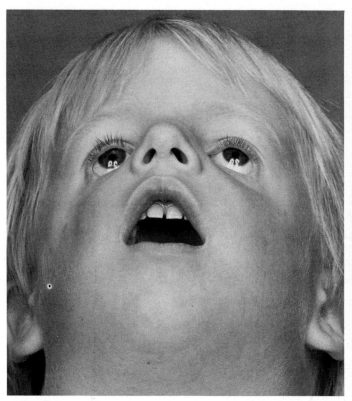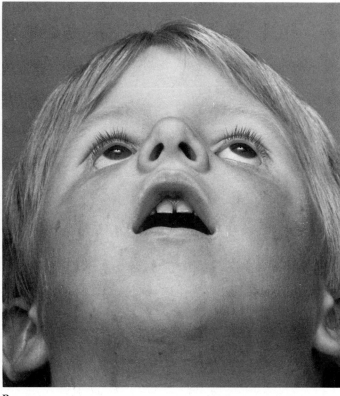

A   B

Fig. 38-1. Five-year-old patient with Treacher Collins syndrome before (A) and after (B) zygomatico-orbital reconstruction with lyocartilage demonstrating a natural contour of the area involved.

3. Homologous lyophilized and sterilized bone and cartilage grafts are used exclusively for surgical reconstruction in all kinds of craniomaxillofacial malformations. These grafts are processed in the tissue bank of the Department of Maxillofacial Surgery at the University of Zurich. The infection rate after the use of lyocartilage is lower than that after an autologous graft. The unique property of lyocartilage processed by our method is its slow transformation into the patient's own bone without resorption. Lyobone is less rapidly resorbed and incorporated than autologous bone and therefore offers more stability. Lyobone is taken from the iliac crest, the calvarium, the femur, the sternum, or the ribs. It is chosen by the surgeon according to the needs of construction or reconstruction. It goes without saying that these materials are not only lyophilized but also sterilized and taken from specially selected donors of a young age group.

4. Craniofacial segments cut with the osteotome are stabilized by miniplates and microplates and by lag or compression screws. Therefore, an intermaxillary fixation can often, but for safety reasons cannot always, be avoided.

Timing of Surgical Treatment

For each craniomaxillofacial malformation there is a special timing protocol for surgical intervention. The timing for mandibulofacial dysostosis is as follows.

Patients with an Isolated Cleft Palate

Palatal closure follows the timing of the Zurich cleft palate treatment at the age of 15 to 18 months. The method used for closure is that of Perko derived from the Widmaier technique. Our convincing speech results after the techniques of palatoplasty were published by van Denmark and associates. Primary orthodontic treatment is not used for patients with isolated cleft palates. An audiologist, who is a member of our treatment team, examines and treats the child according to a speech therapy protocol that is the same as for a child with a cleft palate.

Patients Without a Cleft Palate

Treatment is provided at the age of 2 to 4 years, before the child goes to kindergarten. Construction of the zygomatic arch and bone, the infraorbital and lateral orbital rim and walls, and the lateral parts of the forehead is undertaken at this age using lyocartilage exclusively. At the same time the prolapse of the lateral supraorbital rim is trimmed off using a bur to modify the ovoid form of the orbital aperture. Audiologic examinations with objective audiometry are performed during the first months of life, and hearing aids if necessary are given as soon as possible.

If an elongated coronoid process inhibits the mouth from opening, the process is

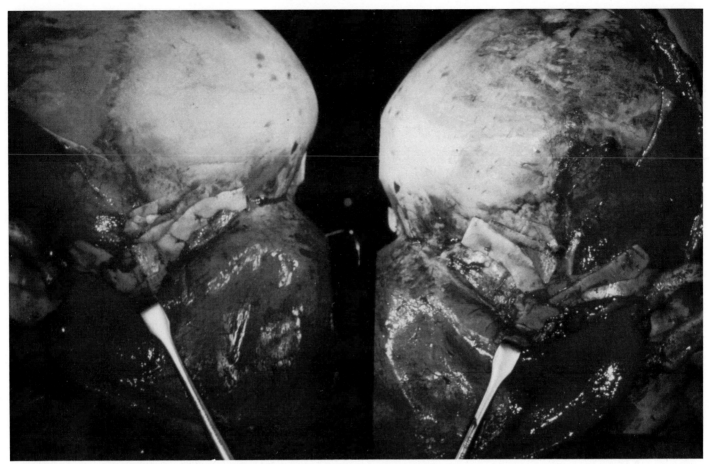

Fig. 38-2. Intraoperative condition of a patient with Treacher Collins syndrome during construction of the lateral orbital rim and the zygomatic arches using slices of lyocartilage.

removed. During the same operation, any ankylosis between the coronoid process and the rudimentary zygomatic arch is removed. Simultaneously the lower eyelid is placed into a normal position by elevation using lyophilized cartilage for infraorbital rim support and lateral canthopexy.

The receded chin prominence is built up with lyocartilage. A simultaneous sliding chin osteotomy is not indicated at this age to avoid damage to the caudally positioned buds of the permanent teeth, located in the chin area. Depilation of the dystopic hairline running in the direction of the angle of the mouth should also be performed at this stage.

Children 6 to 10 Years of Age

Depending on the growth deficiency, the zygomatic and periorbital areas can be repeatedly built up with lyocartilage to achieve good proportion and harmony during growth of the middle third of the face. The indications for these procedures depend on the individual psychological and social needs of the child and the severity of the malformation. Between the ages of 6 and 10 years, orthodontic activator treatment is indicated to develop the hypoplastic mandibular ramus.

Children 12 Years or Older

From the age of 12 years on, orthodontic presurgical treatment takes place 14 months for girls and 16 months for boys before the surgical advancement of the mandible and the chin or a combination of operations on the upper and lower jaw is performed. The mandibular operation may be performed before general growth has ceased because of the obvious lack of further condylar growth in most children. Postsurgical orthodontic follow-up care is necessary until facial growth is complete.

Surgical Procedure
Zygomatic-Orbital Defects

We use a bicoronal incision for exposure. Under direct observation the pathologic anatomy is evaluated. The periosteum is carefully elevated along the rudimentary orbital walls and especially in the infraorbital region. Here multiple periosteal cuts are made vertically in the direction of the upward pull of the lateral canthus. Wherever periosteum is identifiable in the zygomatic area, it is incised in a rectangular pattern to allow maximal expansion of the soft tissues.

Lyophilized rib cartilage is cut into 0.6- to 1.0-mm slices with the help of a dermatome. The zygomatic arch and infraorbital rim are constructed using several layers of lyocartilage, fixed with 0.3-mm wires or absorbable suture material. Finally, the orbital floor and lateral orbital wall are built up and the flattened supraorbital forehead area is recontoured. At this point the prolapse of the lateral supraorbital rim is trimmed off using a bur to modify the ovoid form of the orbital aperture (Figs. 38-1 and 38-2).

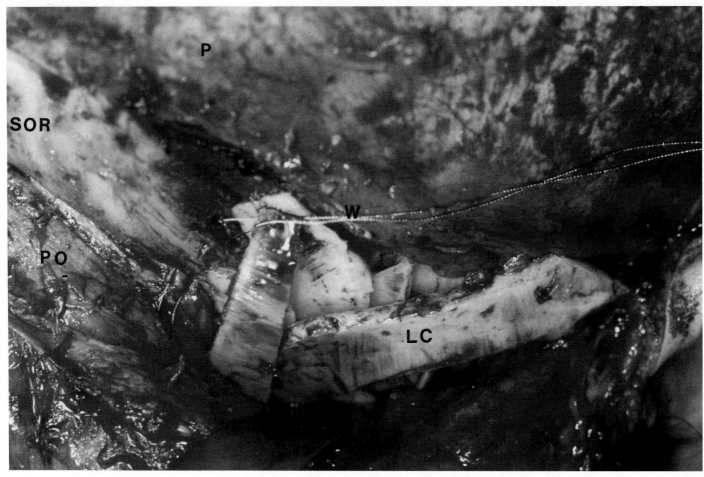

Fig. 38-3. *Intraoperative situation in a young patient with Treacher Collins syndrome. The canthopexy wire (w) is led through two bur holes within the supraorbital rim (SOR). PO = periorbit; P = pericranium; LC = lyocartilage.*

Elevation of Lower Eyelid and Lateral Canthus

The most effective point for upward pulling of the eyelids is identified, and a woven fine wire or a nylon suture is thread through for fixation of the canthus to the orbital rim, if present, or to the sheets of lyocartilage used for construction of the lateral orbital rim. The eyelids and the canthus are always elevated together; this elevation is not stable without simultaneous lower eyelid support by the lyocartilage grafts (Fig. 38-3).

Augmentation of Chin with Lyocartilage and Construction of a Labiomental Groove

The incision is made in the anterior mandibular vestibule, the periosteum is elevated, and two bur holes are made through the most caudal rim of the chin, where no tooth buds are present. For determination of the most favorable location of the bur hole, a cephalometric roentgenogram and orthopantomogram are used. A lyocartilage block is cut and fixed to the bone surface with wires or suture material (Fig. 38-4).

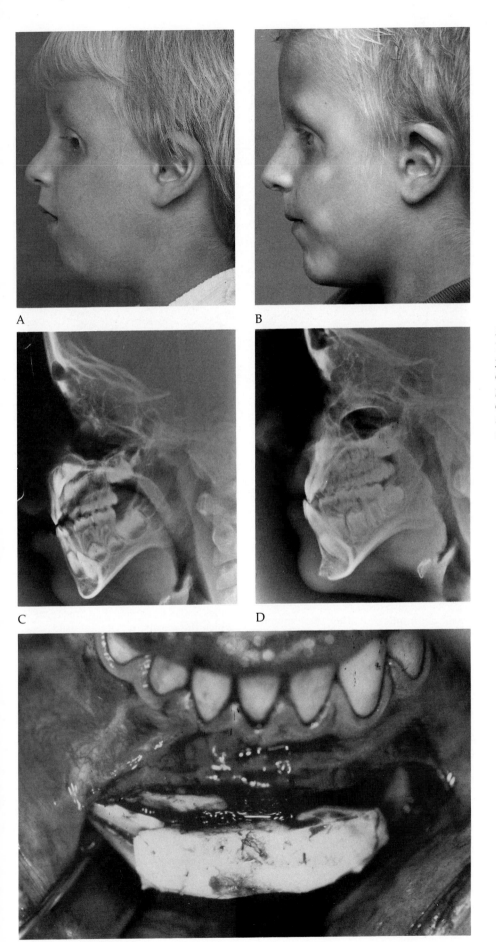

Fig. 38-4. Chin augmentation using lyocartilage. The preoperative view (A) and the condition 6 years postoperatively (B). The preoperative cephalometric roentgenogram (C) shows the caudal position of the tooth buds in the chin region at the age of 5 years. The condition 6 years later (D) shows the ossified lyocartilage seen in the intraoperative photograph (E).

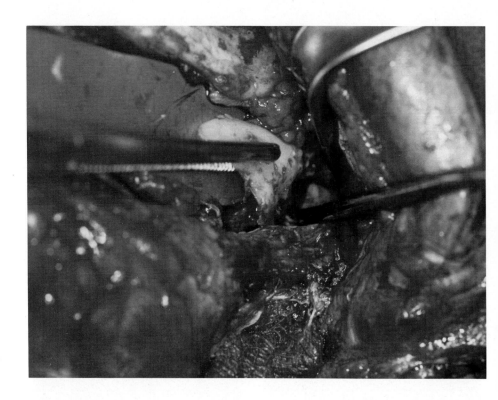

Fig. 38-5. Intraoperative view during removal of the elongated coronoid process.

Removal of Elongated Coronoid Process When Mouth Opening Is Inhibited

Immediately before construction of the zygomatic arch, the coronoid process is palpated within the temporal muscle. The muscle fibers are divided by blunt dissection, and the process is sectioned and removed (Fig. 38-5).

Positioning of Lower and Upper Jaw Depending on the Severity of the Deformity

As soon as orthodontic treatment allows surgical intervention, a cast model operation is performed. This procedure simulates the advancement of the mandible in small deformities or the three-dimensional movement of the whole maxillomandibular complex in more severe deformities (Fig. 38-6A). We have found that it is extremely important to normalize the relation between the length of the upper lip and the position of the maxillary incisors. In severe deformities, the maxilla often has to be raised in the anterior area and tilted downward in the posterior aspect. Simultaneously the mandible is advanced massively. The heavy backward pull of the genioglossus and geniohyoid muscles is eliminated by resection of the posterior mental spine and by interpositioning lyobone into this point (Fig. 38-6G). To ensure the patency of the nasal airways, the inferior turbinate bones must be reduced in instances in which the maxilla has to be raised.

For elongation of the ramus and body of the mandible, long sagittal splitting is used as described by Obwegeser; for maxillary movements, a Le Fort I osteotomy is performed. A Le Fort II osteotomy as advocated by Tessier is rarely indicated and then only in extreme instances of mandibulofacial dysostosis.

Fig. 38-6. Patient with Treacher Collins syndrome who underwent a bimaxillary operation for facial harmony. The cast model operation (A) gives the exact movements of upper and lower jaw. The preoperative (B) and postoperative (C) orthopantomograms detail our technique of segmental fixation using miniplates at the Le Fort I osteotomy level and in the area of the mandibular sagittal splitting (together with positioning screws). The lower wisdom teeth are removed 4–6 months before the operation. The preoperative cephalometric roentgenogram (D) shows the lip incompetence caused by the open bite and the unfavorable relation between the upper lip and the incisors. The postoperative cephalometric roentgenogram (E) reveals the harmony of the facial thirds. ▶

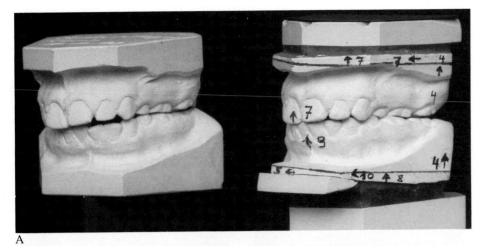

A

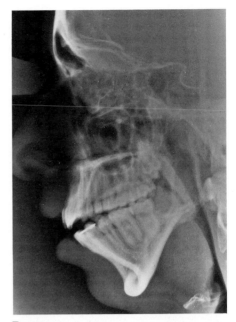

D

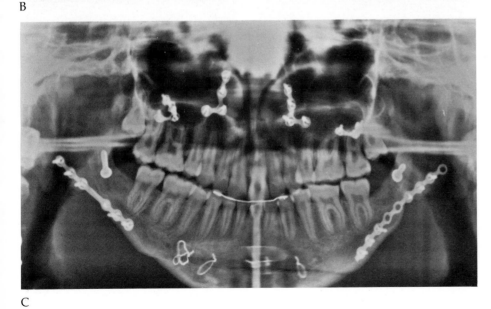

B

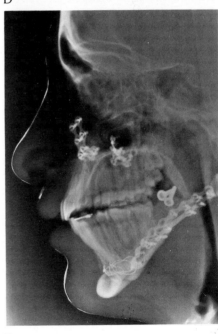

E

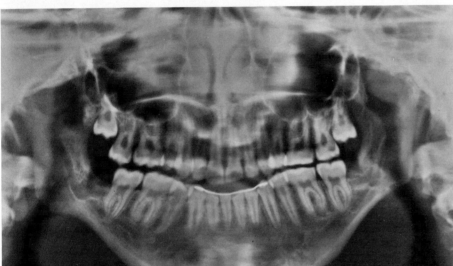

C

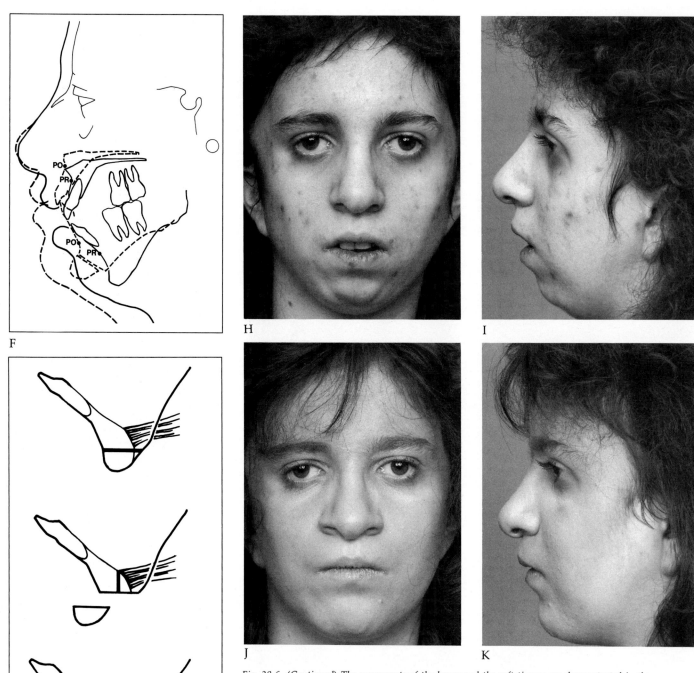

Fig. 38-6. (Continued) *The movements of the bones and the soft tissues are demonstrated in the superpositional drawings of the cephalograms (F). To avoid a relapse caused by the pull of the muscle, the bony origin of the genioglossal and geniohyoid muscles is sectioned by the transoral approach (G) after an osteotomy of the chin prominence, sagittal splitting of the rami, and an interpositional lyobone graft are performed. Wiring is used for fixation. This procedure allows restoration of normal facial appearance in Treacher Collins syndrome, as shown in the preoperative (H, I) and postoperative (J, K) photographs. Further augmentation of the zygoma and a nasal correction were declined by the patient. PR = preoperative; PO = postoperative; solid line = preoperative; dotted line = postoperative.*

Reconstruction of Auricular Deformities

Reconstruction of the various auricular deformities depends on the amount of tissue present. If very few or no auricular remnants exist, we recommend the use of artificial auricles fixed to osseointegrated titanium implants. Auricular reconstruction, if needed, is postponed until adolescence.

Correction of Coloboma

Correction of coloboma should not be performed before construction of the zygoma, which tremendously improves the eyelid position and the oblique axis of the palpebral fissure. In extreme instances of ectropion, the usual Z-plasty corrections are not sufficient and full-thickness skin or composite grafts taken from the rudimentary auricles are necessary for the reconstruction of the lower eyelid.

Nasal Reconstruction

Nasal reconstruction is not always required; it depends on the individual needs of the patient.

Anesthesiologic Considerations

Patients with mandibulofacial dysostosis present special anesthesiologic problems. Only a skilled anesthetist who has mastered blind and fiberoptic intubation should work with these patients. The discrepancy between the size of the upper and the lower jaws sometimes associated with macroglossia and a reduced mouth opening complicates or even prevents laryngoscopy, especially in extreme deformities.

Even fiberoptic intubation is not always feasible because of the dorsal positioning of the tongue and the inability to pass through the extremely narrow angle between the root of the tongue and the trachea. Visibility problems originate from the persistent contact of the mucosa with the tip of the optic device and so impair the anesthetist's view. Preoperative fiberoptic laryngoscopy in a patient who is awake without relaxation has to be performed to predict difficulties with intubation. A tracheotomy setup always should be present during attempts at intubation. Extubation should take place only when the patient is fully awake, and the patient should be monitored continuously for at least 24 hours in an intensive care unit. After long operations, which could cause extensive swelling of the masticatory system, these patients should remain intubated overnight in a specialized intensive care unit.

Suggested Reading

Argenta, L.C., and Iacuobucci, J.J. Treacher Collins syndrome: Present concepts of the disorder and their surgical correction. *World J. Surg.* 13:401, 1989.

Arvystas, M., and Shpintzen, R.J. Craniofacial morphology in Treacher Collins syndrome. *Cleft Palate Craniofac. J.* 28:226, 1991.

Berry, G.A. Note on a congenital defect (coloboma ?) of the lower lid. *Royal London Ophthalmol. Hosp. Rep.* 12:255, 1889.

Normans, A.P. *Congenital Abnormalities in Infancy.* Oxford, England: Blackwell, 1971. P. 352.

Obwegeser, H. The surgical correction of mandibular prognathism and retrognathia with consideration of genioplasty. *Oral Surg.* 10:677, 1957.

Obwegeser, H. Surgical correction of the small or retrodisplaced maxillae. *Plast. Reconstr. Surg.* 4:351, 1969.

Perko, M. Primary closure of the cleft palate using a palatal mucosal flap: An attempt to prevent growth impairment. *J. Maxillofac. Surg.* 2: 40, 1974.

Poswillo, D. The pathogenesis of Treacher Collins syndrome (mandibulo-facial dysostosis). *Br. J. Plast. Surg.* 13:1, 1975.

Rasch, D.K., et al. Anaesthesia for Treacher Collins and Pierre Robin syndrome: A report of three cases. *Can. Anaesth. Soc. J.* 33:363, 1986.

Rogers, B.O. The surgical treatment of mandibulofacial dysostosis (Berry syndrome, Treacher Collins syndrome, Franceschetti-Zwahlen-Klein syndrome). *Clin. Plast. Surg.* 3: 653, 1976.

Sailer, H.F. Transplantation of lyophilized cartilage in maxillo-facial surgery: Experimental foundations and clinical success. Basel: Karger Verlag, 1983.

Sailer, H.F. Insuffiziente Ergebnisse nach Le Fort III-Osteotomie und deren Vermeidung durch die doppelstufige Mittelgesichtsbewegung. *Fortschr. Kiefer Gesichtschir.* 30:102, 1985.

Sailer, H.F. Fortschritte und Schwerpunkte der orthopädischen Kiefer- und Gesichtschirurgie. *Fortschr. Kiefer Gesichtschir.* 33:24, 1990.

Sailer, H.F., and Farmand, M. The Treatment of Otomandibular Dysostosis. In G. Pfeifer (Ed.), *Craniofacial Abnormalities and Clefts of the Lip, Alveolus, and Palate.* New York: Thieme, 1991. P. 102.

Tessier, P., and Tulasne, J.F. Stability in correction of hyperteleorbitism and Treacher Collins syndromes. *Clin. Plast. Surg.* 16:195, 1989.

Van Denmark, D.R., et al. Speech results of the Zurich approach in the treatment of unilateral cleft lip and palate. *Plast. Reconstr. Surg.* 83:605, 1989.

39

Hemifacial Microsomia

Douglas K. Ousterhout   Karin Vargervik

Hemifacial microsomia is a congenital condition characterized by regional hypoplasia of the proximal mandible, the temporomandibular joint, the temporozygomatic arch complex, and the associated soft tissues. Also called the *first and second branchial arch syndrome* or *craniofacial microsomia*, the condition is usually unilateral, although it can be bilateral. Hemifacial microsomia varies widely from relatively minor (Fig. 39-1) to extremely severe deformities involving the entire side of the face, the orbit, the forehead, and the temporal fossa (Fig. 39-2). As a result of the mandibular hypoplasia, there is a compensatory hypoplasia of the maxilla on the affected side and deviation of the mandible toward the side of involvement.

Numerous other conditions may be associated with the basic deformity, including microtia, seventh nerve paralysis (partial, rarely complete), branchial clefts or fistulas, variable orbital deformities, and lipodermoids (Goldenhar syndrome). Occasionally there is contralateral involvement of various degrees.

Although the origin of the condition in humans is not known, studies in animals completed by Poswillo favor an intrauterine factor causing stapedial artery hemorrhage early in embryonic formation. The size of the hemorrhage may be correlated with the degree of the deformity.

Our original classification system, which is based on the deformity of the mandibular ramus, has been modified slightly and brought into conformity with other classification systems reported in the literature. It is as follows:

Type I: A coronoid and condylar process is present but without condylar cartilage. A glenoid fossa may or may not be present, and the joint space is decreased.

Type IIA: A coronoid and condylar process is present but without a condylar neck and cartilage. There is no glenoid fossa.

Type IIB: The condylar process and condyle are absent but the coronoid process is present.

Type III: The ramus is completely absent.

In this chapter attention is directed primarily toward mandibular and maxillary growth management and surgical reconstruction. Chin, nose, temporomandibular, zygomatico-orbital, and soft tissue reconstructions are mentioned only briefly.

Ear reconstruction, removal of the skin tags, repair of branchial clefts and fistulas, and macrostomia are not discussed in this chapter. The theoretical basis of our treatment approach has been presented in detail in *Treatment of Hemifacial Microsomia*, edited by Harvold and associates. Some changes in the surgical procedures originally presented have resulted in new systems for fixation of osteotomies.

The overall goal in treatment of a child with hemifacial microsomia is optimal facial symmetry and aesthetics combined with optimal function as an adult. Therefore, treatment has to achieve the following:

1. An increase in the size and improvement in the contour of the underdeveloped, malformed mandible and associated soft tissues
2. Maintenance or establishment of a functional articulation between the mandible and the temporal bone
3. Correction of secondary deformities of the maxilla, nose, and chin
4. Establishment of a functional dental occlusion
5. An acceptable and improved appearance of the face and dentition

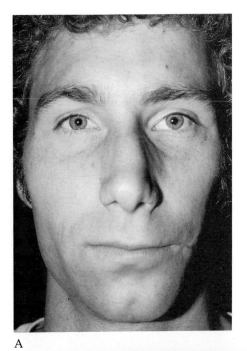

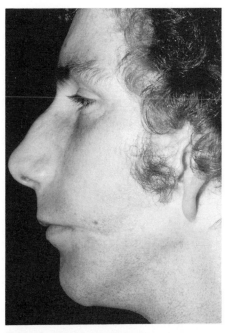

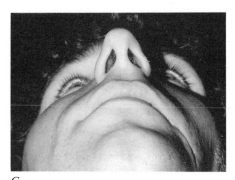

C

Fig. 39-1. Nineteen-year-old patient with type I hemifacial microsomia.

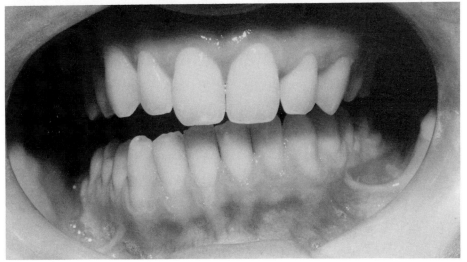

D

The most challenging of these treatment goals is the achievement of symmetry. The patient's system is in balance despite the asymmetries. To successfully bring the mandible into a new relation with the face, mandibular musculature, and dentition requires reprogramming of masticatory muscles and establishment of new functional patterns. This in turn changes the architecture and morphologic structure of the bones with which they are associated. Six rules of muscle-bone interaction apply in this regard. They were tested by Harvold and his colleagues and are as follows:

1. Shifting of any bone to a new position within its muscular system results in reorganization of the shape and trabecular structure of the bone.
2. Changing the muscle activity affects bone morphology.
3. Placing a neutral body within a bone or obstructing development of a bone alters the stress distribution and causes remodeling.
4. Moving a neutral body within a bone changes the distribution and elicits remodeling (e.g., orthodontic tooth movement).
5. Adding a new section to a bone re-

quires the establishment of muscle activity, which sets up and maintains the particular stress system that induces the formation and retention of new bone.
6. A bone loses its potential for bone opposition if muscular influence is removed, but resorption still proceeds.

When these rules are used, a systematic treatment approach to hemifacial microsomia was developed that includes the following steps:

1. Use of a functional appliance to change muscle patterns and in some instances reduce asymmetry in soft tissues, mandible, and maxilla.
2. Placement of a free mandibular bone graft, either as an extension or as an interpositional graft. (Occasionally sagittal split osteotomy of the mandible may be used.)
3. Protection of the bone graft with further neuromuscular adaptation during the period of ossification.
4. Orthodontic or surgical correction of the canted and rotated maxilla.
5. Orthodontic finishing and additional operations on the chin, nose, other bones (such as the cheekbone), and the soft tissues as needed.

Fig. 39-2. Twenty-two-year-old patient with
severe facial deformity secondary to type III
hemifacial (hemicraniofacial) microsomia.

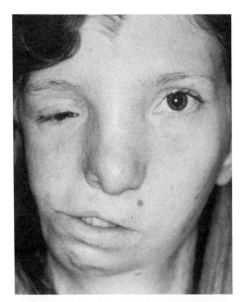
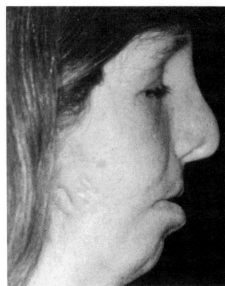
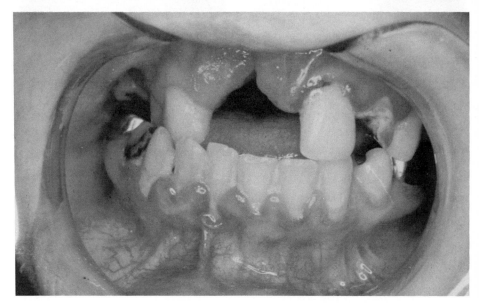

Nonsurgical Treatment

Presurgical Functional Appliance

A functional appliance constructed to hold the affected side of the mandible in a lowered, forward position can stimulate an increase in size of both the abnormal condyle and the short coronoid process. This treatment principle is applied routinely on our young patients during the presurgical growth management phase. Response to this treatment is particularly beneficial to patients with type I deformities, in which both soft tissue and bony asymmetries may improve.

Preparation for Mandibular Reconstruction

Before the operation, the desired new position of the mandible is determined from clinical findings, from cephalometric roentgenograms of the head (lateral, posteroanterior, and oblique 45° projections), and from custom-made scale models. In the surgical procedure, the mandible is mobilized with or without unilateral or bilateral osteotomies, the prefabricated registration splint is inserted, and the graft matrix is placed. The jaws are wired together over the splint with the hooks on the custom-made arch bars.

Postsurgical Treatment

Procedures have been established to maintain the new mandibular position and to establish and maintain new bony

additions. After 6 weeks of interarch fixation, the splint is removed and a thorough cleaning is completed. The arch bars are left in place, and hooks are placed in the splint to allow it to be attached to the maxillary arch wire with elastic bands. Two or more rubber bands are placed between the upper and lower arch bars to limit jaw movement to controlled opening and precise return into the splint, thus protecting the bone-grafted areas from uncontrolled forces. During this process the neuromuscular system is reeducated to new opening and closing patterns by proprioceptive feedback, mainly from the periodontium of the teeth. Consistent jaw

position and patterns of jaw movement are essential for the soft tissue tension and orientation necessary for establishing the periosteal sleeve within which graft revascularization and new bone formation take place.

Correction of Maxillary Deficiencies and Distortions

The hypoplasia and asymmetry of the maxilla can be corrected by a Le Fort I maxillary procedure. In a young child it can be corrected by orthodontic extrusion of the maxillary teeth on the affected side.

Orthodontic Treatment

Orthodontic treatment of a growing child should be focused on control of tooth eruption and prevention or correction of dental alveolar adaptations to the asymmetric position of the maxilla and mandible. There may be delayed tooth eruption and dental irregularities. Crowding of the teeth is common. When the maxillary teeth have reached the mandibular occlusal plane after mandibular reconstruction, conventional orthodontic treatment is necessary to detail the occlusion.

If the surgical procedures on the jaw are not completed until maturity is reached, orthodontic treatment to remove dentoalveolar compensations and to coordinate the dental arches should precede a jaw operation. A relatively short period of final detailing is necessary postoperatively.

Surgical Procedures

For the past 20 years all patients with hemifacial microsomia at the University of California, San Francisco, have been treated according to the protocol described earlier. There is some variation in the timing of surgical intervention, however, which depends on maturational stage and degree of dysfunction. Our protocol requires that surgical treatment be phased with the long-term facial growth management of these patients. The preoperative and postoperative treatment is an essential and integral part of the therapy and is as important as the surgical repositioning and bone grafting for the long-term result. The type of mandibular operation performed depends on which of the two basic types of ramus deformity is to be treated—condyle present or condyle absent.

Condyle Present

When the condyle is present, as in type I and IIA deformities, there is usually some form of temporomandibular joint. There is no articular disk or much of a glenoid fossa, but some form of capsular support and lateral pterygoid muscle is present. In these patients the operation is basically a lengthening of the mandibular ramus by placing an interpositional bone graft within the vertical ramus or by a sagittal split procedure if possible. At present

cranial bone is most often used as graft material, but if a large area needs to be filled an iliac crest graft is usually indicated.

An intraoral approach is used exclusively. This obviates a facial scar and helps avoid injury to the mandibular branch of the facial nerve. A sagittal split osteotomy is used when possible. When this procedure can be completed it avoids a bone graft, and both segments remain vascularized. One must be careful in completing the sagittal split because there may be considerable deformity in the shape of the

ramus and variation in the location of the neurovascular bundle. Adequate roentgenographic evaluation must be completed before careful dissection.

When an interpositional bone graft is to be placed, the approach to the ramus is exactly the same. When the channel retractors are in place, a wire-passing bur is used to make two holes, one each above and below the proposed line of mandibular transection (Fig. 39-3A). A full length of 28-gauge wire (18 inches) is passed through each of these holes and clamped outside the mouth. A long reciprocating

Fig. 39-3A. Condition of the mandible before osteotomy and bone grafting with interpositional bone graft. The dashed line represents the proposed osteotomy. The two small bur holes are made before the osteotomy is completed. B. Postoperative position of the mandible, bone grafts in place and stabilized, and registration bite-block in position.

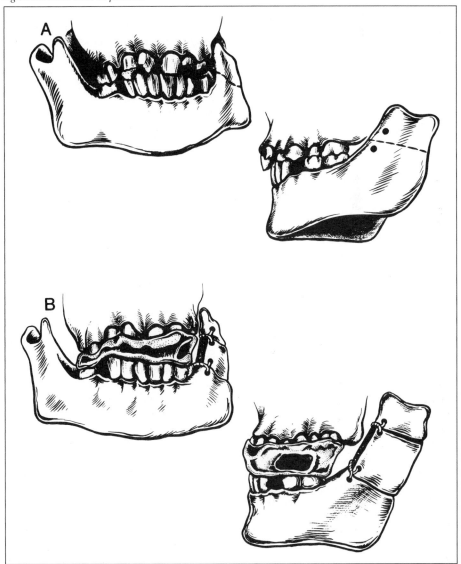

saw is used to complete the osteotomy. Not infrequently the uninvolved side must be moved posteriorly to establish proper midline positioning. If this is the case a sagittal split or a vertical osteotomy is necessary. Usually the osteotomy is completed only on the affected side, however, allowing the condyle on the contralateral side to rotate within the glenoid fossa. This has not caused temporomandibular joint problems in any of our patients.

The mandible is manipulated into the desired position and placed into the prefabricated registration bite-block. This brings the involved side of the mandible down to a lower level and accomplishes the necessary midline rotation. After the mandible is stabilized in the splint to the maxilla with interarch wires, a gap is present at the osteotomy site. The gap is filled with the bone graft using the two wires previously placed for stabilization. It is imperative that before the final vertical height of the bone graft is determined, the "condyle" be in the most superoposterior position (see Fig. 39-3B). When the bone graft is nicely in position and stable, the wounds are closed.

One note of special concern is that occasionally after the horizontal osteotomy is completed on the involved side, the mandible cannot be moved into the desired position. Ligamentous tissues (both the sphenomandibular and the stylomandibular ligaments), muscle, fascia, and periosteal tissues can interfere with this movement. What generally works at this stage is to ensure that the muscles are totally relaxed. If the mandible still is not adequately separated, the strongly built registration bite-block is inserted onto the maxillary teeth. The posterior mandibular teeth are brought into proper position in the splint, and with slow but rather firm pressure under the chin the mandible is brought up into the splint. A rather sharp periosteal elevator can be used to score the soft tissues adjacent to the osteotomy. This may be a slow and frustrating procedure, but eventually the mandible comes into position. As soon as the mandible is in proper position, an anterior fixation wire, usually 28 gauge, is placed. Because of the severe tension, the arch bars must be firmly wired to the teeth. Bonded orthodontic appliances are not strong enough to withstand these forces.

Finally the soft tissues can be closed; running 000 or 4–0 chromic catgut suture is used. A fishhook or J-shaped needle is especially useful. Neither drains nor external dressings have been used, although cold packs over the patient's soft tissues are helpful. The postoperative treatment is the same as for any other mandibular operation in which intermaxillary fixation is used. Because of the large space made on the affected side by lowering the mandible, a large opening can be placed in the registration bite-block. This allows for suctioning in the immediately postoperative period and subsequently for the ingestion of liquid and food.

Condyle Absent

Type IIB and III deformities, in which the condyle is absent, are seen less frequently than types I and IIA. In these more severe types there is more facial deformity, generally of both bone and soft tissue (see Fig. 39-2). Not only is the face more distorted but also there are several unknowns within that distortion. The exact position of the facial nerve and the inferior alveolar neurovascular bundle may be difficult to locate, and extreme care must be taken during the operation to avoid injury to these structures. The operation basically is the placement of a bone graft between the end of the mandible and the cranial base after an appropriate space has been developed. Formerly, most of these deformities were approached extraorally, but now the intraoral route is used, although not exclusively.

In type III deformities there may be little bone posterior to the last molar (Fig. 39-4A). The track, which is developed from the proximal end of the mandible toward the cranial base for placement of the bone graft, is established by blunt dissection; the soft tissues are separated carefully while proceeding cephalically. Extreme care must be taken near the mandibular end not to tear or separate the oral mucosa, particularly around a developing molar, which may be only partially exposed into the oral cavity. It is of course desirable to place the cranial end of the bone graft as close as possible to a symmetric position with the contralateral, normal condyle. In these patients, however, who have more severe deformities, the ipsilateral ear or ear remnants are gen-

erally in an anterior and often inferior position compared with the normal ear. Additionally, the skull may be quite narrow on the affected side. Therefore, obtaining a symmetric relation usually is not possible (see Fig. 39-1). This is a point of considerable difference from what has been described in articles by other authors.

When the first phase of treatment is completed, the mandibular advancement is more of a horizontal rotation than a vertical one, although both movements may be necessary. The ligamentous structures generally are already stretched by the use of the activator appliance that has brought the mandible into a more normal position. The registration bite-block can be inserted easily. In type IIB deformities, or those in which the first-phase activator treatment has not been completed, both a vertical and a horizontal expansion are necessary and the situation is much more difficult. In an occasional patient who has had a macrostomia repair, the scarring can cause interference with the vertical and horizontal movement. In such patients some sort of scar revision, such as a Z-plasty, might be considered.

The bone graft, preferably a costochondral graft, is placed with the contoured cartilage properly directed, firmly against the skull or reconstructed glenoid fossa as an articular cartilage. The bone is stabilized to the mandibular end with particular care. When there is little bone beyond the developing tooth buds, one must be careful not only to secure the new bone adequately but also to avoid injury to a developing tooth bud. At least two-point fixation should be used. Plate or lag screw fixation is, of course, desirable but often is not possible. The bone can overlap the mandibular body, helping to improve symmetry (see Fig. 39-4B). Once the graft is stabilized, the wound can be closed in multiple layers. Drains generally are used in these patients, but they are removed as soon as possible.

Glenoid Fossa

Much has been written about the reconstruction of the zygomatic arch and, particularly, the glenoid fossa. Although the short-term results of such reconstructions have been encouraging, we have found that the only part of the reconstruction that remains is the cartilage and bone of the glenoid fossa reconstruction. Over a

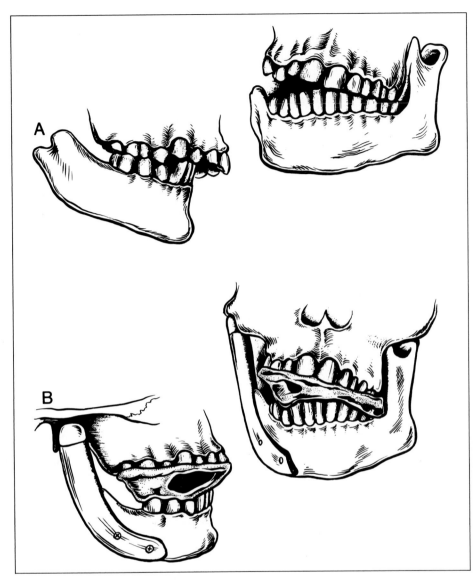

Fig. 39-4A. *Preoperative condition of mandible before placement of end-on or proximal overlapping bone graft. B. Postoperative position of the mandible, bone graft in place and stabilized with lag screws, and registration bite-block in place.*

ally a maxillary operation is not necessary, and correction can be completed with orthodontics alone. Conditions that require a maxillary operation are maxillary rotation; a large, open bite after mandibular reconstruction; maxillary excess on the contralateral side requiring impaction; and a narrow maxilla requiring widening. Older patients in whom both jaws can be operated on simultaneously also require a maxillary operation. A Le Fort I osteotomy should not be done in a developing child lest there be injury to the permanent teeth. Generally the Le Fort I osteotomies are completed after the patient is 14 years of age. Maxillary and mandibular procedures are combined only in older patients as the sequential phases of treatment are adhered to in the growing child.

An acrylic registration splint is always used to ensure proper positioning of the maxilla in relation to the mandible and to the cranium. With plate fixation, postoperative intermaxillary fixation may not be necessary, but the registration biteblock may need to be held in place against the maxillary teeth with elastic bands. This is necessary because there may be some cuspidal interference or other factors that necessitate additional orthodontic treatment before a good occlusal relation can be completed.

Even with internal plate fixation, we generally continue with a degree of third-phase postoperative treatment to maintain maxillary position. This is particularly important in patients with Goldenhar syndrome in whom a cleft palate was present and scarring may affect the long-term results.

Postoperative Care

In patients requiring intermaxillary fixation, nasal endotracheal intubation is used, and the endotracheal tube is left in overnight with the cuff inflated. The patient is kept either in the recovery room or in the intensive care unit overnight. We have always been able to take the tube out the following day because the patients have been alert and able to dispose of their own secretions, including suctioning themselves. Outpatients take antibiotics, generally cephalosporins, for approximately 8 to 10 days after the operation.

period of several years, the zygomatic arch for the most part resorbs entirely. In patients whose proximal mandible is absent, there generally is not a complete zygomatic arch, if there is any at all. There is also little or no evidence of the masseter, medial pterygoid, or temporalis muscle. It seems that the masseter muscle is necessary, at least in part, for the maintenance of the zygomatic arch. We have at least three patients in whom zygomatic arch reconstruction was completed. The early results and even the results 1 and 2 years after reconstruction seemed encouraging, but sometime between 2 and

3 years after the operation, the bone disappeared almost totally, whereas bone and cartilage remnants of the fossa reconstruction remained.

Maxillary Surgery

Once the third phase of treatment is complete and it is established that the mandibular grafts are ossified, maxillary surgery may proceed, provided the maxillary teeth have erupted and most of the craniofacial growth is completed. In general a Le Fort I osteotomy is necessary to reposition the upper dental arch. Occasion-

After completion of the fourth phase of treatment, final orthodontic detailing is finished. During this period of time, other surgical procedures may be performed. Of particular importance is the nose and the nasal septum, which have developed asymmetrically, usually deviated toward the side of involvement. There are also asymmetries of the chin, orbit, and cheek.

Nose

The nose is deviated toward the side of involvement and generally is perpendicular to the plane of the maxilla before the Le Fort I osteotomy. After the Le Fort I procedure is completed, the floor of the nose comes into a more symmetric position, but the septal deviation may not be totally corrected. There may be a need to reduce the size of the turbinate processes as well. A total nasoseptal reconstruction is therefore usually necessary. We have had only a few patients who required only septal straightening and reduction of the turbinate processes.

Chin

In almost all patients the chin is deviated asymmetrically toward the involved side. Again the position of the chin may appear to be perpendicular to the mandibular occlusal plane. Interestingly, however, unlike the septum, after correction of the mandibular position to the midline, the chin is still generally inclined toward the affected side and is generally in a markedly retruded and inferior position. The degree of deformity usually prohibits correction by a chin implant. An asymmetric sliding genioplasty, generally of the jumping form, is the preferred procedure. The techniques for sliding genioplasty have been well described. The range of possible corrections is limited only by the imagination of the surgeon. The operation on the chin is generally completed in conjunction with the operation on the nose.

Other Operations

The other operations, important aspects of the total reconstruction, include reconstruction of the cheek and zygomatic arch, orbital repositioning, otoplasty in all its various forms, and major soft tissue augmentation of the involved side and reduction of the uninvolved side. These operations are no different from those previously described in the literature. Table 39-1 lists the various operations and the suggested timing of treatment.

Table 39-1. Optimal ages for treatment of hemifacial microsomia

Procedure	Age (years)
Excision of preauricular tags and branchial clefts, sinuses, or cysts; correction of macrostomia	1–4
Otoplasty (first of three stages)	6–8
Growth management treatment (start functional appliance)	6–8
Glenoid fossa reconstruction when indicated (type III)	6–14
Mandibular ramus lengthening, when occlusal plane is severely canted (type I and IIA)	7–10
Orthodontic treatment	12–15
Mandibular ramus reconstruction or lengthening (most patients)	13–15
Le Fort I osteotomy	13–15
Sliding genioplasty	14–17
Nasoseptal reconstruction	14–17
Cheek and orbital reconstruction	14–17
Soft tissue reconstruction (generally a free flap)	17–19

Complications

Hemorrhage has not been a problem in any of the mandibular operations. It has, however, been a problem on rare occasions in patients who have undergone a Le Fort I procedure when the internal maxillary artery system has been injured. When this situation occurs, control by exposure of the bleeding internal maxillary artery through the posterior wall of the maxillary sinus has been successful.

Infection has rarely been a major problem, although a bone graft in a patient with a type IIA deformity occurred 2 months postoperatively. In one patient with a severe type III deformity there was a developing molar close to the small amount of residual bone posterior to this molar, which allowed for exposure and contamination of the bone graft.

Sensory nerve deficits, particularly with the mandibular osteotomies, and stretching of the neurovascular bundle have occurred. The lowering of the body of the mandible associated with rotation has caused considerable stretching of the soft tissues on the affected side with a resulting high degree of temporary numbness in the distribution of the mental nerve. Sensation has returned to normal or near-normal within 12 to 15 months after surgical treatment. When the chin procedure is completed, injury to the mental nerve may occur. The injury results from the asymmetry and the amount of advancement required. Certainly numbness following sagittal splitting has been recorded and may be permanent. In three extreme facial deformities, VIIth nerve paralysis has occurred with the lengthening of the mandibular ramus. All the patients recovered completely within one year of the operation.

Results

In 1986 we completed an analysis of the treatment of 25 patients. In 10 of these 25 patients the surgical procedure was completed during the period of growth, and in 15 patients it was performed after cessation of growth (Figs. 39-5 and 39-6).

Of particular interest were patients who were still growing. It was found that the reconstructed mandibular ramus increased in length, but on average there was less growth on that side than in the normal mandibular structures. In 7 of the 10 growing patients, the length increase was similar on the two sides, plus or minus 2 mm, and the established symmetry was maintained. In three patients, however, the asymmetry recurred. This asymmetry was corrected in two of the patients by a second surgical lengthening of the mandible. In the patients who were not growing, there was minimal change during the follow-up period, and the established symmetry was maintained.

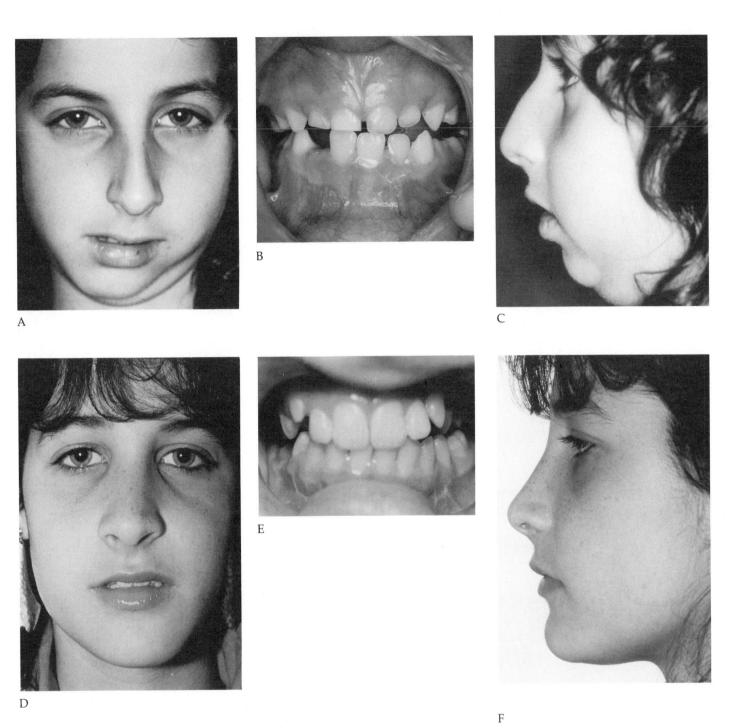

A

B

C

D

E

F

Fig. 39-5A, B, C. Preoperative appearance. The patient is 9 years of age. D, E, F. Postoperative appearance. The patient is 16 years of age. The operations included an interpositional bone graft to the mandible, a Le Fort I osteotomy, nasoseptal reconstruction, and a sliding genioplasty.

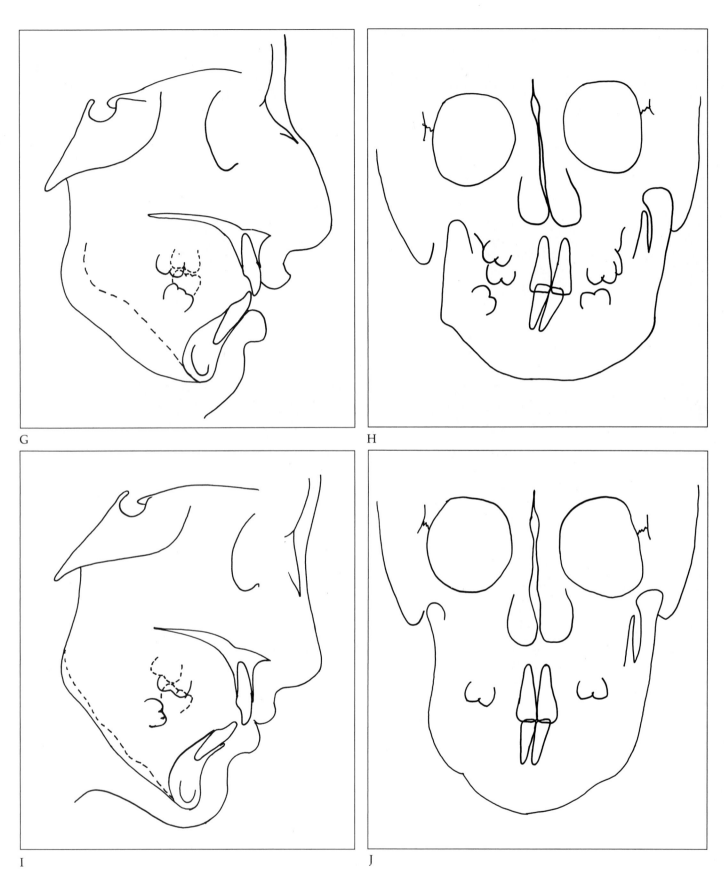

G   H

I   J

Fig. 39-5. (Continued) G. Preoperative lateral cephalometric tracing when the patient was 14 years of age. H. Preoperative posteroanterior cephalometric tracing. I. Lateral cephalometric tracing 3½ years after treatment. Patient is 18 years of age. J. Postoperative posteroanterior cephalometric tracing.

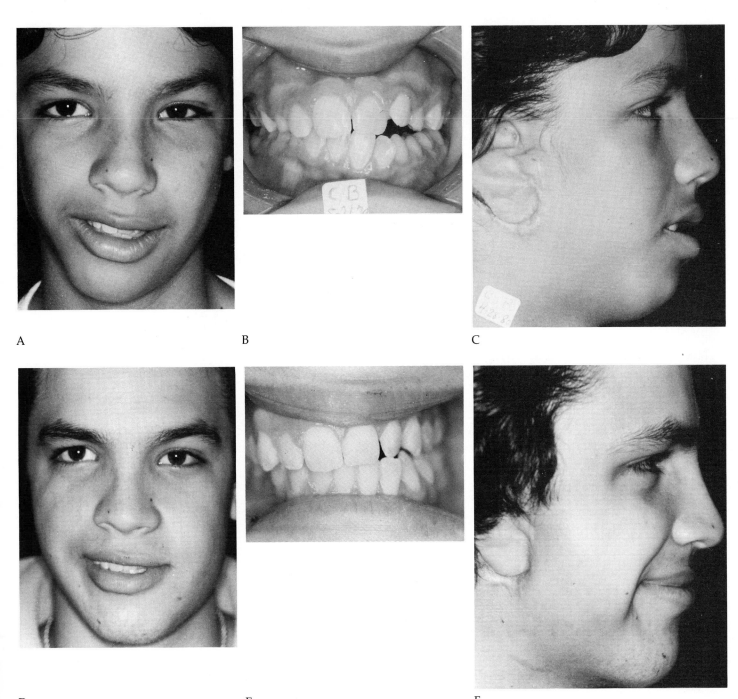

A

B

C

D

E

F

Fig. 39-6.A, B, C. Preoperative appearance. The patient is 12 years of age. D, E, F. Postoperative appearance. The patient is 19 years of age. The operations included an interpositional bone graft to the mandible, a Le Fort I osteotomy, nasoseptal reconstruction, a sliding genioplasty, and a serratus anterior muscle free flap to the right face.

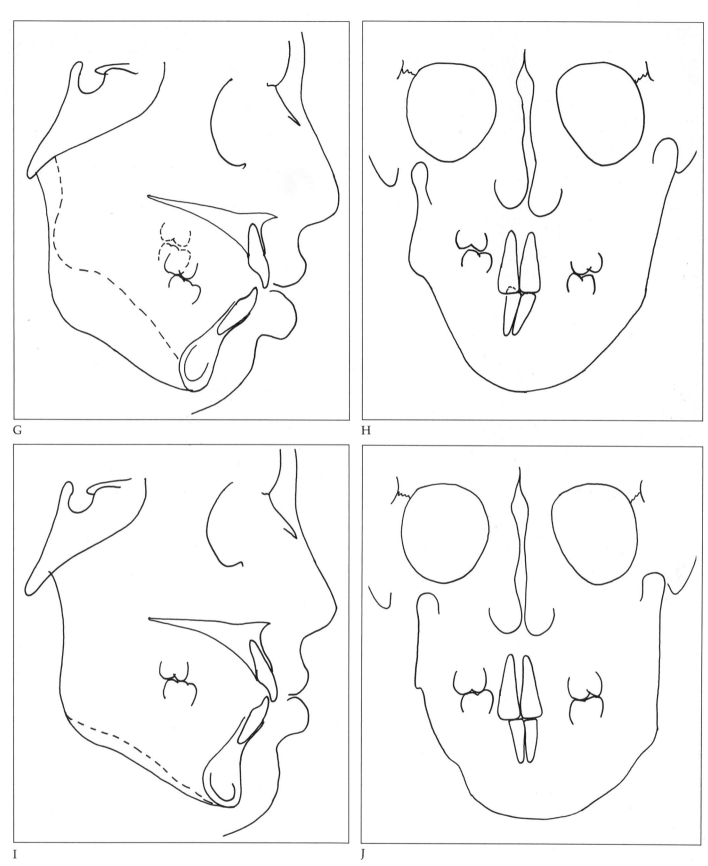

G

H

I

J

Fig. 39-6. (Continued) G. Preoperative lateral cephalometric tracing. The patient is 16 years of age. H. Preoperative posteroanterior cephalometric tracing. I. Lateral cephalometric tracing 1½ years after the operation on the jaw. The patient is 18 years of age. J. Postoperative posteroanterior cephalometric tracing.

Discussion

The treatment approach presented is based on biologic principles that have been tested and proved. The results show a successful outcome in a series of patients followed for many years. The results of this treatment protocol have in general been pleasing, and there has been minimal relapse or unfavorable remodeling. It is a disadvantage that the treatment extends over a long period of time and requires considerable cooperation from the patient. It should be noted, however, that patient cooperation has rarely been a problem.

One of the primary differences between our treatment protocol and that of other centers is that the other centers start the mandibular surgery when the patients are younger. It must be recognized, however, that these patients may require secondary and even tertiary operations on the mandible over a long period of development. Prediction of normal growth on the unaffected side is impossible; more important, normal growth is not achievable without first producing an even more extensive deformity. Bringing the youngster's affected side into an adult position and planning that the mandibular growth will catch up with resulting symmetry is not possible at this time. In addition, the maxilla becomes a problem because the Le Fort I osteotomy cannot be completed for several years. Maxillary orthodontic treatment cannot produce a symmetric maxilla with a flat occlusal plane at the proper level. There has been considerable hope that by releasing the mandibular deformities the growth potential of the adjacent structures would be unlocked. This point is still in need of considerable evaluation. We do not believe that such growth occurs.

The results of treatment when all phases are completed are pleasing. Symmetry, although not perfect, is markedly improved, and the overall facial appearance is quite acceptable.

Of considerable importance in the treatment of these patients is team care. This is a multisystem effort that requires the work of several specialists to obtain optimal results. With such a team working with patient and family, one can anticipate a high degree of success and patient satisfaction.

Suggested Reading

Alpert, B. Soft Tissue Augmentation: Various Methods and how it Can Facilitate Facial Contouring. In D.K. Ousterhout (Ed.), *Aesthetic Contouring of the Craniofacial Skeleton.* Boston: Little, Brown, 1991.

Harvold, E.P. The Theoretical Basis for the Treatment of Hemifacial Microsomia. In E.P. Harvold, K. Vargervik, and G. Chierici (Eds.), *Treatment of Hemifacial Microsomia.* New York: Alan R. Liss, 1983. Pp. 1–37.

Munro, I.R., Chen, Y.R., and Park, B.Y. Simultaneous total correction of temporomandibular joint ankylosis and facial asymmetry. *Plast. Reconstr. Surg.* 77:517, 1986.

Murray, J.E., Kaban, L.B., and Mulliken, J.B. Analysis and treatment of hemifacial microsomia. *Plast. Reconstr. Surg.* 74:186, 1984.

Poswillo, D.E. The pathogenesis of the first and second branchial arch syndrome. *Oral Surg.* 35:302, 1973.

Vargervik, K. Muscle Activity and Bone Formation. In Dixon and Sarnat (Eds.), *Normal and Abnormal Bone Growth: Basic and Clinical Research.* New York: Alan R. Liss, 1983. Pp. 269–279.

Vargervik, K., Ousterhout, D.K., and Farias, M. Factors affecting long-term results in hemifacial microsomia. *Cleft Palate J.* (Suppl. 1) 23: 53, 1986.

Whitaker, L. Aesthetic Alteration of the Malar-Midface Structures. In D.K. Ousterhout (Ed.), *Aesthetic Contouring of the Craniofacial Skeleton.* Boston: Little, Brown, 1991.

Wolfe, S.A. The Chin. In S.A. Wolfe and S. Berkowitz (Eds.), *Plastic Surgery of the Facial Skeleton.* Boston: Little, Brown, 1989.

40

Unilateral Cleft Lip

Janusz Bardach

Reconstructive surgery for unilateral cleft lip requires in-depth knowledge and understanding of the morphologic and functional changes that occur in the affected structures. During reconstructive procedures, we attempt to correct misshapened, misplaced, and malfunctioning structures. In complete unilateral cleft, these structures are the lip, nose, alveolus, and palate. Only with a detailed understanding of the existing deformity can the proper choice and sequence of procedures be devised.

Although the team approach and multidisciplinary management underscore the special role of orthodontists and speech pathologists in the treatment of patients with clefts, it is important to realize that surgical treatment has the greatest impact on the outcome and that the surgeon carries the major responsibility for the most difficult stages of treatment. Close cooperation among the surgeon, orthodontist, and speech pathologist is important in all stages of planning, evaluating, and performing the procedures. It is imperative that surgeons not only consult with orthodontists and speech pathologists but also understand the rationale for the procedures they apply in diagnosis and treatment. To achieve mutual understanding,

I prefer that the orthodontist and speech pathologist participate in my evaluation of patients and observe procedures in the operating room. I attend the patient examination by the orthodontist and speech pathologist and discuss their findings, which influence my decisions about the timing and type of surgical procedure.

Unilateral complete cleft lip, alveolus, and palate requires surgical treatment to correct all affected structures including the lip, nose, alveolus, and palate. In the past, the first operation included repair of the lip with no attempt to correct the nasal deformity or to close the nasolabial fistula. At present, most surgeons attempt to correct the nasal deformity simultaneously with primary cleft lip repair; this procedure is currently referred to by many surgeons as primary lip-nose repair. Salyer, McComb, and Anderl are among the pioneers who attempt radical correction of the nasal deformity at the time of primary lip repair.

Anatomy of Unilateral Cleft Lip

Complete unilateral cleft lip, alveolus, and palate is the most common cleft form,

constituting approximately 50 percent of all clefts. Cleft lip also may appear as an isolated cleft form or in conjunction with cleft of the alveolus without a palatal cleft. In both forms, there is a typical nasal deformity of varying degrees of severity. Cleft lip only and cleft of the lip and alveolus constitute approximately 10 to 12 percent of clefts. Complete unilateral cleft of the lip, alveolus, and palate not only is the most common cleft form but also presents the most difficult treatment problems. Complete unilateral cleft lip, alveolus, and palate may appear in a variety of forms depending on the width of the cleft, the position of the maxillary segments, the type and severity of the nasal deformity, and the degree of hypoplasia of the bony skeleton and soft tissue.

The great variety of cleft forms necessitates an individual approach to each patient (Fig. 40-1). The cleft divides the maxilla, alveolus, and lip into two uneven and asymmetric portions. The larger half includes the premaxilla and the larger portion of the lip. The asymmetry of the bony skeleton and soft tissue also causes functional imbalance because of the different distribution of muscle forces on both sides of the cleft. This functional imbalance results in malpositioning of the max-

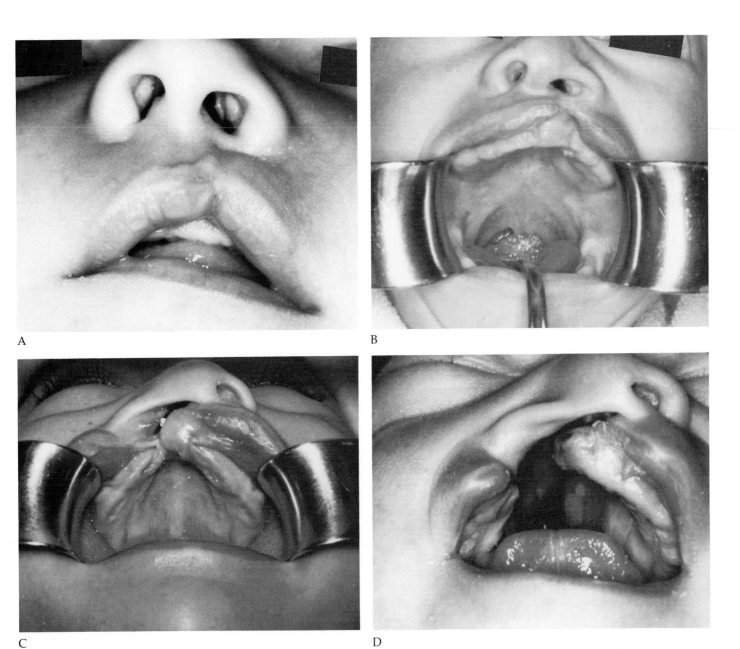

Fig. 40-1A, B, C, D. Various forms of unilateral cleft lip, alveolus, and palate. Note the different types of lip and nasal deformity and the position of the maxillary segments.

illary segments; the large segment is rotated upward and outward, and the small segment may be collapsed and displaced medially. This malpositioning of the maxillary segments is caused by prevalent muscle forces that act on the larger side of the maxilla without counterbalance from the muscle forces on the smaller segment.

The unevenly divided orbicularis oris muscle, with the remaining facial muscles attached to it, contributes greatly to the

functional imbalance that leads to skeletal asymmetry of the maxilla. When the orbicularis muscle is divided completely, as takes place in complete cleft of the lip, alveolus, and palate, the direction of its fibers along the cleft edge changes from horizontal to oblique and vertical (Fig. 40-2). The muscle turns upward along the edge of the cleft and attaches to the maxilla at the base of the ala on the cleft side and at the base of the columella on the noncleft side. The sooner a normal position and symmetry of the orbicularis oris muscle are obtained, the better the posi-

tioning of the maxillary segments. The functional balance produced by lip repair also is beneficial for growth and development of the midface. Malpositioning of the maxillary segments caused by muscle imbalance also results in nasal deformity. Asymmetry of the skeletal base, especially in the frontal plane, leads to imbalance of the nasal base such that the base of the ala on the cleft side is positioned in different planes from the one on the normal side. Division of the orbicularis oris muscle causes displacement of the alar base laterally.

Even the slightest cleft lip may affect the shape of the nose because of displace-

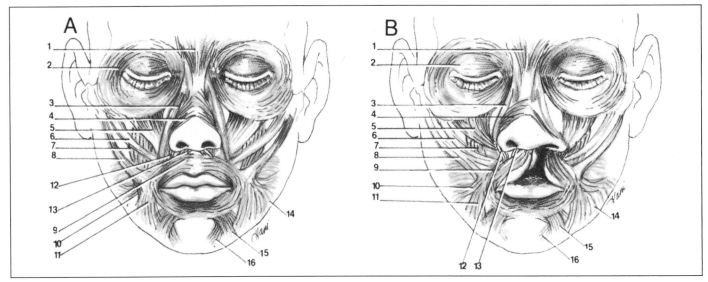

Fig. 40-2. Muscles of facial expression. A. Normal. B. Unilateral cleft lip, alveolus, and palate. 1 = procerus m.; 2 = orbicularis oculi m.; 3 = levator labii superioris alaeque nasi m.; 4 = nasalis m. (compressor naris m.); 5 = levator labii superioris m.; 6 = zygomaticus minor m.; 7 = levator anguli oris m.; 8 = zygomaticus major m.; 9 = orbicularis oris m.; 10 = risorius m.; 11 = depressor anguli oris m.; 12 = nasalis, alar part; 13 = depressor septi m.; 14 = platysma m.; 15 = depressor labii inferioris m.; 16 = mentalis m. (From J. Bardach and K.E. Salyer. Surgical Techniques in Cleft Lip and Palate (2nd ed.). Chicago: Mosby–Year Book, 1991. Reproduced with permission.)

ment of the lower lateral cartilage on the cleft side. As the extent of the cleft lip progresses, so does the severity of the nasal deformity. Complete cleft of the lip, alveolus, and palate with severe malpositioning of the maxillary segments results in nasal deformity that affects the ala, columella, nasal tip, and nasal septum. Collapse and medial displacement of the lesser maxillary segment leads to nasal deformity in which the base of the ala is displaced laterally, backward, and downward. The lower lateral cartilage is deformed; its medial crus is shorter than on the opposite side and its lateral crus is longer and often S-shaped, thus buckling into the nasal passage. The columella is positioned obliquely, and the caudal edge of the septum is deviated to the noncleft side. The septum is usually deviated, resulting in varying degrees of nasal obstruction on the cleft side.

The asymmetry of the nasal structures results from the difference in position of the skeletal base on both sides of the cleft. Because both maxillary segments can be displaced in various planes (frontal, sagittal, and vertical), surgical orthodontic treatment must be applied to produce symmetry of the skeletal platform and

equilibrium of the nasal structures. The sooner symmetry of the maxillary segments can be obtained and a normal position established, the better are the chances of producing a more symmetric configuration of the nares, alae, and nasal tip. It must be understood, however, that primary lip repair combined with orthodontic treatment only seldom corrects the nasal deformity to the degree that no more surgical intervention is necessary. In most instances, deformity of the lower lateral cartilage persists, and correction of the nasal deformity at a later time is indicated.

Alveolar cleft presents another problem that must be considered in discussions of the anatomy of the unilateral cleft lip, alveolus, and palate. Depending on the position of the maxillary segments, an alveolar cleft may vary in dimension; however, the initial width and shape of the alveolar cleft change dramatically after repair of a cleft lip or presurgical orthopedic treatment followed by cleft lip repair. The presence of the alveolar cleft may cause serious problems related to tooth eruption. In many patients, surgical treatment with bone grafting may be needed to produce the conditions necessary for normal

tooth eruption and normal occlusion. Failure to close the alveolar cleft may lead to nasolabial fistulas.

Dysmorphogenesis, especially hypoplasia of the maxillary bone on the cleft side, is another factor that must be seriously considered in evaluating the deformity associated with a unilateral cleft lip and in planning the reconstructive procedure. The degree of hypoplasia cannot be measured. In some instances, it is evident that the most careful correction of the existing deformities does not lead to the expected result because of severe hypoplastic changes in the skeletal structures. These patients usually require not only alveolar bone grafting but also onlay grafting on the anterior maxillary wall to produce symmetry with the opposite side.

Timing of Repair of Cleft Lip

Most surgeons perform cleft lip repair according to the "rule of tens": when the child is in good health, is at least 10 weeks old, weighs at least 10 pounds, and has a hemoglobin count of at least 10 g. Although some surgeons operate on cleft lips during the first hours or days of life, this practice never became popular. Better results can be obtained when the child is approximately 3 months old at the time of the primary operation. In newborn infants proper alignment of the lip segments and closure of the nasal floor presents a difficult problem. I cannot find justification for the urgency of this operation or for recently promoted ideas concerning intrauterine lip repair.

Presurgical Orthopedic Treatment

In patients with complete unilateral cleft lip, alveolus, and palate and in patients with cleft lip and alveolus only, presurgical orthopedic treatment is used to realign the maxillary segments into a normal position before lip repair to improve the balance and symmetry of the skeletal base; to provide better conditions for growth and development of the midportion of the face; to better align the alveolar arch; and subsequently to produce better occlusion. Better positioning of the maxillary segments improves the position of the alar base and facilitates correction of the nasal deformity during primary lip repair. In many cleft palate centers, presurgical orthopedic treatment is considered an important and integral part of the overall treatment plan. In contrast to the opinion that presurgical orthopedic treatment is crucial in establishing proper alignment of the maxillary segments before surgical repair of the cleft lip, many specialists use this technique rarely or not at all. One of the most experienced cleft orthodontists, Olin, presented convincing documentation and long-term results that indicate that presurgical orthopedic therapy is not essential to obtaining proper occlusion, normal midfacial growth, and facial symmetry. In Olin's opinion, proper orthodontic treatment during the stage of mixed dentition with careful follow-up care during permanent dentition allows for correcting malocclusion to the same degree achieved when presurgical orthopedic treatment is used. Huddart, who performed many clinical studies related to the influence of presurgical orthopedic treatment on positioning of the maxillary segments, occlusion, and growth, concluded that this process is helpful but not essential in patient care.

In the past, I used presurgical orthopedic treatment for most patients with unilateral cleft lip, alveolus, and palate, particularly in all patients with wide clefts and all patients with malalignment of the maxillary segments. A large number of patients who had operations at 3 months of age or later did not have presurgical orthopedic treatment, allowing me to observe realignment of the maxillary segments under the influence of lip repair only. Multiple observations of the changes that occurred after surgical treatment convinced me that, in most instances, presurgical orthopedic treatment does not enhance proper alignment of the maxillary segments to a greater degree than surgical treatment alone. I must emphasize that by indicating the influence of surgical treatment on proper alignment of the maxillary segments, I have in mind primary lip repair, which I perform simultaneously with construction of the floor of the nose and construction of a normal sulcus. Those observations stimulated me to abandon presurgical orthopedic treatment, even for wide clefts and for collapse of the minor maxillary segment. Proper surgical treatment and skilled orthodontic care afterward lead to proper alignment of the maxillary segments in the same way that presurgical orthopedic treatment does.

The Operations
Lip Adhesion

At present, two surgical techniques are used most widely in cleft lip surgery—the rotation-advancement technique and the triangular flap technique. One more technique, lip adhesion, must be discussed because there is a long-standing difference of opinion concerning the use of this technique.

Lip adhesion is the first stage of the two-stage lip reconstruction. It precedes the rotation-advancement or triangular flap technique performed in the second stage. This approach, advocated by Randall and by Lesavoy, has definite benefits: Lip segments are sutured together, and the pressure of the reconstructed lip is helpful in realigning the maxillary segments and narrowing the gap between them. Lip adhesion also may be advantageous for an inexperienced surgeon who may feel more secure performing final lip reconstruction when the cleft has already been

closed and the second stage involves correction of the secondary lip-nose deformity rather than a primary cleft lip repair.

Lip adhesion has serious disadvantages, however. When lip adhesion is used, two procedures for lip reconstruction rather than one are planned. Considering the fact that minor corrections may be needed, the total number of operations is always increased by one. The other serious disadvantage is the waste of valuable tissue when the scar resulting from lip adhesion is excised. This waste of tissue is contradictory to one of the dominant principles of the rotation-advancement or triangular flap technique: to save as much tissue as possible because of the tissue deficiency intrinsic to clefts. Lip adhesion does not necessarily enhance the proper alignment of maxillary segments. There are no convincing clinical data demonstrating that lip adhesion is more beneficial or produces better final results than primary lip repair. A study by Salyer proved that there is no difference in the results obtained with or without lip adhesion.

Instead of starting with lip adhesion, I prefer to plan the final reconstructive procedure at the time of primary lip repair, including limited correction of the nasal deformity and closure of the nasolabial fistula. Often this primary repair is also the final one; if correction is needed, however, another operation is performed on the lip.

Rotation-Advancement Technique

In many instances of incomplete cleft lip, I use the rotation-advancement technique, although the triangular flap technique is my preference for complete clefts of the lip, alveolus, and palate and for some incomplete clefts. The rotation-advancement technique as described initially by Millard in 1957 underwent multiple changes in the attempt to perfect surgical results. At the same time, the surgical design of unilateral cleft lip repair became more complicated because of the design of additional flaps. Rotation-advancement became the most popular procedure because of the simplicity of its initial design and the definite advantages it allows.

The advantages and disadvantages of rotation-advancement are clearly summarized by Salyer in the second edition of

Surgical Techniques in Cleft Lip and Palate (1991). According to Salyer, the main advantages of the rotation-advancement technique include the minimal amount of tissue discarded; camouflage of the suture line; construction of a normal-looking cupid's bow; and easy access to the alar base and nasal floor, which can be reconstructed simultaneously with primary lip repair. Salyer also indicated that the technique is flexible and adaptable, allowing improvisation and artistry on the part of the surgeon. Salyer also listed several disadvantages. Among them was frequent contracture of the vertical scar, resulting in secondary deformity such as a notch in the vermilion or shortening of the entire lip in the vertical dimension. In wide unilateral clefts, another disadvantage of the rotation-advancement technique is excessive tension after closure of the cleft defect and advancement of the lateral lip portion medially. In these patients, there also may be difficulty matching the vermilion on both sides. Undermining of the soft tissue on the anterior surface of the maxilla, which in many patients seems to be imperative, may lead to excessive scarring and may contribute to maxillary growth aberrations.

The rotation-advancement technique does not require precise marking and measurements to design the incision lines. The technique is based on the ability of the surgeon to use the basic design and to adjust the tissue as the operation progresses until an acceptable alignment is achieved. I find the use of the rotation-advancement technique extremely practical for incomplete cleft lips. For complete clefts of the lip, alveolus, and palate and especially for wide clefts, I prefer the triangular flap technique for the following reason: Designing the advancement flap on the cleft side and making incisions around the ala to advance it to a position symmetric to the noncleft side often resulted in a small nostril on the cleft side, which in my opinion is the main disadvantage of the rotation-advancement technique. A small nostril may be difficult to avoid because at the time of the operation, after tissue adjustment, it may seem that the nostrils are symmetric and the alar base is placed in a desired position. However, one cannot anticipate how postoperative scarring will affect the growth and development of the nasal structures or when scarring may result in asymmetry, with the nostril and ala

smaller on the cleft side. Surgical correction of a small nostril is more difficult than correction of any other secondary nasal deformity associated with unilateral cleft. For this reason, I use the rotation-advancement technique for incomplete clefts when a small nostril can be easily avoided.

When starting a partial cleft lip repair using the rotation-advancement flap, marking of the highest points of the cupid's bow on the skin-vermilion margin is indicated to ensure that the point at which the vermilion will be sutured together from both lip segments will correspond with the highest point of the cupid's bow on the noncleft side. I usually use a C flap for lengthening the columella because in most incomplete clefts, there is still marked nasal deformity; the columella is shorter on the cleft side, and the alar base is displaced laterally with a flattened ala and an asymmetric nasal tip. Adding the C flap helps reestablish symmetry of the columella and sometimes allows for improving the nasal tip. The alar base is approximated medially to achieve perfect symmetry with the opposite side. The design of the incisions as presented in Figure 40-3 allows variations in the size of the C flap and the way it is used. If there is no need to use a C flap to lengthen the columella on the cleft side, it may be used to fill the gap after advancement of the lateral lip segment (Fig. 40-4). However, I caution surgeons about placing the C flap below the nasal sill and alar base on the cleft side, because it contributes to excessive length of the lateral lip segment. Adjustment of the tissue is needed primarily at the upper portion of the lip when inserting the tip of the lateral lip segment into the gap caused by downward rotation of the medial portion of the lip. This adjustment is crucial in terms of establishing the proper length of the reconstructed lip and avoiding excessive tissue tension after the sutures are placed.

Another step of the operation in which special caution is advised is adjustment of the vermilion in the suture line between the lateral and medial sides. Often the thickness of the vermilion differs on both sides, and to achieve symmetry it may be necessary to perform an additional unequal Z-plasty to produce an equal and symmetric vermilion (Fig. 40-5).

It is important to realize that the results achieved on the operating table are not

always the final ones. Alteration of the result may occur because of postoperative scarring and the growth and development of tissues. As in any technique for cleft lip repair, rotation-advancement must be evaluated in terms of late results and in terms of type, severity, and rate of occurrence of secondary lip deformity. I consider the surgical procedure highly advantageous in selected patients and highly successful when performed by experienced plastic surgeons.

Triangular Flap Technique

Another widely used technique for repair of cleft lip is based on the idea of using a triangular flap design to establish equal vertical dimensions on both lip segments. This technique, developed by Tennison, is based on the construction of equilateral triangular flaps on each side of the defect. These flaps fit the triangular defects on each side of the cleft. The technique has undergone several modifications; the essential ones are described by Randall, Hagerty, and Skoog. The triangular flap technique gained widespread popularity because of its simplicity and precision and the predictability of its results. It can be used for any type of cleft lip. Its design facilitates the achievement of the main goals of reconstruction of the normal anatomy and function of the lip and correction of the nasal deformity.

Goals of the Procedure

Currently primary repair of a cleft lip includes much more than lip repair. The goals defined for this operation must include the reconstructive procedure in which the normal anatomy and function of the lip are restored, a more or less limited correction of the nasal deformity, and closure of the nasolabial fistula. In complete unilateral clefts with malalignment of the maxillary segments, this operation also must aim to achieve realignment of the misplaced segments to form a symmetric skeletal platform for nasal structures. It is expected that a normal alveolar arch will be made after lip reconstruction.

The goals of primary lip repair are lengthening of the lip on both sides of the cleft to produce a vertical dimension symmetric with the normal side; construction of a normal cupid's bow and a normal vermilion; construction of a deep normal sulcus; and arrangement of the orbicularis oris muscle in proper alignment. Simultaneously with the primary lip repair, my

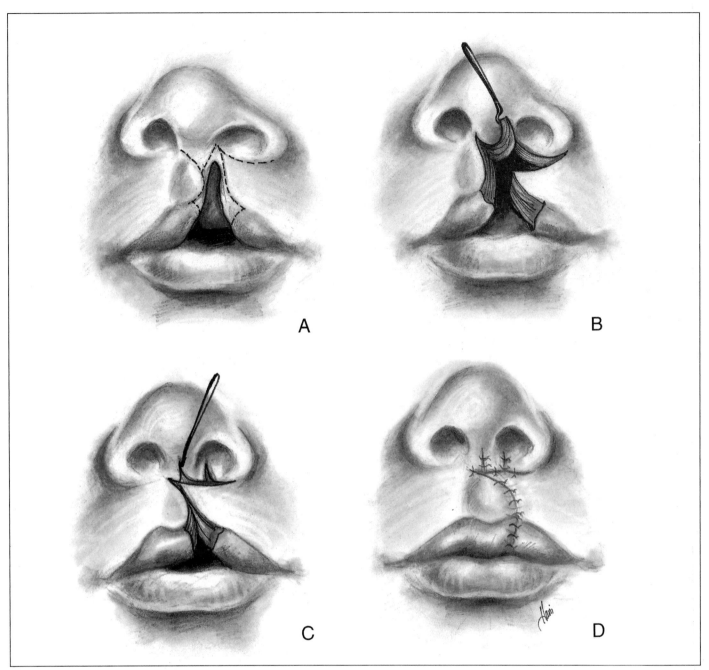

Fig. 40-3. Millard's design of the rotation-advancement technique for incomplete unilateral cleft lip repair.
A. Design of incisions. B. Incisions made and *C* flap raised. C. Approximation of the lip segments. *C* flap
is used for lengthening the columella on the cleft side. D. Final closure of the lip and lengthening of the
columella.

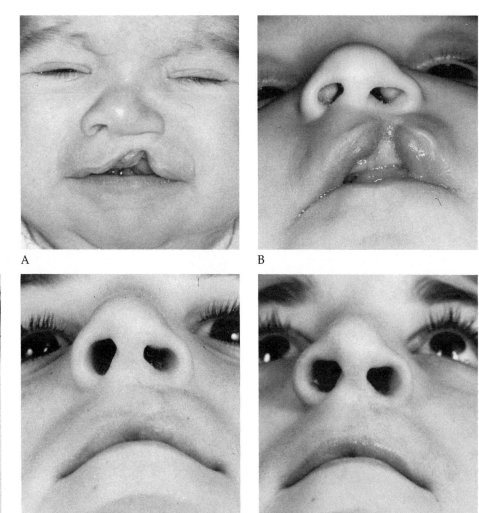

Fig. 40-4A, B. Front and base view of infant with incomplete cleft lip. Note distinct nasal deformity. C. After rotation-advancement cleft lip repair at age 12. D. Base view showing residual nasal deformity on cleft side. E. After correction of the nasal deformity using the Bardach cleft rhinoplastic technique.

A

B

C

D

E

colleagues and I attempt to achieve limited correction of the nasal deformity. This involves construction of the floor of the nose by suturing a mucoperiosteal flap from the lateral nasal wall to a mucoperichondrial flap from the nasal septum and medial approximation of the distorted alar base and straightening of the columella. In contrast to the radical approach to correction of nasal deformity advocated by Salyer, McComb, and Anderl, I do not attempt to reshape and realign the lower lateral cartilage at this stage. Another goal pursued at the time of primary cleft lip repair is two-layer closure of the nasolabial fistula. It cannot easily be achieved in very wide clefts;

however, in narrow and medium-sized clefts, a stable closure is readily obtained. These goals can be achieved using various surgical techniques. My motivation to use the triangular flap technique is based on long-term experience and observation, encompassing secondary lip and nasal deformities after primary repair.

When analyzing the use of any surgical technique, one must pay attention not only to the immediate results but also to secondary deformities, which determine the number of corrective procedures necessary to achieve optimal results with the lip and nose. The proficiency of the technique and of the surgeon can be assessed

by the aesthetic and functional result of primary lip repair and by the secondary deformities and the number of operations necessary to correct them. It is a mistake to assume that surgical technique as described and illustrated by different authors is the most crucial factor in achieving satisfactory results. The surgical technique is only a guideline; the skill, inventiveness, and artistry of the surgeon are the decisive factors in achieving optimal results. Unfortunately, in the literature much more attention is paid to technique than to the proficiency of the surgeon. A few studies have been devoted to exploring the relation between the surgeon and the results obtained.

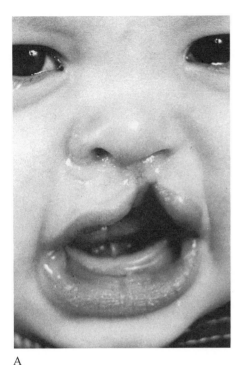

A

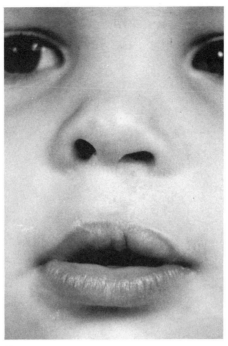

B

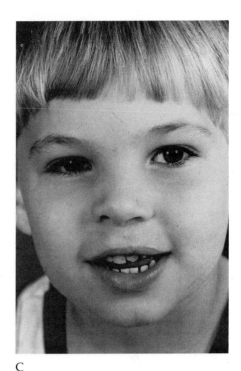

C

Fig. 40-5A. Incomplete cleft lip on the left side. B. After rotation-advancement lip repair. C. When the patient is 5 years of age, the lip and nose are symmetric.

The extent and severity of the cleft determine which goals can be achieved in the primary cleft lip repair. As a rule, I aim to achieve maximal as well as optimal results. However, what is attainable for each patient depends on the form of the cleft, the width of the cleft, the position of the maxillary segments, and the associated nasal deformity.

The results obtained at the time of primary lip repair may undergo changes with growth and development. Understanding the fact that the results of the operation are not permanent must influence one's approach to correction of the secondary deformities. My long-term experience and observations and multiple published studies of late results by my team indicate that the results of primary lip repair may improve with time to the degree that a lip that seems far from perfect immediately after the operation looks good enough after 1 or 2 years so that no corrective operations are required. This observation led to the important decision to refrain from immediate correction of secondary lip deformities. The improvements we observed in the growth and development of the lip may be related to restored muscle balance and lip function.

After lip repair, I recommend massage of the scar on the lip with vitamin E, which softens the scar and efficiently prevents vertical scar contracture. After lip repair is performed using my design and technique, realignment of the maxillary segments into a proper position occurs during the several months after the operation. Realignment of the maxillary segments may lead to some correction of the nasal deformity. However, even perfect positioning of the maxillary segments, bringing them to the same level as the skeletal platform for the alar bases on both sides, cannot entirely correct the existing nasal deformity caused by a misshapen and misplaced lower lateral cartilage.

I provide limited correction of the nasal deformity at the time of primary lip repair, but for most patients another nasal correction at a later time is necessary. Closure of the nasolabial fistula, achieved during primary lip repair, may remain complete, or the fistula may open as the result of maxillary expansion during orthodontic treatment. If the fistula does open, it must be closed, sometimes simultaneously with alveolar bone grafting.

Preoperative Measurements

When using the rotation-advancement technique, preoperative measurements may be helpful; however, they are not necessary because the operation is performed by sight rather than by precise measurements. In contrast, the triangular flap repair requires precise measurements because the entire design is based on these measurements, which are illustrated in Figures 40-6 and 40-7. *Two measurements are crucial.* One of these is the distance between the highest points of the cupid's bow on the noncleft side and the base of the columella on both sides. The difference between those two height measurements (1–5 and 3–4) determines the amount by which the lip must be lengthened to bring the peak of the cupid's bow at the edge of the cleft to the level of the other peak of the cupid's bow. It also determines the amount by which the lesser segment of the lip must be lengthened. The vertical dimension on each side of the cleft is distorted because of the upward curvature of the edges of the lip segments. The measurement described allows the definition of the existing deficiency in the vertical dimension and gives the amount by which it must be length-

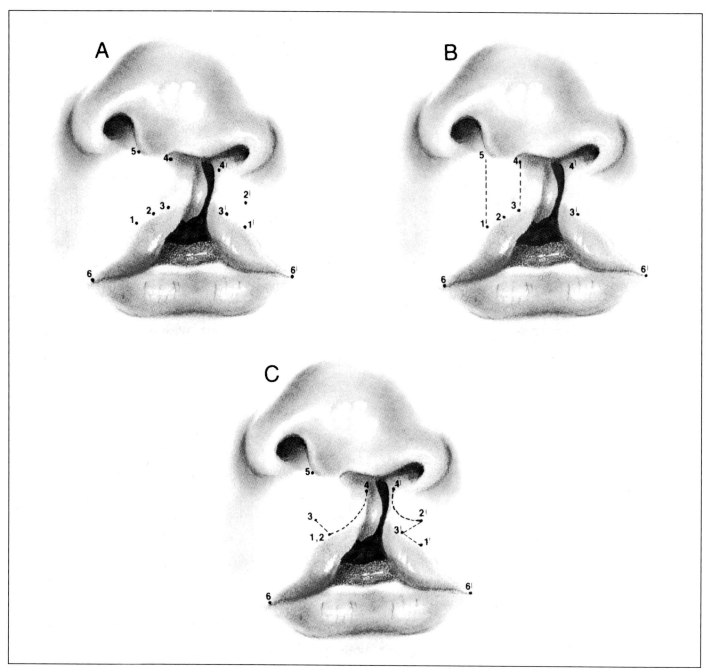

Fig. 40-6. *Unilateral cleft lip repair by the Bardach technique. A. Basic points to be used for measurements and design. First, the peak of the cupid's bow on the noncleft side (1) is established, followed by the lowest point of the cupid's bow (2). The distance between 1 and 2 establishes point 3, which corresponds to the peak of the cupid's bow on the cleft side. Points 4 and 5 are marked on both sides of the base of the columella. These points are the reference points for establishing the difference in height between the peaks of the cupid's bow. Two points, 6 and 6', are marked at both commissures. The distance 1–6 establishes the point corresponding to the peak of the cupid's bow on the cleft side, point 1'. B. Measurements made on the lip determine the difference in height between the two peaks of the cupid's bow and the columellar base. The difference between distances 1–5 and 3–4 establishes the difference in height between the peaks of the cupid's bow. This difference applies to both the cleft and the noncleft sides. Distance 1–5 minus distance 3–4 = x, where x is the difference in height that must be added to establish symmetry of the reconstructed lip. C. Design of the unilateral cleft lip repair using the single triangular flap technique with the Bardach modification. 1,2–3 = 1'–3' = 3'–2', and 1,2–4 = 2'–4'. After the incision is carried from point 3 to point 1,2, a triangular gap is made with arms 1–3 = 2–3. (From J. Bardach and K.E. Salyer.* Surgical Techniques in Cleft Lip and Palate *(2nd ed.). Chicago: Mosby–Year Book, 1991. Reproduced with permission.)*

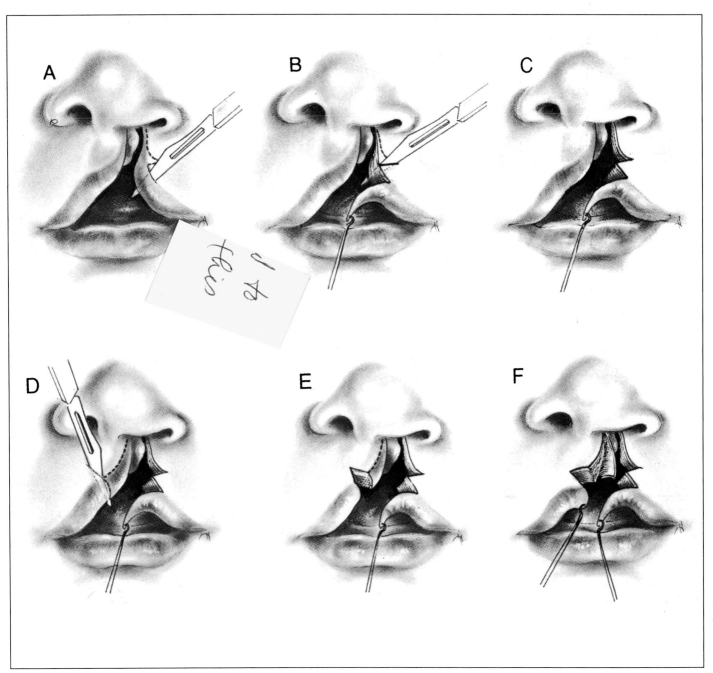

Fig. 40-7A, B, C. The operation starts with dissection of the vermilion flap along the vermilion-cutaneous junction from point 1', continuing upward to point 4'. A No. 11 blade is used for this purpose. D. Incisions are completed on the cleft side. Note the triangular flap and the vermilion flap turned down in the lower portion of the lip. The incision on the noncleft side is carried through and through from point 3 to point 1,2. E. The gap is opened on the noncleft portion of the lip to accommodate the triangular flap from the cleft segment of the lip. F. The incisions on both sides are completed. (From J. Bardach and K.E. Salyer. Surgical Techniques in Cleft Lip and Palate (2nd ed.). Chicago: Mosby–Year Book, 1991. Reproduced with permission.)

ened to achieve a well-balanced and symmetric lip. It is important to realize that the principle of triangular flap repair is based on the use of the same measurement in designing the triangular flap on one side of the cleft and the triangular gap on the other side of the cleft, so that the flap and the gap fit perfectly. Another measurement that allows the determination of the peak of the cupid's bow on the lesser lip segment is achieved by measuring the distance from the commissure to the peak of the cupid's bow on the noncleft side and transferring the same measurement to the lesser segment of the lip, thus establishing the point that corresponds with the peak of the cupid's bow on the noncleft side (1–6 = 3'–6'). This measurement is important because the peak of the cupid's bow on the larger part of the lip is easily visible, whereas the point corresponding to it on the lesser part of the lip must be determined by this measurement.

The measurements used on the lip determine the design of the single triangular flap, which is made in the lower portion of the lip next to the vermilion-cutaneous border. The construction of this single triangular flap lengthens the vertical dimension of the lesser segment of the lip to the same degree that the larger portion of the lip is lengthened at its edge by a through-and-through incision, forming the triangular gap where the flap is inserted. The single triangular flap is used in nearly all complete clefts of the lip, alveolus, and palate, and in some partial clefts of the lip.

Extremely wide clefts of the lip, alveolus, and palate may require a double triangular flap technique when the difference in vertical dimension between the philtral columns is larger than 5 mm. Instead of using one triangular flap, which may place too much tension on the lower portion of the lip and excessively violate the contour of the philtrum, two triangular flaps are used: one in the lower portion of the lip and one in the upper portion, thus distributing the tension along the entire height of the lip. Two smaller triangles are less conspicuous and less disturbing aesthetically.

Long-term experience indicates that in most instances of complete unilateral cleft, the difference in vertical dimension that determines the size of the equilateral triangle in the lesser lip portion and the equilateral gap in the larger lip portion

equals 4 mm. With incomplete clefts, this difference is usually less than 4 mm. The design of the single triangular flap operation is simple enough because it is based on a single measurement, which guides the necessary dimensions for the triangular flap and for the gap in which it will fit. The triangular flap design has one advantage that must be emphasized: Insertion of the triangular flap into the triangular gap efficiently prevents vertical scar contracture when the incisions are carried through and through, and the triangular flap is used not only for skin but also for muscle and mucosa. A mistake often made is designing a triangular flap limited to the skin or skin and muscle and closing the mucosal layer in a straight line. This type of lip closure may lead to vertical scar contracture because there is no triangular flap in the mucosal layer to prevent that contracture.

Avoidance of Incisions in the Sulcus

One principle of unilateral cleft lip repair that I have followed for many years is to perform this operation with no incisions in the sulcus and without undermining the soft tissue on the face of the maxilla. My rationale for avoiding these incisions is based on my experience that they are not necessary for successful lip closure. I have found this to be true even for very wide clefts. I accepted this principle many years ago on the basis of physiologic considerations presented by Walker and associates and on the basis of my experimental studies in rabbits and in beagles, which indicated that the incisions in the sulcus with undermining of soft tissue on the face of the maxilla contribute to aberrations in facial growth. It can be assumed that the growth aberrations result from postoperative scarring following wide soft tissue undermining on the face of the maxilla. There is another reason to avoid incisions in the sulcus and the undermining of soft tissue from the standpoint of facial growth and development: When incisions are made in the sulcus, and the soft tissue from the lesser maxillary segment is undermined, the fibrous band between the alveolar ridge and the lesser lip portion is destroyed, preventing the use of the fibrous band as the pulling force to realign the maxillary segments after lip repair. Incisions in the sulcus and wide undermining of soft tissue enhance the collapse of the lesser maxillary segment, especially when the collapse is evident at the time of primary lip repair.

Treatment of the Nasal Deformity

Serious consideration is always given to the existing nasal deformity, which may be present even in instances of slight cleft lip. In partial cleft lip, the division of the orbicularis oris muscle leads to lateral displacement of the alar base and, consequently, to the horizontal orientation of the nostril and misplacement and deformity of the lower lateral cartilage. On many occasions obtaining an optimal result in cleft lip repair is easier than correction of the existing nasal deformity, even when it is not a severe one. In complete clefts, I always perform limited correction of the nasal deformity simultaneously with lip repair. This limited correction includes construction of the floor of the nose, placement of the alar base in a position symmetric to the opposite side, and straightening of the columella. When performing correction of the nasal deformity, special emphasis is placed on achieving these goals without repositioning or reshaping the lower lateral cartilage and, primarily, on avoiding the construction of a small nostril. A small nostril, which is frequently the result of the rotation-advancement technique used by inexperienced surgeons operating on complete clefts, is difficult and sometimes impossible to correct.

Surgical Technique

Incisions. Preoperative evaluation of the anatomic and functional conditions of the cleft allows detailed planning of the surgical procedure. Even when a surgeon uses the same technique for all types of clefts, an individual approach is necessary because of variation in details that may affect the outcome. In the operating room, before the incision lines are measured and marked, it is necessary to stabilize the endotracheal tube in the midline without distorting the lower lip and the commissures. When the endotracheal tube pulls the lower lip downward, it also distorts the upper lip and interferes with precise measurement.

After the lines of incision are drawn, the operation begins with an incision on the nasal septum along its lower margin, approximately 2 to 3 mm above the lower edge of the septum. The incision is carried along the vermilion-cutaneous border to the peak of the cupid's bow marked as point 1,2 (Fig. 40-8). Using a No. 11 blade, the incision is carried along line 1,2–3

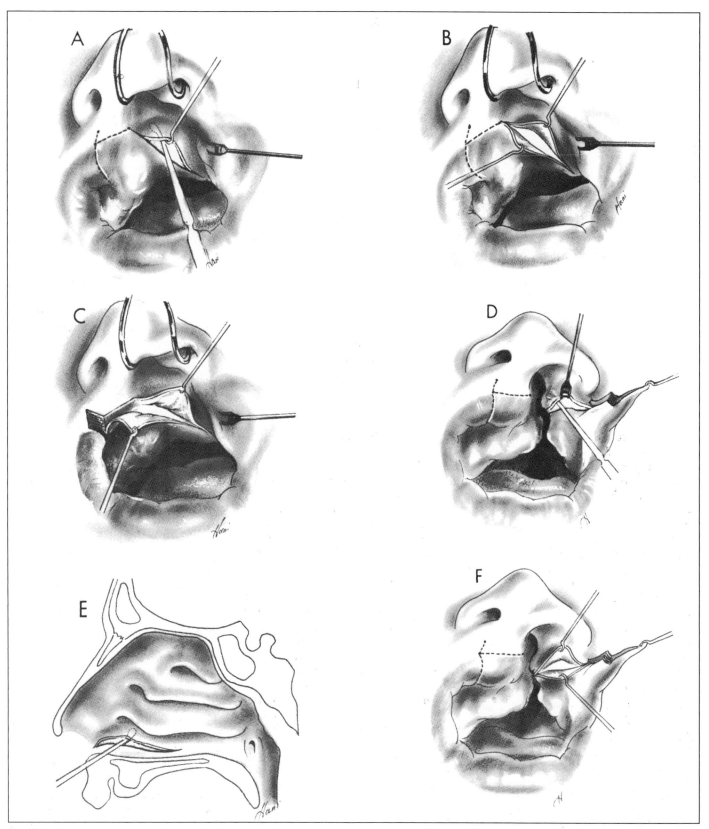

Fig. 40-8. Construction of the nasal floor. A. Undermining of the mucoperichondrial flap on the septum. B. The mucoperichondrial flap on the septum and the turned-down mucoperiosteal flap are raised. C. The incision on the medial lip element and undermining of the flaps are completed. The upper flap is used for construction of the floor of the nose. The lower flap is used partially as a second layer for the nasal floor and for reconstruction of the sulcus. D. Undermining of the mucoperiosteal flap on the lateral nasal wall. E. The area of undermining where the mucoperiosteal flap is made to be used for construction of the nasal floor. F. Upper and lower flaps on the lateral lip element are undermined. The upper flap is used in construction of the nasal floor. The lower flap partially forms the second layer and is used in reconstruction of the sulcus. Note that the Bardach band remains attached to the maxillary segment, and no incision is made in the sulcus on either side. (From J. Bardach and K.E. Salyer. Surgical Techniques in Cleft Lip and Palate (2nd ed.). Chicago: Mosby–Year Book, 1991. Reproduced with permission.)

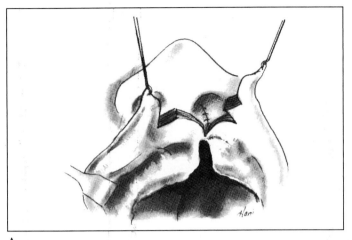
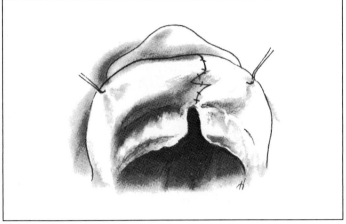

A

B

Fig. 40-9. Final closure of the lip on the inner surface. A. Incisions on the skin correspond to incisions on the muscles and mucosa. B. Closure of muscles and mucosa and construction of the sulcus are performed in the same way as closure of the skin using the triangular flap technique to prevent contracture and secondary deformities of the lip. (From J. Bardach and K.E. Salyer. Surgical Techniques in Cleft Lip and Palate *(2nd ed.). Chicago: Mosby–Year Book, 1991. Reproduced with permission.)*

through the skin, muscle, and mucosa as well as through the vermilion, thus opening a triangular gap in the lower portion of the lip. With a Freer knife, a mucoperichondrial flap is raised on the nasal septum. In the anterior portion of the septum, I continue to raise the mucoperichondrial flap from the septum and also raise a mucoperiosteal flap from the extended alveolar ridge. This flap is turned downward with the epithelium facing the sulcus and is used to close the nasolabial fistula and to construct the sulcus. The mucoperiosteal flap is extended into the mucosal flap made at the edge of the larger lip segment, turned down, and used to close the mucosal layer of the reconstructed lip and to form the sulcus.

Starting the operation with incisions inside the nasal cavity prevents blood from obstructing the operative field on the lip. The incisions on the lateral side of the cleft also are started inside the nasal cavity below the lower turbinate process in the groove between the lateral nasal wall and the palatal plate. The incision is carried through the mucosa and periosteum to the lateral nasal bone, and a mucoperiosteal flap is elevated. The incision is carried along the vermilion-cutaneous border from point 1' to point 4' using a No. 11 blade, producing a vermilion flap that will be used to adjust the final shape of the vermilion.

The next step is incision through the skin, muscle, and mucosa from point 2' to point 3', thus producing the triangular flap in the lower portion of the lip. According to the previous measurements, this flap will fit precisely into the gap made on the noncleft side. From point 2' to point 4', the semicircular incision through the skin, muscle, and mucosa is carried on, increasing vertical extension of the lesser lip segment and providing a close fit for the flap above the gap on the noncleft side. In the incisions on the cleft side, it is important to preserve the fibrous band that extends from the alveolar ridge to the base of the ala. Preservation of this fibrous band ensures the proper direction for realignment of the maxillary segments because it acts synchronously with lip pressure exerted by the reconstructed orbicularis oris muscle. In this technique, no incisions are made in the sulcus and no soft tissue is undermined from the face of the maxilla, for reasons previously explained. This approach does not prevent closure of very wide clefts.

When all incisions are completed, detachment of the orbicularis oris muscle from the alar base on the cleft side and from the base of the columella on the noncleft side is necessary to facilitate horizontal alignment of the muscle fibers on both sides of the cleft before they are sutured together. I do not use muscle flaps as ad-

vocated by Randall, nor do I suture the muscle layer separately.

Verification of Preoperative Measurements. To prevent mismatch of the flaps and to avoid secondary deformities, it is possible to confirm during the operation that the measurements are precise and accurate. After the first incision on the noncleft side, which produces a gap in the lower portion of the lip, the design of the incisions on the lesser lip portion may be repeated to make sure that the dimensions of the triangular flap and the length of the incisions fit perfectly with those on the noncleft side.

Closure of the Cleft. Closure of the cleft starts with construction of the nasal floor by suturing the mucoperichondrial flap from the septum to the mucoperiosteal flap from the lateral nasal wall. These flaps are sutured together with a 4–0 chromic catgut, the knots facing the nasal cavity. Depending on individual conditions, the floor of the nose is extended posteriorly as much as is technically feasible. This one-layer closure is supplemented anteriorly by the second layer of the mucoperiosteal flaps from the alveolar ridge on both sides of the cleft. These flaps are sutured with 4–0 chromic catgut, the knots facing the oral cavity. Sometimes both layers can be approximated by

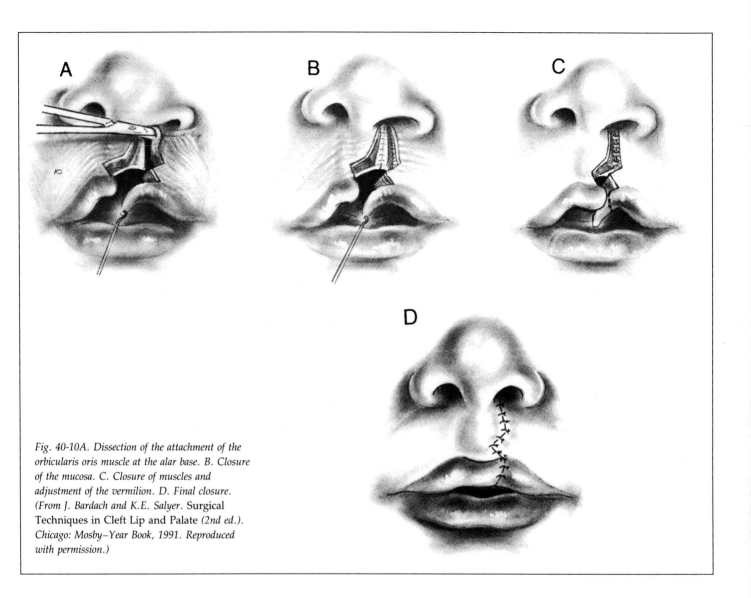

Fig. 40-10A. Dissection of the attachment of the orbicularis oris muscle at the alar base. B. Closure of the mucosa. C. Closure of muscles and adjustment of the vermilion. D. Final closure. (From J. Bardach and K.E. Salyer. Surgical Techniques in Cleft Lip and Palate *(2nd ed.). Chicago: Mosby–Year Book, 1991. Reproduced with permission.)*

a vertical mattress suture to ensure obliteration of the nasolabial fistula and to provide a solid structure for the nasal floor. This type of closure, which is an integral part of my technique for cleft lip repair, not only allows for construction of the nasal floor but also stimulates approximation of the maxillary segments and alveolar ridges and determines the proper alignment of those structures (Figs. 40-9 and 40-10).

Positioning the Nasal Ala. The next step of primary lip repair is the positioning of the nasal ala symmetric to the ala on the opposite side, stabilizing it in this position using deep catgut sutures, and closing the skin with 6–0 nylon. Whenever possible, the nasal sill is recon-

structed; however, this cannot be done successfully in all complete clefts. When the suturing reaches the level of the alar base, the deep suture inserted not only approximates the alar base medially and symmetric to the other side but also is used to straighten the columella. As mentioned earlier, I do not attempt to reposition or reshape the lower lateral cartilage in this operation because I prefer to leave the cartilage untouched, without scars around it, and to correct the remaining nasal deformity when the patient is older.

Before closing the cleft of the lip, I insert one 6–0 nylon suture in the vermilion-cutaneous border. This suture is tied and used to pull both lip segments downward to achieve perfect alignment of the tri-

angular flap within the gap made on the noncleft side. The next two sutures are inserted through skin and muscle, one through the tip of the triangular flap to the tip of the gap in which the flap is inserted, and the second from the corner above the triangular flap to the tip of the flap from the noncleft side. All the remaining sutures through skin and mucosa are mattress sutures of 6–0 nylon.

When skin-muscle closure is completed, I suture the mucosal layer using 4–0 chromic catgut, suturing mucosa and muscle together. By using this type of closure, I avoid separate sutures on the muscle layer; however, I make sure that approximation of the muscle is complete because I insert the sutures through the muscle on both sides of the lip, through

Fig. 40-11A, B. Narrow unilateral cleft lip, alveolus, and palate. Triangular flap technique was used for lip and nose repair. Note symmetry of the cupid's bow. The left nostril is larger than the right. An additional corrective procedure may be needed to narrow the nostril.

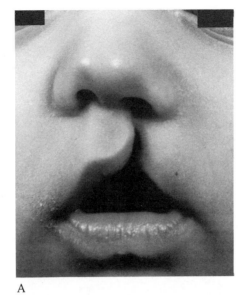

A

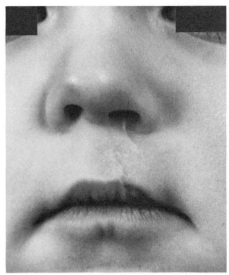

B

Fig. 40-12A. Unilateral cleft lip, alveolus, and palate with a Simonard band. Note malpositioning of the larger maxillary segment and severe nasal deformity. B. After one-stage cleft lip repair using triangular flap technique. The lip and nose were corrected simultaneously. Note symmetry of the cupid's bow and of the lip segments. C. Note horizontal orientation of the left nostril. Additional correction of the nasal deformity is indicated.

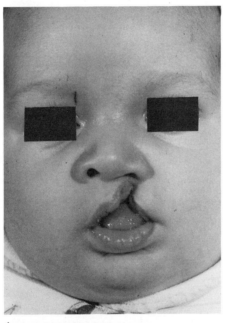

A

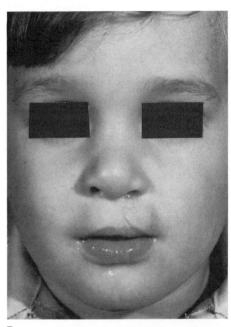

B

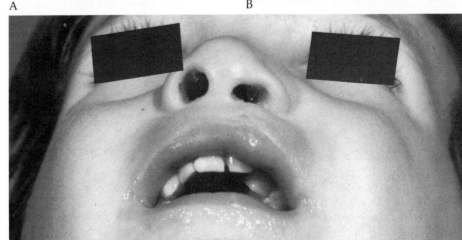

C

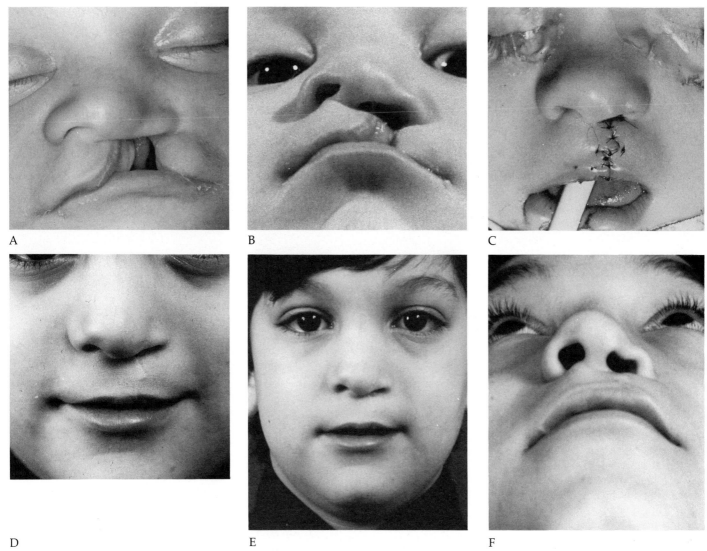

A   B   C

D   E   F

Fig. 40-13A, B. Wide unilateral cleft lip, alveolus, and palate with severe nasal deformity and malpositioning of the lesser maxillary segment. C. Triangular flap technique was used for lip and nose repair. D, E, F. Six years postoperatively. No more corrections were performed. Note symmetry of the vermilion, shape of the cupid's bow, and symmetry of the lip segments. The nose on the left side is distorted, and rhinoplasty for cleft nose is required.

the skin and through the mucosal layers. When closing the mucosal layer, one must be sure to use the same design used for the triangular flap, which includes skin and muscle. Closing the mucosal layer in a straight line may contribute to postoperative vertical scar contracture, which necessitates a corrective operation (Figs. 40-11 and 40-12).

Adjustment of the Vermilion. The last step in lip reconstruction is adjustment of the vermilion, which is usually most trying for inexperienced surgeons. To facilitate adjustment of the vermilion, ex-

cessive vermilion is left on both sides of the cleft. At this point it is important to make sure that the fullness of the vermilion is even on both sides, and to obtain this it may be necessary to reduce some of the excessive vermilion on one side or the other or to interdigitate a vermilion flap. Special attention must be paid to forming a symmetric vermilion in both segments of the lip. Sometimes there is a marked discrepancy between fullness of the vermilion in the two lip segments, vermilion in the lesser segment being hypoplastic, which suggests the use of vermilion from the larger portion to achieve

equilibrium and symmetry of the entire lip (Fig. 40-13).

Summary of Triangular Flap Technique

The triangular flap technique with the modification described in this chapter has many advantages, the most important being the precise preoperative measurements it allows, which determine the design of the triangular flap and other incisions; the simplicity of this operation and of adjusting the details when it is performed; the prevention of postoperative vertical scar contracture; and the decrease

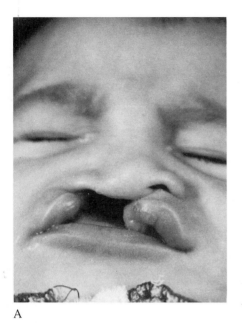

A

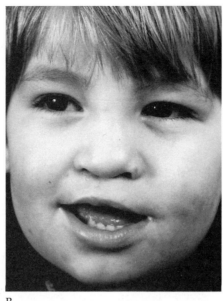

B

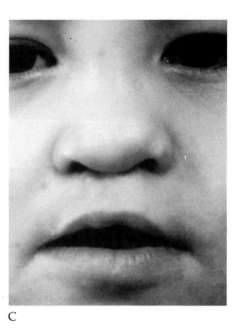

C

Fig. 40-14. *Extremely wide unilateral cleft lip repair with extremely severe nasal deformity. A. Before the operation. B, C. Four years after single operation in which single triangular flap technique was used for the lip-nose repair. Note symmetry of the vermilion, cupid's bow, and lip. There is also symmetry of the nasal ala; however, correction of the existing nasal deformity will be considered in the future.*

in the negative effect of postoperative lip pressure, which results from distribution of the tension of the repaired lip along the suture line. The disadvantages of the triangular flap technique include intraoperative adjustment to achieve a symmetric vermilion and violation of the philtral column. Adjustment of the vermilion is intrinsic to any surgical technique, and thus it cannot be considered a disadvantage specific to the triangular flap technique. Violation of the philtral column is specific to the triangular flap technique, however, and cannot be avoided. However, the zigzag scar is often less noticeable when the remaining lip elements are symmetric and well balanced (Figs. 40-14 and 40-15).

Influence of Cleft Lip Repair on Maxillofacial Growth

Progress in the surgical and multidisciplinary treatment of unilateral complete cleft lip, alveolus, and palate has been accompanied by better understanding of the influence of lip repair on maxillofacial growth. From the late 1940s until the present, many surgeons and researchers have considered cleft palate the major cause of secondary maxillofacial deformities. The existing clinical and experimental data concerning the influence of repair of cleft palate on maxillofacial growth leave many unanswered questions. One of the most important questions is how the influence of repair of cleft palate can be isolated from the influence of lip repair and other surgical procedures performed on young children. Another question not answered is why cleft palate repair is considered the only factor leading to maxillary growth inhibition and cleft lip repair is not considered at all, despite the fact that lip repair is performed before cleft palate repair. Another concern that drew my attention to lip repair was the presence of maxillary growth retardation after operations on the lips of patients who never had a palate repair. Doubts and controversy surrounding the problem of cleft palate repair as the major factor in maxillary growth inhibition stimulated me to design and perform a large series of experimental studies in rabbits and beagles and a clinical study in children with complete unilateral cleft lip, alveolus, and palate. These studies allowed an assemblage of factual material, indicating the role and influence of cleft lip repair as a major factor in maxillofacial growth inhibition causing secondary maxillofacial deformities. I concluded that cleft lip repair and cleft palate repair must be considered the most important factors modulating maxillofacial growth. The realization that cleft lip repair is such an important factor influenced my approach and the principles guiding my surgical technique of lip repair.

Several clinical studies were also performed to evaluate the late results of multidisciplinary management of patients with complete unilateral cleft lip, alveolus, and palate. According to these studies, an average of approximately 1.8 surgical procedures are performed to achieve a highly satisfactory result in lip reconstruction. The corrective procedures were performed most commonly because of a notch in the vermilion, asymmetry of the vermilion, and nasolabial fistulas. The most common secondary deformities prove that adjustment of the vermilion and construction of a symmetric and well-balanced vermilion still present a problem. The number of patients with nasolabial fistulas reflects the impact of maxillary expansion as the primary cause of reappearing fistulas at the time of orthodontic treatment.

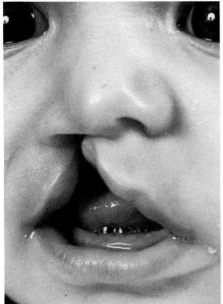

A

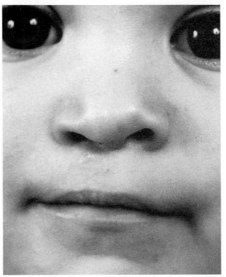

B

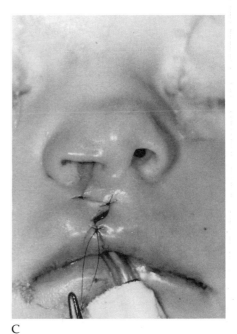

C

Fig. 40-15A. Unilateral cleft of the lip, alveolus, and palate on the right side. B. Design of the triangular flap. C. After insertion of the triangular flap and placement of key sutures. D, E. Three and one-half years postoperatively. No corrective procedures were performed. Note well-balanced and symmetric lip vermilion, well-defined cupid's bow, and minimal nasal deformity.

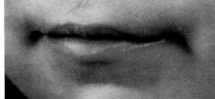

D

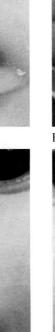

E

Suggested Reading

Anderl, H. Primary Unilateral Cleft Lip and Nose Reconstruction. In J. Bardach and H. Morris (Eds.), *Multidisciplinary Management of Cleft Lip and Palate*. Philadelphia: Saunders, 1990. Pp. 184–196.

Bardach, J., and Cutting, C. Anatomy of the Unilateral and Bilateral Cleft Lip and Nose. In J. Bardach and H. Morris (Eds.), *Multidisciplinary Management of Cleft Lip and Palate*. Philadelphia: Saunders, 1990. Pp. 150–158.

Bardach, J., and Kelly, K.M. The role of animal models in experimental studies of craniofacial growth following cleft lip and palate repair. *Cleft Palate J*. 25:103, 1988.

Bardach, J., and Salyer, K. *Surgical Techniques in Cleft Lip and Palate* (2nd ed.). St. Louis: Mosby–Year Book, 1991.

Fara, M. Anatomy of Unilateral and Bilateral Cleft Lip. In J. Bardach and H. Morris (Eds.), *Multidisciplinary Management of Cleft Lip and Palate*. Philadelphia: Saunders, 1990. Pp. 134–143.

Huddart, A.G. Presurgical Orthopedic Treatment in Unilateral Cleft and Palate. In J. Bardach and H. Morris (Eds.), *Multidisciplinary Management of Cleft Lip and Palate*. Philadelphia: Saunders, 1990. Pp. 574–578.

McComb, H. Primary Unilateral and Bilateral Cleft Lip Nose Reconstruction. In J. Bardach and H. Morris, *Multidisciplinary Management of Cleft Lip and Palate*. Philadelphia: Saunders, 1990. Pp. 197–203.

Millard, D.R., Jr. *Cleft Craft: The Evolution of Its Surgery*. Vol. I. *The Unilateral Deformity*. Boston: Little, Brown, 1976.

Randall, P. Lip Adhesion for Wide Unilateral and Bilateral Clefts of the Lip. In J. Bardach and H.L. Morris (Eds.), *Multidisciplinary Management of Cleft Lip and Palate*. Philadelphia: Saunders, 1990. Pp. 163–165.

Randall, P. Long-Term Results with the Triangular Flap Technique for Unilateral Cleft Lip Repair. In J. Bardach and H. Morris (Eds.), *Multidisciplinary Management of Cleft Lip and Palate*. Philadelphia: Saunders, 1990. Pp. 173–183.

Salyer, K. Primary correction of the unilateral cleft nose: A 15-year experience. *Plast. Reconstr. Surg*. 77:558, 1986.

Salyer, K.E. Unilateral Cleft Lip and Cleft Lip Nasal Reconstruction. In J. Bardach and H. Morris (Eds.), *Multidisciplinary Management of Cleft Lip and Palate*. Philadelphia: Saunders, 1990. Pp. 173–183.

Tennison, C.W. The repair of unilateral cleft lip by the stencil method. *Plast. Reconstr. Surg*. 9:115, 1952.

41

Bilateral Cleft Lip

M. Samuel Noordhoff

Anatomically and embryologically a bilateral cleft lip can be divided into right and left incomplete and complete clefts of the primary and secondary palates. There are many possible bilateral variations from occult to complete, and these variations are marked out on a modified striped Y using numbers that are easily computerized for classification. On careful examination and comparison of both sides, all bilateral clefts have an element of asymmetry. It is important to recognize these variations and record them so that an evaluation of the postoperative result is possible.

General Management

The initial lip repair is usually done when the patient is 3 months of age, provided the baby is gaining weight and is in good physical condition. An adhesion cheiloplasty is occasionally indicated when one side of the cleft is complete and much more deficient in available tissue for repair than is the incomplete opposite side. Most commonly, both sides are operated on at the same time, facilitating a symmetric repair. The palate is operated on when the patient is 1 to $1\frac{1}{2}$ years of age.

The columella is elongated when the child is one year of age or at the age of 4 to 5 years, when better cooperation from the child is possible for adequate postoperative care and follow-up study. The alveolar clefts are grafted with cancellous bone when the patient is 8 to 11 years of age; the timing is determined by the orthodontist before eruption of the permanent canine teeth. Routine speech evaluation is started when the child is $2\frac{1}{2}$ years of age and is continued at 6-month intervals until normal speech is achieved.

Management of the Premaxilla and Prolabium

The patient is seen as soon as possible after birth. Baseline studies are made by the orthodontist, and the baby is fitted with an orthodontic plate to prevent maxillary collapse. Rarely, an active expansion of the maxillary halves is indicated. The use of the passive orthodontic plate along with gentle traction on the premaxilla results in a better positioning of the premaxilla relative to the maxilla, allowing for an easier repair of the lip.

Gentle traction is placed on the premaxilla by using micropore tape across the prolabium attached to orthodontic rubber bands taped to microporous tape on the cheeks. This results in better positioning of the premaxilla and a stretching of the prolabial skin for easier lip repair.

The prolabium varies considerably in size and is always used in reconstruction of the lip, regardless of severity of deficiencies. The premaxilla varies in size and in the extent of protrusion in relation to the maxilla. Deficiencies in the central developing structures—the nasal and vomer bones, the septal cartilage, the columella, the prolabium, and the premaxilla—occur in bilateral clefts as in unilateral clefts. When severe, these deficiencies are categorized as median facial dysplasia. These types of clefts are the most severe and have the poorest results. An example is shown in Figure 41-1.

General Surgical Principles

Minimal dissection is done over the maxilla. All operative incision lines are closed to minimize scarring. The lip should be adequately reconstructed in the primary

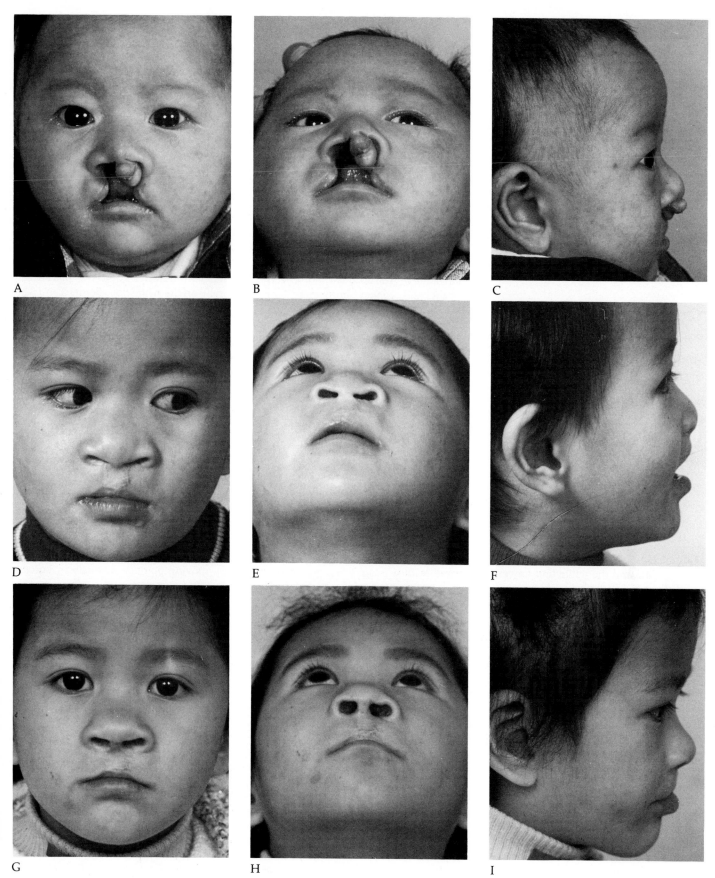

Fig. 41-1A, B, C. Preoperative views at the age of 3 months. Median facial dysgenesis with poorly developed small premaxilla and prolabium. A bilateral cheiloplasty was done at 3 months. D, E, F. Post-operative views at the age of 4 years, when an elongation of the columella was done using the Cronin technique with a dorsal cartilage strut from the ear. G, H, I. Postoperative views one year after elongation of the columella.

repair with minimal need for minor revisions. Muscle continuity is restored unless there is excess tension. All possible excess tissue is banked in the nasal floor. The columella frequently requires elongation at a later date.

For some incomplete bilateral clefts, the rotation advancement principle of repair is used, particularly when there is good muscle penetration into the prolabium from either side. The type of cheiloplasty described is particularly suitable for complete bilateral clefts and is readily modified for all other types of bilateral cleft lips.

Operative Technique

Operative Markings and Evaluation of Lip Pathology

It is important to identify anatomic references for determining incision lines (Fig. 41-2A). The white and dark (red) lines in the figure refer to the lines of the cutaneovermilion and vermilion-mucosal junctions. The red line is always present on both prolabium and lateral lip and is readily seen and marked out with a marking pencil at the time of the operation (Figs. 41-3C and 41-4C).

Lateral Lip

The red line and the white line converge medially at the cleft edge as shown on the patient in Figure 41-4C. Point 2' eventually becomes the base of the future philtral column and is placed on the white line

where the vermilion is the widest. This is also the point at which the red line and the white line start to converge. The most common vermilion width at the base of point 2' is 3 to 4 mm.

The vertical lip length is measured from point 2' to the alar base. The horizontal lip length is measured from point 2' to the commissure. The vermilion, muscle, and mucosa medial to point 2' are used to reconstruct a new cupid's bow, filling out the central part of the lip beneath the prolabium. Moving point 2' medially gives less vermilion and muscle for reconstruction of the central lip and a shorter vertical height and longer horizontal length. Moving point 2' laterally has the opposite effect. There must be enough vermilion, muscle, and mucosa medial to point 2' on the lateral lip to give a full lip under the prolabium and to give parallel red and white lines with a full vermilion in the central part of the lip. If point 2' is too far toward the median, a central peaking effect of the vermilion will result (see Fig. 41-2J).

Prolabial Markings

The red line is marked and the width of vermilion on the prolabium is compared with the width of vermilion at the base of the philtral column (point 2') on the lateral lip. Usually the central prolabial vermilion is only 1 to 2 mm wide, as compared with a 3- to 4-mm width of vermilion at point 2' on the lateral lip. This discrepancy is readily apparent in Figure 41-4C. Whenever the prolabial vermilion is deficient and the prolabial white skin

line is indistinct, a new cupid's bow is constructed (see Figs. 41-2G, H and 41-4). Whenever the central prolabial vermilion is as wide as the lateral vermilion at the base of the philtral column on the lateral lip at point 2', and the prolabial white line is distinct, the prolabial vermilion is left attached to the prolabium and the prolabial vermilion and white skin roll are used for the cupid's bow. An example of this situation is shown in Figures 41-2K and 41-3.

The vertical limb point 3 to point 2 extends from just inside the base of the columella inferiorly. Point 1 is placed centrally on the white line. Points 2 and 3 are placed so that they are about 2 mm higher than point 1 for a new cupid's bow. This results in a prolabium about 5 mm wide and 5 to 9 mm long. The ideal width of the cupid's bow should be determined by racial characteristics and availability of tissue. The cupid's bow should rarely exceed 6 mm in width. A width less than 4 to 5 mm makes the tissue difficult to handle and the face unattractive.

Evaluation of Measurements

The prolabial length of limb point 3 to point 2 is compared with the vertical length of the lateral lip. As a general principle, lateral lip vertical height must match the central prolabial vertical length. Minor adjustments can be made by moving point 2' medially or laterally to achieve lip symmetry. Major changes in lip shortening are made during the surgical procedure after muscle reconstruction (see Fig. 41-2H).

Fig. 41-2. Bilateral cheiloplasty. A. P is the prolabium and PF the prolabial forked flaps. The white line is the cutaneovermilion junction line, and the dark line is the red line of the vermilion-mucosal junction. RV,LV is the vertical lip length as measured from the base of the philtral column on the lateral lip where the vermilion first becomes widest. RH,LH is the horizontal length of the lip as measured from the base of the philtral column to the commissure. The length from points 2 to 3 on the prolabium is transferred to the lateral lip as points 2' to 3' and used as a guideline for lateral lip length. B. L is a mucosal flap elevated from the lateral lip, and T is an inferior turbinate flap based on vestibular skin. Two marking dots are placed on the margin of the intercartilaginous incision to identify the extent of superior rotation of the lower lateral cartilage, shown in D. C. The prolabial incisions are made, freeing the prolabium (P) and its forked flaps (PF). The orbicularis marginalis (OM) flap of white line, vermilion, and mucosa is incised on the right side. The orbicularis peripheralis (OP) muscle is dissected free from skin at a point *from the base of the philtral column to the alar base as shown on the left side. The T and L flaps are elevated based on vestibular skin. D. The lower lateral cartilage (LLC) is elevated by a traction suture in the dome and repositioned in its superior position, held by an intercartilaginous suture at its base to the upper lateral cartilage. The inferior turbinate flap (T) and the mucosal flap (L) resurface the vestibular area. The insert shows an alternative method of support. The LLC is sutured to the upper lateral cartilage and suspension suture is placed at the end of the procedure through the skin tied over a bolus of cotton or gauze. E. The left side shows the L flap attached to the alveolus and folded on itself to be attached to the premaxillary mucosa and periosteum as shown on the completed right side. The floor of the nostril is thus reconstructed, and the pyriform area is completely closed with inferior turbinate and mucosal flaps. F. Another view shows the mucosal flap (L) folded on itself, bridging the alveolar gap for reconstruction of the floor of the nostril. The flap is sutured behind the columella and to the periosteum of the premaxilla.*

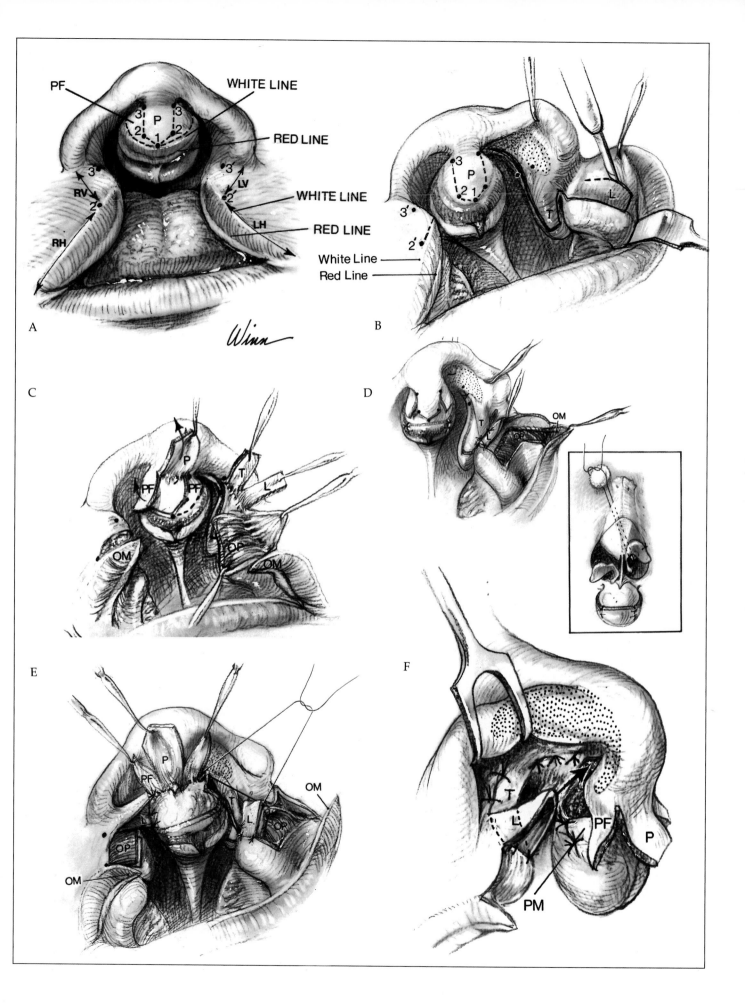

A

B

C

D

E

F

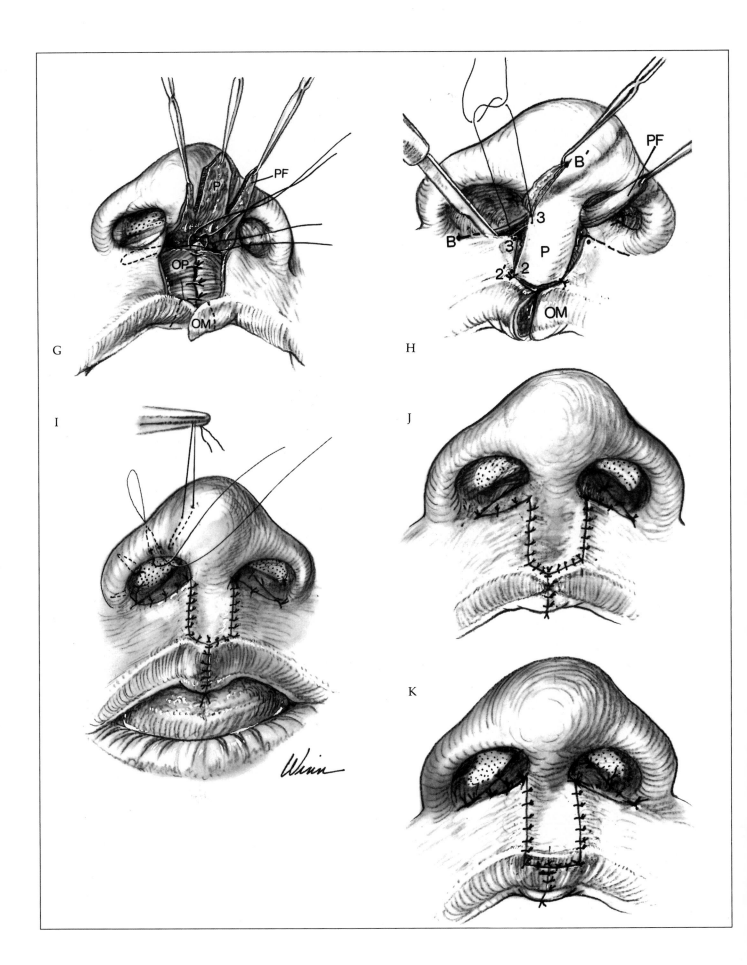

G

H

I

J

K

Fig. 41-2. (Continued) G. The orbicularis peripheralis (OP) is reconstructed in front of the premaxilla and attached to the nasal spine. H. Points 2 and 2' are approximated, and the lateral lip length 2' to 3' is adjusted to that of the prolabial length, point 2 to point 3. The tip (B') of the prolabial forked flap (PF) is inserted to point B. The OM flaps are trimmed to fit beneath the prolabium to reconstruct a new cupid's bow. I. All incision lines are closed with fine absorbable sutures. The LLC is held in position with a traction suture through its dome and leading edge. It is supported in its elevated position with several alar transfixion vestibular monofilament absorbable sutures; these sutures catch the caudal leading edge of the alar cartilage and transfix it to the alar groove as a subcuticular dermal suture tied on the inside of the nostril on the vestibular skin. J. An undesirable peaking effect of the red line occurs centrally when point 2', shown in A, is placed too far medially. K. When the prolabial white skin roll is prominent and its vermilion adequate, they are left attached to the prolabium. (Parts C, D, F, H, J from M.S. Noordhoff. Bilateral Cleft Lip Repair. In J. Bardach and H.L. Morris (Eds.), Multidisciplinary Management of Cleft Lip and Palate. Philadelphia: Saunders, 1990. Pp. 242–246. Reproduced with permission. Parts E and G, from M.S. Noordhoff. Bilateral cleft lip reconstruction. Plast. Reconstr. Surg. 78:45, 1986. Reproduced with permission.)

Anesthesia

Endotracheal anesthesia is carefully monitored with fixation of the endotracheal tube by a sponge moistened with normal saline solution that is packed into the pharynx. Normal saline solution with epinephrine 1:200,000 is used for infiltration into the lateral pyriform and maxillary margins. To prevent distortion of tissues, no other areas are infiltrated.

Incisions and Tissue Mobilization

Lateral Lip

A mucosal flap (L) 0.5 to 0.75 cm wide is elevated from the buccal alveolar sulcus (see Fig. 41-2B). One limb of the incision extends from the pyriform aperture down the inferior edge of the inferior turbinate process and across to the superior edge to dissect an inferior turbinate mucosal flap (T). Both the L and T mucosal flaps are attached to the vestibular skin. The incision extends as an intercartilaginous incision as far as necessary to allow upward mobilization of the lower lateral cartilage and lip. There is no dissection on the maxilla and no elevation of periosteum because freeing only the edge allows for adequate mobilization of tissues. Extensive dissection is unnecessary. After the lateral lip and ala are freed, a flap (OM) from the free edge of the lateral lip is incised for reconstruction of the cupid's

bow (see Fig. 41-2C, right side). This OM flap consists of a 1-mm edge of a white skin roll, vermilion, orbicularis marginalis muscle, and mucosa. A remaining 2- to 4-mm bridge of mucosa between the L flap and the OM incision is incised on the free edge of the lip allowing for dissection of the muscle. The orbicularis peripheralis muscle (OP) is dissected free from the skin in a subdermal plane from point 2' to the base of the ala, extending into the vestibular area of the nose. The orbicularis peripheralis muscle is now free to be mobilized for primary reconstruction of the muscle in front of the premaxilla.

Prolabial Dissection

It is imperative that accurate incisions be made on the prolabium. These incisions are best done by fixing and flattening the prolabium on the premaxilla with a fingertip. A No. 11 blade is laid on the full length of the limb of the incision, making an accurate straight incision. The lateral forked flaps (PF) (see Fig. 41-2C) are incised on the cutaneomucosal junction extending posteriorly on the premaxilla and superiorly posterior to the columella along the line of the cutaneomucosal junction. The prolabium (P) with attached PF is now freely movable for repositioning. The premaxilla is covered with the remaining prolabial mucosa (PM) for about two-thirds of its surface, which gives a buccal alveolar sulcus of adequate depth.

Reconstructive Phase

All incisions have been made and all parts are now ready to be reconstructed. There has been no dissection over the maxilla. In reconstruction the emphasis is on closing all operative areas to minimize scarring.

Alar Cartilage Repositioning and Vestibular Reconstruction

The alar cartilage and nose complex are elevated by a 4–0 nylon suture passed through the dome of the ala and returning near the edge of the alar rim to pull the alar cartilage cephalad (see Fig. 41-2D). This maneuver rotates the alar cartilage superiorly where it is held by an absorbable intercartilaginous suture between the lower lateral alar cartilage at its base near the inferior turbinate flap (T) and the upper lateral cartilage. It is important that no intercartilaginous sutures be placed in the dome area because they will pull the dome of the upper lateral cartilage down; it is normally elevated above the dorsum in this area. The inferior turbinate flap (T) is now rotated into the pyriform area. The donor area of the T flap heals rapidly and can barely be seen when healed. The T flap is sutured to the alveolus and maxilla.

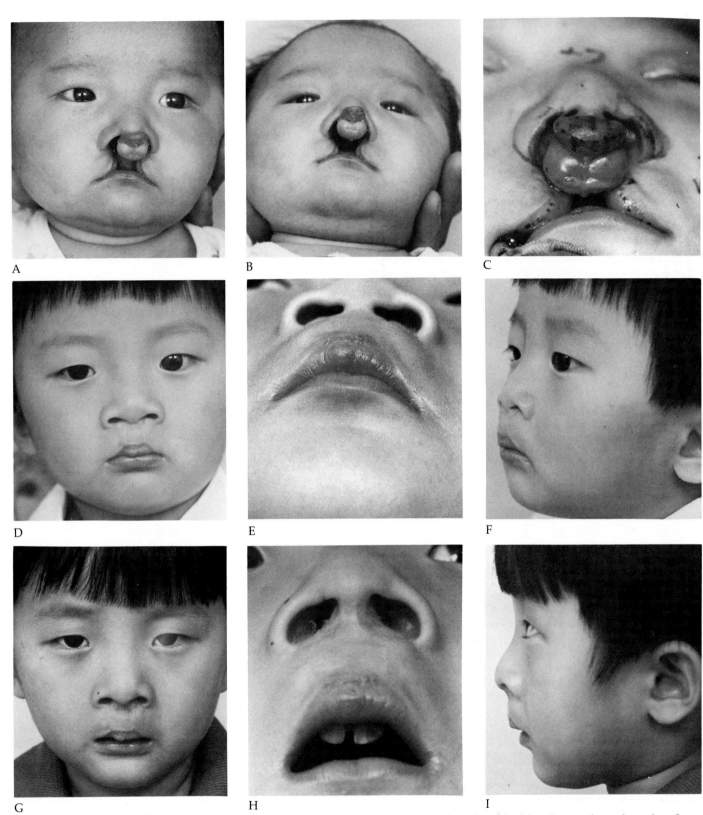

Fig. 41-3A, B. Preoperative views of a bilateral complete cleft of the primary and secondary palate. C. Intraoperative view. The marked-out vermilion mucosal red line with a very narrow lateral lip vermilion of only 2 mm. The lateral vermilion was the same width as the prolabium. A bilateral cheiloplasty was done when the patient was 3 months of age. D, E, F. Postoperative views at the age of 15 months. At the age of $1\frac{1}{2}$ years, a Cronin elongation of the columella with a dorsal cartilage strut from an ear was done. G, H, I. Postoperative views one year after elongation of the columella.

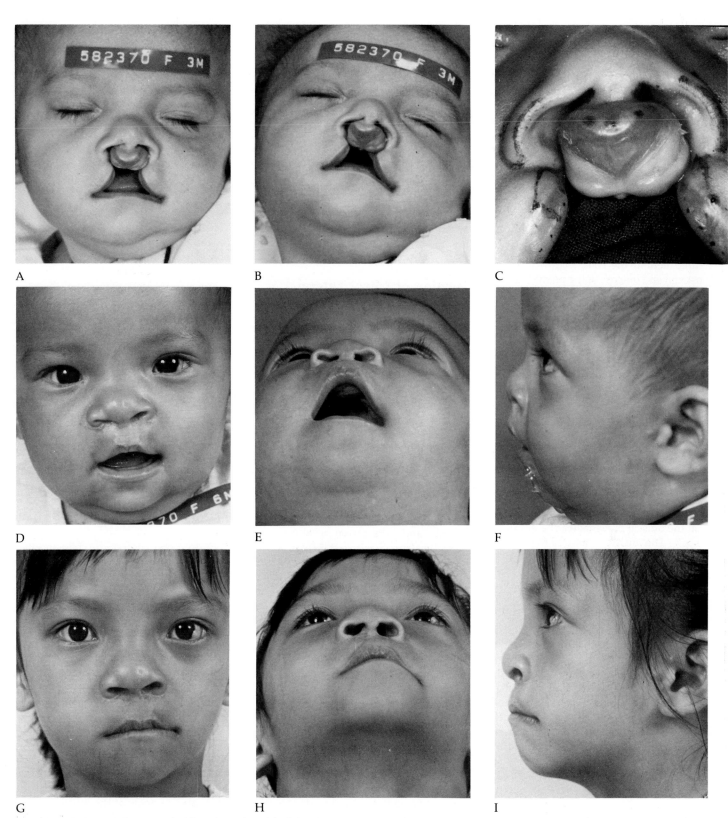

A

B

C

D

E

F

G

H

I

Fig. 41-4A, B. Preoperative views of a bilateral complete cleft of the primary palate. C. Operative markings for a new cupid's bow show the prolabial vermilion width of 1 mm and lateral lip vermilion width at the base of the philtral column of 4 mm. D, E, F. Postoperative views at the age of 5 months, before elongation of the columella. G, H, I. A forked flap elongation of the columella was done when the patient was 5 years of age. Postoperative result one year postoperatively when the patient was 6 years of age. There is an associated left lateral commissure cleft and associated hemifacial microsomia.

The edge of the L flap is also sutured to the alveolus. The remaining two edges of the T and L flaps are sutured to each other, thus effecting a complete mucosal closure of the vestibular area and maxilla to promote healing and to prevent scarring. The alar cartilage is additionally supported in its new position by alar transfixion subcuticular sutures placed at the completion of the procedure (see Fig. 41-2I).

Nasal Floor Reconstruction

The folded-over L flap (see Fig. 41-2E) now bridges the alveolar gap and is sutured behind the columella to the periosteum and mucosa of the premaxilla (see Fig. 41-2F). The tension of the flap is adjusted to reposition the premaxilla centrally. The flap provides for good reconstruction of the nostril floor and bridging of the alveolar gap.

Muscle Reconstruction

The OP with attached posterior mucosa is repositioned in front of the premaxilla with interrupted sutures (see Fig. 41-2G). These sutures must be placed so that points 2′ and 2′ are at the same horizontal level to give an equal, symmetric, balanced lip. It is helpful to place all sutures before tying them so that equal tension on the muscle prevents tearing of muscle fibers. The muscle is sutured to the nasal spine. If necessary, the muscle can be shortened on either side after it is matured to the nasal spine.

Cupid's Bow Reconstruction

Points 2 of the prolabial flap (P) are sutured to comparable points 2′ on the lateral lip with an interrupted subcuticular suture. The orbicularis marginalis flaps (OM) are trimmed to fit centrally beneath the prolabium (see Fig. 41-2H). A key central 7–0 absorbable suture is placed between point 1 on the prolabium and the trimmed OM flaps. A continuous 7–0 absorbable suture is placed between the white skin roll of the OM flap and the prolabium. Similar interrupted sutures are placed in the free edges of the OM flaps to complete wound closure. This procedure should result in a new cupid's bow with an adequate full central lip and parallel white and red lines (see Fig. 41-2I).

Lip Closure and Shortening

The vertical lip measurements made previously are now taken into consideration. If the lip needs to be shortened, it is done by balancing the distance between point 3 and point 2 on the prolabium with the lateral lip (see Fig. 41-2H). A horizontal incision at the appropriate point is made on the lateral skin so the lateral lip can be sutured to the prolabium without tension. The prolabial flap tip point B′ is sutured to point B in the floor of the nostril. All suture lines are closed with fine 7–0 absorbable sutures, which are left in unless there is skin irritation, a rare occurrence.

Fixation of Lower Lateral Alar Cartilage

The remaining 4–0 nylon sutures in the alar domes are placed under tension to hold the alar cartilages in their elevated position. A 4–0 clear absorbable monofilament suture is placed to support the alar cartilage (see Fig. 41-2I). A forceps is used for accurate placement of these sutures; the ala is grasped at the most anterior and inferior caudal edge of the lower lateral cartilage and the corresponding opposite skin surface. The suture is passed from the inside of the vestibule at the edge of cartilage through the alar skin. It is subsequently passed back, catching only the dermis, and exits in the vestibular skin near the alar rim, where it is tied. Two or three of these sutures are used to define the alar crease and to fix the alar cartilage. The sutures cause a dimpling of skin initially, but these dimples flatten out without scarring. Occasionally a suture reaction occurs, necessitating removal of the suture. This type of reaction is not common, and it is believed that these sutures contribute to a more permanent support of the ala than provided by bolster sutures, which usually need to be removed in 5 to 6 days.

Lip Symmetry

At the conclusion of the procedure, there should be a symmetry to the lip with a balanced cupid's bow and a full central lip beneath the prolabium. In addition, there should be a full vermilion of the lip at the base of the philtral column (points 2, 2′) and at the central part of the lip beneath point 1 on the prolabium. If these results are achieved, the red line will parallel the

white line, giving a pleasing lip contour (see Fig. 41-2I). Placing points 2′ too far medially (see Fig. 41-2A) leaves an inadequate vermilion centrally, the result being a peaking of the red line and inadequate vermilion in the central part of the cupid's bow (see Fig. 41-2J). The original prolabial white skin roll and vermilion are left on the prolabium as depicted in Figure 41-2K and shown in the patient in Figure 41-3.

Postoperative Care

The fine 7–0 absorbable sutures are removed only if they cause a suture reaction. The wound is supported with microporous tape, which is changed whenever needed. Finger massage of the lip is started in several weeks and is continued until the wound matures. In addition to the suture support for the alar cartilage, a silicone stent (Koken Co., Ltd., Tokyo, Japan) is used postoperatively. Examples of this type of repair are shown in Figures 41-1 and 41-3 to 41-6. This procedure is equally suitable for the most severe type of bilateral cleft deformity (see Fig. 41-1).

Surgical Correction of Bilateral Cleft Nasal Deformity

Because cooperation of the child and parents is needed during the postoperative care when a nasal stent is used, longation of the columella is done when the patient is 1 year or 4 to 5 years of age. At the age of 4 to 5 years, the lower lateral cartilages are more mature and stronger, and they hold their position better.

If the alar cartilages are severely deficient and soft, an additional delay may be considered. Additional support of the alar base is obtained with subsequent alveolar bone grafting at the age of 8 to 11 years, before eruption of the permanent canines. Correction of the nasal deformity includes (1) repositioning of the lower lateral cartilages, (2) formation of a columella and an angle at the junction of the columella and the lip, (3) narrowing of the floor of the nostrils, (4) reorientation of the nostril from a horizontal to an oblique-vertical position, and (5) narrowing of the dome of the cartilage with a nasal tip projection. One of four surgical procedures

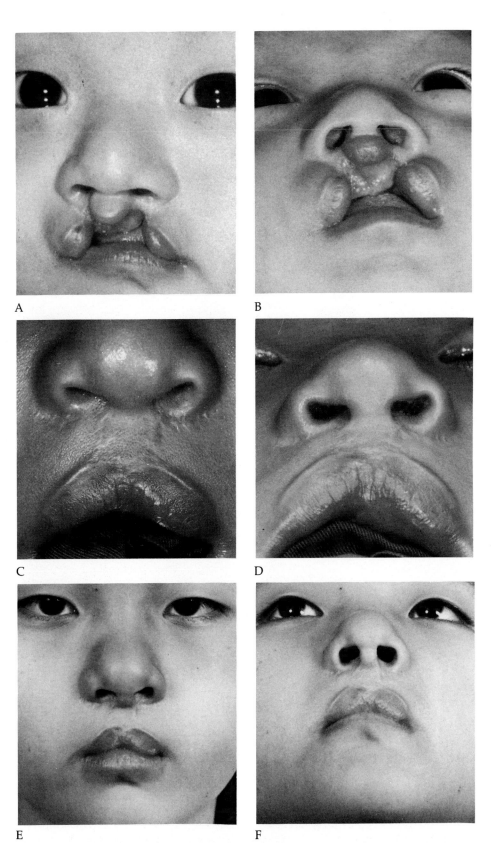

A

B

C

D

E

F

Fig. 41-5A, B. Preoperative views of a bilateral incomplete cleft of the lip. C, D. Postoperative views when the patient was 6½ years of age. Very short columella and small nostrils. An elongation of the columella with an earlobe composite graft was done at this time. E, F. Postoperative views 1½ years after the operation.

can be used in the surgical correction of a bilateral cleft nasal deformity—Cronin elongation, forked flaps from the nasal floor, composite earlobe grafts, or the open-tip approach. All the procedures have their advantages and disadvantages. It is helpful to be familiar with each technique and to choose the most appropriate procedure to correct each type of nasal tip problem encountered.

Elongation of the Columella (Cronin Method)

The incision extends from the short columella across the nasal floor to the ala (Fig. 41-7A). Enough subcutaneous tissue should be included with the skin to form a good columella with adequate bulk. The horizontal flap must be adequately released from the nasal floor and septum to allow for repositioning without tension. The lower lateral alar cartilage is freed from its attachments (see Fig. 41-7B). The lower lateral cartilage is supported with a dorsal cartilage strut taken from the ear or rib when indicated (see Fig. 41-7C) and with alar transfixion sutures (see Fig. 41-7D). The alar base is supported with a 4–0 absorbable suture to the nasal spine. Whenever there is marked narrowing of the alar base, the horizontal lip length must be shortened by removing a small Burow triangle of skin at the nasolabial line or in the vertical lip scar. The technique is most suitable with a wide ala and nostril floor, as shown in Figures 41-1 and 41-3.

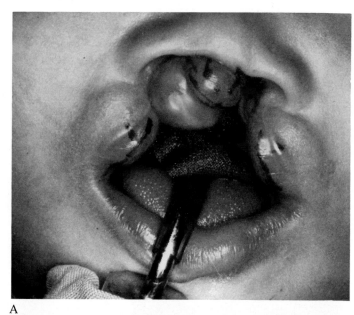

Fig. 41-6A. Bilateral complete cleft of primary and secondary palate with twisted small premaxilla. The vermilion mucosal line is marked by a dot on the white skin roll as the point of the base of the lateral philtral column. A bilateral cheiloplasty was done when the patient was 3 months of age. B, C. Postoperative views at the age of 4 years, 7 months, at which time an open-tip elongation of the columella was done. D. View 6 months postoperatively showing silicone nasal stent. E, F, G. Views 8 months postoperatively after use of the silicone stent was discontinued.

A

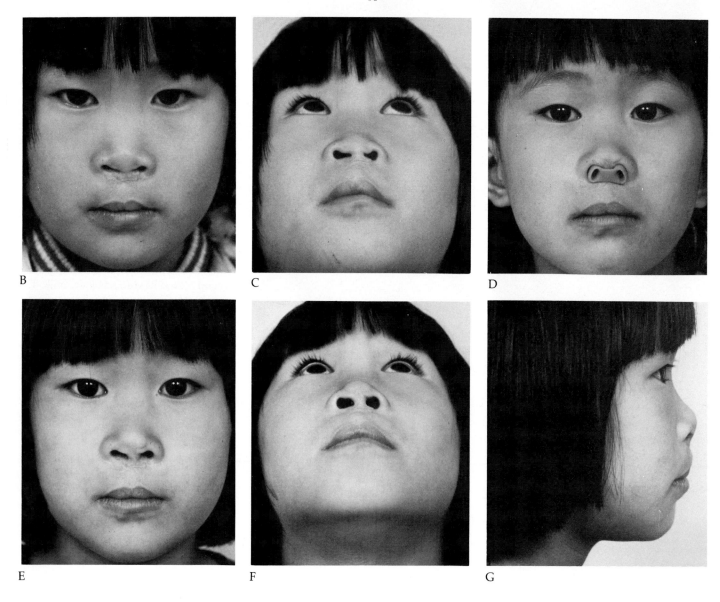

B

C

D

E

F

G

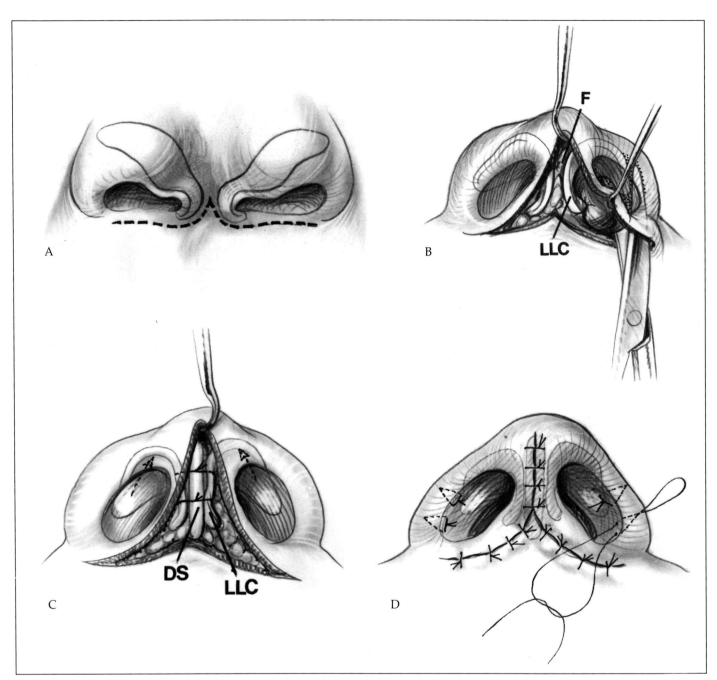

Fig. 41-7. Elongation of the columella (Cronin technique). A. The incision lines extend along the base of the nostril to the columella. It is important to leave intact all attachments of the lip to the nasal spine and premaxilla. B. The dissection of the lower lateral alar cartilage (LLC) must be sufficient to free it from its attachment to the skin, the upper lateral cartilage, and the rim of the maxilla to allow its rotation superiorly. The intercartilaginous fat and fibrous tissue (F) are excised. C. When the cartilage is soft, the lower lateral alar cartilage (LLC) is repositioned and supported with a dorsal cartilage strut (DS) to help support it. D. The LLC is suspended by a traction suture in its dome while alar transfixion sutures are placed to support the cartilage in its new position, similar to those described in Fig. 41-21.

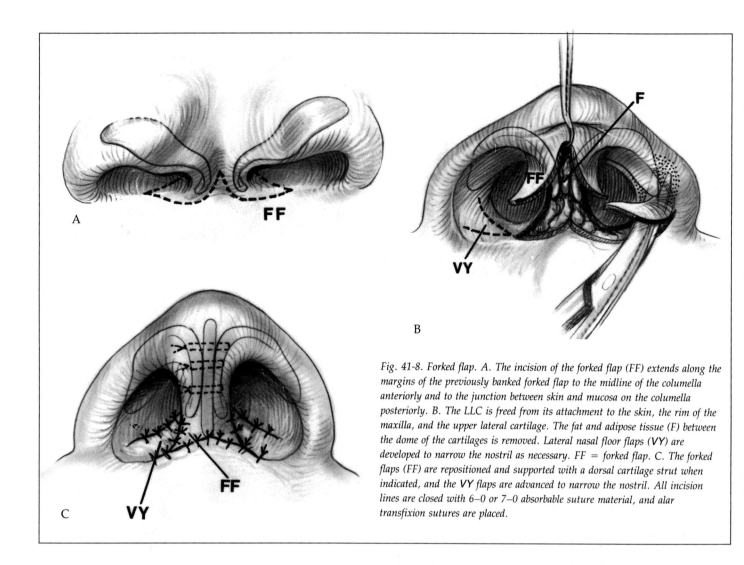

Fig. 41-8. Forked flap. A. The incision of the forked flap (FF) extends along the margins of the previously banked forked flap to the midline of the columella anteriorly and to the junction between skin and mucosa on the columella posteriorly. B. The LLC is freed from its attachment to the skin, the rim of the maxilla, and the upper lateral cartilage. The fat and adipose tissue (F) between the dome of the cartilages is removed. Lateral nasal floor flaps (VY) are developed to narrow the nostril as necessary. FF = forked flap. C. The forked flaps (FF) are repositioned and supported with a dorsal cartilage strut when indicated, and the VY flaps are advanced to narrow the nostril. All incision lines are closed with 6–0 or 7–0 absorbable suture material, and alar transfixion sutures are placed.

Forked Flap Method

Whenever the banked forked flap tissue from the prolabium is adequate and the alae are narrow, the forked flaps are elevated from the floor of the nostril for elongation of the columella (Fig. 41-8). The alar cartilages are freed from attachments to the upper lateral cartilage and pyriform area for adequate mobilization and repositioning. They are also supported in a similar manner with dorsal cartilage struts when indicated and with alar transfixion sutures. Whenever the prolabium is excessively wide and needs to be narrowed, the forked flaps are taken from the lip scar for elongation of the columella. Figure 41-4 is an example of a forked flap elongation of the columella.

Composite Earlobe Graft Technique

The composite earlobe graft technique is best suited when the nostril is small and there is little tissue in the nostril floor available for reconstruction (Fig. 41-9). Because of the necessity for a good take to the composite graft, there is less dissection of the alar cartilage. The repositioning of the lower lateral cartilages is done through an open-tip approach as a second procedure when necessary. Figure 41-5 is an example of the composite earlobe graft procedure.

Open-Tip Method

The open-tip technique is used when the alar base is well positioned (Fig. 41-10). The alar cartilages are released and re-

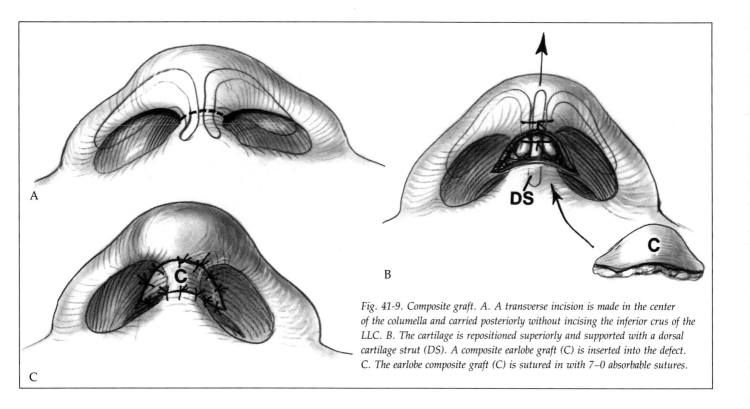

Fig. 41-9. Composite graft. A. A transverse incision is made in the center of the columella and carried posteriorly without incising the inferior crus of the LLC. B. The cartilage is repositioned superiorly and supported with a dorsal cartilage strut (DS). A composite earlobe graft (C) is inserted into the defect. C. The earlobe composite graft (C) is sutured in with 7–0 absorbable sutures.

positioned by direct visualization. There is some swelling of the nasal tip for a period of 6 months during the healing process and scar maturation. The open-tip technique is shown in Figure 41-6.

Postoperative and Follow-up Care

Regardless of the type of procedure, the use of alar transfixion sutures helps to hold the repositioned alar cartilages in their new position. The postoperative use of a silicone prosthesis during scar maturation is extremely beneficial (see Fig. 41-6D). The prosthesis should be used for a period of at least 6 months. Gentle wound massage of the nasal tip and scars also is advocated. Overall good results can be expected in most instances, but they require cooperation among the surgeon, the parents, and the child. The original pathology of the deformity needs to be taken into consideration when the end result is evaluated. A less than satisfactory result can be predicted when there are severe deficiencies of available tissues in the original cleft. Direct visualization of the lower lateral cartilage is helpful in securing an adequate release. This allows for better repositioning and fixation. The

nasal tip has a somewhat bulbous appearance during the time of scar maturation, a period of 6 months, particularly after the open-tip procedure. In all types of procedures for elongation of the columella and reconstruction of the nasal tip, the lower lateral cartilages are fixed to each other at the dome and held in this position by alar transfixion sutures (see Fig. 41-10D).

Suggested Reading

Bardach, J., and Morris, H.L. (Eds.). *Multidisciplinary Management of Cleft Lip and Palate.* Philadelphia: Saunders, 1990.

Bardach, J., Salyer, K., and Noordhoff, M.S. Bilateral Cleft Lip Repair. In J. Bardach and K. Salyer (Eds.), *Surgical Techniques in Cleft Lip and Palate.* Chicago: Mosby–Year Book, 1991. Pp. 113–172.

Cronin, T.D., and Upton, J. Lengthening the columella associated with bilateral cleft lip. *Ann. Plast. Surg.* 1:75, 1978.

Manchester, W.M. The repair of bilateral cleft lip and palate. *Br. J. Surg.* 52:878, 1965.

Manchester, W.M. The repair of double cleft lip as part of an integrated program. *Plast. Reconstr. Surg.* 45:207, 1970.

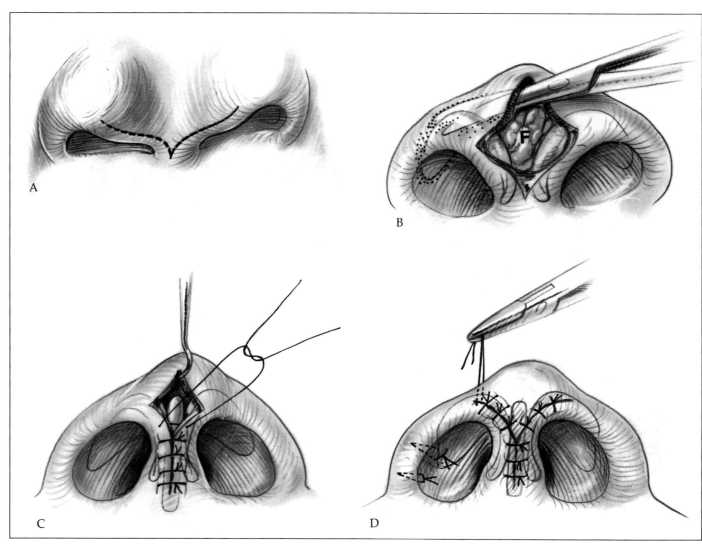

Fig. 41-10. Open tip. A. The incision for open-tip elongation of the columella starts in the midline of the columella and parallels the rim at a distance of one-half the normal width of the columella, about 2 to 3 mm. B. The skin is elevated from the dome and lateral crus of the lower lateral cartilage, freeing it from its fibrous attachment to the rim of the maxilla and the upper lateral cartilage. After the lower lateral cartilages are freed, the fibrofatty tissue (F) is removed to allow repositioning of the LLC. C. The domes of the LLC are rotated superiorly, where they are approximated and held with sutures incorporating a dorsal cartilage strut for support. D. Traction sutures in the domes of the LLC support the LLC in its elevated position while alar transfixion sutures are placed to give it support in its newly elevated position.

Matsuo, K., et al. Repair of cleft lip with non-surgical correction of nasal deformity in the early neonatal period. *Plast. Reconstr. Surg.* 83: 25, 1989.

Millard, D.R., Jr. *Cleft Craft: The Evolution of Its Surgery,* Vol. 2. Boston: Little, Brown, 1977.

Mulliken, J.B. Principles and techniques of bilateral complete cleft lip repair. *Plast. Reconstr. Surg.* 75:477, 1983.

Noordhoff, M.S. Reconstruction of vermilion in unilateral and bilateral cleft lips. *Plast. Reconstr. Surg.* 73:52, 1984.

Noordhoff, M.S. Bilateral Cleft Lip Repair. In J. Bardach and H.L. Morris (Eds.), *Multidisciplinary Management of Cleft Lip and Palate.* Philadelphia: Saunders, 1990. Pp. 242–246.

Noordhoff, M.S., and Cheng, W.S. Median facial dysgenesis in cleft lip and palate. *Ann. Plast. Surg.* 8:83, 1982.

Noordhoff, M.S., Huang, C.S., and Lo, L.J. Median facial dysplasia in unilateral and bilateral cleft lip and palate: A subgroup of median cerebrofacial malformations. *Plast. Reconstr. Surg.* 91:996, 1993.

Noordhoff, M.S., Huang, C.S., and Wu, J. Multidisciplinary Management of Cleft Lip and Palate in Taiwan. In J. Bardach and H.L. Morris (Eds.), *Multidisciplinary Management of Cleft Lip and Palate.* Philadelphia: Saunders, 1990. Pp. 18–26.

42

Primary Correction of the Nasal Deformity Associated with Cleft Lip

Kenneth E. Salyer

Unilateral Cleft Lip Nose

The nasal deformity associated with unilateral cleft lip includes disfigurement and displacement not only of the lower lateral cartilage on the cleft side but also of other elements of the nose—the nasal septum, the columella, the tip, the ala, and sometimes the entire nasal pyramid. An imbalance of the nasal structures results from malpositioning of the maxillary segments, especially the lesser segment on the cleft side. Both segments may be displaced in the frontal, sagittal, and vertical planes, making an asymmetric skeletal base for the nasal structures.

Hypoplasia of the lesser maxillary segment is another important factor that contributes to asymmetry of the skeletal base and nasal structures. Displacement of the maxillary segment on the noncleft side is usually overlooked as a major factor producing skeletal asymmetry. This displacement results from muscle imbalance and potentiates the discrepancy in alignment of the maxillary segments (Fig. 42-1).

Many surgical techniques proposed for correction of the unilateral cleft lip and nasal deformity fail because the procedures are designed to correct only one facet of this deformity without consideration of the complex morphologic and dynamic changes that occur during growth and development of a patient with a cleft. For example, when the lesser maxillary segment is collapsed, producing an imbalance of the nasal structures, correction of the nasal deformity cannot be achieved simply by repositioning the lower lateral cartilage. To achieve good results it is necessary to establish a symmetric skeletal base through orthognathic treatment and bone grafting. The characteristics associated with a unilateral cleft lip and the associated nasal deformity may include any or all of the following:

The columella is shorter on the cleft side.
The columella has an oblique position with its base deviated to the noncleft side.
The lateral crus of the lower lateral cartilage and the adherent skin are drawn into an S-shaped fold.

The lateral crus of the lower lateral cartilage is longer on the cleft side.
The lower lateral cartilage is displaced in the frontal and horizontal (backward and downward) planes.
The nasal tip is displaced in the frontal and horizontal planes following displacement of the lower lateral cartilage.
The tip of the nose is asymmetric.
The vestibular dome is excessively obtuse.
The ala is flattened, resulting in a horizontal orientation of the nostril.
The nostril is smaller or larger than the nostril on the opposite side.
The entire nostril is retropositioned.
The base of the ala is displaced laterally, posteriorly, inferiorly, or in a combination of these directions.
The nasal floor is absent.
The nasal floor is lower on the cleft side.
A nasolabial fistula is present.
The caudal edge of the nasal septum and the anterior nasal spine are deflected into a noncleft vestibule.
The nasal septum is deviated, resulting in varying degrees of nasal obstruction on the cleft side.

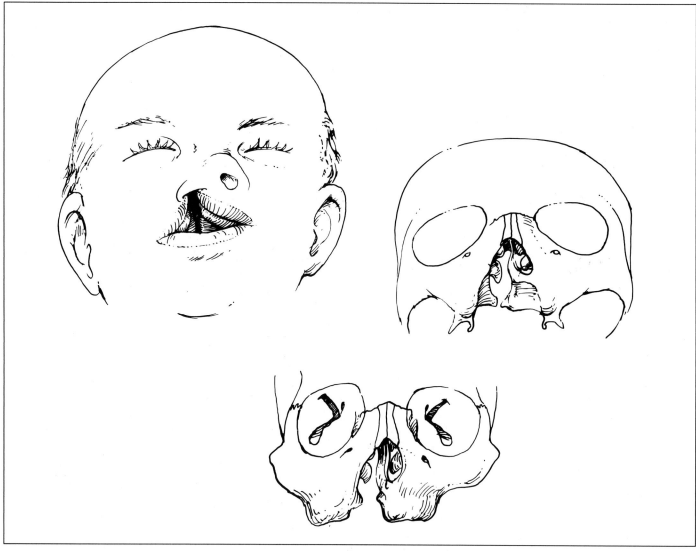

Fig. 42-1. Right unilateral complete cleft lip and cleft palate deformity with underlying skeletal imbalance.

The lower turbinate process on the cleft side is hypertrophic.

The nasal pyramid is asymmetric.

The maxilla is hypoplastic on the cleft side.

The maxillary segment is displaced on the cleft side.

The premaxilla and the maxillary segment are displaced on the noncleft side.

Primary Reconstruction of Unilateral Cleft Nose

The goals of repair of a primary cleft lip and nose are to construct a balanced and symmetric lip and a normal-looking nose. Sometimes these goals are difficult to achieve; we attain them, however, by continually modifying and improving our surgical treatments. Each patient's treatment is individualized. Technique is important, but surgical artistry and individualization are more important.

The nasal deformity associated with a complete unilateral cleft lip, alveolus, and palate involves various anatomic structures: the nasal ala, the alar base, the alar cartilage, the columella, the medial and lateral crura, the nasal dome, and the nasal septum. The position of the maxillary segments contributes greatly to the severity of the nasal deformity and the asymmetry. In a cleft nasal deformity, the lower lateral cartilage on the cleft side is displaced laterally and inferiorly. As a re-

sult, the alar dome is flat and turned downward. The ala on the cleft side also is flat and seems to be longer than the ala on the noncleft side. The floor of the nose is absent.

Correction of the nasal deformity at the time of primary cleft lip repair includes the following (Fig. 42-2):

1. Constructing the nasal floor
2. Providing symmetry to the nasal floor, ala, and dome on both sides
3. Providing symmetric projection of the nasal tip
4. Reshaping the lower lateral cartilage
5. Repositioning the lower lateral cartilage
6. Repositioning the alar base

7. Reshaping the nasal ala
8. Lengthening the columella on the cleft side
9. Straightening the columella
10. Achieving a nostril opening equivalent to the noncleft side
11. Removing nostril webbing from the cleft side

Procedures involving the lower lateral cartilage are beneficial when performed early and delicately. Dissection of the cartilages is performed carefully and without direct exposure of the cartilages. After dissection, the cartilages are shifted and reshaped to produce better projection and symmetry of the nasal tip and a normal contour to the ala. This dissection can best be performed at the primary operation without an external skin incision and without exposure of the alar cartilages. Freeing of the skin, cartilages, and lining with reshaping and repositioning are achieved without exposure. If total correction is not achieved, additional surgical treatment can be performed before the child enters school at the age of 5 years. Important steps for early reconstruction are:

1. Dissection of the lower lateral cartilages, the skin, and the mucosa
2. Shifting and repositioning of the lower lateral cartilages and redraping of the skin and mucosa
3. Construction of a symmetric alar base
4. Construction of a symmetric ala and nasal tip

After it is repositioned on the cleft side, the lower lateral cartilage is stabilized with through-and-through sutures to maintain the new alignment of the cartilage and the shape of the nasal tip and ala. This procedure is performed with Dacron polyester stents.

I am usually able to establish a satisfactory contour of the ala and a symmetric nasal tip. Sometimes, however, some secondary deformities remain that require correction at a later time. Correction of the primary nasal deformity is enhanced by the addition of vertical suspension sutures carried through the alar dome toward the glabella. A Dacron polyester stent is used inside and outside the nasal cavity to mold the desired shape of the nasal tip and ala. The stents, supported by the suspension sutures, facilitate con-struction of the desired shape of the tip and ala. The stents are removed one week postoperatively. Sometimes there is a slight relapse, but usually position and shape are retained.

Presurgical Orthopedic Treatment

I performed cleft reconstruction for 7 years without the use of presurgical orthopedic treatment. For the past 15 years, all my patients with complete unilateral cleft lip and palate have undergone passive presurgical orthopedic treatment as performed by Genecov. This adds an additional element of control and gives better results than are found in patients who have not had orthopedic treatment. The method is modified from that of Hotz.

Surgical Technique

The operation described is based on a modified Millard rotation-advancement technique. When the rotation-advancement procedure is used after rotation of the medial lip element, the C flap is used to lengthen the columella on the cleft side. Often the incision must be extended into the nasal mucosa, but not to the extent that the medial crus of the lower lateral cartilage is exposed. Through this incision dissection between the two medial crura is done with small, curved tenotomy dissection scissors. Dissection is carried over the alar dome, and the skin is undermined over both lower lateral cartilages in the area of the alar dome. The lower lateral cartilage is not exposed, and only the skin overlying it in the dome area is undermined. The attachment of the cartilage to the nasal mucosa in the dome area is maintained, allowing shifting of the entire lower lateral cartilage together with the attached nasal lining. Adjustments are made to position the lower lateral cartilage in symmetry with the normal side so that normal contour and projection of the nasal tip and ala may be established.

Laterally, access to the lower lateral cartilage is achieved through the incision at the alar base. The incision is made in the crease around the base of the ala, in anticipation of the medial shift of the alar base. An attempt is made to minimize this incision. At times it is necessary to carry the incision all the way around the alar base to achieve symmetry. Access to the nose is secondary. The suture line around the ala is hidden in the natural crease. The next incision is carried through the nasal mucosa, as a back-cut, separating the entire ala from its attachment to the maxilla. This incision is made just above the inferior turbinate process. Transection is carried to the nasal process of the maxilla and up into the nasal dome, allowing complete shifting of the nose to gain symmetry (Fig. 42-3A).

Total dissection of the alar base from the underlying bony structure facilitates the approach to the lateral crus of the lower lateral cartilage. Dissection of the orbicularis oris muscle from maxillary segments is performed in the plane above the periosteum, separating the muscular attachment so that it can be repositioned and sutured together with the muscle of the medial lip element. Undermining of the lip at this level does not impair facial growth and development, but it does facilitate reorientation of the orbicularis oris muscle and allows better cosmetic and functional results, eliminating an unnatural muscle bulge on the lip.

Wide dissection of the nasal ala from the bony structures does not have an adverse effect on facial growth. As indicated earlier, this incision is helpful for approaching the lateral crus and dissecting it from the skin, proceeding toward the dorsum and the alar dome, and joining the dissection of the lower lateral cartilage. In this manner, the lower lateral cartilage is freed entirely from the overlying skin. Because the attachment of the lower lateral cartilage to the nasal mucosa is preserved only at the dome level, the lateral and medial crura are totally separated from the skin and nasal mucosa and are easily shifted to the new position. The entire dissection of the lower lateral crus is performed without exposure. Exposure or cutting of cartilage in patients at this age greatly increases the potential for problems (see Fig. 42-3B and C).

Once it has been dissected and mobilized from the skin and nasal mucosa, the lower lateral cartilage is repositioned anteriorly and superiorly to match the position of the lower lateral cartilage on the noncleft side. Special attention is focused on constructing a nasal tip and ala, which are symmetric with respect to the opposite side. On the cleft side, total dissection of the lower lateral cartilage from the

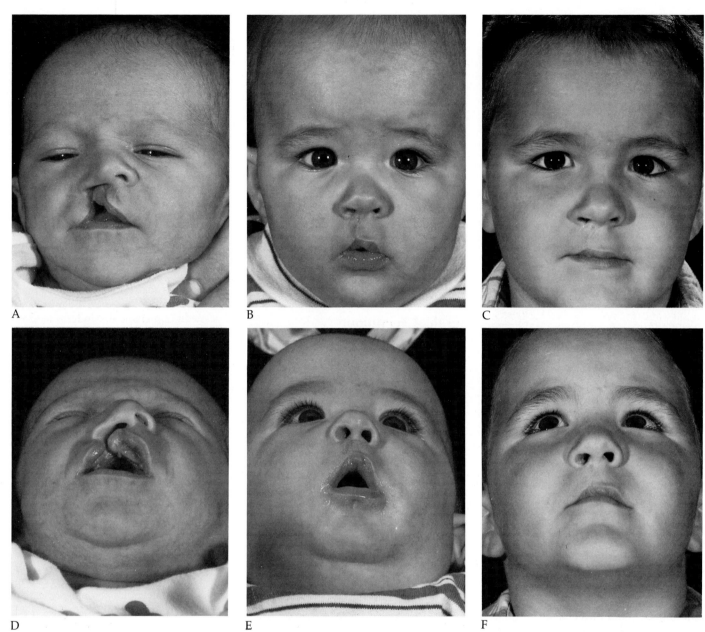

A

B

C

D

E

F

Fig. 42-2A. A 9-day-old infant with right unilateral complete cleft lip and cleft nasal deformity with associated complete cleft of the palate. B. Frontal view 3 months postoperatively. C. Frontal view after primary repair of cleft lip and cleft nose. The patient is 4 years of age. D. A preoperative submental vertex view when the patient is 9 days of age. Marked nasal base asymmetry; distortion of the alar cartilage, columella, nasal tip, and alveolar cleft; and lip incompetence. E. Submental vertex view at 5 months of age after reconstruction gave good symmetry to the nose and the lip with alar webbing on the cleft side. F. Submental vertex view of patient at 4 years of age with good balance and harmony to his lip and nose.

nasal mucosa allows the entire cartilage to be shifted. This maneuver results in a delicately curved dome and eliminates the flat, elongated shape of the lateral crus. When the alar base remains displaced after the entire lower lateral cartilage has shifted, additional dissection is performed. It is not necessary to use an L flap or to line the lateral incision. Once the displaced elements of the lip and nose are entirely freed and are mobile, the first stitch in the muscle of the lip sets up the balance for achieving correction of the nasal and lip deformities. If this stitch is not performed correctly, it is repeated until basic symmetry is achieved.

The repositioned lower lateral cartilage is stabilized with stent sutures through the skin, cartilage, and nasal mucosa. This maneuver produces a contoured shape of the ala, similar to that of the noncleft side. When the maneuvers described do not produce the desired effect, vertical suspension sutures can be used to augment the technique for early nasal reconstruction (see Fig. 42-3D and E).

The nasal floor and sill are built when a mucoperichondrial flap from the septum and a mucoperiosteal flap from the lateral nasal wall are sutured together to form the nasal floor. This procedure corrects and eliminates all nasolabial fistulas. I do not see nasolabial fistulas as a complication today. Once the floor of the nose has been constructed, the alar base is positioned so that it is symmetric with respect to the noncleft side. It is important not to overcorrect when trying to establish a curved shape of the ala. Overcorrection typically results in a nostril that is smaller than the one on the opposite side. It is much easier to decrease nostril size later than to increase it. Correction of a nostril that is too small is a most difficult, if not impossible, task (see Fig. 42-3F and G).

Associated Difficulties

The previously described procedures do not always adequately correct the nasal deformity. Typically the lower lateral cartilage is displaced laterally and inferiorly, the alar dome is flat, and the nostril retains a horizontal orientation.

Secondary correction is usually performed when the patient is 4 to 15 years of age. Correction of the nasal deformity during primary lip repair and any secondary operations should not be so ex-

tensive as to inhibit nasal growth. I have observed excessive scarring and severe secondary deformities in some patients referred to me after overly aggressive operations.

Optimal results for a severe nasal deformity may be achieved through direct exposure of the lower lateral cartilage. The cartilage is shifted, recontoured, and sutured to the cartilage on the noncleft side. The philosophy of the surgeon influences whether this procedure is attempted at the time of primary lip repair or as a secondary procedure. Direct exposure of the lower lateral cartilage also may be performed in infants, whose cartilages are pliable and adaptable. I do not recommend exposure of the lower lateral cartilage at the time of the primary operation.

Recontouring and reshaping of the lower lateral cartilage may be more difficult at older ages when the cartilage is firmer and less flexible. Furthermore, leaving the secondary deformity until the child is 8 to 12 years of age is undesirable, because the patient may experience psychological problems related to self-image. I try to achieve improvement at the time of primary lip repair, keeping in mind that some nasal asymmetry may persist. Results that appear satisfactory at the time of primary lip repair for the nasal deformity do not always continue to be satisfactory as the patient matures, and further surgical treatment may be suggested. The technique I describe here eliminates the severe deformity and leaves only minor deformities in most patients. The results achieved are uniformly good and satisfying. The secondary correction necessary to achieve an attractive face is much less complicated (Figs. 42-4 and 42-5).

Bilateral Cleft Lip Nose

With bilateral cleft lip and palate, the severity of the nasal deformity is proportional to the severity of the bilateral cleft. The more extensive the cleft and the greater the protrusion of the premaxilla, the more severe is the nasal deformity. The nasal deformity is especially severe when there is extensive clefting, severe protrusion, and deviation of the premaxilla to one side. When the prolabium is

small, lip repair may result in secondary nasal deformities caused by a tethering effect of the downward pull on the prolabium. Even with perfectly symmetric partial clefts of the lip with no initial nasal deformity, lip repair must be designed and executed to avoid interference with the normal shape of the nose.

The surgeon must distinguish between symmetric and asymmetric nasal deformities associated with bilateral cleft lip. The nasal deformity is usually symmetric in the incomplete bilateral cleft. The nasal deformity in complete bilateral clefts may be asymmetric because of rotation and deviation of the protruding premaxilla or because of the asymmetry of the cleft. An asymmetric cleft may be present in various forms and combinations, that is, with complete or incomplete cleft of the lip, with unilateral or bilateral cleft of the palate, and with complete or incomplete cleft of the alveolus on one or both sides. In all forms of asymmetric clefts, restoring symmetry of the nasal structures during primary cleft lip repair is important. I always attempt to minimize the primary nasal deformity to ensure continued balanced growth and development of the nasal structures and to provide better conditions for final cleft rhinoplasty.

The characteristics associated with bilateral cleft lip and the related nasal deformity may include any or all of the following:

1. The columella is short; sometimes it seems not to exist, and the prolabium seems to be attached to the nasal tip.
2. The nasal tip is flat and broad.
3. The nasal alae are flat and sometimes drawn in an S shape.
4. The bases of the alae are displaced laterally and sometimes inferiorly and posteriorly.
5. Both nostrils are horizontally oriented.
6. The lower lateral cartilages are severely deformed. The medial crura are short and widely separated at the nasal tip; the lateral crura are flat and elongated; and the dome is angled obtusely.
7. The nasal floor is absent.
8. The columella, caudal end of the septum, and anterior nasal spine are displaced inferiorly relative to the level of the alar bases.
9. The nasal tip and nostrils are asymmetric.

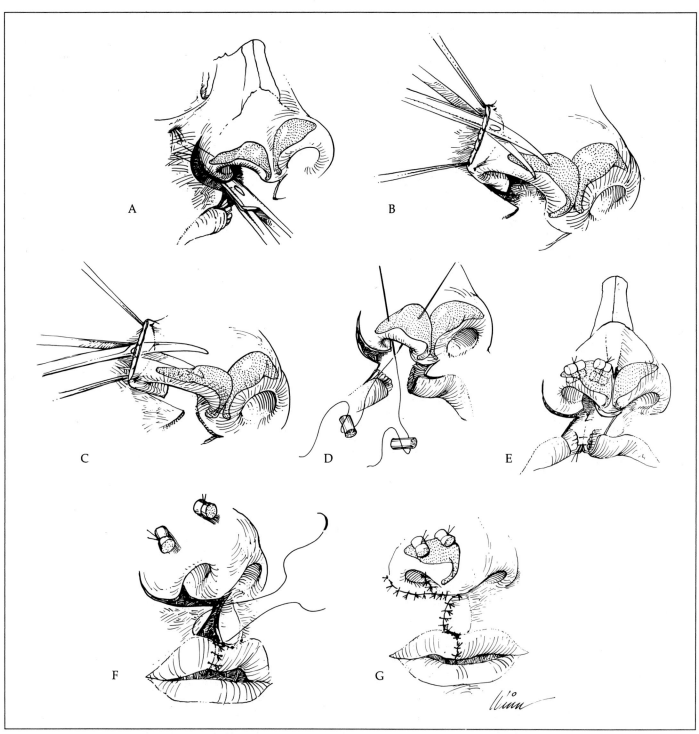

Fig. 42-3. Steps in nasal reconstruction of a unilateral cleft. A. The back-cut is performed just above the inferior turbinate process to separate all the nasal soft tissue from the underlying displaced maxillary segments. This allows reconstruction and repositioning of the nostril into normal relations. B. Dissection, using tenotomy scissors, from the lateral alar incision, separating the remaining portion of the skin envelope from the underlying alar cartilage on the cleft side. C. Dissection at a deeper level, separating the nasal lining from the overlying alar cartilage laterally. At the level of the dome and the genu, the lining is left attached. Although not shown in the illustrations, the muscle is dissected free and the orbicularis oris muscle is sutured. This makes the entire nose and lip symmetric. D. The Dacron polyester stent suture is placed through and through the three structures, readapting these; polypropylene suture is used over Dacron polyester stents placed on both sides of the nose— the lining side and the skin side. E. Early closure of the lip with the nasal alar stent sutured down, readapting and repositioning the underlying alar cartilage on the cleft side. The stents are left in place for one week postoperatively. F. Alignment and closure of the anatomic parts of the vermilion and lip, gaining symmetry, which contributes to the nose as well. G. Closure of the floor of the nose, erring on the side of leaving a slightly larger nostril on the cleft side. A small nostril is impossible to correct secondarily. The remaining portion of the skin of the nose and lip is closed, giving proper balance and symmetry to the cleft nasal deformity.

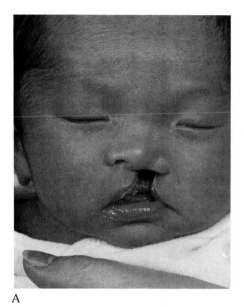
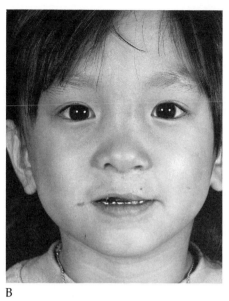
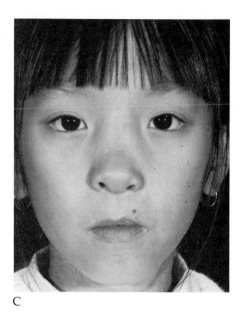

A   B   C

Fig. 42-4A. Preoperative left unilateral complete cleft lip and associated cleft palate in Asian girl. B. Frontal view at 4½ years of age (4 years and 2 months postoperatively). C. Results of primary repair. The patient is 9 years of age.

Fig. 42-5A. Preoperative frontal view at 6 weeks of age showing unilateral complete cleft of the lip with cleft nasal deformity and associated complete cleft palate. B. Patient 15 years of age after primary repair of the cleft lip and cleft nose.

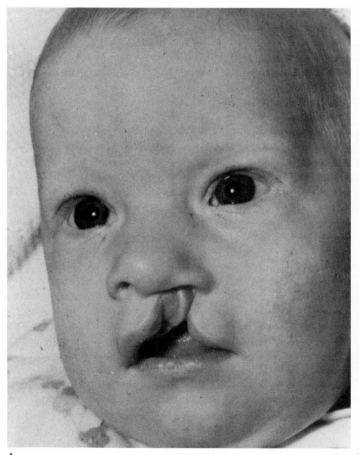
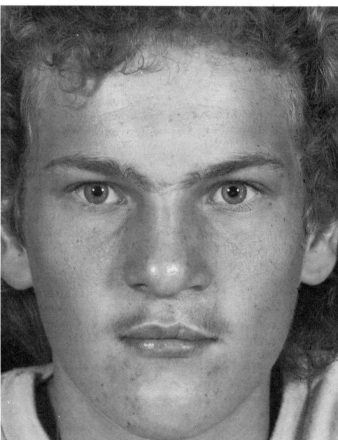

A   B

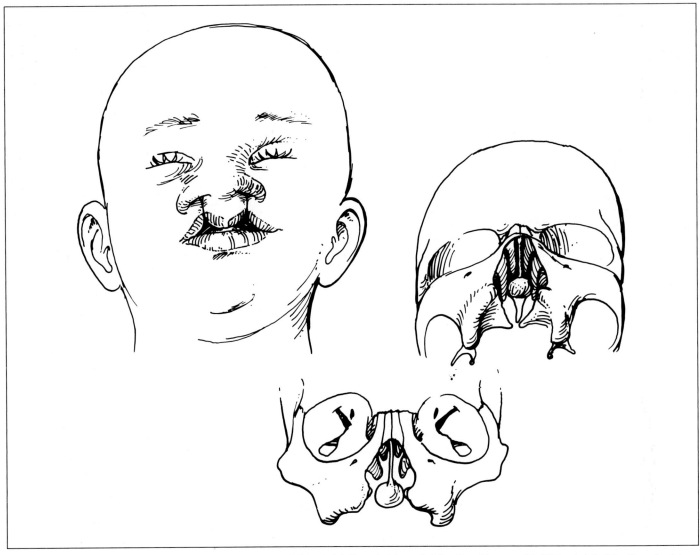

Fig. 42-6. Bilateral cleft lip and cleft nasal deformity with a complete bilateral cleft of the lip and palate. The underlying associated skeletal deformity is shown. A bilateral cleft deformity presents with a complex tissue deficiency, which prevents the surgeon from achieving the desired perfection and always leaves bilateral cleft stigmata.

The described deformities may be present before lip repair and may be found after lip reconstruction. Not all deformities are always present. The preoperative definition and symmetry of the nasal tip and nostrils can be destroyed by a poorly planned or poorly executed operation; however, everything cannot be blamed on poor planning. Even the best design and surgical performance may result in secondary nasal deformities. Correction of a symmetric nasal deformity is easier than correction of an asymmetric deformity (Fig. 42-6).

Presurgical Orthopedic Treatment

Presurgical orthopedic treatment is a matter of preference. Various techniques are used to expand the maxillary segments and to place the protruding premaxilla within the alveolar arch. The orthodontist with whom I work, Edward Genecov, D.D.S., starts presurgical orthopedic treatment as early as possible and uses maxillary segmental expansion when necessary before and after lip repair. Enough space must be made between the maxillary segments within the alveolar arch.

This space must be maintained postoperatively because the premaxilla will move posteriorly because of the pressure of the repaired lip. Lip pressure is the only force that moves the protruding premaxilla posteriorly until it achieves its proper position in the alveolar arch. No other pressure, extraoral or intraoral, is used to achieve alignment.

Most patients with complete bilateral cleft lip, alveolus, and palate are successfully operated on after passive presurgical orthopedic treatment. Active or forceful repositioning of the premaxilla and the maxillary segments may interfere in some manner with anteroposterior facial growth. I know of no studies indicating that treatment techniques based on active and forceful repositioning of the segments are beneficial to maxillofacial growth.

Primary Reconstruction of Bilateral Cleft Nose

Correction of the nasal deformity associated with bilateral cleft lip, alveolus, and palate is performed when the patient is 3 to 5 months of age. The second stage of nose repair is performed when the patient is approximately one year of age. During primary repair of a cleft lip, correction of the nasal deformity includes the following:

1. Reconstruction of the nasal floor and sill
2. Positioning of the alar bases in a symmetric manner
3. Positioning of the skin from the floor of the nose for reconstruction of the columella during final repair (Fig. 42-7)

When the premaxilla protrudes, the surgeon has to decide whether to repair the lip in one or two stages. If it is judged that one operation will pull the columella too much, resulting in excessive lip tension, two stages are used for lip repair. Even using this criterion, sometimes when one-stage lip repair is performed the nasal deformity may be more obvious. This is because of tethering of the nasal tip and wide displacement of the alar bases, which persist until the second stage of repair corrects the deformity at one year of age.

The lower lateral cartilages are restructured and reshaped without being dissected from the nasal lining. Early definition of the nasal tip is established, and the orientation of the nostrils is changed from horizontal to oblique. Accurate planning during primary lip-nose repair is important to achieve good results during the second stage.

Proper assessment before correction of the nasal deformity is essential because the amount of tissue in the nasal floor and the severity of the deformity determine the design of the procedure and its success. In secondary operations, older patients with a short prolabium and a tight lip may require an Abbe flap. This procedure is performed simultaneously with lengthening of the columella using residual prolabial tissue. When the columella is short, it must be lengthened before the lower lateral cartilages are restructured (Fig. 42-8).

During the primary operation the nasal floor is reconstructed, eliminating nasolabial fistulas. The skin flap from the floor of the nose on each side is elevated and sutured to the lateral alar bases so that the width of the floor of the nose is greater than needed when the final correction is performed. This step is a preparation for final correction, which is performed when the child is one year of age. The reason for operating when the child is one year of age is to release the tethered nasal tip and allow better growth and development of the nose. Lengthening of the columella also is beneficial for nasal growth. Repositioning the displaced anatomy with early reconstruction allows for more normal growth.

Stage-2 Nasal Reconstruction

The second operation is designed to rotate the lower lateral cartilages medially and cephalad. Because the cartilages remain attached to the underlying nasal mucosa, repositioning and contouring can be completed without dissection of the lateral crura. This operation, designed to correct the nasal deformity, includes the following:

1. Lengthening of the columella
2. Narrowing of the alar base
3. Projection of the nasal tip
4. Reshaping of the nostril

5. Improvement of the columella-lip angle

The following steps are included in the operation:

1. Lengthening of the columella using skin from the nasal floor.
2. Dissection of the lateral crura of the lower lateral cartilages from the skin and nasal lining. The lining remains attached to the lower lateral cartilages in the alar dome region.
3. Realignment of the lower lateral cartilages by lengthening of the medial crura and shortening of the lateral crura.
4. Transection of the lining between the septum and the columella to facilitate upward rotation of the medial crura and the columellar skin.
5. Transection of the skin and mucosa on the nasal floor to allow medial and superior rotation and lengthening of the columella.
6. Suturing together of the medial and lateral crura at the genu under direct vision and at the appropriate height to establish cartilaginous support for projection of a symmetric nasal tip.
7. Medial and upward rotation of the skin from the nasal floor to narrow the alar bases, which changes the shape of the nostrils from horizontal to oblique.
8. Reshaping and repositioning of the cartilages with stent sutures to maintain all elements in the desired position.

Correction of the nasal deformity is effective when all the steps are performed during the same operation. Correction is less than adequate in operations that lengthen the columella only. The described procedure does not require any cartilage implants or augmentation at a later time. This procedure differs from repair of a unilateral cleft lip and nose, in which cartilage augmentation may correct the existing asymmetry.

The operation described is based on a procedure originally outlined by Cronin, but it involves more than just lengthening of the columella. A key point to this procedure is the exposure achieved by extending the midline incision on the columella to the level of the nasal dome, allowing limited dissection and repositioning of the cartilages under direct vision.

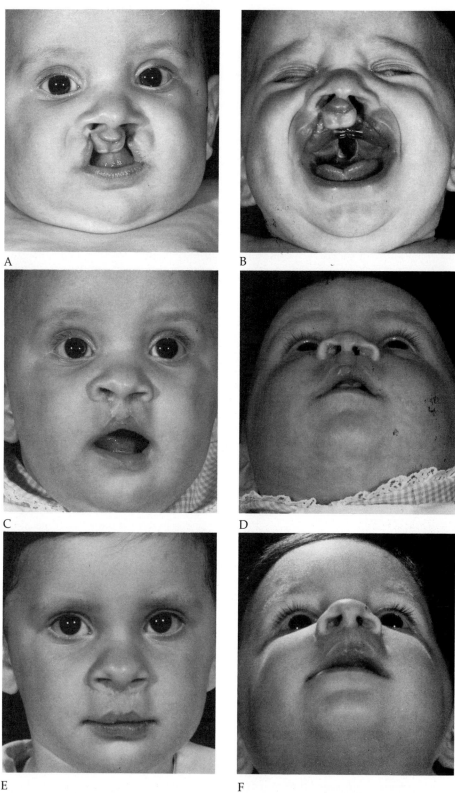

Fig. 42-7A. Preoperative frontal view of bilateral cleft lip and cleft nose in a child 3 months of age. B. Submental vertex view showing the passive orthodontic appliance in place allowing for adjustment of the maxilla after closure of the lip. C. The child is 5 months of age. Postoperative frontal view one month after repair. D. Submental vertex view showing the result after primary lip and primary nasal reconstruction. E. Frontal view after the second stage of reconstruction of the cleft nose. The child is 22 months of age. F. Submental vertex view after the second stage of reconstruction of the cleft nose.

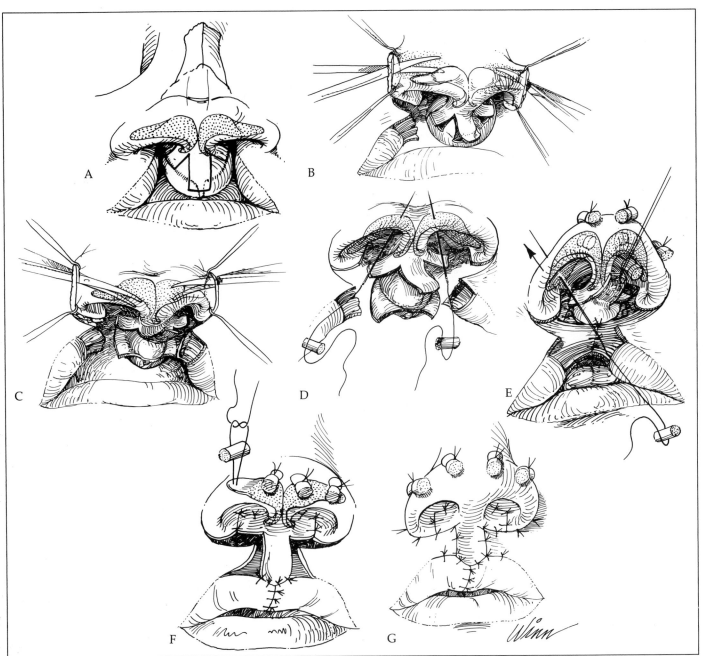

Fig. 42-8. Primary reconstruction of bilateral cleft lip and first stage of reconstruction of cleft nose. A. Depending on the degree of tissue deficiency, one determines the prolabial tissue to be used for the central portion of the lip. Frequently, if tension is present, the entire prolabium should be used. One need not worry about a definitive lip but should be concerned about minimizing tension and scarring and ending up with a long-term desirable result. The most important aspect of the design is to determine before the first operation the ultimate columella. This is done by using tissue of the floor of the nose, not the prolabium, in designing the ultimate procedure. B. Dissection using tenotomy scissors from the lateral alar incision, separating the remaining portion of the skin envelope from the underlying alar cartilage bilaterally on both sides. This is similar to the procedure performed for the unilateral cleft nose. This series of steps may be omitted and may be performed at the secondary procedure, depending on the deformity, the amount of nasal alar tissue, and the degree of tissue deficiency. C. The extension of the tenotomy scissors over the alar cartilage, freeing the skin envelope as needed. D. The insertion of needles attached to Dacron polyester stents with polypropylene suture used to reshape the displaced alar cartilages. E. Additional insertion of stents to reshape and reform the displaced and misshaped nasal elements. F. Final suturing of the floor of the nose to the alar bases is important in determining the ultimate columella. Although the nose is wide and flat at this point, preparation for the ultimate nose is important at the time of the primary procedure and cannot be overemphasized. The use of lateral vermilion flaps below the prolabium is probably the best method for reconstruction of the cupid's bow. There are times when the vermilion-cutaneous junction of the prolabium is maintained instead of the lateral vermilion flaps. G. The final closure of the lip and nose at stage 1. Depending on the degree of tissue deficiency in a bilateral complete cleft, it is anticipated that a second operation will be needed to move the tissue of the floor of the nose into the columellar region. At the same time, the necessary restructuring and repositioning of the alar cartilage is performed to provide early definitive delicate structures of the nose for optimal growth and development.

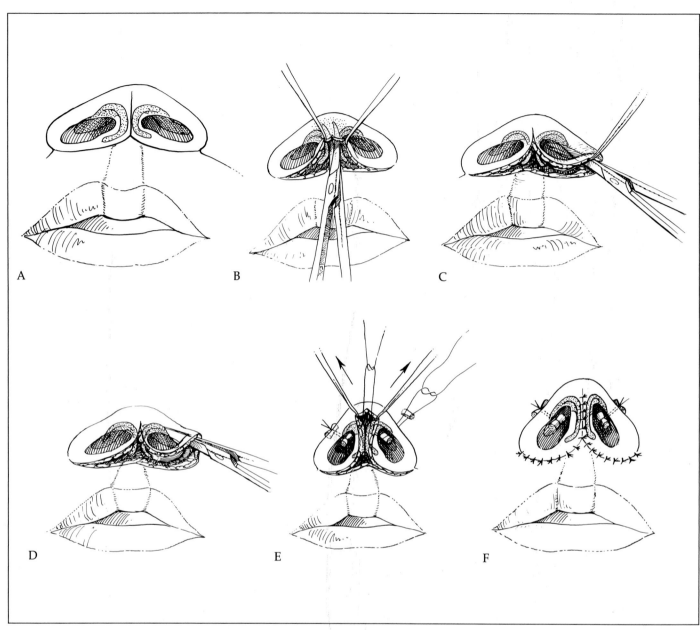

Fig. 42-9A. The initial incision is made at the base of the nose, transecting the nose from the upper lip. The incision is extended up the midline of the columella into the nasal dome. This method allows access to the lower lateral cartilage. Dissection is carried through this incision; an additional incision is made in the floor of the nose, high in the nasal mucosa, forming a bucket-handle flap. Dissection and release of the nasal mucosa are determined by the amount of rotation indicated for each patient. B. With small curved tenotomy scissors, the skin is freed from the medial crus and the nasal dome on both sides. The lower lateral cartilages are identified. The entire skin over the nasal dome and tip is dissected. C. The incision in the lateral alar base exposes the attachment of the soft tissue to the maxillary process for transection. The nasal lining is dissected from the lateral crus of the alar cartilage with tenotomy scissors up to the dome. D. The remaining skin envelope is freed from the underlying alar cartilage. E. The lower lateral cartilage on each side is mobilized, elevated, rotated, and sutured to the other side with 4–0 or 5–0 white braided nylon and using a PS-3 needle. The adjacent skin and alar dome complex with its attached lining is freed laterally so that they can be rotated into the new position, which allows lengthening and projection of the tip and redraping of the shifted underlying cartilaginous structure. Fixation of the skin, cartilage, and lining is secured with through-and-through tie-over stent sutures over Dacron polyester, as described for the unilateral repair. F. The repositioned lower lateral cartilages, fixed in position with closure of the skin, and advancement of the columella and projection of the nasal tip result from shifting of the lower lateral cartilages and suturing them together at the alar dome.

The operation starts with an injection of 1% lidocaine with 1:100,000 epinephrine to facilitate dissection of the lateral crura and eliminate bleeding during the procedure. The incision is carried along the base of the nose, extending down the midline of the columella, along the floor of the nose at the junction of the floor and lip, and around the alar bases along the alar crease. The incision goes through soft tissue, separating the lip and nose (Fig. 42-9A and B).

With the use of small tenotomy scissors, the lining of the floor of the nose is elevated laterally. With slightly larger scissors, the mucosa is transected high along the attachment to the pyriform aperture along the maxilla. The lateral crura are dissected from the skin and nasal mucosa with small tenotomy scissors lateral to the dome. This step is done under direct exposure of the cartilage and results in precise separation of the lateral crura from the skin and nasal mucosa, enabling repositioning and restructuring of the cartilage.

The nasal lining is transected on the floor of the nose, forming bilateral bucket-handle flaps, which allow rotation of the skin medially and superiorly to lengthen the columella. The internal incision on the nasal floor is extended medially so that the medial crura are separated from the membranous septum after transection of the nasal mucosa. Through the midline columellar incision that extends to the alar dome, the skin is dissected from the lower lateral cartilages at the dome area, with care to dissect the skin completely from the underlying cartilage. The nasal mucosa at the alar dome remains attached to the cartilage (see Fig. 42-9C to F).

Once this maneuver is done, white braided 4–0 or 5–0 nylon sutures are used to close the alar domes at the appropriate level and to achieve projection and elevation of the nasal tip. No attempt is made at this stage to resect or cut through the cartilage; the cartilages are shifted, repositioned, and restructured. When the columella is lengthened, a conservative length should be used to balance the size of the nose in anticipation of growth of the nasal structures. There is a tendency for surgeons to make too long a columella.

After the skin, cartilages, and nasal lining are reoriented, through-and-through stent sutures are used to contour the cartilage. Suspension sutures brought through the skin at the glabellar region are used over rubber stents. This method facilitates stabilization of the position of the nasal tip and ala. All incisions are closed subcutaneously with 4–0 and 5–0 chromic catgut suture and with 5–0 or 6–0 nylon or 4–0 polypropylene pullout in the subdermis. Sutures are removed 5 to 6 days postoperatively; the through-and-through stent sutures are left for approximately one week without tension. Petroleum jelly nasal packing is used for 1 or 2 days. A paper tape dressing may be used to stabilize the new shape of the nose (Figs. 42-10 and 42-11).

Conclusion

Correction of the nasal deformity at an early age ensures more normal growth of the lower portion of the nose and minimizes the severity of the deformity. I divide primary cleft nose reconstruction into two stages. The first is performed at 3 months of age; the lip repair is done and the tissue in the nasal floor is set up for the second stage, nasal reconstruction. The second stage, which takes place when the child is one year of age, is still considered part of the primary bilateral

Fig. 42-10A. Preoperative frontal view of bilateral complete cleft lip and cleft nose with associated cleft palate at one month of age. B. Frontal view 4½ years postoperatively after stage 1 and stage 2 operations. The patient is 5 years of age. C. Submental vertex view showing good balance and harmony to the lip and nose after reconstruction.

A

B

C

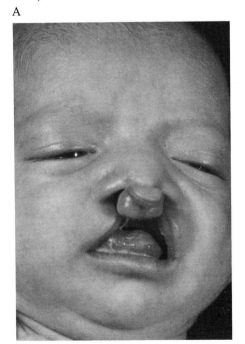
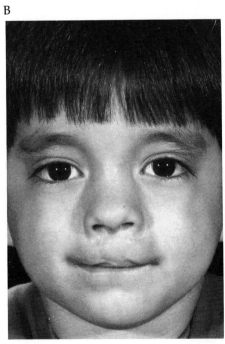
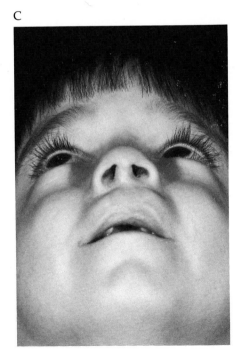

Fig. 42-11A. Frontal view of bilateral cleft lip and palate with cleft nose and no columella. B. Lateral preoperative view at the age of 9 days. C. Frontal view at 13 years of age after primary reconstruction of cleft lip and cleft nose in two stages. D. Lateral view showing good balance and columella-lip angle 12½ years after primary reconstruction. E. Submental vertex view after two-stage reconstruction.

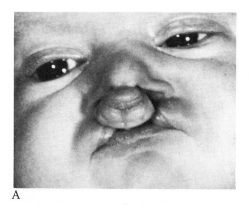

A

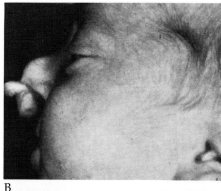

B

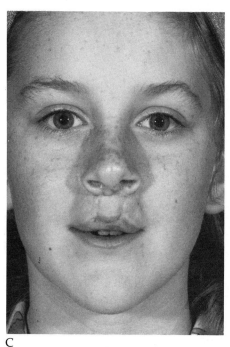

C

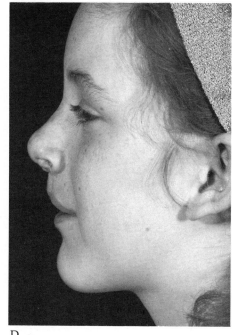

D

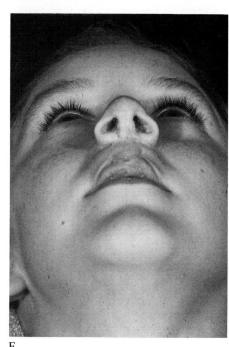

E

cleft nose repair. The columella is lengthened using tissue from the floor of the nose. This tissue is inserted into the nasal floor at the time of primary lip repair to ensure that there will be enough tissue to lengthen the columella. The nasal reconstruction allows for better definition of the nasal tip, narrowing of the alar bases, and orientation of the nostrils in a vertical—not horizontal—position while a patent nasal airway is maintained. Early correction of the nasal deformity ensures a more normal columella-lip angle, with better projection and definition of the lip, while allowing for subsequent growth in more normal anatomic relations. This approach decreases the frequency and severity of secondary deformities that require surgical correction. After two-stage repair of bilateral cleft lips, the columella

grows and remains adequate through the period of facial growth in some patients. Others require additional columellar lengthening or other corrective procedures. As in unilateral cleft nose, almost all bilateral cleft nose deformities require additional surgical treatment by the time most of the primary growth has occurred.

Overall, the results of early reconstruction of cleft nose are beneficial in terms of reducing or minimizing secondary deformities. The results for unilateral complete cleft nose remain far superior to those for bilateral complete cleft nose. State of the art surgery has resolved most of the stigmata of unilateral cleft nose except for subtle nasal deformities. The stigmata of bilateral cleft deformities cannot be adequately corrected. This problem remains for future refinement.

Suggested Reading

Bardach, J.B., and Salyer, K.E. *Surgical Techniques in Cleft Lip and Palate* (2nd ed.). Chicago: Year Book, 1991.

Cronin, T.D., and Denkler, K.A. Correction of the unilateral cleft lip nose. *Plast. Reconstr. Surg.* 82:419, 1988.

Millard, D.R., Jr. *Cleft Craft: The Evolution of Its Surgery,* Vol. I. Boston: Little, Brown, 1976.

Salyer, K.E. *Techniques in Aesthetic Craniofacial Surgery,* New York: Gower Medical Publishing, 1989.

Salyer, K.E. Unilateral Cleft Lip and Cleft Lip Nasal Reconstruction. In J. Bardach and H. Morris (Eds.), *Multidisciplinary Management of Cleft Lip and Palate.* Philadelphia: Saunders, 1990. Pp. 173–184.

43

Cleft Palate

Don LaRossa

Cleft palate or cleft lip, or both, occurs between 1 in 750 and 1 in 1000 live births and is, therefore, the second most common major congenital anomaly. The palate develops from two embryonic shelves that are oriented vertically in the developing fetus. Between the seventh and eleventh months of gestation, the shelves become horizontal and fuse from anterior to posterior. Complete lack of fusion causes a cleft of the palate from the incisive foramen to the uvula. Varying degrees of successful fusion result in lesser degrees of clefting. Fusion of the mucous membranes only results in a submucosal cleft of the palate, the palatal muscles remaining separated. Clinical findings of submucosal cleft palate are a bifid uvula and zona pellucida and a palpable notch of the posterior edge of the hard palate.

The alveolus anterior to the incisive foramen develops with the upper lip structures. Failure of normal fusion of the upper lip on one or both sides, along with failure of fusion of the palate posterior to the incisive foramen, may result in a unilateral or bilateral cleft lip and palate extending from the lip to the uvula. Varying degrees of fusion produce either complete or incomplete clefting, submucosal clefting, or asymmetric clefting.

Timing of Cleft Palate Repair

There is some disagreement regarding the exact timing of cleft palate repair; however, there is general agreement on an age range. It is well accepted that late repair of a cleft palate results in a higher incidence of cleft-related speech problems, such as hypernasality, velopharyngeal incompetence, and nasal escape. Clefts of the lip and palate can be repaired in patients as young as 3 months of age, but because of the risks from bleeding and airway problems, clefts are more commonly repaired when the patient is 6 to 18 months of age. I repair clefts before the patient is one year of age, except in unusual circumstances, such as the Pierre Robin sequence; the Treacher Collins, Apert, or Crouzon syndrome; or other craniofacial syndromes in which patients are at higher risk for airway obstruction. In these situations, I make every attempt to repair the cleft by the time the child is 18 months of age, although repair may have to be delayed until the child is 2 years of age in instances of more severe airway compromise.

Preparation

The patient is in the supine position on the operating table. The table cushions are arranged in a stair-step manner to allow extension of the head. The patient is anesthetized using an endotracheal tube (Ring-Adair-Elwyn Endotracheal Tube, Mallinckrodt Critical Care, Glen Falls, NY) positioned precisely in the midline. A Dingman mouth gag is used to hold the mouth open and to retract the tongue. Tissues are infiltrated with 1% lidocaine with 1:100,000 epinephrine (5 to 7 mg/kg) at the beginning of the procedure. The tissues are infiltrated with 0.25% bupivacaine with epinephrine 1:200,000 at the completion of the procedure for prolonged postoperative pain relief. Oxymetazoline hydrochloride (Afrin) 0.05% nasal drops are placed in each nasal cavity at the start of the procedure to reduce bleeding in the nasal mucous membranes and adenoids. A No. 10Fr nasal oxygen cannula is passed through one nostril into the operative field to aid in visualization by removing pooled blood and fluid from the nasopharynx. I use an overbed instrument table, which allows easy access to all the instruments by the operating surgeon and also allows manipulation of the endotracheal tube by the anesthesiologist to maintain maximal safety. Antibiotics are used prophylactically in all our patients who undergo cleft palate repair.

Furlow Double-Reversing Z-Palatoplasty

Since its introduction in 1980, I have used the Furlow double-reversing Z-palatoplasty for the repair of almost all cleft palates, including very wide ones. Theoretically, it allows a reorientation of the soft palate musculature from an anteroposterior direction to a transverse direction. This normal orientation should facilitate more normal muscular function. Simultaneously, lengthening of the soft palate is achieved through the effects of the Z-plasty. By maintaining the attachment of muscle to mucosa, the dissection is simplified and reduces the risk of injury to the muscle that may occur with an intravelar veloplasty.

Although Furlow considered relaxing incisions to be unnecessary, I use them when needed to obtain a tension-free closure. Von Langenbeck–type incisions are used to maintain as rich a blood supply as possible and to reduce the amount of exposed bone. Not using relaxing incisions does not reduce the amount of bare bone but simply hides it from the surgeon's view.

There may be additional benefits from the Z-plasty. Because the closure is not linear, the amount of shortening secondary to scar contracture may be reduced. Because a Z-plasty produces length at the expense of width, the caliber of the nasal airway is reduced, producing a pharyngoplastic effect. In more than 10 years of follow-up study, patients who had the Furlow operation had a higher incidence of normal speech than did patients who had pushback or intravelar veloplasty procedures.

The Furlow procedure is primarily a method of soft palate closure. The hard palate closure can be performed by a variety of techniques, potentially including a Wardill-Veau-Kilner pushback. A two-flap palatoplasty can be modified to incorporate the double-reversing Z-plasty closure of the soft palate.

Potential shortcomings and disadvantages of the Furlow technique include a greater dissection of muscle than with straight-line repairs, difficulty in closing very wide clefts, and probably a higher incidence of posterior crossbite. The solutions to these problems should be forthcoming as greater experience is achieved at a number of centers.

In an attempt to reduce growth restriction from scar in the alveolar cleft, I do not repair the area at the time of primary palatoplasty. Coupling this factor with an avoidance of horseshoe or W-shaped incisions anteriorly should reduce the amount of scar in this region. Von Langenbeck–type incisions are used when needed but may be avoided altogether in narrow clefts. The residual alveolar fistula is closed at the time of bone grafting in the stage of mixed dentition. These measures seem to have reduced the incidence of severe growth disturbance.

Repair of a Cleft Palate from the Incisive Foramen to the Uvula

Incision Design
The incision lines are drawn on the oral mucous membrane with methylene blue dye and a wood cotton-tipped applicator with a sharpened end (Fig. 43-1). The principle of the operation involves two opposing Z-plasties, one on the oral and one on the nasal surface. The posteriorly based flap on each surface is muscle and mucosa; the anteriorly based flap is mucosa only. Interposition of the flaps reorients the muscle from an anteroposterior direction to a transverse one, reconstructing the levator sling. In most patients, the arms of the Z form a 60° angle; however, the angle depends on the length of the soft palate. As the palate becomes shorter, the angle becomes more obtuse and may approach 90°. Asymmetric angles may be seen when the lengths of the soft palate halves are asymmetric (see Fig. 43-1D). The posteriorly based flap on the oral surface is usually marked on the left side because the left side is easier for a right-handed surgeon to dissect. The posterior margin of the hard palate is identified with a blunt instrument, and the left-sided arm is drawn at an angle approximately 60° to the medial edge of the cleft margin. The incision line is drawn from the estimated location

of the hamulus laterally to near the junction of the hard and soft palates medially. The anteriorly based oral flap is drawn from a point just proximal to the uvula and angled to end near the hamulus laterally. Two posteriorly based uvular flaps are also outlined. This helps to form a more normally shaped uvula and reduces the risk of a bifid uvula.

The medial incision is planned also and should end in a V shape to facilitate the anterior closure. In a complete unilateral cleft of the palate, the medial incisions end at the alveolus. A vomer flap is used to close the nasal side of the hard palate. In bilateral clefts, bilateral vomer flaps are used. Additional mobility of the posterior edge of the vomer flap can be obtained by making a back-cut at the base of the posterior end of the vomer. In wide clefts, lateral relaxing incisions are used. Care should be taken to keep the end of the Z-plasty incisions away from the relaxing incisions to reduce the risk of tearing at this point.

Surgical Technique
The uvular flaps are elevated first with a sharp serrated scissors (Fig. 43-2). Next, the medial margins of the cleft are pared with a No. 12 Bard-Parker or No. 72 Beaver blade. The posteriorly based oral musculomucosal flap is elevated subsequently (Fig. 43-3). An incision is made through the mucosa down to the nasal mucosal surface with a No. 15 Bard-Parker scalpel (Fig. 43-4).

With a No. 64 Beaver blade, the muscle and mucosa are carefully elevated from the nasal mucosa using a combined scraping and cutting motion (Fig. 43-5). Some submucosal tissue and glands are left on the nasal surface if possible to maintain its substance because the muscle is closely adherent to the nasal surface and a nasal flap of mucosa alone would be too thin. The dissection of the musculomucosal flap is continued posteriorly and medially until it is fully elevated.

At this point, the nasal mucosal flap can be cut by stabbing laterally through the nasal mucosa and cutting medially along the reflection of the oral musculomucosal flap through the free medial edge of the soft palate (Fig. 43-6). Despite its thinness, the nasal mucosa is quite tough, and care must be taken not to slide the knife gradually posteriorly. Care must be taken

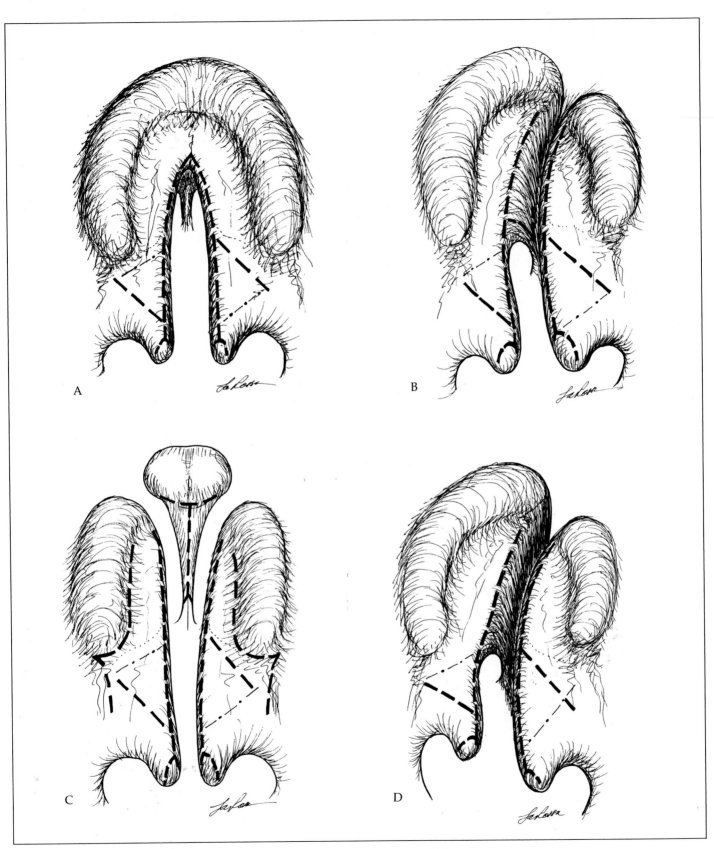

Fig. 43-1. Incision design for repair of various clefts of the palate by the Furlow double-reversing Z-palatoplasty. A. Incomplete cleft of secondary palate. B. Complete unilateral cleft. C. Complete bilateral cleft. D. Asymmetric complete unilateral cleft.

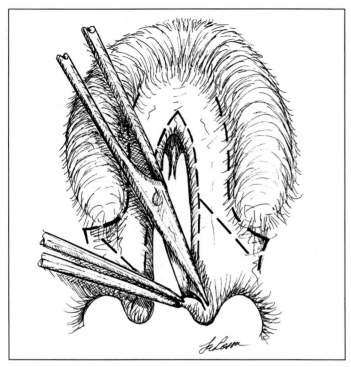

Fig. 43-2. Repair of palate from incisive foramen to uvula. The uvular flaps are elevated.

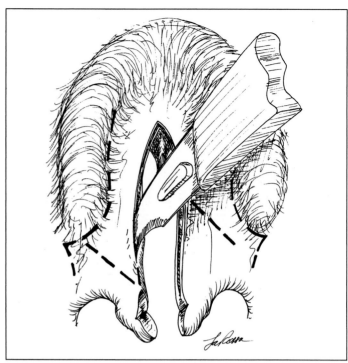

Fig. 43-3. Repair of palate from incisive foramen to uvula. The medial margins of the cleft are pared, and the posteriorly based oral musculomucosal flap is elevated.

Fig. 43-4. Repair of palate from incisive foramen to uvula. The mucosa is incised down to the nasal mucosal surface.

Fig. 43-5. Repair of palate from incisive foramen to uvula. The muscle and mucosa are elevated from the nasal mucosa.

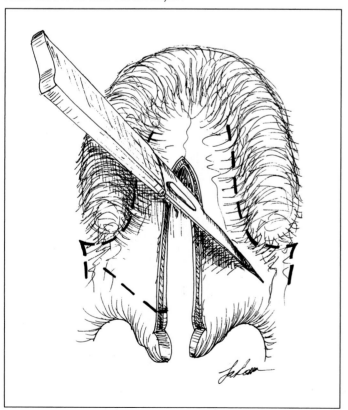

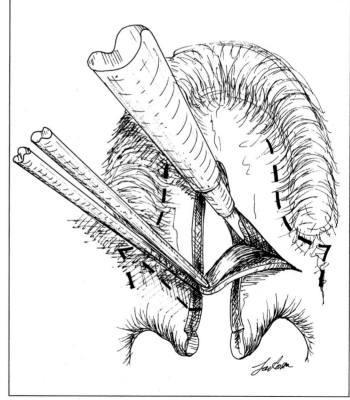

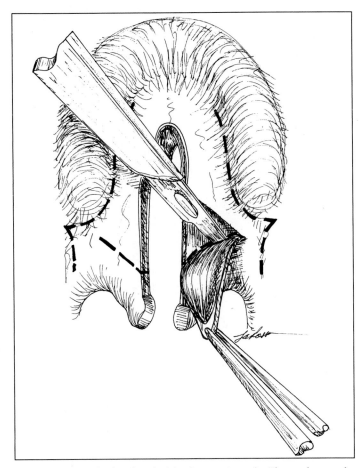

Fig. 43-6. *Repair of palate from incisive foramen to uvula. The nasal mucosal flap is cut.*

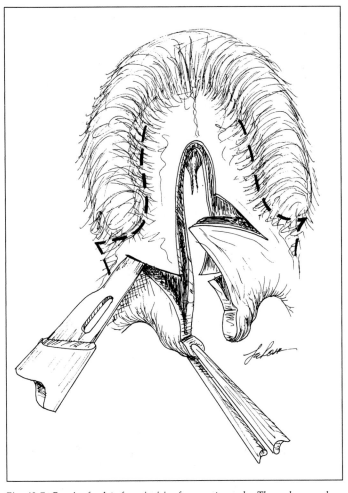

Fig. 43-7. *Repair of palate from incisive foramen to uvula. The oral mucosal flap is elevated.*

laterally to avoid injury to the eustachian tube, which lies directly beneath the lateral extent of this incision. The scissors also can be used to cut this flap, depending on the surgeon's preference.

The oral mucosal flap is elevated next (Fig. 43-7). The incision is made through the mucosa and gradually deepened until the muscle fibers become evident. They will be most superficial at the medial margin of the cleft and gradually become deeper laterally. There is a considerable amount of submucosal fat and glandular material on the oral side.

The flap is elevated from posterior to anterior at the level of the muscle (Fig. 43-8). The nasal musculomucosal flap is cut at this time by the same method of stabbing laterally through the nasal musculomucosal composite and cutting medially along the reflection of the oral mu-

cosal flap, thus completing the dissection of the soft palate flaps (Fig. 43-9).

The oral and nasal mucoperiosteum at the anterior end of the cleft, where the hard and soft palate meet, must be elevated to allow closure of the cleft in this area. The elevation can be done by carefully lifting the tissue from the bony surface of the hard palate from medial to lateral (Fig. 43-10).

An alternative method is to make a stab incision in the oral mucosa at the junction of the alveolus and the mucosa of the hard palate. A Blair palate elevator is introduced and carefully worked to the cleft area from lateral to medial (Fig. 43-11). With bilateral incisions of this type, elevation of the oral mucosa at the cleft apex can be done without difficulty. In wide clefts, relaxing incisions may be needed. In the soft palate area, the incision is

deepened by careful spreading of the scissors in the space of Ernst. When necessary, stretching of the greater palatine vascular pedicle can be done as can infraction of the hamulus to gain additional medial movement of the palatal shelves.

The closure is done with 4–0 chromic catgut suture. The nasal musculomucosal flap is inset first and the closure is completed back to the uvula on the nasal side (Fig. 43-12). The anteriormost portion of the nasal mucosa is closed next because this area is difficult to reach. The nasal mucosal flap is inset, completing the closure on the nasal side. If the nasal mucosal flap does not reach to the apex of the incision, it is closed in a V-Y manner.

The oral closure is done by insetting the oral musculomucosal flap and closing the palate back to the uvula with interrupted sutures (Fig. 43-13). Anteriorly, horizon-

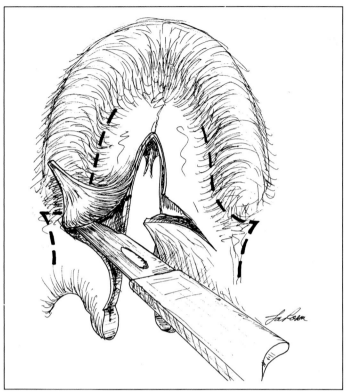

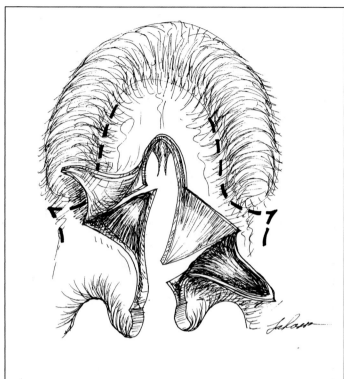

Fig. 43-8. Repair of palate from incisive foramen to uvula. The flap is elevated from posterior to anterior at the level of the muscle.

Fig. 43-9. Repair of palate from incisive foramen to uvula. The dissection is complete.

Fig. 43-10. Repair of palate from incisive foramen to uvula. The oral and nasal mucoperiosteum is elevated by lifting the bony surface of the hard palate from medial to lateral.

Fig. 43-11. Repair of palate from incisive foramen to uvula. Alternative method of elevation of the oral and nasal mucoperiosteum. A stab incision is made in the oral mucosa at the junction of the mucosa of the alveolus and the mucosa of the hard palate.

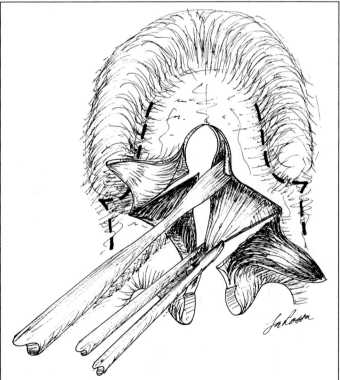

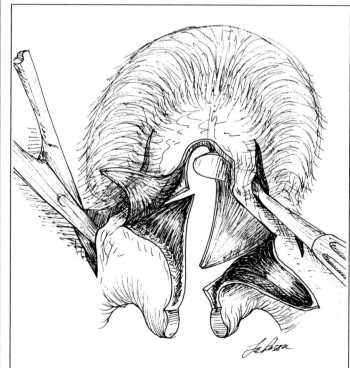

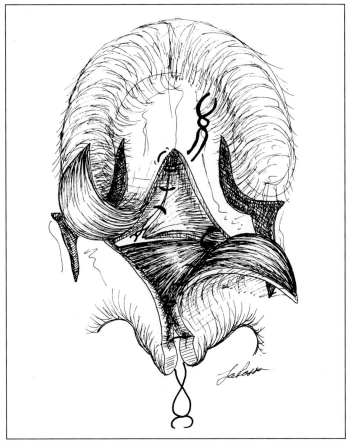

Fig. 43-12. Repair of palate from incisive foramen to uvula. The nasal musculomucosal flap is inset, and the closure is completed back to the uvula on the nasal side.

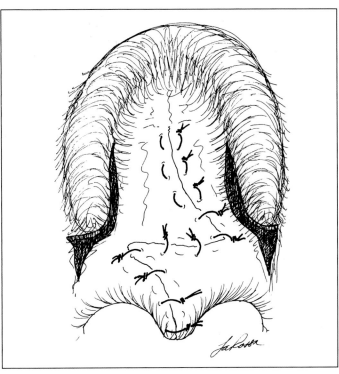

Fig. 43-13. Repair of palate from incisive foramen to uvula. For the oral closure, the oral musculomucosal flap is inset and the palate is closed back to the uvula with interrupted sutures.

tal mattress sutures are used to evert the oral mucoperiosteal edges to obtain a more precise closure and to reduce the risk of fistula formation. The oral mucosal flap is inset last because it is the more friable. As described earlier, the edges can be closed in a V-Y configuration rather than a V if the flap does not comfortably reach the apex of the defect. The relaxing incisions are left open to heal secondarily. If the closure seems tight, the mouth gag can be partially released, which allows the palatal tissues to relax, facilitating the closure.

Repair of a Complete Unilateral Cleft Palate

The soft palate dissection is the same as described for a cleft of the secondary palate. A vomer flap is dissected for closure of the nasal side of the cleft in the hard palate (Fig. 43-14). A Freer elevator works

nicely for flap elevation. The vomer flap is inset first by suturing it beneath the contralateral hard palate mucoperiosteal flap with three or four mattress sutures (Fig. 43-15A and B). They are left untied until the end of the closure. This method facilitates closure of the hard palate mucoperiosteal flaps along the midline. The nasal musculomucosal flap is inset first, and the closure is completed back to the uvula. The nasal mucosal flap is inset second because it is more friable.

In narrower complete clefts, the hard palate mucoperiosteum on the oral and nasal sides may be elevated from the medial margin of the palate, thereby avoiding the use of relaxing incisions (see Fig. 43-15C). Because of the vault-shaped configuration of the hard palate shelves, the mucoperiosteal tissues often can be closed without tension by reflecting them out of the vault and into a more horizontal position.

The oral musculomucosal flap is inset, and the closure is completed back to the uvula (Fig. 43-16). The hard palate mucoperiosteal flaps are closed next, beginning as far anteriorly as possible. The alveolar cleft is left open to allow for growth unimpeded by scar. Horizontal mattress sutures are used to obtain an accurate approximation of the edges. The mucosal flap is inset last because it is the most fragile. Horizontal mattress sutures are used in the hard palate mucoperiosteum to obtain accurate closure.

Repair of a Complete Bilateral Cleft Palate

Bilateral vomer flaps are elevated to close the nasal side (Fig. 43-17). A back-cut can be made to obtain more mobilization (see Fig. 43-1B). Relaxing incisions are almost always needed. As in the unilateral cleft, mattress sutures are used to inset the

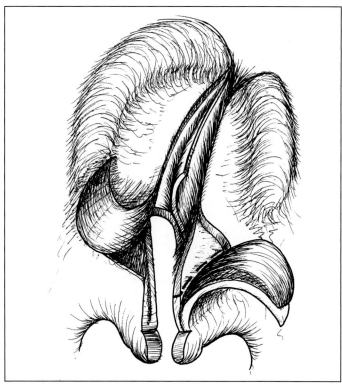

Fig. 43-14. *Repair of a complete unilateral cleft palate by the Furlow double-reversing Z-palatoplasty. Vomer flap is dissected for closure of the nasal side of the cleft in the hard palate.*

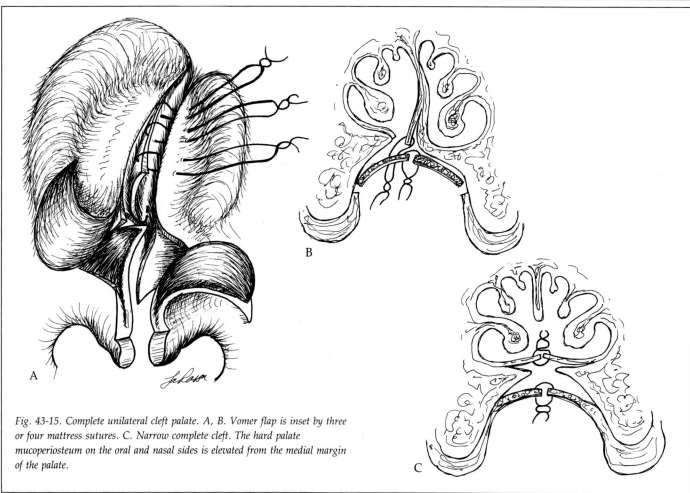

A

B

C

Fig. 43-15. *Complete unilateral cleft palate. A, B. Vomer flap is inset by three or four mattress sutures. C. Narrow complete cleft. The hard palate mucoperiosteum on the oral and nasal sides is elevated from the medial margin of the palate.*

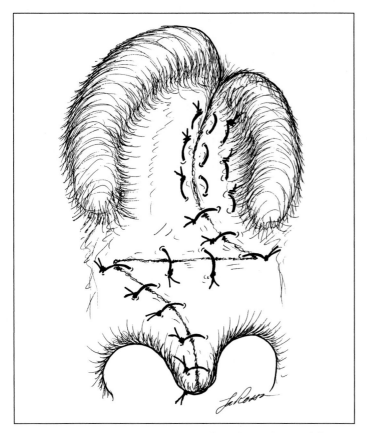

Fig. 43-16. Complete unilateral cleft palate. The oral musculomucosal flap is inset. Closure is completed back to the uvula.

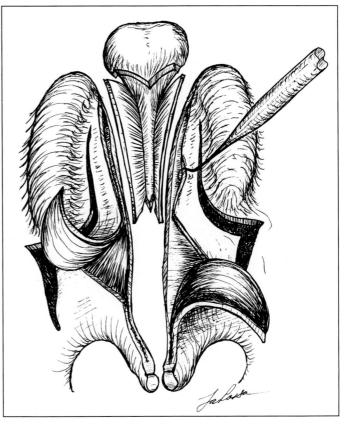

Fig. 43-17. Repair of a complete bilateral cleft palate by the Furlow double-reversing Z-palatoplasty. Bilateral vomer flaps are elevated to close the nasal side.

vomer flaps. They are left untied until the end of the closure (Fig. 43-18). The nasal musculomucosal flap is inset first, and the closure is completed back to the uvula. The nasal mucosal flap is inset next, and the ends of the vomer flap are sutured to it if possible (Fig. 43-19).

The oral musculomucosal flap is inset, and the closure is completed back to the uvula. The hard palate mucoperiosteum is closed from anterior to posterior with horizontal mattress sutures. The mucosal flap is inset at this time; because it is fragile, it is left until close to the end of the procedure. A tapered needle may be needed to prevent tearing. Finally, the vomer mattress sutures are tied down, completing the closure (Fig. 43-20).

Postoperative Care

A suture of 0 gauge black silk is placed through the anterior third of the tongue and taped to the cheek. This facilitates control of the airway should obstruction or bleeding occur in the postoperative period. The suture is removed after 12 to 18 hours if the patient's condition is stable. Arm restraints are used routinely for the first $2\frac{1}{2}$ weeks after the operation to prevent injury from objects or fingers placed in the mouth. Bottle feeding with a cross-cut nipple is allowed immediately after the operation. Pacifiers are not allowed. Strong narcotic medications are avoided to reduce the risk of respiratory depression. Acetaminophen with codeine may be used in limited amounts. Diet is limited to liquids and soft foods for $2\frac{1}{2}$ to 3 weeks postoperatively. Patients are examined 3 weeks postoperatively to assess their healing and at $2\frac{1}{2}$ years of age to assess their speech development and vocal quality. They are evaluated by the surgeon and speech pathologist yearly thereafter, in conjunction with the follow-up plan of the cleft palate team.

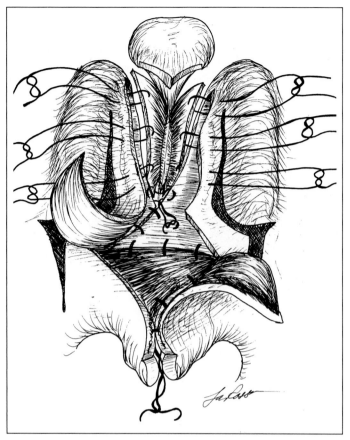

Fig. 43-18. *Complete bilateral cleft palate. Vomer flap is inset with mattress sutures.*

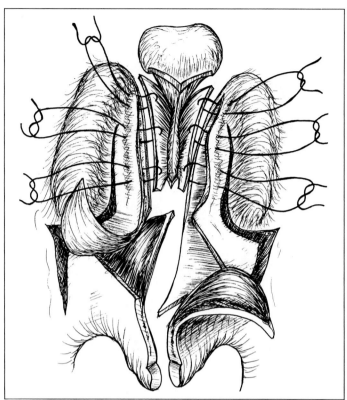

Fig. 43-19. *Complete bilateral cleft palate. Nasal musculomucosal flap is inset first, and the closure is completed back to the uvula. The nasal mucosal flap is inset next. The ends of the vomer flap are sutured to it.*

Fig. 43-20. *Complete bilateral cleft palate. The closure is complete.*

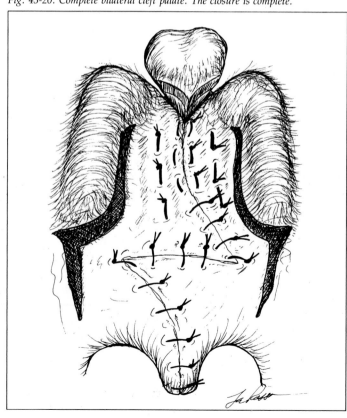

Suggested Reading

Dorf, D.S., and Curtin, J.W. Early cleft palate repair and speech outcome. *Plast. Reconstr. Surg.* 70:74, 1982.

Fogh-Anderson, P. Inheritance of harelip and cleft palate. *Am. J. Hum. Genet.* 22:125, 1970.

Furlow, L., Jr. Cleft palate repair by double reversing Z-plasty. *Plast. Reconstr. Surg.* 78:5, 1986.

Kaplan, E.N. Cleft palate repair at 3 months. *Ann. Plast. Surg.* 7:179, 1981.

LaRossa, D., et al. The Furlow Double Reversing Z-Plasty for Cleft Palate Repair: The First Ten Years of Experience. In J. Bardach and H.L. Morris (Eds.), *Multidisciplinary Management of Cleft Lip and Palate.* Philadelphia: Saunders, 1990. Pp. 337–340.

Randall, P., et al. Cleft palate closure at three to nine months: A preliminary report. *Plast. Reconstr. Surg.* 71:624, 1983.

Randall, P., et al. Experience with the Furlow double reversing Z-plasty for cleft palate repair. *Plast. Reconstr. Surg.* 77:569, 1986.

Stark, R.B. The pathogenesis of harelip and cleft palate. *Plast. Reconstr. Surg.* 13:20, 1954.

44

Secondary Soft Tissue Procedures for Cleft Lip and Palate

Michael B. Lewis

Cleft Lip

The need for secondary operations for cleft lip, or revision, implies a failure of the original, or primary, repair. As in rhinoplasty, a second operation is usually more difficult than the initial one. This is true because each secondary problem is unique and is complicated by deep and superficial scar tissue; often parts are missing that may have been available at the time of the primary operation.

Some revisions are more acceptable than others. Specifically, revisions that do not require intrusion into the original skin and muscle repair have better results than operations that do require such an intrusion. Minor revisions of vermilion and mucosal problems do not disturb these important elements of the original repair and can be done with little or no compromise. Occasionally, as in banking of fork flaps for later columellar lengthening, a secondary operation for a cleft lip is planned as part of the surgical habilitation. The old adage that the primary lip scar is the best lip scar is true. A surgeon performing a primary repair has a tremendous responsibility to preserve necessary tissue elements and to place them

correctly in the repaired lip. If this is done, secondary corrections are usually minor. If these steps are not taken, secondary corrections are more difficult, are usually a compromise, and sometimes are impossible.

It is impossible to describe every secondary cleft lip deformity and the procedures used to revise them. Rather I describe here a general approach to the problem, emphasizing principles, goals, and priorities. Subsequently I describe in some detail the procedures I find reliable in solving particular reproducible secondary problems.

Evaluation of the Deformity

The first step in evaluating a secondary cleft lip deformity is to establish whether the problem is only within the lip or is caused totally or in part by an underlying maxillary deformity or nasal imbalance. Timing of the cleft lip revision in relation to maxillary and nasal correction depends on the particular problem, the age of the patient at presentation, and the desires of the patient or his or her parents. For older patients, I prefer to correct the maxillary

deformity first and, at a second procedure, revise the lip and nose. If the lip is too tight to allow maxillary advancement, lip correction must precede maxillary repair. For younger patients, if I believe it will make a difference, I perform the lip operation in children of almost any age. The only caveat is that a considerable amount of time, 12 to 24 months, be allowed to pass between operations. When looking specifically at the lip, I break the problems down into the following elements:

Scar

Vermilion and mucosa, excess or deficiency

Cupid's bow

Major asymmetry

Muscle

Proportion (lip either too long or too tight)

Often more than one element is affected. How many and which elements are involved determine the procedure or procedures used. There is no algorithm to determine which method is best, since this type of surgery is more an art than a science. Which procedure is done depends greatly on the surgeon's aesthetic sense, training, and experience.

Of course the patient's or the parents' desires must be considered. Frequently they verbalize only dissatisfaction with the scar. Rarely, however, is this what they really mean; they do not have the aesthetic or plastic surgical background to articulate what they mean. A thorough discussion is necessary and usually results in agreement regarding what the problems are and what the goals of surgical treatment should be. The first step in deciding on the surgical plan is to identify what is wrong. Rarely is it the lip scar. More often, other elements of the lip repair are at fault.

Second, it must be determined whether the secondary lip problem can be altered in a positive way without producing other, less acceptable, deformities. It is important at this stage to consider the appearance of a new or replacement scar on the lip, if required, in relation to the improvement the revision might offer in other elements of the lip. Experience is helpful in this regard.

Third, the surgeon must consider the options available and choose the best one. The choice may not be the same for all surgeons. Finally, the timing of revision must be coordinated with the overall needs of the patient.

Secondary Soft Tissue Problems

Table 44-1 lists categories of secondary soft tissue problems and the reconstructive options in order of increasing complexity. Which solution I use depends on the magnitude of the specific problem and what associated lip problems exist. Although they do not literally constitute a secondary lip problem, I discuss the short columella and tethered nasal tip because of the close if not inevitable association of their solution with lip revision.

As mentioned earlier, rarely does the appearance of the primary lip scar alone present a clinically significant secondary problem. The primary scar is almost always narrow, flat, and faded. It may not be located in the ideal position, but a decision to revise such a scar should be based on a prediction of the final appearance of the new scar and the potential of causing additional deformity. In general, scar revision on the lip follows the same rules and principles of scar revision elsewhere. In the more common circum-

Table 44-1. Correction of secondary soft tissue cleft lip deformities

Deformity	Reconstructive options
Scar	Simple revision
	Revision with Z-plasty
	Total lip revision
Mucocutaneous ridge malalignment	Limited reopening and closure with Z-plasty at white roll
	Total lip revision
Vermilion and mucosal excess	Excision at free border
	Excision by inverted T
Vermilion deficiency	V-Y rolldown*
	Cross-lip vermilion flap (Kawamoto)*
	Double pendulum flaps (Kapetansky)*
	Total lip revision*
	Cross-lip flap (Abbe)*
Lip adherent to maxilla (absent sulcus)	Release with advancement of labial-buccal mucosal flaps
	Release with mucosal graft
	Cross-lip flap (Abbe)*
Absent cupid's bow	Sculpting excision above vermilion-cutaneous junction with vermilion advancement
	Quadrilateral vermilion flap (Thomson)*
	Total lip revision
	Cross-lip flap (Abbe)*
Asymmetry (repaired side either too long or too short)	Total lip revision*
Muscle bulges or imbalance	Recreation of cleft with total revision
	Double pendulum flaps (Kapetansky)*
Lip too tight	Cross-lip flap (Abbe)*
Entire lip too long	Full-thickness excision at upper lip-nasal junction to shorten lip
Short columella (bilateral cleft lip)	Fork flap lengthening*
	Prolabium advanced into columella with cross-lip flap (Abbe)*
	Composite ear graft

* Procedure described in detail.

stance in which a replacement scar must be made to solve other secondary lip problems, the position of the scar is often dictated by the needs of the revision. Ideally it should be placed in the position of the philtral ridge, although to do so in some patients would cause problems of asymmetry or lip tightness.

Isolated problems of the mucocutaneous ridge (white roll) at the point where the scar passes from vermilion to the skin are usually treated by limited reopening and closure with a Z-plasty or by direct suturing with a white roll flap. The results of these procedures are sometimes limited by the erythema that persists in the new scar and by wound contraction.

Secondary problems of vermilion and mucosal excess are the easiest to manage because they do not require intrusion into

the skin or muscle scar. In my own primary operations, such excess is the most common cause for revision. Although this revision is basically a straightforward procedure, some guidelines must be followed. If local anesthesia is used, over-inflation of the lip should be avoided because it can interfere with judgment regarding how much to excise. Second, direct excision of the redundant tissue is required. It is impossible to precisely revise the free vermilion border by excising mucosal tissue at any distance. I have seen this done to "hide" the scar with poor results. Finally, no undermining of vermilion or mucosa should be done because this sets up a situation in which swelling and deep scar tissue can recreate the excess. These procedures should not be performed for at least one year after the primary repair. The most common form of excision is in the shape of an inverted T, the vertical limb running up the mucosal surface of the lip.

Deficiencies of the vermilion are often referred to as whistle deformities. Minor problems can be managed nicely with a V-Y rolldown procedure. Major deficiencies, when isolated, require a cross-lip vermilion flap as described by Kawamoto. In central deficiencies in repaired bilateral cleft lips, especially when the lip muscle is not united, the pendulum flap technique of Kapetansky is a good solution. I have found these three procedures useful and reliable. They are described in detail later in the chapter. Of course, vermilion deficiencies associated with other major secondary problems can be solved by total lip revision after reproduction of the cleft or by using an Abbe flap.

Absence of a labial sulcus with adherence of the central lip to the premaxilla is almost always a complication of bilateral cleft lip repair. This problem usually can be solved by release planned in a manner to allow mucosal flap coverage of the premaxilla and reconstruction of the mucosal surface of the central lip by advancement of labial-buccal mucosal flaps. Rarely, a buccal mucosal free graft is required. If other secondary problems demand it, an Abbe flap also can be used to solve this problem. In this situation the original central vermilion and mucosa are used to cover the premaxilla; of course, the Abbe flap brings along its own mucosal surface for the underside of the lip.

Lack, not merely displacement, of a cupid's bow is somewhat uncommon. This is especially so in operations done in the past 15 or 20 years; preservation of cupid's bow elements should have been a part of every unilateral cleft lip repair. Because of the complex relations among vermilion, white roll, and skin and because this area is three-dimensional, reconstruction is difficult and never perfect. Sculpting excisions above the white roll with advancement look good on paper but are often compromised by the new transverse scar above the white roll, the wound contraction that flattens the bow, and the lack of convexity that should be present in this area. Thomson recently described a quadrilateral flap technique of cupid's bow reconstruction that I have found useful but not perfect. It more reliably forms the height of the bow and

provides some three-dimensional qualities but has no white roll associated with it. The Abbe flap is an excellent way of forming a cupid's bow and philtrum but is a more complex procedure. A composite ear graft philtrum and cupid's bow reconstruction can look good in a photograph but rarely does in person.

Asymmetry of the lip results when the repaired side of a unilateral cleft lip or one side of a bilateral cleft lip is either too long or too short. In my experience, reproduction of the cleft with total revision is required to solve this problem. It is therefore important to determine whether the deformity is severe enough to warrant the procedure and the fresh scar that results. Correction of a short lip by the rotation-advancement principle can cause a transverse deficiency, which can be noticeable.

Muscle bulging or muscle imbalance during animation is a difficult problem to resolve completely. I have been totally unsuccessful in trying to treat this problem by approaching it from the mucosal side alone. I therefore resort to surgical reproduction of the cleft with complete revision (Fig. 44-1) if the deformity warrants the correction. Kapetansky's pendulum flap procedure can be used for this problem in bilateral cleft lip.

If lip proportion is such that the lip is too tight in a transverse dimension, additional tissue in the form of an Abbe flap is required. Usually, in these circumstances, the lower lip is quite redundant and its reduction as a result of the Abbe is complementary to the increase in upper lip volume. A deficient or retrusive maxilla can cause or add to the appearance of a tight lip, and this contribution must be evaluated and treated.

If the entire lip is too long, shortening by full-thickness lip excision at the lip and nasal junction should be carried out. To avoid pulling down the nasal base, producing anterior-facing nostrils, the muscle layer should be sutured to the periosteum along the lower border of the pyriform opening and nasal spine.

A short columella requiring reconstruction is a problem seen exclusively in complete bilateral clefts of the primary palate. It is incumbent on the primary surgeon to plan the habilitation to allow reconstruction without reentering the lip repair. Millard's technique of banking fork flaps for

later use in columellar lengthening is my preferred way of handling this situation. Columellar lengthening by any technique is always a compromise. The reconstructed columella never looks normal, and the disturbance of the lip-columella junction is usually a problem. However, the improvement in tip projection and in the separation of the lip and nasal aesthetic units outweighs these negative factors. Attention to particular details of columellar construction and inset can improve the final result. The techniques available for columellar lengthening are listed in Table 44-1. Which method is used depends on the associated problems. If the lip and nose are otherwise perfect, release of the tethered tip with placement of a composite ear graft can be considered; however, this procedure is rarely necessary.

Surgical Procedures

V-Y Vermilion Mucosal Rolldown

Used for minor deficiencies in the vermilion (whistle deformities), the V-Y succeeds more because of the undermining than because of the V-Y geometry involved. In fact, the advancement is usually quite minor and in some instances nonexistent.

In planning and marking (Fig. 44-2), which is always done before local infiltration, the apex of the V is well up the mucosal surface of the lip. The limbs of the V as they approach the free border of the upper lip must be at the extreme margin of the whistle deficiency. I usually continue the limbs beyond the free border, but without further divergence, for another few millimeters.

Undermining or development of the flap takes place at the submucosal-muscular interface. It is important to continue the undermining beyond the imaginary line connecting the ends of the V limbs up to and beyond the vermilion-cutaneous junction. Some limited correction of separation of the orbicularis oris muscle can be carried out by this approach, and theoretically a dermal graft could be placed to add further bulk; in general, however, I do not perform adjunctive procedures.

In closing, precise suturing with limited or no advancement is done. Because this procedure depends in good part on residual and permanent swelling beneath the

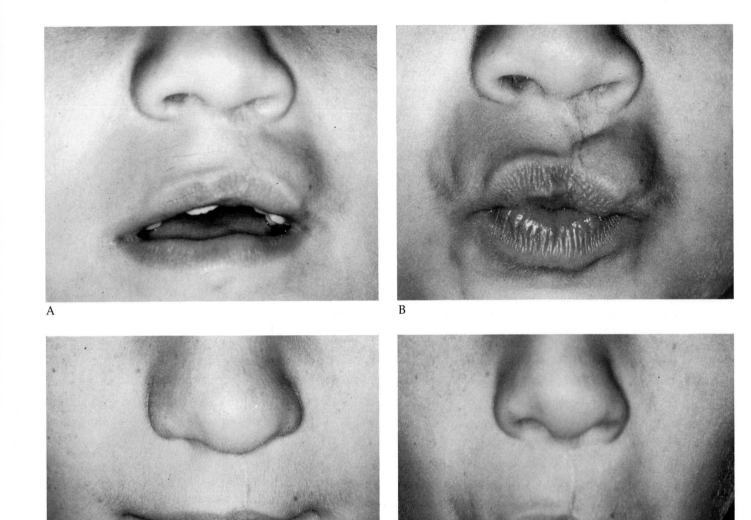

Fig. 44-1A. *Preoperative condition in repose. Lip is short on the repaired side and warrants correction. B. Preoperative condition during animation demonstrating muscle imbalance and bulging. Condition 2 years postoperatively in repose (C) and during animation (D). Revision included surgical reproduction of the cleft with special attention to muscle repositioning during revision.*

flap of the "injured" lip, the outcome is somewhat unpredictable. I have missed on either side. It is unusual for an experienced surgeon to need to reoperate.

Cross-Lip Vermilion Flap

Before Kawamoto described the cross-lip vermilion flap technique, the standard means of correcting larger deficiencies in the vermilion was to use an apron flap from lower lip to upper lip. This procedure, because of its design, reversed the

positions of the vermilion and mucosa in the upper lip. Kawamoto's procedure (Fig. 44-3) is essentially a wide but shallow Abbe flap reconstruction that does not reverse the vermilion-mucosa relation in moving the tissue from the lower to the upper lip. The flap contains no skin. I reserve this procedure for secondary lip problems that have a vermilion deficiency too great to treat by the V-Y rolldown, but in which there are no other secondary lip problems to be solved. It does thin the

lower lip a slight amount, but apparently not as much as the width of the flap might suggest. At the first stage the deficient recipient site of the upper lip is prepared with a transverse incision along the free border of the lip. Care is taken not to have any wet vermilion remain on the external side of the incision. The incision is carried deep enough to allow the edges to separate sufficiently to accept the vermilion flap. This usually means dissection into the subvermilion portion of the orbicularis oris muscle. The lower lip flap is designed with the width necessary to correct the upper lip deficiency. Most of the flap is vermilion; however, depending on the needs of the recipient site, mucosa can be included. The flap contains vermilion,

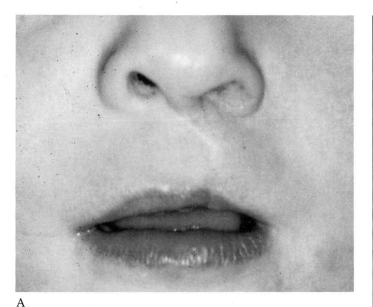

A

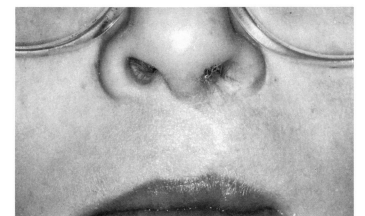

C

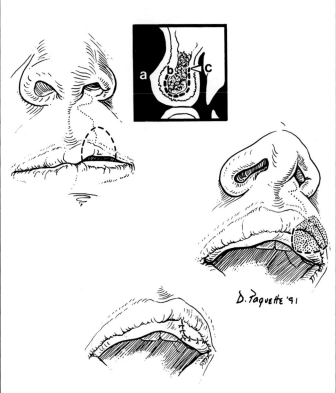

B

Fig. 44-2A. Condition before revision with deficient vermilion evident on the repaired side of the lip. B. Upper left, outline of the mucosal vermilion V-Y rolldown flap. Inset, dashed line indicates level and extent of the flap development from point c to point b. This goes beyond the vermilion-cutaneous junction at point a. Middle right, dotted region demonstrates the extent of undermining. Lower left, closed wound indicating a very short vertical limb of the Y closure. C. Result 2 years after the operation.

subvermilion, and submucosa, but no muscle. There is no need for the flap to contain the labial artery, and it is probably preferable not to include it.

Once the flap is designed, dissection begins at the commissure opposite from most of the upper lip recipient site. Approximately 60 percent of the lower lip transverse dimension is included in the first stage—50 percent for inset and 10 percent for bridging. Meticulous hemostasis of the donor and recipient sites is followed by careful closure of the donor site with fine catgut sutures. The flap is rotated 180° and sutured into place in the upper lip defect with fine catgut sutures.

The end of the flap should be tapered appropriately to reproduce the normal thinning of the upper lip as it approaches the commissure. The second stage, which can be done in 10 days, is usually a little more difficult than the initial stage because residual lip swelling and induration make judgments of dimension less precise. The lower lip flap is continued across the lower lip in the exact dimension it was started, ending in the opposite commissure from where it began. After hemostasis, the donor site is closed similarly to the previous closure. The remaining defect in the upper lip is opened in the same transverse line, and the new end of the flap is shaped appropriately and inset.

A tertiary procedure to properly construct the free border is rarely required, but when it is, it should be put off for 6 to 12 months. The adaptability of this procedure is great. Although it is rare to require the full length of the lower lip in the flap, it is important to take it to ensure a balanced and smooth lower lip.

Cross-Lip (Abbe) Flap

In the recent past, I have heard in public forums a few well-known and respected plastic surgeons indicate they no longer use the Abbe flap. They suggested that manipulation of the maxilla combined with an upper lip procedure alone could solve all the problems an Abbe flap might solve without the need for a lower lip scar and the inevitable inconvenience of having the lips hooked together for 2 weeks. I could not disagree more. Not only can the Abbe procedure rescue a disaster but

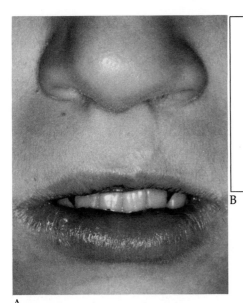

A

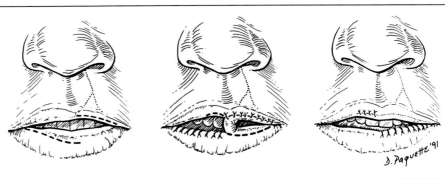

B

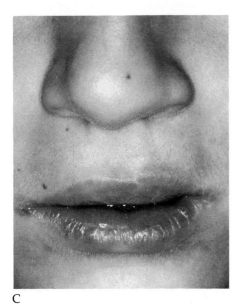

C

Fig. 44-3A. Condition before revision. Vermilion is deficient centrally and on the entire repaired side of the upper lip. Note the generous lower lip vermilion. B. Left, dashed line on upper lip at wet-dry junction. Incision here opens the upper lip to accept the cross-lip vermilion flap. Dashed line on the lower lip marks the external incision of the lower lip flap, which is usually centered on the wet-dry line. About 60 percent of the flap is developed at the first stage. Middle, first stage is completed, and markings for the second stage are indicated. Right, second stage is completed. It is important to continue the lower lip flap to the commissure, even if some tissue will be discarded, to ensure an even, balanced lower lip. C. Result one year after the operation.

also it alone can add the elegance of a natural-looking philtrum, cupid's bow, and central tubercle. Millard has shown us how to get the most from this procedure and has raised the use of the Abbe flap to an art form. Some points of this procedure need emphasis.

The flap should always be taken from the center of the lower lip and placed in the aesthetic center of the upper lip. In its final location it should make up all of the philtral unit, central vermilion tubercle, and central cupid's bow. This can mean removing from the upper lip any original philtral elements that might upset the new aesthetic philtral subunit in the reconstructed upper lip. The shape and dimension of the flap depend on the needs of the upper lip. The flap is usually harvested as a shield shape (Millard) and set into the upper lip unaltered (Fig. 44-4); except for bilateral cleft lip when the philtral skin is advanced to lengthen the columella. In that situation I prefer to square off the end of the shield by amputating the apex (Fig. 44-5). This produces a differently shaped but normal philtral unit. The flap is usually no wider than 10 mm at the free border, but in extreme cases I have taken the flap as wide as 15 mm.

The first step in the procedure is preparation of the recipient site. If the philtrum is being advanced to lengthen the columella, this step is done first. This tissue

is raised quite thick, and the dissection is continued into the membranous septal area, releasing the nasal tip. The tissue is partially tubed and shaped to make the new columella. The columella should not be made too long. After it is constructed, the columella is inset in the new position so that none of it is present in the upper lip. The remaining lip elements on either side of the defect are then balanced. Not uncommonly, I find myself shortening these elements by excision at the junction of the nostril sill and upper lip.

Now the Abbe flap is designed, and appropriate points along the white roll and wet-dry vermilion junction are tattooed. The pedicle can be quite small, which makes insetting easier. The pedicle contains a few millimeters of vermilion and mucosa with some subvermilion musculature and the labial vessels. The exact position of the vessels can be determined easily by their identification when the nonpedicled side is dissected. The donor site in the lower lip is closed first in three layers, and the flap is rotated 180° and inset, each side being closed in three layers. The nonpedicled side is closed first, followed by the pedicled side, beginning with the mucosa. In closing the muscle layer, considerable advancement of the pedicled side of the flap must be done to properly align the cupid's bow and to resist the pulling down from the lower lip.

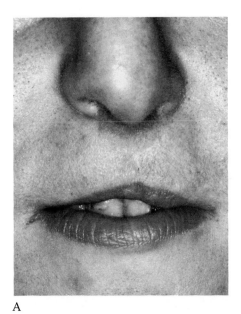

A

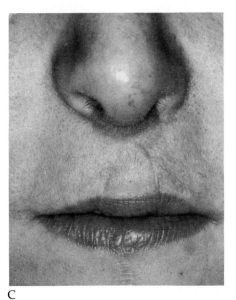

C

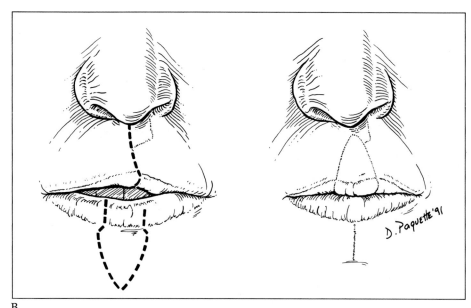

B

Fig. 44-4A. Frontal view before revision in a repaired unilateral cleft left. Absence of the cupid's bow and philtral subunit and a tight vermilion border make this an ideal situation for an Abbe flap. B. Left, dashed line in upper lip marks the aesthetic center of the lip and the line of the full-thickness incision. Dashed lines in the lower lip outline the Abbe flap taken from the anatomic center of the lower lip. Right, completed revision. C. Nine months after division and inset of the Abbe flap.

This operation can be done under local or general anesthesia. If general anesthesia is used, I prefer oral intubation. Nasal tubes prevent adequate, undistorted visualization of the upper lip. The second stage is done 2 to 3 weeks after the first stage. The site of division of the pedicle should be precise to allow adequate tissue for insetting of both upper and lower lip. Attention to detail at this point avoids the need for a third stage.

Double Pendulum Flaps

This procedure, described by Kapetansky in 1971, is ideal for correcting the severe central whistle deformity seen in bilateral cleft lip (Fig. 44-6). Lack of central muscle union and excessive lateral vermilion, which often coexist with the central deficiency, are corrected as well. The arm of each pendulum is the orbicularis oris muscle, and the bob of the pendulum is a long, narrow, triangular portion of lateral vermilion and mucosa. Flaps of vermilion and mucosa are designed beginning medially at the margin of the whistle deficiency extending laterally to within a few millimeters of the commissure. The lateral apex is at the wet-dry junction. An incision is marked between the two medial ends to open up the central defi-

ciency. This should be done in a way that accentuates eventual medial fullness, but only dry vermilion should be external to the incision. The anterior and central incisions are made, and a plane is dissected between subcutaneous tissue and muscle. The posterior incisions are made, and a second plane is developed between the submucosal and muscular layers. These planes must extend cephalad close to the lip-nasal junction to allow proper medial rotation of the pendulum flaps. At this point in the procedure there should be three separate layers draped from above.

The arms of the pendulum are made by excising scar tissue centrally and releasing the orbicularis oris laterally. After meticulous hemostasis, the pendulum flaps are rotated toward each other centrally and the muscle is sutured with a slowly absorbable suture. Just above the vermilion bob, a small cutback is made and suturing is continued. This step helps accentuate the central vermilion peak. Suturing of the vermilion and mucosa is done with interrupted fine catgut sutures. Along the free border of the lip, the vermilion flaps are moved toward one another in a V-Y manner. A good deal of lip swelling results from this procedure, and it can take weeks for total resolution to occur.

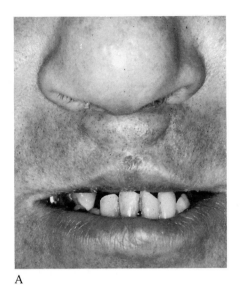

A

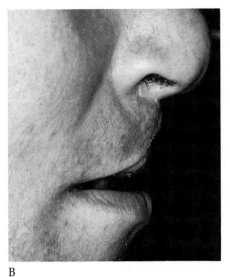

B

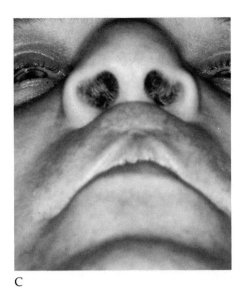

C

Fig. 44-5A, B, C. Preoperative condition. Tight upper lip without a cupid's blow, tethered nasal tip with relatively short columella, and "biscuit" prolabium in upper central lip. D. Shaded area in upper lip indicates the tissue excised to free the prolabium for advancement into the columella and for shortening of the upper lip before acceptance of the Abbe flap. Dashed lines in the lower lip outline the Abbe flap from the anatomic center of the lower lip. The stippled area on the Abbe flap is usually excised in bilateral clefts. E, F, G. Result 3 years after cross-lip flap reconstruction.

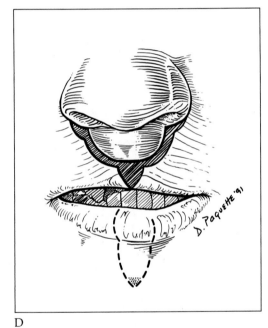

D

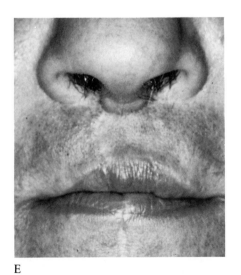

E

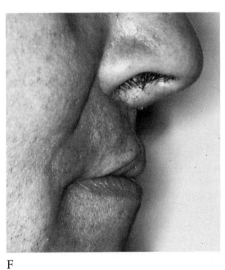

F

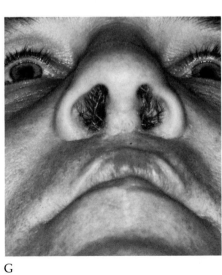

G

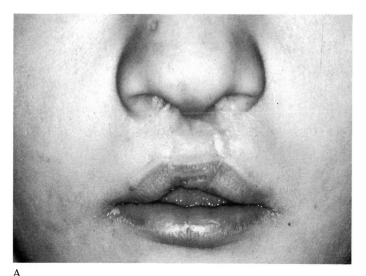

A

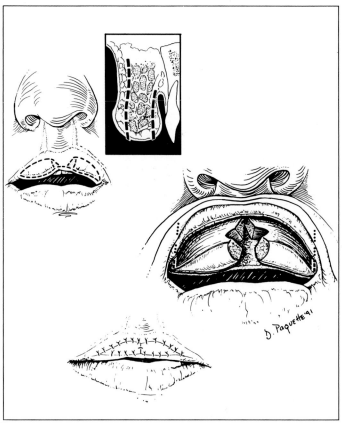

B

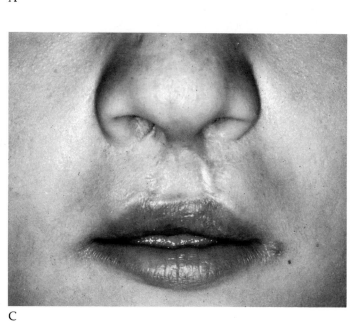

C

Fig. 44-6A. Preoperative condition with central "whistle" deficiency and abundant lateral vermilion. B. Upper left, incisions for pendulum flaps indicated by the dashed lines. Stippled area at central end of each flap is excised. Inset, dashed lines indicate extent and plane of undermining immediately superficial to the orbicularis oris muscle. Center right, pendulum flaps have been fully dissected except for the lateral releasing incision, which is indicated by the dashed, dotted line. Central scar tissue has been removed, and a small cutback into the muscle at the medial edge has been completed. Lower left, completed operation. C. Condition 6 months after the operation.

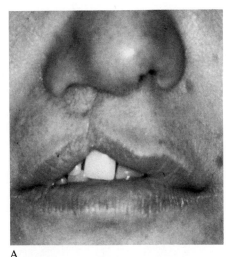

A

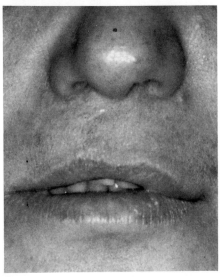

C

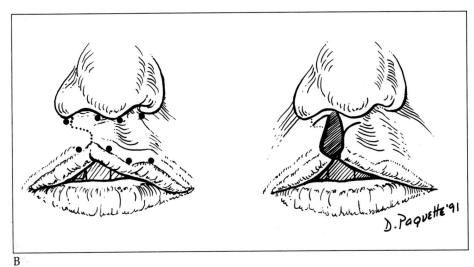

B

Fig. 44-7A. Condition before revision. B. Left, cupid's bow, columella-lip junction, and alar base–lip junction points have been identified and marked. Measurements of the normal and the cleft side determine the amount of lengthening required. Right, Z-plasty outlined to add length in the upper part of the rotation-advancement revision. Shaded tissue (the old scar) has been excised. C. Ten months after lip revision.

Total Lip Revision

An asymmetric, disproportionate secondary cleft lip deformity requires total lip revision for improvement (Fig. 44-7). The first step is to identify the points that will be used to make the height of the cupid's bow on the revised side. The center of the bow and opposite height are marked as well. Symmetric points are marked at the alar base–lip and columellar base–lip junctions on either side of the lip. By comparing measurements from side to side, the needs of the lip revision can be determined. The geometric markings for this are placed, at first, without regard to the old scars. If possible, alterations are made so that all old scars can be removed. I do not hesitate to use Z-plasties to accomplish the goals of lip revision. The exact position of the final scar is not as important as lip balance, proportion, and the cupid's bow. If possible, however, I favor a position for final scar placement as close as possible to the philtral ridge.

Almost always this type of revision requires total reproduction of the cleft by full-thickness dissection. The lip incisions marked on the skin are made in full thickness, producing composite flaps. Unless there is unusual muscle bulging or considerable lip muscle imbalance, I do only minimal separation of the skin and mucosa from the muscle. A three-layered closure is carried out, the key layer being muscle. If only minimal separation of skin and mucosa from the muscle has been done, proper placement of the muscular sutures carries the skin, mucosa, and vermilion to their proper places.

Quadrilateral Vermilion Flap Reconstruction of the Cupid's Bow

Thomson described the technique of quadrilateral vermilion flap reconstruction, which I find useful in shaping a bow when one truly does not exist (Fig. 44-8). As Thomson pointed out, this procedure is based essentially on the principles of the rhomboid transposition flap originally described by Lindburg. Sculpting excision to shape the ipsilateral portion of the central bow is done in a modified rhomboid manner to mimic the opposite, normal side. An adjacent rhomboid flap is outlined in good dry vermilion, developed, and transposed. The flap should be a bit thicker than the tissue excised to help shape the three-dimensional qualities of this area. The donor site of the flap is closed directly. The upper borders of the flap are sutured to the lip with half-buried

A

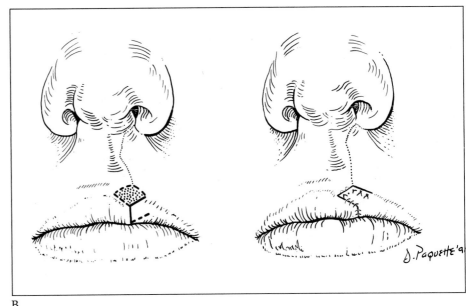

B

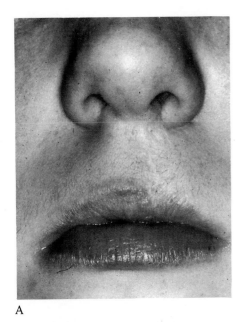

C

Fig. 44-8A. Condition before revision. The cupid's bow on the repaired side is absent, and the vermilion in the area is scarred. B. Left, stippled area indicates sculpting excision of tissue and scar. This is done superficially. Quadrilateral flap is outlined. Right, completed operation with flap donor site closed primarily. C. Result 3 months after operation.

horizontal mattress sutures to eliminate possible suture marks on the skin, which could mar the final result. Fine catgut sutures are used throughout. The limitation of this procedure is that no white role exists at the new junction of vermilion and skin.

Forked Flap Columellar Reconstruction

When the columella needs lengthening and the upper lip needs revision, but not an Abbe flap, the forked flap procedure of Millard is my preferred method of reconstruction (Fig. 44-9). The forked flap is designed in a symmetric way to include lateral prolabial tissue and scar. It is based superiorly at the lip-columella junction and is as long as required. Additional markings are placed to revise the lip as required. This is usually an excellent time to narrow and shape the philtrum, narrow the nostril sills, shorten the lip, repair the muscle, and modify the cupid's bow.

During dissection, the forked flap is elevated quite thickly. Dissection proceeds from the base of this flap into the nose at the membranous septal level on out to and beyond the septal angle. This releases the nasal tip, which naturally springs out into a more normal position.

Making a good-looking columella from a forked flap is not easy. I have found that after suturing the flaps together at the skin level with both a subcuticular and a skin layer, it is helpful to tube the flap partially by adding another suture layer along the eventual upper border of the new columella. This step helps modify the excess width seen from below and the deficiency often seen on profile. Because the ends of the forked flap tend to get pulled back into the lip during healing and maturation, I no longer leave them in the nostril sill area to simulate the columellar flare but rather turn them up toward the caudal end of the septum. A small dog-ear at the tip end of the columellar suture line often needs correction.

During the lip portion of this repair, I suspend the muscle layer to the periosteum around the lower border of the pyriform opening and maxillary spine to prevent lip lengthening and blunting of the lip-columella angle.

Cleft Palate

Discussion of secondary soft tissue operations in the palate area is here confined to closure of oral nasal fistulas. Velo-

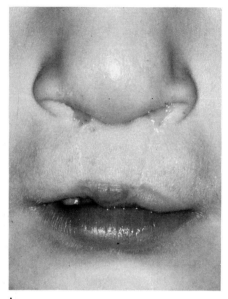

A

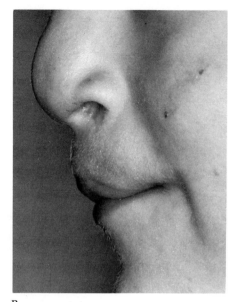

B

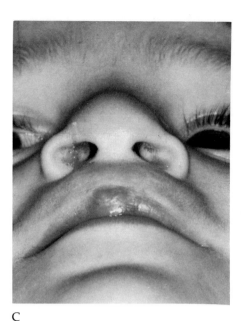

C

Fig. 44-9A, B, C. Condition before forked flap columellar lengthening and lip revision. Note the widened philtrum (prolabium) especially superiorly. Muscle bulging and some asymmetry are also present. D. Upper left, outline of forked flap is indicated by the dashed line. Middle right, forked flap has been elevated, the nasal tip is released, and columellar reconstruction is proceeding. Mattress suture to partially tube the forked flap is shown being placed. Upper philtral tissue is partially dissected to allow muscle repair in the upper half of the lip. Lower left, completed revision. Distal ends of the forked flaps are turned up into the nose to prevent them from being drawn back into the lip during healing. E, F, G. Eighteen months after revision. Note that the columella has not been made too long. Nostril shape is reasonable.

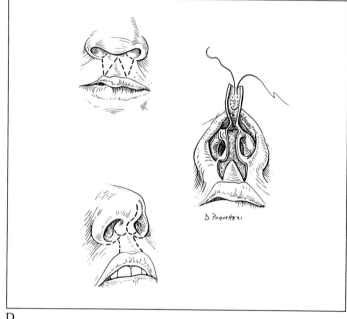

D

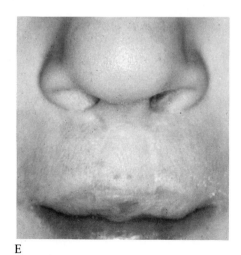

E

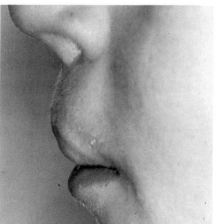

F

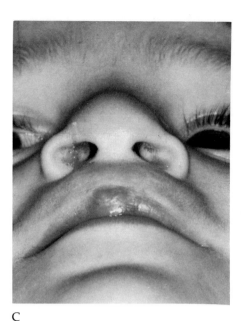

G

Table 44-2. Palatal fistulas

Location	Reconstructive options
Anterior palate (incisive foramen and forward)	Mucoperiosteal flaps of vomer, palate Buccal mucosal flaps Tongue flap
Midpalate	Mucoperiosteal flaps of vomer and palate Tongue flap
Posterior palate (soft palate–hard palate junction and back)	Palate repair redone with or without pharyngeal flap

pharyngeal incompetence is discussed in Chapters 45 to 47. The abnormal communication between the mouth and nasal passages can be a complication of palate repair or an intentional delay of repair in the anterior hard palate. Either way, closure can be difficult. Minimal tissue is available locally and it is often scarred. Visualization of the area is poor, and the narrow space makes manipulation of instruments and sutures difficult. Because secondary closure is so difficult, I repair the hard palate and anterior floor of the nose above the alveolus at the time of lip repair and before soft palate repair. With the lip and alveolus open, visualization is better and manipulation of instruments is less impaired. Evidence that early hard palate closure is more harmful to maxillary growth is not well substantiated, and the only advantage of waiting seems to occur when the hard palate is left open until the age of 12 or 14 years. The speech problem related to delayed hard palate closure is well documented.

Once an oronasal fistula exists, the questions to be answered are if, when, and how it should be repaired. The answers to these questions depend on the presence or absence of symptoms, where the fistula is located, and whether there have been previous attempts at closure.

Symptoms related to fistulas include nasal regurgitation of food; speech problems; drainage of thick mucus from the nose to the mouth, especially during upper respiratory infections; and problems of dental hygiene if the fistula is adjacent to the alveolus and there is accompanying bony deficiency. The smaller the fistula and the more anterior it is, the less likely it is to produce troublesome symptoms.

Not all fistulas need to be or should be closed surgically. Totally asymptomatic fistulas need no treatment. Large fistulas, especially after repeated attempts at closure, might be best treated with a prosthetic obturator. The majority of fistulas, however, should be considered for surgical closure.

Timing of the repair and the technique to be used must be determined (Table 44-2). Anterior fistulas should be repaired at the time of alveolar maxillary bone grafting. The local tissue used to close the fistula is generally the same as would be used to cover the bone graft and should be saved for this combined procedure. The exception to this rule is a very large and symptomatic fistula, which should be closed earlier; the additional scar tissue would make orthodontic correction and later bone grafting more difficult. On one occasion, in an adult with a recalcitrant anterior fistula, I used a tongue flap for closure.

Symptomatic fistulas in the middle and posterior palate should be closed early, especially if they are thought to be causing a speech problem. Timing is influenced by the need for maxillary expansion, and good communication between the surgeon and orthodontist is required. I prefer to close fistulas after expansion because the true tissue needs are more obvious and there is less likelihood of reopening than when the expansion is done after the repair.

Table 44-2 outlines the different techniques of closure that I have used. In general a two-layer closure is preferred, but if local tissue is sparse and scarred, I prefer one good layer of repair to two poor layers. Releasing incisions and the development of true transposition or advancement flaps are often required. Care has to be taken in planning these flaps to avoid producing a fistula elsewhere or shortening the soft palate. Previous pal-

ate dissection and scars must be respected to ensure an adequate blood supply to the local flaps. All flaps should contain mucosa and periosteum, and closure should be tension free.

The use of tissue from off the palate is occasionally necessary. Tongue flaps and buccal and labial mucosal flaps are the usual options. Arterialized musculomucosal flaps have been described; either the buccal artery or the facial artery is used as the vascular pedicle. Additionally, tissue expansion at the edge of the fistula has been described to obtain more tissue for a successful closure. I have not used any of these recently described techniques but have used tongue flaps in difficult, large, or recurrent fistulas.

Tongue flaps are quite versatile and often are the answer to difficult and recurrent fistulas (Fig. 44-10). Local flaps based on the edge of the fistula are turned over to provide nasal closure. This method produces a larger but fresh oral surface defect that is covered by the tongue flap. The dorsal, ipsilateral surface of the tongue is used for the flap. For anterior defects, the flap is based anteriorly, and for posterior defects the flap is based more posteriorly. It should be remembered that the anterior portion of the tongue is more mobile than the posterior part and can more comfortably be positioned within the mouth. The donor site on the tongue can be closed primarily, and the bridging portion of the flap is loosely tubed. Most if not all of the defect on the oral surface of the palate is closed in the first stage. Division and insetting of the flap is usually performed 3 weeks after the first stage. No special splinting or jaw fixation is required when the base of the tongue flap is planned to coincide with the location of the fistula.

Fig. 44-10. Top, anterior fistula in the hard palate and outline of an anteriorly based dorsal tongue flap. Center, local mucoperiosteal turnover flap to make nasal lining is completed. Tongue flap has been developed. Bottom, sagittal view of the dorsal tongue flap in place.

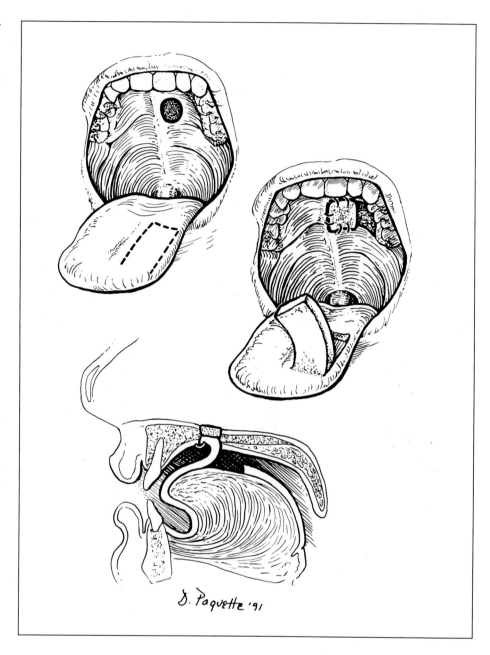

Suggested Reading

Kapetansky, D.I. Double pendulum flaps for whistling deformities in bilateral cleft lips. *Plast. Reconstr. Surg.* 47:321, 1971.

Kawamoto, H.K., Jr. Correction of major defects of vermilion with a cross-lip vermilion flap. *Plast. Reconstr. Surg.* 64:315, 1979.

Millard, D.R., Jr. *Cleft Craft: The Evolution of Its Surgery.* Vol. I. *The Unilateral Deformity.* Boston: Little, Brown, 1976.

Millard, D.R., Jr. *Cleft Craft: The Evolution of Its Surgery.* Vol. II. *Bilateral and Rare Deformities.* Boston: Little, Brown, 1977.

Thomson, H.G., and Hart, N.B. Reconstruction of cupid's bow: A quadrilateral flap technique. *Ann. Plast. Surg.* 22:195, 1989.

45

Velopharyngeal Insufficiency

Bonnie E. Smith   Thomas W. Guyette

Velopharyngeal Function

Normal Velopharyngeal Function

During normal speech production, the velum and pharynx act as a valve that channels airflow and acoustic energy into the oral and nasal cavities. During the production of nasal speech sounds—the consonants m, n, and ng—the velopharynx allows airflow and acoustic energy to enter the nasal cavities, causing resonance in the nasal chambers. During the production of oral speech sounds, including all vowel sounds and consonants other than m, n, and ng, the velum and the pharyngeal walls separate the oral from the nasal cavities. During conversational speech, the velum and pharyngeal walls must move rapidly to open the velopharyngeal port for nasal consonant production and close it for adjacent oral sounds. Given the time taken for velar movement, there is often a spread of nasalization to adjacent oral sounds. The ability to open and close the velopharynx rapidly so that speech has normal oronasal features constitutes velopharyngeal competence.

Air pressures and airflows are important products of the movements of speech sound articulators, including the velopharynx. In the production of most oral consonants, adults who speak normally achieve a peak pressure of approximately 5 to 7 cm H_2O in the oral cavity behind the site of oral constriction, with little nasal airflow. However, oral airflow occurs either in the form of a slow "leak" through a small oral opening, as in the fricative consonant /s/, or through quick release of a complete oral constriction, as in the plosive consonant /p/. It is the turbulent airflow caused by the constriction of the oral cavity that becomes the "noise" typical of the consonant sound.

Air pressure and airflow events are different during the production of nasal consonants. During nasal sounds, oral pressure is low (<1 cm H_2O) because of the large nasal cavity airflow leak, if the nasal cavity and velopharyngeal resistances are normal. The magnitude of nasal airflow ranges from 50 to 200 cc per second during the production of nasal consonants.

Abnormal Velopharyngeal Function

According to Peterson-Falzone, the term *velopharyngeal insufficiency* refers to closure problems related to "space" inadequacies such as when the velum is too short or the nasopharynx is too deep. Velopharyngeal insufficiency can be caused by anything that disturbs the normal space relations between the velum and the nasopharynx. Examples include congenital conditions such as overt cleft palate, submucous cleft palate, and congenitally short soft palate or deep nasopharynx.

Velopharyngeal insufficiency may cause three perceptual (speech) characteristics: hypernasality, nasal emission, and reduced aspiration and frication. The first feature, hypernasality, is the presence of too much nasal resonance, primarily during vowel production. The second perceptual feature, audible nasal emission of air, is produced by turbulent air flowing through the nasal cavities. The third speech symptom associated with velopharyngeal insufficiency is the perception of reduced aspiration and frication during consonant production; that is, consonants are perceived as "weak" because the velopharyngeal leak prohibits the accumulation of sufficient oral pressure to produce turbulent airflow. An impaired velopharyngeal mechanism may have a major impact on the pressure-flow patterns observed during speech. A person with velopharyngeal insufficiency experiences nasal airflow during production of oral consonant sounds, usually decreasing the magnitude of oral pressure.

A person may be judged to have borderline velopharyngeal function, exhibiting hypernasality, nasal emission, or reduced aspiration and frication either inconsistently or mildly. Morris defines two types of borderline velopharyngeal function. The first is the almost but not quite (ABNQ) category. These patients usually demonstrate consistent symptoms that are perceived as mild. It is hypothesized that these patients have a small but consistent velopharyngeal opening during oral speech sounds. The second group is the sometimes but not always (SBNA) category. These patients usually exhibit inconsistent symptoms. For example, they may be hypernasal in conversational speech but able to repeat words and phrases with normal resonance balance. Even on speech samples of the same type, they may exhibit symptoms inconsistently.

Another type of velopharyngeal disturbance occurs when the velopharynx does not open sufficiently during the production of nasal sounds. Causes of such velopharyngeal obstruction include an excessively wide pharyngeal flap and hypertrophy of the adenoids. If the degree of obstruction is great enough, the perceived (speech) characteristic hyponasality results. Hyponasality describes the condition in which not enough acoustic energy can pass into the nasal cavities. In severe instances, audible aspiration during nasal consonants also occurs. In this phenomenon, the nasal consonants, such as /m/ and /n/, acquire characteristics of their oral cognates, such as /b/ and /d/. Aerodynamically, notable velopharyngeal obstruction causes an inability to generate adequate nasal airflows and, therefore, results in increased intraoral pressures during production of nasal consonants. This situation may cause nasal consonants to take on aerodynamic properties more like their corresponding oral consonants.

A mixed type of velopharyngeal disturbance also can occur. In this instance, the velopharyngeal mechanism provides neither adequate closure for oral sounds nor adequate opening for nasal sounds. The resultant speech may be characterized by oronasal resonance balance, which varies between hyper- and hyponasality. This situation may occur after pharyngeal flap operations when a wide flap obstructs airflow during nasal sounds but has lateral ports that cannot be sufficiently closed by pharyngeal wall movement during production of oral sounds.

Diagnosis

Because these patients often have medical or social problems in addition to the velopharyngeal defect, interdisciplinary cleft palate or craniofacial teams plan the comprehensive treatment of people with velopharyngeal insufficiency. Only by planning and careful consideration of all the patient's needs can the most appropriate and beneficial care be delivered.

Important to the management of velopharyngeal insufficiency is the accurate diagnosis of the disorder and its impact on speech production. Techniques or measurements used to assess velopharyngeal function generally can be classified into three categories: (1) perceptual, including listener evaluations of speech production; (2) anatomic, including evaluations of velopharyngeal and nasal structures; and (3) physiologic, including evaluations of velopharyngeal and nasal function. Many measurement approaches provide information in more than one of these areas, and a complete diagnostic evaluation should provide information in each category. Our discussion includes the widely used measurement approaches, highlighting the approaches we use most often.

Patient History

Before testing we take an extensive history, especially noting clefting or velopharyngeal insufficiency in family members, a history of adenotonsillectomy or other orofacial and nasal procedures, a history of feeding or swallowing problems, including nasal regurgitation of liquids, a history of speech problems, and a history of frequent ear infections. If physical management of the velopharyngeal

valve is anticipated, we include questions to determine whether nasal airway obstruction exists, as indicated by the presence of decreased exercise tolerance, eating or swallowing problems, arrested growth, snoring, frequent awakenings at night, decreased sensations of smell and taste, personality change, morning headaches, daytime fatigue, frequent colds, or denasal speech. These responses and the results of the diagnostic tests determine whether the nasal airway needs to be managed to increase patency *before* an additional resistive load such as a pharyngeal flap is introduced into the airway.

What follows is a brief description of commonly used diagnostic instruments in relation to their primary category (perceptual, anatomic, or physiologic) and a discussion of the types of measurements they provide (objective versus subjective, direct versus indirect).

Perceptual Evaluation

Judgments of speech made by a qualified speech-language pathologist form an essential part of the evaluation of velopharyngeal function for speech. These judgments include the results of standardized speech sound (articulation) testing and ratings of oronasal resonance balance.

In children between 1 and 2 years of age, much can be learned about the function of the velopharyngeal mechanism through informal observation and parent reports. Using these means, we are able to establish the child's speech sound repertoire, obtain a general impression of oronasal resonance balance, and refer children for early speech therapy if problems are noted.

We usually begin administering standardized articulation tests when the patient is between 2 and 3 years of age. We complete articulation testing to determine whether speech sound errors related to velopharyngeal insufficiency exist. Such errors include weak production of plosive and fricative consonants, nasal emission of air during consonant sound production, and substitution of compensatory articulations for particular consonant sounds. Assessment of oronasal resonance balance includes judgments regarding the presence or absence of consistent or inconsistent mild, moderate, or severe hypernasality. When the nasal airway is obstructed, mild, moderate, or severe hyponasality may be present.

Once a history is obtained and perceptual testing is completed, we can make decisions about the need for additional assessment of the velopharyngeal valve and the nasal airway. As indicated earlier, instruments for the anatomic evaluation provide information about velopharyngeal and nasal form, and those for the physiologic evaluation provide information about velopharyngeal and nasal function. Many instruments provide information about both form and function.

Anatomic Evaluation

An intraoral examination is our first step in obtaining anatomic information about the velopharyngeal structures. At our center, this examination is often completed by a speech-language pathologist, a surgeon, and a dentist in the course of a team visit. This examination provides information about the presence, location, and size of palatal fistulas and the presence of tonsillar tissue. It also provides impressions about length, movement, and symmetry of the velum and direction, degree, and symmetry of visualized pharyngeal wall movement. In addition, if a corrective operation such as a pharyngeal flap has been performed, the intraoral examination should provide impressions about the width and position of the base of the flap, size of left and right ports, and degree of flap motion. A rhinoscopic examination is generally performed by a team physician to note the presence of hypertrophic turbinates, septal deviation, and nasal congestion or obstruction.

Instrumental approaches that provide direct views of internal body structures such as radiographic and endoscopic studies, sometimes referred to as image-based techniques, are frequently completed to provide additional anatomic information about the velopharynx and nasal cavities. Because they provide direct views of the structures being considered, the measurements being made at rest and at specific moments during movement, cephalometric roentgenograms are discussed with the anatomic evaluation. The techniques of endoscopic and multiview videofluoroscopy are frequently used to provide physiologic (movement) data in addition to anatomic information and therefore are discussed with the physiologic evaluation.

At our center, we obtain direct and quantitative information about the velopharyngeal and nasal structures using cephalometric roentgenography. These lateral view roentgenograms allow us to make observations concerning the structural relations of the velum and posterior pharyngeal wall. Cephalometric roentgenograms are taken at a standard distance of 5 feet from the middle of the skull to the source of radiation. The patient stands at a right angle to the x-ray source.

To evaluate velopharyngeal function, we first obtain a roentgenogram at rest (Fig. 45-1A). A speech sample is elicited from the patient while a second roentgenogram is taken (Fig. 45-1B). Many different samples have been used, including sustained vowels, sustained consonants, and repeated syllables. Our speech sample varies according to the speech skills of the patient being examined; however, it usually includes a sustained /s/ (sssssss) and may include a repeated syllable such as /pipipipipipi/ (peepeepeepeepeepee). Caution should be used when interpreting roentgenograms with sustained vowels and consonants because people who speak normally may not consistently demonstrate complete closure on these speech samples.

Cephalometric measurements commonly used in the evaluation of palatal function include the length of the soft palate, length of velar contact, velar height, velopharyngeal gap, cranial base angle, and depth of the nasopharynx. These measurements are illustrated in Figures 45-1C and D. Palatal length may be measured at rest or during speech. When palatal length is measured at rest, a straight line is drawn between the posterior nasal spine and the tip of the uvula. The "effective" length of the velum also may be obtained. According to Bateman and Mason, this measure is made during an oral speech sample and is defined as the distance between the posterior nasal spine and the distal nasal surface of the velum as measured along the palatal plane. The effective length of the palate would appear to be more closely related to velopharyngeal closure than velar length at rest.

The length of velar contact is defined as the distance between the superior and inferior borders of the velar contact. A long velopharyngeal contact suggests a strong, stable velopharyngeal closure pattern. A short velopharyngeal contact suggests a more borderline or incompetent mechanism.

There is a velopharyngeal gap when no velar contact is made with the posterior pharyngeal wall. The velopharyngeal gap is defined as the distance between the nasal surface of the velum and the posterior pharyngeal wall at the level of the palatal plane. Velar height is defined as the distance from the most superior portion of the soft palate (usually the velar eminence) to the palatal plane. The palatal plane is defined as a line extending in space between the posterior and anterior nasal spine. Most patients with adequate mechanisms can elevate the soft palate up to or above the palatal plane.

Pharyngeal depth is the distance between the posterior nasal spine and the anterior surface of the posterior pharyngeal wall measured along the palatal plane. This distance is used in conjunction with the palatal length measure to make inferences about the structural etiology of velopharyngeal insufficiency.

Another measure of pharyngeal depth is the cranial base angle. This angle is defined by drawing a line from nasion to sella to basion. According to Batemen and Mason, in most people who speak normally, this angle is 130° ± 10°. An angle less than 120° is an indication of a narrow nasopharynx. If the angle is greater than 140°, the patient is likely to have a wide or deep nasopharynx. This information is used in combination with measurements of palatal length to better understand velopharyngeal structures.

Several well-documented limitations of cephalometric measurements include the observation that the cephalometric view represents only one static instant in time and, therefore, does not adequately represent the dynamic aspects of palatal movement. Another limitation is that the cephalometric view is only two-dimensional. Thus closure may be observed on the roentgenogram when lateral openings are present. We find this technique more helpful in determining the structural relations that underlie velopharyngeal insufficiency once it has been diagnosed on the basis of speech and other techniques.

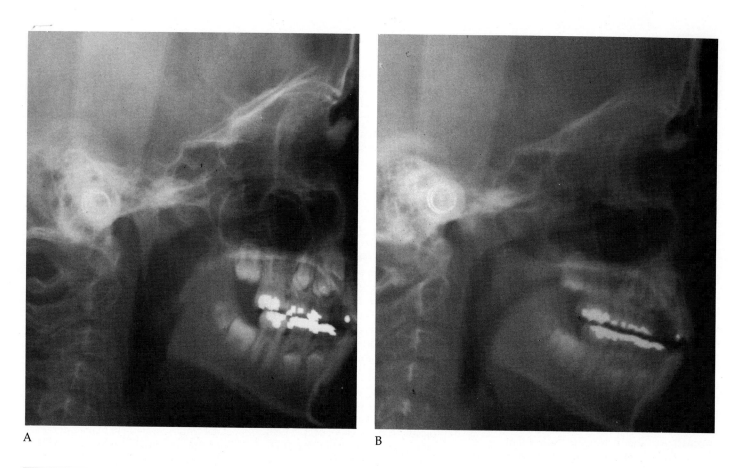

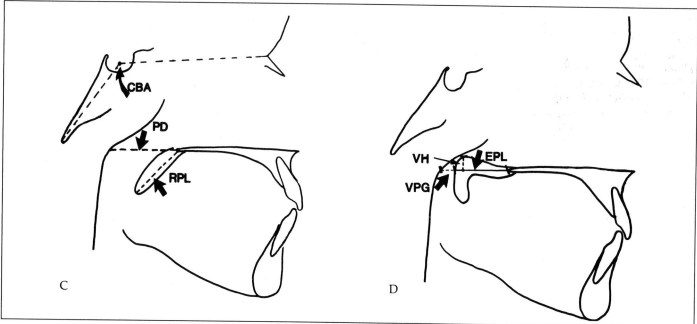

Fig. 45-1A. *Lateral cephalometric roentgenogram during breathing at rest. B. Lateral cephalometric roentgenogram during production of extended /s/. C. Tracing of lateral cephalometric roentgenogram during breathing at rest illustrating measurement of resting palatal length (RPL), pharyngeal depth (PD), and cranial base angle (CBA). D. Tracing of lateral cephalometric roentgenogram during /s/ production illustrating measurement of effective palatal length (EPL), velopharyngeal gap (VPG), and velar height (VH).*

Physiologic Evaluation

After information about velopharyngeal and nasal function is obtained as a result of completing the patient history and perceptual and anatomic evaluations, additional important information can be gained from other tests.

Nasopharyngoscopy and Multiview Videofluoroscopy

Nasopharyngoscopy and multiview videofluoroscopic techniques are used frequently to provide additional anatomic and physiologic information about velopharyngeal function. In providing direct visualization and images of internal structures, these techniques have been used to describe velopharyngeal closure patterns and pharyngeal wall motion. A primary limitation in using these techniques is their inability to provide absolute measurements of structural relations, as is possible using cephalometric roentgenography. A report of Golding-Kushner and colleagues, however, may guide the examiner in interpreting endoscopic and multiview videofluoroscopic images using, in part, ratios as opposed to absolute measurements. This study outlines quantitative (ratio) and qualitative (descriptive) information that can be obtained for the nasopharyngoscopic parameters of velar movement, lateral pharyngeal wall movement, posterior pharyngeal wall and Passavant ridge movement, and the velopharyngeal gap. All ratio data are derived by comparing the position of the structure at the point of maximal movement to the position of the structure at rest.

In multiview videofluoroscopy, ratio data and descriptive information like that obtained for endoscopy also are obtained for the en face (base or Towne) view. In addition, information regarding pharyngeal wall displacement, contour, direction, and symmetry of movement is obtained from the frontal view, and information on velar displacement, direction, contour, and location of movement is obtained from the lateral view.

The speech sample used during both nasopharyngoscopic and multiview fluoroscopic studies should elicit velopharyngeal movements like those that occur in conversational speech. The protocol recommended by Golding-Kushner and associates includes production of sustained consonants, consonant-vowel syllable combinations, and phrases. We also use repeated oral syllables such as /pipipipi-pipi/, repeated nasal syllables such as /mimimimimimi/, and select phrases such as "cut the cupcake" and "mama made lemon jam." Additional samples may be included, but the entire sample should be short enough to limit radiation exposure during videofluoroscopic evaluations.

For nasopharyngoscopic evaluations, the entire velopharyngeal orifice, including lateral and posterior pharyngeal walls, must be seen in each view. An example of nasopharyngoscopic information provided to assess velopharyngeal gap size (quantitative, ratio) and shape (qualitative) is shown in Figure 45-2. Complete closure is represented by 1.0, and 0.0 represents opening during rest. The degree of velopharyngeal opening during various speech tasks is assigned a number in accordance with these values. Qualitatively, gap shapes are described as coronal, sagittal, circular, or other, including irregularly shaped gaps.

Although nasopharyngoscopy provides substantial information about movement of the velum and pharyngeal walls, many factors need to be considered in interpre-

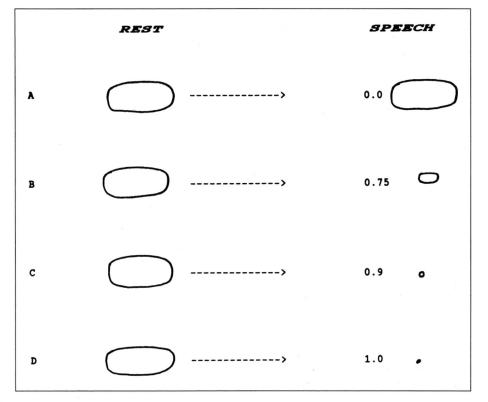

Fig. 45-2. Size of velopharyngeal opening measured by ratio system for nasopharyngoscopic and en face videofluoroscopic views. A. No movement during speech. B. Partial closure during speech. C. Only a bubble without a defined gap during speech. D. Complete closure during speech. (From K.J. Golding-Kushner and the International Working Group. Standardization for the reporting of nasopharyngoscopy and multiview videofluoroscopy: A report from an international working group. Cleft Palate J. 27:337, 1990. Reproduced with permission.)

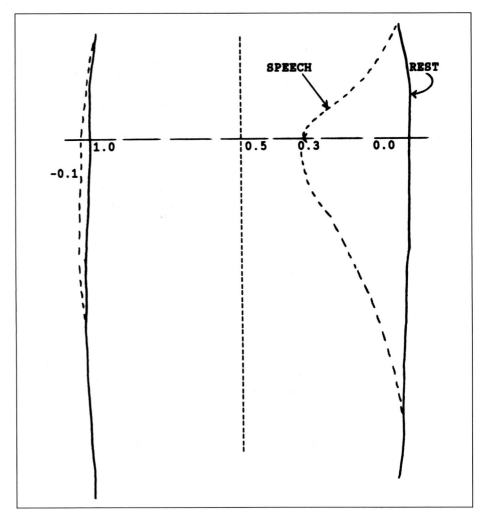

Fig. 45-3. Tracing of frontal videofluoroscopic view of lateral pharyngeal wall displacement using ratio system. (From K.J. Golding-Kushner and the International Working Group. Standardization for the reporting of nasopharyngoscopy and multiview videofluoroscopy: A report from an international working group. Cleft Palate J. 27:337, 1990. Reproduced with permission.)

tation of nasopharyngoscopic images. For example, placement of the endoscope is critical given that some placements do not include all the structures in question, such as the velum, posterior pharyngeal wall, and lateral pharyngeal walls. Inappropriate placement also may result in distorted images. In addition, the examiner cannot reliably detect extremely small velopharyngeal openings or the location (height) of velopharyngeal closure using endoscopy. Endoscopy also frequently involves administration of a topical anesthetic, which may influence nasal or velopharyngeal function. In addition, patient cooperation is critical if adequate information is to be obtained from these approaches.

A multiview videofluoroscopic study typically includes frontal and lateral projections; other views such as an en face (base or Towne) view can be added as indicated by Golding-Kushner and colleagues. Analysis of en face views is similar to that described for nasoendoscopic views. For the frontal view, lateral pharyngeal wall motion, typically in the region of the second cervical vertebra, is analyzed (Fig. 45-3).

In the lateral view, movement of the velum and posterior pharyngeal wall is described (Fig. 45-4). It should be noted that absolute, standardized measurements of palatal length, thickness, and pharyngeal depth cannot be obtained from lateral videofluoroscopic views; only relative (ratio) values of the size of the velopharyngeal opening can be obtained using nasopharyngoscopy or en face view videofluoroscopy, according to Golding-Kushner's group.

Aerodynamic Assessment

We find aerodynamic or pressure-flow evaluation of velopharyngeal function helpful in readily identifying velopharyngeal dysfunction. We use pressure-flow results to assist in distinguishing velopharyngeal insufficiency from dysfunc-

tions of the laryngeal or oral (tongue) valves during speech production. In addition, aerodynamic assessment provides us with valuable information about nasal airway patency, especially important in our planning of surgical management for velopharyngeal insufficiency. Aerodynamic techniques are examples of indirect assessment approaches because they measure the by-products of the processes being evaluated, for example, speech production or nasal respiration. Indirect approaches have also been referred to as signal-based methods.

We use the pressure-flow technique developed by Warren and Dubois to determine the presence and magnitude of velopharyngeal incompetence. The method also can be used to determine whether velopharyngeal obstruction exists (i.e., too little velopharyngeal opening during nasal sounds and nasal respiration). This technique measures simultaneous differential pressure across the velopharyngeal

orifice and the airflow through the orifice during speech production and uses these data to solve the modified hydrokinetic equation:

$$\text{Area (cm}^2) = V/K(2[P_1 - P_2)/d])^{\frac{1}{2}}$$

where V = nasal airflow
       P_1 = oral pressure
       P_2 = nasal pressure
       d = density of air (0.001)

and K = correction factor (0.65)

A pneumotachometer is used to measure airflow, and a differential pressure transducer is used to measure the pressure drop across the velopharynx. The output signals from the pressure-flow transducers may be amplified and conditioned (usually low-pass filtered) and recorded either in analog form (e.g., strip chart) or digitized and stored in a computer file for later analysis.

The interface between the patient and the

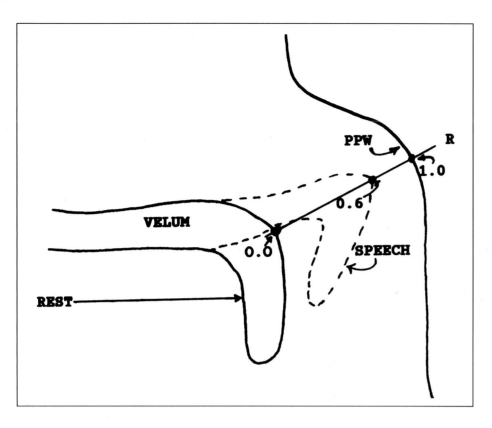

Fig. 45-4. Tracing of lateral videofluoroscopic view of referent line R using ratio measurement system. PPW = posterior pharyngeal wall. (From K.J. Golding-Kushner and the International Working Group. Standardization for the reporting of nasopharyngoscopy and multiview videofluoroscopy: A report from an international working group. Cleft Palate J. 27:337, 1990. Reproduced with permission.)

equipment is illustrated in Figure 45-5. To measure nasal airflow, a tube is inserted into the most open nostril and attached to the flowmeter. Nasal pressure is measured by a pressure probe inserted into the opposite nasal vestibule and connected to the pressure transducer. To measure oral pressure, a small catheter is inserted into the mouth just past the central incisors and attached to the flowmeter. All tube lengths are kept to a minimum to reduce pressure-flow measurement artifacts during speech events.

Once the tubes and probes are in place, we elicit a speech sample. We usually limit the speech sample to consonants that involve bilabial or labiodental closure, given the difficulty involved in measuring pressure behind tongue constrictions. Our typical speech protocol involves repetitions of consonant-vowel syllables such as /pi/, /fi/, /mi/, and /ma/ and repetitions of the word *hamper* during

Fig. 45-5. Interface between patient and equipment during pressure-flow assessment of velopharyngeal function for speech. Airflow tube is inserted into the patient's nasal vestibule (patient's right side in this figure). Nasal pressure probe is inserted into the opposite nasal vestibule. Oral pressure tube is inserted just past incisors. Pressures and flows are transduced to electrical signals, amplified, and displayed, along with the audio signal, on a computer screen.

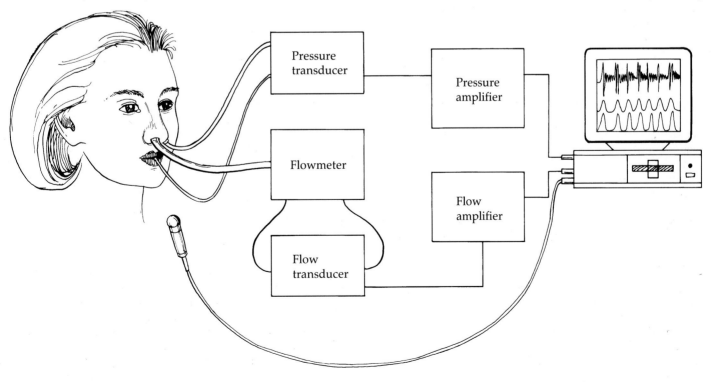

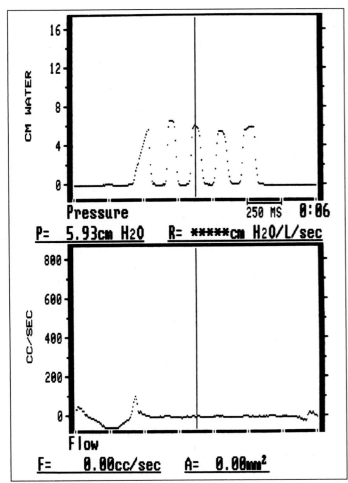

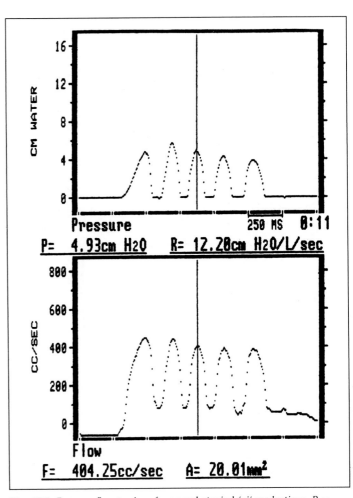

Fig. 45-6. *Representative pressure-flow tracings for several /pi/ productions by an adult who speaks normally. Values are displayed for the location of the cursor at the center of the figure. P = differential pressure; F = airflow rate; R = resistance; and A = cross-sectional area. (From M.L. Andreassen, B.E. Smith, and T.W. Guyette. Pressure-flow measurements for selected oral and nasal sound segments produced by normal adults. Cleft Palate Craniofac. J. 29:1, 1992. Reproduced with permission.)*

Fig. 45-7. *Pressure-flow tracings for several atypical /pi/ productions. P = differential pressure; F = airflow rate; R = resistance; A = cross-sectional area.*

which differential pressures, nasal airflow rates, and velopharyngeal orifice areas are measured. The consonant-vowel samples allow for sampling of both oral and nasal consonants and oral consonants of different types (plosive /p/ and fricative /f/). The word *hamper* is often included because, according to Warren, the nasal-plosive blend /mp/ in *hamper* approximates the degree of velopharyngeal opening and closing that normally occurs in conversational speech.

Once the speech sample has been recorded, pressure-flow tracings are examined. Figure 45-6 shows the graphic record of several /pi/ productions produced by an adult who speaks normally. Pressure values are in the range of 5 to 7

cm H_2O, and no nasal airflow is demonstrated. Figure 45-7 illustrates a similar pressure-flow tracing for a person who does not speak normally. This figure shows reductions of differential pressures and notable nasal airflow rates during /pi/ productions. To obtain an estimate of the size of the velopharyngeal opening for this speaker, pressure and flow values are measured simultaneously from the peak of nasal airflow. In this illustration, the differential pressure is 4.93 cm H_2O, the nasal airflow rate is 404.25 cc per second, and the velopharyngeal orifice area is 20.01 mm^2 at the cursor line.

Figure 45-8 illustrates a graphic record of several /mi/ productions produced by an adult who speaks normally. Pressure

peak values are minimal (<0.50 cm H_2O) given the relatively open velopharyngeal port for this nasal sound segment. Peak nasal airflow values are 100 to 150 cc per second. At the cursor location, the differential pressure is 0.39 cm H_2O, the nasal airflow rate is 127.05 cc per second, and the oronasal opening is 22.36 mm^2 for /mi/.

Figure 45-9 illustrates a similar pressure-flow tracing for a person who does not speak normally. This figure shows increases in differential pressure and reductions in nasal airflow rate, leading to a calculated oronasal opening of only 7.01 mm^2 for the one /mi/ production shown at the cursor location. This decrease in velopharyngeal opening suggests some de-

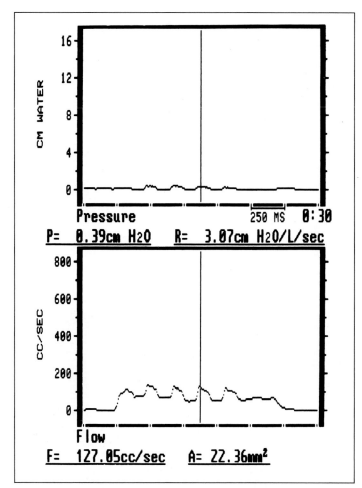

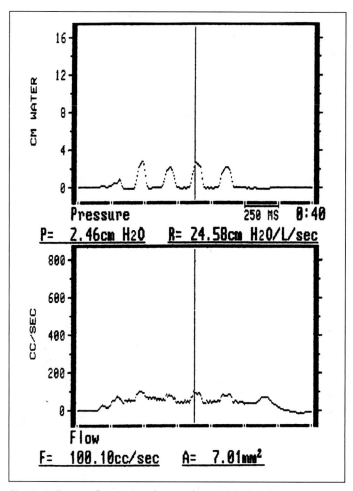

Fig. 45-8. Representative pressure-flow tracings for several /mi/ productions by an adult who speaks normally. P = differential pressure; F = airflow rate; R = resistance; A = cross-sectional area. (From M.L. Andreassen, B.E. Smith, and T.W. Guyette. Pressure-flow measurements for selected oral and nasal sound segments produced by normal adults. Cleft Palate Craniofac. J. 29:1, 1992. Reproduced with permission.)

Fig. 45-9. Pressure-flow tracings for several atypical /mi/ productions. P = differential pressure; F = airflow rate; R = resistance; A = cross-sectional area.

gree of velopharyngeal obstruction (e.g., an obstructive pharyngeal flap) in this speaker.

Typically we use 10 productions of each consonant-vowel syllable and 3 to 6 productions of *hamper* to obtain mean, standard deviation, and range values for differential pressures, nasal airflow rates, and velopharyngeal orifice areas. The timing relations between flow and pressure landmarks during production of *hamper* have been reported by Warren.

On the basis of our pressure-flow clinical and research data for both oral and nasal sound segments produced by adults who speak normally, we use four categories to characterize velopharyngeal physiology

for speech using area estimates—one typical category and three atypical categories (open, closed, and mixed). These velopharyngeal functional categories and their area cutoffs for oral and nasal sound segments are shown in Table 45-1. The typical category represents the physiologic, that is, aerodynamic, characteristics of normal speech for the sounds. Speakers who have velopharyngeal areas greater than those shown for oral sounds would be considered atypical in that their velopharyngeal valves are more open than typical valves. Speakers whose velopharyngeal areas are smaller than those shown for the nasal segments would be considered atypical in that their valves are closed to a greater degree than usually

found in persons with normal speech. The mixed category constitutes speakers who have greater than typical openings for the oral sounds and less than typical openings for the nasal sounds. In interpreting area values, we note that different criteria may exist for different speech protocol items and that the areas provided in Table 45-1 are cutoff values for the specific items tested only.

We use aerodynamic techniques to assess nasal patency also. The measurement of nasal airway patency is important in the clinical management of velopharyngeal insufficiency because the patients may have congenital orofacial and nasal structural defects in addition to the velopharyngeal defects. In addition, these pa-

Table 45-1. Characterization of velopharyngeal valving for speech using selected utterances

Category	X̄ VP area for orals (mm²)				X̄ VP area for nasals (mm²)		
	/pi/ (n = 10)	/fi/ (n = 10)	/pa/ (n = 10)	/p/ in *hamper* (n = 3)	/mi/ (n = 10)	/ma/ (n = 10)	/m/ in *hamper* (n = 3)
1. Typical	≤1	≤1	≤5	≤3	≥20	≥27	≥13
2. Atypical—open	>1	>1	>5	>3	≥20	≥27	≥13
3. Atypical—closed	≤1	≤1	≤5	≤3	<20	<27	<13
4. Atypical—mixed	>1	>1	>5	>3	<20	<27	<13

VP = velopharyngeal.
From M.L. Andreassen, B.E. Smith, and T.W. Guyette. Pressure-flow measurements for selected oral and nasal sound segments produced by normal adults. *Cleft Palate Craniofac. J.* 29:1, 1992. Reproduced with permission.

tients are at risk for airway obstruction secondary to surgical management of their velopharyngeal defects, as in patients with an obstructive pharyngeal flap.

Traditional aerodynamic approaches to assessing nasal airway patency include anterior and posterior rhinomanometry. In these approaches, nasal airway resistance is determined by dividing the airflow rate through the nasal airway by the differential pressure across the airway. In anterior rhinomanometry, the pressure drop is measured across the nasal cavities (from the choanae to the nasal vestibule). In posterior rhinomanometry, the pressure drop is measured across the entire nasal airway, including both velopharynx and nasal cavities. Neither of these methods provides information about the relative contributions of the airway components (velopharyngeal and nasal) to the total nasal airway resistance.

We recommend an aerodynamic approach that partitions the nasal airway into its nasal cavity and velopharyngeal components. In the component approach, the calculation of nasal and velopharyngeal resistances during breathing follows the principles of Ohm's law; that is, in partitioning the nasal airway, the nasal cavities are viewed as two resistors in a parallel circuit. Add to this parallel circuit a resistor in series, the velopharynx, and the result is a combination series-parallel circuit.

For the component approach, the procedure for obtaining nasal cavity resistance

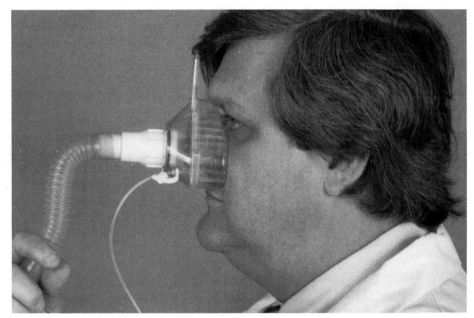

Fig. 45-10. *Patient-to-instrumentation interface for anterior rhinomanometry. The patient wears a nose mask to measure nasal airflow. A pressure probe is inserted into the nostril opposite the one being tested to measure nasal cavity pressure.*

is similar to that described for anterior rhinomanometry (Fig. 45-10). Nasal airflow is collected using a clear anesthesia face mask held gently against the patient's face. Nasal pressure is measured through a catheter secured by tape to the patient's contralateral nostril. The patient is seated and relaxed before the test is begun and is instructed to breathe through the nose in as relaxed a manner as possible. Once a recording of nasal breathing is made, the nasal pressure catheter is inserted into the opposite nostril, and the resistance of the other nostril is measured.

The procedure for measuring velopharyngeal resistance is similar to that described by Warren and DuBois. The patient's most open nasal passage (as determined during the foregoing procedure) is fitted with a clear plastic tube, which is attached to a pneumotachometer screen. A pressure-sensing device is inserted into the patient's opposite nos-

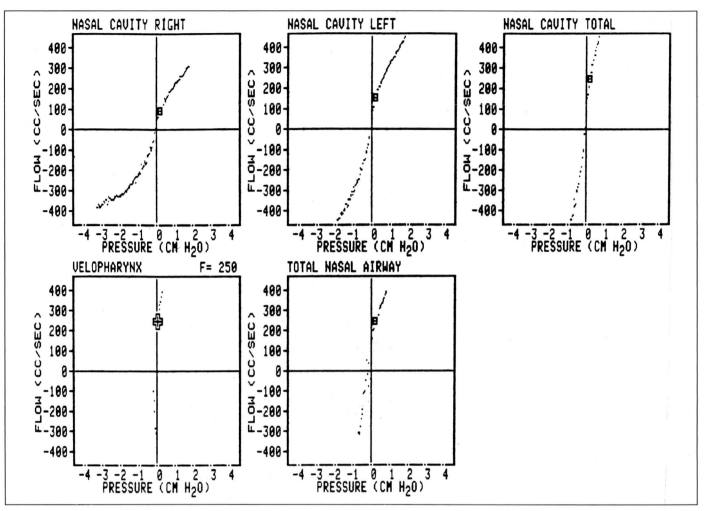

Fig. 45-11. Pressure-flow plots for the right nasal cavity, left nasal cavity, total nasal cavities, velopharynx, and total nasal airway for an adult who breathes normally through the nose.

tril to measure nasal cavity pressure. Oral pressure is measured with a small tube inserted into the patient's mouth just posterior to the lips. The patient-to-instrumentation interface for obtaining velopharyngeal resistance measurements and the instrumentation used in rhinomanometry are shown in Figure 45-5.

After pressure-flow recordings are obtained for the right and left nasal cavities and the velopharynx during nasal respiration, a computer software program (ICS Speech Mastr) allows the examiner to analyze inhalational and exhalational portions of each tracing to obtain graphic displays of inhalational and exhalational pressure-flow plots for the right and left nasal passages, the total nasal cavity, the velopharynx, and the total nasal airway (Fig. 45-11). Average pressures, flows, resistances, and areas are displayed in Table 45-2 along with the percent contribution

Table 45-2. Nasal breathing data (differential pressure, nasal airflow rate, resistance, and cross-sectional area) at 250 cc/sec for an adult who breathes normally and percent contribution of the total nasal cavities and velopharyngeal region to the total nasal airway

	Pressure (cm H_2O)	Flow (cc/sec)	Resistance (cm H_2O/L/sec)	Area (mm²)
Nasal cavity, right	0.23	96.15	2.39	22.03
Nasal cavity, left	0.23	153.85	1.49	35.25
Nasal cavity, total	0.23	250.00	0.92	57.28
Velopharynx	0.08	250.00	0.31	99.05
Total nasal airway	0.31	250.00	1.23	49.59

NCR = 0.92 (75% contribution)
VPR = 0.31 (25% contribution)
NAR = 1.23

Velopharyngeal flow = 250.00 cc per second.
NCR = total nasal cavities; VPR = velopharyngeal region; NAR = total nasal airway.

of the total nasal cavity and velopharynx to the total nasal airway resistance.

Table 45-2 shows such information for an adult who speaks normally. As these data indicate, overall nasal airway resistance is minimal, the nasal cavities contributing most to total airway resistance. Table 45-3 shows similar information for a patient with a pharyngeal flap. The total nasal airway resistance is substantially increased, the greatest contribution coming from the velopharyngeal region. Research and clinical reports suggest that difficulties with nasal respiration arise when the total nasal airway resistance exceeds 3.0 to 4.0 cm H_2O/liter/second. The information in Table 45-3 suggests that this patient has nasal respiration difficulties largely attributable to the pharyngeal flap.

Acoustic Assessment

Acoustic approaches provide indirect, quantitative measurements of velopharyngeal function by measuring changes in nasal resonance (acoustic energy) that occur with greater or lesser degrees of coupling between the oral and nasal cavities. An acoustic instrument developed and used as part of an evaluation of velopharyngeal function is the Nasometer (Kay Elemetrics Corp.). This instrument requires that the patient wear headgear, to which oral and nasal microphones are attached (Fig. 45-12). The patient is instructed to speak; usually a standard phonetically structured passage is read. The Nasometer provides, in real time, the ratio of the acoustic energy from the oral and nasal cavities. In children with velopharyngeal insufficiency, excessive acoustic energy in the nasal cavity is observed during reading of passages containing primarily oral sounds. In children with velopharyngeal obstruction, insufficient acoustic energy in the nasal cavity is observed during reading of passages containing many nasal sounds. Given that they are provided simultaneously with the speech produced, these data can be used as biofeedback in diagnostic or treatment sessions. Additional information concerning the use and the interpretation of Nasometer ratios, as well as levels of functioning, should be considered in conjunction with the results of perceptual, anatomic, and physiologic testing to form a complete picture of velopharyngeal function for speech and, as needed, nasal airway patency.

Table 45-3. Nasal breathing data for a patient who has had a pharyngeal flap operation

	Pressure (cm H_2O)	Flow (cc/sec)	Resistance (cm H_2O/L/sec)	Area (mm^2)
Nasal cavity, right	0.31	64.10	4.84	12.65
Nasal cavity, left	0.31	166.67	1.86	32.90
Nasal cavity, total	0.31	230.77	1.34	45.55
Velopharynx	1.23	230.77	5.33	22.86
Total nasal airway	1.54	230.77	6.67	20.43

NCR = 1.34 (20% contribution)
VPR = 5.33 (80% contribution)
NAR = 6.67

Velopharyngeal flow = 230.77 cc per second.
NCR = total nasal cavities; VPR = velopharyngeal region; NAR = total nasal airway.

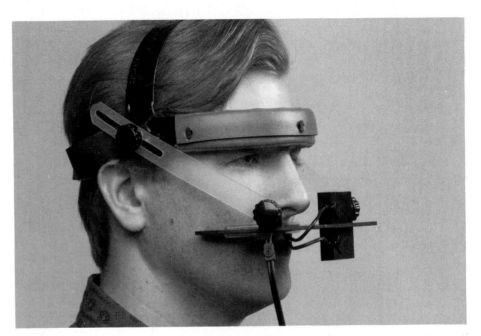

Fig. 45-12. A patient wearing a Nasometer headpiece containing nasal and oral microphones and a sound separator plate. This device allows the speech signal to be displayed as the ratio of nasal to oral-plus-nasal sound energy.

Occasionally perceptual, anatomic, and physiologic tests provide contradictory results. When perceptual testing and patient reports show normal speech but anatomic and physiologic measurements suggest a velopharyngeal disturbance, patients should be retested at regular intervals because of the possibility that future management may be required. When perceptual testing and patient reports reveal abnormal speech but anatomic or physiologic results indicate normal velopharyngeal function, testing, including expanded protocols, should be repeated or trial speech therapy should be initiated in an attempt to identify anatomic or physiologic factors underlying the perceptions of abnormal speech.

Management

Management of velopharyngeal insufficiency includes behavioral (speech therapy) or physical (prosthetic and surgical) approaches. Speech therapy includes techniques intended to improve velopharyngeal function by strengthening the velopharyngeal musculature, increasing the range of motion of these muscles, or improving the skill with which the muscles are used. Speech therapy techniques also have focused on teaching the patient to reduce the degree of hypernasality perceptible in his or her speech by attempting to speak with a more open oral cavity. Some clinicians also have used biofeedback (acoustic and aerodynamic) devices to teach patients to reduce the amount of nasal coupling during speech sound production.

Clinical experience and research reports suggest that speech therapy generally is not effective in improving velopharyngeal insufficiency, except possibly when velopharyngeal dysfunction is inconsistently present or very mild. In these instances, speech therapy should be completed on a trial basis only. These patients frequently eventually require physical management.

Prosthetic management, that is, fabrication of a speech bulb prosthesis, is often considered when surgical intervention is contraindicated. The anterior portion of the speech bulb is constructed of hard plastic and attaches to the patient's maxillary molars. The posterior portion of the device comprises a metal wire that extends backward and follows the contour of the palate, curving upward between the palate and the nasopharynx. On the wire portion between the palate and the nasopharynx, a hard palate "bulb" is fabricated that fills this space and allows for complete velopharyngeal closure. This device may be used as interim treatment for a child who has velopharyngeal insufficiency after primary surgical repair but who is not yet a candidate for a secondary procedure. Prosthetic management also is advised for patients for whom surgical management would likely result in airway obstruction, for whom surgical treatment could not completely obturate the palatal defect, or for whom an operation is otherwise not indicated.

For most patients with velopharyngeal insufficiency, surgical treatment is the recommended form of management. There is some controversy regarding the relation between patient age at the time of primary palatal repair and speech outcome. For example, Dorf and Curtin studied a total of 131 patients and examined speech outcomes when palatal closure was completed early, before one year of age, rather than late, after one year of age. Their results suggest that more normal speech development (defined as an absence of compensatory articulations) exists when palatal closure occurs before a child is 12 months of age. In contrast, a study by Peterson-Falzone of 240 children indicated a notably smaller percentage of compensatory articulations and did not find a dramatic difference between the frequency of children with compensatory articulations in the early versus late surgical groups. These findings indicate that more research is needed to determine whether there is a relation between the patient's age at the time of the operation on the palate and the development of abnormal speech.

For all surgical procedures designed to establish velopharyngeal competence, we need additional data to evaluate surgical outcomes. We suggest that a thorough patient history, perceptual ratings, and anatomic and physiologic measurements be obtained before and at designated intervals after the operation, for example, 6 to 8 weeks, 6 months, 1 year, and 2 years postoperatively, depending on the patient's age, the ease of testing, the cooperation of the patient and the family, growth factors, and surgical results. Comprehensive, regularly completed (longitudinal) evaluations of velopharyngeal and nasal function, as described here and as conducted by cleft palate or craniofacial teams, allow examiners to evaluate not only the outcome of their management techniques but also the adequacy and timing of specific techniques and the adequacy of patient selection procedures. This system may identify factors leading to successful surgical results and thus answer questions regarding how and when velopharyngeal insufficiency should be managed to provide optimal results.

Suggested Reading

Andreassen, M.L., Smith, B.E., and Guyette, T.W. Pressure-flow measurement for selected oral and nasal sound segments produced by normal adults. *Cleft Palate Craniofac. J.* 29:1, 1992.

Bateman, H., and Mason, R. *Applied Anatomy and Physiology of the Speech and Hearing Mechanism.* Springfield, Ill.: Thomas, 1984.

Dorf, D.S., and Curtin, J.W. Early Cleft Palate Repair and Speech Outcome: A Ten-Year Experience. In J. Bardach and H. Morris (Eds.), *Multidisciplinary Management of Cleft Lip and Palate.* Philadelphia: Saunders, 1990. Pp. 341–348.

Golding-Kushner, K.J., and International Working Group. Standardization of the reporting of nasopharyngoscopy and multiview videofluoroscopy: A report from an international working group. *Cleft Palate J.* 27:337, 1990.

McWilliams, B.J., Morris, H.L., and Shelton, R.L. *Cleft Palate Speech.* Philadelphia: Decker, 1990.

Morris, H.L. Types of Velopharyngeal Incompetence. In H. Wentz (Ed.), *Treating Articulation Disorders: For Clinicians by Clinicians.* Baltimore: University Park Press, 1984.

Peterson-Falzone, S.J. Speech Disorders Related to Craniofacial Structural Defects: Parts 1 and 2. In N.J. Lass et al. (Eds.), *Handbook of Speech-Language Pathology and Audiology.* Toronto: Decker, 1988. Pp. 477–591.

Peterson-Falzone, S.J. A Cross-Sectional Analysis of Speech Results Following Palatal Closure. In J. Bardach and H. Morris (Eds.), *Multidisciplinary Management of Cleft Lip and Palate.* Philadelphia: Saunders, 1990. Pp. 750–757.

Smith, B.E., Fiala, J.F., and Guyette, T.W. Partitioning model nasal airway persistence into its nasal cavity and velopharyngeal components. *Cleft Palate J.* 26:327, 1985.

Warren, D.W., et al. A pressure-flow technique for quantifying temporal patterns of palatopharyngeal closure. *Cleft Palate J.* 22:11, 1985.

Warren, D.W., and DuBois, A.B. A pressure-flow technique for assessing velopharyngeal orifice area during continuous speech. *Cleft Palate J.* 1:52, 1964.

46

Pharyngeal Flaps for the Correction of Velopharyngeal Insufficiency

William C. Trier

There may be an advantage to using the inclusive term *velopharyngeal inadequacy* when labeling the clinical entity characterized by hypernasality and nasal escape of air and sound during phonation. *Velopharyngeal incompetency* is the inability to close the velopharyngeal sphincter because of neuromuscular dysfunction. *Velopharyngeal insufficiency* is the inability to close the velopharyngeal sphincter because of an anatomic defect such as a cleft palate, a short palate, or an excessively large pharynx. This discussion is more than a semantic one because, as a number of clinicians argue, the precise nature of velopharyngeal inadequacy may determine the particular treatment. There can be no argument, however, that structural alteration of the velopharyngeal orifice must occur to correct velopharyngeal inadequacy. Management may range from prosthetic devices and speech appliances, such as speech bulbs and palatal lift appliances, to surgical procedures that include pharyngeal wall and palatal augmentation by injection or implantation of various materials, pharyngoplasty, sphincter pharyngoplasty, and the pharyngeal flap operation.

Anatomy and Physiology

Closure of the velopharyngeal sphincter is required for the correct phonation of all vowels and all consonants except for /n/ and /m/ and the blend /ng/. Sphincter closure depends on the contraction of the paired levator veli palatini muscles and the superior pharyngeal constrictor muscle acting as a sphincter. Some reports indicate a role also for the paired palatopharyngeus muscles and the musculus uvulae. Muscle contraction produces both upward and backward movement of the soft palate along with medial movement of the lateral pharyngeal walls. The muscles of the soft palate, with the exception of the tensor veli palatini, are innervated by the pharyngeal plexus from the IXth, Xth, and XIth cranial nerves. The bulbar portion of the XIth cranial nerve—the pharyngeal branch of the vagus nerve—provides motor innervation. Sensation is through the lesser palatine nerve from the glossopharyngeal nerve.

The valvelike, or sphincteric, action of the velopharyngeal orifice is a soft palate–pharyngeal muscle activity. There must

also be an intact hard palate, however, including the alveolar processes of the maxilla. Although unrepaired alveolar clefts are unlikely to cause hypernasality and nasal emission, a fistula of the hard or soft palate or both may be the cause.

Diagnosis

The examination and evaluation of patients with speech disorders that appear to be related to structural abnormalities of the oropharyngeal area are best conducted by an interdisciplinary team composed of speech pathologists, plastic surgeons, otologists, audiologists, and various dental specialists, including orthodontists, pedodontists, prosthodontists, and oral surgeons. In addition, of course, a pediatrician or other primary care physician, social worker, psychologist, and patient care coordinator are, if not essential, at least extremely important to an effective team. All these professionals should have experience and special skills in the evaluation and treatment of patients with orofacial disorders. Examination and evaluation by a representative of each of the disciplines is required, followed by a face-to-face meeting of team members for presentation of findings, recommendations, and agreement on a treatment plan.

Specific diagnostic measures include, of course, the history and physical examination, a speech and language evaluation, and an audiologic evaluation. Except for the last, each team member should carry out not only the evaluation appropriate to his or her discipline but also as complete an examination as possible in other disciplines. The plastic surgeon, for example, should evaluate the patient's speech and defects or abnormalities of the jaws and teeth. This practice not only enhances patient care but also educates team members and leads to improved communication among them.

In addition to the basic evaluation, consideration must be given to special diagnostic studies. In my experience, pressure-flow studies are the most useful because they provide the size of the velopharyngeal orifice in phonation, a clearly objective measurement.

A number of clinicians emphasize nasopharyngoscopy and videofluoroscopy. Both these techniques provide more information regarding the area of velopharyngeal closure than the degree of closure. Both methods, along with pressure-flow studies, require patient cooperation, which decreases in younger children. Videofluoroscopy, of course, carries the additional concern of radiation exposure. There appears to be particular value to nasopharyngoscopy for patients who have undergone previous pharyngeal flap operations or pharyngoplasty whether or not a fistula is present to determine the anatomic location of attempted velopharyngeal closure, the size of the lateral pharyngeal ports in phonation and at rest, and the size and position of the previous pharyngeal flap.

Indications for a Pharyngeal Flap Operation

The ideal candidate for a pharyngeal flap operation is a healthy child with velopharyngeal inadequacy who is older than 4 years, who has normal hearing and intelligence, whose articulation is normal, who has good lateral pharyngeal wall mo-

tion, and who has class I or class II dental occlusion. Relatively few patients, however, have such clear-cut characteristics.

The primary indication for a pharyngeal flap is velopharyngeal inadequacy. Patients about whom there is diagnostic doubt because of faulty articulation should undergo speech remediation and have the operation delayed until the diagnosis is certain. If the velopharyngeal inadequacy is believed to be responsible for the faulty articulation, a worthwhile compromise is fabrication of a temporary speech appliance until articulation is normal and a decision has been made regarding continuing use of the appliance or performing a pharyngeal flap operation. If the patient is in an obturator reduction program, he or she may be able to discard the appliance without requiring an operation.

Patients with health problems may not be candidates for any operative procedure unless the coexisting problems can be corrected. Because of the adverse effect of hearing loss on speech, every effort should be made to provide auditory acuity before or at the same time as the pharyngeal flap operation; tympanostomy tubes may need to be inserted at the time of the flap operation.

As noted, the chief value of nasopharyngoscopy and videofluoroscopy appears to be the determination of the site of velopharyngeal closure and the extent of medial movement of the lateral pharyngeal walls. The less medial pharyngeal wall movement there is, the wider the flap needs to be and the greater the likelihood of hyponasality, denasality, or obstructive sleep apnea. A number of clinicians have noted increased medial movement of the lateral pharyngeal walls in response to a speech appliance. One might conjecture that increased lateral pharyngeal wall motion would result from a pharyngeal flap operation, but there is no clear evidence that it does.

Finally, patients with class III occlusion who are likely to require maxillary advancement should have pharyngeal flap operations postponed until a definite decision regarding an orthognathic operation can be made. A speech appliance should be used until at least a year after maxillary advancement to lessen the likelihood of relapse of the orthognathic correction.

A primary pharyngeal flap operation should *not* be performed at the usual time of a primary palatoplasty, when the patient is between 1 year and 18 months of age. Needless pharyngeal flaps would be provided in 10 to 40 percent of patients, the number of patients reportedly having velopharyngeal inadequacy after palatoplasty. It is reasonable to perform a pharyngeal flap operation at the time of primary palatoplasty if complete palatal repair is not otherwise technically feasible.

A primary pharyngeal flap operation may be performed in a patient older than 2 years of age with an unrepaired cleft or a patient with a submucous cleft palate with velopharyngeal inadequacy. In the latter patient, diagnosis commonly has been made late, and in the former, considerable delay has made it essential to provide an adequate velopharyngeal mechanism as quickly as possible. The wait before an accurate evaluation of speech can be made and the presence of long-standing compensatory articulations that require prompt correction make these patients an exception.

Timing of a Pharyngeal Flap Operation

Depending on the phonologic development of an infant, provision of an adequate velopharyngeal mechanism should be made by the time the patient is 12 months of age. Palatoplasty in an infant with a wide cleft may have to be postponed until the patient is 16 months of age. It is extremely important to achieve uncomplicated repair of the palate, and the wide cleft may make earlier repair difficult. There is clear evidence that narrowing and shortening of the palatal cleft occurs between 3 and 17 months of age.

Speech development may not allow a definite diagnosis of velopharyngeal inadequacy until the patient is 2 to 3 years of age or older. Also, the so-called objective methods of evaluation such as pressure-flow studies, nasopharyngoscopy, and videofluoroscopy may not be possible until the patient is 4 or 5 years of age. Certainly the pharyngeal flap operation, when indicated, is ideally performed shortly before the child is 5 years of age or at any time afterward.

Associated Procedures

There may be associated operations that can be performed under the same induction of anesthesia as the pharyngeal flap operation. Certainly this is an opportunity to examine the middle ear and replace tympanostomy tubes, if necessary, or to perform a myringotomy and insert tympanostomy tubes. In patients who have a cleft lip in addition to a cleft palate, there is an opportunity for lip revision, nose revision, closure of palatal fistulas, and alveolar bone grafting. For technical reasons the pharyngeal flap is performed first, the Dingman mouth gag is removed, and the additional procedures are carried out. Collaboration among the surgical specialists on the cleft palate team—plastic surgeon, otologist, and oral surgeon—can be of great benefit to the patient.

Pharyngeal Flap Operation

Preoperative Care

It has become essentially impossible to admit patients for elective operations on the day before the operation. Insurance companies and funding agencies do not reimburse expenses for an additional day of hospitalization. Patients should have solid food withheld beginning 6 hours before the operation, and may receive clear liquids up to 3 hours before the operation. No oral intake should be permitted after this time. Anemia should be corrected during the preceding weeks. Patients undergoing pharyngeal flap operations should not require a blood transfusion. The patient should have been cleared for surgical treatment well before the scheduled operation as far as general health is concerned. The brief history and physical examination on the morning of the operation should rule out failure to follow instructions for withholding oral intake and presence of upper respiratory, skin, or other acute infections. For a healthy person, a hematocrit reading is the only routine laboratory test required.

Anesthesia

Oral endotracheal anesthesia is used. Although there are some advantages to the use of the anode or guarded endotracheal tube, many anesthesiologists prefer the RAE tube because of its larger lumen and greater ease of insertion. It must be remembered that the RAE tube can be compressed easily by the Dingman mouth gag, and both surgeon and anesthesiologist must ensure an adequate orotracheal airway. The anesthesiologist must be informed that 1:200,000 epinephrine solution, usually in lidocaine, is to be used for hemostatic effect, and the dose of local anesthesia with epinephrine must be agreed on. Epinephrine, 1 to 5 μg per kilogram, is a safe range.

Patient Position

The patient lies in a supine position on the operating table with a rolled towel under the scapulae to provide a degree of neck extension. Sandbags or bags filled with buckshot placed on either side of the head provide stabilization. The commonly available foam plastic ring is not used under the head because it prevents adequate neck extension. The operating table is placed in the head-down or Trendelenburg position.

Technique

The Dingman mouth gag is inserted to retract the tongue and fix the endotracheal tube in place, at the same time holding the jaws open. The surgeon must be certain that the endotracheal tube is not compressed and must be reassured by the anesthesiologist that ventilatory exchange is not compromised.

Roughly half the amount of local anesthetic solution agreed on to be used in the 1½ to 2 hours of the operation is infiltrated into the soft palate. During the ensuing 7 minutes, while awaiting epinephrine effect, the team can review the plan for the operation. For theoretical reasons, I perform intravelar veloplasty at the time of the pharyngeal flap procedure in an effort to improve lateral pharyngeal wall motion. If I have performed the previous palatoplasty with an intravelar veloplasty, or if I am confident that a previous intravelar veloplasty has been performed, I preserve the reconstructed levator sling.

Palatal Splitting

At the end of the 7-minute waiting period, the soft palate is incised in the midline through the palatal raphe if the patient has a submucous cleft or through the midline scar (Fig. 46-1). The oral mucosal surface is divided to the posterior border of the hard palate. The nasal mucous membrane is divided approximately 0.5 cm short of the length of the oral mucous membrane incision so that a good cuff of nasal mucous membrane is retained to which the midline of the distal end of the pharyngeal flap can be sutured.

Outline of Pharyngeal Flap

Division of the soft palate allows generous exposure of the posterior pharyngeal wall cephalad to the adenoidal pad, laterally on each side to the lateral pharyngeal wall, and caudad well below the tubercle of the atlas. Puncture marks of a dye-tipped hypodermic needle held in the jaws of a hemostat outline the flap. The width of the flap is estimated on the basis of the degree of hypernasality present, the width of the posterior pharyngeal wall, and the extent of lateral pharyngeal wall movement. Care is taken in retraction of the mucous membrane of the lateral pharyngeal wall and the soft palate not to make the flap any wider than the lateral border of the posterior pharyngeal wall. For the caudad border of the flap, an estimate is made of the length of the proposed flap so that it reaches without tension from above the tubercle of the atlas to the cuff of nasal mucous membrane at the anterior end of the palate-splitting incision. The posterior pharyngeal wall superficial to the prevertebral fascia is infiltrated with epinephrine in local anesthetic solution.

Preparation of Turn-Back Flaps and Muscle Dissection

With a curved scissors, incisions are made through the mucous membrane laterally on each side from the anterior end of the nasal mucous membrane incision for a distance of 1 to 1.5 cm on each side. The incisions are curved posteriorly and, parallel to the midline incision, are carried posteriorly to the posterior edge of the soft palate (Fig. 46-2).

If it is judged that a previous intravelar veloplasty is adequate, enough scissors dissection around the sling is carried out so that anterior retraction of the sling is possible while the pharyngeal flap is sutured in position. If a formal intravelar veloplasty is to be performed, skin hooks retract the oral mucous membrane and the levator muscles are identified and dissected by scissors from the oral mucous membrane. The insertions into the hard

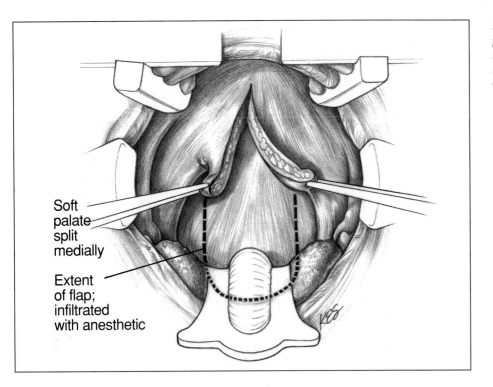

Fig. 46-1. Oral mucous membrane is incised to posterior border of hard palate; nasal mucous membrane is incised 0.5 cm shorter. Two sides of uvula are retracted by skin hooks or Brown-Cushing forceps.

Soft palate split medially

Extent of flap; infiltrated with anesthetic

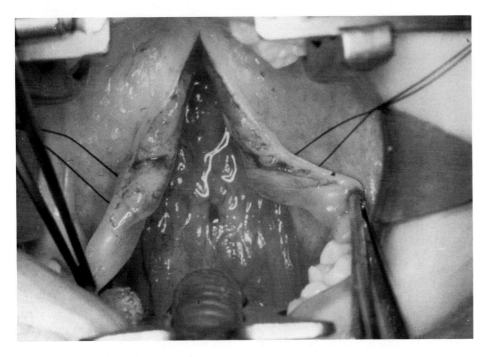

Fig. 46-2. Nasal mucous membrane turn-back flaps are outlined by incisions extending laterally from the anterior end of the nasal mucous incision and posteriorly to the posterior edge of the soft palate. The flaps are about 1 to 1.5 cm wide.

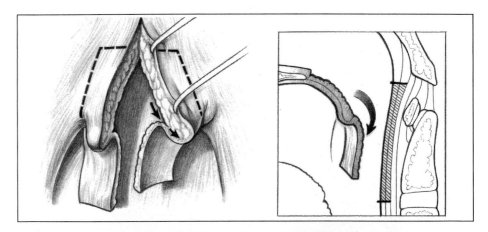

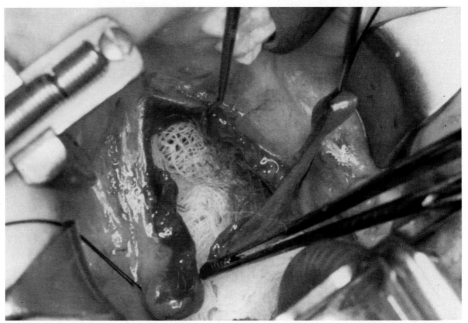

palate are identified and divided so that the muscles can be dissected enough to be drawn medially and posteriorly.

Dissection of Pharyngeal Flap

A 4–0 silk suture is placed through the tip of the pharyngeal flap to be used as a traction suture. Incisions are made just through the mucous membrane of the posterior pharyngeal wall on both sides of the proposed flap (Fig. 46-3A). A transverse mucous membrane incision is made at the distal end of the flap. Before making this incision, it is important to determine again that the flap is of adequate length. An assistant lifts up the blade of the Dingman mouth gag and retracts the lateral wall, first on one side and then the other. A Metzenbaum scissors, concave surface medial or cephalad, is used to cut through the unincised distal corners of the flap and, as the traction suture elevates the tip, to dissect the flap upward in the plane just anterior to the prevertebral fascia (Fig. 46-3B). Dissection continues cephalad until the base of the flap is clearly cephalad to the tubercle of the atlas (Fig. 46-3C). Dissection is done relatively rapidly; the surgeon must be certain not to dissect into the lateral pharyngeal walls, depending on suction of blood and adequate retraction to provide constant visibility of the entire posterior pharyngeal wall. A gauze sponge is inserted into the defect in the posterior pharyngeal wall for a minute or two, and the wound is inspected for bleeding vessels. Little bleeding is usually encountered, but any bleeding points are coagulated with the electrocautery; a Cushing forceps without teeth is used to grasp the bleeding points.

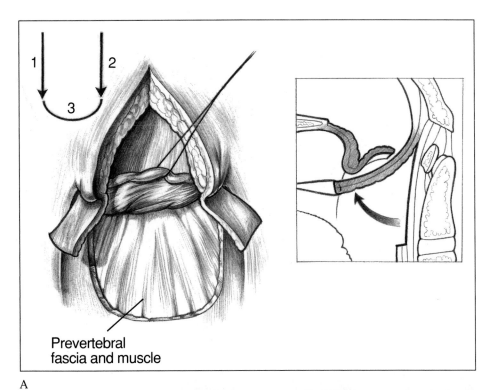

1 2

3

Prevertebral
fascia and muscle

A

Fig. 46-3A. With traction suture in place and a malleable retractor providing adequate exposure of the posterior pharyngeal wall, first on one side and then the other, the lateral incisions are made, followed by a transverse incision at the distal end of the flap. B. The mucous membrane at the corners of the flap is divided with Metzenbaum scissors to connect the two lateral incisions to the transverse incision. The flap includes mucous membrane and pharyngeal constrictor muscle. Prevertebral fascia and the longus colli muscles are exposed. C. The base of the flap must be cephalad to the tubercle of the atlas.

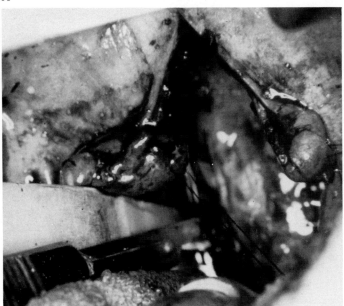

B

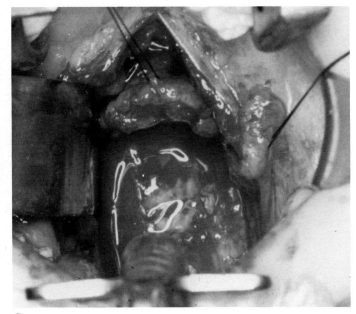

C

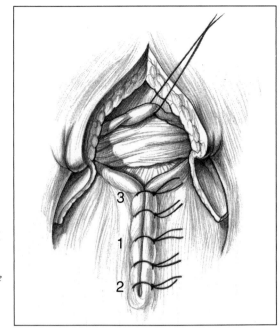

Fig. 46-4. 1. Posterior pharyngeal wall closure is begun at center of vertical defect. 2. The caudal portion of the defect is closed first, followed by the cephalad portion 3. Care is taken not to tear the mucous membrane by attempting to close all the way to the base of the flap.

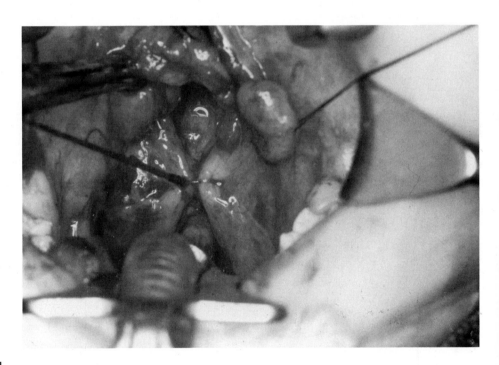

Posterior Pharyngeal Wall Repair

The defect in the posterior pharyngeal wall is closed with interrupted sutures of 000 chromic catgut (Fig. 46-4). I am convinced that patients have less discomfort when the posterior pharyngeal wall is closed. Except for two patients (one in whom dehiscence of the closure occurred, and one in whom closure was simply not possible), it has been easy to approximate the mucous membrane of the posterior pharyngeal wall other than in the area immediately caudad to the base of the pharyngeal flap.

Flap Suture

Two retention mattress sutures of 000 chromic catgut, one on each side, are inserted through the oral mucous membrane anterior to the end of the central incision and are sutured through each distal corner of the flap. These are left untied until just before completion of the operation (Fig. 46-5). An inverted 4–0 chromic catgut suture is inserted between the cuff of the nasal mucous membrane and the center of the distal edge of the pharyngeal flap. As this suture is tied, the silk traction suture is removed. Suture of the corner and sides of the flap to the lateral palatal nasal mucous membrane also is carried out with inverted 4–0 chromic catgut sutures on both sides of the flap. These sutures are carried posteriorly until a lateral port of the proper size remains on each

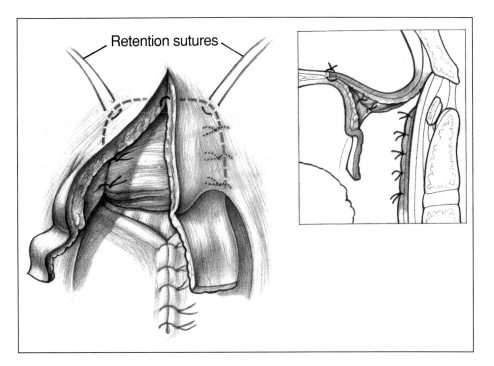

Fig. 46-5. Retention sutures are mattress sutures passed through the oral mucous membrane anterior to the flap that draw the raw undersurface of the flap up and anteriorly. Beginning at the center of the tip of the flap, sutures tied on the nasal surface of the flap approximate the flap to the palatal nasal mucous membrane. Closure is continued posteriorly on each side until a port of the proper size is constructed.

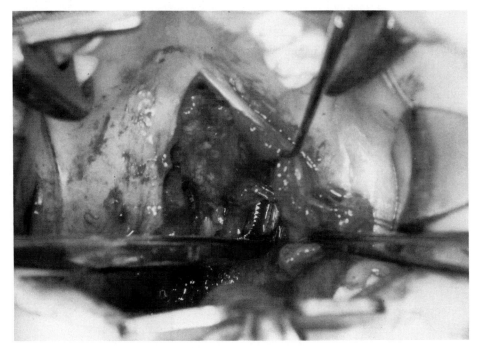

side. The size of the ports is estimated by inserting a right-angled hemostat and judging how wide or narrow a port is made. In a patient with severe hypernasality and poor lateral pharyngeal wall motion, the ports should be smaller. With good lateral pharyngeal wall motion, the ports can be larger. If necessary, the edge of the lateral nasal mucous membrane can be extended posteriorly into the posterior tonsillar pillar.

Suture of Turn-Back Flaps

After the pharyngeal flap is sutured in place, three sutures of 4–0 chromic catgut are used to fix the distal ends of the turn-back flaps to both sides and the center of the base of the pharyngeal flap (Fig. 46-6). The medial edges of the nasal mucous membrane and the turn-back flaps are sutured together beginning at the tip of the uvula and progressing in the direction of the base of the flap.

Levator Muscle Reconstruction

In patients who undergo intravelar veloplasty, muscle approximation is carried out by inserting two mattress sutures of chromic catgut through the oral mucous membrane on each side of the oral surface of the palate, catching the muscle on the opposite side. These sutures, like the retention sutures, are left to be tied until reapproximation of the palate is completed.

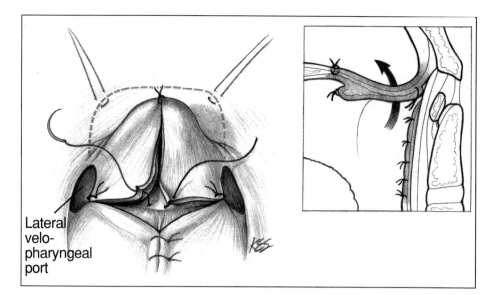

Fig. 46-6. Suture holds tip of uvula together. Ends of turn-back flaps are sutured to each side and center of base of pharyngeal flap. Additional sutures between tip of uvula and base of pharyngeal flap approximate the two turn-back flaps.

Lateral velo-pharyngeal port

Palatal Repair

The oral mucous membrane is approximated with vertical mattress and simple sutures of 4–0 polydioxanone. The two muscle sutures and the two retention sutures are tied (Figs. 46-7 and 46-8). The operative site is inspected for bleeding both before and after the operating table is returned to a level position. The mouth gag is removed. In all children, a suture of 0 gauge or heavier silk is inserted transversely through the thickness of the tongue and remains in place as a traction suture if needed for restoring the airway or to assist in suctioning blood or mucus from the oropharynx for at least the night after the operation.

Postoperative Care and Follow-up Evaluation

An antibiotic—penicillin or cefazolin—is given intravenously just before the operation and intraoperatively but not postoperatively. Maintenance administration of intravenous fluids, usually 5% glucose in one-fourth normal saline solution, is continued until oral fluid intake is adequate in a 24-hour period. Patients are encouraged to drink clear liquids from a cup as soon as they are able after the operation. Straws are not used. Oral intake includes full liquids or a blended diet when tolerated; this diet is continued for 4

weeks. Patients are discharged from the hospital as soon as oral intake is adequate. Children can return to school 2 weeks after the operation, but active athletics or physical education classes are not permitted. Adults can return to all but athletic activity after the same period of time. Full activity and a normal diet are allowed for all patients after 4 weeks.

Patients are seen in the week after discharge from the hospital and a month after the operation. Speech evaluation is carried out 6 months after the operation and annually, along with plastic surgical evaluation, until at least 2 years after the operation for adults and certainly through adolescence for children.

Results

Results of one previous study determined that among 38 patients who had pharyngeal flap operations without intravelar veloplasty, 34 (89.4%) achieved velopharyngeal adequacy, whereas 4 (10.5%) of the patients demonstrated moderate hyponasality. Among 91 patients who underwent intravelar veloplasty at the time of the pharyngeal flap operation, 81 (89%) had velopharyngeal adequacy, but 7 patients (7.7%) had moderate-to-severe hyponasality. Pressure-flow studies in 72 of the latter group of patients revealed adequate velopharyngeal closure in 67 (93%).

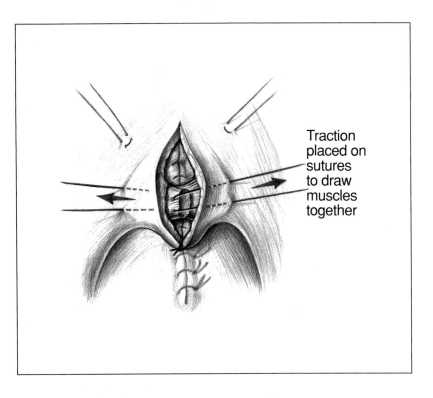

Traction placed on sutures to draw muscles together

Fig. 46-7. Muscle sutures and mattress sutures overlap levator muscles as they are drawn medially and posteriorly.

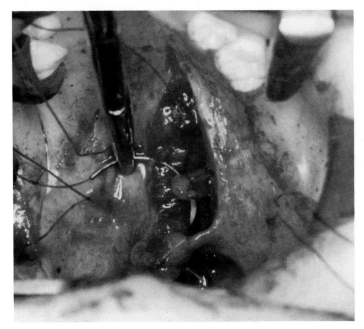

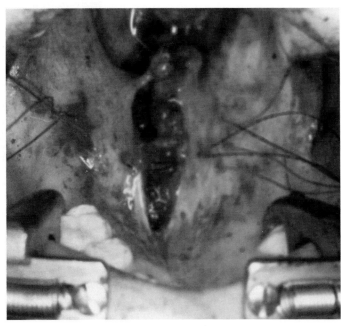

Discussion

The superiorly based, lined, pharyngeal flap attached at a high point provides velopharyngeal adequacy in 89 percent of patients. Although the flap itself is not dynamic, lateral pharyngeal wall motion provides port closure.

A number of surgeons advocate sphincter pharyngoplasty in patients with velopharyngeal incompetency who have limited medial excursion of the lateral pharyngeal wall, as noted earlier in the chapter. Others simply substitute sphincter pharyngoplasty because of personal preference.

Fig. 46-8. Retention sutures and muscle sutures have been tied. Flap and lateral ports lie above the plane of the palate.

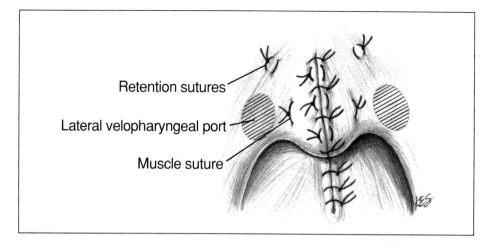

Retention sutures

Lateral velopharyngeal port

Muscle suture

Hypothetically, at least, lining the flap lessens the tubing of the flap that would result in an increase in port size. Some surgeons bury the flap in a pocket in the soft palate; some do not split the palate but turn back a palate-wide flap of nasal mucous membrane. Custom-made flaps, varying in width depending on the degree of inadequacy, have been advocated by some. A technique called *lateral port control* uses catheters as templates around which the lateral ports are sutured. I have never been convinced that precise tailoring of flap width or port dimension can offset the unpredictable effects of wound healing.

An argument has been made for inferiorly based flaps, but a number of partial or complete flap dehiscences have occurred. I have never had a dehiscence of a pharyngeal flap. Hemorrhage also has been reported, but I have never had this event occur. When the patient is in the head-down position, and with careful exposure of the operative area, the few bleeding vessels at the base of the flap or in the posterior pharyngeal wall can be coagulated readily. Except in two patients, posterior pharyngeal wall suture has been accomplished easily.

The most threatening complication of a pharyngeal flap operation is airway obstruction. One study showed an almost universal prevalence of obstructive sleep apnea in the immediately and early postoperative periods. Careful, skilled nursing care is essential, and pediatric patients may require apneic monitoring and even admission to the intensive care unit. One of my patients died of respiratory arrest during the night after the operation; although an autopsy disclosed no cause, it can only be assumed that respiratory distress was not recognized or, if recognized, was not corrected in time. Patients undergoing pharyngeal flap operations should not have routine orders for narcotics or other respiratory depressants.

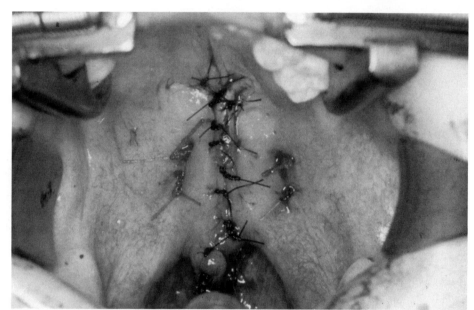

One 16-month-old patient, in whom a pharyngeal flap operation was performed to make primary closure of the palate possible, had persistent obstructive apnea that required flap division. The patient retained adequacy in spite of flap division.

Suggested Reading

Dalston, R.M., and Warren, D.W. The diagnosis of velopharyngeal inadequacy. *Clin. Plast. Surg.* 12:685, 1985.

Davis, D.J., and Bagnall, A.D. Velopharyngeal Incompetence. In J.G. McCarthy (Ed.), *Plastic Surgery*. Philadelphia: Saunders, 1990. Vol. 4, pp. 2903–2921.

Hogan, V.M. A clarification of the surgical goals in cleft palate speech and the introduction of the lateral port control (L.P.C.) pharyngeal flap. *Cleft Palate J.* 10:331, 1973.

Jackson, I.T. Sphincter pharyngoplasty. *Clin. Plast. Surg.* 12:711, 1985.

Kapetansky, D.I. Transverse pharyngeal flap: A dynamic repair for velopharyngeal insufficiency. *Cleft Palate J.* 12:44, 1975.

Owsley, J.Q., Creech, B.J., and Dedo, H.H. Poor speech following the pharyngeal flap operation: Etiology and treatment. *Cleft Palate J.* 9:312, 1972.

Owsley, J.Q., et al. Speech results from the high attached pharyngeal flap operation. *Cleft Palate J.* 7:306, 1970.

Schneider, E., and Shprintzen, D.J. A survey of speech pathologists: Current trends in the diagnosis and management of velopharyngeal insufficiency. *Cleft Palate J.* 17:249, 1980.

Winslow, R.B., et al. The treatment of velopharyngeal incompetency by bilateral island sandwich flap combined with superiorly based pharyngeal flap. *Cleft Palate J.* 11:272, 1974.

47

Sphincter Pharyngoplasty

Roger C. Mixter   Stanley J. Ewanowski

Orticochea developed the sphincter pharyngoplasty in 1959 (Fig. 47-1). Before that time, Passavant, Whitehead, and Sanvanero-Roselli designed manipulations of the posterior pillars of the fauces to elongate the palate. Since the original report by Orticochea in 1970, Reichert, Heller, and Jackson described modifications of the original procedure (Fig. 47-2).

Indications

We use the sphincter pharyngoplasty instead of a pharyngeal flap for velopharyngeal incompetence caused by clefting, neurogenic factors (both congenital and acquired), and postadenotonsillectomy syndrome (Fig. 47-3). We have also used a sphincter pharyngoplasty for definitive treatment of velopharyngeal obstruction in a patient undergoing a pharyngeal flap operation.

Preoperative assessment may include aerodynamic studies, videofluoroscopy, and nasoendoscopy, but a careful speech evaluation is the most important diagnostic tool. Such an evaluation consists of an articulation assessment and a voice evaluation. The exact timing of the op-

eration depends, in large measure, on the results of the speech assessment. Any patient is a candidate for sphincter pharyngoplasty regardless of age if his or her velopharyngeal incompetence is not modifiable by speech therapy. Our patients have ranged in age from $2\frac{1}{2}$ years to 50 years.

Surgical Anatomy and Technique

The patient is placed in the supine position with a rolled towel underneath the shoulders. Preoperative antibiotics are given according to the surgeon's preference. Anesthesia is delivered through a reinforced orotracheal tube. A Dingman mouth gag or its equivalent is placed. The uvula and soft palate are retracted. It may be necessary to split the soft palate to gain additional exposure. The posterior pharyngeal wall below the adenoidal pad and the posterior faucial pillars are infiltrated with 0.5% lidocaine with epinephrine 1:200,000. A pharyngeal pack is placed.

After 15 minutes have elapsed, dissection of the posterior pharyngeal recess is begun. The tonsil is identified, and a vertical incision is begun inferior and just

posterior to the tonsillar pillar. A long-handled knife may facilitate this incision, which is carried superiorly to incorporate the posterior faucial pillar, a continuation of the posterior palatine arch (Fig. 47-4). A second incision is made 1.0 cm medial to the first. The intervening tissue is grasped with a McIndoe tooth forceps. A right-angled dissection scissors is introduced into the most lateral incision and swept medially to incorporate first the pharyngeal constrictors and, more superiorly, the palatopharyngeus muscle (Fig. 47-5). The posteriormost extent of the dissection is just anterior to the deep cervical fascia. After the bridge of tissue has been elevated, the right-angled scissors is used to separate the inferiormost portion of the flap. From this point on the flap is raised from inferior to superior. The palatopharyngeus muscle is identified directly and bluntly dissected. There is frequently an artery traversing from lateral to medial at the proximal pole of the tonsil. Care must be taken to cauterize or ligate this vessel to avoid postoperative bleeding. After the flap has been elevated above the tonsillar fossa, the resultant pharyngeal defect is closed with running 4–0 polyglactin 910. The same dissection is performed on the opposite side.

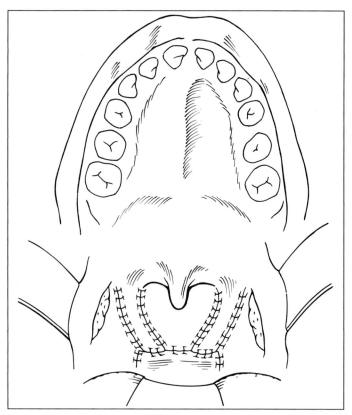

Fig. 47-1. Orticochea's original sphincter pharyngoplasty, 1959.

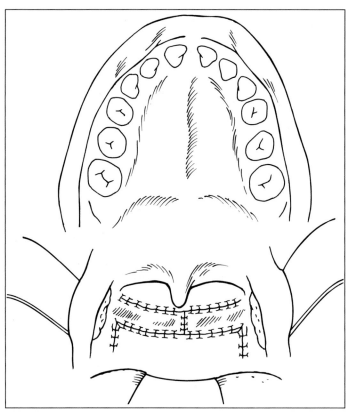

Fig. 47-2. Jackson's modification of the sphincter pharyngoplasty, 1977.

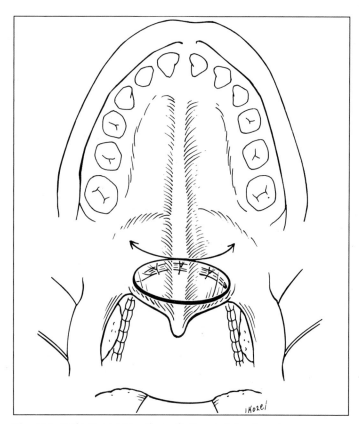

Fig. 47-3. Authors' operation allows adjustment of size of aperture.

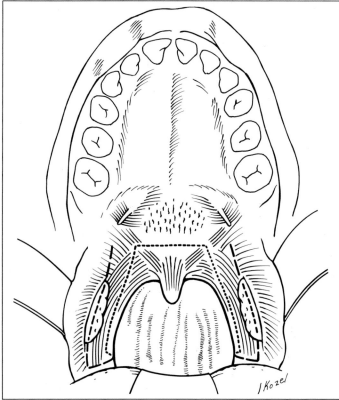

Fig. 47-4. Flap design should include the posterior faucial pillar.

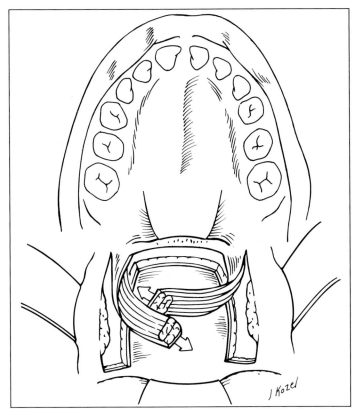

Fig. 47-5. *As much of the palatopharyngeus muscle as possible should be incorporated.*

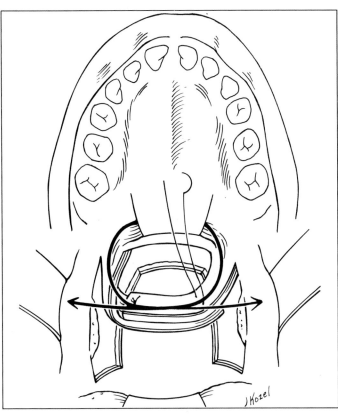

Fig. 47-6. *Aperture size is adjusted to approximately 1.5 cm.*

Attention is turned subsequently to construction of the sphincter. A horizontal incision is made immediately below the adenoidal pad. This incision is deepened to the cervical fascia. Laterally, the incision intersects with the medial vertical flap incision. The flaps are transposed medially, and each flap is rotated to allow approximation of its raw surfaces. The flaps may be tightened to regulate the aperture of the sphincter (Fig. 47-6). Sutures of 4–0 polyglactin 910 are used to approximate the flaps to each other. The interdigitated flaps are secured to the posterior wall of the pharynx immediately below the adenoidal pad (Fig. 47-7). The ideal aperture size is approximately 1.5 cm. Because of the circular nature of the scarring forces, the ultimate aperture size is approximately 1.0 cm. After hemostasis is ensured, the pharyngeal pack is removed, and an endotracheal tube of appropriate size is placed through the nose and into the pharynx to facilitate postoperative suctioning. Postoperative blood loss is usually minimal. Postoperative antibiotics are continued at the discretion of the surgeon. We usually allow resumption of speech therapy within one month

of the operation. The speech-language pathologist is reassured that the maximal benefit from the sphincter may not be attained for 3 to 6 months because the sphincter tightens with healing.

Comparison of Sphincter Pharyngoplasty with the Pharyngeal Flap Operation

Our results corroborate those reported by Orticochea and Jackson. All our patients exhibited improvement in velopharyngeal valving, articulation, nasal resonance, and speech intelligibility after sphincter pharyngoplasty. There was no denasality or hyponasality. A child can undergo sphincter pharyngoplasty at any age without a negative effect on the speech outcome. Sphincter pharyngoplasty works equally well on patients with diverse initial cleft conditions. Given that the speech results after sphincter pharyngoplasty are at least as good as

those after a conventional pharyngeal flap operation, we believe the technical advantages of the procedure should be considered. We find construction of a central port to be easier than constructing lateral ports, as described in the Hogan modification. Because sphincter pharyngoplasty does not disrupt the velum, there is no additional scarring and immobility. Maxillary advancements may be carried out without apparent alteration of the sphincter. Patients do not experience the halitosis from accumulation of nasal secretions that is a frequent embarrassment for people who undergo pharyngeal flap operations. Finally, as mentioned earlier, we have used sphincter pharyngoplasty to treat a patient with nasopharyngeal obstruction following a pharyngeal flap operation. Although the exact cause of the obstruction was unknown, postoperative infection was implicated. Once the obstruction occurs, its treatment is extremely difficult and may involve frequent operations with nasopharyngeal obturation. In our patient we were able to identify the nasopharyngeal passage, open the nasopharyngeal port, and line the resulting raw surfaces with the lat-

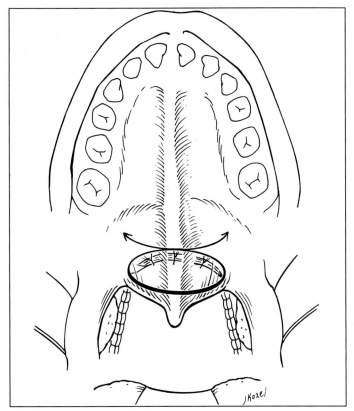

Fig. 47-7. *Sphincter is secured just below the adenoidal pad and thus is not visualized by routine intraoral examination.*

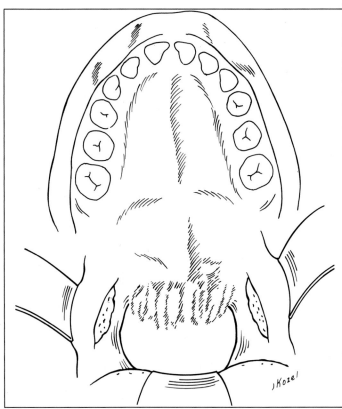

Fig. 47-8. *Nasopharyngeal obstruction after pharyngeal flap operation.*

erally based palatopharyngeal flaps (Figs. 47-8 to 47-10). The patient retained velopharyngeal competence without hyponasality.

Disadvantages and Contraindications

We have seen only one patient on whom a standard sphincter pharyngoplasty could not be performed. The patient was a 6-year-old child with velocardiofacial syndrome in whom the posterior faucial pillars were devoid of useful palatopharyngeus muscle. In addition, because of the well-known medial displacement of the carotid arteries, lateral dissection was somewhat precarious. Our solution was to shorten the palatopharyngeal flaps and to secure them to a superiorly based pharyngeal flap. This patient's postoperative speech was satisfactory.

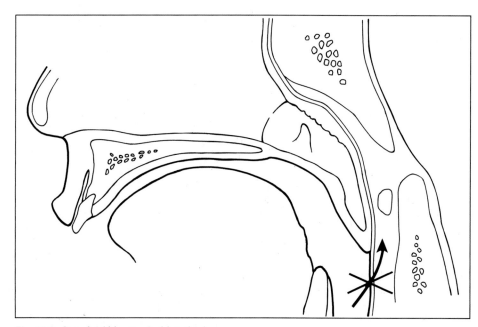

Fig. 47-9. *Care should be exercised lest the deep cervical fascia be violated.*

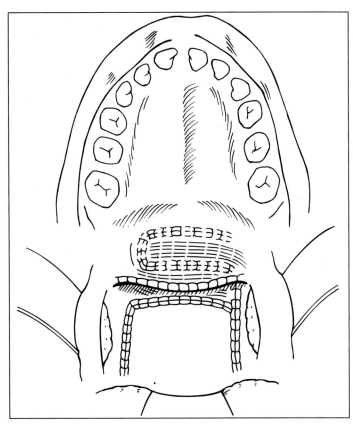

Fig. 47-10. Soft palate is oversewn and raw surfaces are lined by the laterally based flaps.

A concern has been voiced by some that sphincter pharyngoplasties are not modifiable in the event of continuing velopharyngeal incompetence. Although we have not to date had occasion to modify any of our sphincter pharyngoplasties, Jackson commented that it is easily done.

Much criticism has been placed on use of the term *dynamic* applied to sphincter pharyngoplasties. Whereas Orticochea's electromyographic studies implied that the sphincter was dynamic, other investigators have not been able to reproduce his results. Although we have had occasion to observe tightening of the sphincter during speech, we believe the primary benefit is static reduction in the size of the velopharyngeal port. We do believe, however, that lateral wall motion is much less critical for a favorable speech outcome after a sphincter pharyngoplasty than it is after a pharyngeal flap operation.

Conclusion

The sphincter pharyngoplasty is more versatile than the pharyngeal flap. The procedure is technically easy with minimal blood loss. The postoperative speech results are at least equivalent to those obtained with a pharyngeal flap. Finally, a sphincter pharyngoplasty may be useful for postoperative nasopharyngeal obstruction.

Suggested Reading

Heller, A. Pharyngoplasty through cross-palatopharyngeal flap. *J. Maxillofac. Surg.* 3:84, 1975.

Jackson, I.T., and Silverton, J.S. The sphincter pharyngoplasty as a secondary procedure in cleft palates. *Plast. Reconstr. Surg.* 59:518, 1977.

Millard, D.R. *Cleft Craft: The Evolution of Its Surgery.* Vol. III: *Alveolar and Palatal Deformities.* Boston: Little, Brown, 1980.

Mixter, R.C., and Ewanowski, S.J. Presented at the Illinois Cleft Palate Annual Meeting, Chicago, Ill., 1990.

Orticochea, M. Results of the dynamic muscle sphincter operation in cleft palates. *Br. J. Plast. Surg.* 23:108, 1970.

Passavant, G. On the closure of the pharynx in speech. *Virchows Arch.* 46:1, 1869.

Reichert, H. The lateral velo-pharyngoplasty: A new method for the correction of open nasality. *J. Maxillofac. Surg.* 2:95, 1974.

Sanvenero-Roselli, G. Secondary Corrections of Palate. In K. Schuchardt (Ed.), *Treatment of Patients with Clefts of Lip, Alveolus and Palate.* Stuttgart: Thieme, 1966. Pp. 193–198.

Whitehead, W.R. Remarks on a case of extensive cleft of the hard and soft palate, closed at a single operation. *Am. J. Med. Sci.* (n.s.) 62: 114, 1871; *Dent. Cosmos* 13:438, 1871.

48

Orthodontic Management for Patients with Cleft Lip and Palate

Alvaro A. Figueroa   Howard Aduss

Clefts of the primary and secondary palate affect growth and development and affect the position and relations of the maxilla and dentition. These effects are related to the cleft itself and to the scarring subsequent to surgical management. Primary effects on the maxilla that involve malposition of the cleft segment or teeth can be corrected with orthodontic treatment. However, developmental defects related to tissue deficiencies or major displacement of parts require combined orthodontic, surgical, and prosthetic management.

The negative influences of surgical treatment can be minimized in part by use of careful and delicate surgical techniques that respect the growth centers of the maxilla and emphasize minimal undermining of the soft tissues. Adherence to these fundamental concepts in patients with clefts makes it possible to achieve harmonious facial balance with good dental/skeletal relations and normal function (Figs. 48-1 and 48-2).

The orthodontist participates during all stages of patient care: in early management with presurgical maxillary orthopedic treatment; during childhood by aligning the maxillary segments and den-

tition in preparation for bony reconstruction of the cleft maxilla; and later in adolescence, by obtaining ideal dental relations or preparing the dentition for orthognathic surgery or final prosthetic rehabilitation. Throughout the patient's growing years, the orthodontist uses roentgencephalometry to monitor craniofacial growth and dental development. Orthodontists are concerned not only with the position and relations of the teeth but also with the supporting bones—the maxilla and mandible—and their relation to and influence on facial balance and stomatognathic function. Orthodontic treatment can influence the position of the teeth (orthodontic effect), their supporting bones (orthopedic effect), or both. In patients with clefts, positive effects are possible at all stages of treatment from infancy to adulthood.

The rehabilitation of an orofacial cleft crosses the borders of multiple specialties; therefore, discussion of any specialized treatment or focus should be in the context of multidisciplinary management. It should also be remembered that only general guidelines can be given for any approach to treatment. The final treatment of the patient, as mentioned by Pruzansky in his classic 1953 article, should be

highly individualized because not all congenital clefts of the lip and palate are alike; they present with a wide spectrum of anatomic variability and severity.

This chapter presents the various stages in which the orthodontist has a role in the management of cleft lip and palate as practiced at the Craniofacial Center, University of Illinois at Chicago (Table 48-1).

Orthopedic Treatment in Infancy

Orthodontic therapy in infancy takes the form of presurgical orthopedic treatment. Presurgical orthopedic treatment is not routine but is instituted at the request of the surgeon to facilitate closure of a cleft lip or performance of a primary bone graft. The goal of the procedure in unilateral clefts is to bring together and align widely separated segments. In bilateral clefts of the lip and palate, maxillary orthopedic procedures are used to reduce the protrusion of the premaxilla. For the purpose of lip repair, presurgical orthopedic treatment is rarely used at our center. With current techniques, the lip can be repaired primarily without much

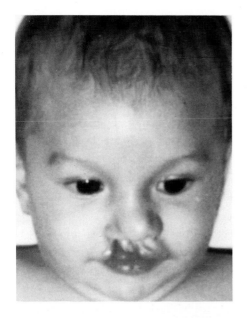

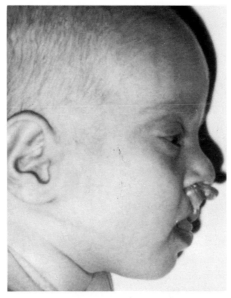

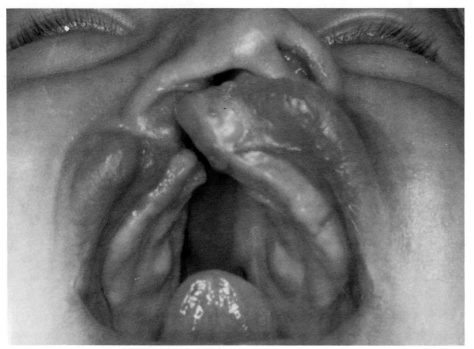

Fig. 48-1. One-month-old infant born with complete right unilateral cleft lip and palate.

difficulty. The lip repair in itself exerts a prompt and marked orthopedic force that results in improvement of the originally displaced maxillary segments (Fig. 48-3).

Surgeons who advocate primary or infant bone grafting are forced to use active presurgical orthopedic treatments to move the segments or passive molding plates that take advantage of the previously mentioned orthopedic force of the repaired lip. The rationale is that it is difficult to cover an alveolar bone graft when the maxillary segments are separated or displaced. At our institution bone grafting procedures are deferred until a later age, when it has been shown that the procedure can be done with the highest degree of success and with no deleterious effects on facial growth.

The only time we use presurgical orthopedic treatment is in bilateral cleft lip with a severely protrusive premaxilla (see Chap. 54). Our protocol does not include feeding plates or other devices to remove the influence of the tongue on cleft width. Adequate feeding techniques, substitute plates, and the possible influence of the tongue on cleft width are overridden by the orthopedic effect of the lip repair (see Fig. 48-3).

After the palate is repaired, we usually do not intervene until the child is in the late primary dentition stage or in transitional dentition. The most important role of the dental specialist during the early stages is to inform the parents of individual differences in dental development and what to expect in their child's development and to emphasize the importance of maintaining a healthy dentition. A regular preventive and restorative program should be carried out by the family's general dentist or a pediatric dental specialist.

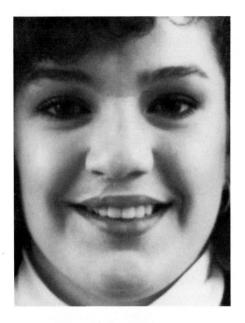

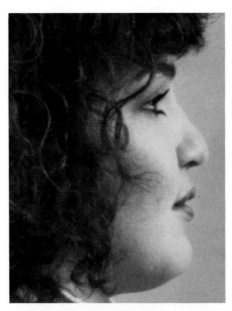

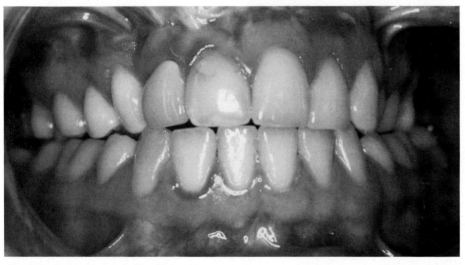

Fig. 48-2. Same patient as in Fig. 48-1 at 18 years of age after rehabilitation for cleft lip and palate.

Table 48-1. Orthodontic treatment of cleft lip and palate

	Dental developmental stages							
	Infancy		Primary		Transitional		Permanent	
Procedure	Yes	No	Yes	No	Yes	No	Yes	No
Presurgical infant orthopedic treatment	X[a]							
Maxillary expansion	X[d]		X[b]		X[c]		X[c]	
Maxillary protraction		X	X[b]		X[b]		X[b]	
Orthodontic treatment		X		X	X[c]		X	

[a]Bilateral cleft lip with protrusive premaxilla.
[b]Occasionally in all cleft types.
[c]Frequently in all cleft types.
[d]Occasionally in bilateral cleft lip and palate.

Orthodontic Treatment in the Primary Dentition

Orthodontic treatment at this stage is limited to correction of functional buccal or lateral crossbite and of an anterior crossbite that might be dental in origin or related to mild or moderate anteroposterior maxillary development.

Posterior Crossbite

The cause of a posterior or buccal crossbite in a patient with a cleft may be dental, skeletal, or both. The most common crossbite associated with cleft lip and palate is that of the canine adjoining the cleft (Fig. 48-4). This crossbite may be caused, in part, by medial movement of the cleft segment after repair of the palate, but it also may be related to the more palatal position of the developing tooth bud as a result of the cleft. Ironically, the crossbite of the maxillary primary canine is generally of no clinical significance because the lower opposing canine moves buccally, and this movement avoids a closing shift (Fig. 48-5). In patients who have a shift, the involved teeth may be equilibrated by grinding and the problem corrected.

A canine crossbite also can be corrected with an expansion appliance. The appliance does not have to exert a great deal of force because there is no bony continuity between the cleft segments. A spring-loaded or quadhelix expander can be used for this procedure (Fig. 48-6). After expansion, the repositioned segments require some type of retention, or they will return to their original position. Additionally, if there is lack of continuity between the cleft segments, there is a good possibility that expansion will result in oronasal communication. The latter necessitates obturation to prevent speech or feeding problems until the alveolar cleft is surgically closed.

To avoid intermittent periods of treatment, long periods with retention appliances, and problems of patient fatigue, the correction of a crossbite can be delayed until the maxillary arch is being orthodontically prepared for a bone graft to reconstruct its anterior surface and alveolus in the area of the cleft (to be discussed later in this chapter). This approach is both therapeutically efficient and cost-effective.

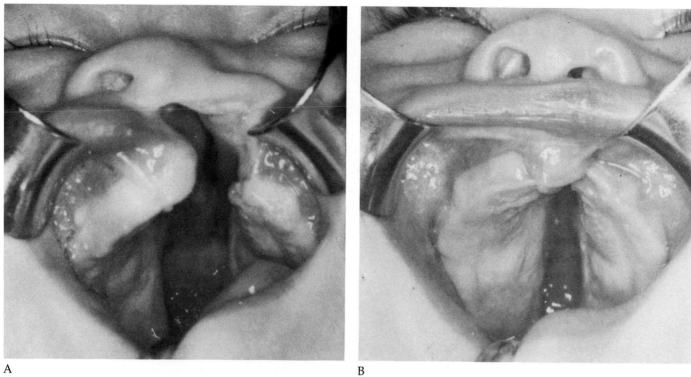

A

B

Fig. 48-3. Restoration of maxillary arch form and narrowing of maxillary and alveolar clefts after lip repair in a patient with complete unilateral cleft lip and palate. Preoperative maxillary orthopedic treatment was not used. A. Preoperatively. B. Postoperatively.

Fig. 48-4. Crossbite of primary canines (arrow) in 4-year-old patient with repaired right unilateral cleft lip and palate in which preoperative orthopedic treatment was not used. Note the ideal dental relations on the side without the cleft.

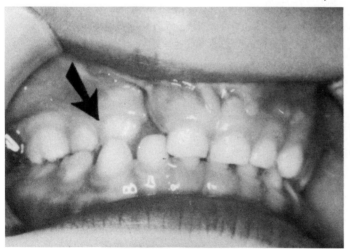 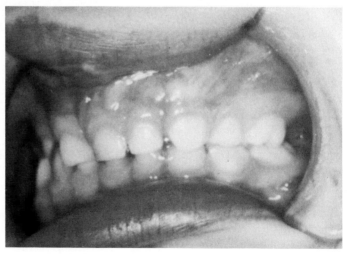

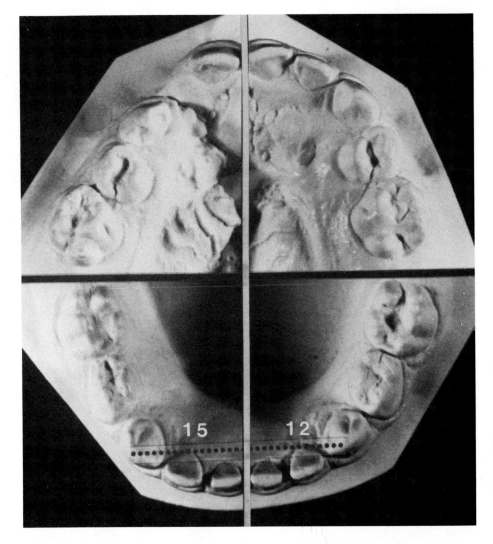

Fig. 48-5. Dental study models of patient shown in Fig. 48-4. Note the increased distance (15 mm) of the right mandibular primary canine from the midline as a result of buccal movement caused by the occlusal relation with the opposing palatally displaced cuspid.

Anterior Crossbite

Anterior crossbites should be carefully evaluated and monitored because of their multiple causes, such as skeletal maxillary hypoplasia, maxillary incisor retroclination, mandibular prognathism, mandibular incisor proclination, or a combination of these factors. It is not uncommon to find a combination of skeletal maxillary deficiency and dental malpositions in the primary dentition of a patient with an orofacial cleft.

If its cause is skeletal and it is not severe in magnitude, the anterior crossbite may be corrected using an orthopedic face mask. This appliance exerts an orthopedic force to the underdeveloped maxilla (Fig. 48-7). This method yields relatively fast results and is more effective during the early childhood and prepubertal years. The overall effects on the facial skeleton are those of maxillary advancement with some mandibular repositioning (Fig. 48-8).

We treat young cleft patients with severe maxillomandibular discrepancies with extreme caution. If longitudinal cephalometric studies reveal an unfavorable growth pattern, treatment of the skeletal imbalance is deferred until a combined orthodontic-surgical treatment plan can be initiated.

Orthodontic Treatment in the Transitional Dentition
Developmental Considerations

According to Bjork and Skieller, after 8 to 10 years of age incremental growth of the maxilla is small in both the transverse and anteroposterior dimensions. It then makes a great deal of sense to defer secondary operations on the maxilla until after this period and thereby avoid the risk of growth inhibition as a result of surgical trauma and scarring.

A developmental guideline that can be used for the timing of secondary surgical procedures on the maxilla, specifically bone graft reconstruction of the area of the cleft and the alveolus, can be found in the dentition. The stability of the reconstructed alveolus depends on the presence of a tooth in the area of the graft. If a lateral incisor adjoins the cleft, it can be moved into the newly placed graft. If the lateral incisor is congenitally missing, the actively erupting canine will preserve the reconstructed alveolus. It is important to remember that orthodontic treatment should not be initiated until root development of the incisors is almost complete. Failure to adhere to this developmental threshold can result in incomplete root formation, root resorption, and an unfavorable crown-to-root ratio for proper attachment of the tooth to its supporting bone (Fig. 48-9).

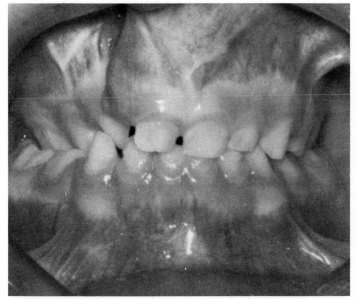

A

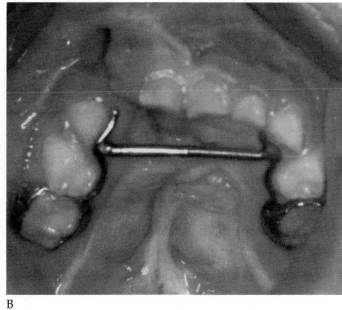

B

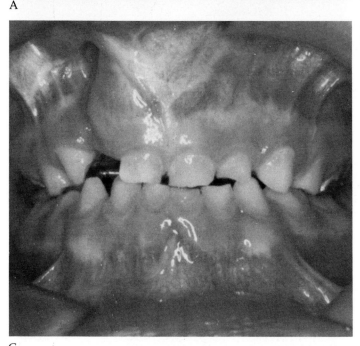

C

Fig. 48-6. Five-year-old patient with repaired right unilateral cleft lip and palate. A. Note crossbite of right buccal segment. B. Spring-loaded expander used to correct crossbite. C. View after crossbite corrected.

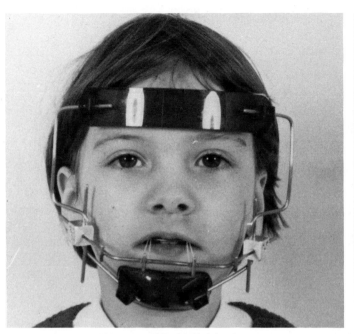

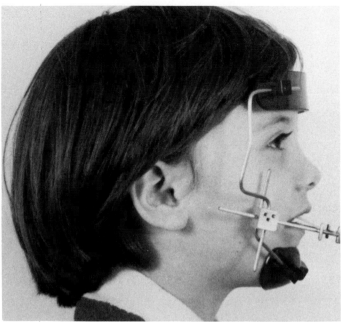

Fig. 48-7. Five-year-old patient with repaired cleft palate wearing an orthopedic face mask for the correction of moderate maxillary hypoplasia and anterior dental crossbite.

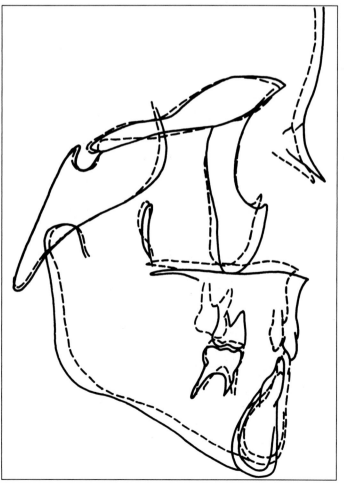

Fig. 48-8. Tracings of patient shown in Fig. 48-7 after 5 months wearing an orthopedic face mask. Note correction of anterior crossbite by advancement of maxilla and downward and backward rotation of mandible. Dashed line = patient age 5 years, 3 months; solid line = patient age 6 years, 4 months.

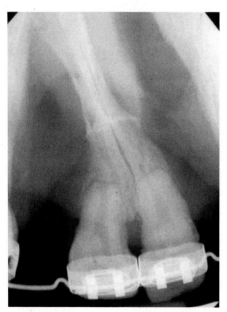

Fig. 48-9. Roentgenogram of maxillary incisors of patient with bilateral cleft lip and palate. Note reduced root lengths and blunting of root apices as a result of tooth movement that began before complete root development and prolonged orthodontic treatment.

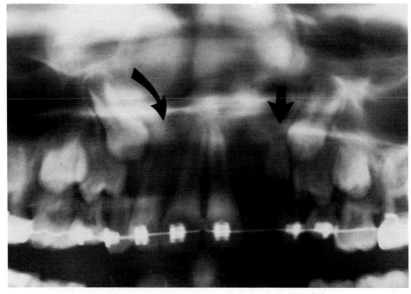
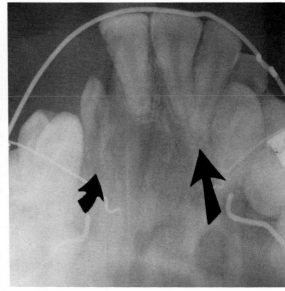

A   B

Fig. 48-10A. Panoramic roentgenogram of 10-year-old patient with complete left unilateral cleft lip and palate. Root development of cleft maxillary lateral incisor (short arrow) is about one-third the length of the contralateral lateral incisor (curved arrow), which has complete root development. B. Occlusal roentgenogram of 11-year-old patient with repaired left unilateral complete cleft lip and palate after orthodontic treatment and bone graft. The cleft lateral incisor erupting through the bone graft has a root with an open apex. Root length is about one-half that of the contralateral incisor, which has complete root formation and closed apex (large arrow).

Initiating orthodontic treatment based on the stage of dental development of the permanent teeth, rather than chronologic age, is particularly appropriate for children with orofacial clefts because these patients frequently have a marked delay in the development and eruption of the permanent teeth. Ranta reported that this delay may be 12 months or longer; his observations have been confirmed in our own patient population (Fig. 48-10). Most important, beginning orthodontic treatment and bony reconstruction of the cleft maxilla on the basis of dental development rather than chronologic age provides a safeguard for the adverse effects of surgical intervention on growth.

The preceding protocol represents a slight but important departure from that presented by Abyholm and associates in 1981, in which the timing of the bone graft to the maxilla was based on the stage of eruption of the permanent maxillary canine, and the success of the procedure was based on the level of alveolar bone around the erupted canine. The protocol used at our center takes advantage of the lateral incisor, if present, to maintain the

bone graft that was placed to restore the alveolus. With the lateral incisor in its proper position, adequate bone for the erupting canine is ensured (Fig. 48-11).

Orthodontic Treatment

Once a developmental basis for the timing of orthodontic treatment and the indications for treatment have been established, consideration can be given to the mechanics of orthodontic treatment during the transitional dentition. The surgical benefit of orthodontic treatment at this stage is that it keeps displaced teeth and segments from interfering with surgical access and flap design during the secondary alveolar bone graft procedure (Fig. 48-12). If the maxillary segments are well aligned and the teeth on either side of the cleft are not in the way of the operation, orthodontic treatment is postponed until after the bone graft.

Orthodontic treatment at this stage takes two forms, orthodontic treatment and orthopedic treatment. The two can be performed simultaneously or in continuity

and are used to address the following common problems:

Collapse of the maxillary arch, especially the canine region
Dental malposition on either side of the cleft
Altered anteroposterior intermaxillary relations

To prepare the maxillary arch for the bone graft, it is necessary to address the first two problems. The last, if present, is deferred until the final phase of orthodontic treatment in adolescence.

When indicated, we accomplish the preparatory phase of orthodontic treatment by means of a fixed segmental edgewise orthodontic appliance. The erupted maxillary incisors, primary cuspids, and permanent first molars are bonded or banded. A sequence of orthodontic arch wires from flexible to rigid is used progressively. This allows rapid correction of dental malpositions and restores arch form in both unilateral and bilateral cleft

Fig. 48-11A. Patient with residual left alveolar cleft at 8 years of age before orthodontic treatment and bone grafting. Note presence of well-developed cleft maxillary lateral incisor (left arrow) and permanent canine with incomplete root formation (right arrow). B. Same patient at 12 years of age after initial orthodontic treatment and bone graft. Note adequate bony support for both the cleft lateral incisor (upper arrow) and the spontaneously erupting permanent canine (lower arrow).

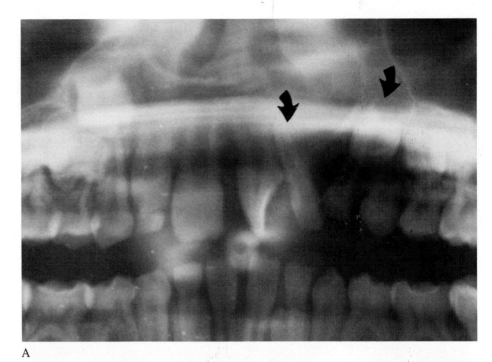

A

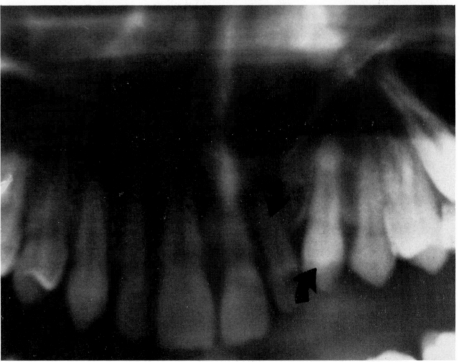

B

lip and palate (Figs. 48-13 and 48-14). In an occasional patient with severe maxillary arch collapse or a markedly scarred palate, a maxillary expander can be used before or at the time of appliance placement (Fig. 48-15). The expansion should be sufficient to correct arch form, correlating it to mandibular arch form. It is not necessary in cleft patients to overexpand the maxilla because there is no bone between the segments. In our experience adequate occlusal relations and the maxillary alveolar bone graft are sufficient to hold the expansion. Overexpansion of the maxilla causes a wider separation of the segments at the alveolar level, making adequate gingival coverage of the graft difficult or impossible (Fig. 48-16).

After the crossbite (anterior or posterior) has been corrected, the incisor teeth are placed in their ideal positions. Orthodontic treatment at this stage is completed rapidly, taking between 6 and 12 months. Before surgical referral, all appliances over the palate are removed; the labial aspect of the orthodontic appliance is maintained for postoperative stability but is segmented to facilitate access to the surgical field.

Orthodontic treatment required after the bone graft can be instituted as soon as the patient is comfortable with intraoral manipulation. If no additional orthodontic treatment is required, the orthodontic appliance is removed and the new position of the maxillary incisors is retained with a bonded lingual wire or a removable maxillary retainer. Prosthetic teeth can be incorporated into the retention plate for cosmetic purposes while the patient awaits additional dental eruption (Fig. 48-17).

Patients treated by this protocol complete the preparatory phase of orthodontic treatment by late childhood or the early teenage years. Although the retention

Fig. 48-12. Complete left cleft lip and palate in a patient 8 years, 8 months of age. Transitional dentition with commonly observed rotation of central incisor adjacent to cleft and crossbite of maxillary cleft segment (arrows). Orthodontic treatment is indicated to correct the crossbite and to align the tooth adjacent to the cleft to facilitate flap design and access to the operative site at the time of secondary alveolar bone grafting. A. Frontal occlusal view. B. Palatal view.

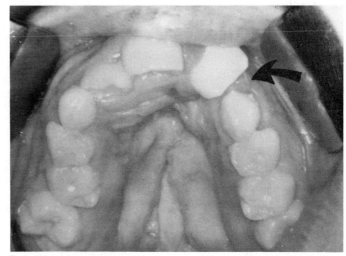

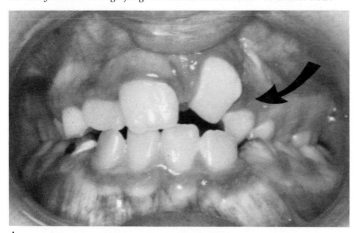

A

B

Fig. 48-13. Patient with complete unilateral left cleft lip and palate in transitional dentition stage before (A, B) and after (C, D) orthodontic treatment in preparation for maxillary alveolar bone grafting. In this patient a labial orthodontic appliance was used to correct arch form and dental malpositions. The occlusal views (B and D) are reversed mirror images.

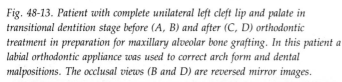

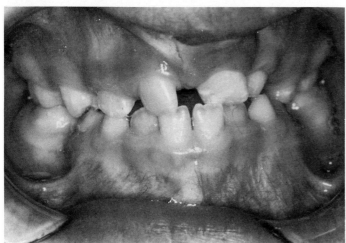

A

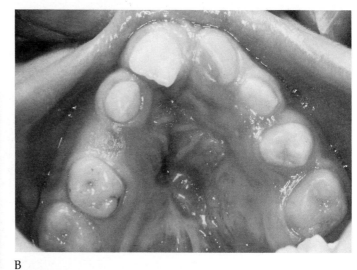

B

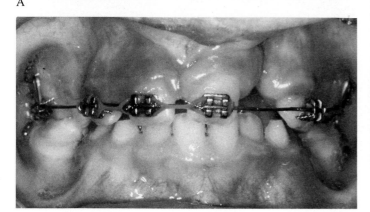

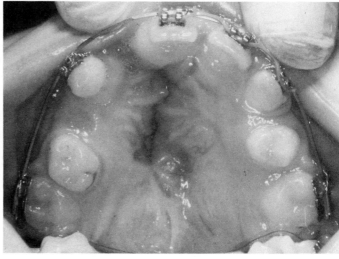

C

D

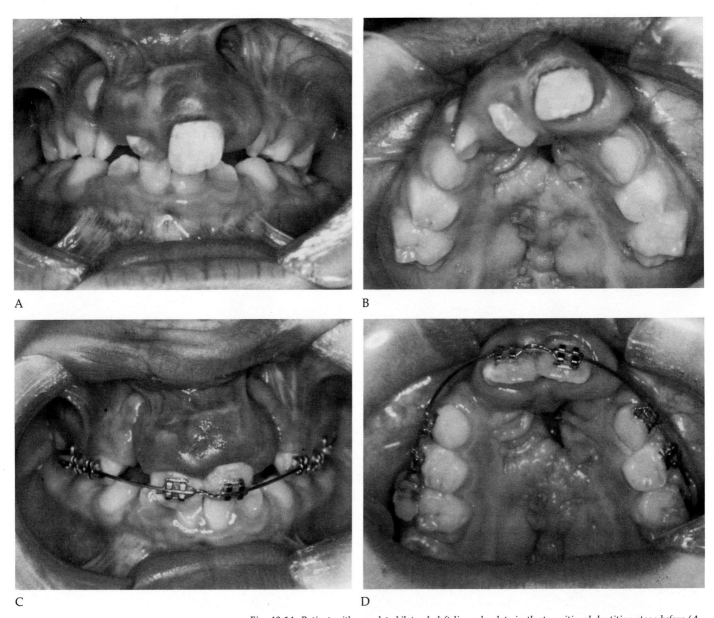

A

B

C

D

Fig. 48-14. Patient with complete bilateral cleft lip and palate in the transitional dentition stage before (A, B) and after (C, D) orthodontic treatment in preparation for maxillary alveolar bone grafting. In this patient a labial orthodontic appliance was used to correct arch form and dental malpositions.

phase is uncomplicated, it is important to monitor the patient's craniofacial growth and dental development regularly, particularly the eruption of the lateral incisor or canine through the cleft (see Figs. 48-10 and 48-11). In most patients teeth erupt spontaneously. Impactions are usually related to severe malposition, crowding of the teeth, or trauma to the teeth during the bone graft procedure. Impacted lateral incisors are usually extracted, and cuspids are surgically uncovered and orthodontically moved into the arch (Fig. 48-18).

Orthodontic Treatment in the Permanent Dentition

In most patients the final stage of orthodontic intervention can be accomplished without difficulty, particularly if the previously defined protocol is followed. Treatment time varies but is usually not different from that of patients who do not have clefts. The goal of this phase of treatment is to provide the patient with ideal occlusal relations for proper function, aesthetics, and long-term stability.

This final phase usually requires a full banded or bonded and fixed appliance complemented by orthodontic auxiliaries necessary to facilitate treatment. At this stage it is quite important to determine the following:

1. The integrity of the dentition and supporting structures
2. Dental arch length (dental crowding)
3. Unusual dental positions such as impacted cuspids or lateral incisors or dental transpositions

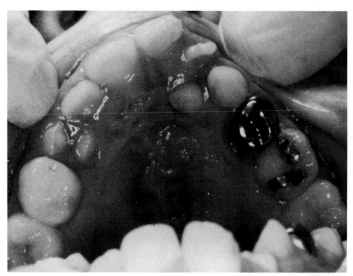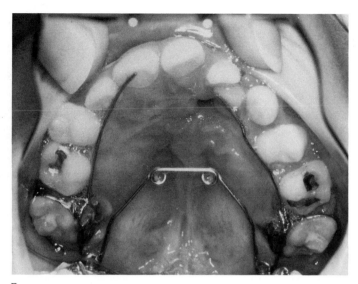

A   B

Fig. 48-15. Views of maxillary arch in patient with complete unilateral cleft lip and palate with transitional dentition before (A) and after (B) expansion with spring-loaded (quadhelix) expander. Note the change in arch form before and after expansion. Also note the change in position of the palatally placed cleft primary incisor caused by the action of the lateral arm of the expander.

Fig. 48-16. Patient with complete right cleft lip and palate after excessive expansion of maxillary segments. Note extremely wide alveolar defect and oronasal fistula. It is contraindicated to expand a maxillary arch to this extent because doing so would make closure of the wide alveolar defect a difficult or impossible surgical task.

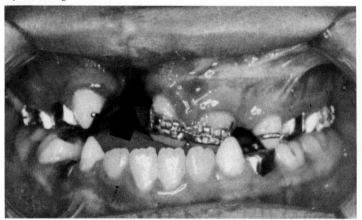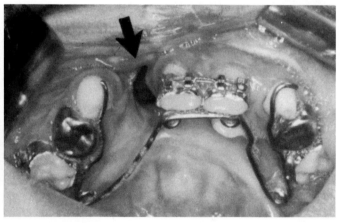

4. Missing teeth that need to be replaced with a prosthesis or closure of residual spaces with orthodontic treatment, especially in the cleft region
5. Anteroposterior and transverse relations of the maxilla and mandible
6. Relation of the dentition and dental arches to each other and to the face

We make every attempt to complete the patient's treatment with class I molar and cuspid occlusal relations and ideal overjet and overbite. If the patient is missing the lateral incisor in the cleft region, a decision is made to close the space and make the cuspid a lateral incisor or to preserve the space for future prosthetic replacement. We prefer to preserve the space and replace the lateral incisor later with a fixed prosthesis or osseointegrated fixture. Our reasoning is that when a maxillary cuspid is moved forward into the lateral incisor position, the cuspid eminence at the pyriform aperture and corner

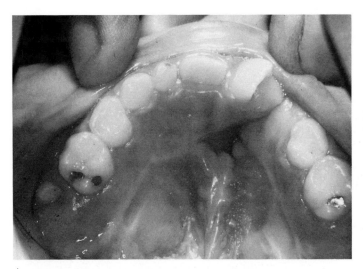

A

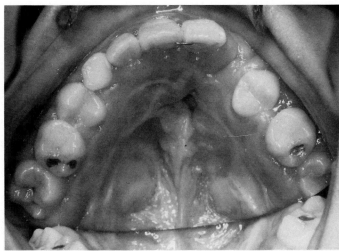

B

Fig. 48-17. Occlusal views of patient with complete unilateral left cleft lip and palate with transitional dentition before (A) and after (B) orthodontic alignment of maxillary arch and reconstruction of alveolar cleft. Note the bonded wire placed behind the maxillary central incisors to stabilize the rotation of the cleft maxillary central incisor. C. Frontal view of same patient wearing temporary maxillary removable retainer with prosthetic tooth replacing missing cleft lateral incisor.

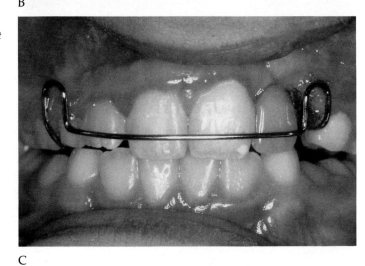

C

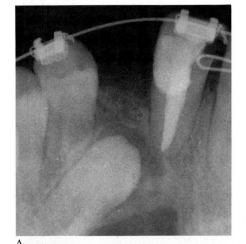

A

Fig. 48-18A. Roentgenogram of patient with complete unilateral cleft lip and palate after maxillary alveolar bone grafting showing abnormal position and eruption path of maxillary cleft permanent canine. B. Palatal view of same patient undergoing orthodontic movement of impacted canine after surgical palatal exposure. C. Patient at completion of orthodontic treatment with aligned canine and good arch form.

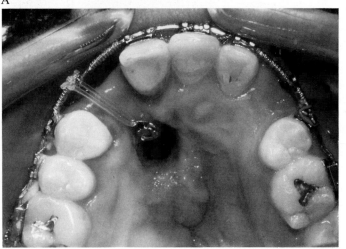

B

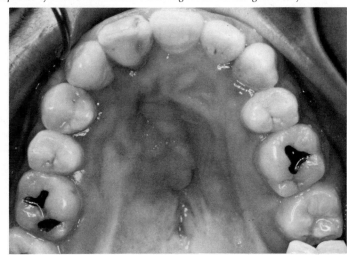

C

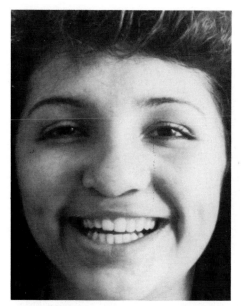

Fig. 48-19. Patient with repaired complete right unilateral cleft lip and palate in which missing cleft maxillary lateral incisor was replaced by moving the canine forward. Note the lack of fullness on the right side of the smile.

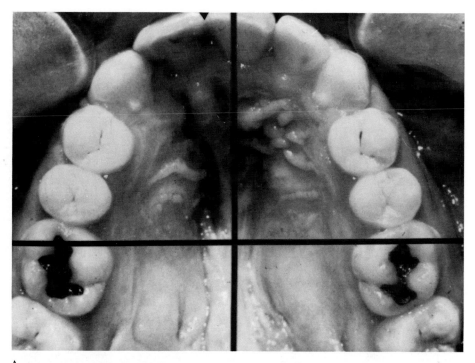

A

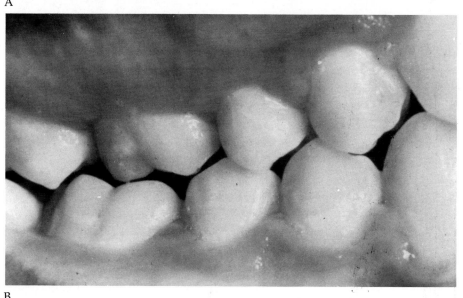

B

Fig. 48-20A. Palatal view of patient with complete right cleft lip and palate in which permanent cuspid was used to replace missing permanent cleft maxillary lateral incisor. Note the deviation of the dental midline toward the cleft side and the asymmetric shape of the arch anteriorly. The vertical line marks the true maxillary skeletal midline. B. Class II dental relations on the cleft side.

of the mouth is lost. In addition, an asymmetric, narrower arch is made on the cleft side, affecting the fullness of the smile (Fig. 48-19). Moving the cuspid forward also can compromise the buccal occlusion on that side (Fig. 48-20).

In patients whose canine tooth has drifted naturally through the bone graft into the position of the lateral incisor and who have excellent buccal occlusion, whose canine root and crown morphology is similar to that of a lateral incisor, or whose oral hygiene is less than optimal, positioning the canine in the lateral incisor position is highly indicated (Fig. 48-21).

If the maxillary alveolar cleft has been properly reconstructed and adequate occlusal relations have been obtained, the long-term stability and retention of these patients' teeth is similar to that of the teeth of patients without clefts. However, special attention has to be given to the retention of severely rotated teeth because of their strong tendency to relapse and to the periodontal status of the teeth in the cleft region. Our current surgical and orthodontic protocol makes it possible to attain occlusal relations that provide excellent function, appearance, and long-term stability (Fig. 48-22).

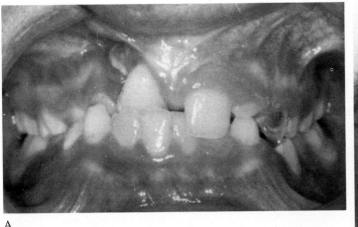

A

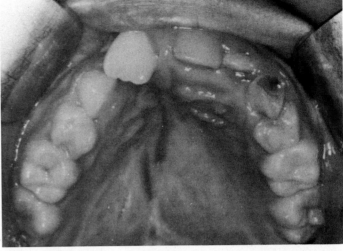

B

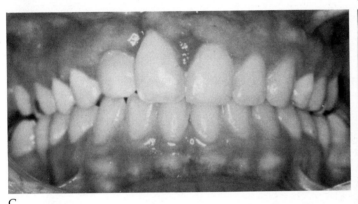

C

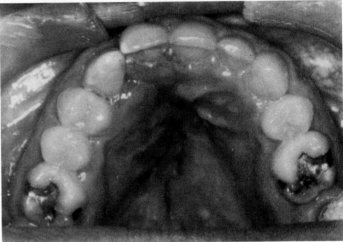

D

Fig. 48-21. Frontal occlusal and maxillary views of patient with complete right unilateral cleft lip and palate before (A, C) and after (B, D) maxillary alveolar bone grafting and orthodontic treatment. Note that the missing right maxillary cleft lateral incisor was replaced by the permanent cuspid. Adequate occlusal and functional results were obtained.

Orthodontic and Orthognathic Surgery for Patients with Clefts

Skeletal and dental discrepancies that are not amenable to orthodontic treatment are managed with a combined orthodontic and orthognathic surgical approach. Orthognathic surgery allows restoration of severely abnormal maxillomandibular relations and provides appropriate support for the overlying soft tissues of the face. This approach yields dramatic functional and aesthetic improvements and provides a better foundation for the final reconstruction of the secondary cleft lip and nasal deformities.

To achieve the goals of a combined orthodontic surgical treatment plan re-

quires close cooperation between the orthodontist and the surgeon over an extended period of time. The planning of orthognathic surgery requires a thorough examination of the face, oral cavity, and temporomandibular joints and the collection and analysis of pertinent records, such as cephalometric and panoramic roentgenograms, dental study models, and photographs. It is beyond the scope of this chapter to cover all these important aspects, but a summary of our approach to these patients is presented and illustrated. The analyses done by the orthodontist and the surgeon are used to arrive at a definitive treatment plan.

All patients are examined before treatment by both surgeon and orthodontist, and all necessary records are obtained. Direct anthropometric measurements and proportions of the face are obtained and

recorded as described by Farkas in 1981. Patients with palatal clefts who are undergoing orthognathic operations are at risk for postoperative velopharyngeal problems; therefore, examination by a speech pathologist is always required. Photographs are obtained while the patient's face is at rest and while the patient is smiling. Lateral and frontal cephalometric roentgenograms are obtained. The lateral roentgenogram is obtained with the lips in repose and the teeth in occlusion. A panoramic roentgenogram is obtained to assess the dentition, the anatomy of the cleft region, and the mandibular rami and condyles. If indicated, other roentgenographic studies are requested, including periapical roentgenograms, temporomandibular joint arthrograms, and computed tomographic scans with three-dimensional reconstruction.

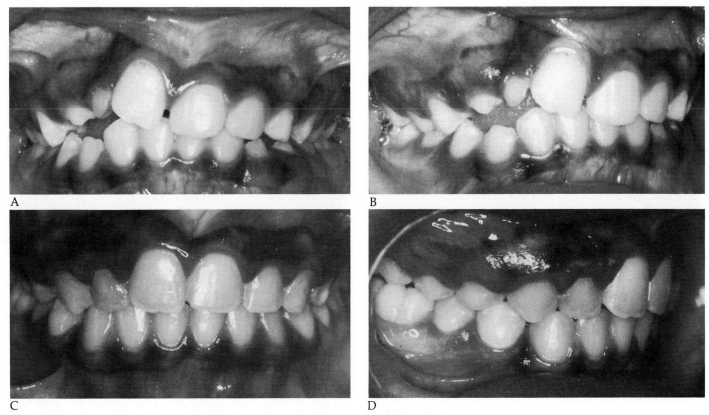

A   B

C   D

Fig. 48-22. Excellent occlusal relations obtained in patient after bone grafting of right maxillary alveolar cleft and full orthodontic treatment. Note that the cleft right permanent maxillary incisor has been preserved. A, B. Before treatment. C, D. After treatment.

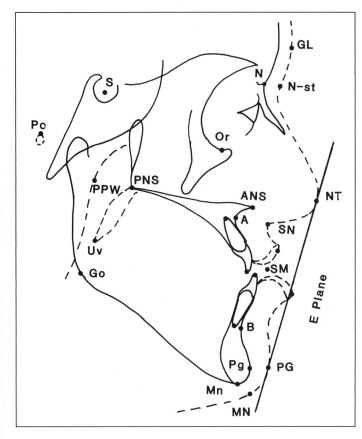

Fig. 48-23. Common cephalometric landmarks. The long axis of the maxillary and mandibular incisors is drawn between the incisal edge and tooth apex. Skeletal: S = sella; N = nasion; Or = orbitale; ANS = anterior nasal spine; PNS = posterior nasal spine; A = point A; B = point B; Pg = pogonion; Mn = menton; Go = gonion; Po = porion. Soft tissues: GL = glabella; N-st = nasion–soft tissue; NT = nasal tip; SN = subnasale; SM = stomion; PG = pogonion; MN = menton; PPW = posterior pharyngeal wall; Uv = uvula tip.

Common landmarks and lateral cephalometric measurements used for analysis are presented in Figure 48-23 and Table 48-2. Prediction tracings to simulate surgical movements are made from the cephalometric roentgenograms (Fig. 48-24).

Dental study models are obtained preoperatively. The study models are used to determine dental positions, the degree of crowding, and interarch relations. When only one jaw is to be operated on and a surgical interdental splint is required, the models are mounted on a hinge articulator to prepare the splint in the laboratory (Fig. 48-25). In patients requiring simultaneous maxillary and mandibular operations, it is imperative that a

Table 48-2. Cephalometric measurements

Soft tissues	Mean ± SD	Skeletal		Dental	
Vertical relations		Vertical relations		Vertical relations	
GL-SN/SN-MN (ratio)	1:1	N-ANS/ANS-Mn (ratio, %)	80 ± 6.00	$\underline{1}$/upper lip (mm)	2.6 ± 1.4
SN-SM/SM-MN (ratio)	1:2			Anteroposterior relations	
Interlabial gap (mm)	0–3	Anteroposterior relations		$\underline{1}$/S-N (degrees)	100.2 ± 5.68
Anteroposterior relations		S-N-A (degrees)	83.9 ± 2.43	$\underline{1}$/ANS-PNS (degrees)	112.1 ± 5.70
N-st-PG/FH (degrees)	90 ± 2	S-N-B (degrees)	81.2 ± 2.63	$\underline{1}$/A-Pg plane (mm)	5.4 ± 2.70
GL-SN-PG (degrees)	−11 ± 4	N-A/FH (degrees)	89.0 ± 3.00	$\overline{1}$/A-Pg plane (mm)	2.7 ± 1.70
Nasolabial angle (degrees)	111.4 ± 11.7	N-Pg/FH (degrees)	87.7 ± 2.60	$\overline{1}$/Mn-Go (degrees)	90.6 ± 5.77
Upper lip–E plane (mm behind)	−6.8 ± 1.9	N-A-Pg (degrees)	3.8 ± 2.19	$\dfrac{1}{\overline{1}}$ (interincisal angle)	135.1 ± 8.30
Lower lip–E plane (mm behind)	−3.9 ± 2.1	Mn-Go/FH (degrees)	22.7 ± 4.30	Velopharyngeal	
				PNS-PPW (mm)	24.2 ± 1.87
				PNS-Uv (mm)	34.5 ± 1.57
				PNS-PPW/PNS-Uv (ratio, %)	70.2 ± 6.99

FH = Frankfort horizontal (Po–Or); $\underline{1}$ = upper incisor; $\overline{1}$ = lower incisor.
Skeletal: S = sella; N = nasion; Or = orbitale; ANS = anterior nasal spine; PNS = posterior nasal spine; A = point A; B = point B; Pg = pogonion; Mn = menton; Go = gonion; Po = porion.
Soft tissues: GL = glabella; N-st = nasion–soft tissue; NT = nasal tip; SN = subnasale; SM = stomion; PG = pogonion; MN = menton; PPW = posterior pharyngeal wall; Uv = uvula tip.

Fig. 48-24A. Prediction tracings from cephalometric roentgenograms showing planned surgical movements with expected soft tissue responses after maxillary advancement and mandibular setback. B. Tracings from preoperative (solid line) and postoperative (dashed line) cephalometric roentgenograms of the patient in Figs. 48-29 and 48-30. Note the similarity of the predicted and actual skeletal and soft tissue changes.

A   B

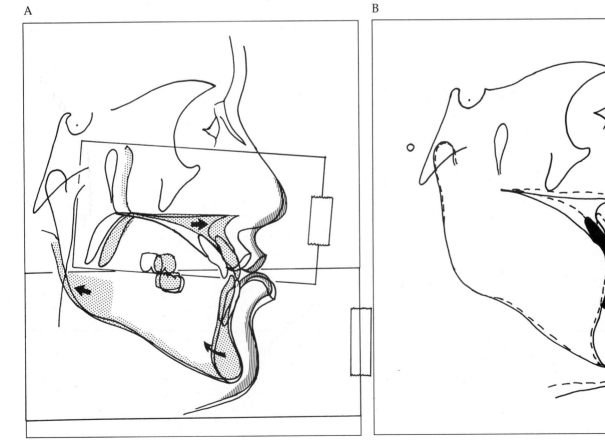

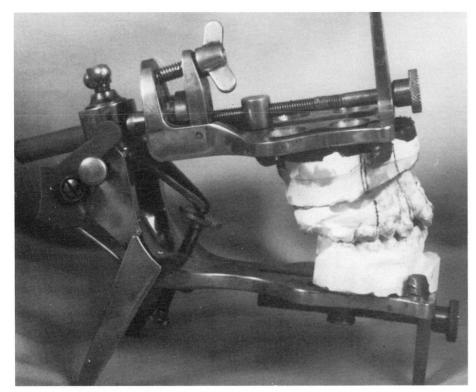

Fig. 48-25. Dental casts mounted on semiadjustable hinge articulator.

face bow transfer be done and the models mounted on an adjustable articulator (Fig. 48-26). On the basis of the clinical examination and cephalometric analysis, the planned operation is performed on the models. In the articulator the maxilla is repositioned and fixed, and an intermediate splint is fabricated. This splint serves as a guide for maxillary position using the mandible that is not operated on as a reference. If required, a final splint is made with the models mounted on a hinge articulator. Patients with clefts usually require expansion at the time of the operation or need other movements, such as closure of the cleft site by bringing the buccal segment forward. If these movements are planned, the use of a final splint is advised to aid postsurgical stability (Fig. 48-27).

If the patient has been followed for a long time and a skeletal disharmony is predicted or noted after the secondary bone grafting stage, the maxilla at the time of intermediate retention (before the final orthodontics or orthognathic surgery)

Fig. 48-26. Dental casts of patient shown in Figs. 48-29 and 48-30 mounted on adjustable articulator using facial and occlusal records obtained from face bow transfer in preparation for double-jaw orthognathic surgery.

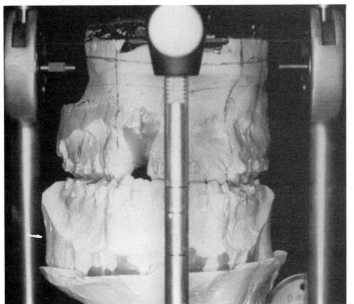

Fig. 48-27. Interdental acrylic occlusal splint used in immediately postoperative phase in which elastic therapy was instituted in patient shown in Figs. 48-29 and 48-30 after segmental two-piece maxillary Le Fort I osteotomy and mandibular setback.

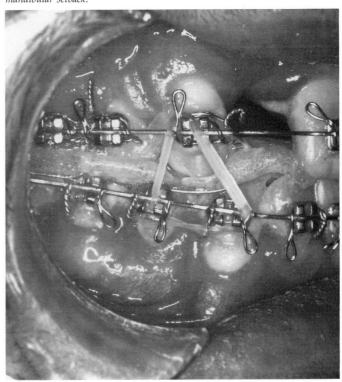

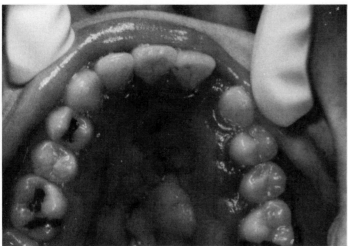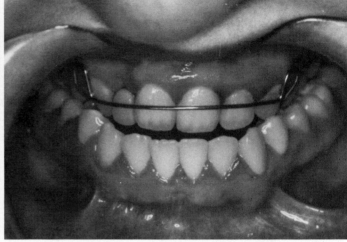

Fig. 48-28. Fourteen-year-old patient with right cleft lip and palate and class III dental and skeletal relations after initial orthodontic treatment and reconstruction of maxillary alveolar cleft. The mirror palatal view on the left side shows a nicely aligned arch in which the space for the missing cleft lateral incisor has been preserved. The frontal occlusal view on the right shows the anterior and posterior transverse discrepancies that require future orthognathic surgical correction. While waiting for further growth and development, the patient wears a temporary removable orthodontic retainer with a prosthetic tooth.

should be in ideal arch alignment to eventually undergo orthognathic surgery (Fig. 48-28). In this way orthodontic preparation is minimized before the operation.

The role of the orthodontist is to position the teeth within their supporting basal bones, to achieve stable dental relations, and to properly align and coordinate the maxillary and mandibular dental arches to allow for ideal dental occlusal relations at the time of and after orthognathic surgery. Additionally the orthodontic appliance is used for intermaxillary fixation during and after the operation. It should be noted that orthodontic preparation for an operation often produces a discrepancy that appears more severe, particularly in the sagittal plane, but the discrepancy is completely corrected when the jaws are surgically repositioned both transversely and anteroposteriorly. Adherence to sound principles of orthodontic and surgical treatment yields ideal occlusal, functional, and aesthetic results (Figs. 48-29 and 48-30).

Suggested Reading

Abyholm, F.E., Bergland, O., and Semb, G. Secondary bone grafting of alveolar clefts. *Scand. J. Plast. Reconstr. Surg.*, 15:127, 1981.

Bjork, A., and Skieller, V. Growth of the maxilla in three dimensions as revealed radiographically by the implant method. *Br. J. Orthod.* 4:53, 1977.

Broadbent, B.H., Sr., Broadbent, B.H., Jr., and Golden, W.H. *Bolton Standards of Dentofacial Developmental Growth.* St. Louis: Mosby, 1975.

Farkas, L.J. Anthropometry of the Head and Face in Medicine. New York: Elsevier, 1981.

Friede, H., and Lennartsson, B. Forward traction of the maxilla in cleft lip and palate patients. *Eur. J. Orthod.* 3:21, 1984.

Jacobs, J.D., and Sinclair, P.M. Principles of orthodontic mechanics in orthognathic surgery cases. *Am. J. Orthod.* 84:399, 1983.

Pruzansky, S. Description, classification, and analysis of unoperated clefts of the lip and palate. *Amer. J. Orthod.*, 39:590, 1953.

Ranta, R. A review of tooth formation in children with cleft lip and palate. *Am. J. Orthod.* 90:11, 1986.

Riolo, M.L., et al. An Atlas of Craniofacial Growth. Monograph No. 2. Craniofacial Growth Series. Center for Human Growth and Development. The University of Michigan, Ann Arbor, Mich., 1974.

Scheideman, G.B., et al. Cephalometric analysis of dentofacial normals. *Am. J. Orthod.* 78:404, 1980.

Subtelny, J.D. A cephalometric study of the growth of the soft palate. *Plast. Reconstr. Surg.* 19:49, 1957.

Subtelny, J.D. Orthodontic Principles in Treatment of Cleft Lip and Palate. In J. Bardach and H.L. Morris (Eds.), *Multidisciplinary Management of Cleft Lip and Palate.* Philadelphia: Saunders, 1990. Pp. 615–636.

Worms, F.W., Isaacson, R.J., and Speidel, T.M. Surgical orthodontic treatment planning: Profile analysis and mandibular surgery. *Angle Orthod.* 46:1, 1976.

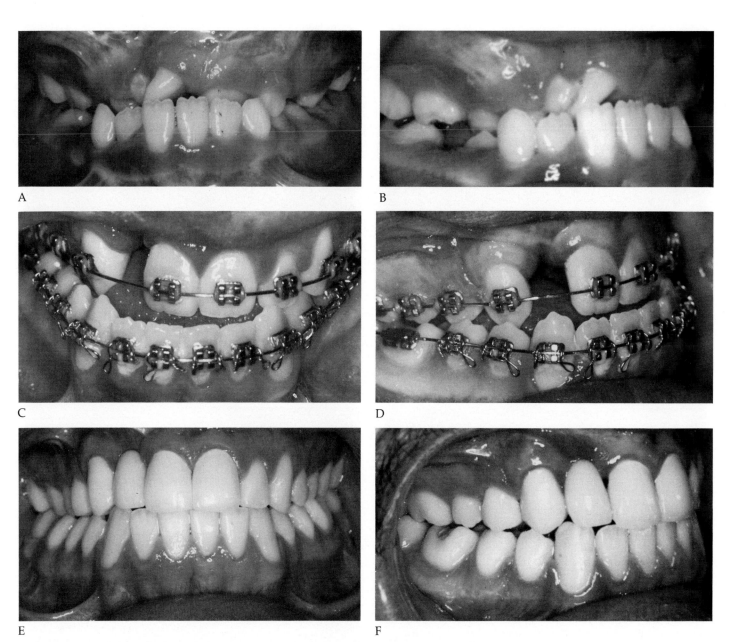

A

B

C

D

E

F

Fig. 48-29. *Frontal and lateral occlusal views of patient with a repaired right unilateral cleft lip and palate with anteroposterior and transverse maxillary deficiency and skeletal and dental class III relations. Preoperative views (A, B), views following orthodontic preparation (C, D), and views after orthognathic surgery (E, F). Note ideal occlusal relations obtained after surgery and fixed prosthetic rehabilitation.*

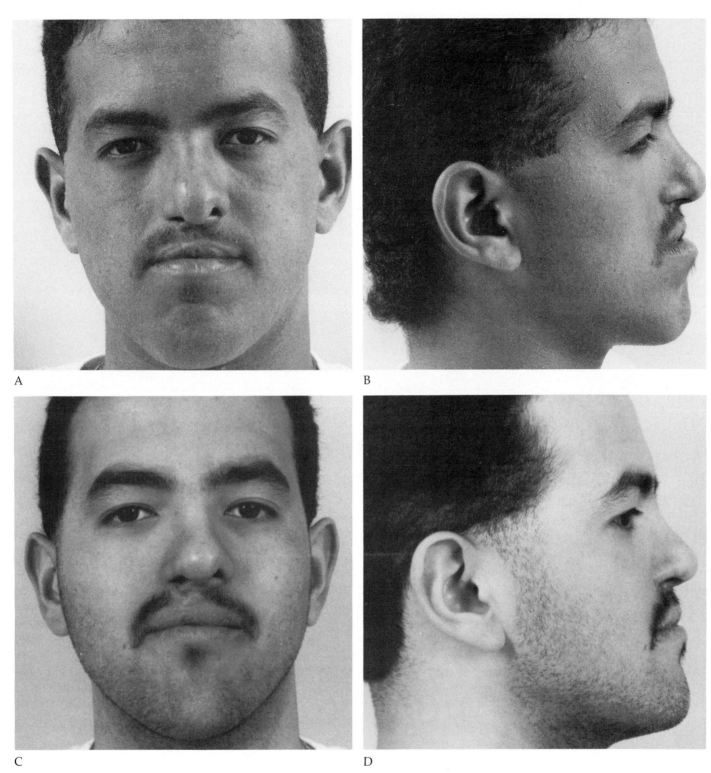

A

B

C

D

Fig. 48-30. Preoperative (A, B) and postoperative (C, D) frontal and lateral facial photographs of patient shown in Fig. 48-29. Note the improvement in nose and lip relations and overall facial balance.

49

Secondary Bone Grafting of Residual Alveolar Clefts

Mimis Cohen

Reconstruction of the alveolar process by secondary bone grafting of the maxillary clefts in the early transitional dentition stage has become a well-accepted procedure. Boyne and Sands are credited as the first to recommend bone grafting of alveolar clefts with particle cancellous bone in conjunction with orthodontic treatment in the mixed dentition stage. Since Boyne and Sands's pioneer report in 1972, several surgeons have demonstrated the value of this approach and have reported excellent long-term results. This technique has been incorporated into the treatment protocols of most cleft teams as an additional procedure to improve the habilitation of patients with residual unilateral or bilateral alveolar clefts and oronasal fistulas.

Goals of Bone Grafting

Several short- and long-term reconstructive and aesthetic goals are achieved with secondary bone grafting of the maxilla and closure of residual alveolar fistulas. The most important ones are summarized in Table 49-1.

Table 49-1. Goals of secondary bone grafting of residual alveolar clefts

Closure of oronasal fistula

Improvement of oral and nasal hygiene

Stabilization of maxillary segments

Preservation of adjacent teeth

Bony support of adjacent teeth

Tooth eruption through graft

Orthodontic movement of teeth

Reduction of need for prosthetic appliances

Improvement of nasal and facial symmetry and appearance

Increased alar support and projection

Improved appearance of alveolus and labial vestibule

Oronasal fistulas, even small ones, result in constant communication between the oral and nasal cavities accompanied by irritation of the nasal mucosa from food and saliva, nasal congestion, and crusting. Furthermore, retention of food particles within the cleft results in halitosis and poor nasal and oral hygiene, leading to caries of the teeth adjacent to the cleft and gingival inflammation. Closure of the oronasal fistula restores the natural barrier between the oral and nasal cavities and effectively eliminates these problems.

In patients with unilateral clefts, permanent stabilization of the maxillary segments is achieved after successful bone grafting. In patients with bilateral clefts, the premaxilla is stabilized with the lateral maxillary segments. Collapse of the orthodontically expanded segments is thus avoided and the need for prolonged wearing of special splints or orthodontic appliances is reduced.

Adequate alveolar bony support is provided to the teeth adjacent to the cleft, ensuring long-term stability and reducing the chances of early loss of these teeth. If the procedure is performed before the eruption of the permanent cleft canine, or even the lateral incisor, an appropriate bony environment is provided for the spontaneous eruption and support of these teeth through the bone graft. Thus more teeth can be preserved, and better long-term oral rehabilitation can be achieved.

The final appearance of the alveolus is also improved and normalized after the bone grafting procedure. The reconstructed alveolar process provides for a

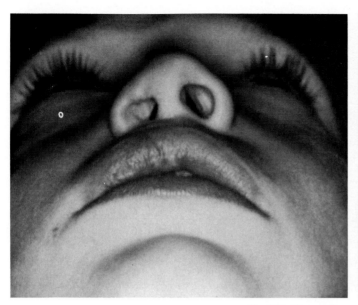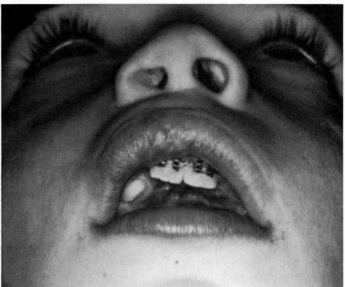

Fig. 49-1. *Preoperative and postoperative views of a 9-year-old patient who underwent closure of right oronasal fistula and bone grafting of the maxilla. Note the improved support of the lip and nasal base after this procedure.*

superior appearance of a bridge or other prosthetic device or the placement of osseointegrated fixtures when permanent teeth are absent. In addition, orthodontic movement of the teeth adjacent to the cleft—to close existing gaps and improve the intraoral appearance without need for prosthetic appliances—is possible with adequate bony support.

In addition to the direct effects of fistula closure and alveolar reconstruction, bone grafting of the maxilla has indirect beneficial effects on facial aesthetics and symmetry; lip support and projection are improved, and a bony platform is provided that raises the alar base on the cleft side to a level symmetric with the unaffected side (Fig. 49-1).

Timing of Bone Grafting

Bone grafting of a cleft maxilla was first reported by von Eiselsberg in 1901 and subsequently by Lexer in 1908 and Drachter in 1914. The technique did not gain popularity until the early 1950s, however, when several surgeons from various European centers almost simultaneously de-

scribed their approach and reported their experience with primary and secondary bone grafting.

Primary bone grafting during the time of lip repair or soon thereafter was introduced in the hope of early maxillary stabilization, subsequent reduction of crossbite and need of orthodontic treatment, and promotion of tooth eruption through the graft. The long-term results of early bone grafting remain controversial. Most early proponents of the technique, including Johanson, of Sweden, abandoned it in favor of secondary bone grafting because of disappointing long-term results, such as pronounced maxillary retrognathia and a high incidence of anterior and lateral crossbites. Currently only a few authors still favor maxillary orthopedic treatment followed by early bone grafting, and report good long-term results with the technique. Most surgeons favor bone grafting during the stage of transitional dentition and agree that this procedure requires close cooperation among specialists, primarily the surgeon and the orthodontist.

The decision for and timing of surgical treatment are based on a combination of developmental, orthodontic, and surgical factors. The dental, rather than the chronologic, age of the patient is a primary factor guiding the decision regarding the timing of a bone grafting procedure. Ideally bone grafting of residual alveolar clefts should be performed at the early transitional stage of dentition—after eruption of the permanent incisors but before eruption of the permanent maxillary canines.

Surgical intervention during the stage of transitional dentition does not seem to have a negative effect on facial growth, because growth of the maxilla is nearly completed by approximately 8 years of age. Semb studied and analyzed the growth of a group of patients with unilateral cleft lip and palate who underwent bone grafting between the ages of 8 and 12 years. She compared their growth with that of a similar group of patients with clefts who did not receive bone grafts. Cephalograms obtained at the ages of 9 and 16 years for all patients were evaluated and analyzed. The conclusion of the study was that maxillary anteroposterior and vertical growth remains unaffected if cancellous alveolar bone grafting is performed after the patients have reached 8 years of age.

At our center my colleagues and I favor orthodontic maxillary arch alignment, when needed, before bone grafting. Teeth on either segment of the maxilla are also aligned by an orthodontist. Thus patients with complete cleft lip and palate undergo bone grafting at the stage of transitional dentition before the eruption of the permanent cleft canine. Patients with clefts only of the lip and alveolus who do not require alignment of the maxillary arch are operated on earlier, before eruption of the permanent cleft lateral incisor. All necessary extractions of deciduous teeth around the area of the cleft are performed at least 6 to 8 weeks before the operation to facilitate the procedure and allow for soft tissue healing and optimal soft tissue conditions. In addition, the patient's oral health is taken into consideration in preparation for the operation, and bone grafting is deferred if gingival inflammation or dental caries is present.

Sources of Bone Grafts

Initially bone grafting of the maxilla was performed simply to stabilize the maxillary segments and to prevent maxillary

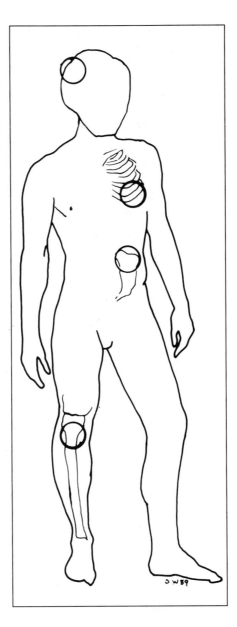

Fig. 49-2. *Cancellous bone from the ilium and the calvarium is used for bone grafting of residual clefts of maxilla and alveolus. A small number of surgeons still demonstrate good results with bone grafts harvested from the rib or tibia.*

collapse and crossbite. Blocks of bone from the ilium or the rib were used for this purpose. With accumulated experience, however, it became apparent that superior results could be obtained when cancellous bone particles only, rather than bony blocks, were used for the reconstruction. These particles represent living tissue that incorporates faster than cortical grafts or blocks of bone, remodels with the rest of the maxilla, and allows for dental eruption through its substance.

Most surgeons use autogenous cancellous bone particles harvested primarily from the ilium or the calvarium with a high rate of success. A few surgeons still favor the use of grafts from the rib or tibia and report almost equally good results (Fig. 49-2).

The superiority of cranial bone grafts in various areas of the maxillofacial skeleton has been demonstrated experimentally and clinically. This superiority, however, had not been demonstrated in the area of residual alveolar clefts. Therefore, my associates and I evaluated our results obtained with both iliac and calvarial cancellous bone grafts to treat alveolar clefts. We found no difference in terms of bone graft incorporation, tooth eruption through the graft, postoperative orthodontic management, or appearance of the alveolus in either group. It seems logical, therefore, to state that in contrast to other areas of the maxillofacial skeleton, the source of the bone graft is not the main factor influencing the success or failure of this procedure. A successful outcome is influenced primarily by adherence to well-established surgical principles and techniques, the use of cancellous bone particles only for the reconstruction, and the coverage of the bone graft with well-vascularized tissues.

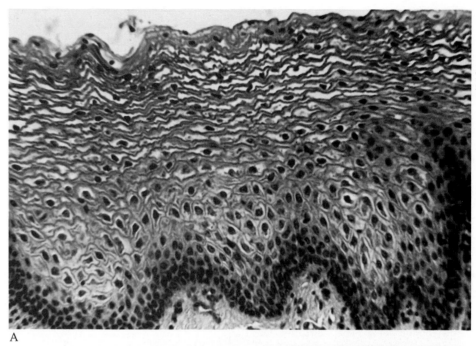

A

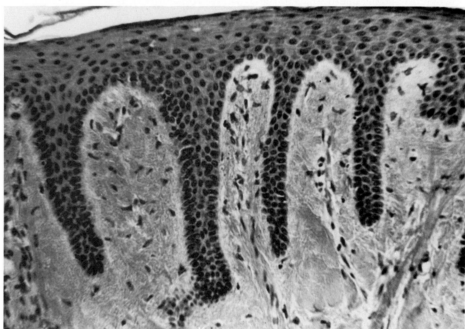

B

Flap Design for Bone Coverage

Little attention had been given to the flap design for soft tissue coverage of the bone grafts, and a variety of local mucosal flaps were described in the literature. Åbyholm in 1981 was the first to emphasize the importance of flap design in secondary bone grafting of maxillary clefts and its importance for the outcome of the reconstruction.

Histologically the gingiva, or masticatory mucosa, consists of a layer of keratinized stratified squamous epithelium and dense and firm lamina propria with immovable attachments to the underlying teeth and bone. Thus a suitable surface to support the masticatory load is provided to protect against mechanical and bacterial damage. The labial and vestibular mucosa, on the other hand, is covered by nonkeratinized epithelium and consists of a thin lamina propria and an abundance of elastic fibers and loose connective tissue. The major portion of the labial mucosa is fixed to the underlying muscles and is highly movable and elastic (Fig. 49-3).

I use gingival mucoperiosteal flaps exclusively for coverage of the bone-grafted maxilla and alveolar process for several reasons. Teeth are "programmed" to erupt through keratinized gingiva and do not erupt normally through labial mucosa. Therefore, if the reconstruction is performed before the eruption of the permanent lateral incisor or canine, one should totally avoid the use of mucosal flaps. Furthermore, the final periodontal condition and the appearance of the al-

veolus is superior when gingival mucoperiosteal flaps are used because tissue of similar texture, thickness, and color to the surroundings is used for the reconstruction (Fig. 49-4).

Surgical Technique

Oral endotracheal anesthesia with a Rae tube is used for the procedure. The tube is taped in the center of the lower lip and

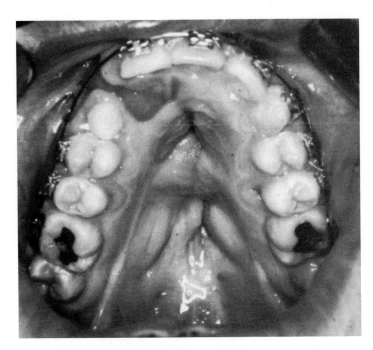

Fig. 49-4. Patient who underwent coverage of bone graft with a labial flap. Note the difference in appearance from the surrounding tissues. The left canine, although present, could not erupt through the flap; surgical uncovering was required.

chin to prevent distortion of the upper lip when a simultaneous lip revision is planned and to avoid compression of the tube by the mouth gag in the event that a palatal fistula coexists and needs to be repaired simultaneously.

The soft tissue defect is evaluated carefully, and its extension into the palate is inspected. The extension of the fistula in the floor of the nose also is evaluated with a nasal speculum. To facilitate this inspection, the nasal cavity on the cleft side is packed with cottonoids soaked in 4% cocaine, which produces vasoconstriction and reduces the swelling of the nasal mucosa. It is mandatory to repair the nasal and palatal portions of the fistula in conjunction with the alveolar repair to achieve complete closure of the fistula and complete soft tissue coverage of the bone graft on both nasal and oral sides.

In patients with unilateral clefts, gingival mucoperiosteal flaps are designed on either side of the cleft (Fig. 49-5). Both flaps are designed inferiorly to the gingival edge to include keratinized gingiva in the area of future tooth eruption. The lateral flap usually extends from the margins of the cleft to the first permanent molar. At this point a back-cut, if necessary, is marked curving upward to the buccal sulcus. This back-cut facilitates medial advancement of the flap and a tension-free closure. Another flap is de-

signed in a similar manner on the medial segment extending from the cleft margin almost to the midline. A back-cut is not necessary on the medial flap because this flap is raised primarily for better exposure of the oronasal fistula and the bony defect of the maxilla. The area of dissection is infiltrated with 1% lidocaine with 1:100,000 epinephrine to achieve vasoconstriction and reduce bleeding during dissection.

Wide exposure of the maxillary cleft is achieved by sharp dissection of the gingival mucoperiosteal flaps. It is vital during this dissection to avoid injuring any unerupted teeth found within the margins of the bony cleft or the thin and friable alveolar bone covering the roots of the teeth around the cleft. The dissection of the lateral flap is carried superiorly to expose the pyriform aperture of the maxilla and the floor of the nose. The medial flap is raised to the nasal spine and the floor of the nose. The nasal mucosa around the fistula is completely freed from scarred surrounding tissues and mobilized to facilitate eversion and closure. As soon as the nasal lining is freed and mobilized within the bony cleft, attention is directed to the palatal fistula to fully expose the extent of the defect of the nasal floor.

A Dingman mouth gag is placed in the mouth, and bilateral palatal mucoperios-

teal flaps are raised sharply on either side of the palatal fistula after infiltration with 1% lidocaine with 1:100,000 epinephrine. The extent of the soft tissue defect of the nasal floor is thus fully visualized.

After meticulous hemostasis, the nasal lining is approximated with interrupted absorbable sutures. The completeness of this closure is evaluated with gentle probing from the nose and with irrigation of normal saline solution into the nostril on the repaired side. Any residual openings are repaired with additional interrupted sutures. In the event that a moderately wide defect is present and complete closure of the nasal floor from the palatal side is not feasible, a superiorly based mucoperiosteal flap is raised from the vomer to facilitate this closure. The palatal mucoperiosteal flaps are approximated together with interrupted absorbable mattress sutures, and the mouth gag is withdrawn.

With these steps, a watertight closure of the nasal floor is achieved, the bony maxillary cleft is completely exposed, all soft tissue and scar are stripped from the margins of the bony cleft, and the palatal fistula is repaired. A soft tissue pocket is thus made to accommodate the bone graft.

Cancellous bone particles harvested from the ilium or the calvarium are used for the

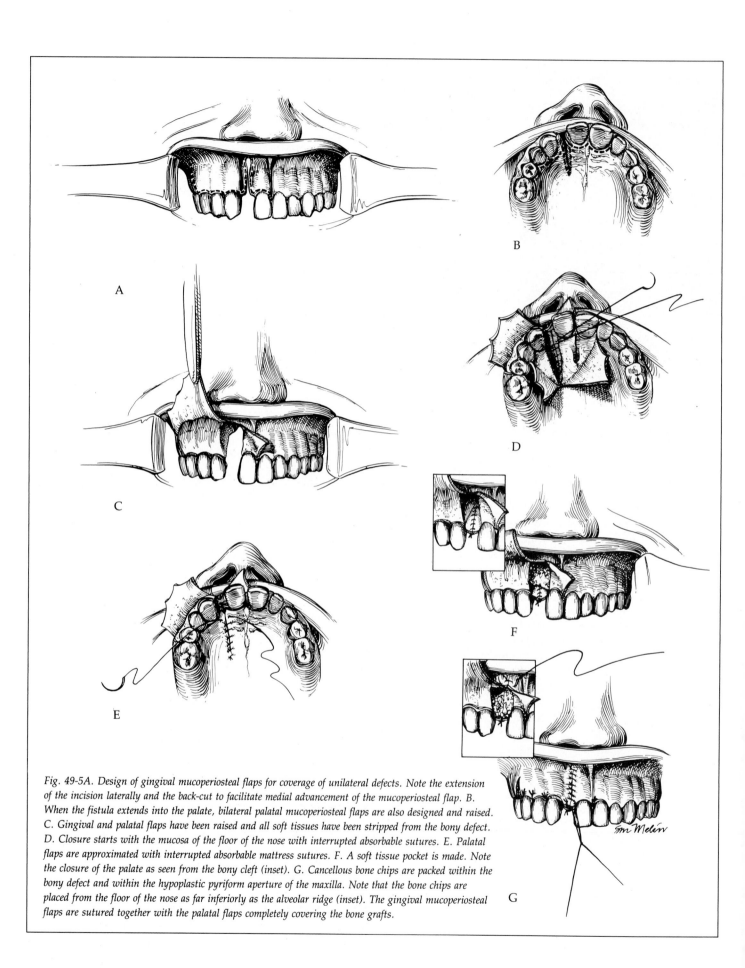

Fig. 49-5A. Design of gingival mucoperiosteal flaps for coverage of unilateral defects. Note the extension of the incision laterally and the back-cut to facilitate medial advancement of the mucoperiosteal flap. B. When the fistula extends into the palate, bilateral palatal mucoperiosteal flaps are also designed and raised. C. Gingival and palatal flaps have been raised and all soft tissues have been stripped from the bony defect. D. Closure starts with the mucosa of the floor of the nose with interrupted absorbable sutures. E. Palatal flaps are approximated with interrupted absorbable mattress sutures. F. A soft tissue pocket is made. Note the closure of the palate as seen from the bony cleft (inset). G. Cancellous bone chips are packed within the bony defect and within the hypoplastic pyriform aperture of the maxilla. Note that the bone chips are placed from the floor of the nose as far inferiorly as the alveolar ridge (inset). The gingival mucoperiosteal flaps are sutured together with the palatal flaps completely covering the bone grafts.

maxillary reconstruction. They are kept in a sponge moistened with normal saline solution to keep the graft from drying out while the soft tissue pocket is prepared. The grafts are packed tightly to fill the bony cleft and to restore the thickness and height of the nasal floor and the maxilla to as close to a normal condition as possible. Unerupted permanent teeth appearing within the bony cleft should be left undisturbed and covered entirely with bony particles. Inferiorly the bone graft should be packed to the level of the alveolar ridge of the maxilla to provide better support to the teeth adjacent to the cleft, to support the teeth that will eventually erupt through the bone graft, and to prevent unattractive notching of the alveolus. Additional bone chips are placed laterally in the area of the hypoplastic pyriform aperture of the maxilla to raise the alar base on the cleft side and to facilitate future correction of the secondary cleft nose deformity. Before soft tissue closure, the bone graft should be molded into position to conform with the contour of the maxilla.

The gingival mucoperiosteal flaps are finally sutured together with interrupted absorbable sutures, providing well-vascularized, tension-free coverage of the bone graft anteriorly. The flaps are also sewn to the previously approximated palatal flaps with interrupted sutures to completely cover the bone graft and the alveolar ridge. The area of the back-cut, if used, is left open and heals secondarily within a few days without problems. Drains or bulky stents have no place in this repair (Fig. 49-6).

Patients with bilateral clefts pose a much more difficult problem for reconstruction because of the deficiency of bone and soft tissue and the increased presence of residual palatal fistulas in addition to the bilateral oronasal fistulas. All procedures, as with unilateral clefts, are performed at the stage of transitional dentition, before the eruption of the permanent canine but after orthodontic alignment of the lateral segments and the premaxilla. In most patients a symmetric arch is achieved with orthodontic treatment only, but sometimes an osteotomy is required to align the premaxilla to the lateral segments. This osteotomy should be performed in conjunction with the bone grafting procedure.

I close both fistulas in the same setting and have never staged the procedure. The design of the lateral gingival mucoperiosteal flaps is similar to that for unilateral clefts; the medial flaps, however, are slightly altered and do not extend to the midline, to avoid complete denudement of the premaxilla from its soft tissue coverage.

The soft tissue deficiency is evident during the closure of the nasal floor and during the closure of the palatal fistulas. As mentioned earlier, one of the prerequisites for successful healing and incorporation of the bone graft is good soft tissue coverage without exposure. For most bilateral clefts, I have used mucoperiosteal flaps from the vomer, based superiorly to achieve a tension-free closure of the nasal floor. Extensive dissection and elevation of the palatal flaps are necessary to achieve good visualization of the nasal floor and to close the palatal fistulas. After soft tissue closure, the bone grafting procedure proceeds as described for unilateral clefts (Fig. 49-7).

Perioperative Care

Broad-spectrum antibiotics are administered perioperatively to all patients. If orthodontic treatment preceded reconstruction and an orthodontic wire is present across the line of the cleft, the wire is not usually removed during the procedure. If the wire is removed to facilitate exposure, however, it is replaced immediately after the procedure to provide additional stability to the teeth and the maxillary segments while the bone graft heals.

A liquid diet is given the night of the operation, and a soft diet is prescribed the day after for 7 to 10 days. The need for maintaining good oral hygiene is emphasized to the patients and their parents. Drains from the donor site, if used, are removed and the patients are discharged to go home, usually the day after the operation. Additional orthodontic treatment, when necessary, is recommended for the end of the healing period, approximately 8 to 12 weeks postoperatively.

Results

Results obtained with this technique have been invariably successful. The associated morbidity or complication rate is low, and with few exceptions the long-term results are very good (Figs. 49-8 to 49-10).

Gingival mucoperiosteal flaps have a broad base and excellent vascularity. When properly designed, released from the surrounding scar tissue, and mobilized, they provide a tension-free closure. Dehiscence of the suture line in this area and bone exposure have been extremely rare in my series of more than 150 patients.

Patients with bilateral residual clefts have a much more difficult problem because of severe soft tissue deficiencies in the alveolus, nasal floor, and palate. With adequate mobilization of the gingival mucoperiosteal flap, a tension-free closure can be achieved (Fig. 49-11). This is not always the case, however, in the repair of nasal mucosa and the palate. I encountered a 10 percent dehiscence rate with partial exposure of the bone graft either in the nose or the anterior palate. This exposure caused partial or complete loss of the graft. In these patients additional bone grafting was performed later. Despite my efforts at placing the bone chips inferior to the alveolar ridge on either side of the cleft, 9 percent of patients had partial resorption of the bone graft, loss of height, and notching of the alveolus. It appears that this degree of clinical and roentgenographic resorption occurs despite efforts at overcorrection during the operation. It has been reported by several other surgeons as well.

Ninety-five percent of the teeth, when present, erupted spontaneously through the bone graft without need for surgical orthodontic assistance. Orthodontic treatment, however, was required in all patients to achieve full alignment of the newly erupted teeth with the adjacent ones, to close existing spaces, and to complete the symmetry of the maxilla.

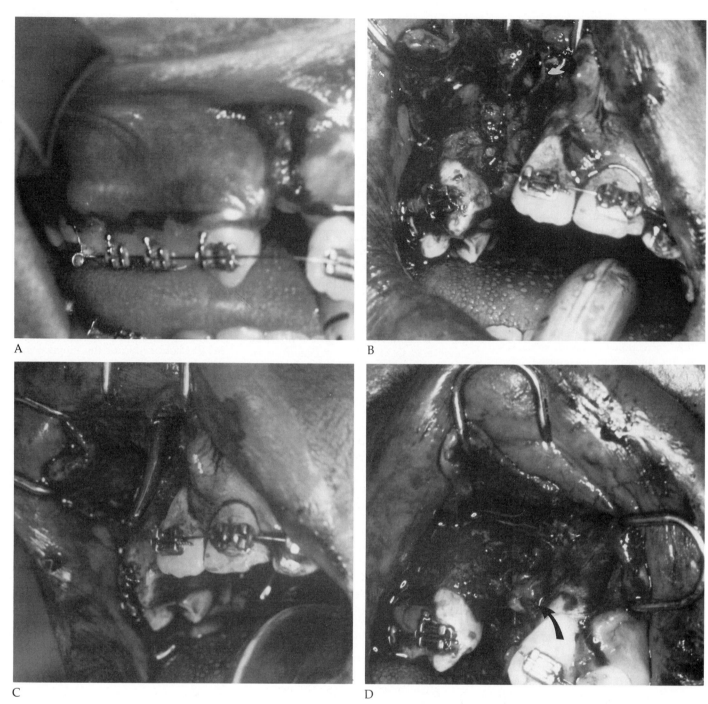

A

B

C

D

Fig. 49-6A. Preoperative markings for gingival mucoperiosteal flaps on either side of oronasal fistula. B. Flaps are elevated and all soft tissues are stripped from the bony cleft. Note the opening in the nasal floor (arrow). C. Hemostat is introduced from the nostril through the fistula to fully delineate extent of the cleft. D. Palatal fistula is repaired (arrow).

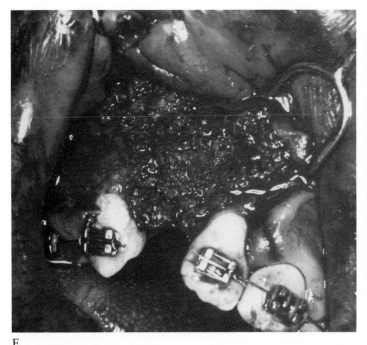

E

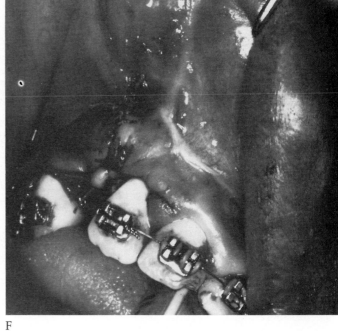

F

Fig. 49-6. (Continued) E. After closure of floor of nose, cancellous bone graft chips are used to pack the defect of the bone. F. Mucoperiosteal flaps are sutured together without tension, providing a well-vascularized coverage over the bone graft.

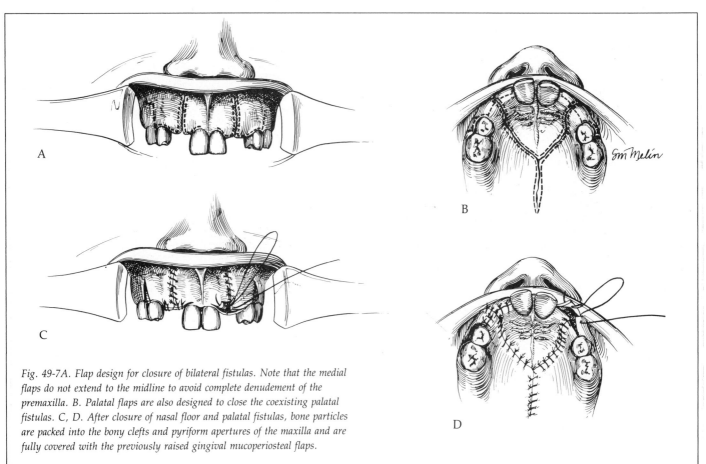

A

B

Jm Melin

C

D

Fig. 49-7A. Flap design for closure of bilateral fistulas. Note that the medial flaps do not extend to the midline to avoid complete denudement of the premaxilla. B. Palatal flaps are also designed to close the coexisting palatal fistulas. C, D. After closure of nasal floor and palatal fistulas, bone particles are packed into the bony clefts and pyriform apertures of the maxilla and are fully covered with the previously raised gingival mucoperiosteal flaps.

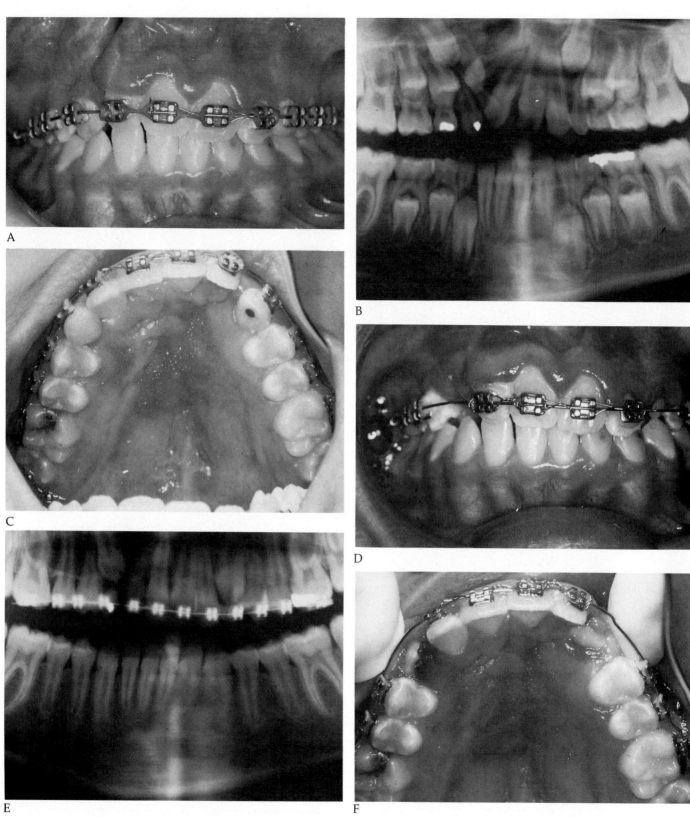

Fig. 49-8A. Patient 10 years, 3 months of age with residual right oronasal
fistula. B. Preoperative roentgenogram demonstrating width of bony cleft. The
permanent cleft canine is still high within the maxilla. C. Preoperative
maxillary occlusal mirror view demonstrating residual cleft. Note the deciduous
canine on the cleft side. D. Postoperative view demonstrating appearance of the
reconstructed alveolus. E. Postoperative roentgenogram. Note the permanent
cleft canine descending through the bone graft. F. Postoperative occlusal mirror
view demonstrating permanent canine spontaneously erupting through bone
graft 13 months postoperatively.

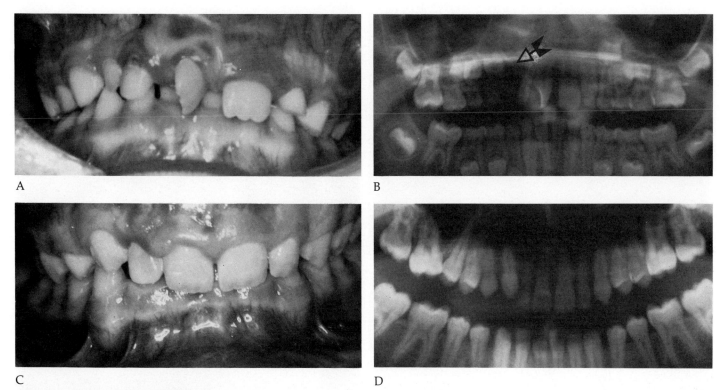

A   B

C   D

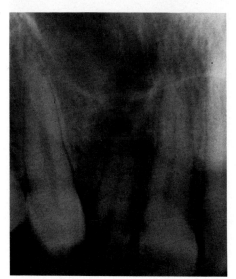

E

Fig. 49-9A. Patient 7 years, 10 months of age with repaired cleft of primary palate only and residual oronasal fistula. B. Preoperative roentgenogram demonstrating large bony defect (arrow) and position of unerupted permanent teeth. C. Final result at 14 years of age after closure of oronasal fistula, bone grafting of maxilla and alveolar cleft, and orthodontic realignment of teeth and arch. D. Postoperative roentgenogram taken at same age as in C. Cleft canine erupted spontaneously through the graft. E. Occlusal roentgenogram of bone-grafted area demonstrating excellent take of bone graft.

Conclusions

A successful outcome with incorporation of bone, little long-term resorption, and spontaneous eruption of the teeth when teeth are present can be expected as long as bone particles alone are used for the reconstruction and the surgeon adheres to some well-established principles. Close cooperation between the surgeon and the orthodontist, timing of the procedure at the stage of transitional dentition, good oral hygiene, complete exposure of the bony cleft, simultaneous closure of co-existing palatal and oronasal fistulas, packing of the bony cleft with cancellous bone particles only, and coverage of the graft with well-vascularized flaps—specifically, gingival mucoperiosteal flaps—are all prerequisites for consistently superior functional and aesthetic results.

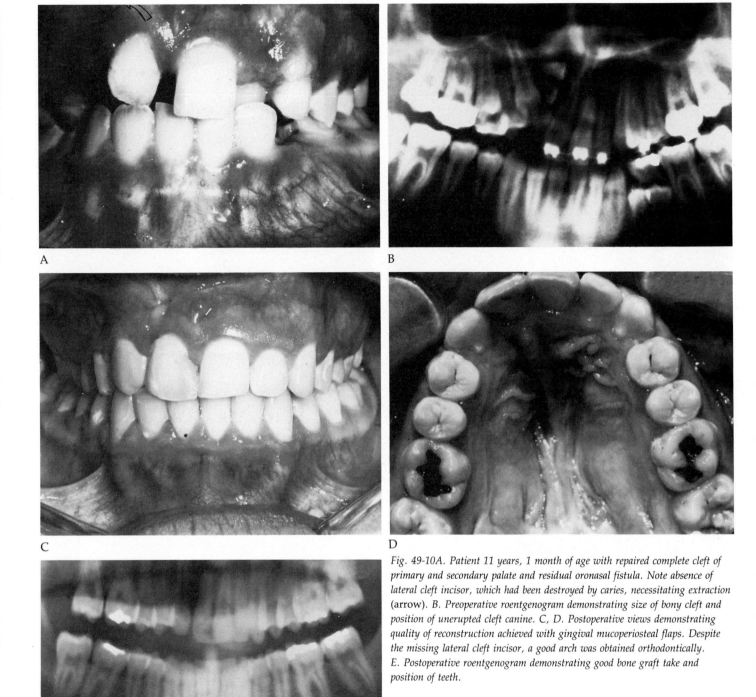

A

B

C

D

Fig. 49-10A. Patient 11 years, 1 month of age with repaired complete cleft of primary and secondary palate and residual oronasal fistula. Note absence of lateral cleft incisor, which had been destroyed by caries, necessitating extraction (arrow). B. Preoperative roentgenogram demonstrating size of bony cleft and position of unerupted cleft canine. C, D. Postoperative views demonstrating quality of reconstruction achieved with gingival mucoperiosteal flaps. Despite the missing lateral cleft incisor, a good arch was obtained orthodontically. E. Postoperative roentgenogram demonstrating good bone graft take and position of teeth.

E

Suggested Reading

Bergland, O., Semb, G., and Åbyholm, F.E. Elimination of the residual alveolar cleft by secondary bone grafting and subsequent orthodontic treatment. *Cleft Palate J.* 23:175, 1986.

Bergland, O., et al. Secondary bone grafting and orthodontic treatment in patients with bilateral complete clefts of the lip and palate. *Ann. Plast. Surg.* 17:460, 1986.

Boyne, P.J., and Sands, N.R. Secondary bone grafting of residual alveolar and palatal clefts. *J. Oral Surg.* 30:87, 1972.

Cohen, M., Figueroa, A.A., and Aduss, H. The role of gingival mucoperiosteal flaps in the repair of alveolar clefts. *Plast. Reconstr. Surg.* 83: 812, 1989.

Cohen, M., et al. Iliac versus cranial bone for secondary grafting of residual alveolar clefts. *Plast. Reconstr. Surg.* 87:423, 1991.

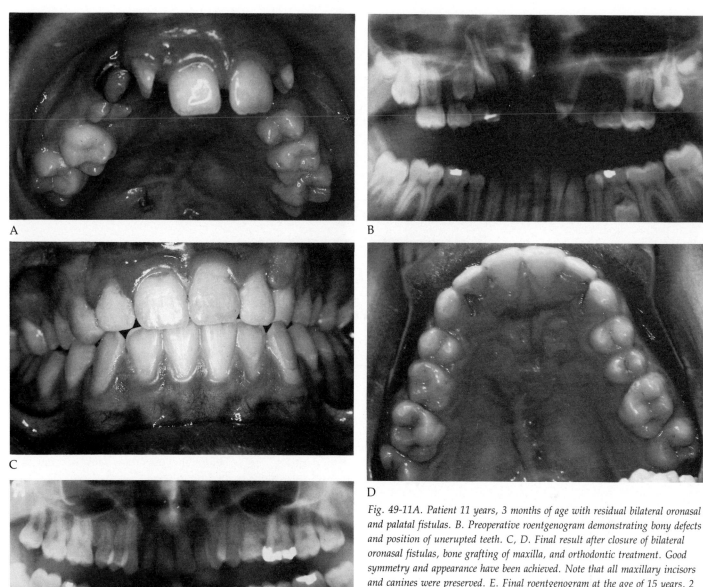

A

B

C

D

Fig. 49-11A. Patient 11 years, 3 months of age with residual bilateral oronasal and palatal fistulas. B. Preoperative roentgenogram demonstrating bony defects and position of unerupted teeth. C, D. Final result after closure of bilateral oronasal fistulas, bone grafting of maxilla, and orthodontic treatment. Good symmetry and appearance have been achieved. Note that all maxillary incisors and canines were preserved. E. Final roentgenogram at the age of 15 years, 2 months, demonstrating good bone graft take and position of erupted teeth.

E

Freihofer, H.P., and Kuijpers-Jagtman, A.M. Early secondary osteoplastic closure of residual alveolar cleft in combination with orthodontic treatment. *J. Craniomaxillofac. Surg.* 17:26, 1989.

Friede, H., and Johanson, B. Adolescent facial morphology on early bone-grafted cleft lip and palate patients. *Scand. J. Plast. Reconstr. Surg.* 16:41, 1982.

Jackson, I.T. Closure of secondary palatal fistulae with intraoral tissue and bone grafting. *Br. J. Plast. Surg.* 25:93, 1972.

Lilja, J., et al. Bone grafting at the stage of mixed dentition in cleft lip and palate patients. *Scand. J. Plast. Reconstr. Surg.* 21:73, 1987.

Rosenstein, S., et al. The case for early bone grafting in cleft lip and palate: A second report. *Plast. Reconstr. Surg.* 87:644, 1991.

Semb, G. Effect of alveolar bone grafting on maxillary growth in unilateral cleft lip and palate patients. *Cleft Palate J.* 25:288, 1988.

Wolfe, S.A., and Berkowitz, S. The use of cranial bone grafts in the closure of alveolar and anterior palatal clefts. *Plast. Reconstr. Surg.* 72: 659, 1983.

50

The Correction of Secondary Skeletal Deformities in Adolescent Patients with Cleft Lip and Palate

Jeffrey C. Posnick

The satisfactory management of patients with cleft lip and palate presents challenging clinical problems to the surgeon and the orthodontist. Orthognathic surgery is often the final therapy to consider in the patient's rehabilitation. It is also the therapy that is most likely to be passed over as "too risky" or to be considered "too big an operation" for a patient who already "has come a long way."

Adding to the difficulties is a lack of information about the exact surgical technique required for each of the cleft types: unilateral cleft lip and palate, bilateral cleft lip and palate, and isolated cleft palate. Because each type may present a different set of residual cleft problems in adolescence, varied surgical techniques are required if a safe orthognathic operation is to be provided for the final reconstruction.

Integrated Team Approach

The care of a patient with a cleft is best delivered by a dedicated cleft lip and palate team that meets to discuss patient protocols and the nature and quality of care of specific patients. It is no longer adequate for individual practitioners, whether surgeons, orthodontists, or speech pathologists, to carry out extensive treatment plans without consideration of a patient's overall care.

The plastic surgeon generally plays a primary role in coordinating the patient's care. The task of the team leader is to transcend his or her own area of expertise and facilitate effective, coordinated care throughout adolescence. The orthodontist may provide preoperative orthopedic treatment in infancy and interceptive orthodontic treatment in childhood. He or she may identify early abnormal growth patterns of the facial skeleton and then carry out final orthodontic treatment in conjunction with orthognathic operations when required. The speech pathologist plays a critical role in speech assessment, performing a clinical examination, assisting with nasoendoscopy, and videofluoroscopy. These procedures may be necessary to characterize both velopharyngeal function and anterior articulation problems that cause sibilant distortion before an orthognathic operation is contemplated. Such evaluation is important because velopharyngeal function tends to deteriorate after a maxillary Le Fort I os-

teotomy with horizontal velopharyngeal advancement. Closure that was adequate before the operation may become borderline afterward, and closure that was borderline may become inadequate. Articulatory distortions caused by malocclusion also are identified and cause-and-effect relations determined. Surgical correction of crossbite, open bite, cleft-dental gaps, residual oronasal fistulas can correct sibilant distortions.

Other team members make contributions to the care of cleft patients. The otolaryngologist and audiologist help prevent and manage middle-ear problems, and the otolaryngologist also assists with potential airway problems. The geneticist helps with the interpretation of additional birth deformities, syndrome analysis and with family planning, both for the parents and for the teenager with a cleft. The social worker assists with self-esteem family, and community-related problems.

Timing of Orthognathic Surgery

Correction of a jaw deformity is usually planned to take place when the skeleton is mature. Maxillofacial growth is generally complete between the ages of 14 and 16 years in girls and 16 and 18 years in boys. Because skeletal growth is variable, however, assessment of each patient must be based on either epiphyseal plate closure documented on hand roentgenograms or cessation of maxillofacial growth documented on sequential cephalometric roentgenograms taken at 6-month intervals.

Only rarely do psychosocial considerations take precedence and require an early operation on the jaw in a patient with a cleft. Wolford showed that when an early operation on the jaw is undertaken in patients with clefts, a revisional jaw operation is required once skeletal maturity is reached. If mandibular hypoplasia is severe and peripheral sleep apnea is documented (Pierre Robin sequence), either a tracheostomy or a mandibular advancement procedure must be performed at an early age and a revisional osteotomy planned for the time of skeletal maturation.

Unilateral Cleft Lip and Palate

Correction of the residual skeletal deformities of an adolescent with unilateral cleft lip and palate (UCLP) challenges the ingenuity and skill of the orthognathic surgeon. In such patients, the central pathology is a degree of maxillary hypoplasia, which may be seen in combination with residual oronasal fistulas, bony defects, and soft tissue scarring. In addition, the maxillary lateral incisor tooth at the cleft site is usually congenitally absent, resulting in a cleft-dental gap.

Residual Deformities

The prevalence of residual clefting deformities in adolescents with UCLP varies widely depending on the center's policy with regard to the staging of reconstruction and on its available surgical expertise. In addition, despite a center's preferred method of management of clefting deformities in infancy, childhood, and early adolescence, a subgroup of patients with UCLP will require orthognathic operations for multiple residual clefting problems.

Maxillary Hypoplasia

The maxilla is often vertically short, causing an edentulous look, and the occlusal plane is often canted. Arch width defi-

ciency causing crossbite may be present in the transverse plane. The maxillary dental midline may be shifted off the facial midline, usually toward the clefted side. The hypoplastic maxilla is retruded in the horizontal plane, causing a concave midface profile, angle class III malocclusion, and a negative overjet. The greater and lesser maxillary segments may vary in their degree of dysplasia, making it difficult to achieve a satisfactory appearance by repositioning the maxilla in one unit rather than with segmental osteotomies.

Residual Oronasal Fistulas

Despite the personal preference for final fistula closure in the stage of mixed dentition prior to the eruption of the permanent canine tooth through the cleft, a patient with UCLP who is a candidate for an orthognathic operation often presents to the orthognathic surgeon with residual labial and palatal fistulas. Previous attempts at closure may have ended in failure or the primary surgeons philosophy for management of the alveolar defect and residual defects may differ. Furthermore, buccal mucosa may have been placed over the cleft site, resulting in a lack of attached gingiva (Keratinized mucosa) in the tooth-bearing surface region.

Residual Bony Defects

As part of the initial cleft deformity, there are large bony defects, not just at the alveolus but throughout the palate and floor of the nose along the cleft site. These defects result in an inferiorly displaced floor of the nose and nasal seal. The cleft adolescent may present to the orthognathic surgeon with these residual bony defects.

Cleft-Dental Gap

The lateral incisor tooth is frequently congenitally absent at the cleft site. A hypoplastic tooth may be present but with inadequate root development or with bony impaction in the cleft. Orthodontic closure of this gap with movement of the canine tooth into the lateral incisor location during the mixed dentition is preferred but only occasionally accomplished. Often with mesial angulation of the canine tooth. The result is often a dental gap at the cleft site between the central incisor and the canine tooth.

Chin Dysplasia

Patients with UCLP frequently breathe through their mouths, resulting in an

open-mouth posture. The addition of a pharyngeal flap in childhood may increase this tendency. The result is a vertically long and retrognathic chin.

Mandibular Dysplasia

True mandibular prognathism in a patient with UCLP is uncommon. Mandibular osteotomy should be limited to facial asymmetries, occlusal plane canting, and the occasional anteroposterior discrepancy.

Surgical Therapy

Rationale

For effective management of the adolescent patient with UCLP who presents with the multiple residual maxillary problems described, I have modified both the classic Le Fort I osteotomy and the previously described techniques. The principal change consists of placement of soft tissue incisions that allow direct exposure for dissection, osteotomies, disimpaction, fistula closure, bone grafting, and application of plate and screw fixation but that do not risk circulation injury to the dento-osseous-musculo-mucosal flaps.

Aided by the increased visibility provided by these incisions, I have incorporated the routine surgical closure of the cleft-dental gap through differential maxillary segmental repositioning. This method of approximating the maxillary segments for closure of the gap also closes up the dead space where the cleft alveolar bone graft exists and approximates the labial and palatal flaps to allow for closure of recalcitrant oronasal fistulas without tension.

Operative Technique

A maxillary vestibular incision is made from one zygomatic buttress to the other without the need for maintenance of labial pedicles (Fig. 50-1). Parallel incisions are made in the region of the residual labial oronasal fistulas, separating the oral and nasal mucosa on each side of the cleft. These incisions are perpendicular to the first incision and follow the line angles of the teeth adjacent to the cleft, generally along the mesial line angle of the canine tooth and the distal line angle of the central incisor. The nasal and palatal mucosae are also sharply incised along the palatal aspect of the fistulas to complete the separation of mucosal layers and facilitate fistula closure.

Through soft tissue subperiosteal dissection, the anterior maxilla on each side is

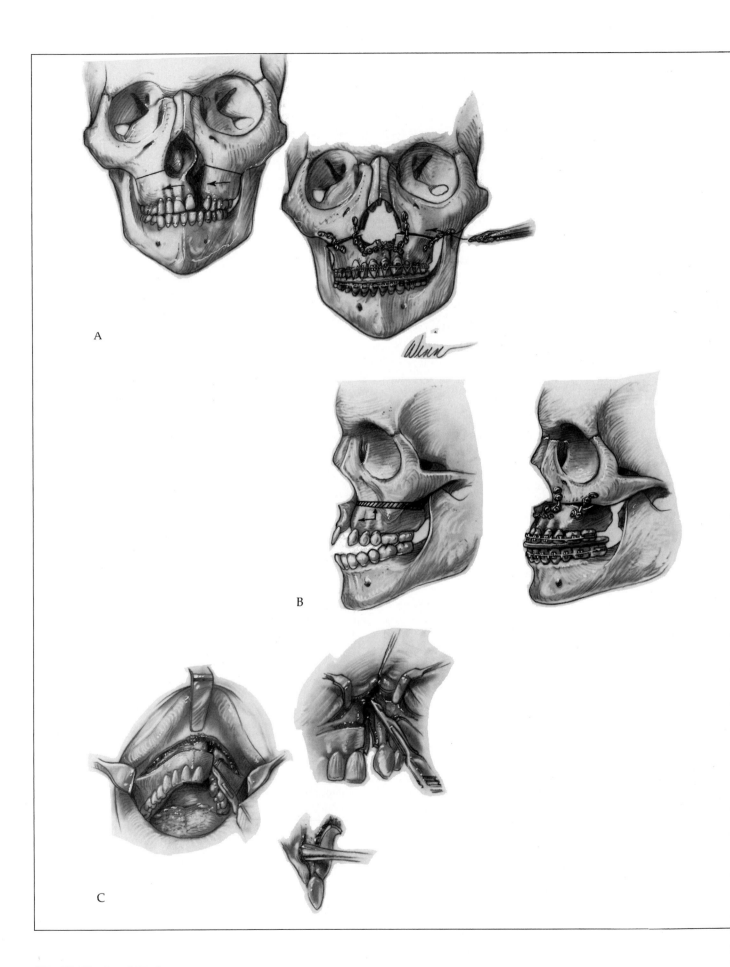

A

B

C

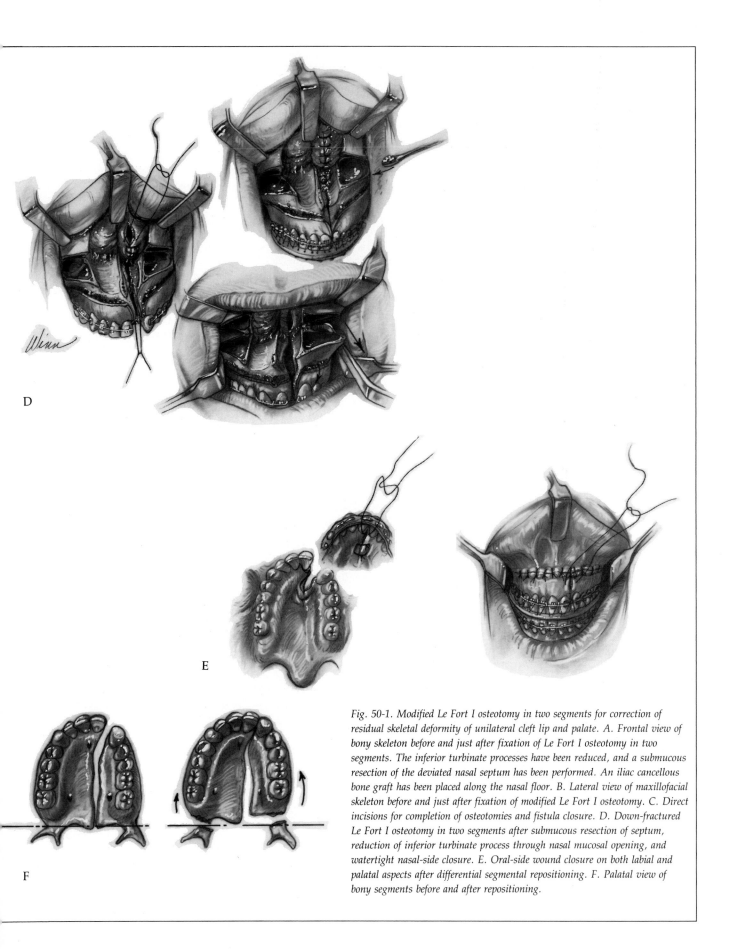

D

E

F

Fig. 50-1. Modified Le Fort I osteotomy in two segments for correction of residual skeletal deformity of unilateral cleft lip and palate. A. Frontal view of bony skeleton before and just after fixation of Le Fort I osteotomy in two segments. The inferior turbinate processes have been reduced, and a submucous resection of the deviated nasal septum has been performed. An iliac cancellous bone graft has been placed along the nasal floor. B. Lateral view of maxillofacial skeleton before and just after fixation of modified Le Fort I osteotomy. C. Direct incisions for completion of osteotomies and fistula closure. D. Down-fractured Le Fort I osteotomy in two segments after submucous resection of septum, reduction of inferior turbinate process through nasal mucosal opening, and watertight nasal-side closure. E. Oral-side wound closure on both labial and palatal aspects after differential segmental repositioning. F. Palatal view of bony segments before and after repositioning.

directly exposed. After retractors have been put in place, horizontal osteotomies are carried out through the lateral, anterior, and medial maxillary walls with a reciprocating saw, as is customary for a Le Fort I osteotomy. The deviated nasal septum is separated from the maxilla with an anterior nasal spine chisel, and the pterygomaxillary sutures are also separated with a chisel in the standard way. The maxilla is down-fractured with finger pressure and disimpacted with Tessier hooks, but no direct pressure is applied to the palatal mucosa, because this would compromise the vascular supply of the flap.

Vomer flaps are elevated and a submucosal resection of the inferior aspect of the vomer and cartilaginous septum is completed. After the enlarged, bulbous, inferior turbinate processes are reduced, the nasal mucosa is sutured along the palatal and labial aspects for a watertight nasal-side closure of the fistula tract.

The down-fractured maxilla usually is in two segments because of the original bony cleft. If it is not, and surgical closure of the cleft-dental gap is required, the segments are separated with a rotary drill. Bony spurs are shaved from the alveolar region along the distal aspect of the central incisor and mesial aspect of the canine tooth to allow good approximation of the segments. Care is taken to avoid penetrating the lamina dura or exposing the dental roots. Any impacted supernumerary teeth in the cleft site are removed at this stage. The maxillary segments are ligated into the prefabricated acrylic occlusal splint.

This procedure closes the cleft-dental gap and the dead space associated with the cleft and approximates the labial and palatal mucosal flaps for adequate oral-side fistula closure. The maxilla and splint are advanced onto the mandible, and intermaxillary fixation (IMF) is applied. The ideal vertical dimension, determined before the operation, is achieved at the maxillary osteotomy site, and titanium bone miniplates are applied at each zygomatic buttress and pyriform aperture. An additional microbone plate frequently is applied across the cleft site (perpendicular to the long axis of the teeth) to stabilize closure of the cleft-dental gap. The IMF is released and the occlusion checked. A few selected sutures may be placed in the palatal mucosa for oral-side fistula closure; however, they are not usually required, because the differential segmental repositioning well approximates the freshened mucosal edges along the palate.

Iliac cancellous bone graft is packed along the floor of the nose and cleft palate beginning posteriorly and eventually filling the nasal sill. The dead space associated with the alveolar cleft has already been closed through the differential segmental repositioning. With the cleft-dental gap surgically closed, the gingival mucosal flaps on the labial aspects are approximated and directly sutured without the need for buccal mucosal rotation flaps.

The jaws are rewired either at the end of the procedure or during the first few days postoperatively, depending on perioperative airway needs, giving increased stability to the horizontal advancement. An alternative is to use training elastics. The prefabricated acrylic splint remains ligated to the maxillary teeth for approximately 8 weeks. The segmental surgical maxillary arch wires are replaced by a continuous one, and orthodontic treatment is resumed.

Results

There are often multiple residual cleft problems in adolescent patients with UCLP. When they present to the orthognathic surgeon they can be resolved by sequencing surgical care and orthodontic treatment using the techniques described here. The modified Le Fort I osteotomy described for a patient with UCLP allows segmental differential repositioning in multiple planes, permitting routine closure of the cleft-dental gap, maxillary cleft dead space, and residual oronasal fistulas. With incision and soft tissue dissection carried out as described, survival of the random-pattern composite dento-osseous-musculo-mucosal flaps is satisfactory without causing undue concern for avascular necrosis or loss of teeth. Dental rehabilitation is frequently achieved without the need for removable or fixed prostheses. Appearance and function are restored with minimal morbidity, enhancing the quality of life for the patient.

Patient Reports
Patient 1
A patient born with a complete cleft of the left lip and palate underwent lip repair at 3 months of age, cleft palate repair with modified von Langenbeck flaps at 18 months, a pharyngoplasty at 6 years, and a cleft lip rhinoplasty at 15 years. Orthodontic brackets were placed when the patient was 15½ years of age to align the maxillary and mandibular teeth on each jaw. Although vertical and horizontal projection of the maxilla was generally adequate, at the age of 18 years the patient was referred for surgical consideration of her multiple residual cleft problems (Fig. 50-2).

Examination revealed a transverse collapse of the greater and lesser maxillary segments with crossbite, a residual perialveolar oronasal fistula, a congenitally missing lateral incisor with a cleft-dental gap, poor alveolar bony support to the teeth adjacent to the cleft, and a shift of the maxillary dental midline of the facial midline with a poor overjet and overbite relation at the incisors.

A modified maxillary Le Fort I osteotomy was performed in two segments with differential repositioning to close the gap and residual oronasal fistulas. The maxillary dental midline was repositioned to match the facial midline, the posterior crossbites were corrected, a positive overjet and an overbite were restored, and periodontal support to the left adjacent teeth was improved. The patient also underwent a vertical reduction and advancement genioplasty.

Two years after the operation the patient had an attractive smile. She did not need prosthetic rehabilitation.

Patient 2
The patient was born with a complete cleft of the left lip and palate. He underwent lip and palatal repair in infancy and sought treatment in adolescence for residual cleft problems (Fig. 50-3). These problems included a left labial and palatal oronasal fistula, maxillary hypoplasia with angle class III malocclusion, lateral crossbite, shift of maxillary dental midline off the facial midline, and a congenitally absent lateral incisor tooth at the cleft site resulting in cleft-dental gap. The patient had a borderline velopharyngeal closure and sibilant distortions secondary to the malocclusion.

Orthodontic brackets were placed approximately one year before the operations on the jaw to level and align the teeth within each maxillary segment and mandible in preparation for the orthognathic operation.

The patient underwent a modified Le Fort I osteotomy in two segments with differential repositioning to close the cleft-dental gap, dead space, and oronasal fistula and to correct his class III malocclusion and overjet and overbite problems. Stabilization was with an iliac bone graft and miniplate and screw fixation, acrylic splinting, and intermaxillary fixation.

One and one-half years after surgical treatment, the patient had improved function and appearance without the need for prosthetic rehabilitation. Speech reassessment confirmed the maintenance of borderline velopharyngeal closure and correction of sibilant distortions. The patient had a minor degree of relapse of the lesser segment.

Bilateral Cleft Lip and Palate
Residual Deformities

Adolescents with bilateral cleft lip and palate (BCLP) presenting for orthognathic operations may have the following multiple residual clefting problems.

Maxillary Dysplasia
The premaxilla may be either vertically long, resulting in a gummy smile, or horizontally short with an edentulous look. The dental midline may differ from the facial midline. There may be a negative overjet, indicating horizontal deficiency. In the transverse plane, the arch width of the lateral segments is generally deficient, with bilateral posterior crossbites and a degree of horizontal deficiency with an angle class III malocclusion.

Residual Oronasal Fistula
Despite a personal preference for fistula closure and bone grafting in the stage of mixed dentition, patients with BCLP who are candidates for orthognathic operations often have residual labial and palatal fistulas with loss of fluid through the nose while drinking and air leakage while speaking. Previous attempts at fistula closure may have failed because of inadequate soft tissue available for wound closure.

Cleft-Dental Gaps
The lateral incisor teeth are most frequently congenitally absent at the cleft site. Rudimentary teeth may also be impacted within the cleft and, if so, are of no functional value. If hypoplastic lateral incisor teeth erupt in the lateral segment, they rarely have adequate root and bone support to become long-term functional teeth. The end result is often a dental gap at the cleft site between the central incisor and canine teeth on each side.

Unless successful alveolar bone grafting and fistula closure was carried out at the stage of mixed dentition followed by orthodontic closure of the cleft-dental gaps; these problems will require orthognathic correction in adolescence.

Residual Bony Defects
Residual bony defects through the alveolus, floor of the nose, and palate are frequent; the result is a mobile premaxilla secured only to the nasal septum.

Chin Dysplasia
Patients with BCLP frequently breathe through their mouths and have an open-mouth posture. The result is a vertically long and retrognathic chin.

Mandibular Dysplasia
True mandibular prognathism in a patient with BCLP is rare. The need for a mandibular osteotomy should be limited to facial asymmetries, occlusal plane canting, and the occasional anteroposterior discrepancy.

Surgical Therapy
Rationale
The one-stage surgical approach for these end-stage clefting problems is appropriate for the neglected or difficult BCLP patient who arrives to the orthognathic surgeon as an adolescent, with maxillary dysplasia, after the eruption of the permanent canine teeth. The technique depends on a thorough understanding of the blood supply of the dento-osseous-musculo-mucosal flaps and preservation of the circulation to the lateral maxillary and premaxillary segments without unduly risking aseptic necrosis and the loss of bone and teeth. The primary modification is incision placement that allows direct exposure for the necessary dissection, segmented disimpaction and repositioning, a layered oronasal fistula closure, effective bone-graft placement, and application of miniplate and screw fixation. The method allows simultaneous surgical closure of the cleft-dental gap on each side through differential maxillary segmental repositioning. The approximated maxillary segments serve to close down the dead space at each cleft site and allow direct approximation of labial and palatal mucosal flaps for successful closure of recalcitrant oronasal fistulas.

Operative Technique
Precise placement of the incisions is critical (Fig. 50-4). The buccal incisions are made in the depth of the vestibules and extend from the zygomatic buttress forward to the location of the residual labial oronasal fistula on each side. The incisions proceed down the mesial line angle of the canine teeth or, if these are missing, the most mesial tooth in each lateral segment. The incisions separate the oral and nasal mucosa along each lateral segment. The incisions in the premaxillary segment are placed adjacent to the distal line angle of the incisor tooth on each side to separate the oral and nasal mucosae. Care is required to prevent any incision into or disruption of the mucosa of the labial vestibule of the premaxilla. The nasal and oral mucosa are sharply incised and separated on the palatal aspect of the premaxilla and of each lateral segment.

Subperiosteal soft tissue dissection provides direct exposure of the anterior maxilla on each side. Osteotomies are performed through the lateral, anterior, and medial maxillary walls with a reciprocating saw, as usual for a Le Fort I osteotomy. The pterygomaxillary sutures are separated with a mallet and chisel. The lateral segments are down-fractured with finger pressure and disimpacted with Tessier hooks to release scar tissue for three-dimensional repositioning. The vomer is rarely attached to the lateral segments, but if it is, an osteotomy is also required before down-fracturing.

After additional dissection and separation of the nasal mucosal flap from the palatal side of the premaxilla, the premaxillary segment is osteotomized from the palatal side to avoid separation of the mucosa of the labial vestibule from the premaxillary bone. This is generally done with a reciprocating saw. It is imperative that the labial mucosa of the vestibule to the premaxilla remain connected to its underlying periosteum and the bone, because blood flows from this pedicle into the premaxillary bone and to the teeth.

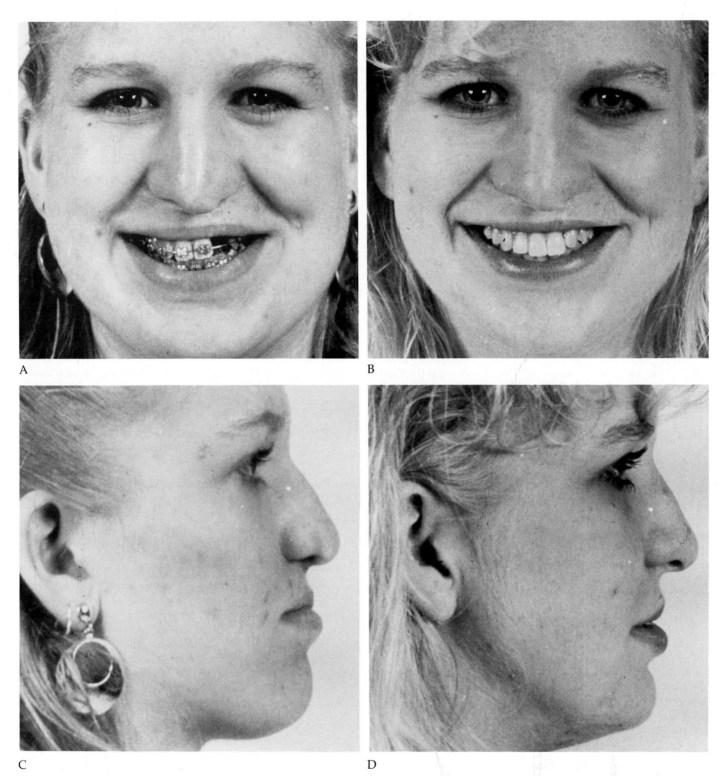

A

B

C

D

Fig. 50-2. Eighteen-year-old patient with UCLP who underwent modified Le Fort I osteotomy in two segments is shown before the operation and 2 years later. A. Preoperative frontal view. B. Postoperative frontal view. C. Preoperative profile view. D. Postoperative profile view. E. Preoperative occlusal view. F. Postoperative occlusal view. G. Preoperative palatal view. H. Postoperative palatal view.

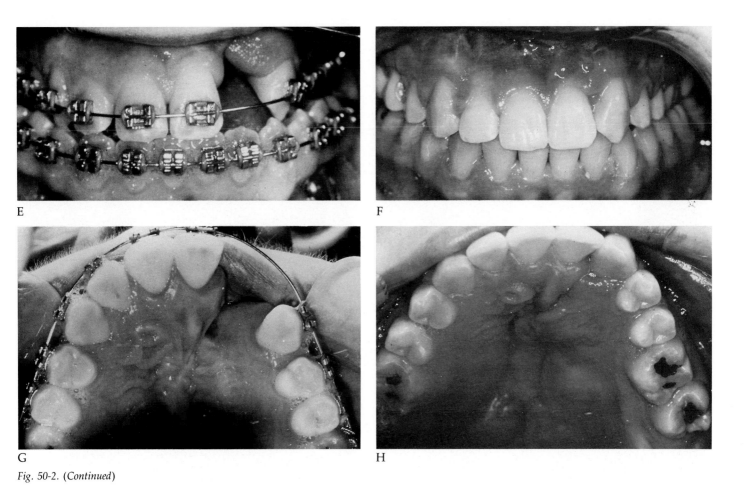

E   F

G   H

Fig. 50-2. (Continued)

The inferior turbinate processes, which are generally enlarged, are reduced with a Mayo scissors to facilitate nasal-side fistula closure. If the nasal septum is deviated, submucosal resection of the inferior aspect of the vomer and cartilage and of the septum is completed. The nasal mucosal lining is sutured for a watertight nasal-side closure on both the left and right palatal and labial aspects. The elevated vomer flaps assist in both the submucosal septal resection and the closure.

The lateral maxillary segments are advanced and ligated into the prefabricated acrylic occlusal splint, along with the premaxillary segment. Through this procedure, the cleft-dental gap on each side and the dead space associated with the bony clefts are closed. It may be necessary, using the rotary drill, to shave a small amount of bone at the alveolar edges to approximate the central incisor and canine tooth on each side. The dif-

ferential segmental advancement approximates the labial and palatal mucosal flaps for adequate oral-side fistula closure. Intermaxillary fixation is applied through the splint. The ideal vertical dimension, determined before the operation, is achieved at the maxillary osteotomy sites to improve the lip-to-tooth relation and the appearance of the smile. Bone miniplates are applied across the osteotomy sites at the zygomatic buttresses and pyriform apertures and secured with titanium screws. The IMF is released and the occlusion checked. Suturing of the palatal mucosa for oral-side fistula closure is generally required, not because the differential segmental repositioning has well approximated the freshened mucosal edges along the palate.

Iliac cancellous bone graft is packed along the floor of the nose and cleft palate on each side, beginning in the posterior area and eventually filling the nasal sill, thus

establishing an appropriate nasal floor level. The dead space associated with each alveolar cleft has already been closed through the segmental repositioning. Iliac bone is also interposed along any bony gap at the anterior maxilla made when the lateral segments are advanced. Finally, with the cleft-dental gaps surgically closed, the gingival mucosal flaps on each side are approximated and directly sutured without the need for buccal mucosal rotation flaps.

The jaws are rewired either at the end of the procedure or during the first few days, depending on perioperative airway needs, to provide increased stability when horizontal advancement is carried out. An alternative is to use training elastics. The splint remains ligated to the maxillary teeth for 8 weeks. A continuous arch wire is then reapplied to the maxilla and active tooth movement reinitiated as required by the treating orthodontist.

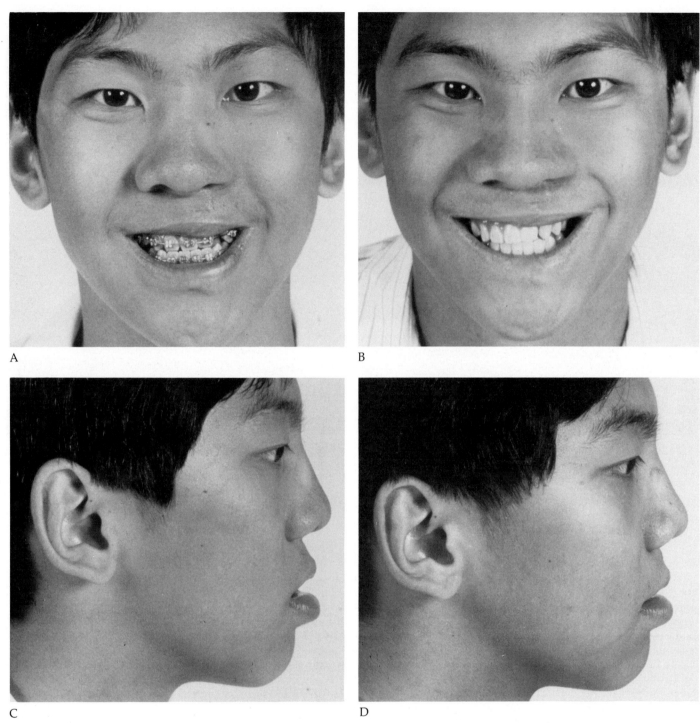

A

B

C

D

Fig. 50-3. *Seventeen-year-old with UCLP who underwent modified Le Fort I osteotomy in two segments seen before and 1½ years after surgical treatment. A. Preoperative frontal view. B. Postoperative frontal view. C. Preoperative profile view. D. Postoperative profile view. E. Preoperative occlusal view. F. Postoperative occlusal view. G. Preoperative palatal view. H. Postoperative palatal view.*

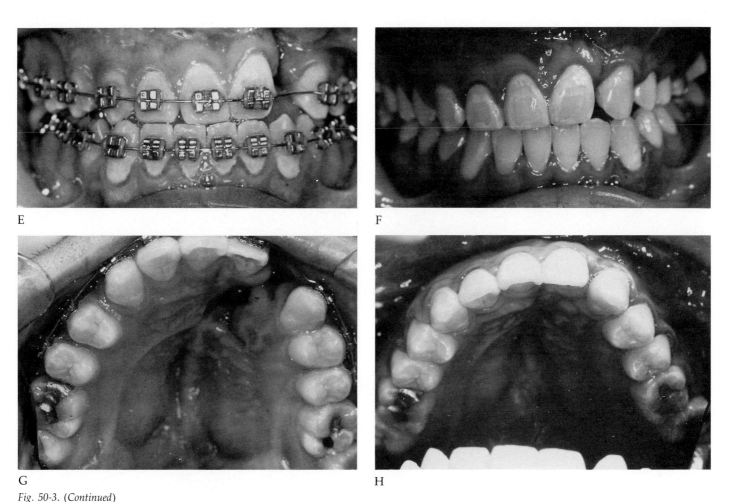

E   F

G   H

Fig. 50-3. (Continued)

Results

The direct exposure provided with the modified Le Fort I osteotomy described for a patient with BCLP allows for differential segmental repositioning that enables closure of cleft-dental gaps, maxillary cleft dead space, and residual oronasal fistulas when they exist in a BCLP adolescent.

Three-dimensional repositioning of the premaxillary segment, when indicated for improved function and appearance, can also be incorporated. Strict adherence to the placement of incisions and flap dissections described allows the safe elevation of these complex composite dento-osseous-musculo-mucosal flaps without undue concern for aseptic necrosis or loss of teeth. Dental rehabilitation is achieved, limiting the need for removable or fixed prosthetic devices. This technique allows for stabilization of the premaxilla and fistula closure in otherwise difficult defects.

Patient Reports

Patient 3

The patient was born with a complete BCLP. She underwent lip and palatal repair in infancy followed by interceptive and then final orthodontic treatment. She was referred for treatment in adolescence with residual clefting problems including a mobile premaxilla, bilateral residual labial and palatal oronasal fistula, alveolar and palatal bony defects, and bilateral cleft-dental gaps in the region of her congenitally missing lateral incisor teeth (Fig. 50-5).

Although the patient had good anterior projection of her maxilla, the residual problems required additional surgical intervention. The options were either closure of the residual fistula with local flaps and combined alveolar bone grafting followed by prosthetic rehabilitation or a cleft-orthognathic operation to anteriorly reposition the lateral maxillary segments

to close the cleft-dental gaps, dead space, and oronasal fistula in one stage without the need for prosthetic rehabilitation. The patient underwent the cleft-orthognathic operation. The aesthetics of her face improved, her fistulas were successfully closed, her maxilla was stabilized, and she did not need prosthetic rehabilitation.

Patient 4

A skeletally mature 16-year-old patient was born with a BCLP (Fig. 50-6). She underwent lip and palatal repair in infancy followed by a pharyngoplasty and two cleft-lip nasal revisions later in childhood. With the permanent dentition in place, she underwent orthodontic alignment of her maxillary and mandibular teeth. Her maxillary lateral incisor teeth were present and aligned within the premaxillary segment. Unfortunately, there was limited alveolar bony support. Her canine teeth and three of four premolar teeth were maintained in the lesser segments

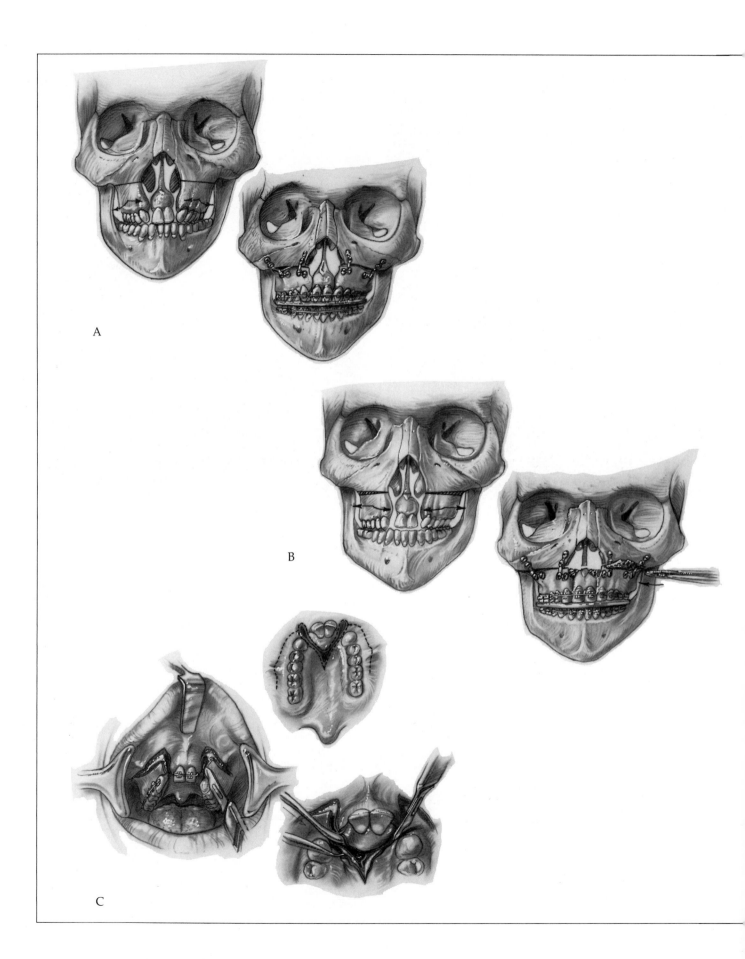

A

B

C

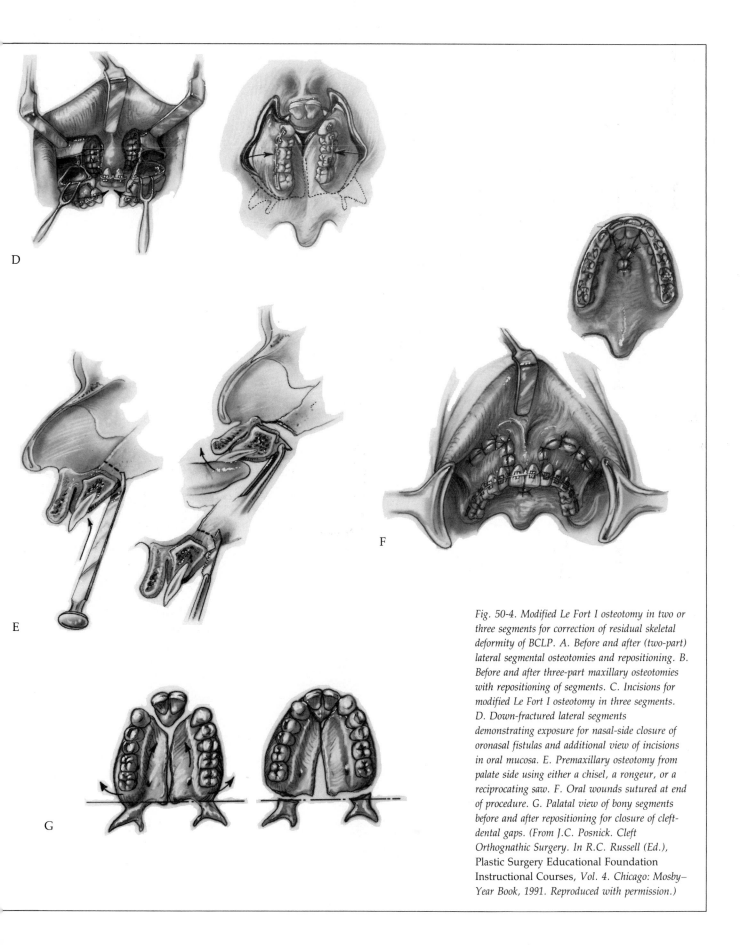

D

E

F

G

Fig. 50-4. Modified Le Fort I osteotomy in two or three segments for correction of residual skeletal deformity of BCLP. A. Before and after (two-part) lateral segmental osteotomies and repositioning. B. Before and after three-part maxillary osteotomies with repositioning of segments. C. Incisions for modified Le Fort I osteotomy in three segments. D. Down-fractured lateral segments demonstrating exposure for nasal-side closure of oronasal fistulas and additional view of incisions in oral mucosa. E. Premaxillary osteotomy from palate side using either a chisel, a rongeur, or a reciprocating saw. F. Oral wounds sutured at end of procedure. G. Palatal view of bony segments before and after repositioning for closure of cleft-dental gaps. (From J.C. Posnick. Cleft Orthognathic Surgery. In R.C. Russell (Ed.), Plastic Surgery Educational Foundation Instructional Courses, Vol. 4. Chicago: Mosby–Year Book, 1991. Reproduced with permission.)

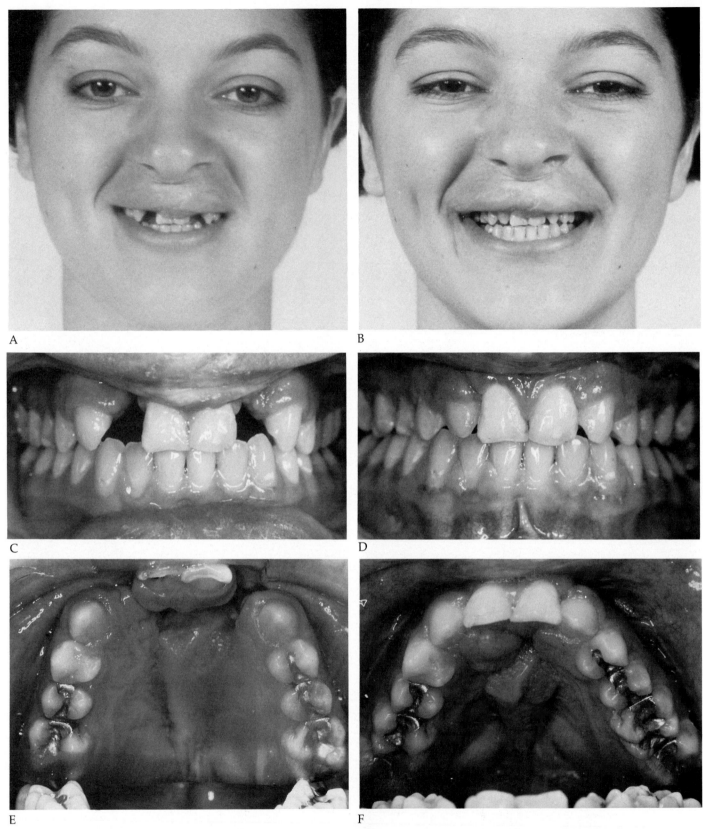

Fig. 50-5. Eighteen-year-old patient with repaired bilateral cleft lip and palate who underwent Le Fort I osteotomy with anterior advancement of lateral segments for closure of cleft-dental gaps, closure of residual perialveolar fistula, and stabilization of mobile premaxilla. Function and appearance were improved without the need for any prosthetic teeth. A. Preoperative frontal view with smile. B. Frontal view with smile 2 years postoperatively. C. Preoperative occlusal view. D. Occlusal view 2 years postoperatively. E. Preoperative palatal view. F. Palatal view 2 years postoperatively. (From J.C. Posnick in discussion of S. Rosenstein et al. Orthognathic surgery in cleft patients treated by early bone grafting. Plast. Reconstr. Surg. 87:840, 1991. Reproduced with permission.)

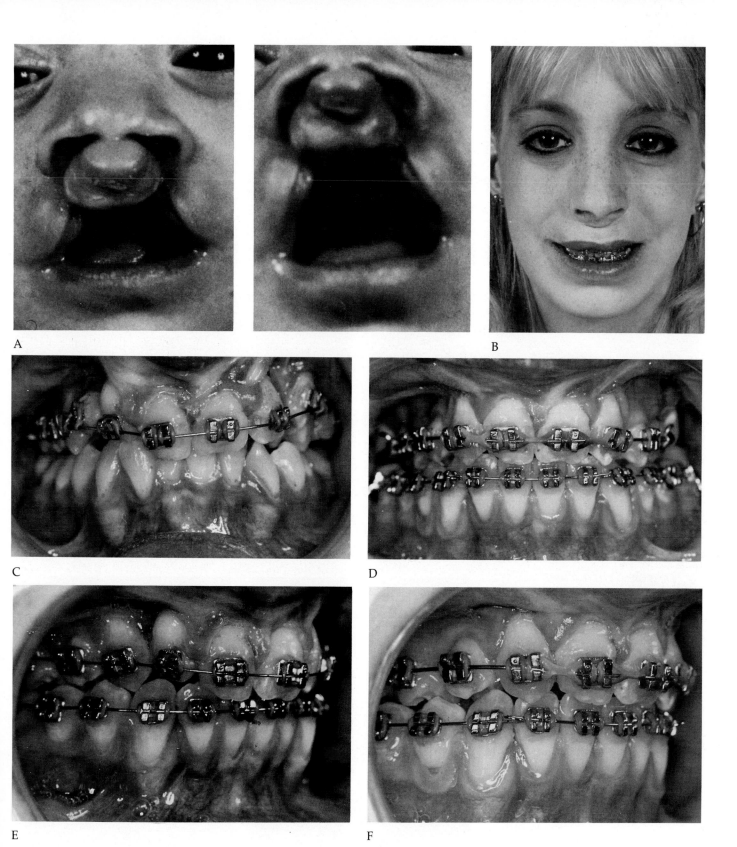

A

B

C

D

E

F

Fig. 50-6. Sixteen-year-old patient with repaired bilateral cleft lip and palate with marked residual oronasal fistula and poor alveolar bone support to teeth adjacent to each cleft. She underwent combined orthodontic and orthognathic surgical treatment with a modified Le Fort I osteotomy to close her fistula and stabilize her premaxilla. A. Initial cleft deformity at 8 weeks of age. B. Six-month postoperative frontal view. C. Preoperative occlusal view. D. Occlusal view six months postoperatively. E. Right lateral occlusal view before operation. F. Right lateral occlusal view after operation.

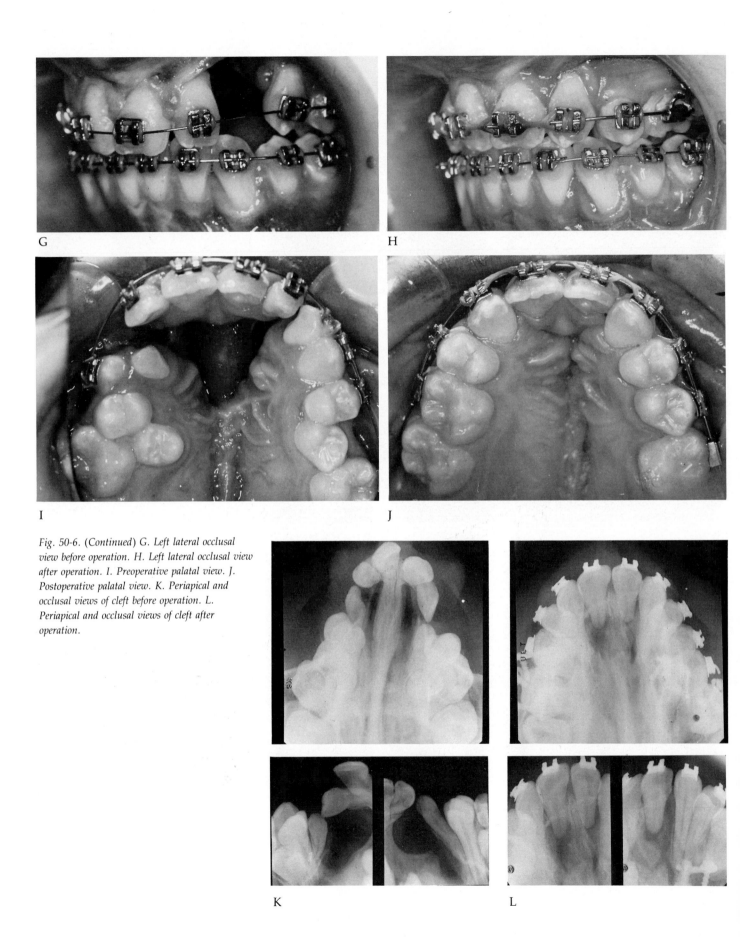

Fig. 50-6. (Continued) G. Left lateral occlusal view before operation. H. Left lateral occlusal view after operation. I. Preoperative palatal view. J. Postoperative palatal view. K. Periapical and occlusal views of cleft before operation. L. Periapical and occlusal views of cleft after operation.

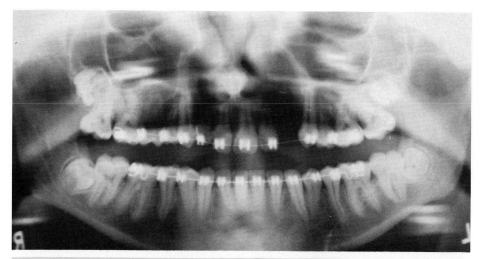

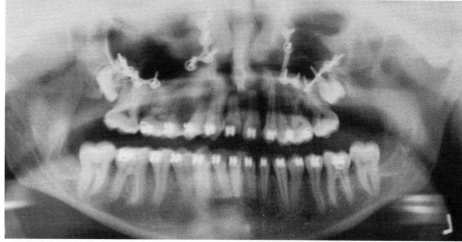

M

Fig. 50-6. (Continued) M. Preoperative and postoperative panoramic views. (From J.C. Posnick and A.P. Dagys. Bilateral cleft deformity: An integrated orthognathic and orthodontic approach. Oral Maxillofac. Clin. North Am. *3:693, 1991. Reproduced with permission.)*

but at the expense of severe alveolar bone resorption along the mesial aspects of the canine tooth within each hypoplastic lateral maxillary segment. A marked oronasal fistula remained in the palate and along each alveolar cleft site. There was residual mobility of the premaxilla and marked velopharyngeal incompetence with regurgitation of fluid while drinking and air while speaking through the large fistula, necessitating a palatal prosthesis. She was referred for surgical consideration of fistula closure.

After discussion with the treating orthodontist and her family, the patient underwent a modified maxillary Le Fort I osteotomy in three segments with differential repositioning. With intraoperative

extraction of the lateral incisor teeth, it was possible to reposition the maxillary lateral segments to close the cleft-dental and alveolar gap at each cleft site. Anterior repositioning of the lateral segments were effective in closing down this maxillary dead space allowing oronasal fistula closure. An iliac bone graft, miniplate fixation, and a prefabricated acrylic splint were used to stabilize the osteotomies.

Six months later, the patient was nearing completion of her postoperative orthodontic treatment. As a result of fistula obliteration, there was marked improvement in her velopharyngeal closure. The patient has improved dental health and self-esteem without the need for a fixed or removable appliance.

Isolated Cleft Palate
Residual Deformities

The following deformities may be present in adolescent patients seeking correction of problems associated with isolated cleft palate.

Maxillary Dysplasia
When maxillary dysplasia occurs, it generally follows one of two patterns. The first is horizontal maxillary retrusion, generally with a minor degree of vertical hypoplasia. The second is vertical maxillary excess with a minor degree of horizontal retrusion. The latter occurs more frequently in people who breathe through their mouths. Often a pharyngeal flap was placed in childhood.

Residual Oronasal Fistulas

There may be a residual fistula in the palate, located in the midline in the region between the incisive foramen and the soft palate.

Residual Bony Defects

The alveolus is not cleft, but generally there are bony defects of the central hard palate.

Chin Dysplasia

Many patients with isolated cleft palate (ICP) breathe through their mouths and have the resulting open-mouth posture. The end result is a vertically long and retrognathic chin. If Pierre Robin sequence is present, a retrognathic mandible and/or chin is also expected.

Mandibular Dysplasia

True mandibular prognathism in a patient with ICP is uncommon. Mandibular retrognathism may be part of a Pierre Robin sequence. The need for a mandibular osteotomy in addition to a maxillary osteotomy is limited.

Surgical Therapy

Rationale

In general, a standard one-unit, down-fractured Le Fort I osteotomy provides an effective way of managing maxillary dysplasia in a patient with ICP. Residual palatal oronasal fistulas are not closed simultaneously with the Le Fort I procedure, because elevation of palatal flaps would be required and could endanger the blood supply to the down-fractured maxilla. The fistula if present, is closed 6 months to 1 year after the orthognathic procedure by either local palatal flaps or, if necessary, an anteriorly based dorsal tongue flap.

Operative Technique

The surgical technique is that of a standard maxillary Le Fort I down-fracture osteotomy. The dissection may be complicated by residual palatal fistulas and the need to separate the oral and nasal layers carefully. Great care is taken to prevent subperiosteal dissection of the palatal mucosal flaps. If they are present, residual fistulas cannot be closed at the same time as the Le Fort I osteotomy because flap circulation would be compromised.

Results

The approach has proved to be an effective method for management of skeletal deformities in adolescents with ICP. No patient I have treated has had postoperative difficulties with avascular necrosis, infection, or loss of teeth.

Patient Reports

Patient 5

A 23-year-old patient who was born with an ICP underwent repair of the cleft palate at 18 months of age and an operation for a superiorly based pharyngeal flap at 12 years of age to correct velopharyngeal incompetence.

She had maxillary hypoplasia, angle class III malocclusion, and velopharyngeal incompetence (Fig. 50-7). After preoperative orthodontic treatment, she underwent a maxillary Le Fort I osteotomy with horizontal advancement, posterior intrusion, and anterior (vertical) extrusion. Bone miniplates and screws were used for stabilization in combination with a prefabricated occlusal splint and intermaxillary fixation. She also underwent a horizontal advancement genioplasty. Postoperatively, the patient required a revision of her superiorly based pharyngeal flap for the management of velopharyngeal incompetence.

Conclusion

Care is best delivered to a patient with a cleft by a dedicated cleft lip and palate team. Sequencing operations and orthodontic treatment can resolve the multiple end-stage residual skeletal cleft problems that adolescent patients may present with. Each cleft type—UCLP, BCLP, and ICP—presents unique challenges requiring varied surgical techniques for safe orthognathic surgery. For patients with UCLP or BCLP, the modified Le Fort I osteotomy described allows differential segmental repositioning and routine closure of residual cleft-dental gaps, dead space, and recalcitrant oronasal fistulas. When orthognathic surgical treatment is required for a patient with ICP, the surgical technique is standard.

Dental rehabilitation and improvements in both function and appearance are achieved with only limited need for removable or fixed prostheses. Over the long term, these surgical refinements in cleft rehabilitation should allow for a more normal quality of life for the patient.

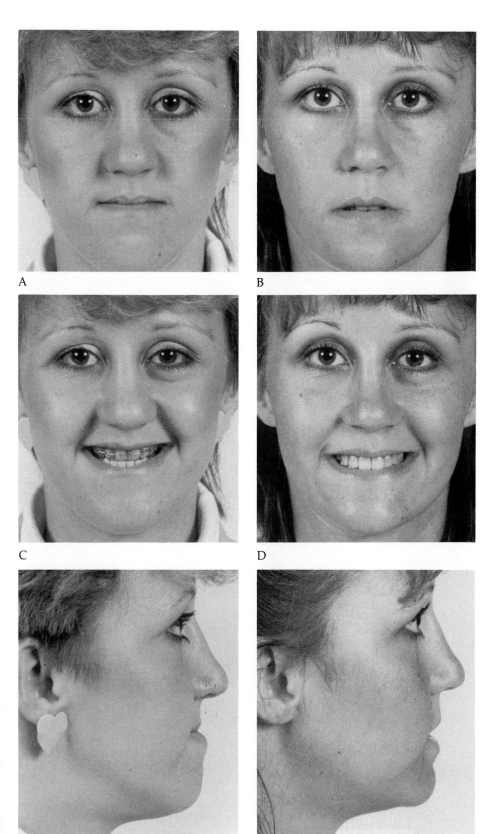

Fig. 50-7. Twenty-three-year-old patient born with isolated cleft palate. She underwent a maxillary Le Fort I osteotomy with horizontal advancement and a vertical reduction and horizontal advancement genioplasty.
A. Preoperative frontal view in repose.
B. Postoperative frontal view in repose.
C. Preoperative frontal view with smile.
D. Postoperative frontal view with smile.
E. Preoperative profile. F. Postoperative profile.

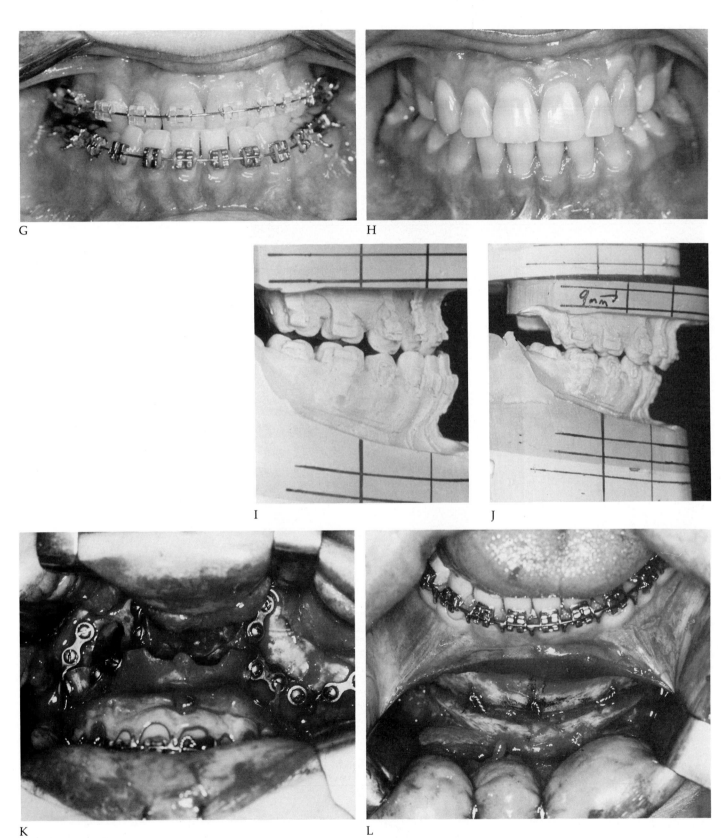

Fig. 50-7. (Continued) G. Preoperative occlusal view. H. Postoperative occlusal view. I. Articulated dental model ready for model operation. J. Maxilla advanced and ready for splint reconstruction on articulator. K. Intraoperative view of Le Fort I osteotomy stabilized with titanium miniplates and screws. L. Intraoperative view of vertically reduced and horizontally advanced genioplasty stabilized with three direct transosseous wires.

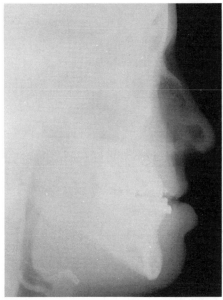
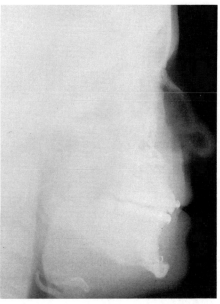

M   N

Fig. 50-7. (Continued) M. Preoperative lateral cephalometric roentgenogram. N. Postoperative lateral cephalometric roentgenogram. (Parts I, J, and K from J.C. Posnick and M.P. Ewing. The Role of Plate and Screw Fixation in the Treatment of Cleft Lip and Palate Jaw Deformities. In J.S. Gruss, P.N. Manson, and M.J. Yaremchuk (eds.), Rigid Fixation of the Craniomaxillofacial Skeleton. *Stoneham, Mass.: Butterworth-Heinemann, 1992. Reproduced with permission.)*

Suggested Reading

Obwegeser, H.L. Surgical Correction of Maxillary Deformities. In W.C. Grabb, S.W. Resenstein, and K.R. Brock (Eds.), *Cleft Lip and Palate.* Boston: Little, Brown, 1969.

Posnick, J.C. Cleft Orthognathic Surgery in the Cleft Patient. In R.C. Russel (Ed.), *Instructional Courses.* Plastic Surgery Education Foundation and C.V. Mosby Co., 1991.

Posnick, J.C. Orthognathic surgery in cleft patients treated by early bone grafting. *Plast. Reconstr. Surg.* 87:840, 1991.

Posnick, J.C. The Use of Rigid Fixation in the Treatment of Jaw Deformities in Patients with Cleft Lip and Palate. In J.S. Gruss, P.M. Manson, and M.J. Yarmachuk (Eds.), *Rigid Fixation of the Craniomaxillofacial Skeleton.* London: Butterworth, 1992. In press.

Posnick, J.C., and Thompson, B. Modification of the maxillary Le Fort I osteotomy in cleft-orthognathic surgery: The unilateral cleft lip and palate deformity. *J. Oral Maxillofac. Surg.* 50:666, 1992.

Posnick, J.C., and Thompson, B. Modification of the maxillary Le Fort I osteotomy in cleft-orthognathic surgery: The bilateral cleft lip and palate deformity. *J. Oral Maxillofac. Surg.* 51:2, 1993.

Posnick, J.C., and Dagys A.P. Skeletal stability and release patterns after Le Fort I maxillary osteotomy fixed with miniplates: The unilateral cleft lip and palate deformity. *Plast. Reconstr. Surg.* In press.

Posnick, J.C., and Dagys, A.P. Orthognathic Surgery in the Bilateral Cleft Patient: An Integrated Surgical and Orthodontic Approach. In J.W. Hudson (Ed.), *Oral Maxillofacial Surgical Clinics of North America.* Philadelphia: Saunders, 1991. Pp. 693–710.

Posnick, J.C., and Ewing, M. Skeletal stability after Le Fort I maxillary advancement in patients with unilateral cleft lip and palate. *Plast. Reconstr. Surg.* 85:706, 1990.

Posnick, J.C., and Taylor, M. Skeletal stability and relapse patterns after Le Fort I osteotomy using miniplate fixation in patients with isolated cleft palate. *Plast. Reconstr. Surg.* In press.

Posnick, J.C., Witzel, M.A., and Dagys, A.P. Management of Jaw Deformities in the Cleft Patient. In J. Bardach and H.L. Morris (Eds.), *Multidisciplinary Management of Cleft Lip and Palate.* Philadelphia: Saunders, 1990. P. 530.

Ross, R.B. Treatment variables affecting facial growth in complete unilateral cleft lip and palate: An overview of treatment and facial growth. *Cleft Palate J.* 24:75, 1987.

Tessier, P., and Tulanse, J.F. Secondary repair of cleft lip deformity. *Clin. Plast. Surg.* 11:747, 1984.

51

Secondary Correction of the Nasal Deformity Associated with Cleft Lip

Mimis Cohen

Better understanding of the anatomy involved and the improved surgical techniques of primary repair of unilateral and bilateral cleft lip, which incorporate simultaneous correction of the coexisting nasal deformity, have resulted in a superior outcome with a lesser degree of residual nasal deformity. Most surgeons agree, however, that despite efforts to correct nasal asymmetry during the initial cleft lip repair, with various degrees of undermining and repositioning of the alar cartilage and nostrils, a secondary procedure is still almost invariably required for functional and aesthetic purposes. Definitive correction of a cleft-lip nasal deformity remains a challenge for reconstructive surgeons. Despite the great number of procedures and modifications for correction of the residual functional and aesthetic deformities, a single perfect operation does not exist to treat all deformities.

The nasal deformity associated with a cleft lip is caused by factors intrinsic to the nasal structures, such as a deformed, depressed, and laterally deflected lower alar cartilage; a deviated septum; an asymmetric nasal tip, columella, and nostril; and asymmetric and deviated nasal bones and nasal pyramid. Furthermore, the de-

formity is accentuated by extrinsic skeletal factors, such as maxillary hypoplasia of the lesser maxillary segment, a coexisting cleft of the maxilla, and the subsequent lack of bony support of the nasal base. The severity of the primary nasal deformity varies among patients; and depends on the initial cleft lip deformity (unilateral or bilateral, complete or incomplete). The severity of the secondary deformity also varies, depending on the initial deformity and the degree of nasal correction performed when the cleft lip was repaired or during subsequent revisions. In addition, previous procedures and scarring produce a variable degree of iatrogenic deformity that also needs to be taken into consideration. It is therefore imperative for the surgeon to analyze each patient extensively, to examine the existing deformity, and to individualize the surgical procedure for successful management of both the functional and the aesthetic residual deformities.

Timing of the Procedure

I prefer to defer the final correction of the nasal deformity until after orthodontic realignment of the maxilla; bone grafting of

the hypoplastic maxilla, maxillary cleft, and alveolus; and closure of the coexisting oronasal fistula(s). There are several distinct advantages to this approach.

1. In patients with unilateral clefts, the maxillary platform assumes a symmetric position after realignment of its segments and bone grafting of the maxillary cleft and the hypoplastic area of the pyriform aperture. The depressed, unsupported nostril is raised also to a level similar to that of the contralateral side.
2. In patients with bilateral clefts, after the premaxilla is realigned with the lateral segments and the maxillary clefts are bone grafted, both nostrils are supported and raised and the nasolabial angle is improved.
3. After closure of residual oronasal fistulas and reestablishment of the natural barrier between the oral and nasal cavities, regurgitation of food and saliva is controlled and irritation of the nasal mucosa is eliminated. A more accurate evaluation of the intranasal abnormalities is feasible, leading to more appropriate and successful management of the various components of any coexisting airway obstruction.

Preoperative Evaluation and Planning

All patients undergo an extensive preoperative examination to evaluate and record the extent of the aesthetic deformity and functional nasal pathology. The external nasal deformity must be evaluated for deviations and asymmetries in the vertical, horizontal, and coronal planes (Fig. 51-1). The degree of deviation and asymmetry of the nasal pyramid, the nasal width, the position of the dorsum, the asymmetry in tip projection, the lack of tip projection, the asymmetry of the nasal base, the shape and size of the nostrils, the condition of the columella, the presence of a skin web within the vestibule of the nostril, and the presence and location of external or internal scars should be recorded.

Intranasal evaluation with a nasal speculum, with adequate lighting, is incorporated into the evaluation of all patients. Intranasal abnormalities, including scars, obstructions, septal deviation, previous resection of septal cartilage, and turbinate hypertrophy, and the condition of the nasal mucosa are recorded. Additionally,

each patient undergoes subjective and objective evaluation of airway patency. In the event that nasal swelling and drainage is present caused by a cold or allergies, a solution of epinephrine is instilled into the nasal cavities to produce vasoconstriction, reduce nasal swelling, facilitate the examination, and provide for a more accurate evaluation. The level of intranasal obstruction also must be evaluated. In most patients, the airway obstruction is caused primarily by a septal deviation. In some patients the hypertrophic inferior turbinates are also responsible for the obstruction. Nostril collapse and intranasal scarring might contribute to the obstruction. Additionally, one should not forget that a number of patients with cleft lip and palate have a pharyngeal flap in place, which might contribute partially to the airway obstruction. With an accurate and detailed preoperative evaluation, the surgeon is able to identify the degree and level of airway obstruction and treat the patient accordingly.

Rhinomanometry is useful in the pre- and postoperative evaluation of patients with secondary nasal deformities of cleft lip.

This test provides an objective, functional assessment of the magnitude of nasal airway obstruction before and after surgical treatment. Described and illustrated in Chap. 45, this approach measures the resistance of each nasal cavity and the resistance of the velopharyngeal region. From these data, resistances for the total nasal cavity and total nasal airway are obtained. This information allows the craniofacial team to determine which region—nasal cavities or velopharynx or both—is contributing to the nasal obstruction and facilitates surgical planning. Furthermore, comparison of pre- and postoperative rhinomanometric values allows the team to quantify objectively the degree of surgical correction with respect to airway patency. Finally, standardized photographs, including worm's eye views and oblique views, are obtained from all patients to assist in the final evaluation and planning of the corrective procedure.

Surgical Technique
Nasal Deformity from a Unilateral Cleft Lip

Open rhinoplasty is extremely helpful in the management of residual nasal deformities from cleft lip. I use this approach in most patients, with the exception of those who have only minor residual deformities. With this approach, I can directly visualize and appreciate the degree of deformity and correct it accordingly. Accurate repositioning of the tip and placement of cartilaginous grafts are also greatly facilitated. The coexisting septal deviation also can be treated accurately by this approach, without the need for other incisions in the nasal mucosa. Finally, additional length for the columella can be provided when necessary if a V-shaped columellar incision is used and subsequently closed in a Y shape. This incision heals better than a midcolumellar incision and, if closed carefully, leaves a barely visible scar a few months after the procedure.

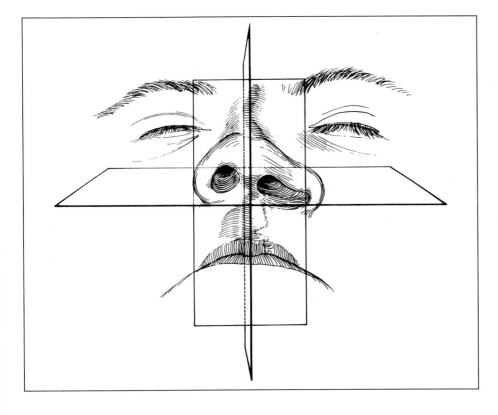

Fig. 51-1. Residual nasal deformity associated with unilateral cleft lip has variable degree of deviation and asymmetry in sagittal, horizontal, and coronal planes.

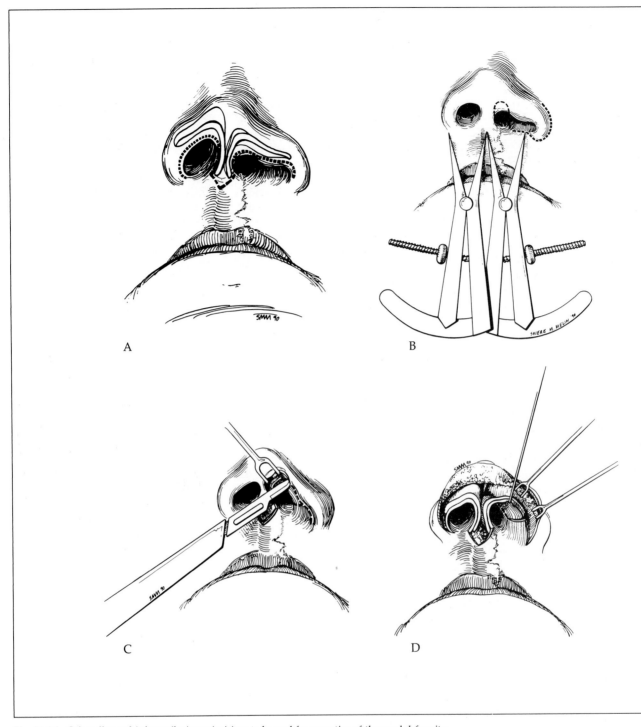

Fig. 51-2A. Columellar and infracartilaginous incisions to be used for correction of the nasal deformity with an open approach. B. The widths of the bases of the noncleft and cleft nostrils are measured and compared. C. After the columellar incision has been completed and the medial crura of the alar cartilages identified, the cartilages are exposed with bilateral infracartilaginous incisions. D. The lateral crus of the affected nostril is dissected free along with its lining to facilitate medial and superior mobilization of this cartilage. E. The domes are secured in a symmetric position with few interrupted clear nylon sutures. F. Any discrepancies between the alar cartilages are corrected with partial cartilage resections, scoring, or the addition of cartilaginous grafts. G. When additional tip projection is necessary, tip grafts alone or in combination with struts between the medial crura are used. All grafts are secured in position with clear nylon sutures. H. At the completion of the operation, the intranasal defect and the columellar incision are closed in a V-Y manner. If the base of the nose has been repositioned, the defect is closed primarily with fine stitches.

Before marking the incisions, I place a double hook in the nostrils and apply traction to lift the nostrils at a symmetric level. A V-shaped incision is marked on the columella with the apex at the lip-columella junction. The surgeon should avoid extending the incision on the lip to prevent unwanted lengthening of the lip after V to Y closure of the incision. A horizontal extension of 2 to 3 mm is marked on either side of the V within the nostrils (Fig. 51-2A). The width of the base of the

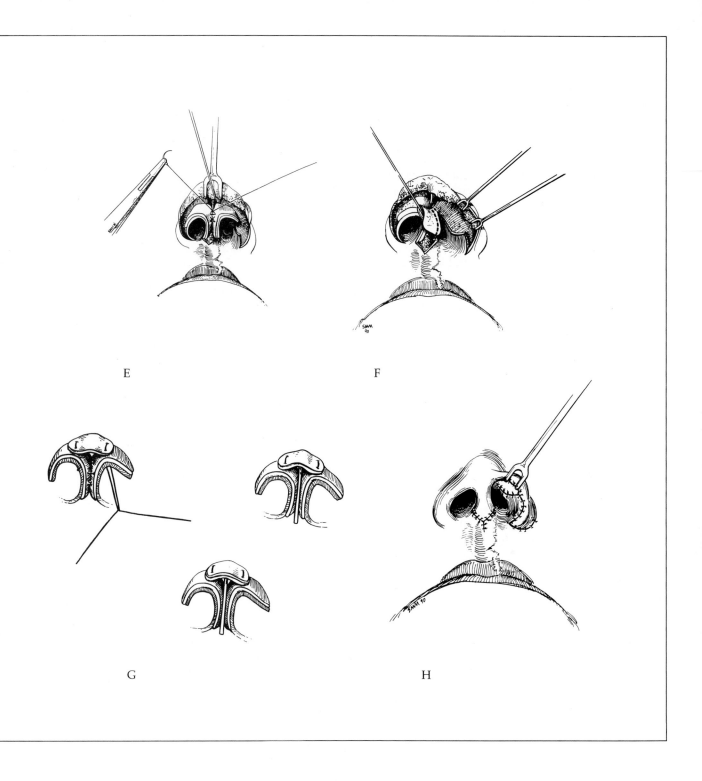

E

F

G

H

noncleft nostril is measured with callipers, recorded, and compared with the width of the base of the nostril on the cleft side (Fig. 51-2B).

The nasal cavities are packed with cottonoids soaked in 4% cocaine solution. After appropriate skin preparation, all areas of proposed incisions are infiltrated with a small amount of 1% lidocaine solution with 1:100,000 epinephrine. An

additional small amount is injected under the tip and dorsum of the nose and along the areas of osteotomies when needed. When a septoplasty or turbinectomies are planned, I also infiltrate either side of the mucoperichondrium of the septum and the mucoperiosteum of the inferior turbinate processes.

The initial columellar incision is carried as designed on the V and its horizontal ex-

tensions within each nostril. This incision should be done with caution to avoid injuring the medial crura of the alar cartilages, which lie very superficially in this area. As soon as the medial crura are identified, the columellar skin is elevated with sharp dissection. The columellar skin and the alar cartilages are placed under tension using single hooks. Thus the caudal margin of the alar cartilage is identified. An infracartilaginous incision is carried from medial to lateral to expose these structures completely (see Fig. 51-2C). The same incision and dissection are carried out on the opposite side. The domes, the entire surface of the alar and upper lateral cartilages, and the cartilaginous and bony framework of the nasal dorsum are then skeletonized and exposed. Any remaining fibrofatty tissue over and between the alar cartilages is removed. The asymmetry and malposition of the domes and of the medial and lateral crura of the alar cartilages can then be evaluated and corrected under direct vision.

When small discrepancies are present between the alar cartilages, I mobilize the depressed dome and suture it to the contralateral one with a few interrupted 5–0 clear nylon sutures to reposition and elevate the depressed dome and achieve nasal tip symmetry. When the depression is more significant, with lateral flaring of the lateral crus, this maneuver alone is not sufficient to produce long-lasting symmetry, because the lateral crus on the cleft side is tethered during medial mobilization of the dome. A lining deficiency also might be present. In these patients, I dissect the lateral crus with its mucosal lining as a flap based medially, as described by Potter and Cronin (see Fig. 51-2D). This is easily achieved by extending the lateral infracartilaginous incision around the lateral border of the alar cartilage and back along its cephalic border. With this maneuver, the alar cartilage can be freely mobilized in a more medial and superior position and sutured to the contralateral alar cartilage. Thus additional height is gained in the area of the medial crus and the domes are secured at an equal height to produce symmetry (see Fig. 51-2E). The residual lateral mucosal defect left after this mobilization is usually closed in a V-Y manner.

If there is a considerable shortage of lining because of scarring or resection from previous procedures, I use a composite graft from the ear to resurface this intranasal defect. The advantage of using a composite graft rather than skin grafts is that the underlying cartilage acts as a splint and prevents contracture of the skin graft. Any additional asymmetry between the alar cartilages is corrected with appropriate partial cartilage resections and scoring or with the addition of cartilaginous grafts (see Fig. 51-2F).

In many patients the tip of the nose lacks projection, or additional projection is judged necessary for superior aesthetic results. A cartilaginous strut harvested from the septum is used in these patients to provide support to the tip and increase projection. A pocket is dissected between the medial crura to the area of the nasal spine, and all fibrofatty tissue between the crura is removed. The graft is designed to be long enough to extend from the nasal spine to just above the nasal tip. It is secured to the medial crura with 2 or 3 permanent 5–0 clear nylon sutures. One should keep in mind that the medial crura of the alar cartilages have a natural flare. All sutures should be placed through the cephalic border of these cartilages to retain the flaring of the caudal margins of the medial crura. Additional tip projection and improved tip contour, when necessary, are achieved with the addition of tip grafts as described by Peck. One or two layers of conchal cartilage strips measuring approximately 0.8 cm by 0.4 cm are secured in place with interrupted 5–0 clear nylon sutures. Any residual depressions of the alar cartilages are also corrected with small local cartilaginous grafts, and asymmetries of the upper lateral cartilage are managed by limited resections or placement of additional grafts (see Fig. 51-2G).

A great degree of deviation of the nasal bony pyramid is corrected by bilateral low osteotomies through the pyriform aperture of the maxilla. Septal deviations are also appropriately corrected. The nasal skin is draped over the reconstructed bony and cartilaginous skeleton. The columellar incision is closed in a V to Y manner, which provides a gain of 0.5 to 0.8 cm in length for the columella. All skin incisions are closed with precision with 6–0 nylon sutures with caution to make sure the skin edges are everted, thus avoiding unsightly depressions or irregularities. All incisions in the nasal vestibule are closed with a few interrupted 5–0 absorbable sutures.

As soon as the incisions are closed, attention is directed to the symmetry of the nasal base. Small discrepancies in size are corrected by local excisions in the floor of the nostril. These excisions involve skin only and should be closed with care to avoid notching in the area of the nostril sill. For greater discrepancies, I completely detach the cleft-side nostril and set

it in a more appropriate position and level. With accurate preoperative evaluation and measurement, one is able not only to correct the nostril flaring but also to reposition the entire nostril in a symmetric plane with the noncleft side. If the circumference of the nostril is found to be greater than that of the noncleft-side nostril, in addition to the repositioning an appropriate resection is carried out (see Fig. 51-2H). A more difficult condition to correct is a cleft-side nostril that is smaller than the normal nostril. In such a patient, the nostril is completely detached and an appropriate composite graft from the ear is applied. All additional skin incisions are closed with 6–0 nylon sutures.

Correction of Airway Obstruction

The information gained from preoperative clinical and rhinomanometric evaluation assists the surgeon in formulating and individualizing a plan of action for the correction of airway obstruction. Attention is directed primarily toward the septum and the inferior turbinate processes and secondarily, if necessary, to a potentially obstructing pharyngeal flap.

When an open rhinoplasty is used, the septum is exposed through its caudal and superior borders after lateral reflection of the medial crura of the alar cartilages. The dissection starts with a knife until the surface of the cartilage is identified. The mucoperichondrium on either side of the septum is dissected from the cartilage with a Freer elevator to completely expose the surface of the cartilage up to the perpendicular plate of the ethmoid bone, the crest of the maxilla, the vomer, and the anterior nasal spine. Thus the septal anatomy and configuration are visualized and managed directly (Fig. 51-3).

In most patients with nasal deformities from a unilateral cleft lip there is some degree of deviation of the septum. In some patients only the deviated caudal portion of the septum needs to be managed, but in most patients the entire septum requires attention to alleviate nasal airway obstruction.

The caudal portion of the septum typically deviates toward the noncleft side. To reposition the caudal portion in the midline, one should completely free this portion of the septum from the nasal spine

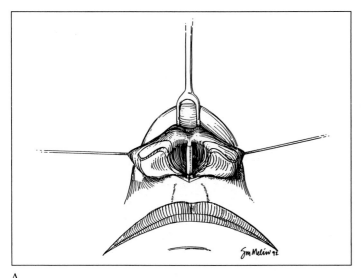

A

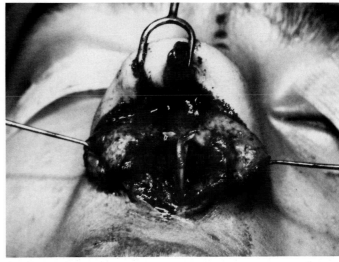

B

Fig. 51-3. When an open rhinoplasty is used, the septum is exposed through its caudal and superior border after lateral reflection of the medial crura of the alar cartilages.

and the maxilla and score the concave surface of the cartilage (Fig. 51-4).

If the septal deformity is severe and cannot be corrected by repositioning of the septum and scoring, a resection should be performed leaving an L-shaped portion of the septum for nasal support. Additional obstructive factors might be present, such as a deviated perpendicular plate and bony spears in the crest of the maxilla. Such bony irregularities are treated by direct excision. The residual mucoperichondrial pocket is irrigated to remove any debris and closed with two interrupted through-and-through absorbable sutures.

Hypertrophy of the inferior turbinate processes must be evaluated and treated accordingly. After injection of a few cc's of 1% lidocaine with 1:100,000 epinephrine solution, local vasoconstriction and reduction of excess swelling occurs. This enables the surgeon to evaluate the degree of hypertrophy and design the appropriate procedure for its treatment.

Obstruction caused primarily by mucosal swelling can be relieved by excision of the redundant mucosa. However, when inferior turbinate hypertrophy is caused by mucosal swelling and bony hypertrophy, an en bloc resection of the inferior portion of the turbinate process should include redundant mucosa and bone. The surgeon should carefully evaluate the remaining portion of the turbinate process

and remove any additional segment causing obstruction. These resections, however, should be done with extreme care to avoid overresection of the inferior turbinate process that may lead to atrophic rhinitis. All visible bleeding points should be cauterized. If an obstruction persists, an outfracture of the remaining portion of the turbinate process may be helpful.

Preoperative rhinomanometric studies provide invaluable information about possible additional airway obstruction caused by a pharyngeal flap. In the event that this obstruction is clinically significant, it is managed in the same setting. A Dingman mouth gag is placed and a silk suture is used to retract the soft palate anteriorly. The ports on either side of the flap are visualized. Red rubber catheters are passed from each nostril through the ports. They assist in retracting the palate forward and fully visualizing the size of each port and the area of scarring. Only completely obstructing pharyngeal flaps complicated with episodes of sleep apnea are totally transected. In most instances, the ports are widened with partial tissue excisions, release of contracted scars, and careful resurfacing of all residual raw surfaces with Z-plasties or other local mucosal flaps.

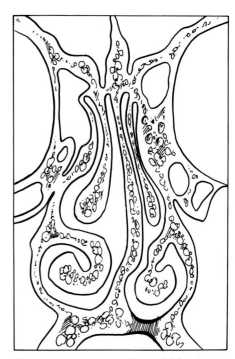

Fig. 51-4. Most patients with nasal deformity from unilateral cleft lip have some degree of septal deviation and inferior turbinate hypertrophy. Shaded area, lower right, demonstrates the bone grafted maxilla and nasal floor.

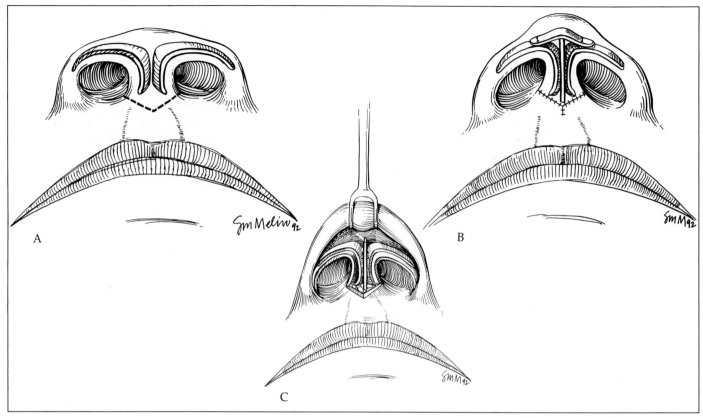

Nasal Deformity from a Bilateral Cleft Lip

The nasal deformity from a bilateral cleft lip differs distinctly from a unilateral deformity. In symmetric bilateral clefts the nose is relatively symmetric without deviation; the nose is flat, lacking projection; the columella is short; and the nostrils flare laterally with a longitudinal rather than an oblique inclination. Patients with bilateral asymmetric clefts have a variable degree of asymmetry and deviation. The deformity is more severe in patients with complete bilateral clefts and less severe in patients with incomplete bilateral clefts.

When planning for correction of the nasal deformity from a bilateral cleft lip, the surgeon should evaluate the adequacy of skin coverage or the need for additional skin in the area of the columella. With improved surgical techniques for management of the primary lip deformity and incorporation of a columella-lengthening procedure in the treatment plan (see Chap. 41), fewer patients require additional columellar skin lengthening during the final correction of the nasal deformity. When needed, however, a forked flap from the lip is incorporated into the de-

Fig. 51-5A. Incisions for correction of nasal deformity of bilateral cleft lip by an open approach. B. After skeletonization of the nose from the soft tissues and excision of the fibrofatty tissue between the medial crura of the alar cartilages, the domes are secured in place with interrupted clear nylon sutures. If additional projection is needed, cartilage tip grafts and struts are used. C. At the completion of the operations, the columellar incision is closed in a V to Y manner. All intranasal incisions are closed with absorbable sutures.

sign of open rhinoplasty to provide for the additional skin coverage of the columella.

I approach the nasal deformities associated with bilateral cleft lips as I do the deformities of unilateral clefts, primarily by open rhinoplasty. I use a V columellar incision and evaluate and address tip projection after skeletonization of the soft tissues. In most patients this is achieved by excision of all fibrofatty tissues present between the domes and the medial crura and medial mobilization of the domes and the lateral crura. Clear 5–0 nylon sutures are used to stabilize the domes in their new position. Additional projection is achieved as described for unilateral deformities by placement of a columellar strut of septal cartilage and onlay cartilage tip grafts. All grafts are secured in place with permanent clear sutures. When irregularities or asymmetries of the alar cartilages or the upper lateral cartilages are observed, they are corrected by local re-

section, additional grafting, or scoring (Fig. 51-5).

Bilateral osteotomies are indicated when the nasal pyramid is found to be wide or when skeletal asymmetry is present. Additionally, in a number of patients with nasal deformities from bilateral cleft lip a dorsal augmentation with onlay cartilage or bone grafts is necessary to increase projection and improve facial harmony. Most patients are treated by an onlay septal cartilage graft, but when a considerable augmentation is necessary, I prefer to use a bone graft taken from the calvarium or ilium.

The columellar incision is closed with interrupted 6–0 nylon sutures in a V to Y manner. This method usually increases the columellar length by an average of 0.7 cm. The intranasal incisions are closed with a few interrupted absorbable sutures. Excess flaring of the nostrils may persist despite medial mobilization of the

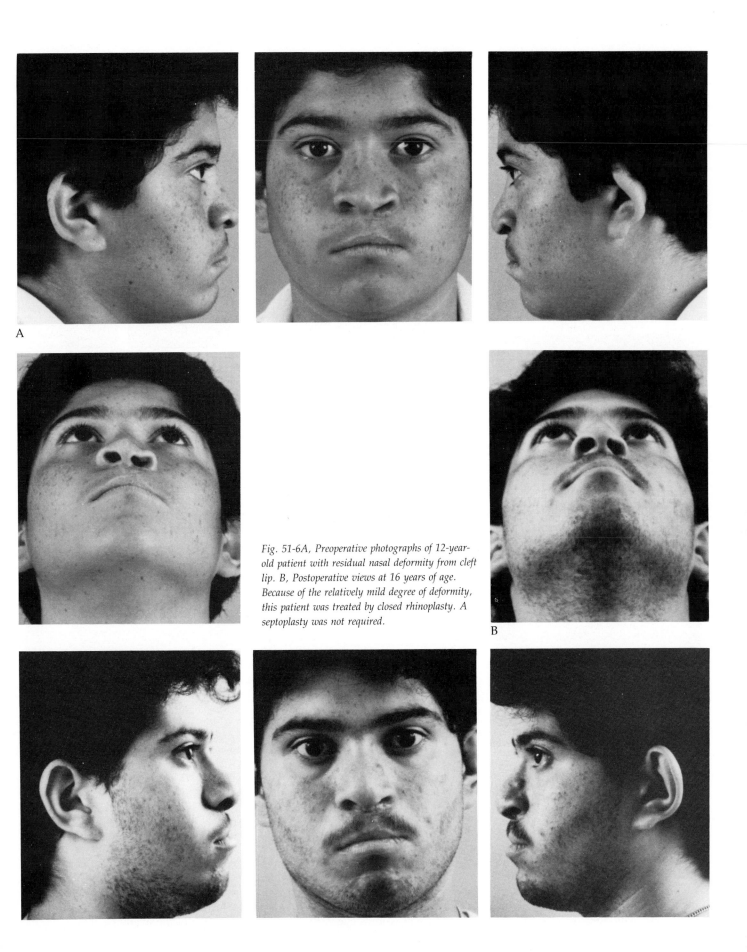

A

Fig. 51-6A, Preoperative photographs of 12-year-
old patient with residual nasal deformity from cleft
lip. B, Postoperative views at 16 years of age.
Because of the relatively mild degree of deformity,
this patient was treated by closed rhinoplasty. A
septoplasty was not required.

B

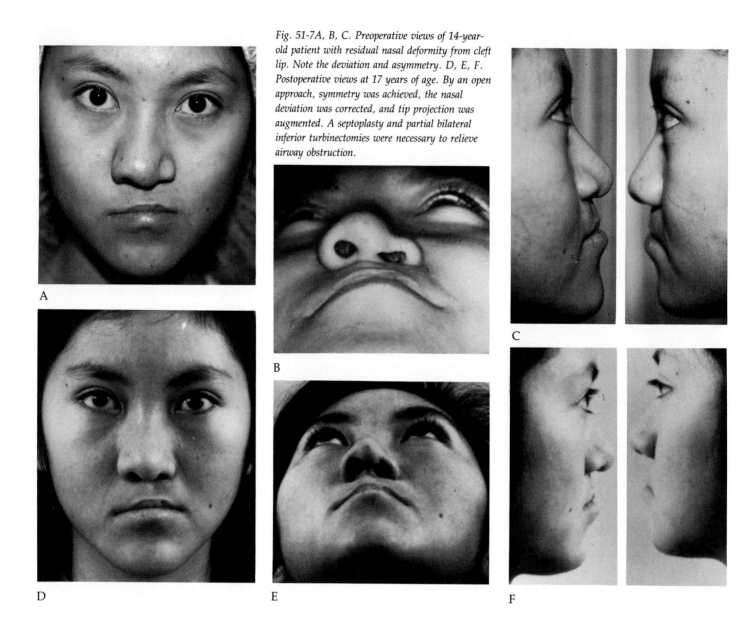

Fig. 51-7A, B, C. Preoperative views of 14-year-old patient with residual nasal deformity from cleft lip. Note the deviation and asymmetry. D, E, F. Postoperative views at 17 years of age. By an open approach, symmetry was achieved, the nasal deviation was corrected, and tip projection was augmented. A septoplasty and partial bilateral inferior turbinectomies were necessary to relieve airway obstruction.

A

B

C

D

E

F

lateral alar cartilage and increased nasal tip projection with grafts. In these patients the shape and size of the nostrils can be additionally modified with appropriate alar resections. These resections are designed according to the deformity and can be symmetric or asymmetric as needed.

Results

More than 100 patients with residual unilateral nasal deformities associated with

cleft lip and 20 patients with bilateral deformities were treated according to this protocol with a high rate of aesthetic and functional improvement.

In most instances symmetry, projection, and improvement of appearance were achieved with a single procedure. Ten percent of patients required minor operations to correct minor residual asymmetries. Fifteen percent of patients had good projection and symmetry in all other views but had some residual asymmetry in the base or worm's eye view, but they

declined further surgical therapy (Figs. 51-6 to 51-10).

Invariably patients who had undergone multiple previous procedures with extensive tissue resections and scarring had worse results than patients who presented with minimal nasal scarring. This was because most of these patients had multiple skin or nasal vestibule scars and contractures and insufficient skin, lining, or cartilage. A few had previous reconstructions with alloplastic implants, which caused additional scarring and thinning of the overlying skin.

Fig. 51-8A, B, C. Preoperative views of 17-year-old patient with residual nasal deformity from cleft lip. D, E. Intraoperative views. Note the considerable deviation of the dorsum and the caudal septum. F, G. Considerable discrepancy between the alar cartilages was managed by medial mobilization, suturing, and a tip graft. A septoplasty and midline repositioning of the caudal septum also were performed.

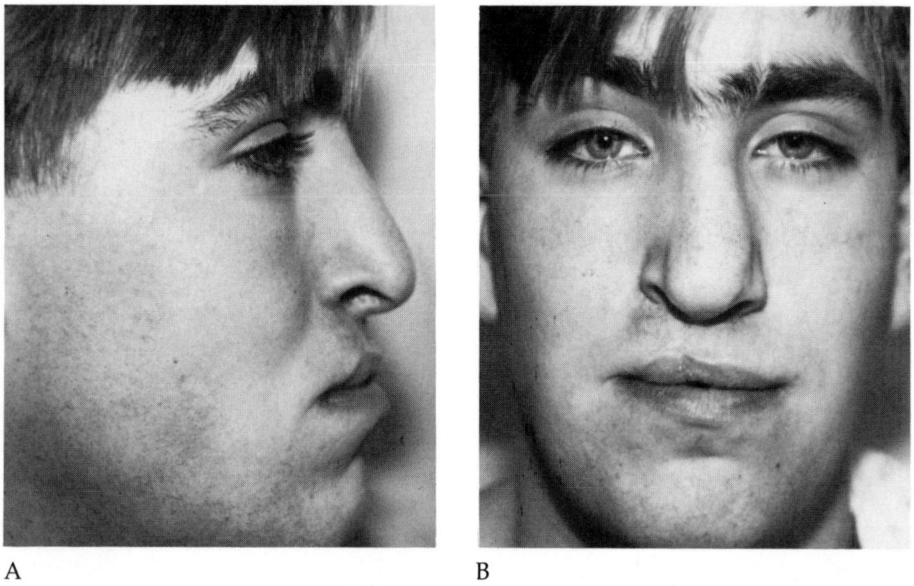

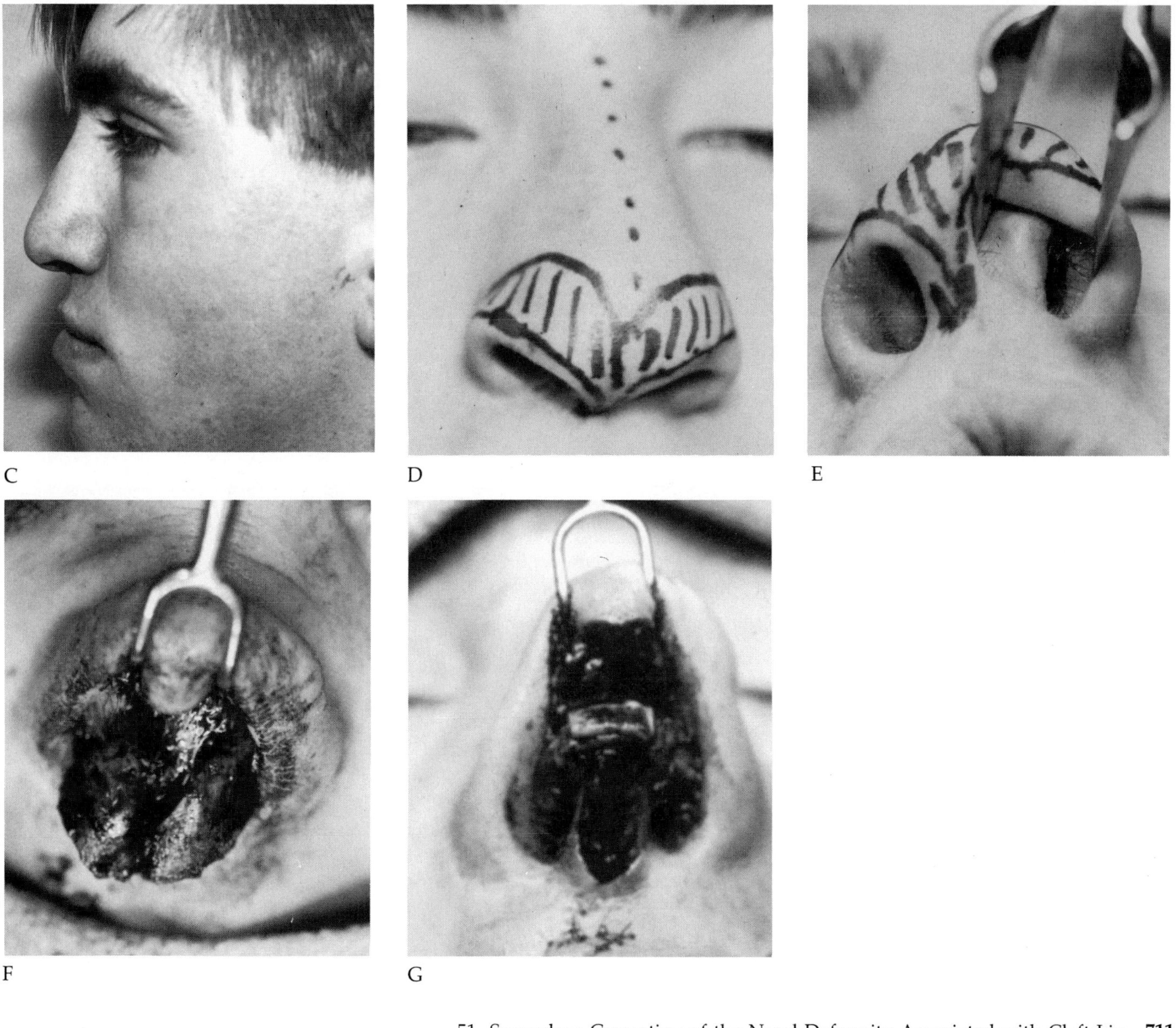

Fig. 51-8. (Continued) H, I. Postoperative views demonstrating good symmetry, correction of nasal and septal deviation, and adequate tip projection.

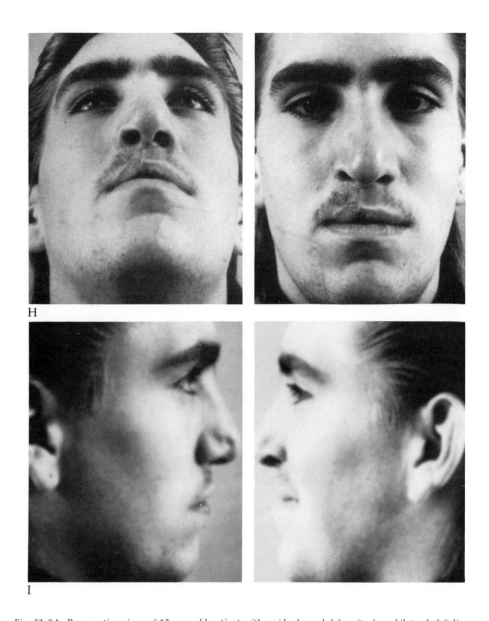

Fig. 51-9A. Preoperative views of 13-year-old patient with residual nasal deformity from bilateral cleft lip. Note the lack of projection, the nasal base, and the horizontal inclination of the nostrils. B, Postoperative views after open rhinoplasty when the patient was 16 years of age. Note the improved tip projection, narrowing of the nasal base, and change in the inclination of the nostrils. ▶

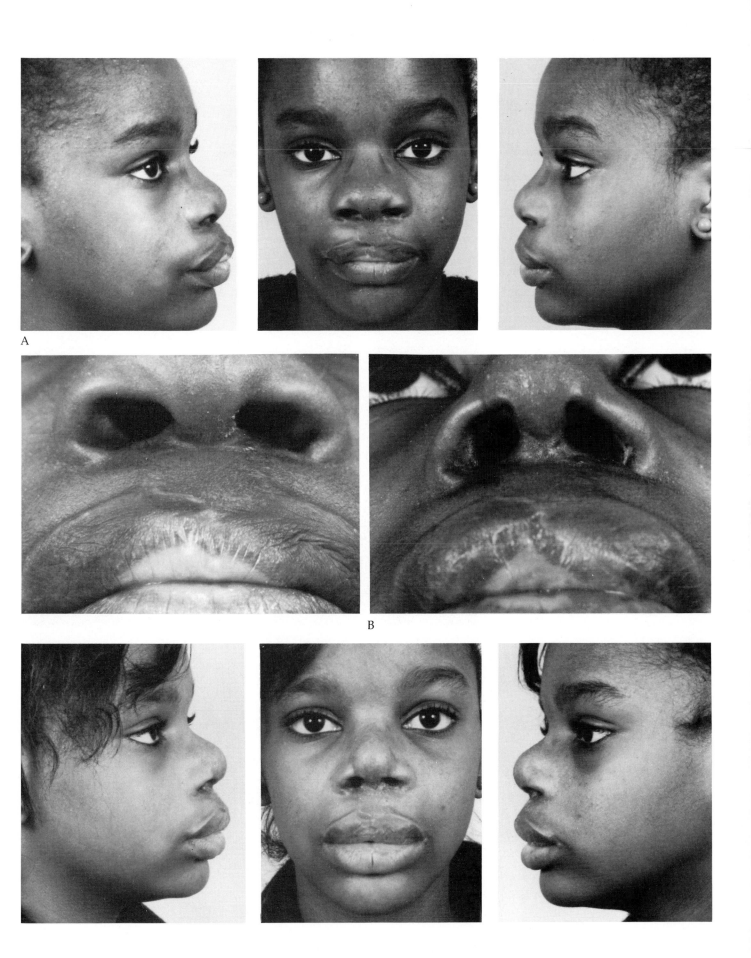

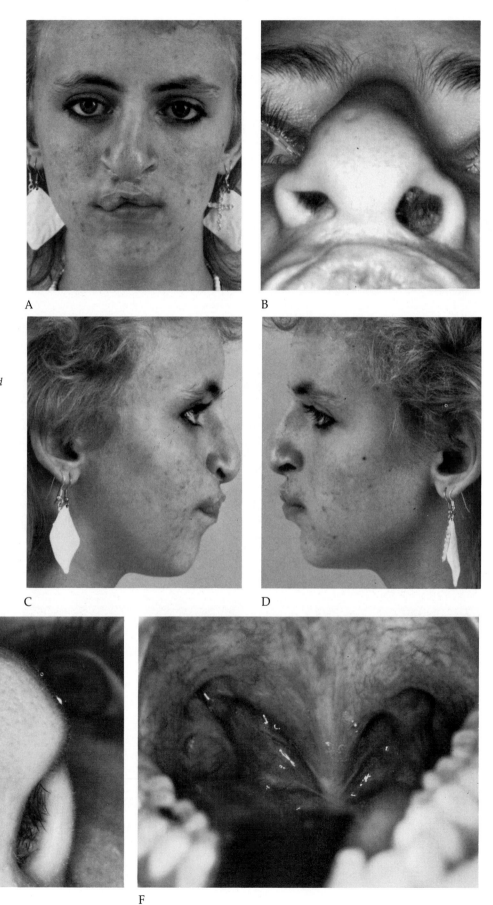

Fig. 51-10A, B, C, D. Preoperative views of 16-year-old patient with residual nasal deformity from bilateral cleft lip. Note the nasal deviation, lack of tip projection, and asymmetry in the shape and position of the nostrils. E, F. This patient had near-total obstruction of the right nostril from previous scarring and an obstructing pharyngeal flap.

A

B

C

D

E

F

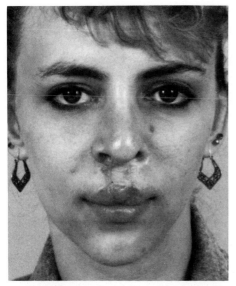

G

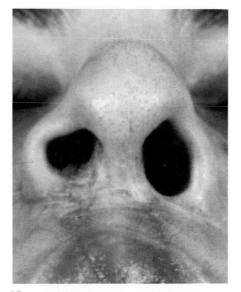

H

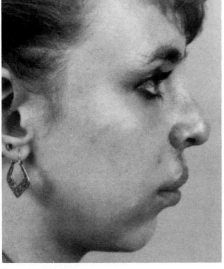

I

Fig. 51-10. (Continued) G, H, I, J. Postoperative views after open rhinoplasty, lip revision, and revision of ports of pharyngeal flap. Note the improvement in symmetry and tip projection and the correction of nasal deviation. Nostril obstruction was managed with release of the scar and applications of a composite graft from the ear. Despite improvement, some residual discrepancy of symmetry is visible in the worm's eye view (H).

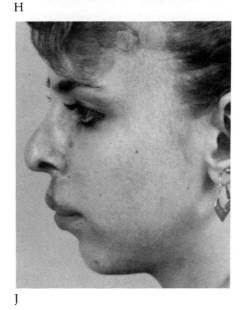

J

All patients requiring septoplasty with or without turbinectomies or revision of pharyngeal flaps to correct airway obstruction had a substantial improvement in airway patency. This improvement was evaluated clinically, but was confirmed with objective rhinomanometric evaluation. A typical example of this evaluation with comparison of pre- and postoperative rhinomanometric data is shown in Figures 51-11 and 51-12 and Tables 51-1 to 51-4.

Conclusion

The initial correction of the nasal deformities associated with cleft lip should be performed along with the cleft lip repair. Additional procedures should be undertaken with care and in a conservative manner. All incisions should be carefully planned, and overresection of soft tissue or cartilage should be avoided.

The definitive correction of the residual nasal deformity from a cleft lip should be deferred until after orthodontic realignment of the maxillary segments and bone grafting of the coexisting oronasal fistulas. Functional and aesthetic reconstruction should be addressed simultaneously. An open rhinoplasty provides direct exposure and visualization of the deformity and facilitates accurate repositioning of the alar cartilages and reconstruction with liberal use of autogenous cartilage or bone grafts. Septal deviations, when present, also can be addressed by this approach. Osteotomies should be performed when necessary to align the nasal skeleton. Finally, ancillary procedures to improve airway patency, such as partial inferior turbinectomies and, when necessary, revisions of obstructing pharyngeal flaps, should be incorporated into the treatment protocol.

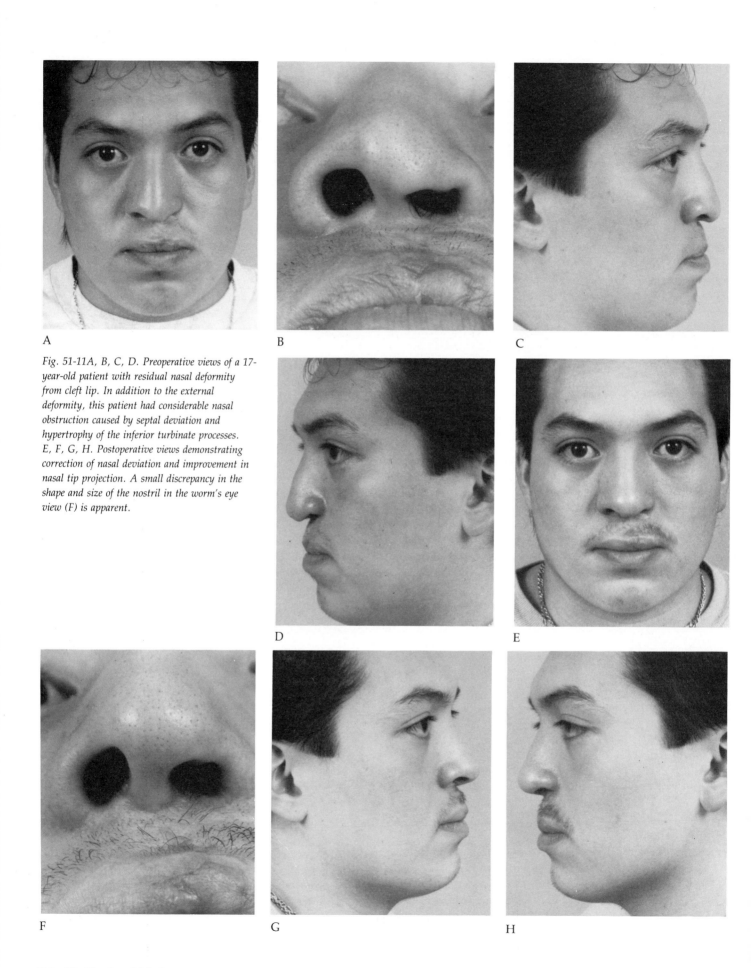

A

B

C

Fig. 51-11A, B, C, D. Preoperative views of a 17-year-old patient with residual nasal deformity from cleft lip. In addition to the external deformity, this patient had considerable nasal obstruction caused by septal deviation and hypertrophy of the inferior turbinate processes. E, F, G, H. Postoperative views demonstrating correction of nasal deviation and improvement in nasal tip projection. A small discrepancy in the shape and size of the nostril in the worm's eye view (F) is apparent.

D

E

F

G

H

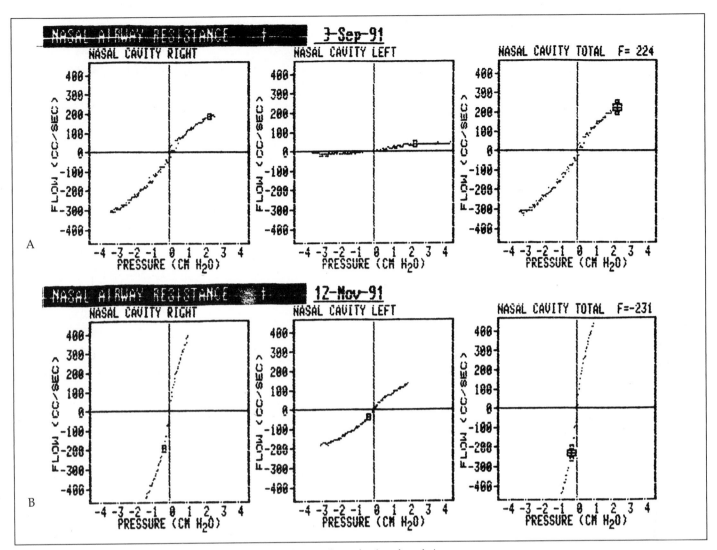

Fig. 51-12. Rhinometric evaluation of patient in Fig. 51-11. A. Preoperative evaluation of nasal airway resistance. Pressure-flow graphic record demonstrates clinically significant airway obstruction. B. Postoperative evaluation of nasal airway resistance. Pressure-flow graphic record demonstrates improvement in patency of both right and left nasal cavities.

Table 51-1. Preoperative pressure-flow data during inhalation at a flow rate of 0.22 L/sec

	Pressure (cm H₂O)	Flow (cc/sec)	Resistance (cm H₂O/L/sec)	Area (mm²)
Nasal cavity, right	−1.73	−205.13	8.43	17.14
Nasal cavity, left	−1.73	−19.23	89.96	1.61
Nasal cavity, total	−1.73	−224.36	7.71	18.75
Velopharynx	*****	*******	*****	*****
Total nasal airway	−1.73	−224.36	7.71	18.75

NCR = 7.71

$$VPR = \frac{*****}{NAR = \overline{7.71}}$$

Nasal cavity total flow = −224.36 cc per second.
NCR = total nasal cavities; VPR = velopharyngeal region; NAR = total nasal airway.

Table 51-2. Preoperative pressure-flow data during exhalation at a flow rate of 0.22 L/sec

	Pressure (cm H$_2$O)	Flow (cc/sec)	Resistance (cm H$_2$O/L/sec)	Area (mm^2)
Nasal cavity, right	2.38	185.90	12.80	13.24
Nasal cavity, left	2.38	38.46	61.88	2.74
Nasal cavity, total	2.38	224.36	10.61	15.98
Velopharynx	*****	*******	*****	*****
Total nasal airway	2.38	224.36	10.61	15.98

NCR = 10.61
VPR = *****
NAR = $\overline{10.61}$

Nasal cavity total flow = 224.36 cc per second.
NCR = total nasal cavities; VPR = velopharyngeal region; NAR = total nasal airway.

Table 51-3. Postoperative pressure-flow data during inhalation at a flow rate of 0.24 L/sec

	Pressure (cm H$_2$O)	Flow (cc/sec)	Resistance (cm H$_2$O/L/sec)	Area (mm^2)
Nasal cavity, right	−0.31	−192.31	1.61	37.96
Nasal cavity, left	−0.31	−38.46	8.06	7.59
Nasal cavity, total	−0.31	−230.77	1.34	45.55
Velopharynx	*****	*******	*****	*****
Total nasal airway	−0.31	−230.77	1.34	45.55

NCR = 1.34
VPR = *****
NAR = $\overline{1.34}$

Nasal cavity total flow = −230.77 cc per second.
NCR = total nasal cavities; VPR = velopharyngeal region; NAR = total nasal airway.

Table 51-4. Postoperative pressure-flow data during exhalation at a flow rate of 0.24 L/sec

	Pressure (cm H$_2$O)	Flow (cc/sec)	Resistance (cm H$_2$O/L/sec)	Area (mm^2)
Nasal cavity, right	0.38	192.31	1.98	34.28
Nasal cavity, left	0.38	44.87	8.47	8.00
Nasal cavity, total	0.38	237.18	1.60	42.28
Velopharynx	*****	*******	*****	*****
Total nasal airway	0.38	237.18	1.60	42.28

NCR = 1.60
VPR = *****
NAR = $\overline{1.60}$

Nasal cavity total flow = 237.18 cc per second.
NCR = total nasal cavities; VPR = velopharyngeal region; NAR = total nasal airway.

Suggested Reading

Bardach, J., et al. *Surgical Techniques in Cleft Lip and Palate* (2nd ed.). St. Louis: Mosby, 1991.

Black, P.U., Hartrampf, C.R., Jr., and Beegle, P. Cleft lip type nasal deformity: Definitive repair. *Ann. Plast. Surg.* 12:128, 1984.

Chen, K-T., and Noordhoff, M.S. Open tip rhinoplasty. *Ann. Plast. Surg.* 28:119, 1992.

Cronin, T.D., and Denkler, K.A. Correction of the unilateral cleft lip nose. *Plast. Reconstr. Surg.* 82:419, 1988.

Gorney, M. Rehabilitation for the post-cleft nasolabial stigmas. *Clin. Plast. Surg.* 15:73, 1988.

Gruber, R.P. Primary Rhinoplasty: The Open Approach. In L.M. Vistness (Ed.), *Procedures in Plastic and Reconstructive Surgery.* Boston: Little, Brown, 1991.

Millard, D.R., Jr. *Cleft Craft.* Vol. I. *The Unilateral Deformity.* Boston: Little, Brown, 1976.

Millard, D.R., Jr. *Cleft Craft.* Vol. II. *Bilateral and Rare Deformities.* Boston: Little, Brown, 1977.

Nishimura, Y., and Kumoi, T. External septorhinoplasty in the cleft lip nose. *Ann. Plast. Surg.* 27:526, 1992.

Ortiz-Monasterio, F., and Olmedo, A. Cleft Lip Nose. In T. Rees, D. Baker, and N. Tablal (Eds.), *Rhinoplasty: Problems and Controversies.* St. Louis: Mosby, 1988.

Thompson, H.G. The residual unilateral cleft lip nasal deformity: A three-phase correction technique. *Plast. Reconstr. Surg.* 76:36, 1985.

Tschopp, H.M. "The open sky rhinoplasty" for correction of secondary cleft lip nose deformity. *Scand. J. Plast. Surg.* 22:153, 1988.

52

Maxillary Deformities: Orthognathic Surgery

James A. Lehman, Jr.

Correction of facial imbalance and malocclusion associated with maxillary deformities can be achieved by a number of osteotomies and, occasionally, by onlay procedures. In the past it was common to treat maxillary deformities with procedures on the mandible because of concern about the stability of maxillary osteotomies. As a result, the aesthetic and functional results often were compromised. Today maxillary osteotomies combined with rigid fixation are stable, and one should use them to approach deformities of the upper jaw.

The goals of any surgical procedure on the maxilla are to obtain a stable functional occlusion and good facial aesthetics. This chapter presents a commonsense approach to maxillary deformities. Rather than attempt to describe all the osteotomies available, the focus is on procedures that have been found to be reliable, safe, and technically simple. The technical aspects are presented to enable the surgeon to complete the procedures with a minimal amount of effort. Procedures that move the maxilla as a single unit are usually preferred because of stability and technical ease. Complex procedures with multiple segmentation of the maxilla are usually unnecessary and increase the risk of complications.

Preoperative Planning

The correction of the skeletal, soft tissue, and dental disharmonies associated with maxillary deformities requires careful preoperative treatment planning. This is the key to good results in all orthognathic operations. Initially it is important to develop an understanding of the problem as the patient perceives it. This assessment should be followed by a clinical examination, photographs, cephalometric roentgenograms, panoramic roentgenograms, and dental models.

Skeletal and soft tissue analyses are important. The cephalometric measurements of primary concern are those that evaluate the anteroposterior position of the maxilla in relation to the cranial base. In addition, it is important to assess the amount of protrusion or retrusion of the maxillary dentition and the anterior vertical facial height.

The soft tissue analysis should take into account lip posture and the relation of the lip to the central incisors. This factor is important, especially in vertical movement of the maxilla. The nasolabial angle should be measured because its position can be altered by movement of the maxilla. The soft tissue changes associated

with skeletal movement of the maxilla have been documented.

Dental models are important in the evaluation of dentoalveolar malformations. After presurgical orthodontia they provide the basis for fabrication of a surgical splint. Model surgery is of little value when surgical procedures are performed on only one jaw with an intact dental arch. If the maxilla is to be segmented, model surgery is required to construct the appropriate surgical splint.

A percentage of patients undergoing maxillary surgical procedures have cleft lip and palate deformities in association with their maxillary deformity. Some of these patients have a pharyngeal flap. The management of the pharyngeal flap is a controversial issue. Certainly a tracheostomy is not an acceptable solution. The best approach is to divide the flap, leaving the bulk of the flap attached to the palate; this allows the maxilla to move without any restriction. In my experience only 50 percent of the patients so treated had velopharyngeal incompetence and required reconstruction of the pharyngeal flap.

With this overall evaluation of the patient, an appropriate treatment plan to solve the skeletal and soft tissue problems can be formulated. The plan also takes into consideration the patient's own concerns.

Presurgical Orthodontic Treatment

A close working relationship with an orthodontist is extremely important in planning the treatment of all dentofacial deformities. In maxillary osteotomies the amount of maxillary movement needs to be coordinated between the surgeon and the orthodontist in relation to the clinical examination and the cephalometric findings.

Presurgical orthodontic treatment is a prerequisite for almost all maxillary osteotomies. It may be as simple as the insertion of a tooth tissue–borne appliance for rapid palatal expansion or as complex as 12 to 18 months of full orthodontic treatment. Full orthodontic treatment is usually necessary to align the dental arches and eliminate crowding and dental compensations. This process may require extractions. The purpose is to achieve two arches that are compatible in the postsurgical position. Orthodontic movements that attempt to close open-bite deformities should be avoided, and orthodontic movements that accentuate open bites should be completed before the operation so that the open bite can be corrected surgically.

Rigid Fixation

Plates and screws for the fixation of maxillary fractures and osteotomies were first introduced in the late 1970s. The greatest advantage is safety; the patient does not need to be in intermaxillary fixation postoperatively. Rigid fixation of the bone fragments also promotes faster bone healing and greater resistance to infection. Without intermaxillary fixation there is improved nutrition, which enhances wound healing, and early jaw motion is beneficial to function. The major disadvantage is that one must be technically precise because there is no leeway for orthodontic correction of discrepancies.

In maxillary osteotomies, the maxilla is moved to a new position and must remain

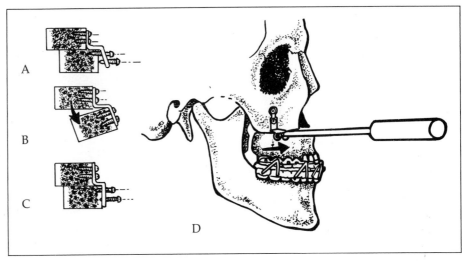

Fig. 52-1A. A compression-type force will be applied if the fixation plate is not flush with the bone. B. This situation can cause movement of the bone and resultant open bite. C. Proper contouring of the plate before insertion of the screw. D. Application of plate for Le Fort I osteotomy with advancement with teeth in intermaxillary fixation.

there while the plates and screws are applied passively. The plates must be bent to fit flat with the surface of the maxilla (Fig. 52-1). Most miniplate systems have soft, malleable templates that can be pressed across the osteotomy, and these templates can be used as the benchmark for bending the permanent plate. If the plate is not lying flush with the underlying bone as the screw is tightened, the position of the maxilla will change (see Fig. 52-1).

The plates should be placed where the bone is thick enough to accommodate the self-tapping screws. In anterior segmental osteotomies the plates can be fixed directly across the osteotomy sites (Fig. 52-2). In a Le Fort I osteotomy the plates should be inserted at the pyriform margin and the zygomaticomaxillary buttress where the bone is thickest (Fig. 52-3). It is important to use four plates with four screws in each plate. L- or T-shaped plates are best to maximize fixation. Plates that are too long are palpable in the infraorbital area. If the patient has a cleft, a fifth plate should be used across the alveolar cleft (see Fig. 52-3).

After the osteotomy is completed, the maxilla is positioned and placed into in-

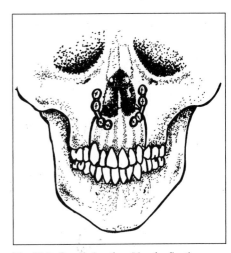

Fig. 52-2. One choice of position for fixation plates in anterior segmental osteotomy.

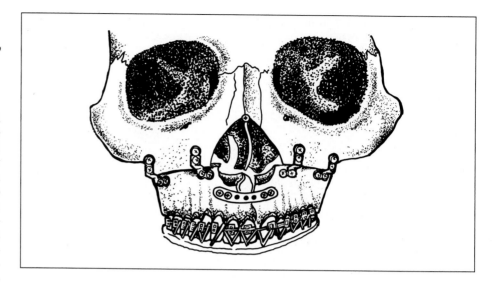

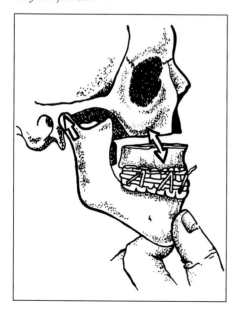

Fig. 52-3. Usual position for the four fixation plates in a Le Fort I osteotomy. L- or T-shaped plates are preferred. A fifth plate should be used to stabilize the two segments in a patient with a cleft.

termaxillary fixation using the occlusal splint as the guide for the occlusion. The maxillary-mandibular complex is moved up and down to ensure there are no bony interferences and that the condyles are in the glenoid fossa (Fig. 52-4). Failure to seat the condyles properly results in a malocclusion when the intermaxillary fixation is released. After the first two plates are fixed, the intermaxillary fixation is removed and the mandible rotated to ensure that it occludes properly with the maxilla in the centric position. If it does not occlude properly at this time, the plates should be removed. After removal of bony interferences, the maxilla is repositioned. The foregoing steps are repeated. If the occlusion is good, intermaxillary fixation is replaced and the final two plates are applied.

At the completion of the procedure, the intermaxillary fixation is removed. There is no point in maintaining intermaxillary fixation if rigid fixation is used. The Le Fort II osteotomy requires fixation at the

Fig. 52-4. After the maxilla is placed into intermaxillary fixation, the maxillary-mandibular unit should be rotated up and down to see that the condyles are seated in the fossa and there are no bony interferences.

frontonasal region with a T-shaped plate and either a straight plate at the infraorbital rim or an L-shaped plate in the zygomaticomaxillary buttress.

Surgical Procedures

Maxillary Expansion

With the increased interest in adult orthodontic treatment, problems with transverse maxillary width in nongrowing patients have been encountered with greater frequency by orthodontists. Attempts at rapid palatal expansion in adults have usually resulted in failure. With maturity the zygomaticomaxillary buttress resists expansion, and attempts at rapid palatal expansion result in tipping of teeth, bending of alveolar bone, inability to open the midpalatal suture, pressure necrosis of the palatal mucosa, and relapse. It has been demonstrated in adults that a lateral osteotomy of the zygomaticomaxillary buttress combined with a rapid palatal expansion appliance allows for successful expansion of the maxilla.

Before the operation a rapid palatal expansion device is cemented to the maxillary first premolar and first molar teeth. This should be a tooth tissue–borne appliance. Using general anesthesia in an outpatient setting, the surgeon makes an incision in the upper buccal sulcus through the mucoperiosteum from the first molar to the first molar. The mucoperiosteum is elevated superiorly and lat-

erally, exposing the pyriform aperture, anterior nasal floor, anterior lateral maxilla, and zygomatic buttress. A horizontal osteotomy is made with a power saw through the lateral wall of the maxilla, approximately 4 to 5 mm above the apices of the teeth from the inferior lateral aspect of the pyriform aperture to the inferior aspect of the junction of the maxillary tuberosity and the pterygoid plate (Fig. 52-5). The anterior portion of the lateral nasal wall is included after elevation of the nasal mucosa. Sectioning of the pterygomaxillary suture is unnecessary. Expansion of the anterior part of the maxilla can be started by inserting a thin osteotome between the roots of the central incisors (Fig. 52-6), but this is not a necessary part of the procedure. Care must be taken not to cut so deep as to sever the transseptal fibers linking the central incisors. Doing so makes it difficult for the orthodontist to bring these teeth into approximation.

In patients with ossification of the midpalatal suture (30% of all patients), a midpalatal osteotomy is performed in addition to the procedure described. After a thin osteotome is placed between the roots of the central incisors, the osteotome is turned 90° and malleted down the length of the hard palate in the submucosal plane (see Fig. 52-6). After closure of the buccal mucosa, the palatal expansion appliance is activated four one-quarter turns (Fig. 52-7). The palatal appliance normally is activated one one-quarter turn twice a day until the desired amount of expansion is achieved.

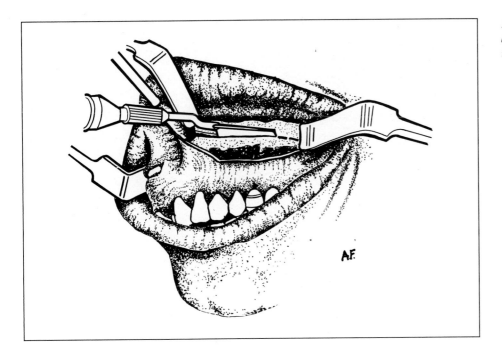

Fig. 52-5. The transverse osteotomy is made with a reciprocating saw from the pyriform aperture through the zygomaticomaxillary buttress.

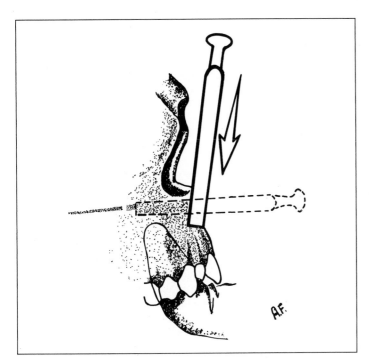

Fig. 52-6. Thin osteotome is placed between central incisors and hammered to start expansion. Dotted osteotome shows position of osteotomy to section the midpalatal suture if necessary.

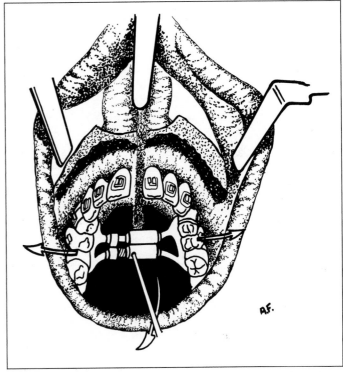

Fig. 52-7. Activation of palatal expansion appliance at conclusion of procedure.

52. Maxillary Deformities: Orthognathic Surgery   **723**

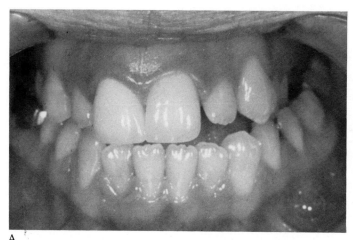

A

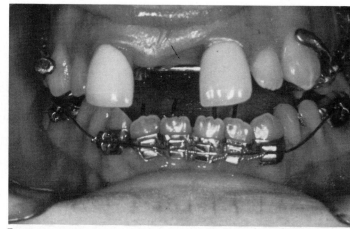

B

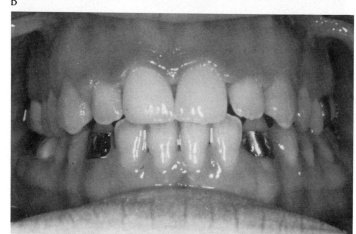

C

Fig. 52-8A. Bilateral maxillary crossbite in class I occlusion. B. After completion of expansion. C. Final result one year after completion of orthodontic treatment.

The maxilla is always overexpanded in anticipation of some relapse owing to lateral tipping of the teeth. Expansion is usually completed in approximately 3 weeks, and at this point the appliance is stabilized with a wire or acrylic device. The expanded segments are retained for 3 to 4 months, but other orthodontic procedures can be initiated after the appliance is stabilized.

In maxillary deformities the primary candidate for a lateral maxillary osteotomy and rapid palatal expansion is a patient who does not require vertical or sagittal repositioning of the maxilla (Fig. 52-8). It should be noted that segmentation of the maxilla increases the risk of skeletal, dental, and periodontal complications that do not exist when the maxilla is not segmented. This is another reason to consider rapid palatal expansion as a preliminary procedure before an orthognathic operation in patients with marked skeletal arch discrepancies (Fig. 52-9).

Maxillary Osteotomies

Maxillary osteotomies can be segmental or total in relation to the dental alveolar arch. The choice of osteotomy depends on the extent of the maxillary deformity, the type of malocclusion, and the involvement of other structures, such as the nose, orbital rims, and malar bones, in the deformity.

Segmental dentoalveolar osteotomies have the advantage that the procedure is performed only in the part of the dental arch that is deformed. These can be anterior or posterior but are of limited use today. The only segmental osteotomy that is still occasionally useful is the anterior segmental osteotomy.

When the deformity extends beyond the dentoalveolar segment, total maxillary osteotomies are required. These osteotomies follow the classic lines of fracture described by Le Fort. Discussion here is lim-

ited to the Le Fort I and Le Fort II osteotomies. Most maxillary skeletal deformities can be corrected with a Le Fort I osteotomy. The down-fractured Le Fort I segment may be moved forward, backward, upward, or downward depending on the problem (Fig. 52-10). One can also correct for pitch, roll, and yaw at the same time (Fig. 52-11). In addition, segmentation of the maxilla may be used to correct disproportion in the transverse or anteroposterior plane (Fig. 52-12).

Anterior Segmental Osteotomy

Before it was realized that the entire maxilla could be mobilized and repositioned based on its palatal blood supply, segmental osteotomies of the maxilla were popular. These osteotomies could involve the anterior segment or the posterior segments. The versatility of the multiple-segment Le Fort I osteotomy has practically

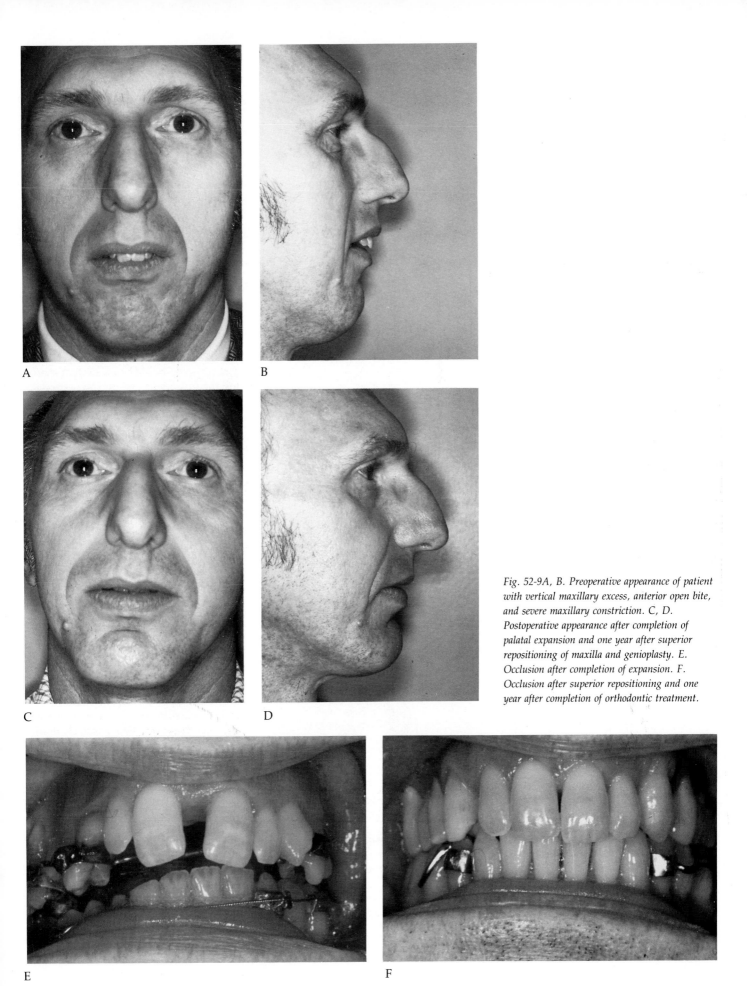

A

B

C

D

E

F

Fig. 52-9A, B. Preoperative appearance of patient with vertical maxillary excess, anterior open bite, and severe maxillary constriction. C, D. Postoperative appearance after completion of palatal expansion and one year after superior repositioning of maxilla and genioplasty. E. Occlusion after completion of expansion. F. Occlusion after superior repositioning and one year after completion of orthodontic treatment.

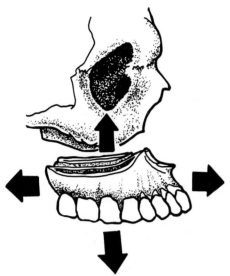

Fig. 52-10. The Le Fort I osteotomy allows movement in four directions.

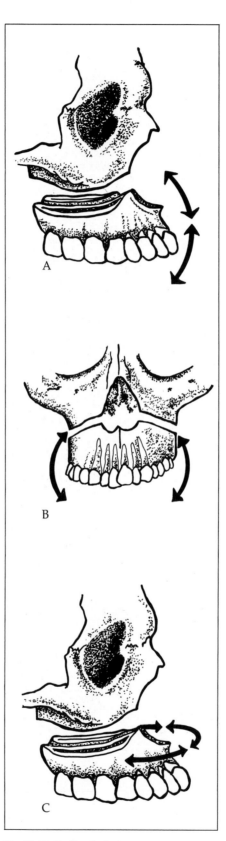

Fig. 52-11. Besides the basic movements, the Le Fort I osteotomy allows for multidimensional movement of the maxilla, which includes pitch (A), roll (B), and yaw (C).

eliminated the isolated anterior and posterior segmental osteotomies from clinical use. The isolated anterior segmental osteotomy is useful in class II, division I patients with a good functional posterior occlusion, prominent upper lip and teeth, and a well-aligned mandibular arch (Fig. 52-13).

The down-fracturing technique offers the best access to the anterior maxilla so that it can be repositioned posteriorly or superiorly or both. The first bicuspid is extracted, and a horizontal buccal sulcus incision is connected to the vertical incision line at the extraction site (Fig. 52-14A). The mucosa is elevated from the anterior and lateral chest walls of the nasal cavity. Bone is removed vertically from the extraction sites. The osteotomy is carried into the pyriform aperture, and a transpalatal osteotomy is completed through the vertical osteotomy sites with the power bur (Fig. 52-14B). The anterior maxilla is down-fractured with the aid of an osteotome. Using a bur, the appropriate amount of bone is removed from the palatal and vertical osteotomy sites to obtain the desired posterior movement (see Fig. 52-14C). The palatal mucosa is preserved to maintain the blood supply to the anterior segment. When superior movement is required, a portion of the septum is also removed. After the segment is moved into the desired position,

a rigid fixation plate is applied to each side (see Fig. 52-14D). In some patients the segment can be fixed to the arch wire. The incisions are closed with 4–0 polyglactin 910.

Le Fort I Osteotomy

The Le Fort I osteotomy is the cornerstone of the treatment of maxillary deformities. The basic osteotomy can be modified depending on the direction of movement. These modifications are addressed in separate sections. Movement of more than 10 to 12 mm in any one direction is not recommended. Deformities in the maxilla that require that much movement should be under consideration for a combined maxillary and mandibular operation.

The surgeon should be aware that changing the position of the maxilla, especially in a vertical direction, can alter the patient's facial appearance considerably. This change may not always be accepted positively. The older the patient, the more difficulty he or she has in adapting to the change regardless of the aesthetic improvement. This issue should be discussed with the patient.

To appreciate the overall aesthetic requirement, it is important in maxillary operations to be able to see the entire face (Fig. 52-15A). After the endotracheal tube is in place it can be secured with a nasal septal suture or a plastic drape, which allows the surgeon access to the entire face. The upper buccal sulcus is infiltrated with 1% lidocaine with epinephrine, and the nose is packed with 5% cocaine to reduce bleeding. The incision is made in the upper buccal sulcus about 5 mm above the mucogingival junction from first molar to first molar. A cuff of mucosa is developed inferiorly to assist in wound closure. The periosteum is elevated over the anterior maxilla up to the infraorbital nerve and over the zygomaticomaxillary buttress to accommodate the fixation plates (see Fig. 52-15B).

The nasal mucosa is elevated from the floor of the nose and from the septum medially. The osteotomy line is marked with a no. 2 pencil from the inferior lateral aspect of the pyriform aperture horizontally over the zygomaticomaxillary buttress. The line should be 4 to 6 mm above the apices of the teeth to prevent injury to the teeth and to allow room for screw placement.

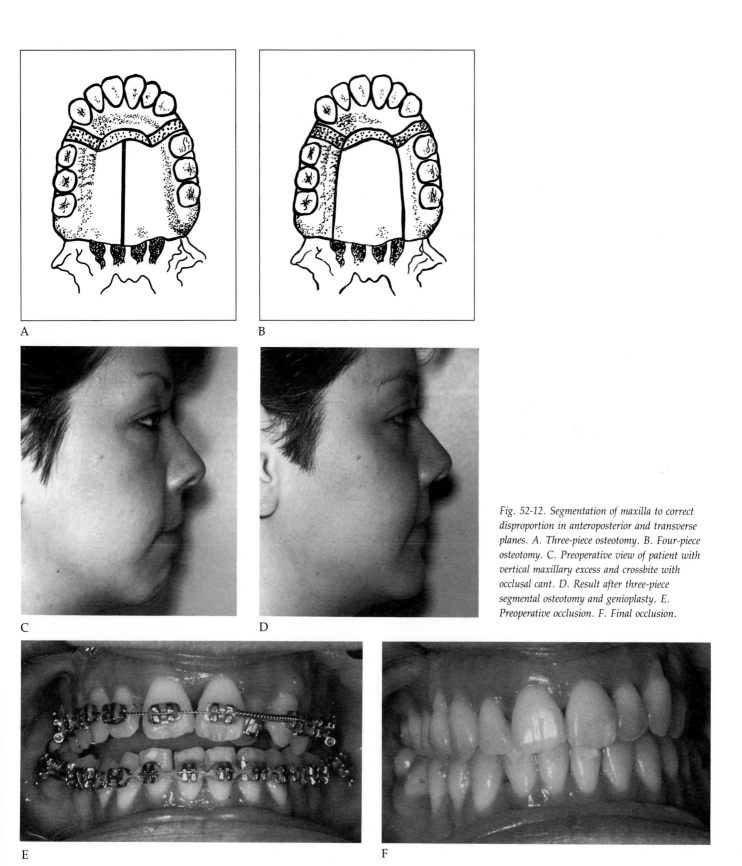

Fig. 52-12. *Segmentation of maxilla to correct disproportion in anteroposterior and transverse planes. A. Three-piece osteotomy. B. Four-piece osteotomy. C. Preoperative view of patient with vertical maxillary excess and crossbite with occlusal cant. D. Result after three-piece segmental osteotomy and genioplasty. E. Preoperative occlusion. F. Final occlusion.*

A

B

C

D

E

F

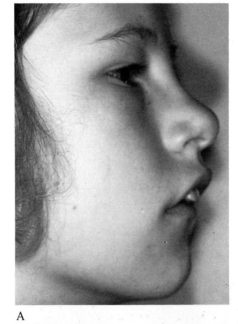

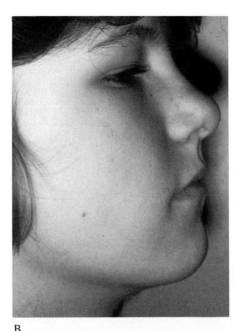

Fig. 52-13A. Preoperative lateral view showing protrusion of upper lip and excessive incisor exposure. B. Postoperative view after extraction of first bicuspid and setback of anterior maxilla. C. Preoperative dental occlusion. D. Postoperative occlusion.

A

B

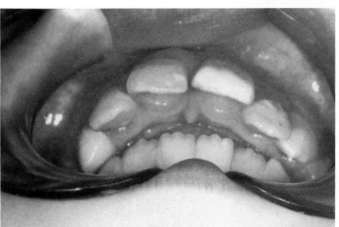

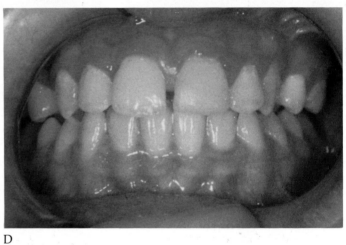

C

D

The reciprocating saw is used to complete the osteotomy on both sides (see Fig. 52-15C). The nasal septum is cut; the saw cuts away from the side with the endotracheal tube (see Fig. 52-15D). A thin curved osteotome is used to separate the maxillary buttress from the pterygoid plates. The osteotome should be kept below the level of the horizontal osteotomy cut to avoid injury to branches of the internal maxillary vessel (see Fig. 52-15E).

At this point one is ready for the down-fracture. A sponge is placed on the anterior teeth. Using both thumbs, the surgeon forces the maxilla downward (see Fig. 52-15F). The maxilla should break free quite easily if the osteotomies have been completed properly. A Rowe max-

illary forceps is used to mobilize the maxilla (see Fig. 52-15G). No matter what direction the maxilla is to be moved in, it must be freed to the point at which it can be positioned with a forceps. Mobilization also can be facilitated by placing a heavy periosteal elevator behind the maxillary tuberosity and levering forward. An attempt is made to preserve the descending palatine vessels, but the maxilla survives if both vessels are ligated.

Bony projections and interferences along the lateral nasal wall and in the area of the tuberosity are removed with a rongeur or power bur. The maxilla can now be moved and should fit easily into its new position. The interdental splint is inserted and the teeth placed into inter-

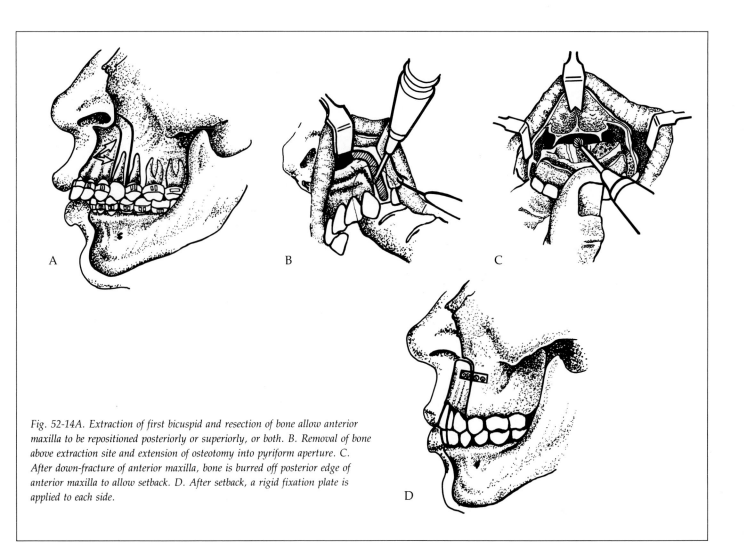

Fig. 52-14A. Extraction of first bicuspid and resection of bone allow anterior maxilla to be repositioned posteriorly or superiorly, or both. B. Removal of bone above extraction site and extension of osteotomy into pyriform aperture. C. After down-fracture of anterior maxilla, bone is burred off posterior edge of anterior maxilla to allow setback. D. After setback, a rigid fixation plate is applied to each side.

maxillary fixation. The maxillary mandibular unit is rotated to be sure the condyles are in the glenoid fossa and there are no interferences. The fixation plates are applied as previously described (see Fig. 52-15H).

Le Fort I Osteotomy with Forward Movement

Patients with maxillary retrusion usually demonstrate flattening of the midface, a sunken appearance of the upper lip, and prominence of the mandible. There is usually a class III malocclusion. Correction requires a Le Fort I osteotomy with advancement (Fig. 52-16). Bone grafts are no longer required with rigid fixation. Hydroxyapatite can be used with advancements greater than 7 mm or in patients with clefts.

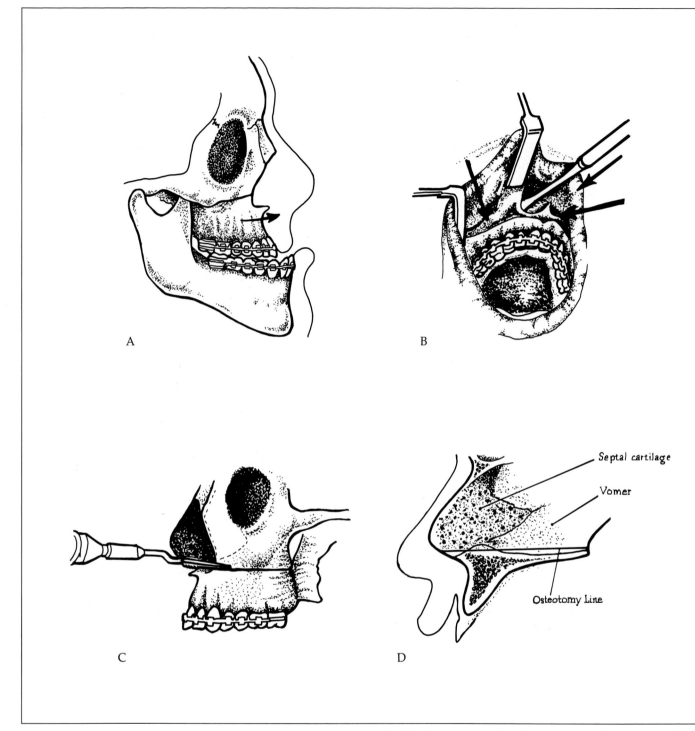

Fig. 52-15A. *Basic osteotomy line for advancement. B. Elevation of periosteum from anterior maxilla and nasal floor. Arrow shows where fixation plates are to be placed. C. Transverse osteotomy made with reciprocating saw. D. Position of septal osteotomy. E. Curved osteotome separating buttress from pterygoid plates. Osteotome should be kept below level of transverse osteotomy. F. Down-fracture of maxilla. G. Mobilization of maxilla with Rowe forceps. H. Rigid fixation plates applied. In the past, bone grafts were placed behind the maxillary tuberosity (arrow). This step is not necessary with rigid fixation.*

Labels on figure D: Septal cartilage, Vomer, Osteotomy Line

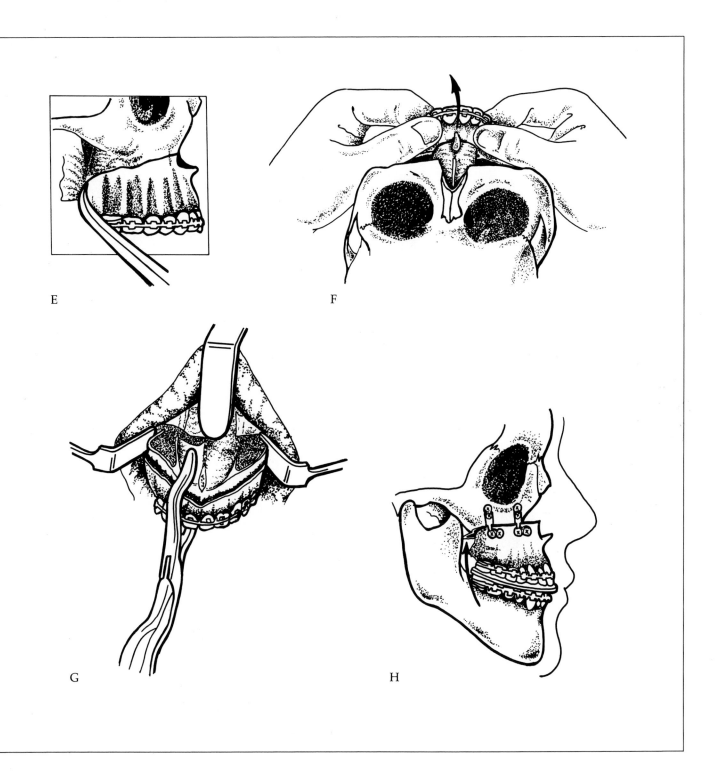

E

F

G

H

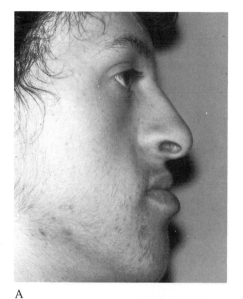

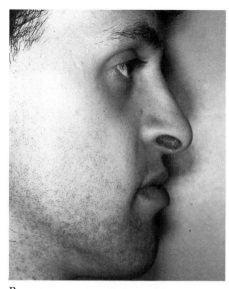

Fig. 52-16A. *Preoperative profile of patient with maxillary retrusion showing flattened midface and sunken upper lip. B. Nine years after treatment showing improved facial contour. C. Preoperative class III malocclusion. D. Final occlusion.*

A

B

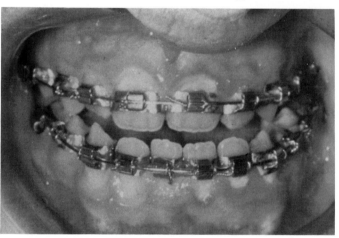

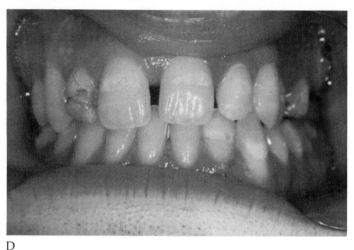

C

D

Le Fort I Osteotomy with Posterior Movement

Posterior movement of the maxilla is indicated in horizontal maxillary excess and can be combined with superior repositioning to obtain a class I occlusion (Fig. 52-17). Posterior repositioning of the maxilla can be accomplished with the maxilla in the down-fractured position. The maxilla can be moved 5 to 7 mm posteriorly by reducing the superior and posterior aspects of the maxillary tuberosities (Fig. 52-18A). Impacted third molars can be removed easily at the same time. The amount of bone to be removed is determined preoperatively; the bone is removed from the posterior aspect of the tuberosity with a power bur (see Fig. 52-18B). The maxilla is placed in intermaxillary fixation with the occlusal splint, and

the maxillary-mandibular unit is rotated into proper position and fixed in the usual manner.

Le Fort I Osteotomy with Superior Repositioning

Superior movement of the maxilla is one of the most common uses of the Le Fort II osteotomy. Maxillary vertical excess is characterized by excessive display of the maxillary central teeth with the lips in repose and an associated lip incompetence. There may be an anterior open bite, and usually there is a class II malocclusion. The most important factor in determining the amount of superior maxillary movement is the clinical assessment of the amount of maxillary incisor show with the lips in repose. The normal value is 2 to 4 mm. Subtracting 2 mm from the

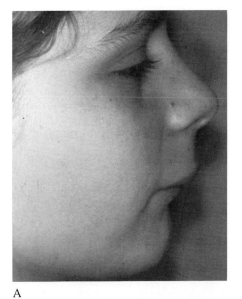

A

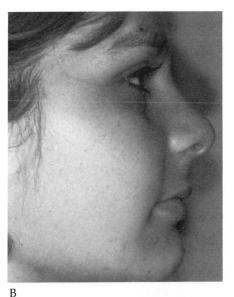

B

Fig. 52-17A. Preoperative profile showing
protrusion of upper lip and maxilla. B. Improved
profile after setback of maxilla. C. Preoperative
occlusion. D. Final occlusion.

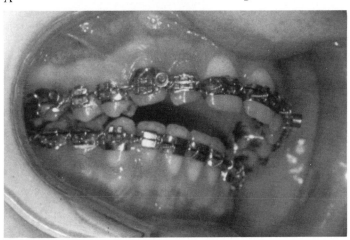

C

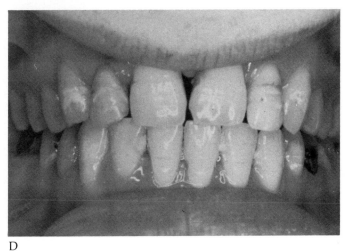

D

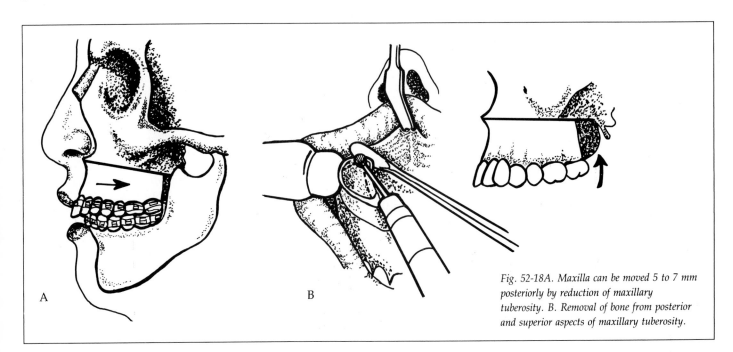

A

B

Fig. 52-18A. Maxilla can be moved 5 to 7 mm
posteriorly by reduction of maxillary
tuberosity. B. Removal of bone from posterior
and superior aspects of maxillary tuberosity.

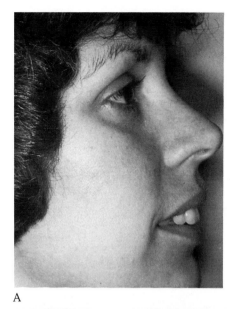

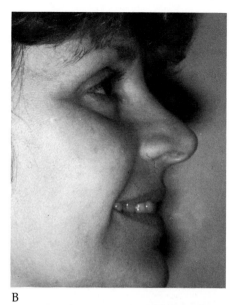

A

B

Fig. 52-19A. Preoperative view showing maxillary vertical excess. B. Final result after superior repositioning of maxilla 7 mm and posterior movement 4 mm. C. Preoperative occlusion. D. Final occlusion.

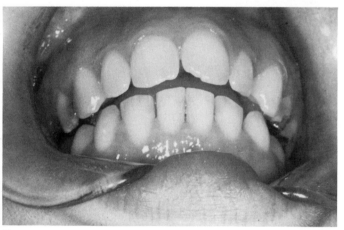

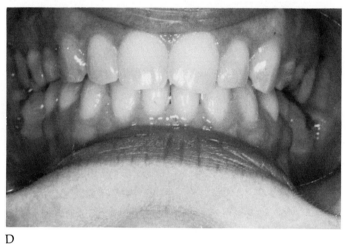

C

D

amount of dental show leaves the amount of maxillary reduction. It is better to err on the conservative side so that the patient does not have an edentulous look postoperatively (Fig. 52-19).

Superior movement of the maxilla is frequently accompanied by anterior or posterior movement to achieve a class I occlusion (Fig. 52-20A). After completion of the horizontal osteotomy, a second osteotomy is measured with a caliper to be 1 mm less than the desired reduction to avoid overcorrection (see Fig. 52-20B). As an additional evaluation of accuracy, one can measure the external distance from the medial canthus to the arch wire. The second osteotomy parallels the first, and the segment of bone is removed (see Fig. 52-20C). The procedure continues as previously described (see Fig. 52-20D). Once

the down-fracture is completed, the remaining excess bone medially and posteriorly is removed with a rongeur (see Fig. 52-20E). A corresponding amount of bone and cartilage also must be removed from the septum to avoid buckling (see Fig. 52-20F). It may be necessary to reduce the inferior turbinate processes to allow for unimpeded cephalad movement of the maxilla (see Fig. 52-20G). This is usually not a problem unless the maxilla is moved upward more than 5 to 6 mm. Careful cautery of the mucosal edges is important to avoid postoperative bleeding. Once the proper vertical position of the maxilla is obtained (using external measurements), the rigid fixation plates are placed as previously described. The Le Fort I osteotomy can be used to correct an open bite deformity by intruding the posterior aspect of the Le Fort I segment.

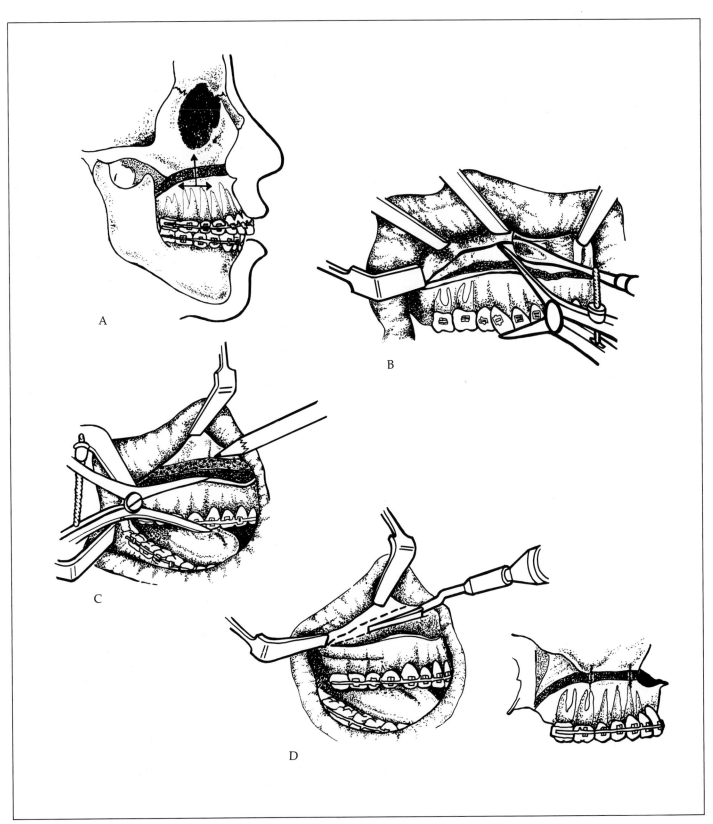

Fig. 52-20A. Superior repositioning of maxilla is frequently accompanied by anterior or posterior movement to achieve a class I occlusion. B. Measuring first osteotomy line and elevating periosteum from pyriform aperture. C. Marking second osteotomy line with pencil. Shaded area to be removed. D. Osteotomies completed with power bur, and shaded area removed.

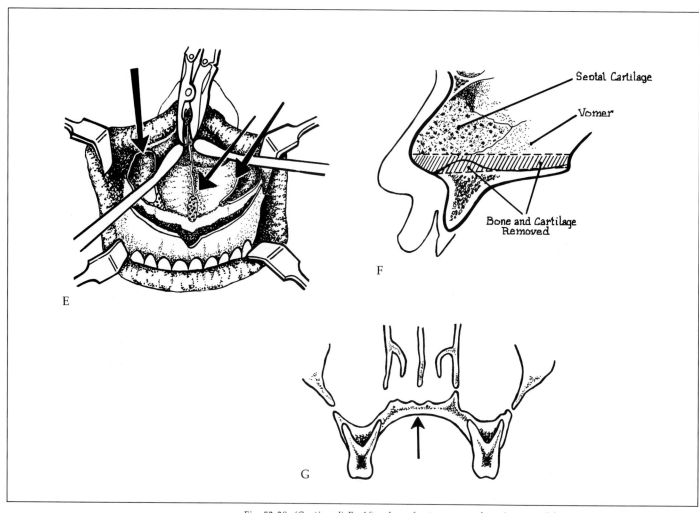

Fig. 52-20. (Continued) E. After down-fracture, excess bone is removed from vomerine ridge, lateral nasal wall, lateral wall of maxilla, and posterior tuberosity with a rongeur. F. Area of bone and cartilage to be removed from septum should be slightly greater than the extent of vertical movement to avoid buckling of septum. G. Coronal view showing how large inferior turbinate processes can impede superior movement.

Le Fort I Osteotomy with Downward Movement

Vertical maxillary deficiency usually manifests in a short lower half of the face; a lack of exposure of the maxillary teeth, giving an edentulous look; accentuated nasolabial folds; and a deep labiomental sulcus. There is usually a class II malocclusion with a deep overbite. To reestablish the proper relation between the upper lip and the maxillary incisors and to correct the vertical deficiency, it is necessary to perform a Le Fort I osteotomy with inferior displacement. The spaces along the osteotomy sites are filled with bone grafts or hydroxyapatite. Hydroxyapatite is preferred because it does not resorb and there is no donor site morbidity (Fig. 52-21).

In marking the osteotomy in a patient with a short face, the line may have to extend well up on the zygomaticomaxillary buttress to avoid injury to the apices of the teeth and give room for screw placement (Fig. 52-22A). The same external reference points used for superior repositioning can be used as guidelines for inferior repositioning.

After completion of the down-fracture, the teeth are placed in intermaxillary fix-ation with the splint. After it is ensured that the condyles are seated in the fossa, the desired amount of downward movement is measured, and a block of hydroxyapatite is inserted (see Fig. 52-22B). In a short face it is best to overcorrect slightly because of the tendency toward relapse and because a little extra tooth exposure gives a more youthful appearance. Before rigid fixation, drill holes are placed above and below the osteotomy line and titanium wires are inserted to hold the hydroxyapatite in place (see Fig. 52-22B). Hydroxyapatite cannot be fixed with screws because it shatters. After insertion of the blocks of hydroxyapatite of appro-

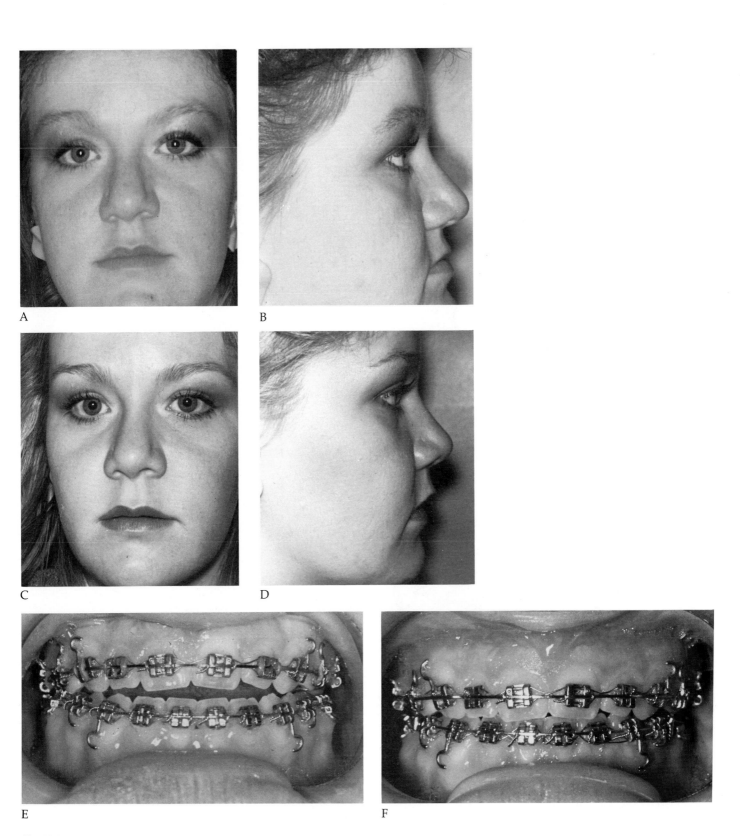

A

B

C

D

E

F

Fig. 52-21A, B. Preoperative views of patient with vertical maxillary deficiency demonstrating short lower face and edentulous look. C, D. Postoperative result after inferior repositioning of 4 mm and reduction genioplasty. E. Preoperative occlusion. F. Postoperative occlusion.

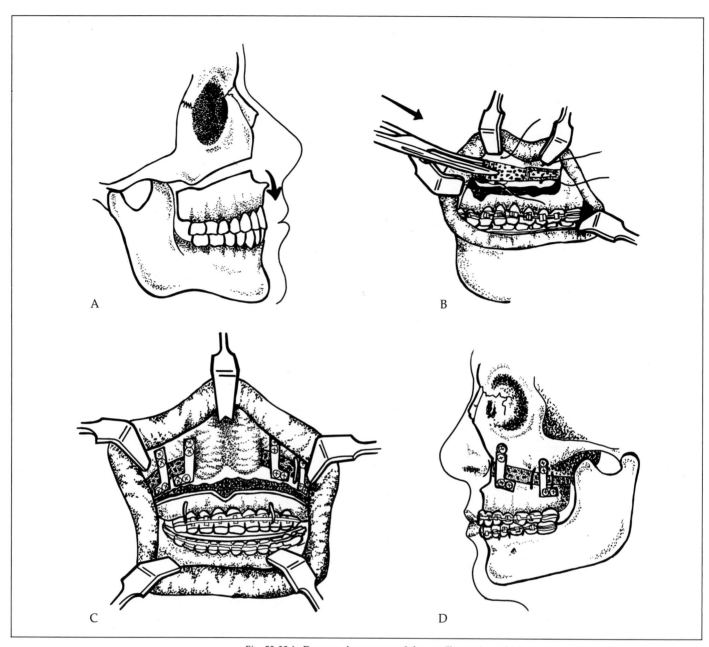

Fig. 52-22A. *Downward movement of the maxilla requires a high placement of the osteotomy line on the maxilla. B. Wires inserted in drill holes before insertion of hydroxyapatite blocks. C. Rigid fixation with four plates. D. Wires and plates for fixation of hydroxyapatite and bone.*

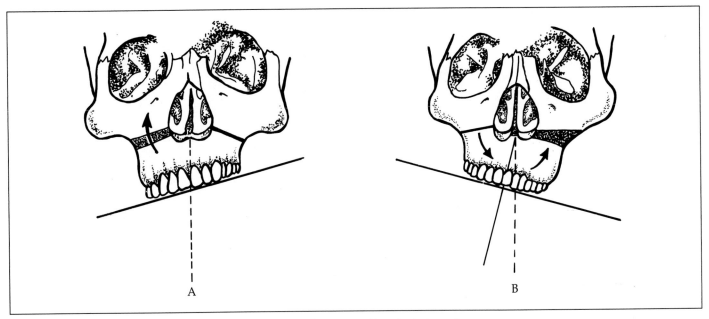

Fig. 52-23A. Leveling of maxilla can be achieved by removal of excess bone on one side and osteotomy of the other. B. Combined reduction of excess on one side and vertical lengthening on the other to level maxilla and bring dental midline to the skeletal midline.

priate size, the fixation plates are applied (see Fig. 52-22C). Once fixation is complete, the wires are twisted down to prevent slippage of the blocks (see Fig. 52-22D). If bone is used, it can be held to one of the plates with a screw rather than with wires.

Leveling of the Maxilla

Vertical maxillary asymmetry is usually associated with hemifacial microsomia, condylar hyperplasia, vascular anomalies, or Romberg disease. The occlusal plane has a cant because of the asymmetric growth. Surgical correction can be achieved by reduction of the vertical excess on one side (Fig. 52-23A), lengthening of the vertical deficiency on one side, or a combination of both (see Fig. 52-23B). The maxillary tooth-to-lip relation is the determining factor in the selection of the technique. The plan should be to have 2 to 4 mm of exposure of the maxillary central incisors at the completion of the operation. It is usually necessary to combine this procedure with bilateral mandibular osteotomies.

Le Fort II Osteotomy

Nasomaxillary hypoplasia involves the nasomaxillary complex with or without involvement of the dentoalveolar segment. The cause may be trauma, cleft lip and palate, or Binder syndrome. Binder syndrome covers a large number of patients with nasomaxillary hypoplasia and has certain identifying features. There is foreshortening of the nose with a short columella and crescent-shaped nostrils. The upper lip is long and there is a lack of definition of the philtrum. The nasal spine and floor of the pyriform fossa cannot be palpated, and there is absence of the anterior nasal spine on roentgenograms.

Nasomaxillary hypoplasia that does not involve the dentoalveolar segment can be treated by augmentation of the anterior maxilla with alloplastic material and an associated rhinoplasty. With involvement of the dentoalveolar segment, a Le Fort II osteotomy with or without grafting is required (Fig. 52-24).

The surgical procedure (Fig. 52-25A) requires an incision in the upper buccal sulcus similar to the Le Fort I osteotomy and a coronal scalp incision. The coronal incision is used to expose the frontonasal and orbital areas. Occasionally infraorbital incisions may be needed to facilitate exposure, but paranasal incisions should be avoided. An osteotomy is made across the nasofrontal suture and continued down behind the lacrimal sac and onto the floor of the orbit, crossing the orbital rim medial to the infraorbital nerve (see Fig. 52-25B). If the hypoplasia extends more laterally, the osteotomy can cross the orbital rim lateral to the nerve (Fig. 52-25C). The osteotomy extends vertically down the maxilla; from this point, working through the buccal sulcus incision, the lateral and posterior parts of the osteotomy are completed like the Le Fort I procedure.

An osteotome is placed in the nasoglabellar area and directed backward and downward to separate the maxilla from the base of the skull (see Fig. 52-25D). The maxilla is down-fractured and mobilized with a Rowe forceps. After separation the maxilla is advanced and rotated according to the presurgical plan and secured with rigid fixation (see Fig. 52-25E). Bony gaps can be filled with hydroxyapatite. The intraoral incisions are closed in a routine manner. Staples are an excellent alternative for rapid closure of the scalp incision.

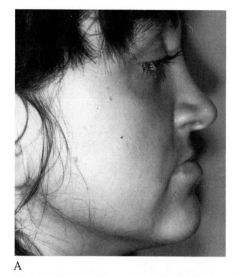
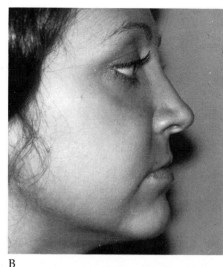

Fig. 52-24A. Preoperative profile of patient with nasomaxillary hypoplasia and class III occlusion caused by trauma. B. Facial contour after Le Fort II osteotomy and bone graft. C. Preoperative occlusion. D. Final occlusion.

A

B

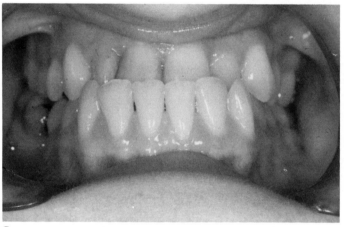
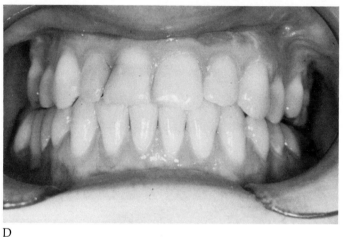

C

D

Complications

Complications in maxillary surgery include infection, hemorrhage, nonunion, delayed union, loss of bony segments, loss of tooth vitality, periodontal problems, relapse, and residual malocclusions. Infection, hemorrhage, and nonunion are extremely rare in maxillary surgery. Delayed union can occur, especially in patients with clefts, but with rigid fixation this is no longer an issue. Loss of a bony segment in the maxilla can occur with multiple segmentation but is most common in patients with bilateral clefts having a Le Fort I operation with advancement. There is usually loss of vascularity to the premaxilla. When avascular necrosis occurs, it usually causes loss of gingiva, exposure of bone, and loss of the two central incisors. Treatment includes antibiotics and debridement. Sub-

sequently the patient requires prosthodontic restoration.

Overimpaction of the maxilla is a technical problem that relates to presurgical planning. One should err on the conservative side. Relapse is most likely to occur with forward and downward movement of the maxilla. With rigid fixation this is less of a problem. Sometimes what appears as a skeletal relapse is actually a dental relapse, and it is important that the teeth are upright in the alveolar bone so that the correction can be maximized with the skeletal movement rendering the teeth stable.

Malocclusion in the immediately postoperative period is usually related to failure to position the condyles properly at the time of the fixation. When this problem is discovered, the patient needs to be returned to the operating room for repositioning of the maxilla.

Suggested Reading

Bell, W.H., Proffit, W.R., and White, R.P. *Surgical Correction of Dentofacial Deformities.* Philadelphia: Saunders, 1980. Vol. 1, pp. 234–683.

Lehman, J.A. The soft tissue manifestations of aesthetic defects of the jaws: Diagnosis and treatment. *Clin. Plast. Surg.* 14:767, 1987.

Lehman, J.A., Jr. (Ed.). Orthognathic surgery. *Clin. Plast. Surg.* 16:633, 1989.

McCarthy, J.G., et al. Surgery of the Jaws. In J.G. McCarthy (Ed.), *Plastic Surgery.* Philadelphia: Saunders, 1990. Pp. 1108–1474.

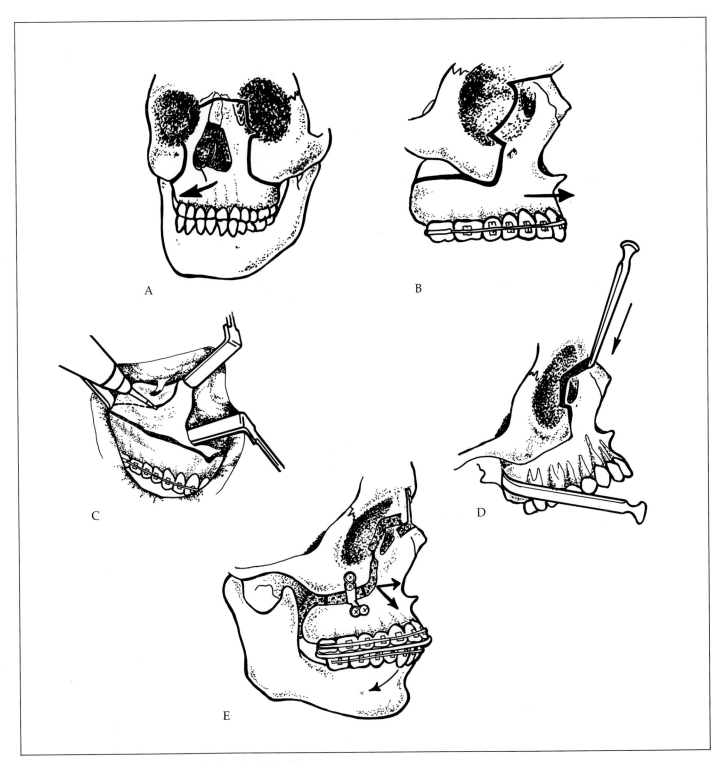

Fig. 52-25A. *Frontal view showing osteotomy lines for Le Fort II osteotomy.*
B. Profile view of osteotomy lines. C. Continuing osteotomy from orbital rim
transversely across posterior maxilla. D. Osteotome in nasoglabellar area
dividing maxilla from base of skull. E. Le Fort II segment moved forward and
downward. Hydroxyapatite inserted in gaps and rigid fixation plate applied.

53

Mandibular Deformities: Orthognathic Surgery

H. P. M. Freihofer

Orthognathic surgery started 150 years ago when von Langenbeck performed an osteoplastic horizontal section of the maxilla and Hullihen performed his often-cited osteotomy of an anterior segment in the lower jaw. In the textbook by Reichenbach and Köle published in 1970, about 40 different osteotomies of the lower jaw were presented. Many of them now are not worth more than a historical footnote. Today, a surgeon perfects only a few techniques to use on most of his or her patients. A few procedures, however, are held in reserve for exceptional problems. With every surgeon making a personal choice, it is not surprising to note an abundance of articles describing techniques and results.

This chapter presents my personal selection. Although I cannot include all possible techniques, I attempt to be complete in dealing with the basic deformities. I discuss operations commonly considered part of orthognathic mandibular surgery, but I stop short of discussing reconstructive surgery, for example, in craniofacial microsomia or condylar hyperplasia. Reconstructive measures in secondary posttraumatic operations also are not discussed. Because these deformities often lie on the border of routine orthognathic

operations, however, the link is easily seen. Finally, it does not seem appropriate to discuss the basics of the planning of these osteotomies.

Timing

Although my concepts of timing generally are not contradicted by other authors, some series and patient reports have been found that did not follow these concepts, although the results were successful. My philosophy for orthognathic operations on the mandible is presented, but the reader has to bear in mind that some arguments and situations may force the surgeon to deviate from the general rules.

The patients under discussion have developmental deformities of the lower jaw. They do not have a syndrome, and the deformity usually begins to manifest toward the end of the patient's first decade of life. The deformity increases until growth stops. That point, therefore, is the time to operate with the least likelihood of relapse or pseudorelapse caused by residual growth. A study of 100 patients showed that it is usually the additional growth of the mandible that negatively influences the results of an osteotomy in young patients.

Patients with angle class II deformities can be operated on relatively early. Certainly if the deformity is caused by the lower jaw, it has not grown sufficiently. After the osteotomy the jaw will not grow much more, and if it does, the growth is in the same direction as that of the operation. Thus further growth "prevents" a relapse of the deformity. For practical reasons, I suggest deferring the osteotomy until the second molar has erupted.

Angle class III deformities present a completely different problem. Additional growth of the mandible causes a pseudorelapse. In one study my colleagues and I found that only 13 of 31 patients younger than 18 years of age retained their results unchanged. Seventeen showed readvancement of the mandible; in one the bite opened. These results are in sharp contrast to those obtained in adults, and there is no reasonable explanation except residual growth of the mandible. On the basis of our study, we recommend operating on girls when they are at least 17 years of age and on boys after the age of 18 years.

It is evident that the rules have to be adapted the moment an asymmetry becomes apparent. In an asymmetric class

II deformity, one side grows more than the other. It is reasonable to assume that the first side grows normally; therefore, the 17- or 18-year rule should be applied if one does not want to incur an increased risk of relapse of the asymmetry. In prognathic asymmetries, it is wise to wait even longer. One side grows normally, but the other side grows more. Often growth stops only at the age of 19 to 21 years.

In summary, if one opts for one corrective operation only, the timing depends on the type of deformity. If one operates too early there is considerable probability that some sort of relapse will need to be corrected later. There are completely different rules of timing when planning treatment of a syndrome. These are not discussed in this chapter.

Of course, cooperation with an orthodontist is necessary. A number of patients are better treated orthodontically only, but some patients need only a surgeon. For patients who need to be treated by both, the question arises as to who treats first. I prefer that the surgeon begin treatment and that the orthodontist continue it. In some instances the orthodontist can correct a partial relapse of the deformity after surgical treatment. However, there are also reasons to opt for the other sequence. Class II deformities can be treated early and successfully by orthodontists. The orthodontist can always start his or her part of the treatment earlier, thus winning time for the patient. Finally, sometimes the form of the arches is so incongruent that a reasonable operation cannot be done without preoperative preparation. Each patient has to be considered individually. It is my suspicion that too many patients are treated by a team, thereby increasing the duration and costs of treatment when a simple solution also would have brought satisfactory results.

Chin Correction

Reshaping of the chin prominence is an extremely important part of orthognathic surgery of the lower jaw. It often serves to enhance the results of "functional" mandibular surgery but sometimes has to replace it.

Indications

Four types of chin correction can be distinguished. *Simple genioplasty* corrects the deformity in its totality, such as retrogenia in a patient with an occlusion clearly in Angle class I and no vertical problem with the upper jaw. *Complementary genioplasty* improves on the results obtained by osteotomy of the jaw. The chin moves in the same direction as the jaw, as in the correction of an Angle class II deformity, by advancement of the jaw and additional chin advancement.

In a *genioplasty as a compromise*, instead of correcting the deformity where it should be done, for example rotating the mandible because of asymmetry, only a chin translation is done to disguise the deformity. In a *harmonizing genioplasty* chin movement is opposite to movement of the mandible. For example, a class III deformity is corrected by shortening of the mandible, but the chin recedes too much, whereas a good occlusion is obtained. Therefore, a simultaneous lengthening of the chin must be done (Fig. 53-1).

Techniques and Results

Advancement Genioplasty

Two types of advancement genioplasty can be distinguished, the sliding osteotomy first described by Obwegeser in 1957 and 1958 and the jumping osteotomy described by Converse and Shapiro in 1952. Either may be used depending on the amount of movement required. For both it is essential that the chin segment remain vascularized by keeping it pedicled on the posterior muscle attachments. Both are best done through a marginal incision, which has less morbidity than a vestibular one. The sliding osteotomy can be stabilized by wire; for fixation of the jumping osteotomy, miniplates are preferred. The results are quite similar for both techniques, the ratio of soft tissue to hard tissue movement being 3:5 to 3:4. More important, chin advancements could be achieved by the double-step technique. Although acceptable results have been reported, I do not use the double-step technique because it is more difficult to stabilize; often considerable bone resorption is seen, and the form of the chin prominence often is not pleasant in the frontal view if no other measures such as additional grafting are taken. Chin augmentation with alloplastic materials is not performed in my department.

Reduction Genioplasty

There are two techniques of reduction genioplasty—the slice or wedge osteotomy (Fig. 53-2) and the sliding back osteotomy. The sliding osteotomy gives better results. The sliding osteotomy reduces the chin in an anteroposterior direction but simultaneously augments it vertically (Fig. 53-3). The ratio of soft tissue to hard tissue contour change is far less than in advancement. The method is less predictable, and the result is only to be obtained if the soft tissues remain attached to the lower border of the chin. Grinding of the lower border is not done because it produces squat chins almost with certainty and because it has little effect, probably because of the necessity of detaching the soft tissues from the chin point during the operation.

Asymmetric Corrections

Transpositions can be obtained in the sliding manner. Here again the attachment of the soft tissues (not only the posterior muscles) to the chin point is important. If the soft tissues are detached, considerable overcorrection is needed to obtain the effect desired. For correction of vertical asymmetries, either wedge excisions or the propeller genioplasty described by Sailer in 1983 can be used (Fig. 53-4). No numerical data on hard-to-soft-tissue ratios can be found for any of these corrections. Again, grinding is used only for minor corrections because its effect is not predictable.

Anterior Segmental Osteotomy

Segmental osteotomies can be useful for the correction of occlusal discrepancies, because this operation may be considered minor.

Indications

Four different types of osteotomies can be distinguished according to the direction of movement of the segment. Receding of the segment with or without extraction of bicuspids is used for the correction of an anterior angle class III relation, in which the labiomental fold is practically filled and the chin prominence is well positioned vertically and horizontally (Figs. 53-1 and 53-5). Lowering of the segment

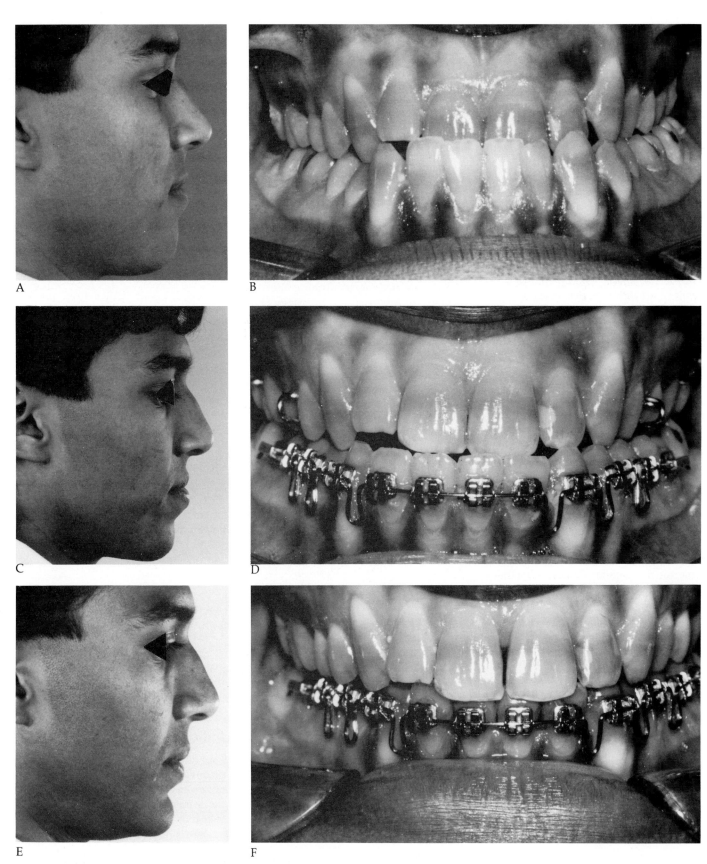

Fig. 53-1. Preorthodontic (A, B), preoperative (C, D), and postoperative (E, F) views of patient with dentoalveolar prognathism without prognathism of base. Mandibular retropositioning by sagittal splitting and simultaneous chin advancement resulted in a good profile. The same result could have been achieved by retropositioning of the lower anterior segment far more easily.

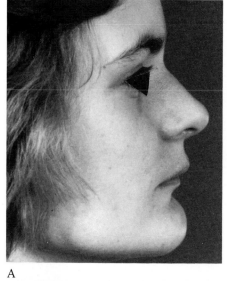

A

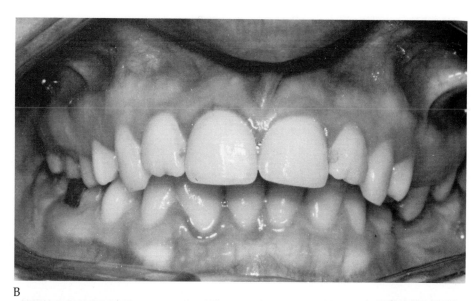

B

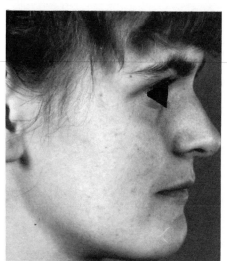

C

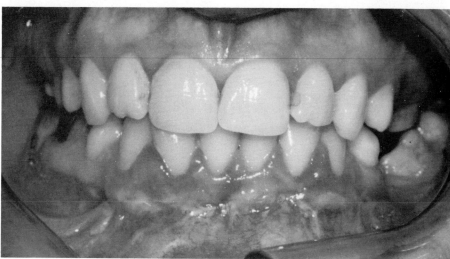

D

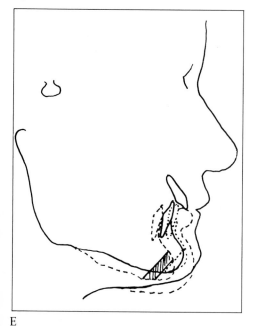

E

Fig. 53-2. Preoperative (A, B) and postoperative (C, D) views of patient with dentoalveolar retrognathia without retrognathia of base of jaw. E. Lengthening of the mandible with simultaneous reduction of the chin results in a good occlusion but a somewhat unnatural profile line. An advancement of the lower anterior segment alone would have been the better solution aesthetically.

is used for the correction of a deep overbite, often in combination with total mandibular movement or an anterior maxillary osteotomy. Advancement of the segment is indicated for a retruded lower lip with good vertical and horizontal positioning of the chin (see Fig. 53-2). Raising of the segment is, of course, indicated for closure of an anterior open bite and is almost always combined with an osteotomy of the chin prominence for filling the defect (Fig. 53-6).

Techniques and Results

The following principles apply to all anterior segmental osteotomies. The oper-

ation is rather minor, and patients recover quickly. Stabilization and fixation are achieved by an arch bar and direct wire osteosynthesis without intermaxillary fixation or plating. The results on average are satisfactory. Usually the bony segments stabilize well, whereas the dental axes tend to move slightly in the postoperative period. If the planning was correct, the overall results are rewarding, and surprising aesthetic effects may be obtained. The specific risks are damage to the mental nerve, depending mainly on the position of the vertical bone cut (the farther back the cut the riskier is the operation) and damage to or devitalization

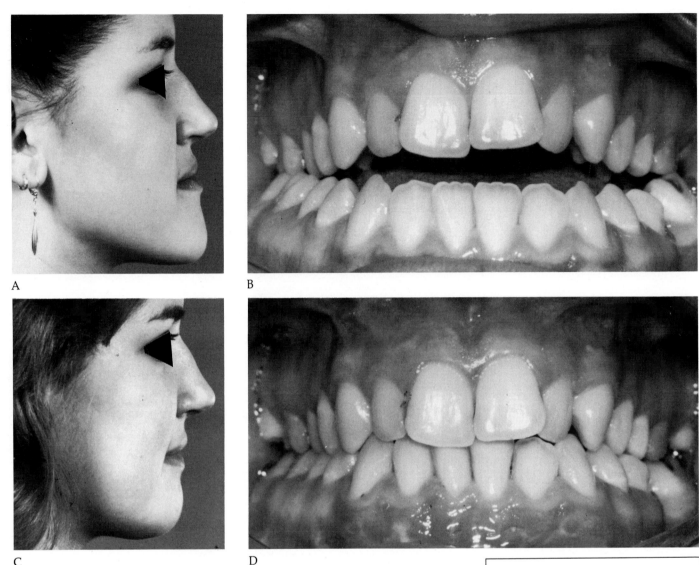

A   B

C   D

Fig. 53-3. Preoperative (A, B) and postoperative (C, D) views of patient with prognathic open bite corrected by sagittal split osteotomy, sliding chin reduction, and paranasal onlays. Although the occlusion is stable, the chin looks a little squat, as often happens with chin reductions (E).

of the teeth, especially those adjacent to the vertical bone cuts.

Receding and Lowering of the Segment

For these two directions of movement, no additional comment seems necessary. It may be appropriate to add, however, that the lower anterior segment, in whichever direction it may be moved, can be segmented additionally in the midline, as measured by Heiss in 1963, if this would improve occlusion. The relapse rate is 0 to 10 percent (Fig. 53-7).

Advancement of the Segment

The main drawback of advancement is the production of a bony defect in the alveolar process. This can be left as it is or filled with either autologous or banked bone. With all techniques, there is the risk of a defect in the alveolar process with or without pockets along the roots of adjacent teeth. This implies a risk for backward rotation of the advanced segment. I have proposed a modification that can be applied when an extraction gap is present. The alveolar process can be split sagittally; thus the segment is advanced maintaining bone contact at the site of the vertical osteotomy, grafting becomes optional, stabilization is improved, and the chance of relapse is reduced considerably (Fig. 53-8).

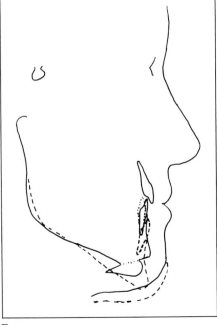

E

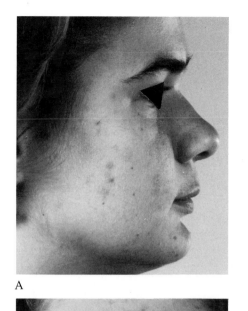

A

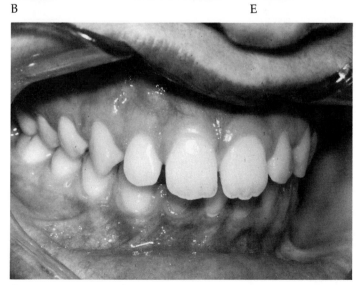

B

C

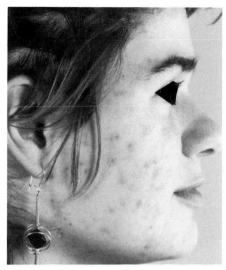

D

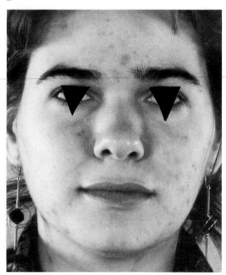

E

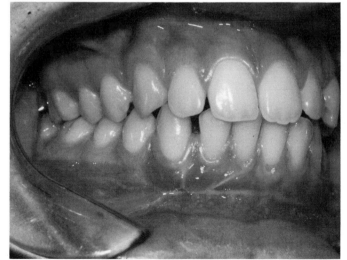

F

Fig. 53-4. Preoperative (A, B, C) and postoperative (D, E, F) views of patient with left condylar hypertrophy. Treatment was simultaneous right sagittal split, left condylectomy, and condylar reconstruction with costochondral graft and propeller genioplasty. Surprisingly symmetric result.

Raising of the Segment

The principle of raising the segment is to use the detached chin prominence for grafting of the defect developing between the mandibular base and the raised segment. This requires considerable height of the mandible. Köle reported no relapses, but Aarnes reported a 20 percent relapse rate with this technique. Even the less favorable report represents quite a success for the closure of an open bite, as discussed later in this chapter. Although the occlusal results are satisfactory, the aesthetic effect may be a problem. Improvements may be obtained easily, because preoperatively the appearance usually is not satisfactory at all. To obtain a good profile line can be difficult. The chin segment harvested may be just large enough to bridge the defect, but not thick and broad enough to provide satisfactory projection of the chin prominence. Furthermore, resorption is increased because this chin segment cannot remain pedicled on muscle unless the continuity of the base of the mandible is (temporarily) broken, a solution that does not seem worthwhile to me.

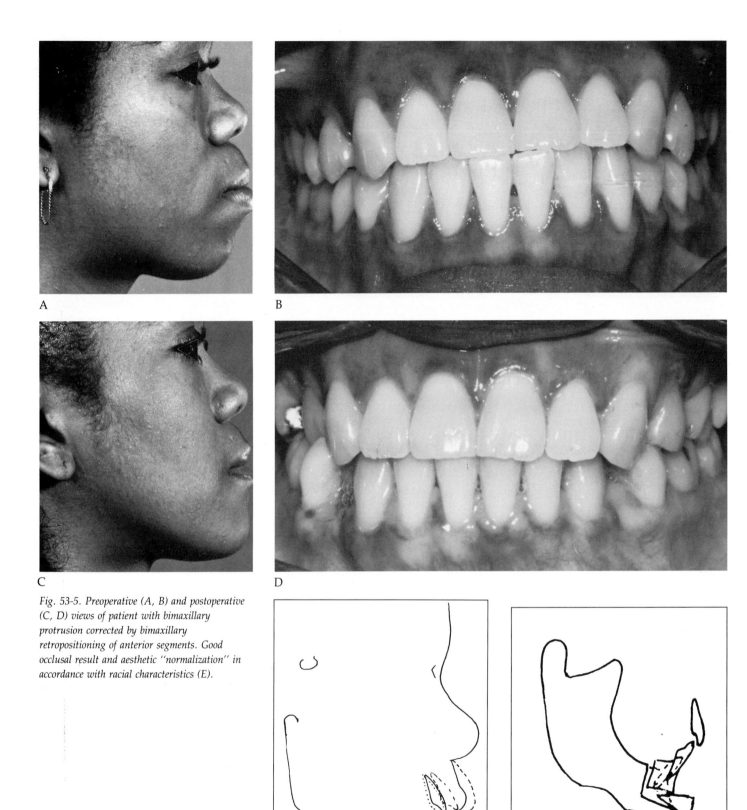

A

B

C

D

Fig. 53-5. Preoperative (A, B) and postoperative (C, D) views of patient with bimaxillary protrusion corrected by bimaxillary retropositioning of anterior segments. Good occlusal result and aesthetic "normalization" in accordance with racial characteristics (E).

E

Fig. 53-6. Closure of open bite by anterior segmental osteotomy with grafting of chin prominence according to Köle.

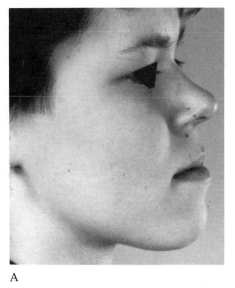

A

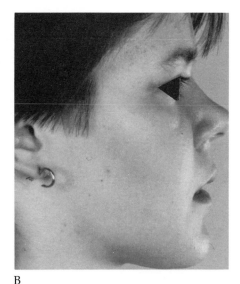

B

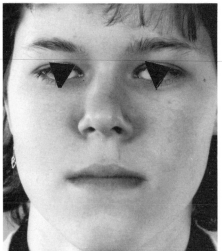

C

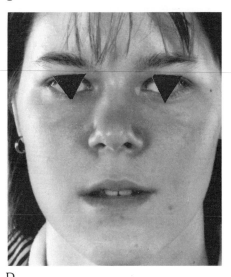

D

Fig. 53-7. Preoperative (A, B) and postoperative (C, D) views of patient with dentoalveolar prognathism without prognathic base of lower jaw. Good correction with retropositioning of lower alveolar segment and paranasal onlays.

Mandibular Body and Ramus Osteotomy

I strongly favor one type of osteotomy for all total mandibular movements—Obwegeser's sagittal splitting of the rami. As mentioned before, another type of osteotomy can be used in exceptional situations.

Indications

The previous statement leads to the conclusion that the indication for sagittal splitting is apparent in practically all patients in whom movement of the whole mandible is necessary, be it advancement, shortening, or rotation to close an open bite with or without additional horizontal movement. If additional widening or narrowing is needed, I use a median osteotomy conforming to the principle of Trauner's operation. It may be desirable to close an open bite by rotating only the anterior part of the mandible. To do this a modification of the sagittal body osteotomy described by Mehnert can be used.

Techniques and Results

Lengthening of the Mandible

The technique has been described countless times and it is certainly one of the best known osteotomies of the face (Fig. 53-9). There is therefore no need to go into detail. In addition, many modifications have been described, the most popular doubtlessly being Dal Pont's and Hunsuck's and their variations.

I have tried most of the variations but adhere basically to Obwegeser's design and technique. The one modification I use quite routinely is the grinding of the cortex of the anterior oblique line as proposed by Spiessl. Dal Pont's modification is applied only in patients with an ad-

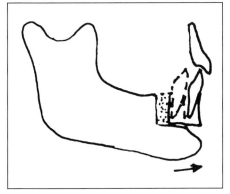

Fig. 53-8. Sagittal sliding of alveolar process for advancement of anterior segment without bone grafting. This is possible only in selected patients. In all others, the Pichler basal technique has to be used.

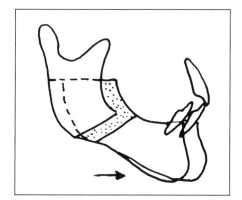

Fig. 53-9. Lengthening of mandible by sagittal splitting of rami according to Obwegeser. Risk of (partial) relapse is moderate.

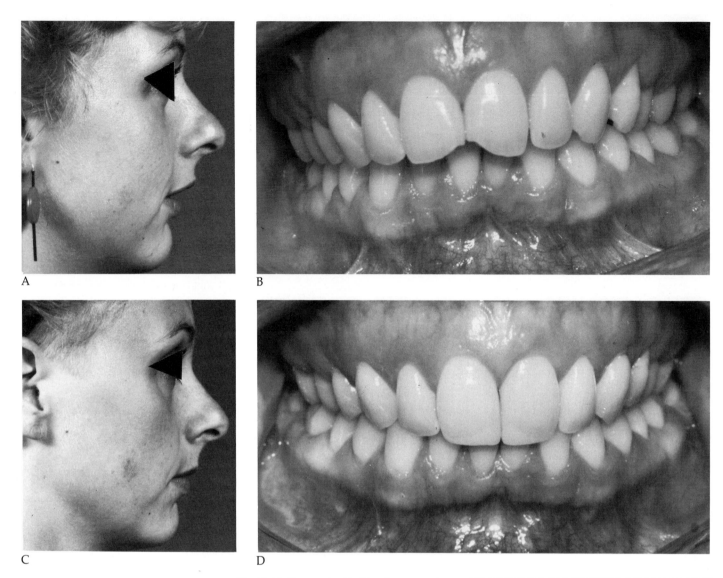

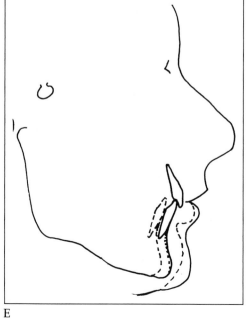

Fig. 53-10. Preoperative (A, B) and postoperative (C, D) views of patient with mandibular retrusion corrected with advancement of the lower jaw. Occlusion is perfect, but the profile is still markedly retrognathic. A combination of a segmental osteotomy repositioning the anterior segment with a lengthening of the lower jaw by twice that amount or additional genioplasty had been indicated (E).

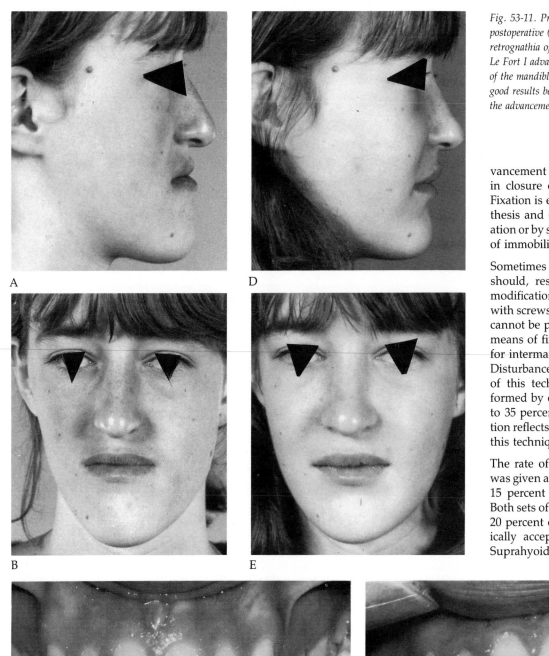

A

D

B

E

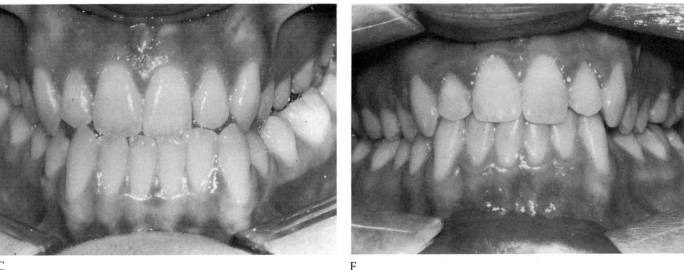

C

F

Fig. 53-11. Preoperative (A, B, C) and postoperative (D, E, F) views of patient with retrognathia of the maxilla. She should have had a Le Fort I advancement osteotomy. The shortening of the mandible by a sagittal split osteotomy gave good results because paranasal onlays simulated the advancement of the maxilla.

vancement of two bicuspids or more and in closure of severe class II open bites. Fixation is either by direct wire osteosynthesis and 6 weeks of intermaxillary fixation or by screws or plates with one week of immobilization.

Sometimes splitting does not occur as it should, resulting in a sort of Hunsuck modification. In these instances fixation with screws may be excluded. It therefore cannot be predicted with certainty which means of fixation is best unless one opts for intermaxillary fixation in all patients. Disturbances of sensibility are a problem of this technique even when it is performed by experienced surgeons. The 10 to 35 percent incidence of this complication reflects the wide range of results with this technique.

The rate of clinically significant relapses was given as 12 percent by MacIntosh and 15 percent by Freihofer and Petresevic. Both sets of authors reported that another 20 percent of patients had minimal, clinically acceptable relapses (Figs. 53-10). Suprahyoid myotomy has been sug-

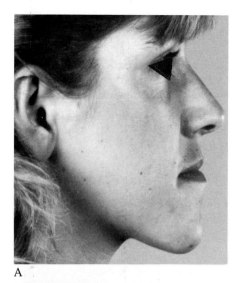

A

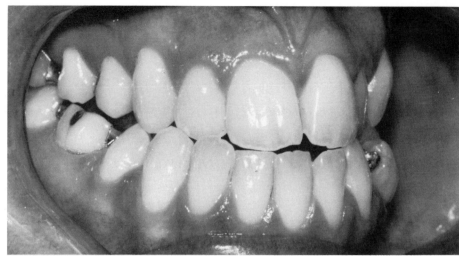

B

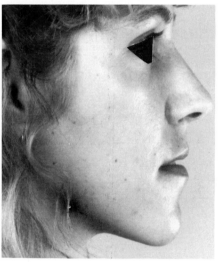

C

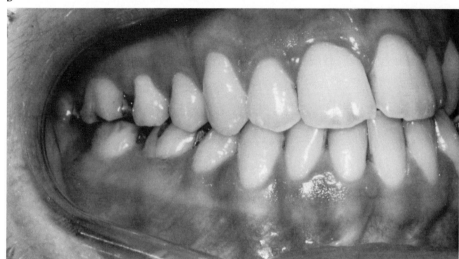

D

Fig. 53-12. Preoperative (A, B) and postoperative (C, D) views of patient with prognathism corrected by retropositioning of the mandible with a sagittal split procedure. The occlusion is good but the profile line is not, because the anterior teeth were not positioned with the correct inclination on the mandibular base. Had this condition been decompensated by orthodontic treatment before surgical intervention, the result would have been much more rewarding.

gested to reduce the relapse rate, but neither Freihofer and Petreśević nor MacIntosh found evidence that it works. Mommaerts and Hadjianghelou reported a 45 percent rate of skeletal relapse. They postulated that fixation with wire is considerably inferior to fixation with screws, a statement contradicted by Watzke and Turvey.

Retropositioning of the Mandible

Basically everything said concerning the technique of lengthening of the mandible and the results obtained applies to retropositioning (Figs. 53-11 and 53-12). The relapse rate is different, however. Pepersack and Chausse in 1978 reported a relapse rate of 27 percent, 9 percent of which represented extremely poor occlu-

sions. MacIntosh in 1981 reported a 31 percent relapse rate and an 11 percent rate of extremely poor occlusions. There are more reports, of course, but comparison is often difficult because the age of the patients is not specified. Age, however, plays an important role in relapse. The question of whether or not skeletal suspension decreases the risk of relapse is not answered definitively, but there are indications that it does. Segments are fixed by either perimandibular wires, plates or screws. If direct wire osteo-

syntheses are used, there is no need to place them on the inferior border.

Rotation of the Mandible

In rotations of the mandible for horizontal asymmetry, no special technical aspects are emphasized. Numerical results of series cannot be found in the literature. Clinical experience demonstrates that splitting is usually not difficult, but fixation with screws often has been discouraged because the segments have no contact planes—only a point of contact. In

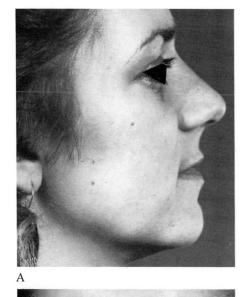

A

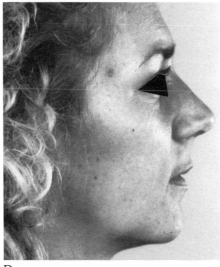

D

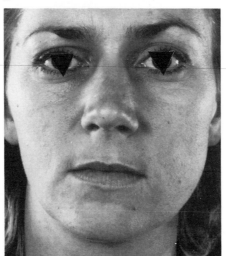

B

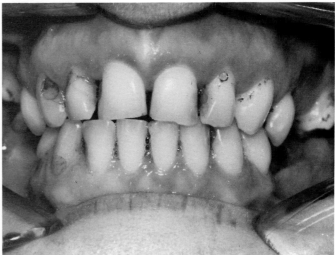

E

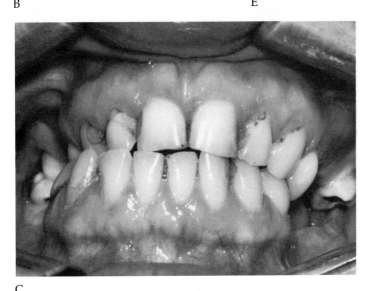

C

F

Fig. 53-13. Preoperative (A, B, C) and postoperative (D, E, F) views of patient with prognathic asymmetry corrected by sagittal splitting. Good alignment of midline but residual asymmetry of chin prominence and cheeks.

these patients we prefer wire fixation because there seems to be less tendency to displace the condyle.

The final result is difficult to predict. Although placement of the mandibular midline in the facial midline should not be too much of a problem, it remains questionable whether the lateral parts of the cheek become symmetric as well. This is often not the case either because of a slightly different form on the two sides of the mandibular body and angle or because of different thicknesses of the soft tissue cover. One should not guarantee a symmetric outcome in one operation (Fig. 53-13).

Use of rotations of the mandible to close a vertical open bite is questionable. Greebe showed that counterclockwise rotation of the mandible has an adverse effect on the stability of the result. This kind of movement is most often needed for correction of a class II open bite. It is therefore not surprising that the few results published are not good. Manz and Hadjianghelou reported a 90 percent relapse rate for class II open bite, 75 percent for class I, and 65 percent for class III. MacIntosh had similar results (Figs. 53-14, 53-15, and 53-16).

Enlargement or Narrowing of the Mandibular Dental Arch

A vertical osteotomy or ostectomy is performed in the midline of the mandible. It is not carried through to the lower border, however, but stops short of it. The chin prominence is cut off horizontally or in a V shape. The tooth-bearing part is moved according to plan and splinted, and the chin prominence is reattached to act as a bridge over the osteotomy. By this procedure, which is basically Trauner's description with an intraoral approach, additional stabilization at the lower border can be obtained. Although there are no published numerical results for this procedure, the impression is that the results are quite acceptable. Less satisfactory outcomes are probably caused by insufficient stabilization and fixation.

Movement of the Anterior Part of the Mandible

In exceptional instances a body osteotomy of the mandible is indicated. I prefer a modification of Mehnert's and Delaire's sagittal osteotomy of the mandibular body. Interdentally the osteotomy is strictly transversely vertical; below the apices of the teeth it becomes sagittal. In contrast to older procedures, however, the cut passes from anterior lateral to posterior medial, and an attempt is made to have the anterior bone cut just in front of the mental foramen. In this way the risk of injury to the mental nerve is reduced. Fixation is obtained by an arch bar on the teeth and a miniplate on the lower border of the mandible. Bone grafting is usually not necessary because of the sagittal bone cut. In appropriate instances even self-retention can be obtained by tilting the posterior segments slightly inward apically. My impression, based on a few operations, is that this procedure is more stable in corrections of an anterior open bite than of sagittal splitting of the ramus and additionally has the desired effect of changing the curve of Spee (Fig. 53-17).

Combinations

Often a simple osteotomy of the mandible cannot manage all problems. Combinations of different osteotomies are then

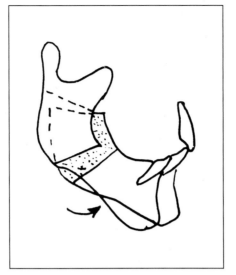

Fig. 53-14. Lengthening of mandible and closure of open bite by Obwegeser osteotomy with counterclockwise rotation. The probability of relapse is considerable.

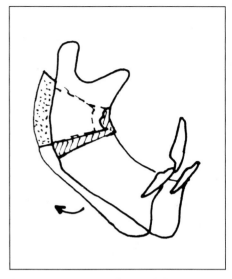

Fig. 53-15. Shortening of mandible by Obwegeser osteotomy with simultaneous clockwise rotation. Probability of relapse is small.

considered. Most often the movement of the whole mandible is combined with a chin osteotomy, mobilization of the lower anterior segment, or repositioning of the maxilla.

Combination of Sagittal Split Osteotomy and Chin Repositioning

This combination presents no specific technical difficulties. In class III profiles it is rarely necessary. The preoperative impression of an excessively high mandible or the absence of a sufficient labiomental fold is often caused by the forced position of the lips when the patient tries to close the mouth. The moment the lips are relaxed, a good profile line of the mandible is seen in most patients. This line simply has to be relocated by sagittal splitting of the mandible without additional measures (see Fig. 53-11). On the other hand, advancement of the chin often must be associated with lengthening of the mandible (see Fig. 53-10). The necessity of that procedure can be evaluated preoperatively by asking the patient to protrude the mandible.

Three aspects have to be considered. In some areas people with a tendency toward class II profiles predominate, in others there is a tendency to class III profiles. This predominance influences the decision of whether or not to perform a chin

advancement. One of the advantages of advancing the chin is that even if there is considerable relapse of the lengthening of the mandible, the patient remains aesthetically improved. When doing a chin advancement, one has to take care not to shorten the anterior mandible too much. Not only will the proportions be less good than hoped for but also too sharp a labiomental fold might develop, which might cause the chin to look too pointed even though in analysis the position of the chin would be correct in the anteroposterior dimension.

Most difficult is the combination of rotation of the mandible and of the chin prominence in instances of asymmetry (see Fig. 53-4). To predict where the chin prominence will be after rotation of the mandible is quite difficult. But evaluation of the position of the chin during the operation also is unreliable, even if all drapes are removed temporarily. The evaluation sometimes proves to be wrong postoperatively. This is an additional reason that one should not promise correction of asymmetry in one operation.

Combination of Sagittal Split Osteotomy with Mobilization of the Lower Anterior Segment

This combination is sometimes indicated in marked distoclusion with a deep bite.

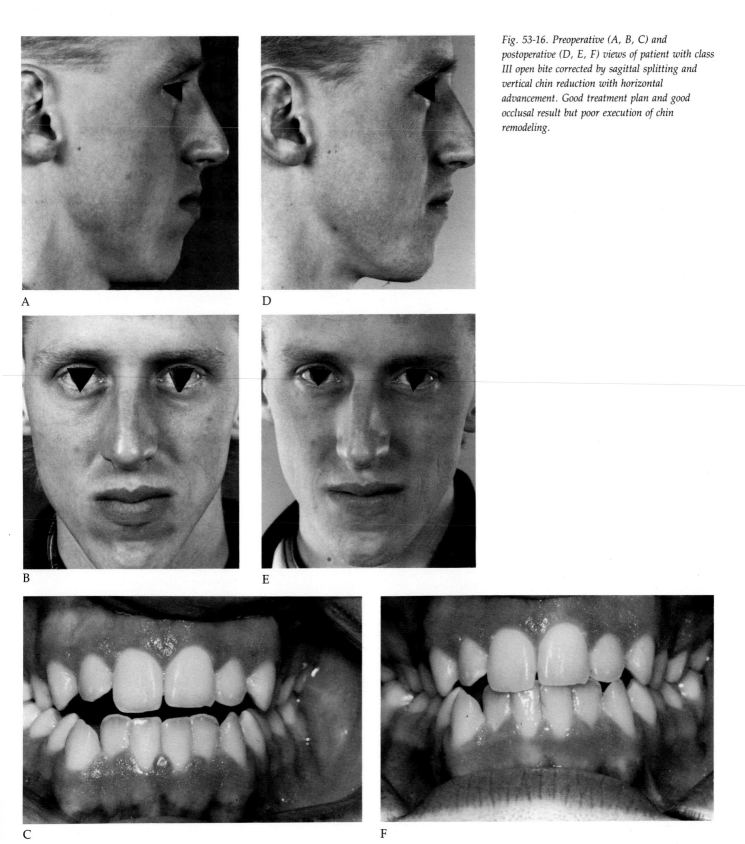

Fig. 53-16. Preoperative (A, B, C) and postoperative (D, E, F) views of patient with class III open bite corrected by sagittal splitting and vertical chin reduction with horizontal advancement. Good treatment plan and good occlusal result but poor execution of chin remodeling.

A

D

B

E

C

F

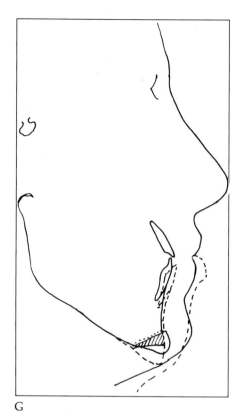

G

Fig. 53-16. (Continued) It should have been advanced much more with a Converse-type genioplasty (G).

Most of the problems have already been described. There is, however, an additional problem—fixation. Depending on the size of the anterior segment, there may be only a few molars for intermaxillary fixation, making the fixation quite unreliable. There are two remedies: The anterior segment is fixed so solidly to the base of the mandible that this segment also can be used for intermaxillary fixation, or the osteotomy at the angle is osteosynthesized with bicortical screws or monocortical plates, making intermaxillary fixation superfluous.

Combination of Sagittal Split Osteotomy with Osteotomy of the Upper Jaw

Many combinations of osteotomies of the upper and lower jaw are used. Advancement of the upper jaw with retropositioning of the lower jaw and raising of the upper jaw with advancement of the mandible are the combinations used most fre-

quently. The diagnoses are prognathism with retromaxillism and class II long face (Fig. 53-18). Special conditions that need this kind of surgery, such as hemifacial microsomia or cleft lip, alveolus, and palate, are not discussed here.

I prefer to mobilize the maxilla first and position it definitively with the aid of an intermediate wafer. The sequelae are the problems of movement of the two jaws separately. As a rule the maxilla remains in the chosen position, and the mandible has a tendency to relapse. Former class III deformities show better results than class II deformities.

Discussion

Several points mentioned are open to discussion. Planning consists of four components: The patient's wishes are important of course, but they are not followed absolutely. I prefer to discuss the various outcomes, trying to persuade the patient by good arguments. The importance of timing for any osteotomy in young patients has already been discussed. The model operation is proof that the plan is feasible and provides the amounts of movement required with considerable accuracy. The prediction tracing has a special place in preoperative planning. Although I like to have it to confirm that my treatment plan is reasonable, the tracing is by no means reliable. I therefore use only the simplest sketch to provide a general idea of what the result could be. I show this sketch to the patient.

Possible complications and the probability of an outcome other than expected also must be discussed. The percentages of relapse are considerable for some of these procedures. It is not a surprise, therefore, that I try to avoid total mandibular movements as much as possible, applying acceptable alternatives. These alternatives exist for all conditions except asymmetry of the mandible. Often this condition has to be corrected by rotation of the mandible. Retropositioning of the mandible is replaced by a Le Fort I advancement osteotomy of the upper jaw. I am not concerned with the different angulations measured on the cephalometric roentgenogram. The decision is made on the basis of aesthetic concerns. It is well demonstrated that the Le Fort I osteotomy is a reliable procedure.

To replace advancement of the mandible, I reposition the maxilla superiorly. This is also a reliable procedure. The mandible follows with a counterclockwise autorotation. This procedure "lengthens" the mandible horizontally. Discrepancies of up to about the width of a premolar can be corrected in this way, if need be in combination with a chin advancement. In severe distocclusions, such as bird faces, total mandibular advancement cannot be avoided; only the amount of movement necessary can be influenced.

Segmental osteotomies of the lower jaw are quite reliable. They also may be considered minor operations in the context of orthognathic surgery. However, they are adequate in only a small number of patients. Combining segmental osteotomies with genioplasty increases the number of indications, but the height of the anterior mandible must be considerable as long as one does not want to apply intermaxillary fixation, which is basically unnecessary.

Remodeling procedures on the mandible are done only exceptionally. Resection of the lower border may be considered; the drawbacks are discussed in the section on chin osteotomies. Augmentations with onlays of autologous bone must be discouraged. The percentage of resorption is high. Augmentation by sandwiching is usually applicable in the area of the chin only, as long as one does not accept an increased risk of damaging the mandibular nerve. Onlays with autologous or lyophilized cartilage may be quite successful. Alloplastic materials are not used in my department.

Fig. 53-17. Modification of body osteotomy for closure of anterior open bite without bone grafting.

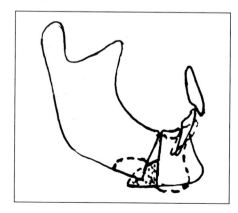

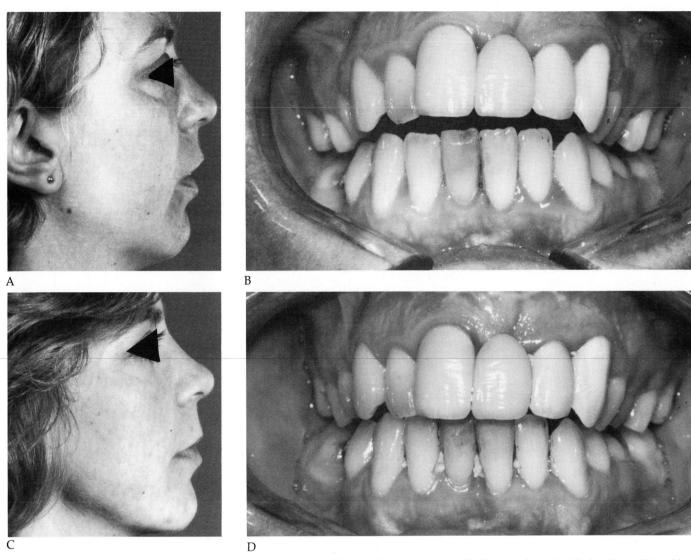

Fig. 53-18. Preoperative (A, B) and postoperative (C, D) views of patient with class II open bite and long face. Good aesthetic result after cranial displacement of upper jaw and lengthening of lower jaw. A counterclockwise rotation was avoided by the maxillary repositioning; vertical occlusal relapse therefore was minimal (E).

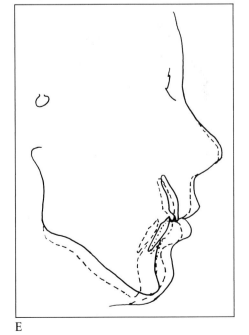

Conclusions

Most mandibular deformities can be treated by a small number of techniques and combinations thereof. In young patients timing plays an important role in that too early an operation can result in a pseudorelapse caused by growth of the mandible. Chin advancements and seg-

mental osteotomies show reliable results. Because all total mandibular movements are unreliable to some extent, it is advisable first to explore alternatives. The most difficult operations to plan and perform are for mandibular asymmetries, because the results are not always predictable. Secondary corrections are the rule rather than the exception in these patients.

Suggested Reading

Bell, W.H., and Dann, J.J. Correction of dentofacial deformities by surgery of the anterior part of the jaws. *Am. J. Orthod.* 64:162, 1973.

Freihofer, H.P.M. The timing of facial osteotomies in children and adolescents. *Clin. Plast. Surg.* 8:445, 1982.

Freihofer, H.P.M. Latitude and limitation of midface movements. *Br. J. Oral Maxillofac. Surg.* 22:393, 1984.

Freihofer, H.P.M. Soft Tissue Contours after Osteotomies. In D.K. Ousterhout (Ed.), *Aesthetic Contouring of the Cranio-Facial Skeleton.* Boston: Little, Brown, 1991.

Köle, H. Surgical operations on the alveolar ridge to correct occlusal abnormalities. *Oral Surg.* 12:277, 1959.

MacIntosh, R.B. Experience with the sagittal osteotomy of the mandibular ramus. *J. Max.-Fac. Surg.* 9:151, 1981.

Obwegeser, H.L. The surgical correction of mandibular prognathism and retrogenia with consideration of genioplasty. *Oral Surg.* 10:677, 1957.

Obwegeser, H.L., and Hadjianghelou, O. Two ways to correct bird-face deformity. *Oral Surg.* 64:507, 1987.

Pepersack, W.J. Tooth vitality after alveolar segmental osteotomy. *J. Max.-Fac. Surg.* 1:85, 1973.

54

Prosthetic Management for Patients with Cleft Lip and Palate

David J. Reisberg

The use of prostheses has a long history and a prominent role in cleft lip and palate habilitation. Descriptions of obturators to cover palatal defects can be traced to Lusitanus and Paré in the sixteenth century, and Fabricius of Aquapendente described a presurgical orthopedic device for cleft lip repair in 1619. Indeed, the original name of the American Cleft Palate Association was the American Academy of Cleft Palate Prosthesis.

The prosthodontist is an active member of the cleft team, providing care from a patient's infancy to young adulthood. This care is directed toward the preservation of valuable hard and soft tissue structures, enhancement of surgical results, and achievement of normal speech and appearance. Today, prosthetic treatment is tempered by the timely application of sophisticated surgical and orthodontic procedures. It is no longer relegated to the role of a salvage procedure for multiple surgical failures, as in years gone by, but is applied as a standard of care to achieve predictable results in close cooperation with other medical and dental specialists. Although the prosthodontist's role may have decreased in degree, it certainly has not diminished in importance.

My prosthodontic protocol has evolved during 15 years of experience and has been influenced by such authorities as Sam Pruzansky and Henry Gold. The craniofacial team at my center has learned from growth and development research performed at our own and other institutions and has developed a treatment sequence that meets our patients' needs and is sensitive to the ordeal with which they and their families are faced.

Some centers advocate the routine placement of an acrylic resin palatal plate within hours after the birth of a child with a cleft palate. Such a prosthesis obturates the palatal cleft to assist feeding. I have found such an appliance to be unnecessary. Most infants with palatal clefts can swallow without serious problems. The only requirements are detailed instructions from an experienced nursing staff and the instilling of confidence in the parents.

Other authors have described the use of similarly designed palatal prostheses for the purpose of aligning and stabilizing palatal segments before surgical repair of complete clefts of the lip and palate or even primary bone grafting at the alveolar cleft site after lip repair. However, there are no convincing long-term results demonstrating that these early procedures do much to enhance the status of a patient with a cleft.

Premaxillary Positioning Appliance

One of the most confounding problems encountered in cleft care is the management of the protrusive premaxilla in a patient with bilateral cleft lip (Fig. 54-1). Successful lip repair in such patients is a challenge to even the most talented surgeons.

Several approaches have been described to position the premaxillary segment in a more favorable relation for lip repair. Among these have been extraoral traction, oral pinning and traction, premaxillary surgical setback, and premaxillary excision. At our center, my associates and I have encountered several technical and philosophical problems with these procedures.

The "bonnet technique" for extraoral traction is cumbersome and uncomfortable for the infant, especially during the

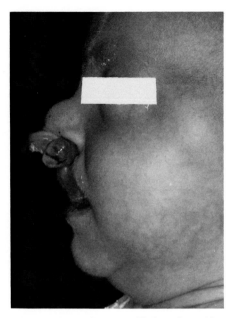

Fig. 54-1. *Protrusive premaxilla in patient with bilateral cleft lip and palate.*

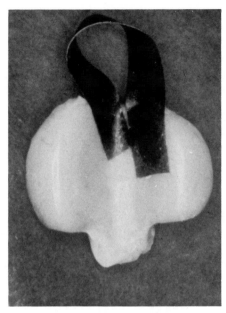

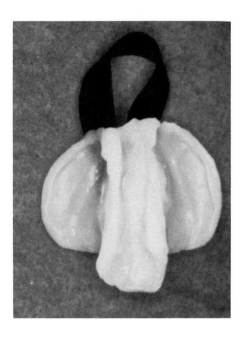

Fig. 54-2. *Premaxillary Positioning Appliance.*

hot summer months. In addition, parents complain of its conspicuousness and the tendency for the traction band to shift from its ideal position, across the premaxilla and prolabium, with normal head movement of the infant. In patients whose premaxilla has deviated laterally, it was also difficult to move the premaxillary segment toward the midline.

Oral pinning and traction are not favored because of the possible interference with maxillary growth and the development of tooth buds. Furthermore, the long-term effects of this procedure on facial growth have not been documented. Although guidelines for the application of premaxillary setback have been suggested, interference with midfacial growth remains a concern. Excision of the premaxilla has been performed in selected cases. It is a drastic procedure that should be avoided because it produces serious problems in dentition, dental arch development, facial aesthetics, closure of oronasal fistulae, and definitive dental habilitation.

I use a conservative prosthetic approach toward positioning the premaxillary segment. Treatment is initiated only at the request of the plastic surgeon when a more favorable position of the premaxilla is necessary before lip repair. Treatment usually begins within the first weeks after birth.

The purpose of the Premaxillary Positioning Appliance is to move the premaxilla downward and backward to a more favorable position so the cleft lip may be surgically repaired with less tension along the suture lines and thus better cosmetic results. It is not an attempt to align the maxillary dental arch in an ideal relationship; little evidence exists to show long-term benefit to the patient from such an early procedure. My preliminary cephalometric evaluations confirm that the appliance achieves its intended purpose without adverse effects on facial growth.

An acrylic resin palatal plate provides anchorage for the prosthetic appliance. The tissue side of the plate is fitted with a resilient denture-lining material that engages the anatomic undercuts of the palatal cleft for retention. Additional retention is achieved by the use of denture adhesive. A latex rubber strip the same width as the prolabium is attached to the polished surface of the palatal plate with cyanoacrylate and looped over the prolabium to provide 5 g of traction (Figs. 54-2 and 54-3). The position of the strip may be adjusted to draw the premaxillary segment straight back and down or toward one side. An expansion screw may be incorporated into the plate if the palatal segments must be moved laterally to allow retraction of the premaxilla.

The patient is seen every week for adjustment or replacement of the traction strip to ensure an adequate, low-grade force in a downward and backward direction. The anterior portion of the plate may need to be relieved to accommodate the premaxilla as it moves back.

We have recently begun substituting an orthodontic elastomeric chain with a section of resilient denture lining material over the prolabium for the latex rubber strip and attaching it to orthodontic buttons instead of using cyanoacrylate. This modification increases adjustability of the appliance and reduces the frequency of follow-up visits for the patient.

The prosthesis is worn continuously and is removed only for cleaning. A surgical evaluation is made every month. Repair of the lip is performed when the surgeon believes that the premaxillary segment has been positioned adequately, usually after 3 to 4 months of treatment. It is not necessary to remake the palatal plate because of growth during this period.

This intraoral prosthetic approach has several advantages. It is a noninvasive technique and allows the parents to participate actively in the treatment of their child. This involvement helps to abate the parents' anxieties about the delay of the lip repair. They understand the reason for

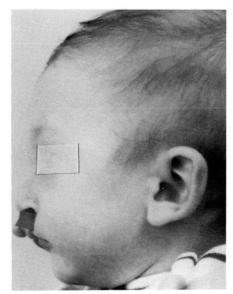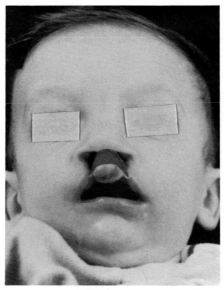

Fig. 54-3. Appliance worn by patient. Note improved position of premaxilla over a period of a few weeks.

the delay and can see their child's condition improve as prosthetic treatment proceeds (see Fig. 54-3). During this period of prosthetic management, facial growth is occurring. In addition to retraction of the premaxilla, the lateral palatal shelves are growing forward to narrow the cleft width; thus more soft tissue is available for the cleft lip repair. Parental cooperation is absolutely necessary to ensure success of this treatment.

Articulation Development Prosthesis

Research plays an important role at the center. Work by Debra Dorf, a speech and language pathologist and Howard Aduss, an orthodontist have shown that early cleft palate repair—before the onset of meaningful speech sounds, before one year of age—results in near-normal speech articulation and has no negative effect on facial growth. Most of my patients with cleft palate are treated by this early repair protocol. Sometimes, however, palatal repair must be delayed. The child's health may preclude surgical intervention, or adequate soft tissue may not be available to repair an excessively wide cleft (Fig. 54-4). In such patients, an Articulation Development Prosthesis is used.

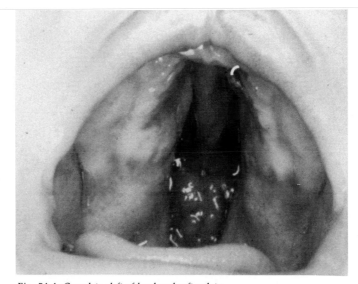

Fig. 54-4. Complete cleft of hard and soft palate.

The prosthesis obturates the palatal cleft and simulates palatopharyngeal valving to establish normal oral anatomy before surgical repair. It is used for speech articulation development, although in appearance it may resemble an orthopedic or feeding appliance.

The child is referred for prosthetic management by the plastic surgeon and the speech and language pathologist as soon as it is determined the palatal repair will be delayed. An acrylic resin palatal plate with a palatopharyngeal extension is fab-

ricated. It may be lined with resilient denture material in the alveolar and hard palate areas to ensure comfort and fit to the soft tissue. The plate does not extend up into the cleft to avoid impeding any medial growth of the palatal shelves (Fig. 54-5). The prosthesis is retained with denture adhesive and is removed only for daily cleaning (Fig. 54-6). The patient is seen monthly for prosthetic and surgical evaluations until such time as the surgeon believes surgical repair may be safely and successfully performed.

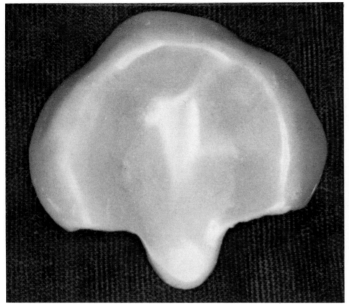 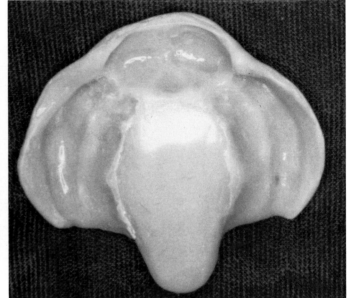

Fig. 54-5. Articulation Development Prosthesis.

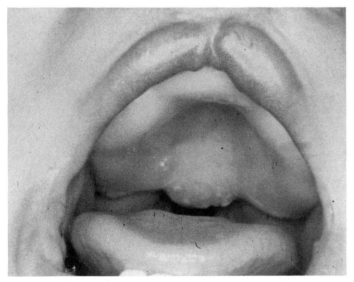

Fig. 54-6. Prosthesis in mouth.

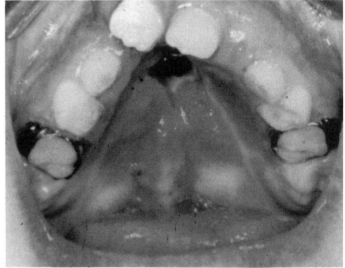

Fig. 54-7. Large oronasal communication in anterior hard palate.

My experience with the articulation development prosthesis has been favorable. Patients who successfully wear the prosthesis require limited, if any, speech therapy. The younger the patients are at the time of placement of the prosthesis, the more readily they adjust to it. Parental cooperation is an absolute requirement for success, especially during the first 2 to 3 days of wear.

General Dental Care

Regular dental care is important for anyone, but it takes on added importance for patients with clefts. The condition of the dentition can determine the outcome of prosthetic treatment and the degree to which this treatment is necessary. Functional prostheses such as obturators and palatal lifts rely on healthy dentition for support, stability, and retention. Fixed or removable partial dentures for tooth replacement are less complex when the dentition is healthy and fewer teeth are involved in the prosthesis. Because prosthetic treatment may be necessary even at an early age, the health of the primary and mixed dentitions as well as that of the adult dentition is important.

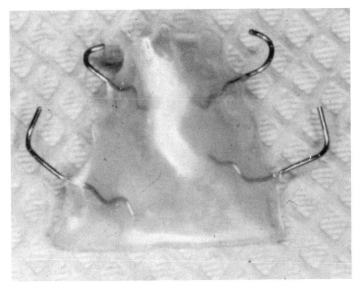

Fig. 54-8. Removable palatal obturator made of acrylic resin with wrought-wire clasps.

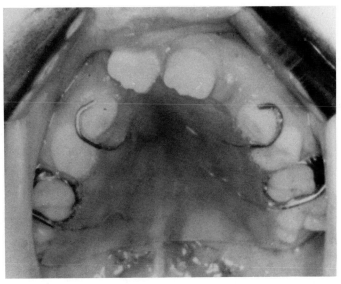

Fig. 54-9. Palatal obturator in place. Composite resin and orthodontic bands on cuspids and molars for retention of clasps.

Patients with clefts should begin regular visits to the dentist by about 2½ years of age. The initial visits are merely to acclimate the child to the dental environment, although some patients may require aggressive caries management even at this early age. The pattern of regular dental visits should continue through adolescence and into adulthood to ensure prosthetic success and general oral health. The prosthodontist works closely with the pediatric and general dentists to provide comprehensive treatment and continuity of dental care.

Palatal Obturator

Oronasal openings in the palate are caused by delay in surgical repair of a cleft or by a fistula at a previously repaired surgical site. The communication may be a frank opening or a narrow fissure in which contact with the nasal cavity may not be readily apparent (Fig. 54-7). In either situation, the opening may extend through the alveolus and into the labial vestibule. The problem is primarily one of function.

In most situations, feeding is not compromised. The patient learns to obturate the defect with the tongue and control the expression of food or liquid into the nasal cavity. Hypernasal speech and compensatory articulations are of greater concern.

Surgical repair of these areas is preferable, but it is not always possible. The opening may be so large that adequate soft tissue is not available for closure, or the patient's medical condition may preclude an operation. Repair may be deferred until orthodontic treatment is completed, or the patient or parents may simply be weary of treatment at that time and choose to defer surgical closure to a later date.

Fabrication of a palatal obturator should begin at the direction of the speech and language pathologist. For children and adolescents, the obturator consists of a removable palatal plate of acrylic resin with wrought wire stainless steel clasps for retention to several teeth (Fig. 54-8). Because of the unfavorable contours of some abutment teeth, orthodontic bands or brackets or composite resin dental restorative material may be added to these teeth to ensure adequate retention of the prosthesis. The palatal obturator closes a static opening in the fixed tissue of the hard palate (Fig. 54-9). It provides normal oral anatomy and allows normal function. The patient may still require therapy to correct preexisting speech problems. Missing teeth may be incorporated onto the obturator for functional and cosmetic considerations (Figs. 54-10 to 54-12). In some patients, the obturator may be fixed in the mouth by cementing it to teeth (Fig. 54-13).

The obturator is easy to adjust and modify as the patient grows, teeth exfoliate, and other teeth erupt. At a later date, if required, a definitive palatal obturator is made of cast chromium-cobalt with acrylic resin in the cleft and tooth areas. This design offers more strength and support for long-term use. When adequate retention of the obturator cannot be obtained from the teeth and residual palatal structures, the anatomic configuration of the palatal opening may be engaged with a resilient material such as silicone rubber to help retain the prosthesis (Figs. 54-14 to 54-16).

It may not be readily apparent whether a patient would benefit from a palatal obturator, especially if he or she has a small anterior fistula. My associates and I have developed a simple technique that allows the speech pathologist to obturate a palatal fistula for diagnostic purposes without having to actually make an obturator.

HolliHesive (Hollister, Inc., Libertyville, Ill. 60048) is a self-adhesive, flexible skin preparation that is a component of a colostomy system. This material has been approved for intraoral use. A piece of HolliHesive slightly larger than the fistula is cut from a larger sheet, and the protective backing from each side is removed. A piece of gauze or facial tissue is used to dry the soft tissue surrounding the fistula, and the patch is pressed into

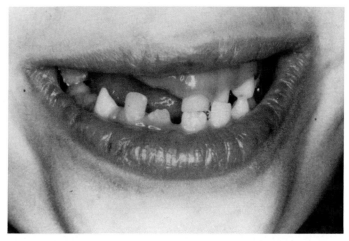

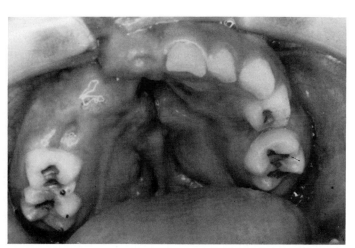

Fig. 54-10. Residual oronasal fistula with missing teeth.

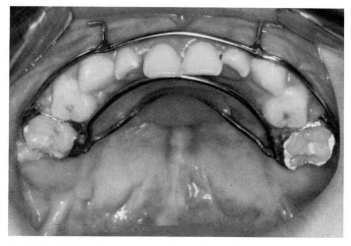

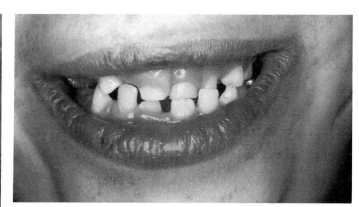

Fig. 54-12. Addition of teeth to obturator for functional and cosmetic improvement.

Fig. 54-11. Palatal obturator to close fistula.

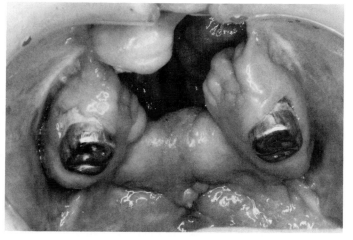

Fig. 54-13. Palatal obturator cemented to teeth. Labial wire also present for orthodontic purposes.

Fig. 54-14. Large residual cleft of hard palate. Patient has inadequate number of teeth for retention of prosthesis.

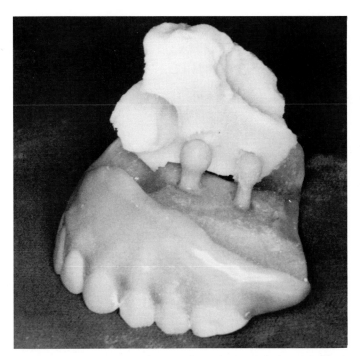

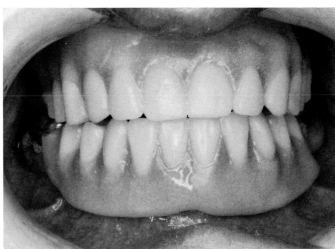

Fig. 54-16. Obturator in place.

Fig. 54-15. Silicone rubber obturator attaches to denture and engages undercut areas within nasal cavity for retention.

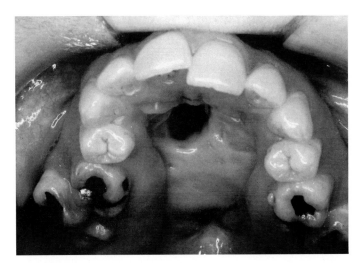

Fig. 54-17. Residual palatal opening.

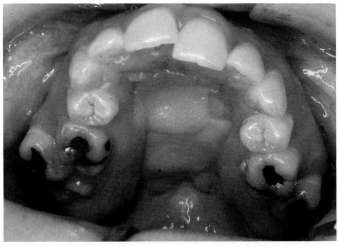

Fig. 54-18. HolliHesive in place obturating the defect.

place with a wet finger. The margins may be smoothed and thinned by wiping from the HolliHesive toward the soft tissue with a wet finger (Figs. 54-17 and 54-18). This technique allows quick evaluation of speech and, if need be, provides temporary obturation until a prosthesis can be made or an operation performed.

The material is slowly dissolved by saliva or other warm liquids over the period of a day, but it remains sufficiently intact during this time. It is removed before sleep to prevent possible aspiration by lifting of a margin and peeling off.

Palatopharyngeal Obturator

For some patients, surgical repair of a cleft of the soft palate is deferred, because there is a compromising medical condition or because of excessive width of the cleft. The result is palatopharyngeal insufficiency, which causes hypernasality and contributes to compensatory speech articulation. Sometimes, even after surgical repair, a palatal insufficiency may persist. If a pharyngeal flap procedure is not performed, similar speech problems exist. A palatopharyngeal obturator is used to correct this problem.

This prosthesis differs from a palatal obturator in that the tissues of the soft palate and pharyngeal walls move to some degree during function. The palatopharyngeal obturator must account for the dynamics of these structures to achieve closure between the oral and nasal cavities. At rest, there is a gap between the obturator and residual palatal and pharyngeal soft tissues. This allows nasal breathing and proper pronunciation of nasal consonants and provides for patient comfort. During speech or swallowing, the residual tissues contact the obturator to separate the oral and nasal cavities (Figs. 54-19 to 54-24).

Palatal Lift

A surgically repaired soft palate may have proper anatomic length yet may remain neuromuscularly compromised. During function, the soft palate may not elevate adequately to achieve palatopharyngeal closure (Fig. 54-25). A palatal lift prosthesis raises the soft palate to the level necessary to achieve such closure (Figs. 54-26 and 54-27).

The prosthesis works best with a flaccid soft palate that is easily elevated. A more turgid palate offers resistance to elevation and may produce a downward rebound effect causing the prosthesis to dislodge.

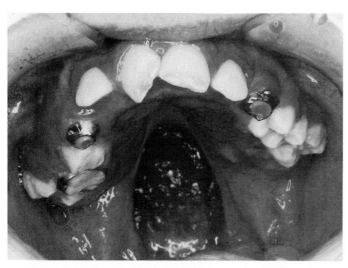

Fig. 54-19. Unrepaired cleft of hard and soft palates.

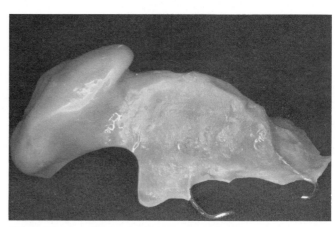

Fig. 54-20. Palatopharyngeal obturator.

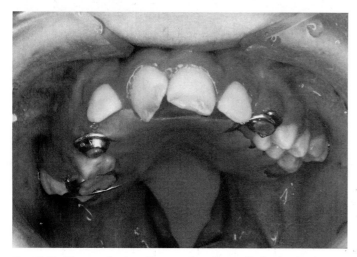

Fig. 54-21. Obturator in place. Note gapping when residual soft palate is at rest.

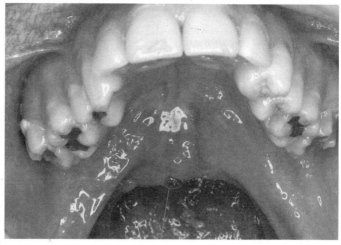

Fig. 54-22. Palatopharyngeal insufficiency following surgical repair of soft palate.

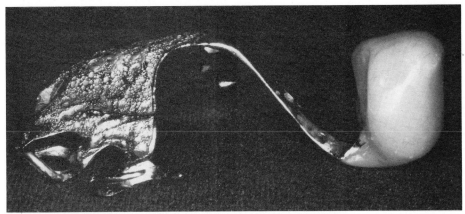

Fig. 54-23. Palatopharyngeal obturator.

Fig. 54-24. Obturator in place.

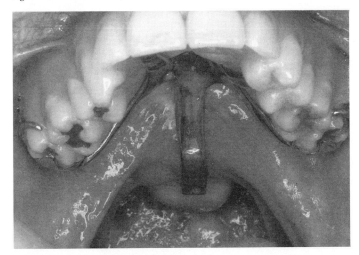

Fig. 54-25. Repaired cleft palate during phonation. Although palatal length is adequate, palatopharyngeal incompetency exists.

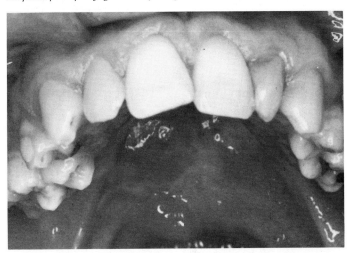

Fig. 54-26. Palatal lift prosthesis.

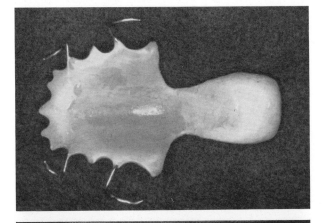

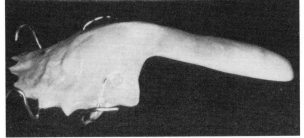

Fig. 54-27. Prosthesis in place. Note multiple clasps for retention and elevated position of soft palate to achieve palatopharyngeal closure.

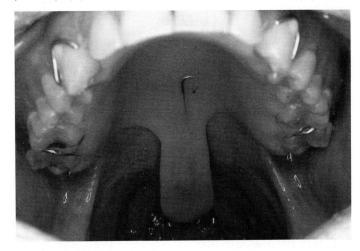

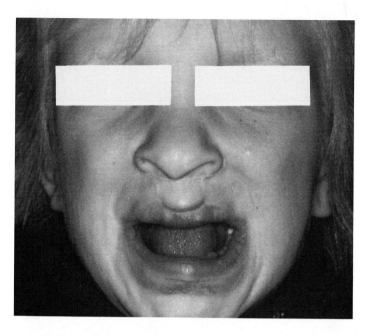

Fig. 54-28. *Patient with EEC syndrome. Note repaired bilateral cleft lip.*

Fig. 54-29. *Patient with EEC syndrome. Note anterior residual oronasal fistula and multiple congenitally missing teeth.*

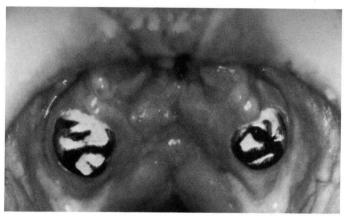 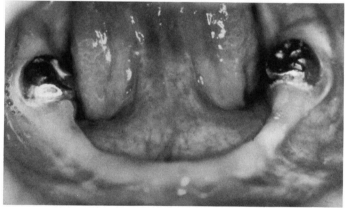

The hard palate portion of the prosthesis clasps to multiple natural teeth for retention of the cantilevered pharyngeal extension. For this reason, the success of the palatal lift relies on healthy dentition. The prosthesis may stimulate palatal and pharyngeal wall movement so that after a period of wear, patients may achieve adequate palatopharyngeal closure without the prosthesis or at least may become better candidates for a pharyngeal flap procedure.

Tooth Replacement

Consideration for prosthetic replacement of teeth begins when the patient is about 5 years of age. Children start formal education and actively socialize with their peers at that age. By this time, their levels of motivation and cooperation are adequate for treatment.

Early tooth replacement may involve simply adding denture teeth to an acrylic resin palatal plate, which may or may not serve to obturate a palatal opening. Modifications are necessary as the patient grows, the dentition changes, and orthodontic treatment is initiated. Some patients have other congenital anomalies as part of a syndrome. Such is the case in EEC syndrome, in which a patient with a cleft has ectrodactyly and ectodermal dysplasia. As a result of the latter, the patient is missing most or all teeth, and removable dentures are indicated (Figs. 54-28 to 54-31). Every effort should be made to retain whatever teeth are present to help preserve alveolar bone and improve prosthetic support. The dentures are worn over these teeth, usually with little or no tooth modification, and must be remade approximately every 3 years because of orofacial growth.

Removable dentures are also seen commonly in middle-aged or elderly patients with clefts. These patients were born too early to benefit from present-day treatment and scientific surgical techniques. Many have poor nose and lip repairs, collapsed dental arches, neglected dentitions, and poor quality of speech (Figs. 54-32 and 54-33). However, they are usually unwilling, at their age, to undergo further surgical treatment, speech therapy, or more extensive and expensive prosthodontic treatment.

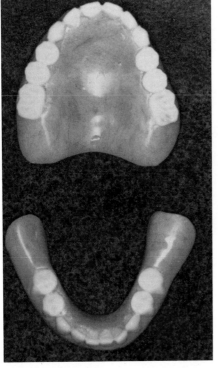

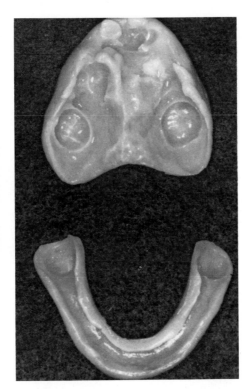

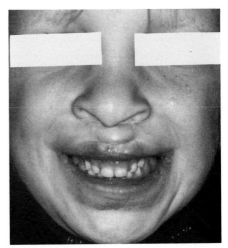

Fig. 54-31. Patient with EEC syndrome with dentures in place.

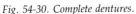

Fig. 54-30. Complete dentures.

Maxillary lateral incisors are the teeth most commonly missing because of a cleft. In addition, supernumerary teeth or maxillary cuspids may be impacted adjacent to the cleft. Once orthodontic treatment begins, the orthodontist and prosthodontist must determine the fate of these teeth. The teeth should be preserved if their presence will contribute to development of the alveolus or if they may erupt later and be guided into a useful position in the dental arch. However, if no such contribution can be made and they are of no use for prosthodontic purposes, these teeth should be removed. It is also important for the orthodontist and prosthodontist to anticipate the final orthodontic result with regard to the position of the maxillary dental midline, occlusal relations, tooth positions, and width of edentulous spaces to achieve the optimal aesthetic and functional prosthetic results. The definitive dental prosthesis for a patient with a cleft not only should restore missing teeth for cosmetic and functional purposes but also should help stabilize segments of the clefted dental arch and retain the teeth in their postorthodontic position.

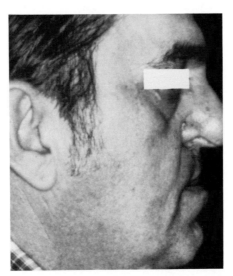

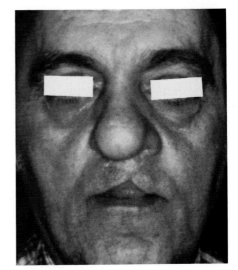

Fig. 54-32. Adult patient with a cleft. Note poor surgical result of lip and nose.

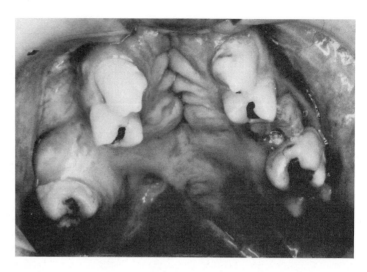

Fig. 54-33. Adult patient with a cleft. Note collapsed dental arch and multiple missing teeth.

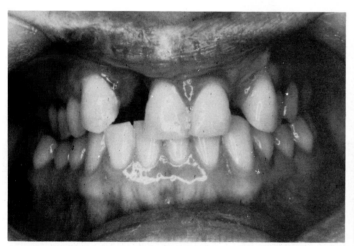

A

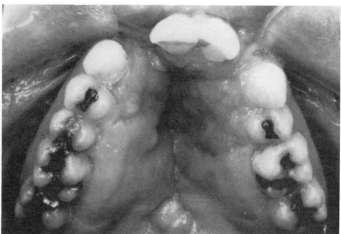

Fig. 54-34A. Bilateral cleft with extremely mobile premaxilla. B. Roentgenogram confirms lack of bone in cleft sites.

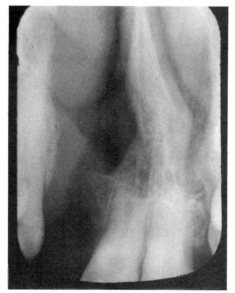

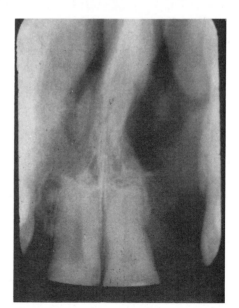

B

Current trends favor a fixed rather than a removable dental prosthesis for tooth replacement in patients with clefts. Although either may provide good aesthetic results and allow for proper oral hygiene, the fixed prosthesis more closely resembles the natural dentition and provides better function and comfort. There is also a considerable psychological benefit to patients who may feel a fixed prosthesis is a permanent, lifelike part of them, as opposed to a removable prosthesis, which may be associated with artificial dentures and old age.

Unilateral clefts are less involved than bilateral ones, and therefore easier to restore prosthetically. The dental arch is more intact and the maxillary segments are more stable. The orthodontic result is often better.

In bilateral clefts, the independent premaxilla poses several problems. Orthognathic and orthodontic management may be required to achieve a normal horizontal and vertical relation. In some patients, the premaxilla may be horizontally mobile or even vertically depressible, factors that compromise arch stability and may complicate prosthetic restoration. A removable prosthesis may be indicated in such a patient (Figs. 54-34 and 54-35).

Bony support for teeth adjacent to the cleft (usually the distal of the central incisors and mesial of the cuspids) is often compromised by the cleft. When restoring such a case with a fixed dental prosthesis, the rule is to use two teeth on each side of the edentulous cleft as abutments for the prosthesis.

In some patients, the potential abutment adjacent to the cleft may need to be extracted because of a severe lack of bony support or may require surgery to improve the periodontal condition so it may be retained. In such situations, an additional tooth on each side of the cleft should be added as an abutment to ensure adequate support, stability, and retention of the fixed prosthesis. The abutment teeth are drilled down and crowns with the tooth replacement attached are cemented over the prepartions. This procedure should be delayed until the patient is at least 18 years of age to allow the dental pulp to recede so that the abutment teeth may be adequately prepared without danger of pulpal exposure (Figs. 54-36 to 54-38).

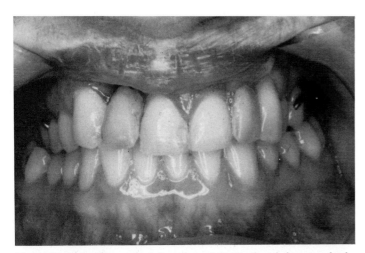

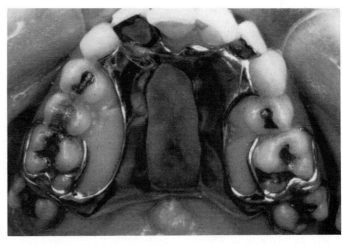

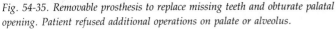

Fig. 54-35. Removable prosthesis to replace missing teeth and obturate palatal opening. Patient refused additional operations on palate or alveolus.

Fig. 54-36. Bilateral cleft after orthodontic treatment.

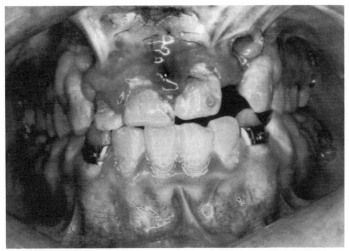

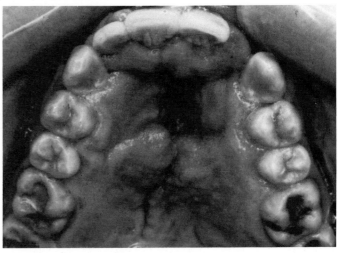

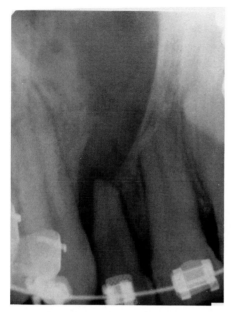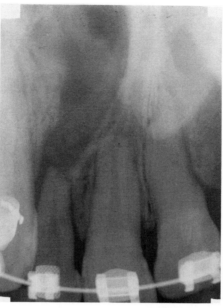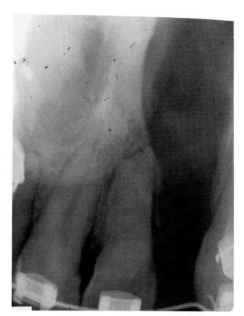

Fig. 54-37. Poor bony support for maxillary left lateral incisor. Tooth was extracted. Note lack of bone at cleft sites.

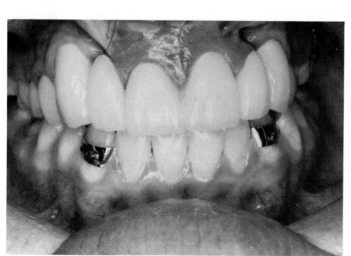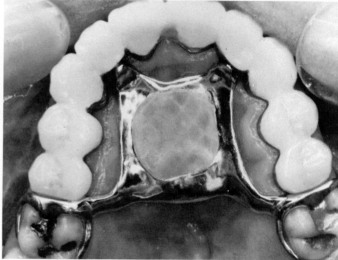

Fig. 54-38. Definitive fixed prosthesis. Second premolars added as abutments because of compromised bony support on cuspids. Removable prosthesis used to obturate palatal opening.

Fig. 54-39. Bone-grafted alveolar cleft.

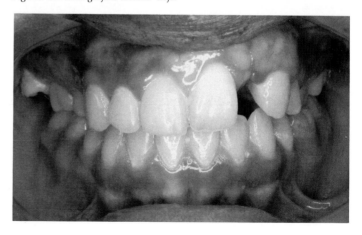

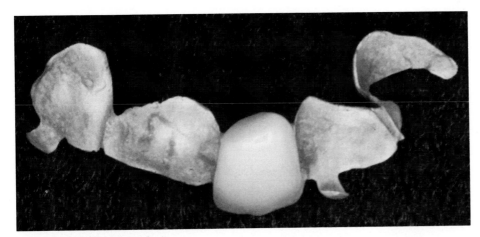

Fig. 54-40. Resin-bonded prosthesis.

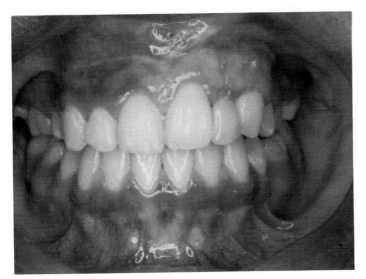
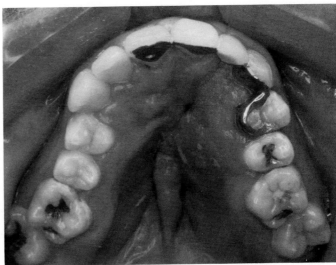

Fig. 54-41. Prosthesis cemented in place.

Bone grafting of the alveolar cleft has become the standard of care in cleft management. It is an excellent means of ensuring stability of the maxillary arch. This is especially true of bilateral clefts, in which a mobile premaxilla can cause failure of the dental prosthesis.

Once the alveolar cleft is bone grafted, special prosthodontic considerations for clefts are eliminated and the treatment becomes conventional tooth replacement. A less extensive dental prosthesis is required. Bone grafting also allows for eruption of impacted teeth into a normal position on the dental arch, which contributes to more conservative prosthodontic treatment. There is even a technique for autotransplantation of a tooth to the bone-grafted alveolus, but it has yet to gain widespread popularity.

When a bone graft is used, replacement of missing teeth may be achieved with a resin-bonded bridge. This type of fixed prosthesis requires less tooth preparation than a conventional fixed bridge and is cemented only to the palatal aspect of the abutment teeth. This is a more conservative approach to definitive tooth replacement and may be performed when the patient is younger (Figs. 54-39 to 54-41). In clefts where a malformed lateral incisor or supernumerary tooth is present or when a cuspid has been surgically or orthodontically moved into the lateral position, the tooth may be "lateralized" by adding composite resin dental restorative material to the incisal edge.

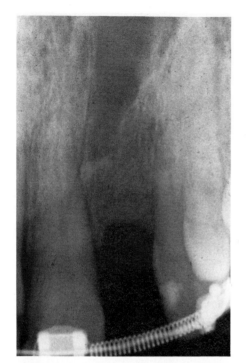

Fig. 54-42. X-ray of bone grafted cleft site.

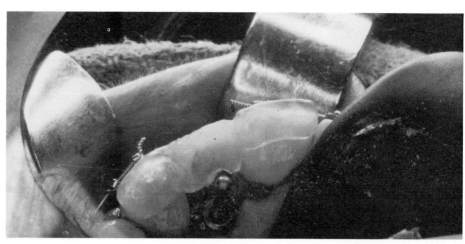

Fig. 54-43. Placement of implant into prepared site in alveolar bone. Note use of implant positioner.

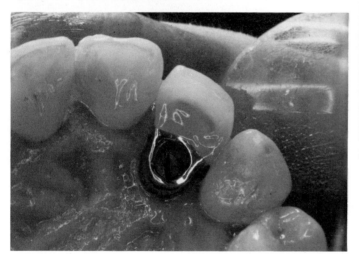

Fig. 54-44. Occlusal view of restoration screwed into implant.

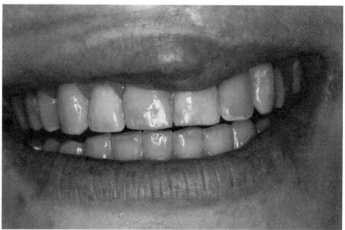

Fig. 54-45. Frontal view of completed restoration.

Osseointegration and Dental Implants

Although dental implants have been used for hundreds of years, they have become a reliable technique for tooth replacement only in the past 25 years in Europe and in the past decade in North America. Their use and predictability were greatly enhanced through the work of Dr. P-I. Branemark of Göteborg, Sweden. A detailed discussion of this technique may be found in Chap. 73.

Osseointegrated implants may be placed in bone-grafted alveolar cleft sites and used to retain a fixed dental prosthesis (Fig. 54-42). Before a stage I operation, the prosthodontist makes an acrylic-resin positioner. This positioner is used by the surgeon to guide the placement of the implant to its optimal position and angulation in the edentulous space (Fig. 54-43). The site is closed with gingival tissue for 6 to 9 months while osseointegration occurs. A variation of this procedure has been described in which the implant is first placed in tibial bone. During the same procedure, a bone graft containing the implant is placed in the cleft site. This technique is popular in Sweden but has had limited use in the United States. At stage II, the implant is exposed into the oral cavity. After several weeks of soft tissue healing, the tooth replacement is attached to the implant (Figs. 54-44 and 54-45).

Dental implants may also be used in cases of oligodontia or anodontia to retain a dental prosthesis. Bone grafting may be necessary to provide adequate support for the implants (Figs. 54-46 to 54-49).

Clinical reports have been published describing the use of dental implants in children to retain fixed or removable dental prostheses. There are, however, not yet enough long-term data on the effects of growth and development to consider these procedures as the standard of care.

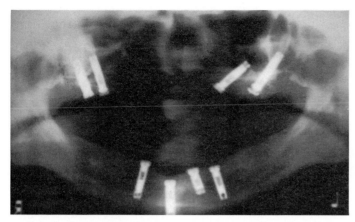

Fig. 54-46. Radiograph following bilateral cranial bone grafts to maxillary segments and placement of osseointegrated dental implants. (Same patient as in Fig. 54-14.)

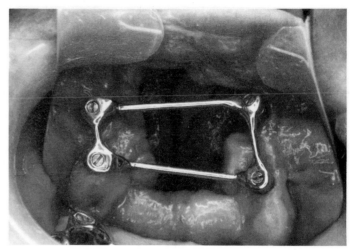

Fig. 54-47. Gold bars connecting implants.

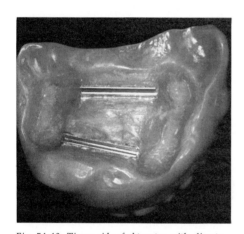

Fig. 54-48. Tissue side of obturator with clips to engage gold bars for retention of obturator.

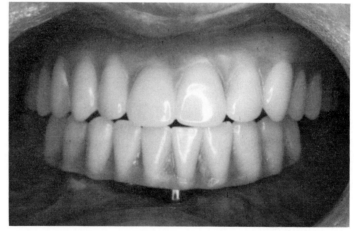

Fig. 54-49. Completed restoration. Note that mandible has been restored with fixed implant prosthesis.

Suggested Reading

Chierici, G. Cleft Palate Habilitation. In J. Beumer, T.A. Curtis, and D.N. Firtell (Eds.), *Maxillofacial Rehabilitation: Prosthodontic and Surgical Considerations* (1st ed.). St. Louis: Mosby, 1979. Pp. 292–310.

Dorf, D.S., Reisberg, D.J., and Gold, H.O. Early prosthetic management of cleft palate: Articulation development prosthesis—a preliminary report. *J. Prosthet. Dent.* 53:222, 1985.

Guckes, A.D., et al. Using endosseous dental implants for patients with ectodermal dysplasia. *J. Am. Dent. Assoc.* 122:59, 1991.

Raamstad, T. Post-orthodontic retention and post-prosthodontic occlusion in adult complete unilateral and bilateral cleft subjects. *Cleft Palate J.* 10:34, 1973.

Reisberg, D.J., Figueroa, A., and Gold, H.O. An intraoral appliance for management of the protrusive premaxilla in bilateral cleft lip. *Cleft Palate J.* 25:53, 1988.

Reisberg, D.J., Figueroa, A., and Heffez, L. Osseointegration in cleft habilitation. *J. Prosthodontics.* In press.

Reisberg, D.J., Gold, H.O., and Dorf, D.S. A technique for obturating palatal fistulas. *Cleft Palate J.* 22:286, 1985.

Verdi, F.J., et al. Use of the Branemark implant in the cleft palate patient. *Cleft Palate J.* 28:301, 1991.

Worthington, P., and Branemark, P.I. (Eds.). *Advanced Osseointegration Surgery: Application in the Maxillofacial Region.* Chicago: Quintessence, 1992.

55

Congenital Deformities of the External Ear

Kunihiro Kurihara

The auricle, which protrudes at an angle of about 30° from the temple, is an oval structure. Its anterior surface has multiple ridges and depressions formed by the underlying cartilage. The auricle develops rapidly in the first 3 years of life to attain 80 to 85 percent of its adult size. Growing slowly thereafter, it reaches about 90 percent of the adult size at 8 to 10 years of age. Deformities of the auricle present at birth undergo slight changes in the first 3 years but change little after that. Not infrequently, the deformity or defect of the auricle is accompanied by deformities or hypoplasia of the temporal, maxillary, and mandibular bones on the ipsilateral side.

Anatomy

The auricle in adults is 6.0 to 7.5 cm long; the width is 55 to 60 percent of the length. The superior margin of the auricle is at the level of the eyebrow. The angle between the vertical axis of the auricle, which tilts posteriorly, and the vertical axis of the face varies greatly among individuals, from 15° to 25° (±6.2°). The vertical axis of the auricle is thus not always parallel to the dorsum of the nose,

but deviates 15° (±7.5°) from the line of the dorsum nasi (Fig. 55-1).

The elastic auricular cartilage is 1 to 3 mm thick and somewhat pliable (Fig. 55-2). The anterior surface of the auricle is covered with skin and a thin layer of subcutaneous tissue. Its posterior surface has a rather thick layer of soft tissue composed of subcutaneous tissue and the auricular muscles.

A cross section of the auricle at the level of the external auditory meatus (Fig. 55-3) shows the opening of the external auditory meatus anterior to the conchal cavity, over which the tragus juts out as if to shield it. Posterior and opposite to the tragus, the concha rises almost vertically to end in the antihelix. More posteriorly, across the concave surface from the antihelical ridge, are the scapha and the helix, which turns back like an overhang. Thus the auricle may be represented as a stepped structure with a slope of about 30° from the temporal area.

Muscles

In humans the auricular muscles, divided into intrinsic muscles and extrinsic muscles, have almost no motor function but serve to fix the auricle in position.

Extrinsic Muscles

The superior auricular muscle, the largest of the auricular muscles, arises with a broad base at the galeal aponeurosis. It narrows and tapers caudally and inserts into the posterior surface of the triangular fossa. The anterior auricular muscle arises from the superficial layer of the temporal fascia, located anterior to the auricle, and inserts on the helical spine. The posterior auricular muscle arises at the aponeurosis on the lateral surface of the mastoid process, extends anteriorly almost horizontally, and inserts on the conchal process (Fig. 55-4).

Intrinsic Muscles

The intrinsic muscles arise and end at the auricular cartilage. In humans they have lost their motor function and, together with the ligaments, serve as supporting tissue. There are six intrinsic auricular muscles: the major auricular, the lesser auricular, the tragus, the antitragus, the transverse auricular, and the oblique auricular. These muscles all are innervated by the facial nerve.

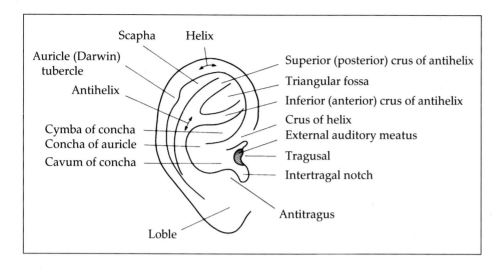

Fig. 55-1. Anterior surface of auricle.

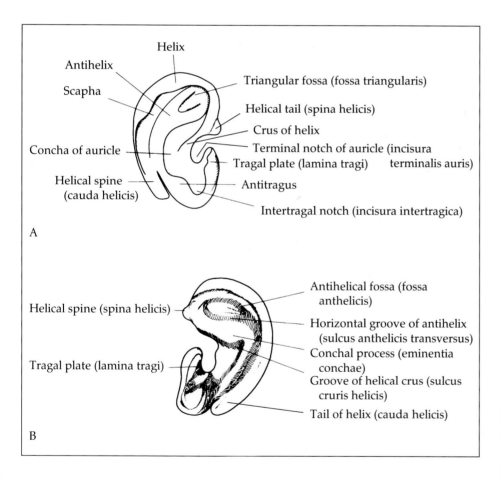

Fig. 55-2A. Anterior surface of cartilage of right auricle. B. Posterior surface of cartilage of right auricle.

Sensory Nerve Supply of the Auricle

The auricle is innervated by branches of the trigeminal, vagus, and cervical nerves. The greater auricular nerve is a cervical nerve distributed over almost all of the posterior surface of the auricle and the lateral portion of the anterior surface of the auricle. The lesser occipital nerve is distributed around the temporomandibular groove at the posterior surface of the auricle. The auriculotemporal nerve derives from the mandibular branch of the trigeminal nerve and is distributed over the tragus and helix at the anterior surface of the auricle. The external auditory canal branch, a branch of the auriculotemporal nerve, is distributed over the skin of the external auditory meatus. The auricular branch of the vagus nerve (Arnold nerve) is distributed over the posterior surface of the auricle and the posterior wall of the external auditory meatus (Fig. 55-5).

Embryology

In the fifth week of gestation, several processes, which eventually become the auricle, arise from the mesenchyme of the posterior margin of the first branchial cleft between the first branchial arch (mandibular arch) and the second branchial arch (hyoid arch). Thomson in 1884 first reported that most of the auricle derives from the hyoid arch and only the tragus arises from the mandibular arch. He wrote that three processes (ear hillocks) appear on both the mandibular and hyoid arches, which are adjacent to the mandibular cleft, and the auricle is formed from these processes. Streeter in 1922 related auriculogenesis to the developmental horizons. At horizon XVI (32 to 35

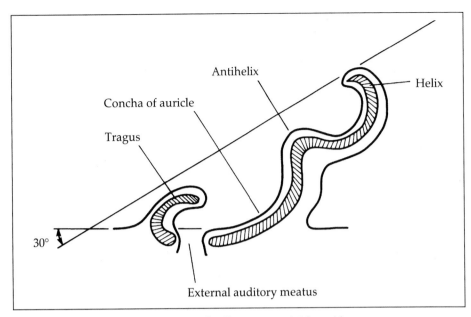

Fig. 55-3. Horizontal section through external auditory meatus of right auricle.

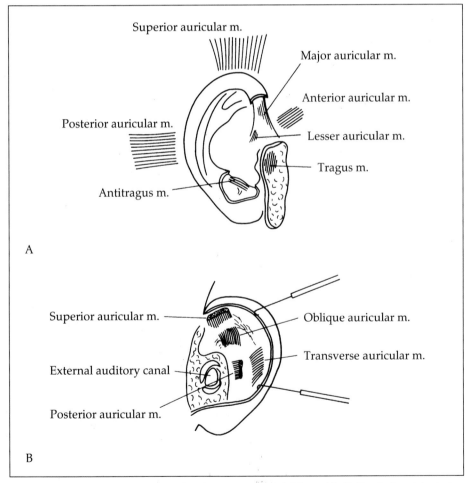

Fig. 55-4A. Extrinsic and intrinsic muscles of anterior surface of right auricle. B. Extrinsic and intrinsic muscles of posterior surface of right auricle.

days of gestation), prominences on the first and second branchial arches develop into ear hillocks.

With the development of the face, the ear hillocks undergo fusion and deviation at horizon XVII and horizon XIX (37 to 40 days of gestation), and the auricle forms at horizon XXII (60 days of gestation). He proposed the so-called upper series of auriculogenesis in which the auricle rotates from the front of the face toward the back as it develops. More recently, Wood-Jones and I-Chuan agreed with the findings of Thomson, that is, that the auricle rotates toward the front. They called this mode of development the lower series, in which most of the auricle arises from the hyoid arch and only the tragus arises from the mandibular arch.

Midera in 1982 used scanning electron microscopy to observe that ear hillocks arise at horizon XV through horizon XVI (33 to 35 days of gestation). He observed that there are three hillocks at both the mandibular and hyoid arches. He also observed that the auricle rotates with the development of the head and neck in the same direction as described by Wood-Jones and I-Chuan until it takes the form of a human auricle at horizon XX (46 days of gestation).

The Deformities and Their Treatment
Prominent Ear

In examining a normal ear from behind, one notes that the concha forms a 90° angle with the head (auriculotemporal angle). The scapha likewise forms an angle of approximately 90° with the concha. The rim of the helix turns slightly outward. The angle between the scapha and the concha, formed by the antihelix, may become obtuse, causing the auricle to protrude. With an excessively cupped concha, rolling of the protuberant part of the posterior conchal wall posteriorly is also a major factor in the prominence of the auricle. This deformity occurs in either one or both auricles and in all or part of the auricle. The cause of prominent ears is unknown; although many patients have morphologic similarities with paternal or maternal families, there are no hereditary tendencies.

Treatment

It is crucial to identify the part of the auricle responsible for the protrusion. Good results can be expected if an operative procedure or a combination of several procedures is chosen according to the patient's need. Reconstruction of the antihelix, concha, and scapha is necessary, but overcorrection or construction of an antihelix that is too sharp produces the opposite effect. In general, the external ear is most pleasing to the eye if the helix protrudes outside the antihelix. On the contrary, if the antihelix protrudes from the rim, the ear looks unnatural.

Skin Excision with or Without Excision of Cartilage.

A reconstructive operation consisting of resection of cartilage from the concha and a skin excision was first reported by Ely in 1881. The method involves a full-thickness resection of the auricle. Luchett in 1910 reported on a reconstructive procedure for a poorly delivered antihelix in which the cartilage was resected along the expected line of the antihelix and a mattress suture was placed to allow the margins of the resected cartilage to stand out. This report has been the basis of the present practice of resecting skin and cartilage. To prevent a sharp antihelix, Barsky, Young, and McDowell modified the initial procedure.

Preoperatively, and with the patient in a sitting position, the antihelix is accentuated by pushing the auricular rim posteriorly by hand (Fig. 55-6). The proposed line of the antihelix is traced (Fig. 55-7), and key points are projected and marked on the posterior auricular skin and cartilage. A spindle- or dumbbell-shaped skin excision 15 mm in maximal width is made on the posterior surface of the auricle. Because the elevation of the antihelix becomes steeper as tension produced by the skin sutures increases, the width of excised skin is kept to a minimum at first and increased later, if necessary. A skin excision at the earlobe or the posterior side of the helix is avoided because this frequently causes an unnatural appearance of the lobe. Skin excision around the auriculotemporal sulcus is done sparingly because this might lead to a shallow sulcus and an unnatural protrusion of the posterior wall of the conchal cavity.

Supraperichondrial undermining is done on almost the entire posterior surface of the auricle. Two incisions, 2 mm apart,

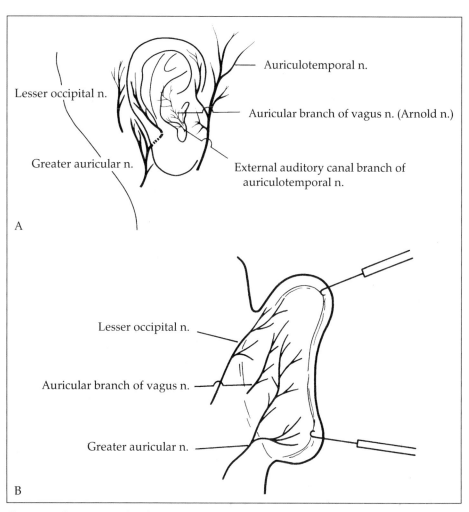

Fig. 55-5A. *Sensory nerve distribution of anterior surface of right auricle. B. Sensory nerve distribution of posterior surface of right auricle.*

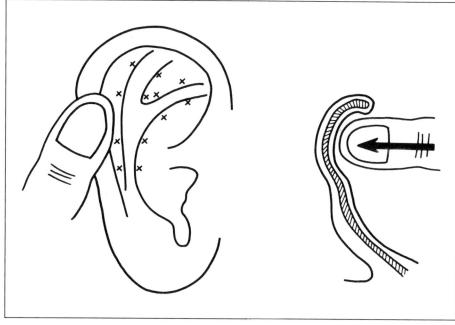

Fig. 55-6. *Identification of line of antihelix while ear is manipulated into ideal position.*

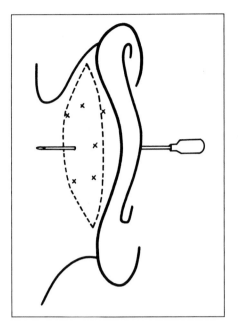

Fig. 55-7. Tracing of antihelical line to posterior surface with needle dipped in ink.

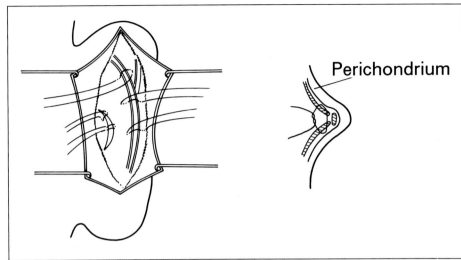

Fig. 55-8. Incision in cartilage along antihelical line. Mattress sutures are placed along tattoo marks.

Fig. 55-9A. Prominent ear in 8-year-old girl. B. One year after otoplasty.

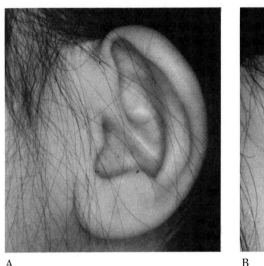

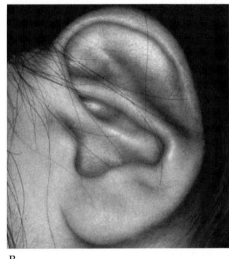

A   B

Fig. 55-10. Skin excision and mattress suture method. Suture needle passed through full thickness of cartilage only.

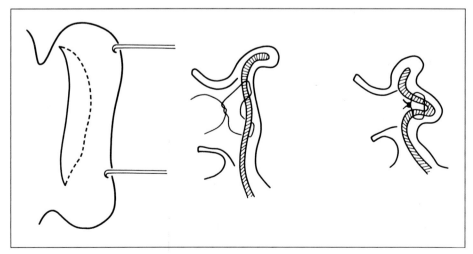

are placed on the auricular cartilage along the traced antihelical line. The anterior perichondrium is conserved to prevent construction of a sharp antihelix. Vertical mattress sutures are placed at three or four sites to form an antihelix. The needle should be passed through the full thickness of the auricular cartilage but not through the anterior perichondrium (Figs. 55-8 and 55-9).

Skin Excision and Mattress Suture.
Monks in 1881 introduced a method of correcting prominent ears by skin excision alone, without cartilage incision or excision. Several other authors subsequently devised similar procedures. This operation is recommended only for relatively mild deformities.

The proposed antihelix is formed by pushing the auricular rim posteriorly. The line of the antihelix and anterior and posterior crura are traced, and an elliptic or dumbbell-shaped skin excision of a maximal width of 15 mm is performed on the posterior surface of the auricle. Mattress sutures are placed at three or four sites along the traced antihelical line. It is important that the suture needle pass through the full thickness of the auricular cartilage without producing a skin dimple on the anterior surface. Nonabsorbable suture such as 4–0 nylon is used for the suturing (Figs. 55-10 and 55-11).

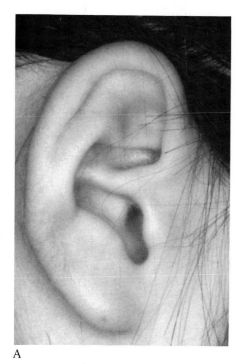

A

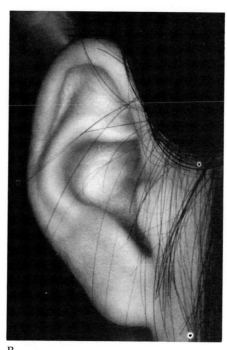

B

Fig. 55-11A. Prominent right ear in 14-year-old girl. B. Six months after otoplasty with mattress sutures.

Fig. 55-12. Skin excision and bending of cartilage by rasping. Posterior approach.

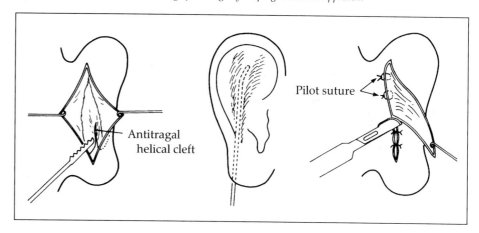

Bending of Cartilage by Rasping.

Converse and Stark tried to modify the cartilage spring by scraping the posterior surface of the cartilage in the area of the antihelix with a wire brush. Stenstrom, expanding on the work of Gibson and Davis, devised an otoplastic procedure that involves scraping the anterior surface of the auricular perichondrium and cartilage. This otoplasty is widely used today.

In the Stenstrom otoplasty the posterior surface of the auricle is widely exposed by an elliptic skin excision. The skin is retracted as far as the anterior surface of the auricle. The perichondrium and cartilage are scraped under direct vision. Currently, a rasp is inserted to the anterior surface of the auricle through a posterior opening in the area of the tail of the helix without exposing the anterior surface of the auricle. After subcutaneous undermining, the perichondrium and cartilage are scraped down with a special rasp. The degree of the cartilage spring broken by rasping is determined as the operation proceeds by pressing on the helix. The antihelix protrudes at the rasped portion of the cartilage because of the tension of the skin closure on the posterior surface of the auricle. I do not preexcise posterior auricular skin. After cartilage repositioning, an appropriate width of skin is ex-

cised to produce the desired appearance of the antihelix (Figs. 55-12 and 55-13).

Postoperatively, to avoid hematoma formation and support the newly formed contour of the ear, a compression dressing with cotton and gauze is applied. It is removed 3 to 4 days after the operation. An excessive postauricular skin excision should be avoided to prevent closure under tension and ear deformity. Rough subcutaneous undermining of the anterior surface of the auricle could lead to skin necrosis and should be avoided.

Stahl Ear

Stahl ear is an auricular deformity with peculiar morphologic characteristics. Although it has been described as rare, it is not rare in Asia, particularly in Japan (Fig. 55-14). Stahl ear has been classified into three types based on morphologic characteristics. In type I, the crus frucata of the antihelix protrudes to hide the triangular fossa and the scapha. In type II, a third crus extends posteriorly from the antihelix. A wide scapha forms above this structure. In type III, the superior crus of the antihelix shows a nodular extension, and the helix is narrow.

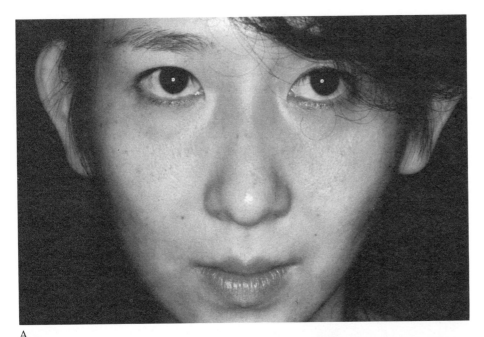

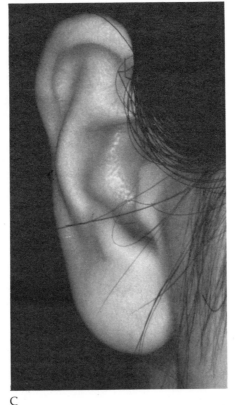

Etiology

Hereditary factors play a major part, but the mode of inheritance is not clear. Patients tend to inherit the trait from their fathers. Pressure on an abnormal cartilaginous protrusion that extends posteriorly from the antihelix—the so-called third crus of the antihelix—forms a nearly normal scapha. This characteristic finding in Stahl ear shows that the deformity is only a morphologic abnormality without a defect of auricular components.

Treatment

Treatment of a Relatively Well-Shaped Helix with a Third Crus.
The deformity of the third crus can be corrected easily. A nearly normal scapha and helical protrusion can be reproduced by pressing the third crus by hand. This type of deformity is treated by chondrotomy of the deformed portion of the auricle. I favor a skin incision parallel to the helix on the posterior surface of the auricle. The anterior skin is elevated over the perichondrium, and the region of the third crus is exposed.

Several incisions 2 mm across are placed along the axis of the third crus on the perichondrium and cartilage. Incisions are also placed on the scapha depending on the patient's condition. It is crucial in this procedure to limit the depth of cartilage incisions to two-thirds of the thickness of

B   C

Fig. 55-13A. Twenty-one-year-old woman with bilateral prominent ears. B. Right ear shows poorly developed helix and antihelix. C. Postoperative appearance demonstrating well-formed antihelix and posterior repositioning of right ear.

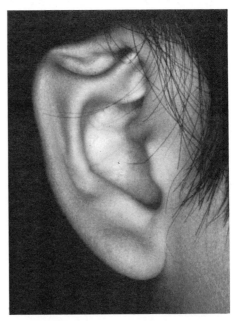

Fig. 55-14. Typical Stahl ear with third crus.

the cartilage and to preserve the integrity of the anterior perichondrium. The rationale for this technique is based on the elongation of the posterior side of the cartilage and the contractile power of the perichondrium on the anterior side. This effect cannot be obtained if the incision is carried through the full thickness of the auricular cartilage, including the anterior perichondrium. To maintain the corrected form obtained by chondrotomy, a rolled piece of gauze is inserted into the scapha and the posterior surface of the auricle, and a bolster through-and-through suture is placed. The bolster suture is kept in place for about 2 weeks, until connective tissue forms at the site of the cartilaginous defect and the anterior perichondrium is stabilized in its contracted form, thus preventing a recurrence of the deformity (Figs. 55-15 and 55-16).

Treatment of Flat Helix, with Unrolled Helix but Without Third Crus Deformity. In these patients the helix needs reconstruction. The free margin of the helix is longer than the outer margin of the auricle and the helix does not fold in. Because in normally sloped auricles the free margin of the helix is shorter than the outer margin of the auricle, a full-thickness, wedge-shaped excision of the auricle is made in the region of the third crus. A fan-shaped excision greatly shortens the helical rim and allows construction of a normal-looking helical rim (Figs. 55-17 and 55-18).

Cryptotia

Features
Cryptotia is a congenital auricular deformity in which the upper portion of the auricle creeps into the space beneath the skin of the temple but can be drawn out when one pulls on this portion of the helical rim. The helix, scapha, and antihelix come into view. When the helical rim is released, however, the upper auricle creeps back under the temporal skin, and the temporoauricular angle at the upper part of the auricle is lost. The degree of deformity varies among individuals. The helix, scapha, and antihelix are nearly normal in form in some people, but they look as if they are folded in others. This deformity is common among Asians, particularly among the Japanese, whereas it is extremely rare in Caucasians (Fig. 55-19).

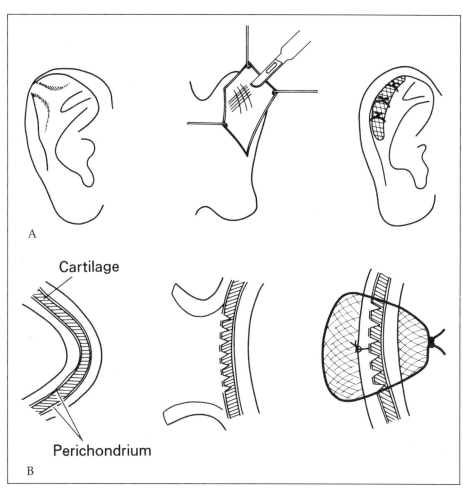

Fig. 55-15A. Posterior perichondrium and cartilage incision along third crus. B. Correction of third crus by incision of posterior perichondrium, elongation of cartilage, and construction of anterior perichondrium. Bolster suture is placed for 2 weeks.

Etiology
The incidence of cryptotia in Japan is 0.26 to 0.28 percent. Several etiologic theories have been suggested, but none of them is applicable in all instances. Maldevelopment of the external auricular muscles and ligaments seems to be a predisposing factor. Because the various parts of the auricle form at about the same time, it is possible that the upper auricle is pulled by the superior auricular muscles and ligaments into the temporal region after formation of all the parts. This theory is corroborated by the fact that the contour of the helix and scapha has been confirmed at the time of the operation to be developed almost normally, even in instances in which these areas appeared to be underdeveloped. It seems reasonable, therefore, to assume that the upper part of the auricle undergoes secondary deformity after its formation because of the abnormal position it has maintained for a prolonged period of time.

Treatment

Conservative Treatment. In mild instances the cartilage is hardly deformed, and the upper auricle does not creep into the temporal region immediately after its release. Such deformities are treated conservatively. A gauze pad is placed at the

Fig. 55-16A. Twelve-year-old boy with Stahl ear and a prominent third crus. B. Postoperative view.

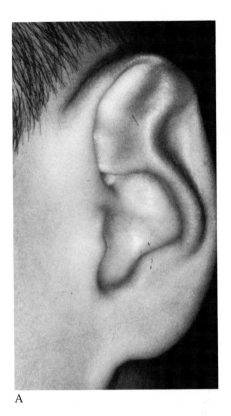

A

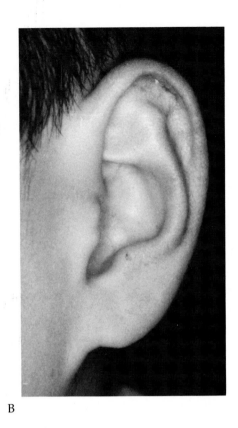

B

Fig. 55-17. Wedge-shaped excision for correction of underdeveloped helix. AA' = outer rim length. BB' = helical rim length. (From J.F. North and N.R.G. Broadbent. Correcting the flat helix. Br. J. Plast. Surg. 30:310, 1977. Reproduced with permission.)

AA' ≦ BB

AA' > BB'

portion of the auriculotemporal sulcus where the buried part of the auricle is drawn out. The auricle is fixed with adhesive tape in the corrected position. A spring splint is sometimes used. The desired effect is achieved after 3 to 4 weeks of immobilization. The younger the child when conservative treatment is initiated, the better are the results (Fig. 55-20).

Buried-Suture Method.
Conservative treatment does not produce any improvement if the patient is older. For such patients, a pursestring suture is placed on the soft tissue at the upper part of the auricle to lift the auricle. Severing of the fibrous tissue that pulls the auricle into the temporal pocket, through a small postauricular incision, makes this treatment reliable. The buried-suture method is indicated for a few patients with relatively minor deformities.

Local Flap Without Skin Graft.
In some patients the buried cartilage under the temporal skin is deformed, without shortage of the absolute amount of cartilage. The deformity can be corrected by incisions or excisions of cartilage at the protrusion deformity. When the connective tissue causing the folding of auricular cartilage is severed, the auricular cartilage expands until it takes a nearly normal shape. As the contracted cartilage expands, shortage of the skin, which is deficient on both the anterior and the posterior surfaces of the buried portion of the auricle, becomes more pronounced. Thus

it becomes necessary to cover the exposed auricular cartilage with a large local skin flap while repairing the temporal portion with a skin graft. To cover a skin defect produced on the posterior surface of the auricle, Kubo and Holmes used a flap from the temporal region (Figs. 55-21 and 55-22). Sercer and Cowan used a flap from the auriculotemporal sulcus, and Ogino and Tani added a skin graft to this procedure (Fig. 55-23).

I prefer the following technique. The buried portion of the auricle is drawn out by hand, and a skin incision is placed on the

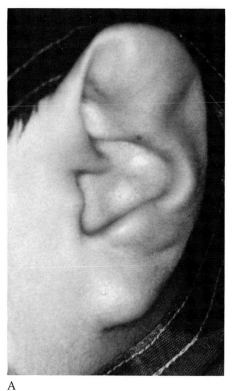

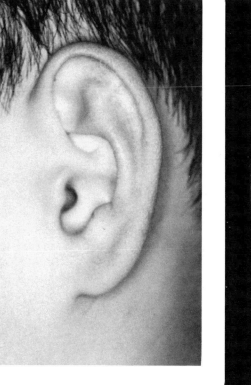

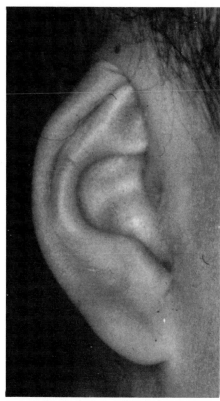

A

B

*Fig. 55-18A. Shell ear deformity with unrolled
helical rim. B. Postoperative view.*

*Fig. 55-19. Cryptotia. Auriculotemporal sulcus is
lost. Upper part of auricle has crept under the
temporal skin.*

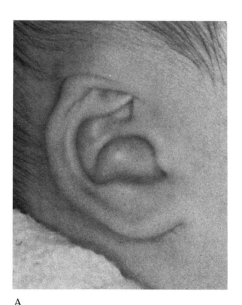

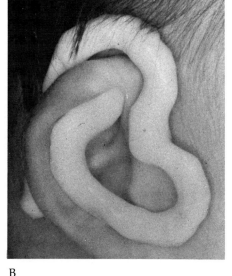

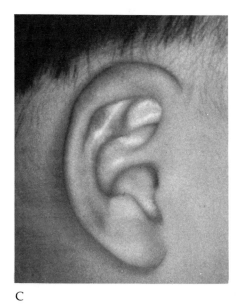

A

B

C

*Fig. 55-20A. Right cryptotia in 4-month-old baby. B. Conservative treatment with wire splint covered
with felt. C. Eight months after treatment with wire splint. Ear is kept in normal position.*

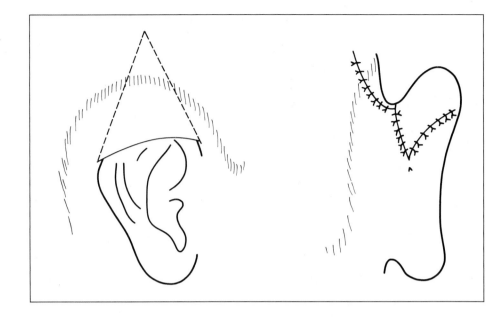

Fig. 55-21. Retroauricular skin defect covered with triangular temporal skin flap (Kubo, 1933).

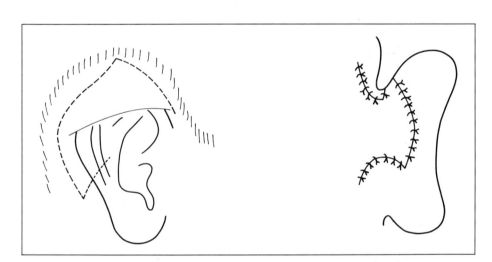

Fig. 55-22. Temporal skin flap method (Holmes, 1949).

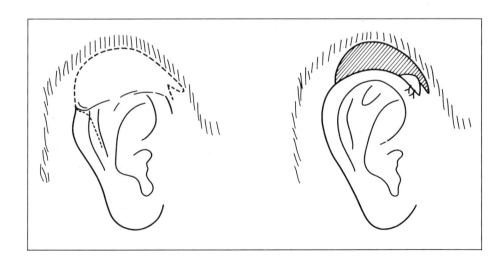

Fig. 55-23. Temporal skin flap and skin graft (Tani, 1961).

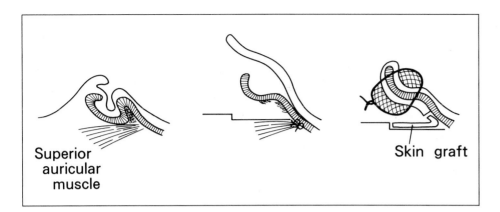

Fig. 55-24. *Author's approach for correction of cryptotia with release of auricular cartilage, transposition of superior auricular muscle, and coverage with skin flap and skin graft.*

Superior auricular muscle

Skin graft

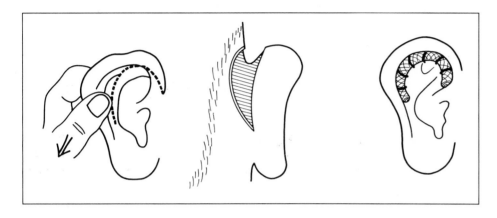

Fig. 55-25. *Dotted line shows incision along auriculotemporal sulcus. Lined area is covered with skin graft.*

auriculotemporal sulcus. The skin from the posterior and through the anterior surface of the auricle is elevated to the concha. Because the skin and subcutaneous tissue of the anterior surface of the auricle are thin, undermining should be done with care to avoid tears or perforations. The superior auricular muscle inserting into the antihelical fossa and transverse antihelical sulcus is severed at its insertion. The transverse and oblique auricular muscles are resected. This allows the auricular cartilage to unfold and expand and the helix, scapha, and antihelix to be brought into position. The isolated superior auricular muscle is sutured onto the conchal process so that the upper auricle is fixed in a protruding position. The auricular cartilage is covered with auricular and temporal skin flaps. It is important to restore the free margin of the auricular cartilage, that is, the auricular rim, from easily becoming folded. To achieve tight adherence of the covering skin flap to the auricular cartilage, prevent hematomas, and form a scapha, the

area is packed with a rolled piece of gauze, and a bolster through-and-through suture is placed. The postauricular skin defect is closed with a full-thickness skin graft. The ear is covered with a bulky dressing, which is removed after 4 to 5 days. The bolster sutures are removed 2 weeks after the operation (Figs. 55-24 to 55-26).

Cup Ear

The cause of cup ear is underdevelopment of the antihelix. The upper portion of the helix and the scapha are bent downward at the level of the auricular tubercle. The vertical height of the auricle appears shortened, but it is found to be nearly normal when the helix is unfolded. The deformity encompasses a wide range of abnormalities from a simple bending of the upper auricle to a small and cupped auricle with underdevelopment of the helix and antihelix. Cup ear is generally divided into a folding type and a cupped type. Tanzer classified it into types I to III, subdividing type II into types IIa and

IIb. In type I and type IIa, the auricle can be reconstructed to a nearly normal shape by unfolding of the helical and antihelical cartilages. No supplemental skin is necessary. Type IIb and type III deformities, however, with the tissue deficiencies and abnormal position of the whole auricle, belong to the category of microtia (Figs. 55-27 to 55-30).

Etiology

Mild deformities are considered to result embryologically from the underdevelopment of the fourth hillock, which is formed from the hyoid arch. In more severe deformities, hillocks such as the fifth from the hyoid arch and the second and third from the mandibular arch are also underdeveloped. Microtia is an extreme form of cup ear. There is no evidence of familial occurrence or hereditary factors.

Treatment

Restoring the Antihelix with a Mattress Suture. In the folded-type cup ear, there is usually no hypoplasia of the au-

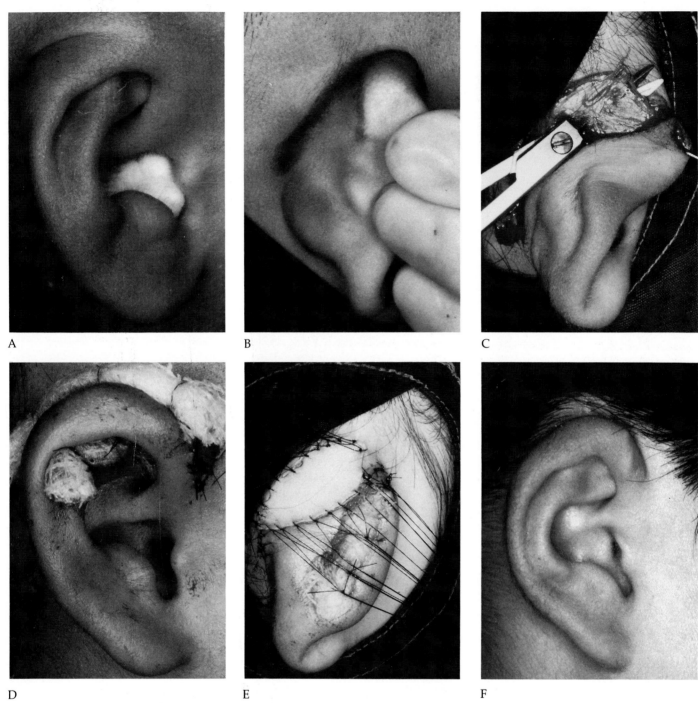

A

B

C

D

E

F

Fig. 55-26A. Right cryptotia. B. Skin incision along auriculotemporal sulcus. C. Superior auricular muscle to be divided. D. Rolled gauze is packed into scapha and fixed with bolster sutures. E. Postauricular skin defect is covered with skin graft. F. One and one-half years after the operation.

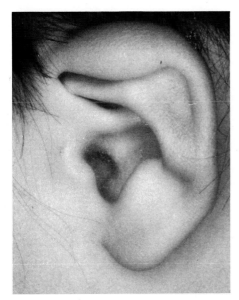

Fig. 55-27. Folded type of cup ear, type I.

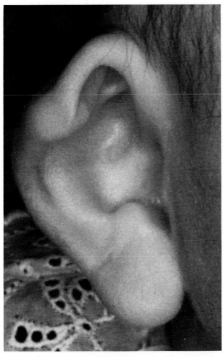

Fig. 55-28. Cup ear. Type IIa with mild deformities of helix and scapha.

Fig. 55-29. Cup ear. Type IIb.

Fig. 55-30. Constricted type of cup ear. Type III.

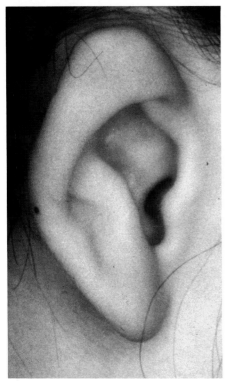

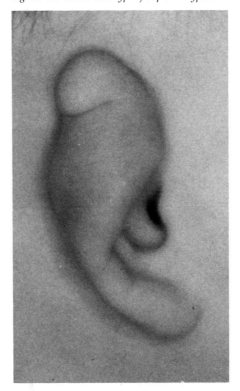

ricular cartilage. The antihelix can be reconstructed, as in prominent ear, with mattress sutures through the posterior surface of the auricular deformity and by building the upper part of the auricle, which is bent superiorly and posteriorly.

Lengthening or Radiating the Helical Cartilage. To extend the hypoplastic helical cartilage in type II cup ear, Tanzer suggested the use of a banner flap from the folded helical crura that is sutured to the cut edge of the helix. This expands the helical cartilage and increases the height of the auricle. The technique, however, is only indicated in a few instances.

The curled helical rim can be expanded with several radial incisions dividing the cartilage in multiple rays. Each ray is kept uncurled with mattress sutures. In severe deformities, a cartilage graft from the rib is used to reconstruct the ear. The cartilaginous frame is then covered by a post-auricular skin flap (Fig. 55-31).

Microtia

Features

Microtia is classified as follows. In type I the auricular components are present, but they are all miniaturized in the manner of a cup ear. In type II the auricular components partially remain. In type III most of the auricular components are lacking. In type IV there are no auricular components or tissues (anotia) (Figs. 55-32 to 55-35).

Microtia is frequently accompanied by other abnormalities, particularly asymmetry of the face caused by the underdevelopment of the ipsilateral temporal, maxillary, and mandibular bones. These anomalies result from underdevelopment of the first and second branchial arches. The severity of the deformity ranges from an externally unnoticeable mild deformity to hemifacial microsomia. Atresia of the external auditory meatus and hearing defects may be present. Embryologically, the external auditory meatus and internal ear are formed from different organs, and the internal ear is usually well-developed in instances of microtia accompanied by closure of the external auditory meatus. If the external auditory meatus is closed bilaterally, however, early reconstruction of the external auditory meatus is necessary to correct the impaired airborne conduction.

Fig. 55-31A. Right cup ear type IIb planned for lengthening vertical height with rib cartilage graft. B. Carved rib cartilage. C. Ear divided into upper and lower portions by full-thickness horizontal incision. Rib graft in place. This will be covered by a postauricular skin flap. D. One year after operation.

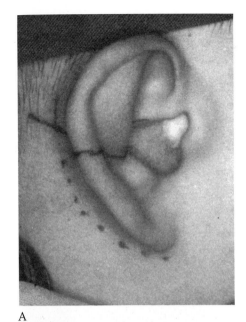

A

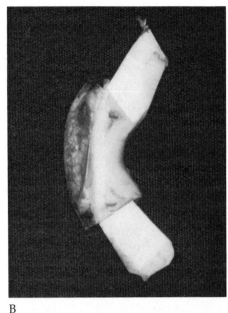

B

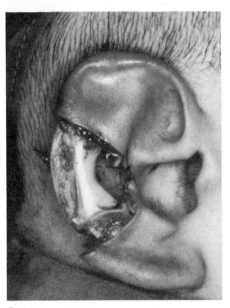

C

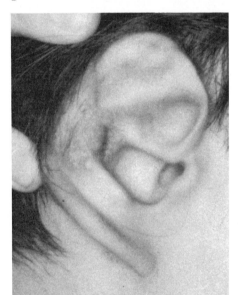

D

Etiology

In the fifth week of gestation, three ear hillocks appear on both the mandibular and hyoid arches, with which the formation of the auricle begins. Microtia has been observed in 7- to 8-week-old embryos, but the cause is still obscure. The incidence is one in every 6,000 to 10,000 births, and the male-female ratio is 2:1. Microtia occurs more frequently on the right side, the right-left ratio being 2:1. The number of bilateral instances is one-sixth the number of unilateral instances.

Treatment

General Principles. Type I microtia and type IIa cup ear deformities are reconstructed by local skin flaps and expansion of the existing auricular cartilage. Stephenson expanded the helix by placing radiating incisions on the helical cartilage. He placed a mattress suture behind each ray of the cartilage to keep it erect, thereby expanding the helix while using Lembert sutures to form the antihelix. Musgrave used a cartilage graft taken from the concha to prevent uneven margins of helix and expanded the graft to a fan shape to enhance the supportive strength. Kislov divided the auricle into upper and lower parts and inserted an auriculotemporal flap to extend its length. In some patients he slid the auricular cartilage upward without dividing it into two parts for support of the auricle.

Reconstruction of the total auricle was first done in the sixteenth century. Dieffenbach in 1840 introduced a reconstructive procedure that used a temporal skin flap. Subsequently ivory and silicone were used in reconstruction, but none of the procedures was satisfactory. The present reconstruction of the whole auricle with the use of costal cartilages was initiated by Tanzer, who described a procedure for reconstructing the auricular frame with a costal cartilage graft.

Two-Stage Method. Stage I. We favor auricular reconstruction when the child is 8 to 10 years of age. Treatment is deferred because at this time the costal cartilages have matured and the temporal region has been developed, and the auricle on the healthy side has attained about 90 percent of adult size.

The shape of the auricle to be reconstructed is determined preoperatively by tracing the auricle on the healthy side on a roentgenographic film. The position and axis of the auricle are determined by using the temporal hairline, the dorsal nasal line, and the level of the eyebrow as reference points. Because it is extremely difficult to shift the vertical axis of the auricle forward or backward after the operation, the vertical axis of the auricle to be reconstructed must be determined carefully. The earlobe is constructed from tissue of the residual auricle, except in patients with anotia. The site of the transposition of the lobule is determined by consulting the tracing (Figs. 55-36 and 55-37).

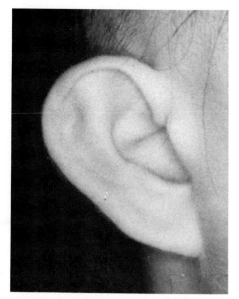

Fig. 55-32. Right microtia, type I.

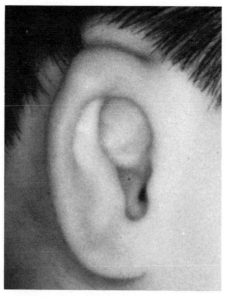

Fig. 55-33. Right microtia, type II.

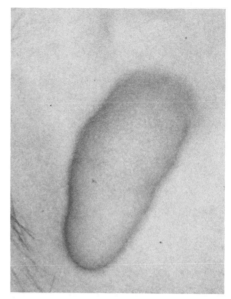

Fig. 55-34. Right microtia, type III.

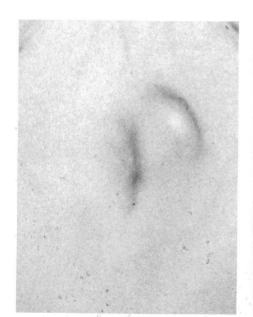

Fig. 55-35. Right microtia, type IV (anotia).

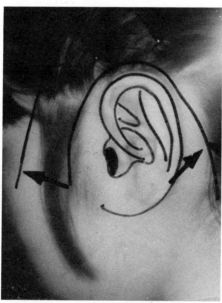

Fig. 55-36. Tracing using roentgenographic film. Arrow shows dorsal nasal line and temporal hairline.

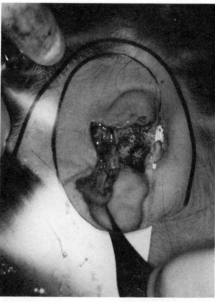

Fig. 55-37. Auricular axis and site of transposed earlobe are determined by consulting tracing on roentgenographic film.

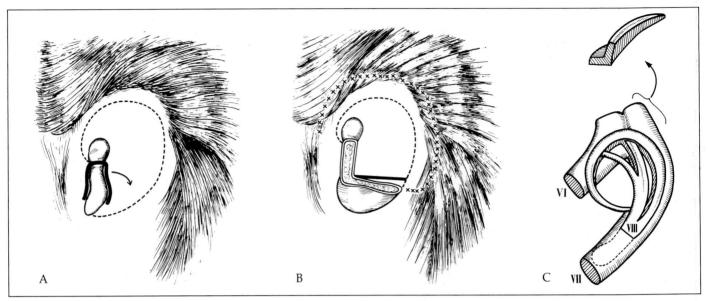

Fig. 55-38A, B. Contour of ear is marked on temporal skin. Inferior portion of remnant is dissected and rotated to form the earlobe. Skin pocket is undermined beyond margin of the cartilaginous frame, which has been rotated into place. Solid line = incision. Broken line = proposed position of the framework. XXXX = area of undermining extending the outline of the framework. C. Cartilaginous framework. Arrow shows construction of tragus with additional piece of cartilage.

Fig. 55-40. Base block is made with cartilage, and helix and antihelix are made with cartilage of the eighth rib.

Fig. 55-39. Template is used to cut cartilaginous frame of sixth and seventh ribs.

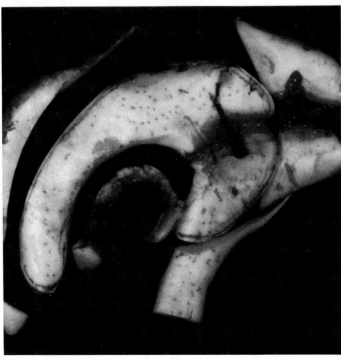

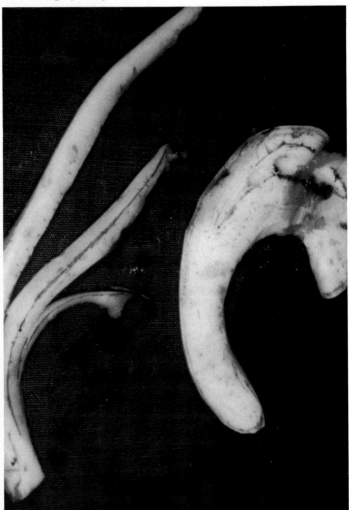

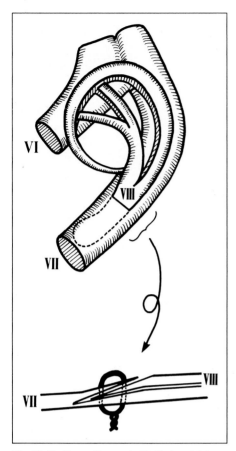

Fig. 55-41. *Descending part of helix is cut into base block to simulate the smooth contour of the auricle.*

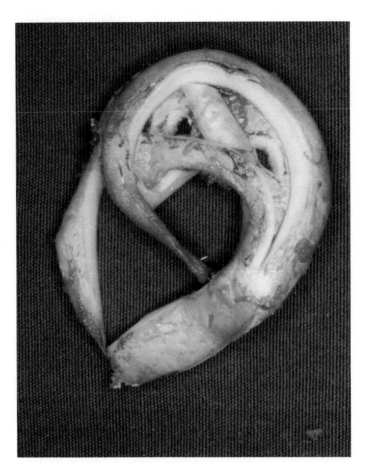

Fig. 55-42. *Completed cartilaginous frame.*

The remnant cartilage is excised, except in the tragus and external auditory meatus. After excision of the cartilage, a temporal pocket is made into which the costal cartilage is transplanted. The skin is widely undermined subcutaneously at the thinner layer, with conservation of a section of subdermal plexus about 2 cm wider than the cartilage frame. The auricular frame is constructed with the sixth, seventh, and eighth costal cartilages. The perichondrium of the costal cartilages is left in place on the chest wall to prevent a chest deformity. The sixth and seventh costal cartilages are used to construct the base of the auricular frame, and the eighth costal cartilage is used to make the helix and antihelix. The piece of costal cartilage harvested from the eighth rib should be long enough to form a helix from its crus to the concha.

The cartilages are constructed into a frame and secured with fine steel wire or 4–0 nylon. The steel wire is always tied on the posterior surface of the auricle and buried within the cartilage by a small stab cut on the cartilage where the wire is tied. The tail of the cartilaginous frame is inserted into the lobule. Before skin closure, the axis and position of the cartilage frame are reconfirmed by consulting the tracing on the roentgenogram of the healthy auricle. A continuous suction drain is inserted through a stab wound in the posterior temporal area, and the skin is closed with interrupted nylon sutures. If any irregularity or sharp edge appears, it should be corrected before wound closure. A sterile drape is applied over the operative field to prevent a leak, produce an airtight seal, and allow for continuous observation of the reconstructed area. A suction drain is left in place for about one week after the operation. I have not seen hematomas or major skin losses with this technique. The foregoing procedure builds the foundation of the auricle in preparation for the second stage of the reconstruction (Figs. 55-38 to 55-45).

Fig. 55-43. *Continuous suction drain in place under frame. Contour of constructed ear is immediately appreciated.*

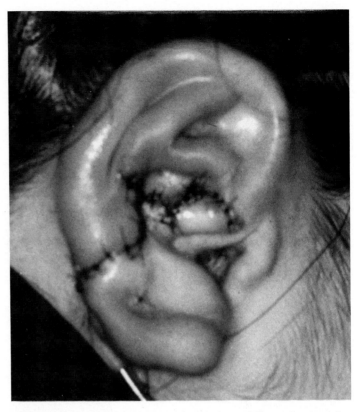

Fig. 55-44. *Sterile drape is applied over ear to achieve airtight seal.*

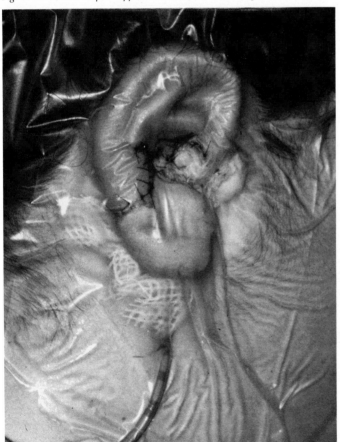

Fig. 55-45. *Postoperative dressing. Suction drain is left in place for one week.*

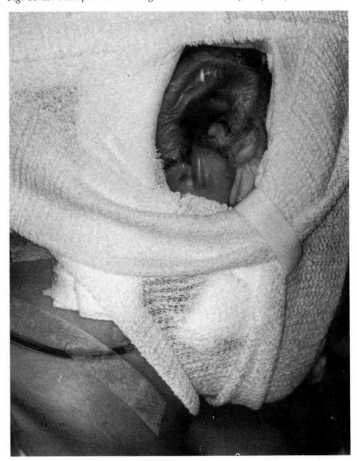

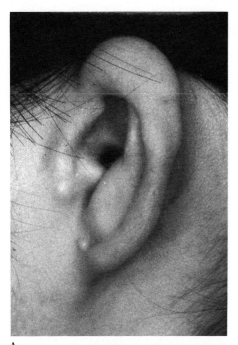
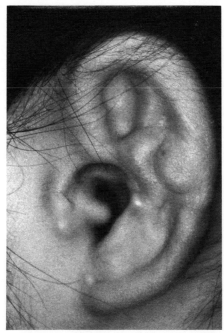

A

B

Fig. 55-46A. Type II left microtia in 13-year-old girl. B. Two years after total ear reconstruction with rib cartilage graft.

Fig. 55-47A. Type III left microtia in 9-year-old girl. B. One and one-half years after total ear reconstruction.

A

B

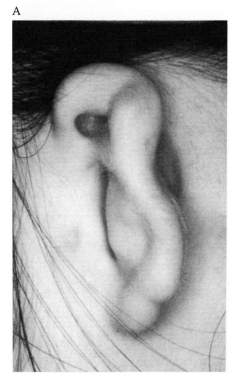
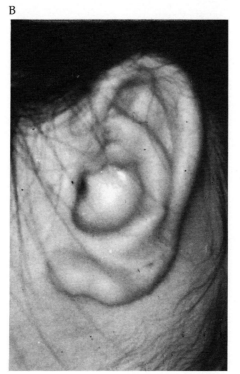

Stage II (Elevation of the Auricle). The second-stage operation is performed about 6 months after the first. The skin incision to elevate the auricle is made a few millimeters outside the lateral edge of the cartilaginous frame so that the final scar is not visible. Care is taken to avoid the temporal hairline. The posterior surface of the auricle is elevated to the conchal cavity with extreme caution to avoid cartilage exposure. The resultant skin defect is covered by a full-thickness skin graft. A tie-over dressing is used to fix the skin graft in position. The second-stage operation is limited to manipulation at the posterior surface of the auricle (Figs. 55-46 to 55-50).

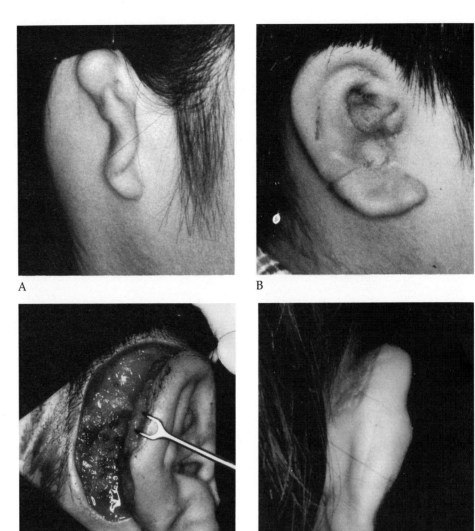

Fig. 55-48A. Type III right microtia in 8-year-old boy. B. Three months after first-stage operation with rib cartilage graft. C. Second-stage operation. Auricle is elevated without exposing grafted cartilage. D. Posterior view shows good projection of auricle and auriculotemporal sulcus.

Cleft Lobe

Features

Cleft lobe is classified into four types. In type I a vertical cleft divides the lobe into anterior and posterior parts. In type II a horizontal cleft divides the lobe into superior and inferior parts. Type III is a mixed cleft with vertical and horizontal parts. Type IV is characterized by dysplasia or absence of the earlobe; most of the lobular tissue is lost. Clefts of the earlobe are rare congenital deformities, but they are frequently seen in Asians, particularly in the Japanese (Figs. 55-51 to 55-55).

Treatment

Because the lobular tissues are scarce, multidimensional reconstruction should be planned with care to avoid the loss of tissue. Passow and Claus used a step incision to prevent a notch deformity at the site of cleft closure (Fig. 55-56). When the cleft is treated by a method based on the tetrahedral Z-plasty advocated by Furnas, a notch frequently occurs at the lateral margin of the lobe. I favor a three-dimensional reconstruction by full-thickness Z-plasty of the lobe combined with a V-Y-plasty of its lateral aspect. In closing the anterior and posterior surfaces of a cleft lobe by Z-plasty, the tissue on the cleft side is maintained at the external margin of the auricle (helix), and after closure of the Z-flaps, the maintained tissue is cut into the lateral aspect of the auricle. A postoperative notch is avoided if this method is used, because the suture line between the anterior and posterior surfaces of the auricle and that on the external margin do not coincide. The direction and size of the Z-flap and the direction of the supporting flap at the cleft edge are adjusted according to the position of the cleft and the size of the lobe (Figs. 55-57 to 55-59).

Fig. 55-49A. Type III right microtia in 10-year-old boy. B. Three years after reconstruction.

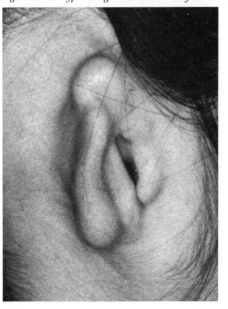

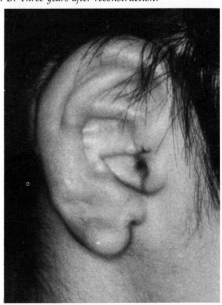

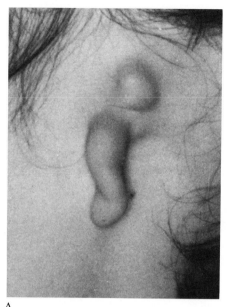

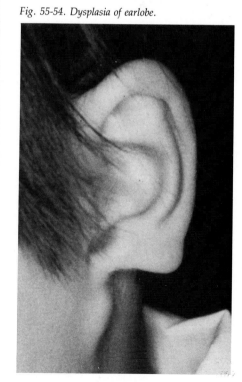

Fig. 55-50A. Type III left microtia in 9-year-old boy. B. Two years after total ear reconstruction.

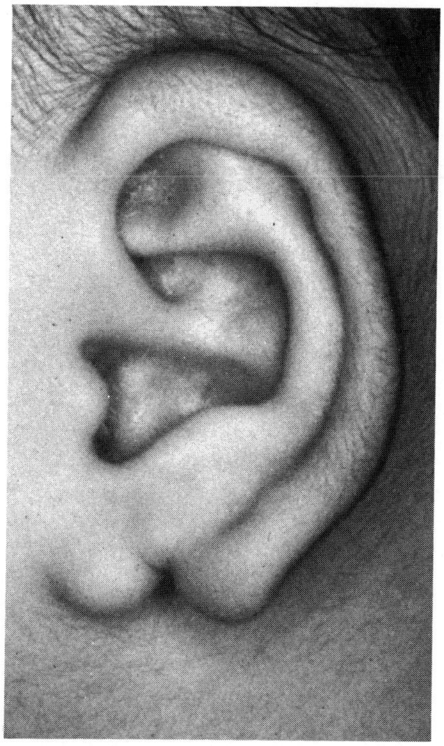

Fig. 55-51. Vertical cleft of earlobe.

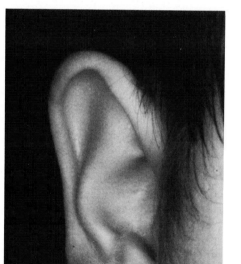

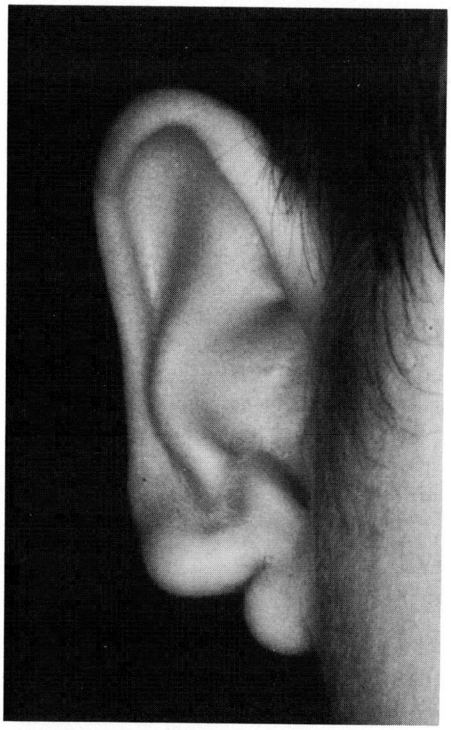

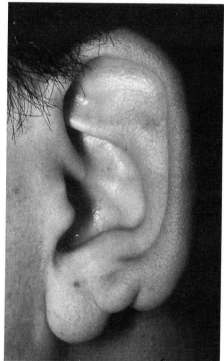

Fig. 55-54. Dysplasia of earlobe.

Fig. 55-52. Horizontal cleft of earlobe.

Fig. 55-53. Mixed cleft of earlobe.

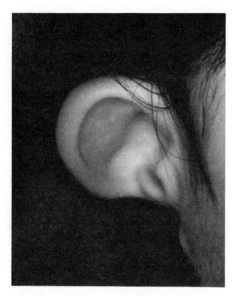

Fig. 55-55. *Defect of earlobe (defect of caudal half of ear).*

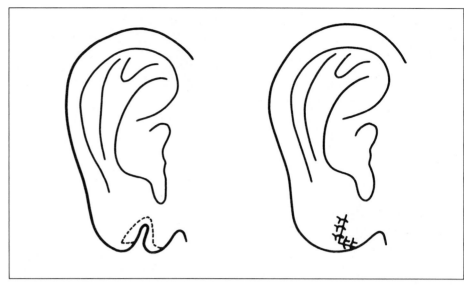

Fig. 55-56. *Step incision by method of Passow and Claus (1923).*

Fig. 55-57. *Three-dimensional reconstruction. Full-thickness Z-plasty on anterior and posterior surface and V-Y-plasty on lateral surface.*

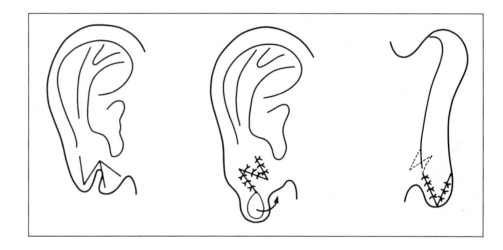

Suggested Reading

Brent, B. The correction of microtia with autogenous cartilage grafts. I. The classic deformity. *Plast. Reconstr. Surg.* 66:1, 1980.

Davis, J.S., and Kitlowski, E.A. Abnormal prominence of the ear: A method of readjustment. *Surgery* 2:835, 1937.

Fukuda, O., and Yamada, A. Reconstruction of the microtic ear with autogenous cartilage. *Clin. Plast. Surg.* 5:351, 1978.

Kislov, R. Surgical correction of the cupped ear. *Plast. Reconstr. Surg.* 48:121, 1971.

Kubo, I. Taschenohr. und Otoplastik. *Jpn. J. Otolaryngol.* 6:105, 1933.

Luckett, W.H. A new operation for prominent ear based on the anatomy of the deformity. *Surg. Gynecol. Obstet.* 10:635, 1910.

Midera, J. A study on auricular development using scanning electron microscope. *J. Jpn. Plast. Reconstr. Surg.* 2:1, 1982.

Monks, G.H. Operation for correcting the deformity due to prominent ear. *Boston Med. Surg. J.* 124:84, 1891.

Passow, V.A. Die Operatinen am Gehörorgan und an der Tonsillen. Chirugische Opertionslehre Band II, s. 7, vom Ambrosius Barth, Leipzig, 1923.

Stenstrom, S.J., and Heftner, J. The Stenstrom otoplasty. *Clin. Plast. Surg.* 5:465, 1978.

Tani, T., Hosokawa, C., and Akazawa, A. Operative procedure for cryptotia. *Jpn. J. Plast. Reconstr. Surg.* 6:121, 1963.

Tanzer, R.C. Total reconstruction of the external ear. *Plast. Reconstr. Surg.* 23:1, 1959.

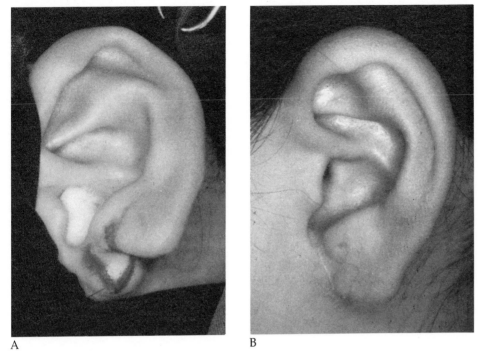

A   B

Fig. 55-58A. Left cleft lobe. B. Two years after operation.

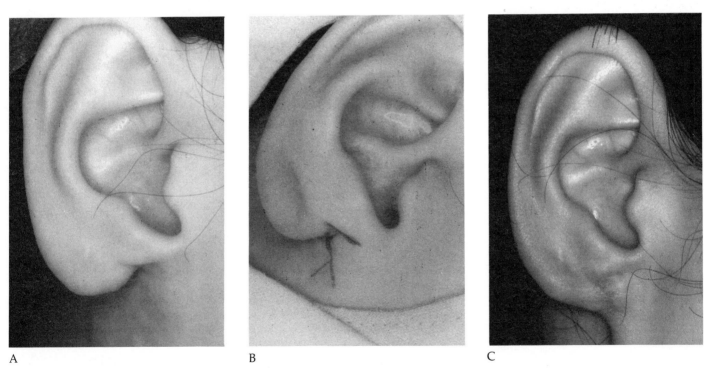

A   B   C

Fig. 55-59A. Left cleft lobe (absent caudal portion). B. Three-dimensional repair. C. Six months after operation.

56

Congenital Ptosis of the Eyelid

Allen M. Putterman

External Levator Resection Procedure

The primary operation to correct congenital blepharoptosis is an external levator resection procedure. This is performed on patients who have 4 mm or more of levator function, as measured by the excursion of the upper lid from downgaze to upgaze. The procedure is not done on patients with minimal amounts of congenital ptosis (1.5 to 2.5 mm) whose upper eyelids elevate to a normal level after instillation of 10% phenylephrine. These patients undergo a Muller muscle–conjunctival resection.

The procedure is performed with the use of general anesthesia in young children and with local anesthesia in some teenagers and most adults. Topical tetracaine is applied over the eye, and a scleral lens is inserted under the eyelids to protect the eye. A methylene blue marking pen is used to draw a line at the site of the proposed lid crease. The site of this line is determined preoperatively by careful measurement of the margin-crease dis-

Supported in part by core grant 1792 from the National Eye Institute, Bethesda, Md., and by an unrestricted research grant from Research and Preventive Blindness, Inc., New York, N.Y.

tance on the opposite normal upper eyelid. (While drawing this line, the surgeon should stretch the skin by pulling the eyebrow upward to the point where the lashes are in a normal position.) The line begins above the punctum nasally and extends to the lateral canthus temporally.

Two percent lidocaine with epinephrine is injected subcutaneously between the lashes and the lid crease line to a level approximately 1 cm above the line. A No. 15 Bard-Parker blade is used to incise skin over the lid crease line (Fig. 56-1A). A 4–0 black silk traction suture is placed through the skin, orbicularis, and superficial tarsus at the center of the lid adjacent to the lashes.

The next step is to enter the suborbicularis space. This is accomplished by pulling the lid downward with the traction suture while a forceps grasping the central orbicularis oculi muscle at the skin incision site is pulled upward and outward. This maneuver tents the central orbicularis, which is severed with a Westcott scissors aimed superiorly and inward. Once this cut in the orbicularis muscle is made, the surgeon should visualize a hole beneath the orbicularis, which is the suborbicularis space. The Westcott scissors is inserted into the space and its blades are

spread apart to enlarge the opening. As the surgeon keeps the traction suture pulled downward and the central orbicularis muscle pulled upward and outward, the inner blade of the Westcott scissors is placed into the central orbicularis opening and is slid under the orbicularis muscle from the opening to the temporal end of the lid while the outer blade is over the external orbicularis. The scissors is pulled outward and the orbicularis is severed (see Fig. 56-1B). (This should allow the surgeon to cut only orbicularis muscle because the orbicularis comes forward with this maneuver while the conjunctiva, the Muller muscle, the levator muscle, and the orbital septum stay deep surrounding the globe.) A similar cut is made from the central orbicularis muscle to the nasal end of the lid.

Blunt dissection with cotton-tipped applicators should allow visualization of the orbital fat and orbital septum. The orbital septum is grasped with a forceps. The surgeon verifies septal tissue by pulling downward and feeling resistance and by palpating the attachment of septum to the orbital roof. Once identified, this structure is pulled outward with a toothed forceps, and a Westcott scissors penetrates the loose connective tissue between the orbital septum and the levator aponeurosis (see Fig. 56-1C). As long as the scissors is kept adjacent to the edge of the septum, injury to the levator is eliminated. Once this loose connective tissue is opened, orbital fat should herniate forward. At this point, the surgeon should be able to visualize both the levator aponeurosis and the orbital septum and to sever the remaining loose connective tissues nasally and temporally to visualize the entire horizontal dimension of the levator aponeurosis. A 4–0 black silk traction suture is placed through the central end of the orbital septum. The prolapsed orbital fat is excised.

If the procedure is performed using local anesthesia, the lid is everted with a Desmarres retractor, and approximately 1 ml of 2% lidocaine with epinephrine is injected subconjunctivally across the lid adjacent to the superior tarsal border. (When general anesthesia is used, this step is unnecessary.) A Westcott scissors is pushed into the nasal aspect of the external levator aponeurosis, and the lid is everted to allow visualization of the tips of the scissors over conjunctiva just above the tarsus about 5 mm temporal to the medial canthus. The scissors is spread slightly, and a No. 15 Bard-Parker blade is used to incise the conjunctiva, the Muller muscle, and the levator aponeurosis over the tips of the scissors. The scissors should penetrate through this opening and be spread slightly to enlarge it (see Fig. 56-1D). A similar opening is made at the temporal end of the lid approximately 5 mm nasal to the lateral canthus.

A levator ptosis clamp, which I originally developed for an internal-external levator resection, is inserted into the temporal opening from externally to internally, and the blade of the clamp is placed through the nasal opening internally to externally (see Fig. 56-1E). The 4–0 black silk traction suture is pulled downward while the clamp is secured by tightening of the screw. (It is important that the clamp be applied above the superior tarsal border securing the conjunctiva, the Muller muscle, and the levator aponeurosis.) A No. 15 Bard-Parker blade is run over the distal end of the clamp to sever the conjunctiva, the Muller muscle, and the levator aponeurosis from the superior tarsal border (see Fig. 56-1F). The handle of the clamp is removed from one end of the clamp blades and is inserted onto the opposite side so that the handle points downward.

The clamp is flipped over to expose the conjunctival surface.

A sharp iris scissors is used to dissect the conjunctiva from its firm attachments to the Muller muscle, and the conjunctiva is severed from the clamp (see Fig. 56-1G). The conjunctiva is dissected from the Muller muscle to the superior fornix. A cotton-tipped applicator is used to dissect bluntly between the conjunctiva and the tenon capsule if a large levator resection is planned.

In the next step, the iris scissors is used to dissect skin from the orbicularis muscle over the tarsus. The dissection should begin approximately 2 mm above the lashes and extend to the skin incision site. The pretarsal orbicularis muscle is excised, and bleeding is controlled by a disposable cautery. The conjunctiva is reunited to the superior tarsal border with a continuous 6–0 polyglactin 910 suture (see Fig. 56-1H).

If a large levator resection (greater than 13 mm) is to be performed, the horns of the levator muscle are cut to allow enough levator to come forward for the proposed amount of resection. A bony eyelid plate is inserted between the conjunctiva and the tenon capsule on one surface and the levator and the Muller muscle on the other surface. A Desmarres retractor is used to pull skin and orbicularis muscle upward; this should allow visualization of attachments of the lateral and medial levator to the medial and lateral orbit. The horns consist of attachments of both levator and Whitnall ligaments to this area. A Westcott scissors is directed straight upward over the temporal end of the lid to cut the temporal horn (see Fig. 56-1I,J). (It is important to avoid injury to the lacrimal gland, which should be visualized during this maneuver.) In a similar manner, the surgeon severs the nasal horn by directing the scissors straight upward. An attempt is made to protect the superior oblique tendon and the bony eyelid plate lying over this tendon by the vertical direction of the scissors (see Fig. 56-1I,J).

When the horns have been severed enough to deliver the amount of levator to be resected, as determined by the formula for the margin limbal distance, any remaining external and internal attachments are cleaned off. If a large levator resection is expected, there are usually attachments between the superior rectus

muscle and the levator muscle. To dissect these attachments, the surgeon uses a cotton-tipped applicator to pull the conjunctiva downward while pulling the Muller muscle and the levator upward and outward. A Westcott scissors spreads any attachments between the levator and superior rectus muscles, and the blades of the scissors are spread apart (see Fig. 56-1K). The loose attachments between the superior rectus and levator muscles should be seen and can be severed easily by pushing the Westcott scissors through them. (Cutting the loose attachments should be avoided because it is possible to injure the superior rectus muscle.) The lower skin edge is placed over the tarsus to determine the site of the proposed lid crease. This maneuver also determines the site where the sutures should be placed into the tarsus. Usually this site is 1 to 2 mm below the superior tarsal border, but it varies depending on the site of the proposed lid crease. When the skin flap is applied over the tarsus, the lashes should be in an appropriate position.

A 6–0 polyglactin 910 suture is placed centrally through the tarsus at this site, and each arm of the suture is passed through the levator internally to externally at the site determined by the margin limbal distance formula (see Fig. 56-1L). A measurement is made from the distal end of the clamp to the area where the needle has passed through the levator muscle to make sure that the measurement obtained from the formula is correct (see Fig. 56-1M). The suture arms are tied with the first tie of a surgeon's knot over a 4–0 black silk releasing suture.

If the procedure is performed using local anesthesia, the contact lens is removed and the patient is placed in an upright position so that the surgeon can judge the lid level. If general anesthesia is used, the position of the upper lid in relation to the cornea is checked and related to the Berke table to ascertain where the lid level should be in correspondence with the amount of preoperative levator function. If the lid is too high or low, the 4–0 black silk releasing suture is pulled outward to release the knot, and the suture arms are placed through the levator above or below the first insertion site until the desired lid level is achieved. When the desired lid level is achieved, nasal and temporal sutures are placed through the tarsus and through the levator muscle, and

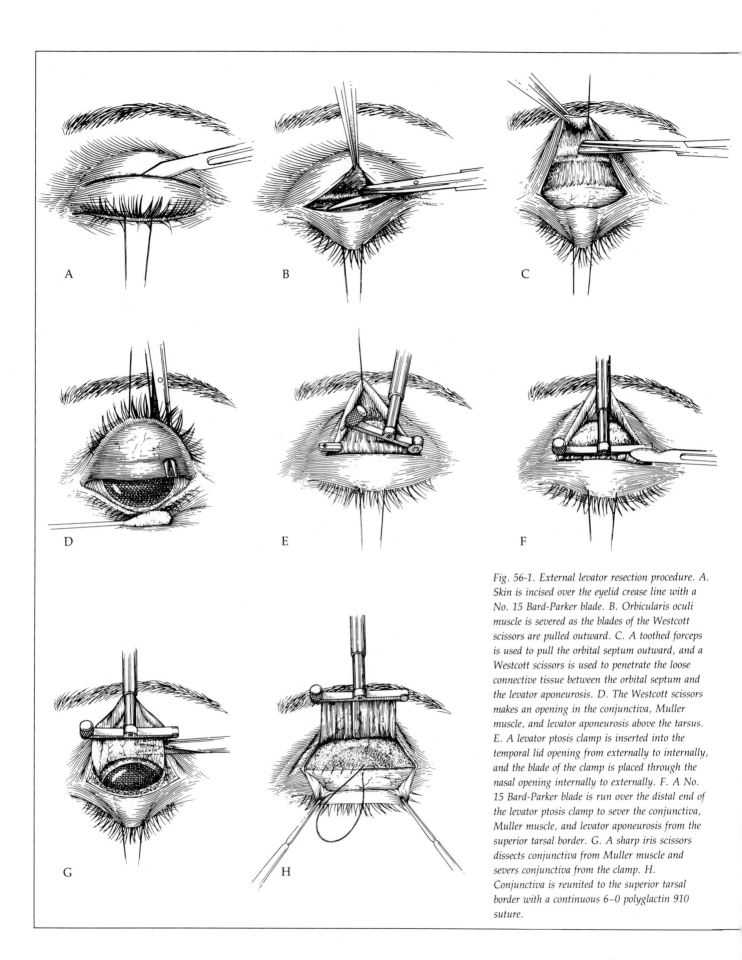

Fig. 56-1. External levator resection procedure. A. Skin is incised over the eyelid crease line with a No. 15 Bard-Parker blade. B. Orbicularis oculi muscle is severed as the blades of the Westcott scissors are pulled outward. C. A toothed forceps is used to pull the orbital septum outward, and a Westcott scissors is used to penetrate the loose connective tissue between the orbital septum and the levator aponeurosis. D. The Westcott scissors makes an opening in the conjunctiva, Muller muscle, and levator aponeurosis above the tarsus. E. A levator ptosis clamp is inserted into the temporal lid opening from externally to internally, and the blade of the clamp is placed through the nasal opening internally to externally. F. A No. 15 Bard-Parker blade is run over the distal end of the levator ptosis clamp to sever the conjunctiva, Muller muscle, and levator aponeurosis from the superior tarsal border. G. A sharp iris scissors dissects conjunctiva from Muller muscle and severs conjunctiva from the clamp. H. Conjunctiva is reunited to the superior tarsal border with a continuous 6–0 polyglactin 910 suture.

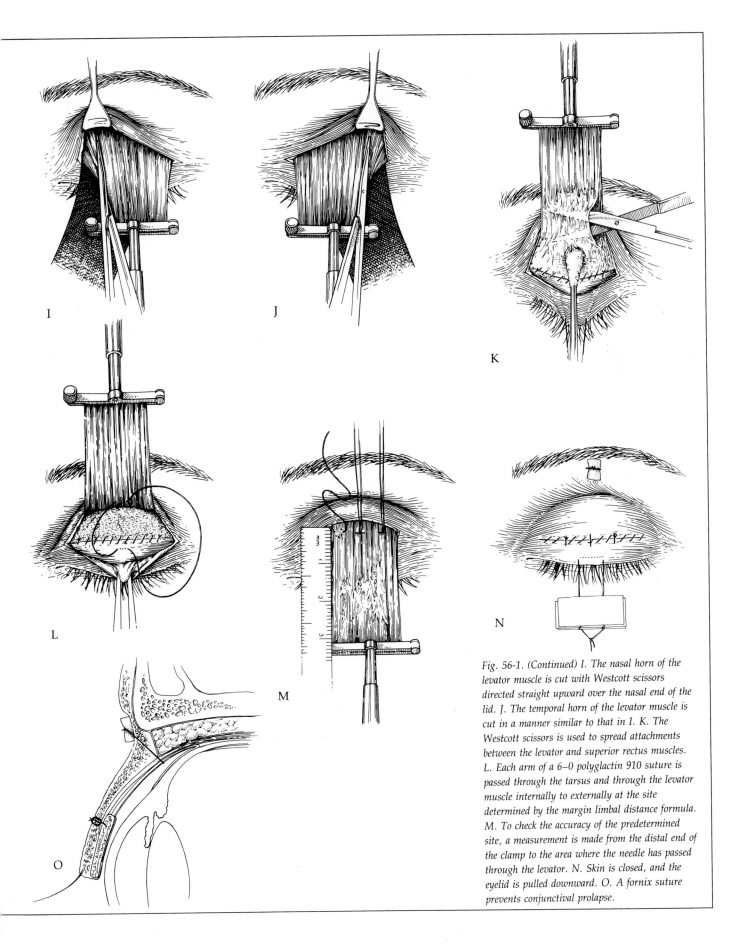

Fig. 56-1. (Continued) I. The nasal horn of the
levator muscle is cut with Westcott scissors
directed straight upward over the nasal end of the
lid. J. The temporal horn of the levator muscle is
cut in a manner similar to that in I. K. The
Westcott scissors is used to spread attachments
between the levator and superior rectus muscles.
L. Each arm of a 6–0 polyglactin 910 suture is
passed through the tarsus and through the levator
muscle internally to externally at the site
determined by the margin limbal distance formula.
M. To check the accuracy of the predetermined
site, a measurement is made from the distal end of
the clamp to the area where the needle has passed
through the levator. N. Skin is closed, and the
eyelid is pulled downward. O. A fornix suture
prevents conjunctival prolapse.

the arms are tied over 4–0 black silk releasing sutures. The lid arch is judged and corrected until it is at an appropriate level. When the lid arch is at the appropriate level, the sutures are tied permanently with approximately four knots but are not cut. Each arm of the suture is placed through adjacent superior and inferior skin edges, and when these sutures are tied, a lid crease is formed (see Fig. 56-1N and O). If the procedure is performed on a patient from whom sutures can be removed, a 6–0 black silk running suture is used to unite the skin. If it is performed on a child from whom sutures cannot be removed, a 5–0 or 6–0 plain catgut suture is run continuously to unite the skin.

If a moderate or large levator resection is performed, a 4–0 double-armed black silk suture is placed through the temporal-central conjunctiva near the superior fornix and is exited through skin. Tying this suture over a cotton pledget helps avoid the complication of conjunctival prolapse (see Fig. 56-1N and O).

At the end of the procedure the contact lens is removed and the lid is pulled downward with the traction suture, which is taped to the cheek. The purpose of this step is to allow the orbital septum to reattach to the levator as high as possible in the hope that this will eliminate postoperative lagophthalmos. A dressing of an eye patch, 4-inch by 4-inch fluffs, and microfoam tape is applied to the eyelids.

On the first postoperative day, the patch and the 4–0 black silk suture are removed. The patient takes systemic antibiotics for one week, and a topical antibiotic is applied to the eye and the sutures twice a day for one week. Artificial tears and ophthalmic ointment are used as needed for the control of exposure keratopathy.

Autogenous Fascia Lata Frontalis Sling

Congenital ptosis with less than 4 mm of levator function, as measured by the excursion of the upper lid from downgaze to upgaze, is best treated with an autogenous fascia lata frontalis sling. This procedure is especially advantageous for patients with bilateral ptosis and poor levator function. In patients who have unilateral congenital ptosis with less than 4 mm of levator function, the choice of a supermaximal levator resection versus an autogenous fascia lata frontalis sling must be considered. I usually choose the supermaximal levator resection if the more normal lid is also slightly ptotic because it is difficult to obtain a high lid level with this procedure in patients with poor levator function. If the normal lid has a high level, an autogenous fascia lata frontalis sling is indicated. If this procedure is done unilaterally, asymmetric results usually are obtained; therefore, I generally excise the levator muscle and perform an autogenous fascia lata frontalis sling on the normal lid also, to ensure symmetry.

Preserved fascia lata is also available. However, the success rate with preserved fascia lata is not as high as with autogenous fascia lata; therefore, the extra effort in obtaining tissue from the leg is warranted.

Obtaining Fascia Lata

An assistant elevates the patient's foot and prepares the leg from 7 cm below to 25 cm above the knee. The leg is lowered over a sterile towel and the foot is taped to the operating table in an inwardly rotated position. The leg is draped to expose the area from the top of the knee to approximately 15 cm above the knee over its lateral internal position. With a marking pen, the surgeon places an X over the draped head of the tibia and over the anterior superior iliac spine of the pelvic bone. A towel is placed so that one edge is at each mark, and a line is drawn from the X at the head of the tibia to the X at the anterior superior iliac spine. A horizontal line is drawn 2.5 cm above the top of the kneecap over the vertical line. Another horizontal line is drawn 3.2 cm above the first horizontal line, and the distance between the horizontal lines is the position of the leg incision (Fig. 56-2A).

A No. 15 Bard-Parker blade is used to make an incision through the skin between the horizontally marked lines. A Westcott scissors is used to dissect subcutaneous tissue until the thick, white, glistening fascia lata is reached. The fascia lata is exposed additionally by blunt dissection with the surgeon's gloved finger; it is wiped with a 4-inch by 4-inch gauze strip to the top of the kneecap in one direction and superiorly to approximately 15 cm above the knee, at which point resistance is met. Dissection is also carried out medially and laterally. Rake and Desmarres retractors are used to separate the wound. The fascia lata is picked up with forceps approximately 1.2 cm above the top of the kneecap, and a horizontal cut is made. A Westcott scissors is used to make a vertical cut over the more superior aspect of the fascia lata (see Fig. 56-2B). Another cut is made approximately 12 mm from the first cut and parallel to it. The rake and Desmarres retractors are repositioned, and these cuts are carried superiorly as far as possible. A slightly open Metzenbaum scissors is used to engage the superoinferior edge of the fascia lata incision, and the scissors is pushed superiorly as far as possible until resistance is met (see Fig. 56-2C). A similar cut is made approximately 1.5 cm from the first cut. The edge of the fascia lata nearest the knee is threaded through a Crawford fascia lata stripper. The end of the fascia lata is grasped with a hemostat, and the fascia lata stripper is pushed superiorly until resistance is met (see Fig. 56-2D). (At least 15 cm of fascia lata should be measured on the stripper at this point.) The lock is released from the stripper, and the fascia lata is cut at its superior end by rapidly closing the fascia lata stripper. The rake and Desmarres retractors are reinserted, and a horizontal cut is made through the fascia lata at the end of the original fascia lata cut nearest the knee.

A Westcott scissors is used to make a vertical cut in the fascia lata parallel to and approximately 12 mm from the cut edge of the first fascia lata resection (see Fig. 56-2E). A Metzenbaum scissors is used to extend this vertical cut as high up as possible and approximately 1.5 cm from the original edge. The Crawford fascia lata stripper is used to obtain a second strip of fascia lata. A Westcott scissors is used to dissect any tissue attached to the fascia lata until it is completely clean. A Westcott scissors is used to make strips of the fascia lata that are about 3 mm wide and 15 cm long. A 4–0 black silk suture is placed on each end of the fascia lata.

Placement of Fascia Lata Within the Eyelids

In all operations, scleral lenses are placed over both eyes to protect them. An ellipse of skin is removed to avoid a redundant skin fold postoperatively except in patients with blepharophimosis. A methylene blue marking pen is used to draw a line approximately 7 mm above the lid margin from the lateral to the medial canthus. One blade of a forceps grasps this line, and the second blade pinches the skin more superiorly until the excessive skin can be pinched together without raising the eyelid. Usually only 7 mm of skin needs to be removed.

Marks are made for placement of the fascia lata incisions in the lids. One mark is placed just above the punctum and slightly temporal to it. A second mark is made at the central aspect of the eyelid, and the third mark is made temporally several millimeters nasal to the lateral canthus. All these marks are approximately 3 mm in horizontal dimension and about 2 to 3 mm above the lid margin. The distance between the temporal and central marks should be equal to the distance between the nasal and central marks. The wooden end of each of two cotton-tipped applicators is used to pick up the skin at both the nasal and central marks and to push the lid upward to see what kind of lift occurs in this area. The skin at the central and temporal marks is engaged with the same applicators to determine the lift of the temporal aspect of the lid. A central brow mark is made 1 cm above the top of the brow and directly over the central lid mark. A nasal brow mark is made a few millimeters above the top of the brow and slightly nasal to the nasal lid mark. Last, a temporal brow mark is made a few millimeters above the top of the temporal brow and slightly temporal to a temporal lid mark. Each of the brow marks is approximately 8 mm long. The distance between the temporal and central brow marks should equal the distance between the central and nasal marks.

A No. 15 Bard-Parker blade is used to make an incision through the skin and orbicularis oculi muscle over the eyelid marks above the lid margins. The knife is also used to incise the outlined ellipse of skin to be resected. A Westcott scissors is used to dissect the outlined area of skin. Bleeding is controlled with a disposable cautery. A 5–0 polyglactin 910 suture is placed through the superficial tarsus at each of the lid incision sites. An incision is made through each of the brow marks through the skin and frontalis muscle down to the periosteum (see Fig. 56-2F).

Bleeding is controlled by cotton-tipped applicators in each of these sites.

A Wright needle is inserted through the nasal brow incision and directed to the nasal lid incision under the orbicularis muscle. As the needle passes the superior orbital rim, it takes a slightly inward turn so that the fascia lata is pulled several millimeters behind the superior orbital rim to prevent the lid from pulling away from the eye postoperatively. The 4–0 silk suture at one end of the fascia lata strip is threaded into the hole of the Wright needle until several millimeters of fascia lata also passes through the needle opening (see Fig. 56-2G). Balanced salt solution is applied to wet the fascia lata, allowing it to slide more easily, and the needle is withdrawn to insert the fascia between the nasal lid and nasal brow incision sites. (The 4–0 silk suture at the brow incision site is clamped to the drape to prevent the fascia lata from moving during the rest of the insertion procedures.)

The Wright needle is inserted through the central lid incision passing just adjacent to the edge of the tarsus until it emerges from the nasal lid incision (see Fig. 56-2H). The other end of the 4–0 silk suture at the fascia lata is placed in the eye of the needle, and the needle is withdrawn to place the fascia between the nasal and central lid incisions. The Wright needle is passed through the nasal brow incision site, aimed toward the central lid incision site; again, a slightly inward turn is taken over the superior orbital rim. The fascia is inserted from the central lid to nasal brow sites (see Fig. 56-2I). The 4–0 silk suture is attached to the drape, and the exposed fascia is covered with a wet 4-inch by 4-inch gauze pad. The other fascia lata strip is placed in a similar manner, first from the temporal brow to temporal lid incisions and then from the temporal lid to central lid sites. Last, it is inserted from central lid to temporal brow (see Fig. 56-2I).

In placement of the fascia lata in the eyelid incisions, care is taken to place the fascia between the polyglactin 910 sutures. The polyglactin 910 sutures are drawn up and tied in triplicate to secure the fascia lata to the tarsus at the three lid incision sites. Several 5–0 plain interrupted sutures are placed at each of these lid skin incision areas to close them completely

and cover the fascia lata. The area in which an ellipse of skin has been resected is closed with a continuous 5–0 plain catgut suture run nasally to temporally. A 5–0 polyglactin 910 suture is laid over the nasal and temporal brow incision areas. The first tie of a surgeon's knot is made with the fascia lata over the nasal and temporal brow incision sites, and the fascia is drawn up and tied until the upper lid margin rests approximately 1 mm beneath the top of the cornea and the lid margin has a curvilinear arch. The polyglactin 910 suture that passes underneath the nasal brow incision site is tied with several knots over the first tie of the fascia lata strip, and the second tie of fascia lata is performed over the tied polyglactin 910 suture. The polyglactin 910 suture is tied again with several knots over the second tie of the fascia lata to secure it additionally, and each arm of the suture is passed through each edge of the fascia lata and tied on each side of the fascia lata to secure the knot additionally. The temporal fascia and polyglactin 910 suture are tied in a similar manner.

The Wright needle is passed from the central brow incision under the frontalis muscle to the nasal brow incision. One end of the fascia lata is slid into the needle, and the needle is withdrawn. In a similar manner, fascia is slid from temporal to central brow. The excessive fascia lata emanating from the nasal and temporal brow incisions is excised. A 4–0 polyglactin 910 suture is passed through the periosteum and frontalis muscle at the central brow incision site. A hemostat is attached to each end of the fascia lata that emanates from the central brow site, and the ends are pulled up until the upper lid elevates to the top of the cornea and the arch of the upper lid is acceptable (see Fig. 56-2J). At this point, the 4–0 polyglactin 910 suture passing out of the central brow is tied over the two strips of fascia lata on each side and the needles are passed through the fascia lata and tied again to additionally secure the fascia to the central brow periosteum and the frontalis muscle. The redundant fascia lata is excised. The brow incision sites are closed with subcutaneous 5–0 polyglycolic acid interrupted sutures, and 5–0 plain catgut is run continuously to close the skin.

A 4–0 black silk suture is passed through the skin and the orbicularis muscle of the central lower lid margin, and each arm is

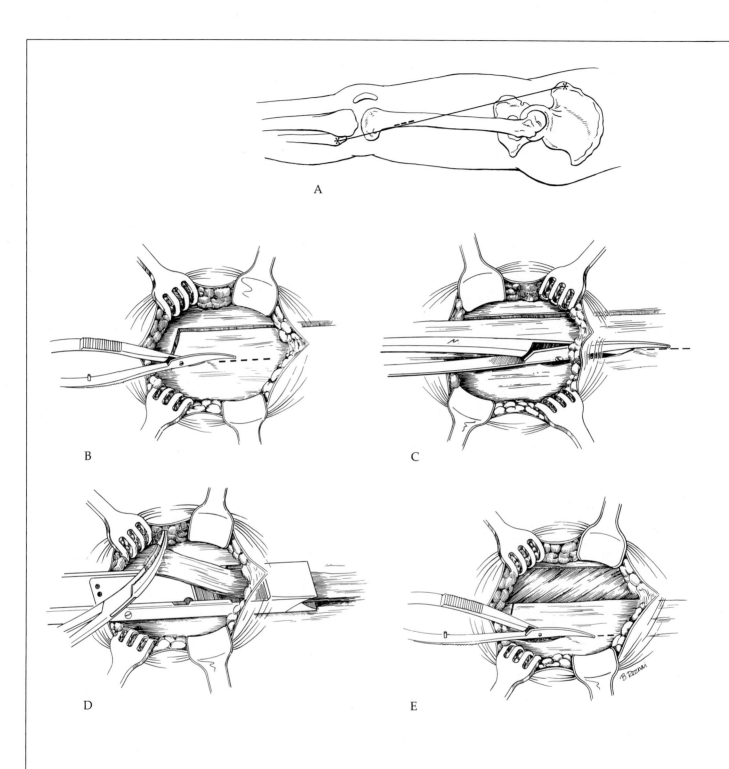

Fig. 56-2. Autogenous fascia lata frontalis sling. A. The site of the leg incision is calculated. B. A Westcott scissors is used to make a vertical cut over the more superior aspect of the fascia lata. C. A Metzenbaum scissors is used to engage the superoinferior edge of the fascia lata incision; the scissors is pushed superiorly as far as possible. D. The end of the fascia lata is grasped with a hemostat, and the fascia lata stripper is pushed superiorly until resistance is met. E. A Westcott scissors is used to make a vertical cut in the inferior fascia lata strip.

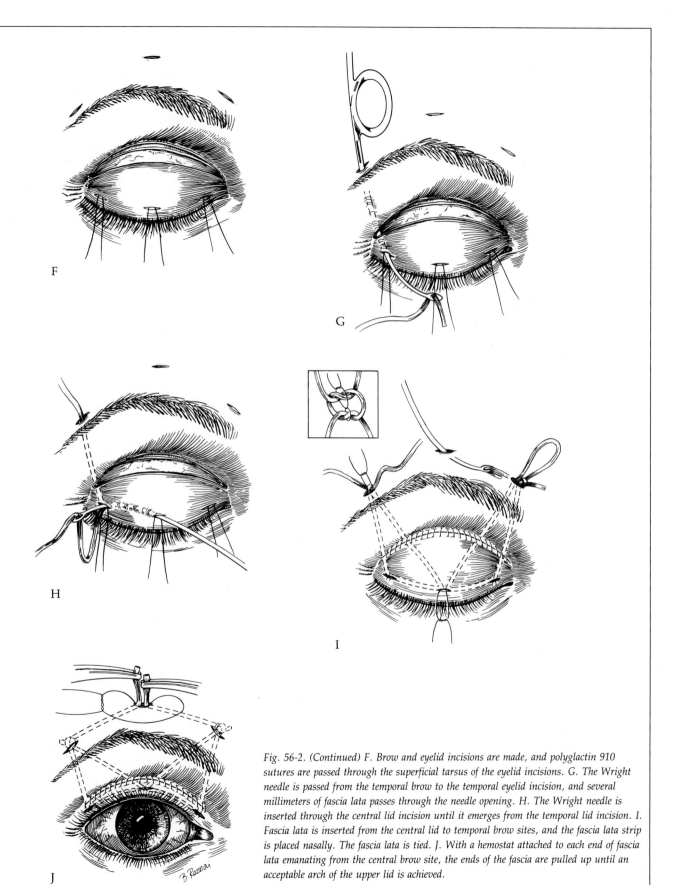

Fig. 56-2. (Continued) F. Brow and eyelid incisions are made, and polyglactin 910 sutures are passed through the superficial tarsus of the eyelid incisions. G. The Wright needle is passed from the temporal brow to the temporal eyelid incision, and several millimeters of fascia lata passes through the needle opening. H. The Wright needle is inserted through the central lid incision until it emerges from the temporal lid incision. I. Fascia lata is inserted from the central lid to temporal brow sites, and the fascia lata strip is placed nasally. The fascia lata is tied. J. With a hemostat attached to each end of fascia lata emanating from the central brow site, the ends of the fascia are pulled up until an acceptable arch of the upper lid is achieved.

passed above the central brow skin incision site. When this suture is drawn up and tied, the lower lid is elevated to the upper lid margin to support the upper lid and to protect the cornea. A pressure dressing is applied over the eyelids. The dressing is changed one day postoperatively; two days postoperatively the tarsorrhaphy sutures are removed. The patient uses multiple instillations of ophthalmic lubricating ointment over the cornea to control exposure keratopathy.

Suggested Reading

Berke, R.N. Results of resection of the levator muscle through a skin incision in congenital ptosis. *Arch. Ophthalmol.* 61:177, 1959.

Epstein, G.A., and Putterman, A.M. Supermaximum levator resection for severe unilateral congenital blepharoptosis. *Ophthalmic Surg.* 15:971, 1984.

Putterman, A.M. A clamp for the transconjunctival isolation and transcutaneous resection of the levator palpebrae superioris muscle operation. *Am. J. Ophthalmol.* 78:533, 1974.

Putterman, A.M., and Fett, D.R. Muller's muscle in the treatment of upper eyelid ptosis: A ten-year study. *Ophthalmic Surg.* 17:354, 1986.

Sarver, B.L., and Putterman, A.M. Margin limbal distance to determine amount of levator resection. *Arch. Ophthalmol.* 103:354, 1985.

57

Congenital Masses and Sinuses of the Head and Neck

Diane V. Dado

Congenital masses and sinuses in the head and neck region can be divided into developmental defects that present laterally and those that occur in the midline. In the head and face, the most common lateral masses and sinuses include external angular dermoid cysts, ear tags, and periauricular sinuses. In the neck there are branchial cleft cysts, sinuses, and fistulas and masses from fibrosis of the sternocleidomastoid muscle as in torticollis; also, there are vascular malformations, including hemangiomas and lymphangiomas. Congenital midline lesions in the head and face presenting in infancy are of ectodermal, neurogenic, or mesodermal embryologic origin and include dermoid cysts or sinus tracts, encephaloceles and gliomas, and again, vascular malformations. In the neck any midline lesion is considered of thyroglossal duct origin until proved otherwise. As with all congenital problems, a clear understanding of the embryology and anatomy is essential for accurate diagnosis and correct surgical management.

Lateral Masses and Sinuses of the Head and Neck

External Angular Dermoid Cysts

Angular dermoid cysts occur around the orbit, most commonly at the upper outer quadrant, just under the brow line. This area is the line of embryonic fusion for the naso-optic groove, and the dermoid cyst is thought to be composed of ectoderm that becomes trapped below. The cyst wall is composed of squamous epithelium and the cyst content is a soft cheesy material composed of the secretions of the hair follicle and sweat and sebaceous glands in the cyst wall. These cysts frequently are not identified until several months after birth; by this time they can be as large as $1\frac{1}{2}$ to 2 cm in diameter, are slightly mobile, and are not attached to the skin. The cyst is situated beneath the orbicularis oculi muscle and can have an attachment to the periosteum below in the area of the frontozygomatic suture. A sinus tract is not present.

Surgical removal is accomplished through an incision within or just below the lateral brow. The muscle fibers are spread apart, and the cyst is freed up from surrounding tissue and cut away from the periosteum to be removed intact. Electric cautery stops any bleeding that may arise from the emissary vein that passes through the suture line from the anterior cranial fossa. Frequently there is a palpable depression in the bone, but when the muscle fibers are sutured as a separate layer over it, the depression is usually not visually discernible after the operation and remodels after the pressure from the cyst is gone. The cyst is closed with interrupted 5–0 clear nylon buried intradermal sutures and a pull-out running 4–0 nylon subcuticular stitch held in place with a sterile adhesive strip. The incision heals extremely well in this area. Complete removal of the cyst ensures there will be no recurrence and eliminates the potential for secondary infection.

Ear Tags

Tags of skin with underlying cartilage are thought to be remnants of accessory auricular hillocks from the developing ear as it migrates from the original site of the otic

809

placode in the upper neck to its final dorsolateral position. The tags therefore occur most frequently just in front of the ear but can occur on the lateral cheek or neck and can be multiple. Although they usually occur without any other anomalies, ear tags are often present in patients with hemifacial microsomia. Many newborn infants with smaller tags are treated in the nursery with sutures tied around the base of the tags. This treatment is inadequate; as protrusive from the skin surface as the tags are, there is underlying cartilage that can be deep to the skin surface. The ligature converts a larger tag to a smaller bump or pit that still may require an operation because of the residual cartilage base.

Outpatient excision can be accomplished with short general anesthesia. Local tissue infiltration with epinephrine is usual, as is magnification to help identify the cartilaginous stalk in the subcutaneous tissue. An elliptic incision is made around the base of the tag, and dissection proceeds until the entire cartilage remnant is freed up. Dissecting immediately on the cartilage prevents any injury to branches of the facial nerve, which are quite superficial in an infant. Buried absorbable sutures in the subcutaneous pocket are used to obliterate any dead space, and the wound is closed with buried intradermal sutures and a pull-out running subcutaneous suture held in place with a sterile adhesive strip. Vertical incisions in this area heal with a fine-line scar that is well hidden.

Preauricular Sinuses

Another common congenital problem around the ear is a preauricular sinus, reported in approximately 1 to 5 percent of infants. These sinuses are distinct from first branchial cleft anomalies and are thought to be caused by incomplete fusion of the first branchial arch hillocks or ectodermal folds sequestered during the infolding of these hillocks. Preauricular sinuses are frequently bilateral (up to 50 percent of the time) and more common in blacks and Asians. The sinuses can be inherited as an incomplete dominant trait with variable penetrance. The external opening of the tract is usually above the tragus, at the anterior margin of the ascending limb of the helix (Fig. 57-1). The sinus can end several millimeters from the skin surface or can pass deeply and

branch around the auricular structures, although it does not open into the external auditory canal. The tract is lined with stratified squamous epithelium, and the surrounding connective tissue may have a hair follicle and sweat and sebaceous glands.

Preauricular sinuses can remain asymptomatic for many years, but they are prone to infection. The usual course is repeated episodes followed by an attempt at excision, which is often incomplete because of the indistinct tissue planes left after inflammation and scarring. Often there remains a boggy mass of granulation tissue covered by thin, discolored epithelium and containing a residual epithelium-lined tract that is prone to recurrent infection. Local incision and drainage of this sinus is insufficient. Wide excision of the granulation tissue should be done with unroofing of the epithelial covering. The wound should be allowed to heal by secondary intention. After several months, the residual tract can be excised.

Prophylactic excision of the sinus tract is therefore recommended to avoid this difficult problem. Again, short general anesthesia is best for children. The area is infiltrated with an epinephrine solution, and loop magnification is used. Although often discussed, injection of the small tract with methylene blue can stain the surrounding tissue as well, particularly if the tract is unintentionally opened during

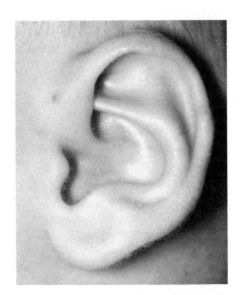

Fig. 57-1. Typical location of external opening of preauricular sinus.

dissection. A better alternative to aid identification of the tract is to pass a small lacrimal probe through the orifice and begin dissection around the stented tract with an elliptic skin incision. As dissection proceeds, the probe can be passed farther and the skin orifice sutured around the probe with silk. To ensure complete removal, a bit of helical cartilage at the base is included with the specimen. The dissection in these patients needs to be meticulous because incomplete excisions can cause recurrent episodes of infection in as many as 30 percent of patients.

Branchial Cleft Cysts, Sinuses, and Fistulas

The etiology of branchial cleft anomalies is not totally understood. The anomalies are generally thought to be caused by incomplete closure of the branchial clefts and pouches with rupture of the branchial plate. Twenty-five to thirty percent of these anomalies are bilateral, and they can be familial. Cysts, which are most common, have no internal or external opening. Sinuses have either an external (more common) or internal opening. An internal opening may not be clinically apparent if it drains freely. A sinus can become infected, however, and if it does, the diagnosis may be made when the patient complains of a foul taste in his or her mouth. Complete pharyngocutaneous fistulas are open externally and internally. Cysts and the lower portions of sinuses and fistulas are lined with squamous epithelium. The upper portions of the tracts can be lined with a ciliated columnar epithelium from which mucous secretions may be produced. The cyst and tract walls have subepithelial lymphoid tissue, and fluid within the cyst contains cholesterol crystals. Although congenital in origin, branchiogenic cysts and fistulas are often not noticed or treated at birth but rather after secondary infections and drainage occur from the fistulas or cyst enlargement occurs because of secretions from the lining of the cysts.

First Branchial Cleft Anomalies

First branchial cleft anomalies are relatively rare. In type I anomalies, the cyst is lined with squamous epithelium (ectodermal origin) without skin append-

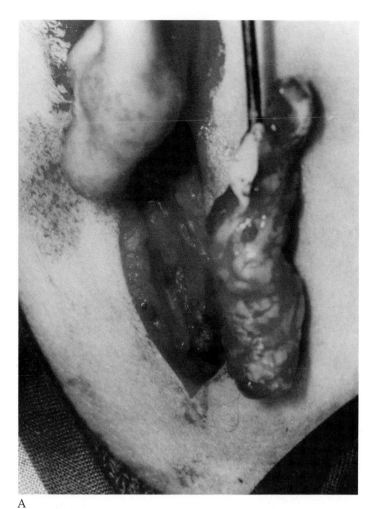

A

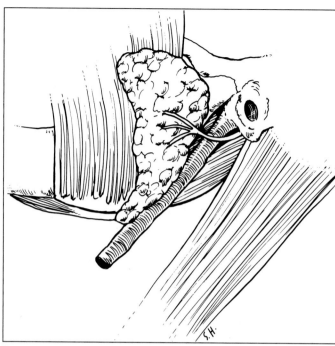

B

Fig. 57-2A. Type II cervicoaural fistula at excision. B. Anatomic relation to mandible, facial nerve, and parotid gland.

ages. It presents as a mass behind the ear and tracks under the concha, parallel to the external auditory meatus, and ends at the tympanic membrane. In type II anomalies (cervicoaural fistulas), the tract begins as a fistulous opening in the concha or external auditory canal and passes along the posterior ramus of the mandible to end as an infected cystic mass or fistulous opening below the angle of the mandible. It can pass in front of or behind the facial nerve and often traverses the parotid gland (Fig. 57-2). This tract is lined with keratinizing squamous epithelium, and hair follicles, apocrine sweat glands, and sebaceous glands may be present. Identification of this tract and drainage from the ear after chronic otitis media is ruled out confirm the diagnosis of first branchial cleft fistula. Complete excision is required, again with magnification and local infiltration with an epinephrine solution to achieve good hemostasis so that the lower branches of the

facial nerve are identified and not injured. Recurrent infections are caused by an incorrect diagnosis followed by incision and drainage of an infected mass or by performing an incomplete excision.

Second Branchial Cleft Anomalies

Developmental defects of the second branchial arch derivatives are the most common of branchial arch anomalies. Sinuses and external fistulas present with drainage from the external opening. This orifice is located at the anterior border of the sternocleidomastoid muscle, $1\frac{1}{2}$ to 3 inches from the sternoclavicular joint. The tract passes upward, beneath the anterior border of the muscle and through the platysma muscle from which it receives an investing layer of muscle. The tract lies on the internal jugular vein, passes superficial to the XIIth cranial

nerve and the internal laryngeal nerve and deep to the posterior belly of the digastric muscle. The tract passes between the internal and external carotid arteries, continues deep to the occipital artery, superficial to the glossopharyngeal nerve, and over that nerve and through the superior constrictor muscle into the palatopharyngeus muscle, which also contributes muscle fibers to its sheath (Fig. 57-3). The tract pierces the pharyngeal wall on the anterior aspect of the posterior pillar of the tonsillar fauces. Although the relation to the carotid vessels is emphasized, the tract does not run particularly close to them; it is, rather, more intimately associated with the jugular vein. The external opening is often noticed at birth but dismissed until recurrent, chronic infections prompt a consultation for treatment. Sometimes an ectopic, skin-covered cartilage tag may be near the opening.

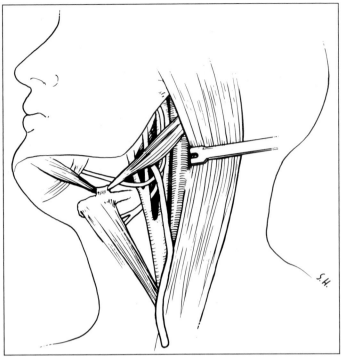

Fig. 57-3. Anatomy of second branchial arch fistulous tract.

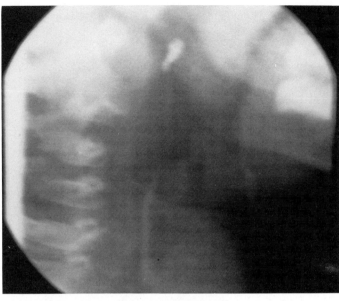

Fig. 57-4. Sinogram of second branchial arch fistula.

Second branchial arch cysts lie on the surface of the carotid sheath, deep to the anterior border of the sternocleidomastoid muscle. They present externally as enlarging, painless, mobile masses in the lateral neck, usually at the junction of the upper and middle thirds of the sternocleidomastoid muscle, slightly higher than the external opening of a sinus tract. They most often present during the second or third decade of life. When they enlarge, these cysts can track up to the base of the skull or forward and inward toward the pharyngeal wall between the hypoglossal nerve and the posterior belly of the digastric muscle and between the internal and external carotid arteries.

The ideal treatment of cysts, sinuses, and fistulas is excision of the entire cyst or tract before infection occurs. Although the history and location of the external opening or mass are diagnostic, a sinogram can be done in questionable instances or to demonstrate the more extensive nature of the lesion to parents or patients when explaining the operation (Fig. 57-4).

At the time of the operation, local infiltration with an epinephrine solution helps to achieve a dry field. The sinus tract is cannulated with a ureteric catheter, which is sutured to the orifice at the skin level with a silk suture for traction. This often passes the entire length of the tract, even into the posterior pharynx. The catheter stiffens the tract, making dissection much easier. Even if it is opened unintentionally, the tract still can be followed for its entire length (Fig. 57-5A). Injection with methylene blue, even diluted, can stain surrounding tissues blue if the tract is opened and does not aid dissection or identification of the tract.

Sinus tracts are best removed with one or more horizontal incisions made in a stepladder manner in the natural creases of the neck. These scars heal well and are hidden. There is no indication for a long vertical incision along the sternocleidomastoid muscle, which can heal with an unsightly, thickened scar. The first incision is an ellipse made in the direction of a neck crease around the orifice. Dissection proceeds as high as possible through this incision. If necessary, a second incision higher up in the neck (usually around the level of the hyoid) is made to remove completely the upper portion of the fistulous tract. The tract is threaded from the first to the second incision. If the dissection stays immediately on the wall of the tract, there is little bleeding and a low risk of injury to any of the nerves. The tract is ligated at its opening to the pharynx with catgut sutures, and the incisions are closed in layers with buried intradermal sutures and pull-out subcuticular nylon sutures (Fig. 57-5B). A wick-type drain is kept in place for the first 24 hours or until any drainage diminishes. If excision is not complete, recurrent drainage and infection can result, necessitating a secondary and much more difficult operation because of scarred, indistinct tissue planes around the residual tract.

The second branchial arch cyst is also excised through a horizontal incision in a neck crease overlying the mass. Dissection proceeds through the platysma muscle and stays immediately on the cyst wall. In this manner, the operation is rapid, safe, and bloodless, and injury to surrounding structures is avoided.

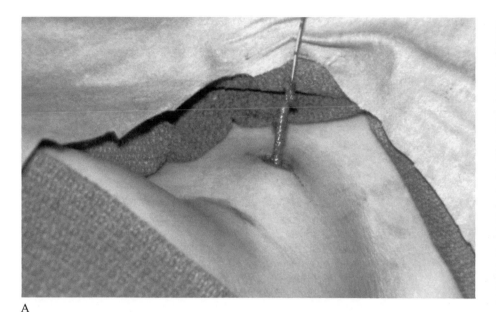

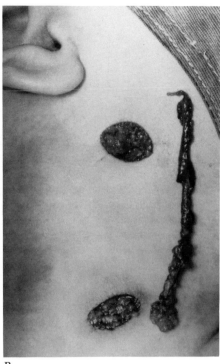

A

Fig. 57-5A. Initial dissection of second branchial arch fistula with ureteric catheter in place as stent. B. Excised second branchial arch fistula after removal through two small "stepladder" incisions in the neck.

B

Third and Fourth Branchial Arch Anomalies

Anomalies of the third and fourth branchial arch are relatively rare but present in a similar way to cysts and tracts of the second branchial arch. The external opening is within the lower third of the sternocleidomastoid muscle at its anterior border. The course of the tract is similar to that of the second branchial arch except that it passes posterior to the carotid arteries rather than between them, below the glossopharyngeal nerve. It pierces the thyrohyoid membrane above the internal branch of the superior laryngeal nerve to open into the pyriform fossa.

Clinically it may not be easy to distinguish between second and third branchial arch anomalies. However, the treatment of cysts and fistulas is identical; the same surgical principles are applied. No fourth branchial arch fistulas have been described to date, but the possibility of a complete fistula is reasonable. Because of its embryology, a fistula would open at the lower end of the sternocleidomastoid muscle (Fig. 57-6) and descend under the subclavian artery on the right and the arch of the aorta on the left (both are derivatives of the fourth branchial arch) and ascend to open internally into the cervical

Fig. 57-6. Patient with history of recurrent drainage and infection through small skin opening at base of sternocleidomastoid muscle. Skin pit present at birth. Parents have refused surgical treatment or diagnostic studies thus far. Opening is consistent with a fourth branchial arch fistula.

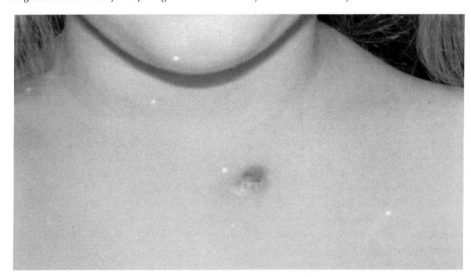

esophagus, pyriform sinus, or larynx. Fourth branchial arch cysts have been described and can occur anywhere in the mediastinum.

Other Lateral Neck Masses

In addition to cysts from the branchial apparatus, the differential diagnosis of congenital masses in the lateral neck includes the fibrosis of the sternocleidomastoid muscle associated with torticollis and the usual variants of vascular malformations seen in infancy and childhood. An infant with muscular torticollis usually presents with a fusiform, nontender, firm mass that consists of fibrotic muscle fibers. This mass usually resolves in about 6 months. No surgical treatment is required, nor should any be done. If no resolution oc-

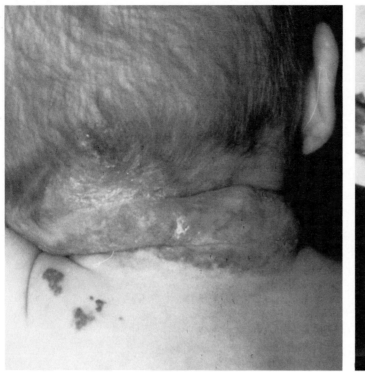
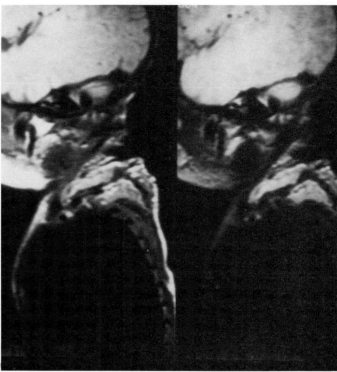

A   B

Fig. 57-7A. Infant with external and laryngeal hemangioma with stridor. B. Magnetic resonance image of same patient. Hemangioma involves all the tissues in the neck.

curs and there is a progressive tilting of the head, surgical release is indicated to prevent the plagiocephaly and facial deformity associated with progressive torticollis. This surgical release is accomplished by making a transverse incision in a neck crease just above the clavicle and dividing both heads of the sternocleidomastoid muscle. The mass dissipates and does not require primary excision. A neck splint may be necessary for a short period of time after the operation to hold the head and neck in proper alignment.

Vascular malformations and lymphangiomas are located in the head and neck region in more than half of patients. Vascular malformations in the lateral neck are treated in the same manner as malformations in other areas of the body but with some exceptions and precautions. The visible external component of a hemangioma or vascular malformation in the neck frequently has a hidden deep component, and it is not unusual for the mass to involve all the neck structures including the esophagus and trachea. In a child with an external hemangioma and mild stridor from hemangiomatous in-

volvement of the trachea, it is unwise to attempt to cauterize the lesions endoscopically in the belief that these lesions are coincidental with the external lesion (Fig. 57-7A). Often this means the hemangioma passes through all the tissue planes in the neck. An endoscopic operation actually may stimulate bleeding within the lesion, and uncontrollable bleeding within the airway could ensue with dire consequences. Magnetic resonance imaging (MRI) can help define the extent of the lesion in these patients (Fig. 57-7B). To shrink the hemangioma in the esophagus or trachea, medical treatment with a short course of systemic steroids is more appropriate than any heroic and perhaps fruitless surgical maneuvers. Edgerton's recommendation of 20 mg of prednisone every other day for several weeks with rapid subsequent tapering of the dose often shrinks the lesion sufficiently, and natural involution occurs afterward.

Lymphangiomas and cystic hygromas can be difficult to treat successfully. The multiloculated and cavernous masses frequently occur about the neck and if large

enough can produce airway obstruction from compression. Rarely, an emergency tracheostomy and debulking are necessary in a newborn infant (Fig. 57-8). Surgical excision is the treatment of choice and is more easily performed if infection has not occurred. Complete extirpation is often impossible, but gross debulking of all visible lymphangiomatous tissue can be done with satisfactory results and a low rate of recurrence.

Midline Masses and Sinuses of the Head and Neck

In the neck, the most common midline lesions are caused by cysts or sinuses of the thyroglossal duct remnant. Development of the thyroid gland begins with epithelial proliferation at the tuberculum impar, at the foramen cecum of the tongue. The thyroid primordium, which is a tubular structure, descends along the neck anterior to the hyoid bone and larynx. Not yet fully formed the hyoid bone is still pieces of cartilage that later fuse in

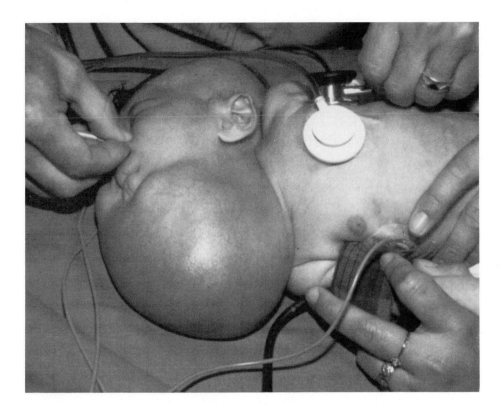

Fig. 57-8. *Infant born with massive cystic hygroma required emergency tracheostomy and debulking.*

the midline. Partial or complete failure of obliteration of this thyroglossal duct remnant results in thyroglossal duct cysts, sinuses, or fistulas. Because of the intimate relation between the duct and the hyoid bone, the tract may pass in front of, behind, or through the body of the hyoid bone (Fig. 57-9A). This fact is of critical importance in the surgical management of these problems. Thyroglossal duct cysts present as a mass at or near the midline of the neck usually after an increase in size secondary to a recent upper respiratory tract infection. The cyst probably forms after the tract, which at an earlier age remained open, became infected, and closed, allowing secretions to accumulate. The mass moves up and down with swallowing. Although it can become clinically apparent at any age, the mass usually presents in the second decade of life.

Thyroglossal duct cysts manifest as draining sinuses from spontaneous rupture of an infected cyst caused by previous incomplete excision or incision and drainage of an infected cyst. The latter only makes complete surgical excision more difficult. An infected cyst is best treated by systemic antibiotics and warm packs.

Only after resolution of the infection should surgical treatment be undertaken. The preoperative evaluation should include a thyroid scan to ensure that the only thyroid tissue present is not within the cyst wall. Additionally, the thyroid gland can be located anywhere along the path of migration of the duct from the foramen cecum (a lingual thyroid) to the mediastinum. Knowledge of this location prevents unintentional removal or injury during the operation.

The operation is performed with the patient's neck slightly hyperextended and the patient's shoulders on a soft roll. Access to the base of the tongue should be maintained. Local infiltration of an epinephrine solution is used for hemostasis. An elliptic incision is made around the sinus tract within a neck crease, or a straight incision is made over the cyst (Fig. 57-9B and C). The cyst is beneath the platysma muscle between the sternohyoid muscles and the skin. The platysma muscle must be opened to dissect around the cyst wall. Dissection proceeds to free up the tract from the surrounding tissue with gentle traction. Below the hyoid bone, the tract is relatively easy to iden-

tify, and dissection does not require cannulation as performed for branchial cleft sinus tracts. The recommendation of Sistrunk in 1920 to remove the tract with a central segment of hyoid bone is still valid today and helps ensure complete excision. Dissection proceeds upward with removal of the entire tract, including a bit of lingual tissue (Fig. 57-9D). Above the hyoid bone, a grossly identifiable tract is often difficult to see, so a central core of tissue up to the foramen cecum is removed. This includes some tissue between the mylohyoid muscle and some geniohyoglossus muscle. The surgeon can place a finger in the patient's mouth and push downward on the foramen cecum to make this final dissection easier through the neck incision. A wick-type drain is used for 24 hours or until drainage diminishes, and the wound is closed in layers approximating the geniohyoglossus muscle fibers. The split hyoid bone can be left as is. If complete excision of the cysts and tract is performed in this manner, recurrence rates are low.

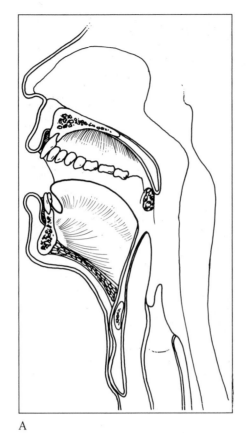

A

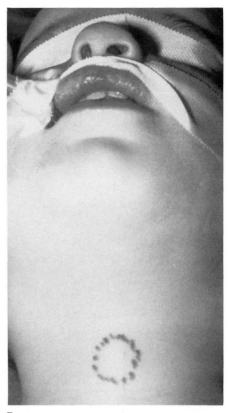

B

Fig. 57-9A. Anatomic relation of thyroglossal duct remnant to surrounding structures in neck. B. Marker notes position of thyroglossal duct cyst in neck of patient during operation. C. Traction reveals extent of thyroglossal duct tract. D. Thyroglossal duct cyst and tract during dissection.

Midline Lesions of the Face

Midline Dermoid Cysts

A midline dermoid cyst classically presents as a fine pit with one or several fine hairs in the center along the mid-dorsal line of the nose or occasionally in the medial canthal area just off the midline. This pit extends inward, into the cyst, and may consist of a short tract or a very long one. These cysts can occur anywhere along the midaxial line, however, from the calvarium to the upper lip. If the stalk is long, it can track upward in front of or behind the nasal bones to a cyst that can be buried in the septum, at the glabella, in the ethmoid or sphenoid bone, or through the cranial bones toward the hypophysis. The cystic dilatation, which is filled with a cheesy material from secretions of the epithelial lining with its adnexal structures, is often not superficial and may not be readily apparent. The foramen cecum is normally obliterated and seals off the dural projection during embryonic life. If there is not complete obliteration, a pathway exists along which ectodermal and glial elements or encephaloceles can exist. Thus there is a potential for intradermal extension of these dermoid cysts; extension probably occurs in approximately 1 percent of patients.

The origin of the lesion is unclear and could be superficial or cranial. Cysts with a superficial origin may arise from an aberration in the development of the ectodermal derivatives. Cysts with deep extensions appear to arise from persistence of the medial ectodermal portion of the developing septum.

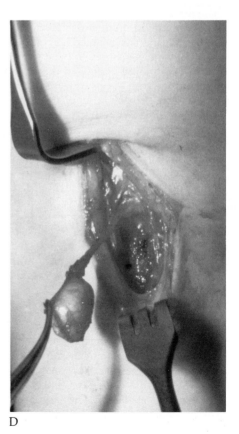

C

D

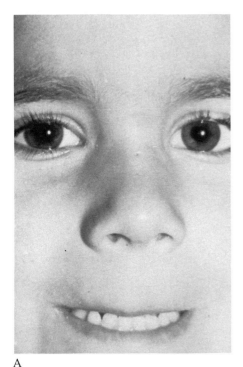

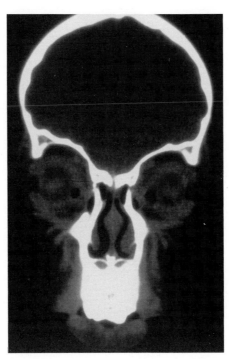

Fig. 57-10A. Patient with pit of dermoid cyst on dorsum of nose. B. Computed tomogram of same patient reveals patent foramen cecum.

Midline dermoid cysts are often misdiagnosed and misunderstood. The potential for intracranial extension dictates that a preoperative evaluation include computed tomography (CT) with 1.5- to 3-mm cuts made at the appropriate level or MRI. When the cyst is without intracranial extension, there may be widening of the nasal septum, a bifid septum, splayed nasal bones, bony destruction or pressure erosion in the frontal area, or a large cystic space identified with the ethmoids. If there is an intracranial component, the foramen cecum is usually enlarged. Cystic dilatation of the anterior crista galli may be visualized as well. If a defect in the bone is identified, a neurosurgeon should be called into the operating room. Most often the tract ends as a fibrous band without an actual dural opening, but rarely it extends intracranially (Figs. 57-10 and 57-11). Any midline, nontraumatic mass should be assumed to have an intracranial extension until proved otherwise. In a recent study of 70 children with solitary calvarial masses, 41 masses were dermoid cysts; 5 of these had considerable intracranial extension, and 10 extended just to the dura.

Complete excision of the entire tract is essential to prevent recurrence. As with all sinus tracts and fistulas about the head and neck, recurrence is often associated with infection and makes complete extirpation of the lesion much more difficult because of secondary inflammatory scarring and a lack of distinct tissue planes.

Excision of nasal dermoid cysts is accomplished with the use of magnification and, again, local infiltration of the tissues with epinephrine to aid hemostasis and visualization of the tract. A lacrimal probe often can be inserted into the pit and excision begun with an ellipse of skin around the orifice (Fig. 57-12A). The direction of the incision varies with the location of the pit. Just above the alar cartilages, a horizontal incision works well. A vertical incision can be made along the middle of the dorsum of the nose. At the glabellar area, it is best to ask the patient to wrinkle up the nose, because there are both vertical and horizontal wrinkle lines in the area. In this manner, the incision can be made to follow one of these creases. Dissection proceeds along the tract with a slight amount of traction. If there is too much traction, the tract tears, making continued dissection difficult. If the tract pass is between the alar cartilages, a gap exists after removal and several sutures can pull the domes of the cartilage together. Rarely, if the tract passes superiorly from the lower nose, a second incision may be necessary for the glabellar area (see Fig. 58-12B). Splayed nasal bones do not need correction. With the mass effect gone, the nasal bones usually remold.

Encephaloceles and Gliomas

Tumors of neurogenic origin are usually not as subtle in their presentation as dermoid cysts are. These tumors, too, are present at birth but are more obvious because of the usual markedly wide nose or medial canthal region (encephalocele, Fig. 57-13) or protrusive mass in this area (glioma, Fig. 57-14A). The encephalocele deformity of the nasal bones is more marked than the deformity from dermoid cysts, and there may be associated hypertelorism. Encephaloceles and gliomas are caused by a herniation of neural tissue into the prenasal space. This space, which is present during frontonasal development, is bounded by the anterior wall of the cartilaginous nasal capsule, the nasal bones and nasofrontal fontanelle, and the dura mater. It is anterior to the nasal capsule. The relation between the neuroectoderm and surface ectoderm is very close during embryologic development. When the foramen cecum closes, the intracranial structures become separated from the nose. Persistent herniation in this area causes an encephalocele (herniation of the meninges and sometimes of brain tissue) or glioma (tissue derived from glial tissue on a stalk, connecting to the area of the foramen cecum but without connection to the brain or its covering, having already been walled-off from its connection with the cranial base).

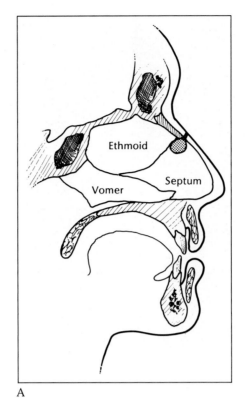

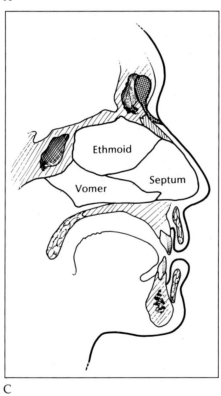

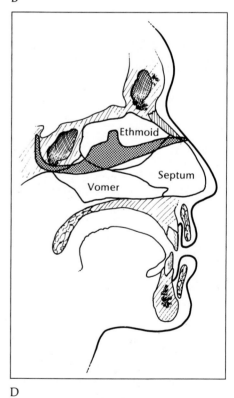

Fig. 57-11A. Dermoid cyst confined to superficial nasal structures. B. Dermoid cysts can pass through nasal bones. C. Dermoid cysts can pass upward to involve the frontal bone. D. Dermoid cysts can have intracranial extension.

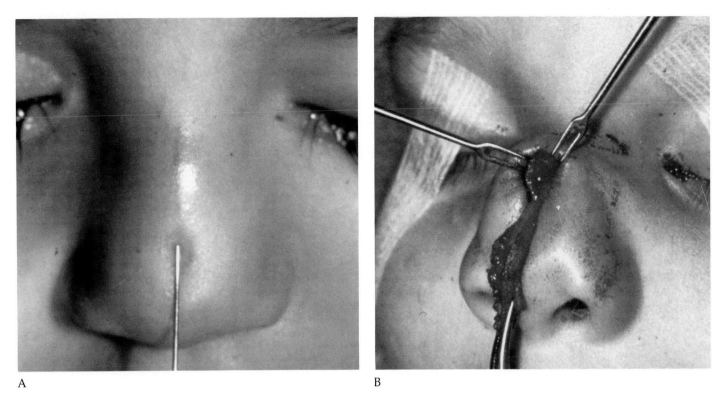

A   B

Fig. 57-12A. Lacrimal probe helps determine extent and direction of the stalk of a dermoid cyst. B. Same patient with dermoid cyst excised.

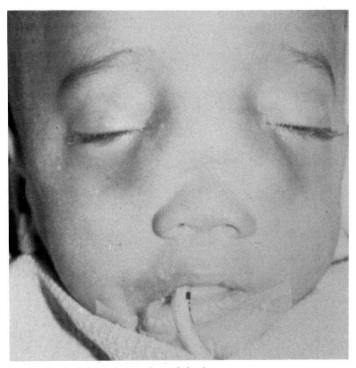

Fig. 57-13. Typical appearance of encephalocele.

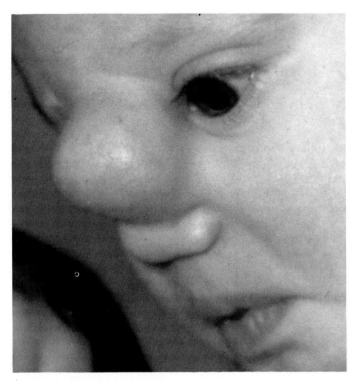

A

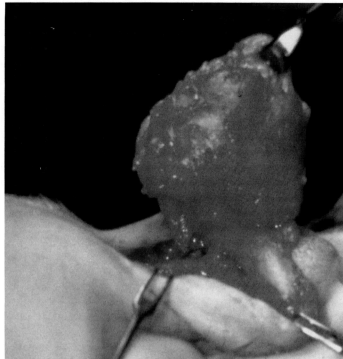

B

Fig. 57-14A. *Infant with glioma of nose. B. Glioma of nose at excision. C. Splayed nasal bones after glioma has been excised. These bones often remodel after the mass is removed.*

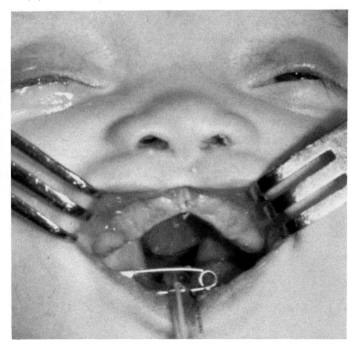

Fig. 57-15. *Encephalocele projecting through floor of anterior cranial fossa into a cleft palate.*

C

The differential diagnosis of a mass in the midline includes a dermoid cyst, an encephalocele, a glioma, or a vascular malformation. As previously described, dermoid cysts often present as relatively small cysts with a central pit and hair. A glioma is firm and not particularly compressible. An encephalocele is usually more diffuse than a glioma; it is compressible and pulsates or increases in size with a Valsalva maneuver (crying and straining). This is because this saclike structure, which is lined with ependymal cells, has circulating cerebrospinal fluid and is in continuity with the fluid in the brain ventricles.

The preoperative evaluation of these tumors is more extensive than that for dermoid cysts. In addition to roentgenography and CT, a neurologic examination may be appropriate, and because of the mass effect on the orbits, an ophthalmologic examination, including a check for lacrimal duct patency, is necessary. Computed tomography definitively differentiates between an encephalocele and a glioma. If an encephalocele is present, there is a defect in the floor of the cranial fossa. Rarely, the encephalocele originates farther back, and the projection through the floor of the anterior cranial fossa is into the nose or through a cleft palate (Fig. 57-15). The size of the bony defect is unrelated to the size of the encephalocele; small encephaloceles may protrude through larger defects, and large encephaloceles may pass through small openings.

Surgical correction should be done in infancy because it can be more difficult if deferred. The encephalocele may continue to enlarge, and skin coverage may be thin and fragile. Gliomas are best excised at this time as well. If the gliomas are intranasal, an external incision may or may not be necessary. Dissection at the base of the stalk can produce an opening in the dura. This needs to be closed with a snug primary repair or a patch if the opening is too large or a larger rent occurs. A good choice of graft within the operating field is temporalis fascia removed through an incision behind the temporal hairline. The splayed nasal bones remodel after the mass effect of the lesion is gone and do not usually need repair at this time. Because the excess cutaneous covering associated with gliomas tends to shrink, vigorous trimming is not necessary at this primary operation.

Suggested Reading

Chami, R.G., and Apesos, J. Treatment of asymptomatic preauricular sinuses. *Ann. Plast. Surg.* 23:406, 1989.

Littlewood, A.H.M. Congenital nasal dermoids, cysts and fistulae. *Br. J. Plast. Surg.* 14: 169, 1961.

Ruge, J.R., et al. Scalp and calvarial masses of infants and children. *Neurosurgery* 22:1037, 1988.

Sistrunk, W.E. The surgical treatment of cysts of the thyroglossal tract. *Ann. Surg.* 71:121, 1920.

Wilson, C.P. Lateral cysts and fistulae of the neck of developmental origin. *Ann. R. Coll. Surg. Engl.* 17:1, 1955.

58

Facial Reanimation: Cross-Face Nerve Grafting and Muscle Transplantation

Ronald M. Zuker

The concept of facial reanimation has given new hope for restoration of social acceptability to patients with facial paralysis. Until recently facial paralysis affected patients' self-confidence, professional advancement, social interaction, and enjoyment of life. Surgical intervention has met with considerable success. Regional muscle transfers, static suspensions, and local adjustments can provide corneal protection, facial symmetry at rest, and possibly even a degree of voluntary movement. The facial nerve not only controls the eyelids and mouth, however, but also is the main instrument for emotional expression by way of facial animation. It is in this area that cross-face nerve grafting and muscle transplantation have made a substantial contribution.

The transplantation of a single skeletal muscle cannot be expected to reproduce the intricate and coordinated movements of the facial musculature. Muscle transplantation can, however, be directed toward oral commissure and upper lip activation. In some circumstances, eyelid function also can be reconstructed. It is the lack of commissure and upper lip activation, however, that is the most obvious deformity in facial paralysis. It is precisely this problem that muscle trans-

plantation addresses most effectively.

The technical advances of microvascular surgery whereby a muscle is transplanted to a new site have allowed a new approach to facial paralysis. In this procedure, the main activity of the facial musculature can be replaced by a muscle or a segment of a muscle transferred from another part of the body. Its viability is ensured by microvascular anastomosis, and its innervation is achieved by precise microneural repairs. Thus the muscle selected for transfer must have an appropriate vascular and neural supply. The muscle can be positioned to produce the precise directional movement required. Its tension can be adjusted to allow for greater excursion. The new muscle in most instances can be innervated by the VIIth nerve. In this way, movement synchronous with the normal side and spontaneous with facial expression can be achieved.

The use of the VIIth nerve is central to the success of the procedure. In some situations there is unilateral muscle absence resulting from trauma or surgical excision. The specific motor nerve supplying the missing muscle is available on the ipsilateral side and can be used to innervate a transplanted muscle. If the nerve stump is very proximal, such as in the vi-

cinity of the stylomastoid foramen, it may be impossible to select the specific site of the stump that will provide the precise innervation desired, such as elevation of the upper lip and commissure. In such situations it may be better to disregard the ipsilateral facial nerve.

Most patients with long-standing facial paralysis have a functional or anatomic absence of facial nerves and facial muscles. This occurs in congenital facial palsy and in the acquired paralysis following Bell palsy or surgical intervention, such as excision of an acoustic neuroma. In the acquired situations, the proximal nerve is irretrievably damaged. Also, because of the prolonged lack of innervation, the facial musculature served by the damaged nerve loses its ability to recover function. Thus not only must the facial musculature be replaced, but also additional neural input must be supplied. To achieve this additional VIIth nerve input, a cross-face nerve graft is used. This procedure, which is described here in detail, sets the stage for the muscle transplant, which in turn is innervated by this graft. The use of the VIIth nerve ensures spontaneous activity of the muscle with facial expressions, specifically smiles. These operations are spaced approximately one year apart so that the time for muscle reinner-

Table 58-1. Reanimation of facial paralysis

Condition	Procedure
Ipsilateral VIIth nerve available	Muscle transplant (with VIIth nerve stump)
Ipsilateral VIIth nerve not available	Cross-face nerve graft and muscle transplant
Bilateral VIIth nerve not available	Muscle transplant (with other motor nerve)

vation is minimized.

In some situations the facial paralysis is bilateral on either a congenital basis, as in Möbius syndrome, or an acquired basis, as in bilateral acoustic neuromas. Because no VIIth nerve input is available, no spontaneous movement with facial expression is possible. However, a degree of facial animation still can be achieved with muscle transplantation. The muscle is innervated by another regional motor nerve such as a segment of the nerve to the masseter muscle (V), a fascicle of the hypoglossal nerve (XII), or a fascicle of the accessory nerve (XI), as outlined in Table 58-1.

Indications and Timing

The indications for microsurgical facial reanimation include a degree of facial paralysis that substantially affects the professional or social activities of the patient. The potential gains of the reconstruction must be weighed against the risks of a prolonged operation, several days of hospitalization and postsurgical recovery, and the rehabilitative phase. A realistic appraisal of what is possible must coincide with the patient's expectations if success is to be achieved.

Because the reconstruction may involve two procedures spaced one year apart, careful consideration must be given to the timing of the intervention. Reconstruction should begin when no further recovery from the facial paralysis is anticipated. Although results seem to be better among younger patients, reconstruction can be carried out with benefit in patients in the fifth or sixth decade of life. In children it is desirable to have the reconstruction completed by the time the child enters the first grade. Thus the muscle transplant procedure should be planned for when the child is 5 years of age; this allows approximately one year for function to improve gradually and to plateau. At this age the vessels are of adequate size and

the child can participate effectively in postsurgical symmetry and strengthening rehabilitative measures.

If needed to activate the muscle transplant, a cross-face nerve graft should be done about one year before the muscle transplant or when the child is 4 years of age. Children tolerate the complex and often prolonged surgical procedure extremely well at this early age. Of course the timing of surgical intervention is influenced by the age at presentation or referral.

Preoperative Planning

Each patient must be evaluated to assess the severity of the paralysis and the functional and social limitations this has imposed. Ancillary procedures for protection of the cornea and of eyelid function may be necessary, but their discussion is beyond the scope of this chapter. The oral configuration is studied carefully. Measurements on the normal side are made; specific note is made of midline deviation at rest and with activation. The extent of excursion on the normal side is noted, and particular attention is paid to the direction of commissure and upper lip movement. In this way, the extent of movement and the direction of movement to be reconstructed can be planned. The vasculature at the recipient site is assessed by palpation or Doppler ultrasonography. Preference for muscle revascularization is given to the facial vessels; however, if these are not available, the superficial temporal vessels may be used. In unusual instances, vein grafting to vessels in the neck may be necessary.

The motor nerve that will innervate the muscle is of critical importance. The decision must be made preoperatively regarding which nerve will be used. It is preferable to use the ipsilateral zygomatic or buccal branches of the facial nerve if these are available. If this potential does

not exist, a stage-setting cross-face nerve graft is necessary. In this situation two nerve repairs are required for innervation to enter the muscle. Because a huge amount of axon deletion occurs across these nerve repairs, this procedure is less reliable than direct muscle innervation with a single nerve repair. In bilateral facial paralysis in which no facial nerve is available on either side, the motor nerve to the masseter muscle or a single fascicle of the hypoglossal nerve or of the accessory nerve may be selected. In bilateral congenital facial palsy (Möbius syndrome), other cranial nerves are often involved, and thus the selection of a normal motor nerve that will not leave an additional deficit is critical.

It is important to note that the hypoglossal nerve (XII) is frequently involved to some extent. If it is, it should be avoided and a different nerve selected, such as a portion of the nerve to the masseter muscle (V) or a portion of the accessory nerve (XI). Clearly a thorough discussion of the complexity of the procedure and of the potential outcome must be undertaken with the patient.

Cross-Face Nerve Grafting

A cross-face nerve graft is necessary in unilateral facial paralysis to provide facial nerve (VII) input from the contralateral side (Fig. 58-1). Through a preauricular incision on the normal side with extension to the mastoid region, a cheek flap is raised above the level of the parotid fascia. The branches of the facial nerve are identified as they pass anteriorly, exiting the parotid at its most anterior margin. Because muscle relaxants are not used, these facial nerve branches can be stimulated and their specific response observed. Particular attention is directed toward the zygomatic and buccal branches. Three to five fascicles are selected for transection, leaving sufficient nerve input to power the musculature on the normal side. A tunnel is made across the face, aided by incisions in both nasal vestibules and the preauricular area on the paralyzed side. This tunnel is placed just above the upper lip and deep to the mucosa of the nasal vestibule. On the paralyzed side it courses upward toward the infraorbital margin over the body of the

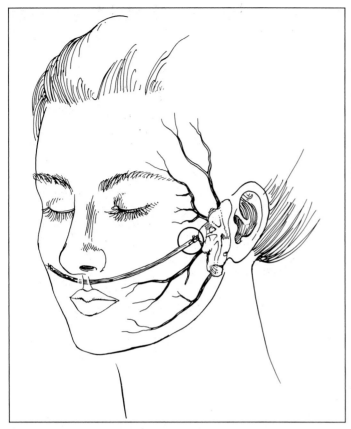

Fig. 58-1. *Cross-face nerve graft in position, sutured to a branch of the facial nerve on normal side and banked in the pretragal region on the paralyzed side.*

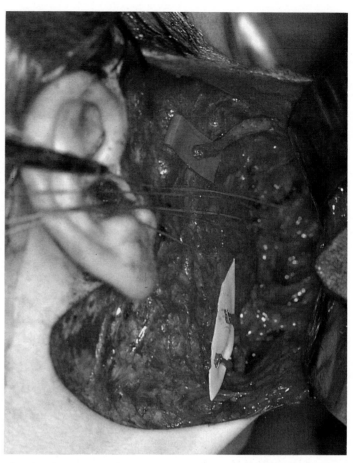

Fig. 58-2. *Preparation of face for muscle transplantation. Note nerve graft at top and recipient facial vessels below.*

maxilla and zygoma. It continues to the pretragal region on the paralyzed side. The nerve graft is placed in this position so that it need not be disturbed when the muscle transplant is inserted.

When the sural nerve is harvested, it is reversed in its direction and placed in the tunnel. A fascicular nerve repair with 11–0 nylon sutures is effected between these selected branches of the facial nerve on the normal side and the sural nerve graft. The stump of the sural nerve graft is positioned and anchored in the pretragal region. Reinnervation of this nerve graft can be followed using the Tinel sign; it generally reaches the stump of the graft in 9 to 12 months. At this time, muscle transplantation can be carried out using this nerve graft to innervate the muscle.

Muscle Transplantation

As in all free tissue transfers, the transplantation of skeletal muscle for facial reanimation can be divided into three stages—preparation of the recipient site, elevation of the donor muscle, and muscle transplantation with revascularization and reinnervation. The site of muscle insertion and direction of movement should be planned preoperatively to achieve symmetry with the normal side. The recipient site is prepared through a preauricular incision with a submandibular extension to the midpoint of the mandibular body. A cheek flap is elevated at the junction of the fascia and subcutaneous tissue. A subcutaneous pocket is thereby made that extends to the commissure and residual musculature of the upper lip and to the inferior portion of the zygoma and zygomatic arch.

Accurate anchoring of the muscle to the commissure and upper lip is extremely important. To avoid lip eversion, anchoring sutures should be placed on the deep surface of the residual orbicularis musculature. Four sutures are usually necessary. The first is placed at the commissure itself. The second is placed below and slightly medially at the lateral border of the lower lip to reproduce a commissural fold. The third and fourth sutures are placed in the upper lip to construct a nasolabial fold. Occasionally additional sutures in the upper lip are necessary to accomplish this anchoring.

After the anchoring sutures are placed, the site of the muscle origin is prepared. This site varies from individual to individual, but it generally involves the lower margin of the maxilla and zygoma and the anterior segment of the zygomatic arch. The muscle should lie flush with the bone to avoid an unnatural bulge. Thus the inferior portion of the bony structures involved should be cleared to the periosteum to provide the appropriate location for the anchoring origin sutures.

The motor nerve to be used is identified. This may be the zygomatic or buccal branches of the ipsilateral facial nerve, the previously placed cross-face nerve graft, or another regional motor nerve for which there is no facial nerve bilaterally. If a segment of the hypoglossal nerve is to be used, it is identified in the neck using the digastric muscle as a guide and dissected into the tongue musculature itself. A single fascicle is identified, transected, and reflected back laterally toward the surface for ease in the nerve repair. If the motor nerve to the masseter muscle is to be used, it is identified as it courses beneath the midportion of the zygomatic arch before entering the deep surface of the masseter muscle itself. It is important to evaluate the fascicular pattern of the distal segment of the nerve to be used. Normal-appearing fascicles must be used, and in a transfacial nerve graft this should be confirmed by quick section. The largest, least fibrotic, and healthiest-appearing fascicle of the cross-face nerve graft should be selected to innervate the transplant.

The next step involves preparation of the recipient vessels. Generally, the facial artery and vein are available. These are readily located on the external surface of the midportion of the mandibular body. The artery courses anteriorly toward the oral commissure, whereas the vein courses superiorly. The vessels are dissected into the cheek, transected distally, and reflected posteriorly. Usually, this procedure puts the vessels in an excellent position for the microvascular anastomoses (Fig. 58-2). If the facial vessels are not available, the superficial temporal vessels can be used; in unusual circumstances vein grafting to the neck may be necessary.

Isolation of the donor muscle usually can be simultaneous with the facial dissection. Many muscles have been used, including the pectoralis minor, latissimus dorsi, serratus anterior, rectus abdominis, and extensor digitorum brevis. At the Hospital for Sick Children, the preferred muscle currently is a segmental section of the gracilis. The gracilis muscle has a neurovascular pedicle that is ideal for free tissue transfer. The problem of excess bulk can be avoided by using a small segment of the gracilis, the precise size required. There is no functional donor deficit, and the resultant donor scar in the proximal thigh is quite acceptable. The muscle is easily identified in its superficial position just posterior to the adductor longus, whose tendon of origin is easily palpated with the hip abducted and externally rotated. The dominant pedicle is located 8 to 12 cm from the origin, consisting of a central artery and paired venae comitantes. It can be traced to its origin from the profunda femoris artery, which provides a vascular pedicle of 6 to 7 cm. The motor nerve of the gracilis muscle is a branch of the obturator nerve; it enters the muscle just proximal to the vascular pedicle at a 45° angle. The motor nerve is easily traced proximally to the inguinal ligament by retracting the adductor longus muscle.

After the neurovascular pedicle is isolated, the segment of the muscle to be used is freed circumferentially. This is usually about a 10-cm length centered on the neurovascular pedicle. Once the pedicle and muscle are isolated, the fascicular pattern of the motor nerve is noted proximal to the site of predicted nerve repair. The two to four fascicles present at this level are individually stimulated, and the segmental contraction of the gracilis muscle is noted. Different fascicles lead to contraction of different segments of the muscle. Approximately one-third of the circumference of the muscle is needed to produce the appropriate amount of movement and avoid excessive bulk. The anterior third of the muscle is generally selected, and the fascicle that stimulates this segment is identified. This is the key fascicle to be repaired and should be marked. The muscle is divided longitudinally along the plane of differential contraction. Great care is taken not to separate the muscle that is to be transferred from its vascular supply. The length of muscle needed is estimated from the facial dissection. The distance from the commissure to the lower part of the zygoma, matching the direction of the normal side, is recorded. Generally, this distance is approximately 7 cm on the lower border and 4 cm on the upper border. The segment of muscle is marked on the gracilis muscle in its stretched position. This is accomplished by abducting the hip and extending the knee. Sutures are placed at 2-cm intervals from the pedicle. The segment of gracilis muscle required is removed along with its vascular pedicle and motor nerve (Fig. 58-3). It is important to take an additional 1 cm of muscle on either end to provide sufficient tissue for muscle fixation. The remainder of the gracilis muscle is left in situ, and the wound is closed in layers. The muscle is transferred to the face for final contouring and insertion (Fig. 58-4).

The bulk of the muscle to be placed at the commissure is reduced by removal of a wedge. This end of the muscle is closed with mattress sutures. These sutures are used to help anchor the muscle to the commissure and upper lip. The mattress sutures must be evenly spaced and should number one more than the anchoring sutures in the face. These anchoring sutures are passed through the muscle and tied over the previously placed mattress sutures. This method securely fixes the muscle to the commissure and upper lip area (Fig. 58-5). The origin of the transplanted muscle is secured to the inferior border of the maxilla and zygoma and to the anterior portion of the zygomatic arch. This is done with the muscle in its physiologically stretched position. The sutures previously placed at 2-cm intervals aid the surgeon in producing appropriate tension. The position of the muscle thus replicates the normal position of the zygomaticus major muscle.

Once the muscle is accurately positioned and secured to the periosteum of the maxilla and zygoma, the vascular repairs can be carried out. If the facial vessels are used, excellent positioning can be achieved. End-to-end microvascular anastomosis of a single artery and a single vein is carried out. Finally, the critical nerve repair is done under high magnification. A fascicular nerve repair is carried out between the recipient nerve in the face and the selected fascicles of the motor nerve to the gracilis muscle. The cheek flap is carefully replaced and the wound closed.

Postoperatively it may be helpful to reduce the tension on both the origin and the insertion of the muscle. This can be done with a hooked device placed in the oral commissure and secured in the scalp or on a biteplate (Fig. 58-6). The hook remains in place for about 10 days, although

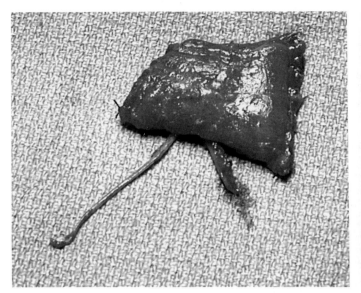

Fig. 58-3. Section of gracilis muscle harvested for transplantation.

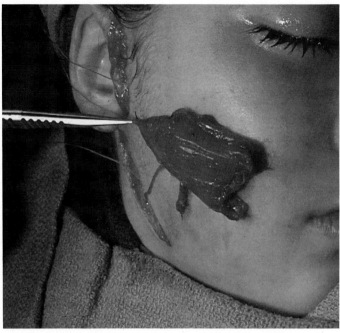

Fig. 58-4. Transplanted segmental gracilis muscle positioned on face.

Fig. 58-5A. Gracilis muscle transplant in position at completion of microanastomosis and neurorrhaphy.
B. Suture fixation of segmental gracilis muscle to anchoring sites at commissure and upper lip.

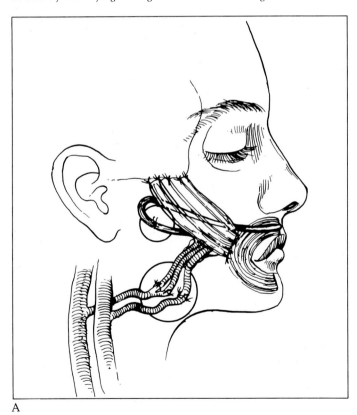

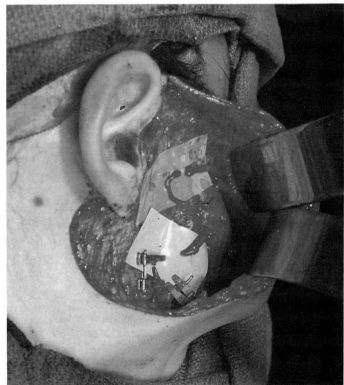

A

B

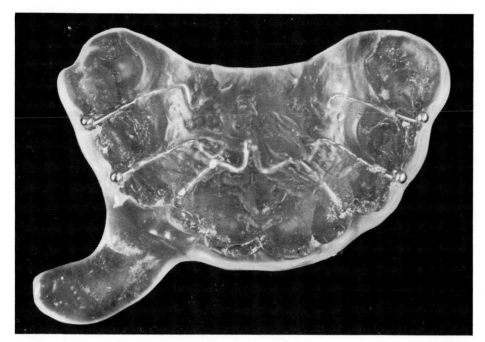

Fig. 58-6. Hooked device on biteplate to reduce tension on muscle.

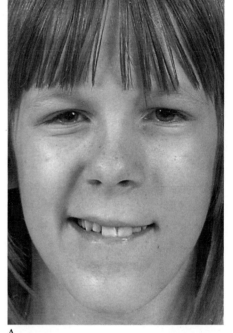

A

it can be removed for eating and speaking. After muscle transplantation, reinnervation generally takes place within 3 to 4 months when an ipsilateral motor nerve is used or 6 to 9 months when a cross-face nerve graft is used.

Once reinnervation begins, an active exercise program helps to maximize strength, excursion, and coordination. The patient does the exercises in front of a mirror and actively tries to achieve symmetric movement. Each side is activated independently and then both together. Biofeedback techniques also can be helpful. Current machines are compact and easy to use. The electrodes are placed directly above the transferred muscle. With contraction, a visual or auditory signal is produced signifying adequate movement. The threshold can be adjusted upward as muscle strength increases. The device is also useful for retraining the nerve-muscle complex to produce the desired movement. Contraction of the muscle with a smile is indicated by the visual or auditory signal. Thus improvement in the symmetry of facial movement also can be achieved. Functional improvement after muscle transfer can occur for up to 2 years (Fig. 58-7).

Fig. 58-7A. Congenital facial paralysis. B. After cross-face nerve grafting and muscle transplantation (at rest). C. With smile and activation of muscle.

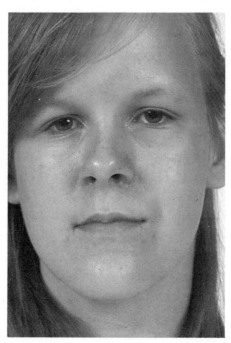

B

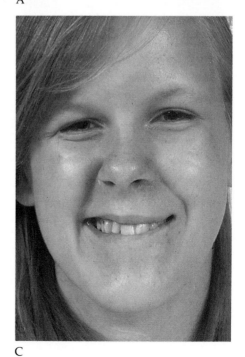

C

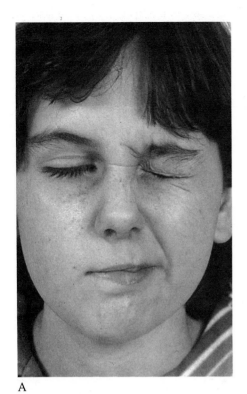
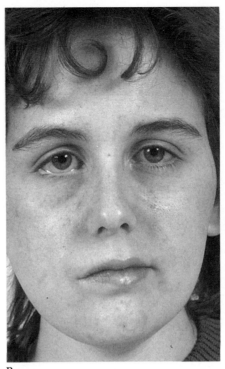
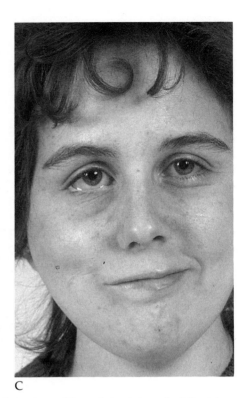

A B C

Fig. 58-8A. Acquired facial paralysis. B. After cross-face nerve grafting and muscle transplantation (at rest). C. With smile and activation of muscle.

Results

The results of functional muscle transfer for facial reanimation have improved steadily. Using smaller segments of muscle eliminates the problem of excess bulk. Placing the muscle flush with the bone has reduced the bulge and the irregularity of contour. Of critical importance is the secure anchoring of the muscle insertion into the commissure and upper lip. Anchorage to dermal elements leads to lip eversion and distortion. This problem can be avoided by anchoring the muscle on the undersurface of the residual orbicularis oculi muscle or the undersurface of any residual zygomaticus muscle. The muscle origin also must be securely anchored to the periosteum of the maxilla, zygoma, and zygomatic arch. The orientation of the transferred muscle must be symmetric to the orientation of similar muscle groups on the normal side. This generally simulates the zygomaticus major muscle, but alterations may be necessary because smiling patterns vary from person to person. It has been most encouraging to assess the results of cross-face nerve grafting and muscle transplantation. Despite the great reduction in

axons present in the nerve to the end muscle, the number remaining seems to be sufficient to allow for adequate power and excursion to match the normal side.

After muscle transfer, the philtral midline should return to the normal position, because the imbalance of muscle power pulling it toward the normal side is reduced. Muscle excursion is generally just under 10 mm, or about 15 percent of the length of the muscle used. This length seems to be adequate for the production of a symmetric smile. Of particular note has been the spontaneity of movement on the affected side. This is expected with the use of the ipsilateral VIIth nerve and has been borne out with the use of the cross-face nerve grafts (Fig. 58-8). The speed of impulse passage, even across a cross-face nerve graft, leads to virtually synchronous activity. With the use of biofeedback techniques and with the patient exercising in front of a mirror, more symmetric movement can be achieved. The overall result is a dramatic improvement in a patient's ability to express emotions through smiling in a synchronous and spontaneous manner.

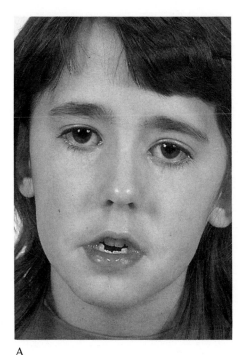
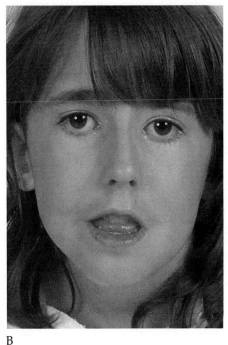
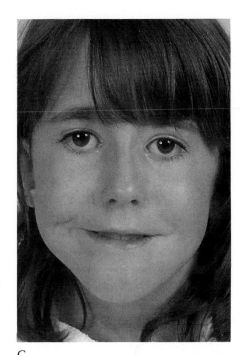

A   B   C

Fig. 58-9A. Möbius syndrome. B. After muscle transplantation (at rest). C. With smile and activation of muscle.

When motor nerves other than the VIIth nerve are used, this spontaneity of activity with emotional expression is not as evident. This result is not unexpected; it may take years for the patterns of spontaneity to be established. Even so, the voluntary movement produced for patients with Möbius syndrome has been of enormous benefit in facilitating facial movement for emotional expression during face-to-face communication (Fig. 58-9). This change is reflected in improved interpersonal skills and self-esteem.

Conclusion

The introduction of microsurgical techniques of reconstruction after facial paralysis has added considerably to surgeons' ability to treat this most devastating problem. There is now an important reconstructive option whereby a new muscle can be inserted to provide facial movement. This may require a stage-setting cross-face nerve graft if no nerve is available on the involved side. Although the procedures are complex and technically demanding, the results have been most gratifying. Further refinements undoubtedly will be forthcoming, but the concept of microsurgical muscle replace-

ment provides renewed hope for patients with facial paralysis.

Suggested Reading

Harii, K., Ohmori, K., and Torii, S. Free gracilis muscle transplantation with microneurovascular anastomoses for the treatment of facial paralysis. *Plast. Reconstr. Surg.* 57:113, 1976.

Harii, K. Microneurovascular free muscle transplantation for reanimation of facial paralysis. *Clin. Plast. Surg.* 6:361, 1979.

Manktelow, R.T., and Zuker, R.M. Muscle transplantation by fascicular territory. *Plast. Reconstr. Surg.* 73:751, 1984.

Manktelow, R.T. *Microvascular Reconstruction.* Heidelberg: Springer, 1986. P. 128.

O'Brien, B.M., Franklin, J.D., and Morrison, W.A. Cross facial nerve grafts and microneurovascular free transfer for long established facial paralysis. *Br. J. Plast. Surg.* 33:202, 1980.

Zuker, R.M. Facial paralysis in children. *Clin. Plast. Surg.* 17:95, 1990.

Zuker, R.M. Microvascular Management of Facial Palsy. In J.L. Marsh (Ed.), *Current Therapy in Plastic and Reconstructive Surgery.* Toronto: Decker, 1989. Vol. I, pp. 157–162.

Zuker, R.M., and Manktelow, R.T. A smile for the Mobius syndrome patient. *Ann. Plast. Surg.* 22:188, 1989.

Index

Index

This index covers all three volumes. Volume I contains pages 1–829; Volume II contains pages 830–1411; Volume III contains pages 1413–2258.

Note: Page numbers in italics indicate figures; those followed by t indicate tables.

Abbe (cross-lip) flap, 609–610, *611–613*
Abbe lip-switch, 909, *909*, *910*
Abdominal contour operations, 2165–2185
  abdominal blood supply and, combining
    abdominoplasty with suction-assisted
    lipectomy and, 2170, *2171*
  complications of, 2181–2184
    abdominolipoplasty and, 2181–2182
    full abdominoplasty with suction-assisted
      lipectomy and, 2182–2184
  contraindications to, 2169
  history of, *2166–2168*, 2167
  indications for, 2167, 2169, *2169*
  lipectomy and, 236–237
    belt, 2172
    in men, 2172
    multiple procedures and, 2172
  patient evaluation, selection, and planning
    for, 2169–2170, 2170t
  surgical instrumentation and procedure
    for, 2172–2181, *2173*
    abdominoplasty with suction-assisted
      lipectomy and, 2177–2178, *2180*, 2171t
    miniabdominoplasty and, 2172–2174,
      2175, *2176*
    modified abdominoplasty and,
      2175–2177, *2177–2179*
    suction-assisted lipectomy and, 2172,
      2174
    umbilicoplasty and, 2178, 2181,
      2181–2183
    variations in, 2172
Abdominal wall reconstruction, 1349–1359
  complex defects and, 1352
  donor sites for, 1353, *1353–1356*, 1355,
    1357, *1358*
  incisions for, 1352
  partial-thickness wounds and, 1350
  problem assessment and, 1349–1350
  prosthetic sheeting in, 1352–1353
  surgical anatomy and, 1351–1352, *1353*
  systematic approach for, 1357, 1359, 1359t
  tissue expansion in, 1350–1351, *1351*

Abdominolipoplasty, complications of,
  2181–2182
Abdominoplasty, *2204*, *2205*. *See also*
  Abdominal contour operations
Abscess, stitch, eyelid operations in Oriental
  patients and, *2072*, *2074*, 2075
Accelerated fractionation, 949, *950*, 951
Accelerated hyperfractionation, 951
Accessory abductor pollicis longus tendon
  transfer, free tendon graft and, 1596
Acne conglobata, 394–395
Acoustic assessment, multiview, 630, *630*
Acral lentiginous melanomas, 344
Acrosyndactyly, 1434, 1441, 1444, *1444*
Actinic keratosis, 309–310, *310*
Activities, therapeutic, in hand rehabilitation,
  1748
Adenoid cystic carcinoma, of salivary glands,
  1037–1038, *1038*
Adenomas, pleomorphic (benign mixed
  tumor), of salivary glands, 1035, 1036t,
  1037
Adhesion, mentosternal, burn wounds of
  neck and, 427
Adolescents
  correction of secondary skeletal deformities
    in patients with clefts and. *See*
    Orthognathic surgery, correction of
    secondary skeletal deformities in
    adolescent patients with clefts and
  facial fractures in. *See* Facial fractures, in
    children and adolescents
Adrenergic block, skin flaps and, 69
Advancement flaps, 57
  for fingertip injuries with exposed bone,
    1496–1501
    Atasony-Kleinert volar V-Y advancement
      flaps, 1497, *1498–1499*
    Kutler lateral V-Y flaps, 1497–1498, *1500*,
      1501
    volar advancement flaps, 1500–1501,
      1504, *1505*

Aerodynamic assessment, multiview,
  624–630, *625–629*, 628t–630t
Aesthetic evaluation, for lipectomy, *228*,
  228–230, *229*
Aesthetic facial surgery. *See also*
  Blepharoplasty; Brow-lift; Facial
  rejuvenation; Forehead-lift; Perioral
  rejuvenation; Rhinoplasty
  in African-Americans, 2050–2058
    aging and, *2053*, 2053–2054, *2054*
    cheiloplasty, 2058, *2058*
    dermabrasion and chemical peel for,
      2052, 2052–2053
    facial and scalp hair and, 2050–2051,
      2051
    rhinoplasty, 2054–2057, 2055t, *2055–2057*
    scarring and, 2051–2052
  in Oriental patients, 2059–2086
    augmentation rhinoplasty. *See*
      Rhinoplasty, in Oriental patients
    complications and suboptimal results
      with, 2083, 2085, *2086*, 2086
    eyelid operations. *See* Eyelid operations,
      in Oriental patients
    postoperative care and, 2083
Aesthetic measurements, cephalometric,
  478–481, *478–481*
Aesthetics
  facial. *See* Facial aesthetics; Facial
    rejuvenation, aesthetic considerations
    in
  following suction-assisted lipectomy, 2199
  termination of lipectomy and, 235
Aesthetic units, of face, 416, *417*
African-Americans, aesthetic facial surgery
  in. *See* Aesthetic facial surgery, in
  African-Americans
Age. *See also specific age groups*
  as indication for breast reduction, 2143,
    2144
  of scar, scar revision and, 35
  scar formation and, 34
  wound healing and, 30, *30*

Aging
   of African-Americans, *2053*, 2053–2054, *2054*
   facial rejuvenation and. *See* Facial rejuvenation
   wound healing and, 9
Aile ptosique, in Oriental patients, 2083, *2084*
Airway management, craniomaxillofacial surgery and, 138
Airway obstruction, associated with cleft lip, secondary correction of, 706–707, *707*
Ala, hanging (hooded), secondary rhinoplasty for, 2040, *2045*, *2046*
Alar base
   narrowing of, in Oriental patients, 2082, *2082*
   resection of, in African-Americans, 2055, *2055*, *2056*
Alar border, retraction of, secondary rhinoplasty for, 2040, 2043, *2047*
Alar cartilage
   fixation of, for bilateral cleft lip repair, 574
   repositioning, for bilateral cleft lip repair, 571, 574
   resection of, in rhinoplasty, 2012–2013, *2013*
Alar wedge resection, in rhinoplasty, 2017, *2017*
Albumin, lipectomy and, 230, 230t, *231*
Alcohol use, as risk factor for oropharyngeal carcinoma, 922
Allergies, following blepharoplasty, 1936
Allografts, 53
   bone, in lower extremity reconstruction, *1802*, 1802–1803
   of nerves, 133–134
Alloplastic materials
   for arthroplasty, in temporomandibular joint deformities, 1227
   in craniomaxillofacial surgery, 148
   for secondary reconstruction of soft tissue deformity associated with orbital fractures, 1199–1200, 1205–1206, *1205–1207*
Alpha-adrenoreceptor block, skin flaps and, 69
Altered fractionation. *See* Radiation therapy, altered fractionation and
Alveolar bone fractures, 1172, *1173*
Alveolar clefts, secondary bone grafting of, 669–679
   flap design for bone coverage and, 672, *672*, *673*
   goals of, 669t, 669–670, *670*
   perioperative care and, 675
   results with, 675, *678–680*
   sources of grafts for, 671, *671*
   surgical technique for, 672–673, *674*, 675, *676–677*
   timing of, 670–671
Alveolar process fractures, in children and adolescents, 1198
Amblyopia
   anisometropic, hemangiomas and, 355
   deprivation, hemangiomas and, 355, *356*
Amputation(s)
   of foot, foot reconstruction and, 1824, *1826*, 1827
   of hand parts, care of amputated parts and, 1481–1482, *1483*
   immediate, lower extremity fractures and, 1770
   replantation and. *See* Replantation
   revision, hand reconstruction and, 1677, 1680

Amputation neuromas, 304–305
Anesthesia, 14–20, 15t
   for augmentation mammaplasty, 2103–2104
   bilateral cleft lip repair, 571
   for eyelid operations in Oriental patients, 2065
   for facial rejuvenation, 1885–1886
      in men, 1904
   hypotensive, for breast reduction, 2118
   for lipectomy, 230
   local, physiochemical properties of agents for, 15
   for management of nasal fractures, 1129–1130
   in mandibular dysostosis, 535
   for pharyngeal flap operation, 634
   for prophylactic subcutaneous mastectomy, 1277
   regional blocks of head and neck, 16–18, *16–19*
   for suction-assisted lipectomy of thigh, 2238
   topical, of mucous membranes, 18–19
   toxicity of, 19–20
Angiofibromas, facial, 299, *299*
Angiogenesis, in wound healing, 5
Angiography, of diabetic foot, 1842
Angiokeratomas, 300, *300*
   circumscriptum, 300
   corporis diffusum, 300
   Mibelli, 300
   papular, 300
   of scrotum, 300
Angiolipomas, of skin, 300
Angiosomes, 60
Anisometropic amblyopia, hemangiomas and, 355
Ankles
   lipectomy and, 238
   suction-assisted lipectomy of. *See* Suction-assisted lipectomy, of calf and ankle
Ankylosis, of temporomandibular joint, 1224–1226, *1225*
Anterior segmental osteotomies
   for mandibular deformities, 743, 745
      indications for, 735, *739*, 743
      techniques and results of, 745, *750*
   for maxillary deformities, 724, *726*, 726, *728*, *729*
   sagittal split osteotomy combined with, for mandibular deformities, 756
Antibiotics
   following lipectomy, 240
   for hand infections, 1467, 1468t, 1469
   prophylactic, hand injuries and, 1488
Anxiety, lipectomy and, 227
Apert syndrome
   bipartition in, 514, *514*
   Le Fort III osteotomy in, 160, *161–162*, 162
   single-stage frontomaxillary advancement in, 163, *163*
   3-D computed tomography in, 272–273, *273*, *274*
   two-stage craniomaxillary procedure in, 162
Apocrine hidrocystomas (apocrine cystadenomas), 303, *303*
Aponeurotic ptosis, traumatic, 1101–1102, *1102–1104*
Areola. *See also* Areolar reconstruction; Nipple-areolar complex
   marking of
      for breast reduction, 2119
      for reduction mammaplasty, 2132, *2132*

Areolar reconstruction, 1342–1348, *1343*
   with tattooing, 1344–1348
      secondary reconstruction and, 1348
      skate technique for, 1344, *1345*, 1346
      tattooing and, 1346–1348, *1348*
   TRAM flap breast reconstruction and, 1335, *1336–1338*
Arginine, wound healing and, 10
Argon lasers, 256–262
   for other superficial vascular lesions, 259, *260–261*
   for port-wine stains, 257, *257*, *258*, 259
   for strawberry hemangiomas, 259–262, *261–263*
Arm. *See* Forearm; Upper extremities
Arterial ulcers, of leg, 1830–1831, *1831*, 1831t
Arteries
   anatomic, dynamic and potential territories of, 60, *60*
   trunk, 60
Arterioles, of skin flaps, 67
Arteriovenous anastomoses, of skin flaps, 67t, 67–68
Arteriovenous malformations, of skin, 370–372, *373*
Arthritis
   infectious, wrist pain and, 1730t–1731t
   osteoarthritis, wrist pain and, 1730t–1731t
   post-traumatic, wrist pain and, 1730t–1731t
   pyogenic, of hands, 1473, 1477
   rheumatoid
      in hands. *See* Hand(s), rheumatoid arthritis in
      in wrist. *See* Wrist, rheumatoid arthritis in
   wrist pain and, 1738–1739, 1739t
Arthrodesis, for fractures of hand and wrist, 1520
Arthrography
   in temporomandibular joint deformities, 1223
   in wrist pain, 1728
Arthroplasty
   for fractures of hand and wrist, 1520, *1529*
   of proximal interphalangeal joint, hand rehabilitation following, 1759–1760
   for rheumatoid arthritis of wrist, 1712
   in temporomandibular joint deformities, 1227–1228
      alloplastic materials and, 1227
      autogenous materials and, 1227–1228, *1228*
Arthroscopy
   in temporomandibular joint deformities, 1224
   in wrist pain, 1732
Arthrotomy, in temporomandibular joint deformities, *1226*, 1226–1227
Articular fractures, hand rehabilitation following, 1759
Articulation development prosthesis, in cleft lip and palate, *761*, 761–762, *762*
Arytenoid cartilage, 1008, *1010*
Asphalt, burns caused by, 451, *451*
Asymmetry
   of breasts, breast reduction for. *See* Breast reduction
   eyelid operations in Oriental patients and, 2072, *2072*
   facial, cephalometrics and, 485
   of lids, following blepharoplasty, 1936, *1936*
   of skin, blepharoplasty and, 1921

Augmentation
  of breast. See Augmentation mammaplasty
  in facial rejuvenation, 1979–1981, *1981*, *1982*
  of upper lip, 1995
Augmentation mammaplasty, 2099t, 2099–2112
  anatomy and, 2101
  anesthesia and, 2103
  asymmetries requiring augmentation and reduction and, 2122–2123, *2124*, *2125*
  capsular contractures and, 2101, 2101t
  complications of, 2112
    autoimmune disorders, 2112
    capsular contracture, 2112
    hematoma, 2112
    malposition, 2112
  history of, 2100
  implants for, 2100–2101
    with foam coating, 2100
    gel-filled, 2100
    inflatable, 2100
    textured silicone, 2100–2101
  informed consent for, 2101–2103, *2102*, *2103*
  patient selection for, 2104, *2105–2110*
  preferred techniques for, 2106–2108, *2110*, 2110–2112, *2111*
  surgical plan and, 2103–2104
  surgical procedure for, 2103–2104
Auricle, sensory supply of, 773, *775*
Autogenous materials
  for arthroplasty, in temporomandibular joint deformities, 1227–1228, *1228*
  for immediate breast reconstruction following mastectomy, *1290*, *1291*, 1291–1292
Autoimmune disorders, augmentation mammaplasty and, 2112
Avascular necrosis, of wrist, 1730t–1731t. *See also* Keinböck disease
  scaphoid, 1744
Avulsion injuries, of nail bed, treatment of, 1495, *1495*
Awake stimulation, nerve grafting and, 1616, 1618, *1618*
Axial pattern flaps, for soft tissue coverage of hand and upper extremity, 1648, 1650, *1650*, *1651*
Axial plane, for computed tomography imaging, in maxillofacial trauma, 1073
Axilla, burn wounds of, 434, *436*
Axonotmesis, 1603
Axoplasmic transport, peripheral nerve injuries and, 1598

Bacteriologic factors, in osteomyelitis, 1810
Barnard procedure, Freeman modification of, 917, *917*, *918*
Basal cell carcinomas
  of eyelids, 324, 330–331
  of hand and nail bed, 1456
  of skin, 316–319
    histology of, 316, *317*
    morphea-like (sclerosing), 316
    nodular, 316
    pigmented, 316
    recurrence of, 318–319
    superficial, 316
    treatment of, 316, 318
    of upper limb, 320, *322*
Basal cell nevus syndrome, 312, *313*, 315

Bazex syndrome, 315
Beard sicosis, 394, *394*
Becker melanosis, 305
Belt lipectomy, 2172
Benign mixed tumor (pleomorphic adenoma), of salivary glands, 1035, 1036t, *1037*
Beta-adrenoreceptor blockers, skin flaps and, 69
Beta-adrenoreceptor stimulators, skin flaps and, 69
Biofeedback, in hand rehabilitation, 1751
Biohazards, of lipectomy, 220
Biopsy, in oropharyngeal carcinoma, 927
Bipartition, in Apert syndrome, 514, *514*
Bites, human, of hand, 1490
Bleeding, management of, in maxillofacial trauma, 1062–1063, *1063*
Bleomycin, in oropharyngeal carcinoma, 940, 940t, 942, 943t
Blepharitis, following blepharoplasty, 1936
Blepharoplasty, 1920–1940, 1968–1976
  anatomic deformity and, 1921–1923
    skin and, 1921–1923, *1921–1923*
  anatomy and, 1968, *1969*
  for atonic lower lids, 1939
  complications of, 1934–1938, 1976
    allergy, 1936
    asymmetry, 1936, *1936*
    blepharitis, 1936
    corneal abrasion, 1937–1938
    dermatologic, 1938
    ectropion, 1935, *1935*
    edema and induration, 1937
    enophthalmos, 1937
    entropion, 1937
    epiphora, 1935–1936
    epithelial tunnels, 1938
    glaucoma, 1938
    hematoma, 1937
    hypertrophic scars, 1938
    inclusion cysts, 1938
    infection, 1936
    keratoconjunctivitis sicca, 1934–1935
    lagophthalmos, 1938
    loss of eyelashes, 1937
    numbness, 1936, *1936*
    patient dissatisfaction, 1934
    ptosis, 1936
    skeletonized appearance, 1937
    skin slough, 1936, *1936*
    skin wrinkling, 1938
    visual, 1938
    web scars, 1938
    wound separation, 1936
  for ectropion, 1972, *1974–1976*, 1975
  for entropion, 1975, 1976, *1977*
  for exophthalmos, 1940
  for festoons, 1939, *1940*
  history of, 1920
  for lateral canthal wrinkles, 1938–1939, *1939*
  lower lid, 1924–1928
    surgical technique for, 1925–1928, *1928–1933*
    undermining techniques for, 1924–1925
  postoperative care and, 1934
  psychological evaluation for, 1920–1921
  for ptosis, 1968–1972, *1970–1973*
  surgical technique for, 1924–1934
  transconjunctival, 1941–1947
    advantages of, 1945, *1945*, *1946*
    aesthetic considerations in, 1941

Blepharoplasty, transconjunctival—*Continued*
    anatomic and physiologic considerations in, 1941
    complications of, 1944
    skin flap technique combined with, 1946–1947, *1947*
    technique for, 1941, *1942–1945*, 1943–1944
  upper lid, 1924
    skin markings and local anesthesia for, 1924, *1924–1927*
    variations in surgical technique for, 1928, 1934
      direct fat excision, 1934, *1934*
      orbital bone contouring, 1934
      subconjunctival approach, 1928
      upper lid fold definition and, 1928
    for xanthelasma, 1939
Blindness, disturbances, 1938
Blood
  viscosity of, 68–69
Blood flow, dermal, control of, 68
Blood supply
  of bone, 102–103
  skin grafting and, 47
  of tendons, 121–122
  wound healing and, 7
Blood transfusions, for leg ulcers, 1835
Blow-out fractures, roentgenographic appearance of, 1080–1082, *1081*
Blue nevi, 307
Blunt suction-assisted lipectomy. *See* Suction-assisted lipectomy
Body contouring
  abdominal. *See* Abdominal contour operations
  of lower extremity. *See* Calf implantation; Suction-assisted lipectomy
  suction-assisted lipectomy for. *See* Suction-assisted lipectomy
  of trunk and limbs, 2201–2214
    cellulite and, 2201–2202, *2202*
    complete lower body lift for, 2214, *2216–2218*
    medial thigh-lift for. *See* Thigh-lifts, medial
    superficial fascial system and, 2201–2202, *2202*
    surgical implications of, 2203, 2205
    transverse flank-thigh-buttock-lift for. *See* Transverse flank-thigh-buttock-lift
  of upper extremities. *See* Upper extremities, brachioplasty and brachial suction-assisted lipectomy and
Body temperature, maintaining, lipectomy and, 230
Boeck sarcoids, of hands, 1463
Bone(s). *See also* Fractures; *specific fractures*
  assessment of, for blepharoplasty, *1923*, 1924
  of hand, evaluation of, 1485
  hand reconstruction and, 1660–1661, *1663*, *1664*, 1665
  healing of, 1809–1810. *See* Bone grafts, bone healing and
    inflammatory phase of, 1809
    remodeling phase of, 1809
    reparative phase of, 1809
  remodeling of, 104
  repair of diabetic foot and, 1857–1858
Bone cysts, solitary, of hands, 1466

Bone grafting
    alveolar clefts and. *See* Alveolar clefts,
        secondary bone grafting of
    cancellous, in lower extremity
        reconstruction, 1800–1802, *1801*
    closed, in lower extremity reconstruction,
        1801, 1801–1802
    maxillary fractures and, 1162, *1162*
    orbital fractures and, 1207, *1209*
Bone grafts, 102–112
    anatomy of bone and, 102–103
        macroscopic, 102–103
        microscopic, 103
    autogenous, 105t, 105–112
        calvarium as donor site for, 108, 110–111
        ilium as donor site for, 105t, 105–107
        lower extremity as donor site for, 105t,
          111–112
        radial forearm as donor site for, 105t, 112
        rib as donor site for, 105t, 107–108
    autografts, 104–105
        cancellous bone, 104
        cortical bone, 104
        mechanical strength of, 104
        onlay grafts, 104–105
        vascularized, 105, 105t
    bone healing and, 103–104
        bone remodeling and, 104
        contribution of host and graft to, 103
        of fractures, 103
        incorporation of bone grafts and, 103
        osteoconduction and, 104
        osteoinduction and, 104
    cranial, in craniomaxillofacial surgery,
        145–146, *147*, 148
    future of, 112
    mandibular reconstruction with, 183, 185,
        186–187, 187
Bone marrow, 102
Bone plates, for mandibular fractures,
    1170–1172, *1171–1173*. *See also* Rigid
    fixation, for maxillary deformities
Bone scans, in wrist pain, 1728–1729,
    1732–1733
Bone substitutes, 113–118
    biologic and mechanical properties of, 116,
        117–119, 118
    clinical considerations with, 113–116,
        114–116
    future considerations with, 118
    general considerations with, 113
Bone wiring, for mandibular fractures, 1170,
    1170
Bony defects. *See also* Fractures; *specific
    anatomic sites and types of fractures*
    bilateral cleft lip and palate and, 687
    isolated cleft palate and, 698
    unilateral cleft lip and palate and, 683
Boutonnière deformity
    rheumatoid arthritis and, 1717–1718
    treatment of, 1574–1575, *1575, 1576*
Bowen disease, *314–315*, 315–316, 1456
Boyes sublimis transfer, *1584, 1585, 1586*
Brachial plexus injuries, hand rehabilitation
    and, 1758
Brachioplasty. *See* Upper extremities,
    brachioplasty and brachial suction-
    assisted lipectomy and
Brachycephaly, 151, *152–153*, 500, 508–509,
    509, 510
Brachytherapy, 951–954
    of base of tongue, 953
    hyperthermia with, 954
    interstitial, 951–952, *952*

Brachytherapy—*Continued*
    intracavitary, 952
    isotopes and source placement for,
        951–953, *952*, 953t
    of pharyngeal wall, 953
    plesiotherapy, 952, *952*
    salvage therapy for recurrent disease
        using, 953–954
    of soft palate, 953
    of tonsils, 953
Bracing, functional, hand and wrist fractures
    and, 1508, *1509*
Braided sutures, 22, 22t
Branchial arch syndrome, first and second.
    See First and second branchial arch
    syndrome; Hemifacial microsomia
    (craniofacial microsomia)
Branchial cleft anomalies
    first, 810–811, *811*
    fourth, 813, *813*
    second, 811–812, *812, 813*
    third, 813
Branchial cleft cysts/sinuses/fistulas, 810, *810*
Brand tendon transfers, *1594*, 1594–1595
Breast(s)
    burn wounds of, 434–435, *437, 438, 439*
    male, lipectomy and, 237–238, *238–239*
    malposition of, augmentation
        mammaplasty and, 2112
    prophylactic subcutaneous mastectomy
        and. *See* Prophylactic subcutaneous
        mastectomy
    reconstruction using soft tissue expansion,
        210–211, *211*
Breast augmentation. *See* Augmentation
    mammaplasty
Breast reconstruction. *See also* Areolar
    reconstruction; Nipple reconstruction
    delayed, with autogenous tissue,
        1309–1322
        abdominal characteristics and, 1310
        body habitus and, 1310
        latissimus dorsi flap reconstruction and.
          See Latissimus dorsi flaps, breast
          reconstruction using
        mastectomy defect and, 1309–1310
        opposite breast and, 1310
        patient evaluation for, 1309–1310
        practical considerations and, 1310
        TRAM flap reconstruction and. *See*
          Transverse rectus abdominis (TRAM)
          flap breast reconstruction
    delayed, with tissue expansion, 1301–1302
    with free tissue transfer, 1324–1341
        buttock flaps for. *See* Buttock flap breast
          reconstruction
        free TRAM flaps for. *See* Transverse
          rectus abdominis (TRAM) flap breast
          reconstruction, using free TRAM flaps
        initial consultation for, 1326–1327
        lateral thigh flaps for, 1339, *1339, 1340*,
          1341
        relationship with oncologic surgeon and,
          1325–1326, *1326*
        selection of technique for, 1327
        team for, 1325
        timing of, 1325
    immediate, following mastectomy,
        1283–1294
        aesthetic advantages of, 1284
        autogenous tissue reconstruction for,
          1290, 1291, 1291–1292
        availability of, 1284

Breast reconstruction, immediate—*Continued*
    complications of, 1293
        economy of, 1283
        interaction with general surgeon and,
          1284
        latissimus dorsi flap reconstruction for,
          1292
        oncologic considerations and, 1294
        postoperative care and, 1292–1293
        preoperative considerations for,
          1284–1285, *1286*
        psychological aspects of, 1283, 1284
        secondary procedures, 1293–1294
        selection of appropriate technique for,
          1285
        soft tissue expansion for, 1289, 1291
        submuscular implant reconstruction for,
          1287–1289, *1287–1289*
        surgical considerations common to all
          techniques for, 1285, 1287
        with tissue expansion, 1300–1301, *1301*
        total breast cancer cure and, 1284
    with tissue expansion, 1289, 1291,
        1295–1308
        complications of, 1306–1308
        delayed, technique for, 1301–1302
        expanders for, 1296–1298, *1297–1299*
        goals of, 1295
        immediate, technique for, 1300–1301,
          1301
        after modified radical mastectomy, 1305,
          1306
        patient selection for, 1295–1296, *1296*
        postoperative care and, 1302
        after radical mastectomy, 1302, 1305
        replacement of expander with permanent
          implant and, 1302, *1303–1305*
        results with, 1302, 1305–1306, *1306, 1307*
        after simple or subcutaneous
          mastectomy, 1306, *1307*
        strategy for, 1298, *1299*, 1300, *1300*
Breast reduction. *See also* Reduction
    mammaplasty
    inferior pedicle, 2114–2123
        adjuncts in, 2118–2119
        in asymmetries requiring augmentation
          and reduction, 2122–2123, *2124, 2125*
        contraindications to, 2115
        examination and consultation for,
          2114–2115
        marking for, *2115*, 2115–2116, *2116*,
          2119–2120, *2121*
        postoperative care and, 2119, *2119, 2120*
        surgical technique for, 2117–2118, *2118*
        in unilateral macromastia, 2119–2122,
          2121–2123
    by liposuction and vertical mammaplasty,
        2143–2155
        choice of technique for, 2143–2147,
          2145–2146
        deepithelialization and, 2147
        indications for, 2143, *2144*
        liposuction, 2147–2148, *2152, 2153*
        marking for, 2147, *2148–2151*
        results with, 2152–2153, *2154–2156*
        surgical technique for, 2147–2148, *2147*
Breast volume, breast reduction and, 2122,
    2122, 2123
Bronchogenic cysts, 303
Bronchopleural fistulas, closure of,
    intrathoracic transposition of soft
    tissue for, 1273

Brow-lift, 1958–1967
  anatomy and, 1958–1966, *1959*
  definition of brow position and, 1958
  direct, of Lewis, 1965
  patient evaluation for, 1958
  surgical technique for, *1959*, 1959–1966,
    1960
    anterior hairline approach, 1962,
      1964–1965
    for coronal forehead-lift, 1961–1962,
      1961–1964
    direct brow-lift of Lewis, 1965
    direct forehead skin excision approach,
      1965
    extended facelift approach, 1966
    internal brow pexy, 1965, *1966, 1967*
    placement os incision and, 1959–1961,
      1961
    subcutaneous approach, 1964–1965, *1965*
    subgaleal approach, 1962, 1964
    suprabrow excision, 1965
    temporal-lift, *1667*, 1966
Buried suture method, for eyelid operations
  in Oriental patients, 2070, *2071*
Burkhalter (extensor indicis proprius) tendon
  transfer, 1587, *1588*
Burns
  chemical. *See* Chemical burns
  electrical. *See* Electrical burns
  radiation. *See* Radiation injuries
  thermal. *See* Thermal burns
Burn wounds, 407–415
  excision of
    burn physiology and, 408–409
    control of hemorrhage and, 411
    early, appearance and use of structure
      and, 409
    early, mortality and, 408
    radiation injuries and, 454
    scar revision and, 417
    technique of, 409, *410*, 411, *411*
    timing of, 407–408
  of extremities and trunk, reconstruction of,
    429–440, *430*
    of axilla, 434, *436*
    of breast, 434–435, *437, 438, 439*
    of hand, 431, *431–435, 433*–434
    of lower extremity, *439*, 439–440, *440*
    principles of, 430–431
    of trunk, 434
    of wrist and elbow, 434
    Z-plasty for, 431
  grafting of, 411–415
    control of hemorrhage and, 411
    dermatomes and, 414
    difficult burn areas and, 414
    donor site management and, 412, *412,
      413*
    dressings and postoperative care and,
      414, 414–415, *415*
    techniques for, 413–414
  of head and neck, reconstruction of,
    416–428
    aesthetic units and, 416, *417*
    ear burns, 418, 420–422
    eyebrow burns, 422–423
    eyelid burns, 423–424
    forehead burns, 418, *420*
    materials for, 417
    mouth burns, 426
    neck burns, 426–428
    nose burns, 424–425
    priorities in, 417

Burn wounds, of head and neck—*Continued*
    scalp burns, 418
    scar excision and, 417
    timing of, 416–417
    tissue expansion and, 417, *417*
Buttock flap breast reconstruction, 1335–1338
  anatomy and, 1335–1336, *1339*
  anatomy and flap elevation and,
    1337–1338, *1339*
  flap dissection and, 1336
  inferior gluteal flaps for, 1336–1337
Buttress plates, for hand and wrist fractures,
  1519, *1527*

Café au lait macules, 306
Calf, lipectomy of, 238
  suction-assisted. *See* Suction-assisted
    lipectomy, of calf and ankle
Calf implantation, 2250, 2252–2256
  anatomy and, 2250, 2252, *2252*
  complications of, 2255
  implants for, 2253, 2255, *2255–2257*
  indications for, 2252
  technique for, 2252–2253, *2252–2254*
  with underdevelopment of leg caused by
    poliomyelitis or clubfoot, 2255–2256,
    2258
Calvarium grafts, 108, 110–111
  nonvascularized, 108, *110*
  vascularized, 108, 111, *111*
Cambium, 102
Canaliculi, 103
Cancellous bone, 102
  grafts of, 104
Cannulas
  for lipectomy, 220, *220*
Canthal reconstruction
  lateral, surgical technique for, 875
  medial, surgical technique for, 874–875,
    875–877
Canthal wrinkles. *See* Crow's feet
Canthopexy, 142, 144
  lateral, 142, 144, *145*
  medial, 144, *145*
Canthus, lateral, elevation of, 530, *530*
Capillaries, of skin flaps, 67
Capillary-cavernous hemangiomas, 353, *355*
Capillary hemangiomas
  argon laser therapy for, 257, *257, 258,* 259
  lobulated (pyogenic granulomas), 353, 355,
    356
Capillary-lymphatic malformations, of skin,
  363, 363–365
Capillary malformations, of skin, 360–363
Capitate fractures, 1742–1743
  background of, 1742
  diagnosis of, 1742
  treatment of, 1742–1743
Capsular contractures, augmentation
  mammaplasty and, 2101, 2101t, 2112
Capsular injury, wrist pain and. *See* Wrist
  pain, capsular
Carbon dioxide lasers, 253–255, *254, 255*
Carboplatinum, in oropharyngeal carcinoma,
  940, 940t
Carcinomas
  adenoid cystic, of salivary glands,
    1037–1038, *1038*
  basal cell. *See* Basal cell carcinomas
  mucoepidermoid, of salivary glands, 1037,
    1038
  orbital. *See* Orbital carcinomas

Carcinomas—*Continued*
  oropharyngeal. *See* Oropharyngeal
    carcinomas
  of paranasal sinuses. *See* Paranasal sinuses,
    carcinoma of
  in situ, of skin, *314–315,* 315–316
  squamous cell. *See* Squamous cell
    carcinomas
Cardiovascular system, thermal burns and,
  405
Carpal bossing, 1744
Carpal collapse patterns, wrist pain and,
  1737, *1737*
Carpal tunnel syndrome, 1734–1735
  diagnosis of, 1735
  hand rehabilitation and, 1757–1758, *1758*
  presentation of, 1734–1735
  treatment of, 1735
Carpometacarpal joints
  anatomy of, 1532
  of fingers, ligament injuries of, 1541–1542
  of thumb, ligament injuries of, 1542
Cartilage(s)
  laryngeal, 1008, *1009, 1010*
  wrist pain and. *See* Wrist pain, cartilage
    and
Cartilage grafts, 88t, 91–92, *92*
  in rhinoplasty, 2009, 2018
    dorsal, 2018, *2018*
    lateral wall, 2018, *2018*
    placement of, 2016, *2016*
    tip, 2018, *2019*
  uses of, 92
Casting techniques, for nasal fractures, 1133,
  1134
Catgut sutures, 21, 22t
Caudal septum, rhinoplasty and, 2011–2012
Cavernous hemangiomas (deep dermal and
  subcutaneous vascular channels), 353,
  354
Cavernous lymphangiomas, 368, *379*
Cellular proliferation, in wound healing, 4–5
Cellulite
  treatment of, 239
  trunk- and thigh-lifts and, 2201–2202, *2202*
Cellulitis, dissecting, of scalp, 392, *393*
Centigray (cGy), 945
Cephalometrics, 475–485, *476, 477*
  aesthetic measurements using, 478–481,
    478–481
  functional measurements using, 478, *478*
  methods of, 476–477
  reasons for using, 475–476
  roentgenograms and, 477
  treatment planning and, 481–485
    asymmetries and, 485
    for mandibular advancement or setback,
      481, *482,* 483
    for maxillary advancement, 483
    problems of vertical dimension and, 483,
      484, 485
  in velopharyngeal insufficiency, 621, *622*
Charles procedure, for lymphedema, 380
CHART (continuous hyperfractionated
  accelerated radiation therapy), 951
Cheek dissection, in facial rejuvenation, *1887,*
  1887–1888
Cheek implants, 1915
Cheek injuries, 1092–1098, *1097*
  anatomy and, 1092–1093, *1094*
  management of, 1093, *1095, 1096*
Cheiloplasty, 2058, *2058*
  Dieffenbach, May modification of, 915, *915,
    916*

Chemical burns, 448–451
  clinical evaluation of, 449
  management of, 449–451, *450*, *451*
  pathophysiology of, 449
Chemical peel
  in African-Americans, 2051, 2052
  in facial rejuvenation, 1987–1989, *1988*, 1988t
Chemotherapy
  adjuvant (maintenance), 943
    in oropharyngeal carcinoma, 943t, 943–944
  in basal cell carcinoma, of skin, 318
  concurrent, 940
    in oropharyngeal carcinoma, 942–943, 943t
  head and neck prostheses for patients treated by, 1028
  induction (neoadjuvant), 940
    in oropharyngeal carcinoma, 941t, 941–942
  in laryngeal cancer, 1016–1017
  for malignant melanomas, 348–349
  multiagent, in oropharyngeal carcinoma, 940
  for oropharyngeal carcinoma, 939–944
    adjuvant, 943t, 943–944
    concurrent radiation therapy and, 942–943, 943t
    induction, 941t, 941–942
    organ preservation and, 942
    primary, 940–941
    recurrent and metastatic disease, 939
    single-agent, 939–940, 940t
  primary, in oropharyngeal carcinoma, 940–941
  for salivary gland tumors, 1044
Cherry hemangiomas (senile hemangiomas), 300
Chest wall anomalies, 1233–1238
  embryology of, 1233, *1234*
  pectus deformities. *See* Pectus deformities
  Poland anomaly, 1233, *1234–1236*, 1235–1237
Chest wall reconstruction, 1248–1266. *See also* Breast reconstruction
  anterior and lateral chest wall defects and, 1257, 1259, *1262–1265*
  flaps for, 1249–1252, *1250*, *1251*
    latissimus dorsi, 1250–1251
    omentum, 1252
    pectoralis major, 1249
    rectus abdominis, 1251–1252
    serratus anterior, 1249–1250
    trapezius, 1251
  infected median sternotomy and, *1252*, 1252–1259
    symptoms and signs of, 1253
    treatment of, *1253*, 1253–1254, *1254–1256*, 1257, *1258–1261*
  intrathoracic transposition of soft tissue in, 1268–1275
    bronchopleural fistula closure and, 1273
    esophageal repair and, 1270
    indications for, 1268–1269, 1269t
    latissimus dorsi flaps for, 1269–1270, *1270*
    pectoralis major flaps for, 1269, *1269*
    rectus abdominis flaps for, 1270
    reinforcement of suture lines of heart and great vessels and, 1270, *1271–1272*
    results with, 1273, 1275t
    serratus anterior flaps for, 1269, *1270*
    surgical procedure for, 1273, *1274*

Chest wall reconstruction—*Continued*
  posterior chest wall defects and, 1259, *1265–1267*
  principles of, 1248–1249, 1249t
Children. *See also* Infants; Orthognathic surgery, correction of secondary skeletal deformities in adolescent patients with clefts and
  facial fractures in. *See* Facial fractures, in children and adolescents
  mandibular fractures in, surgical techniques for, 1176
  scar revision in, 36
  6 to 10 years of age, mandibular dysostosis in, timing of treatment of, 529
  12 years or older, mandibular dysostosis in, timing of treatment of, 529
Chin
  augmentation of, with lyocartilage, 530, *531*
  postoperative care of, in hemifacial microsomia, 542
Chin correction, 743
  advancement genioplasty for, technique and results of, 743
  asymmetric, technique and results of, 743, *748*
  indications for, 743, *744*
  reduction genioplasty for, technique and results of, 743, *745–747*
  sagittal split osteotomy combined with, for mandibular deformities, 756
Chin dysplasia
  bilateral cleft lip and palate and, 687
  isolated cleft palate and, 698
  unilateral cleft lip and palate and, 683
Chordee, 1397
Choroid syringomas (eccrine mixed tumors), 304
Circumdental wiring, for mandibular fractures, 1168, *1168*
Cisplatin, in oropharyngeal carcinoma, 940, 940t, 942
Clasped thumb deformity, 1449, *1453*, 1453t
Clawing, of fingers, tendon transfers for, 1592–1593
Cleft(s), alveolar. *See* Alveolar clefts
Cleft-dental gaps
  bilateral cleft lip and palate and, 687
  unilateral cleft lip and palate and, 683
Cleft earlobes, 796
  features of, 796, *797*, *798*
  treatment of, 796, *798*, *799*
Cleft lip. *See also* Facial clefts
  bilateral, 566–574
    alar cartilage repositioning and vestibular reconstruction in, 571, 574
    anesthesia and, 571
    correction of secondary skeletal deformities in adolescents with, 687, 689, 691, *692–697*, 697
    cupid's bow reconstruction in, 574
    fixation of lower lateral alar cartilage in, 574
    general management of, 566
    incisions and tissue mobilization in, 571
    lip closure and shortening in, 574
    lip symmetry in, 574
    management of premaxilla and prolabium in, 566, *567*
    muscle reconstruction in, 574
    nasal floor reconstruction in, 574
    postoperative care and, 574, *576*

Cleft lip, bilateral—*Continued*
    secondary correction of nasal deformity from, *708*, 708–709
    surgical markings and evaluation of lip pathology and, 568, *569–570*, *572*
  correction of secondary skeletal deformities in adolescent patients with. *See* Orthognathic surgery, correction of secondary skeletal deformities in adolescent patients with clefts and
  nasal deformity associated with. *See* Nasal clefts
  orthodontic management of. *See* Orthodontic treatment, in cleft lip and palate
  prosthetic management of. *See* Prosthodontics, in cleft lip and palate
  secondary soft tissue procedures for, 605–615
    cross-lip (Abbe) flap, 609–610, *611–613*
    cross-lip vermilion flap, 608–609, *610–611*
    double pendulum flaps, 611, *613*
    evaluation of deformity for, 605–606
    forked flap columellar reconstruction, 615, *616*
    quadrilateral vermilion flap reconstruction of cupid's bow, 614–615, *615*
    secondary soft tissue problems and, 606t, 606–607, *608–609*
    total lip revision, 614, *614*
    V-Y vermilion mucosal rolldown, 607–608, *609*
  unilateral, 548–564
    anatomy of, 548–550, *549*, *550*
    correction of secondary skeletal deformities in adolescents with, 683–687, *684–685*, *688–691*
    influence of repair on maxillofacial growth, 564
    lip adhesion in, 551
    preoperative orthopedic treatment of, 551
    rotation-advancement technique in, 551–552, *553–555*
    secondary correction of nasal deformity from, 703–706, *704*
    timing of repair of, 550–551
    triangular flap technique in. *See* Triangular flap technique
Cleft palate, 595–603. *See also* Facial clefts
  bilateral, correction of secondary skeletal deformities in adolescents with, 687, 689, 691, *692–697*, 697
  correction of secondary skeletal deformities in adolescent patients with. *See* Orthognathic surgery, correction of secondary skeletal deformities in adolescent patients with clefts and
  Furlow double-reversing Z-plasty for. *See* Furlow double-reversing Z-plasty
  isolated, correction of secondary skeletal deformities in adolescents with, 697–698
  with mandibular dysostosis, treatment of, 528
  orthodontic management of. *See* Orthodontic treatment, in cleft lip and palate
  preparation for repair of, 595–596
  prosthetic management of. *See* Prosthodontics, in cleft lip and palate

Cleft palate—*Continued*
  secondary soft tissue procedures for, 615, 617, 617t, 618
  timing of repair of, 595
  unilateral, correction of secondary skeletal deformities in adolescents with, 683–687, *684–685, 688–691*
Cleft palate team. *See* Craniofacial team
Clinodactyly, 1439, *1439, 1440,* 1441
Cloverleaf skull, 512
Clubfoot, underdevelopment of leg caused by, calf implantation and, 2255–2256, *2258*
Clubhand, radial, 1445, *1447, 1447, 1447*
Coaptation, nerve grafting and, 132, *132*
Cocaine, for topical anesthesia of mucous membranes, 18–19
Cohesion, among craniofacial team members, 473
Collagen
  injections of, for perioral rejuvenation, 1996
  matrix formation and, 5
Collagen remodeling, in wound healing, 5
Collecting venules, of skin flaps, 67
Coloboma, correction of, 535
Columella
  elongation of, in bilateral cleft nasal deformity repair, 575, *577*
  forked flap reconstruction of, 615, *616*
  lengthening of, in Oriental patients, 2082, *2083, 2084*
  short, cleft lip and, 606t, 607
Comminuted fractures
  mandibular, *1174, 1175,* 1175–1176
  nasal, treatment of, 1133, *1133,* 1134
Complete lower body lift, 2214, *2216–2218*
Composite grafts, 52–53
  composite earlobe graft technique and, for bilateral cleft nasal deformity repair, 578, *579*
Compound fractures, mandibular, 1174
Compound nevi, 350
Compression (tension-band) plates and wires, for hand and wrist fractures, *1524–1526, 1528–1529*
Computed tomography
  in maxillofacial trauma, 1073–1074
    basic principles of, 1073
    equipment for, 1073
    interpretation of, 1073–1074
    multiplanar imaging and, 1073–1074
    standard planes and, 1073
    techniques for, 1073
    three-dimensional imaging and, 1074
  in oropharyngeal carcinoma, 926, *926*
  in temporomandibular joint deformities, 1223–1224
  three-dimensional. *See* 3-D computed tomography
    craniomaxillofacial surgery and, 138, *139–141*
Condylar process fractures, of ascending ramus, 1176–1177
  closed reduction of, 1176
  open reduction of, 1176–1177, *1178, 1179*
Conflict, among craniofacial team members, 473
Congenital nevi, 306, *307*
Conjunctival edema, following eyelid operations in Oriental patients, 2075
Connective tissue, nevi of, 299

Consensus, among craniofacial team members, 473
Constriction ring syndrome, 1441, 1442t, *1443,* 1443–1444
Contact guidance, peripheral nerve injuries and, 1599–1601, *1600–1602*
Contamination, nerve grafting and, 129
Continuous hyperfractionated accelerated radiation therapy (CHART), 951
Continuous passive motion, in hand rehabilitation, 1751, *1752*
Continuous-wave, argon-pumped, tunable dye lasers, 264
Contour deformities, of jaws, mandibular fractures and, 1177
Contractures
  capsular, augmentation mammaplasty and, 2101, 2101t, 2112
  Dupuytren. *See* Dupuytren contracture incisions for, 1419, *1420*
  treatment of, pressure sores and, 1375
Convalescence, following lipectomy, 240
Converging triangular flaps. *See* Z-plasty
Copper, wound healing and, 9
Copper vapor lasers, 263–264
Corneal abrasion, following blepharoplasty, 1937–1938
Corner-lift, *1992,* 1992–1993
  nasolabial furrow excision and, 1993, *1993*
  results with, 1993
  technique for, 1993
Coronal craniosynostosis
  bilateral, 151, *152–153*
  unilateral, 148, *150,* 151
Coronal flaps, in craniomaxillofacial surgery, 138, *141*
Coronal plane, for computed tomography imaging, in maxillofacial trauma, 1073
Coronoid process
  elongated, removal of, 532, *532*
  fractures of, of ascending ramus, 1176
Corrosive agents, burns caused by, 449
Cortical bone, 102
  grafts of, 104
Cortisone injections, rebound, hemangiomas and, 359, *360*
Counseling, of patient, soft tissue expansion and, 202, 204
Cranial dysostosis, history of, 499–500, *500, 501,* 501t
Cranialization, for frontal sinus fractures, 1114, *1114–1118*
Craniofacial dysostosis, 512–514
  Apert syndrome and bipartition and, 514, *514*
  in infants, 512–513, *513*
Craniofacial embryology, 459–469
  molecular determinants of development and, 466–469
    epithelial-mesenchymal interactions and, 468
    homeobox-containing genes, 468
    molecular genetic approaches and, 468–469
    regulatory signaling molecules, 466–468
  origins and early migrations of facial tissues and, 459, *460, 461*
  pharyngeal arches and, 462–463, *462–466,* 465–466
Craniofacial microsomia, *See* Hemifacial microsomia (craniofacial microsomia; first and second branchial arch syndrome)

Craniofacial reconstruction, fixation principles in, 193, 195, *195–200*
Craniofacial team, 471–473
  correction of secondary skeletal deformities in adolescent patients with clefts and, 682
  dynamics of, 472–473
  effective team care and, 473
  members of, 472
Craniofacial trauma, craniomaxillofacial surgery in, 163–165
  acute trauma and, 163–164, *164–165*
  post-traumatic deformity and, 165, *166*
Craniomaxillofacial surgery, 135–168
  airway management and, 138
  alloplastic material in, 148
  canthopexy, 142, 144
    lateral, 142, 144, *145*
    medial, 144, *145*
  coronal flap, 138, *141*
  cranial bone grafts in, 145–146, *147,* 148
  in craniofacial trauma, 163–165
    acute, 163–164, *164–165*
    post-traumatic deformity and, 165, *166*
  in craniosynostosis, 148–151
  in Crouzon and Apert syndromes, 160–163
  galeal frontalis musculofascial flap and, 142, *144*
  in hypertelorism, 151, 154
  infection as complication of, 166, 168
  management of temporalis muscle and, 141, *142*
  plate and screw fixation and, 141–142, *143*
  team and, 135
  in telecanthus, 159–160
  temporal galea in, 144–145, *146–147*
  three-dimensional computed tomographic imaging and, 138, *139–141*
  timing of, 135–136, *136–137*
  in tumors of base of skull, 165–166, *167*
Craniosynostosis, 148–151, 499–512
  coronal
    bilateral, 151, *152–153*
    unilateral, 148, *150,* 151
  history of, 499–500, *500, 501,* 501t
  Kleeblattschädel, 151
  lambdoid, isolated, 151
  malformations associated with, 512
  metopic, 151, *154–155*
  pansuture, 151
  rare and complex forms of, 511–512
  sagittal, 148, *149*
  simple, 500–511
    classification of, 500–501, *502–510,* 503–504, 506, 508–509
    evaluation of treatment of, 509, 511, 511t
    indications for treatment of, 511
Credentials, for laser use, 267
Cricoid cartilage, 1008
Cronin method, 575, *577*
Crooked nose, secondary rhinoplasty for, 2040, *2041*
Crossbite
  anterior, orthodontic treatment in primary dentition for, 652, *654*
  posterior, orthodontic treatment in primary dentition for, 650, *651–653*
Cross-face nerve grafting, 823–824, *824*
Cross-finger flaps, for fingertip injuries with exposed bone, 1498, *1502, 1503*
Cross-lip (Abbe) flap, 609–610, *611–613*
Cross-lip vermilion flap, 608–609, *610–611*
Cross tunneling, in lipectomy, 235

Crouzon syndrome
    Le Fort III osteotomy in, 160, *161–162,* 162
    single-stage frontomaxillary advancement
        in, 163, *163*
    two-stage craniomaxillary procedure in, 162
Crow's feet, correction of
    blepharoplasty for, 1938–1939, *1939*
    dissection for, 1891, *1892*
    planning, 1882–1883
Cryosurgical therapy, in basal cell carcinoma,
        of skin, 316, 318
Cryptotia, 783
    etiology of, 783
    features of, 783, *787*
    treatment of
        buried-suture method for, 780
        conservative, 783–784, *785*
        local flap without skin graft for, 784–787,
            786–787
Cultured epithelial grafts, 54–55
Cup ear, 787, 789, *787*
    etiology of, 787
    treatment of
        lengthening or radiating helical cartilage,
            789
        restoring antihelix with mattress suture,
            787, 789
Cupid's bow
    absence of, cleft lip and, 606t, 607
    quadrilateral vermilion flap reconstruction
        of, 614–615, *615*
    reconstruction of, for bilateral cleft lip
        repair, 574
Curettage, in basal cell carcinoma, of skin,
        316
Cutaneous appendages, tumors of, 301–304
    with apocrine differentiation, 303, *303*
    of eccrine differentiation, 303–304, *304*
    with follicular differentiation, *301,* 301–302,
        302
    with sebaceous differentiation, *302,*
        302–303
Cutaneous horns, 310–311, *311*
Cutaneous meningiomas, 305
Cutaneous scapular artery, 73
Cutis marmorata telangiectasia, 363
Cutting cautery, for breast reduction, 2119
Cyclic adenosine monophosphate,
        craniofacial development and, 466–467
Cylindromas, 303
Cyst(s)
    bone, solitary, of hands, 1466
    branchial cleft, 810, *810*
    bronchogenic, 303
    dermoid. *See* Dermoid cysts
        of cutaneous appendages, 301
    epidermoid, 301
        of hands, 1454–1455
    hair, eruptive, vellus, 301
    inclusion (milia), 301, *301*
        following blepharoplasty, 1938
    pilar (tricholemmal), 301
    post-traumatic, wrist pain and, 1730t–1731t
    synovial, of hands, 1463
Cystadenomas
    apocrine (apocrine hidrocystomas), 303,
        303
    lymphomatosum, papillary (Warthin
        tumor), 1035, 1036t, 1037, *1037*
Cystoides (lymphangioma hygroma), 368, *379*

Dardour flap, 2091, *2091*
Debridement
    of hand injuries, 1488–1489
    hand reconstruction and, 1659
    of leg ulcers, 1833
Decubitus ulcers. *See* Pressure sores
Deepithelialization, breast reduction and,
        2147
Deep venous thrombosis, following suction-
        assisted lipectomy, 2199
Delay phenomenon, skin flaps and, 69
Deltopectoral flap, for oropharyngeal
        reconstruction, 961, *964–965*
Dental care, in cleft lip and palate,
        prosthodontics and, 762–763
Dental pulp, necrosis of, mandibular
        fractures and, 1177
Dental rehabilitation, following mandibular
        reconstruction, 998, *999*
Dentition
    permanent, orthodontic treatment for clefts
        in, 658–659, 661, *661,* 662
    primary. *See* Primary dentition, orthodontic
        treatment for clefts in
    transitional. *See* Transitional dentition,
        orthodontic treatment for clefts in
Dependency, of craniofacial team members,
        473
Depressor septi nasi muscle, anatomy of,
        2077
Deprivation amblyopia, hemangiomas and,
        355, *356*
Dermabrasion
    aesthetic facial surgery in African-
        Americans and, *2052,* 2052–2053
    in facial rejuvenation, 1989, *1989*
    for perioral rejuvenation, *1994,* 1994–1995
        postoperative care and, 1995
        results with, 1995
        technique for, 1994–1995
    for scar revision, 41, *41*
Dermal grafts, 88t, 90, *90*
    fat, 53
    uses of, 90
Dermal melanocytosis, 307
Dermatocrurolipectomy, inner thigh-plasty
        with. *See* Inner thigh-plasty, with
        liposuction or dermatocrurolipectomy
Dermatofibromas, 299
Dermatomes, burn wound grafting and, 414
Dermatosis papulosa nigra, 295, *297*
Dermofasciectomy, with full-thickness skin
        graft, for Dupuytren contracture,
        1722–1723, *1723–1726,* 1725, 1727
Dermoid cysts
    angular, external, 809
    of cutaneous appendages, 301
    midline, 816–817, *817–819*
Dermolevator attachment, blepharoplasty
        and, 1921
Desmoid tumors, of skin, 200
Devascularization, hand reconstruction and,
        1672, *1673*
Dexon (polyglycolic acid) sutures, 7, 21, 22t
Diabetic foot, 1839–1859
    perioperative evaluation of, 1839–1843
        neurologic studies in, *1842,* 1842–1843,
            1843
        roentgenographic, 1839–1840, *1840, 1841*
        vascular studies in, 1840–1842
    reconstruction of. *See* Foot reconstruction,
        of diabetic foot
Dieffenbach cheiloplasty, May modification
        of, 915, *915, 916*

Digits. *See also* Finger(s); Hand(s); Thumb(s)
    supernumerary, rudimentary, 305
Discrimination sensibility, of hand,
        evaluation of, 1746
Dislocations
    of finger dorsal metacarpophalangeal joint,
        1540, *1542*
    perilunate, 1546–1547, *1547, 1548*
    of wrist, 1737, *1738*
Displacement, of nose, following rhinoplasty
        in Oriental patients, 2083
Disseminated superficial actinic
        porokeratosis, 312, *313*
Distal interphalangeal joint, incisions for
        exposure of, 1422, *1422*
Distant flaps, 57, *59*
    local, 1505, *1507*
Distraction osteogenesis, in lower extremity
        reconstruction, 1805–1806
    follow up and, 1806
    technique and fixation and, 1805–1806,
        1806, 1807
Donor sites
    for abdominal muscle flaps, for abdominal
        wall reconstruction, 1353, *1353–1356,*
        1355, 1357, *1358*
    for bone grafts, 105t, 105–108, 110–111, 112
    for flaps, 72
    for flexor tendon grafting, *123,* 123–124
    for free tissue transfer, selection of,
        968–969
    management of, burn wounds and, 412,
        412, 413
    repair of, complications of, 70
    for skin grafts, 48–49, *49*
        healing of, 55
    for tendon grafts, *123,* 123–124
    for toe-to-hand transplantation, morbidity
        of, 1709
Doppler studies, of diabetic foot, 1841, 1842
Dorsal augmentation, in rhinoplasty, in
        African-Americans, 2055
Dorsalis pedis free vascularized flaps, 986t,
        994
Dorsal resection, for rhinoplasty, 2010–2011,
        2012
Dorsal rolls, lipectomy and, 235
Double eyelid operation. *See* Eyelid
        operations, in Oriental patients
Double pendulum flaps, 611, *613*
Drainage. *See* Surgical drainage, for
        lymphedema
Dressings
    burn wound grafting and, *414,* 414–415,
        415
    for facial rejuvenation, 1895
    for leg ulcers, 1833–1834
        occlusive, 1836
    following lipectomy, 240
Drug(s), skin flaps and, 69
Drug therapy. *See also specific drugs and drug
        types*
    for leg ulcers, 1835
    following lipectomy, 240
    for lymphedema, 376
Dupuytren contracture, *1720–1722,* 1720–1727
    etiology and pathophysiology of, 1721
    incisions for, 1419, *1420*
    natural history of, 1721
    treatment of, 1721–1727, *1723*
        dermofasciectomy with full-thickness
            skin graft in, 1722–1723, *1723–1726,*
            1725, 1727
        triamcinolone in, 1722
Dysphagia, free tissue techniques and, 981

Ear(s)
    anatomy and, 1098
    burns of, 418, 420–422
        classification of, 418, 420
        treatment of, 420–422, *421–423*
    deformities of, reconstruction of, 535
    external. *See* External ear
    injuries of, 1098–1099
    management of, 1098–1099, *1099*
    reconstruction using soft tissue expansion, 210
Earlobe(s), cleft, 792
    features of, 792, *793, 794*
    treatment of, 792, *794, 795*
Earlobe graft, for bilateral cleft nasal deformity repair, 578, *579*
Earlobe incision, for facial rejuvenation, 1876
Ear tags, 809–810
Eccrine hidrocystomas, 303
Eccrine mixed tumors (choroid syringomas), 304
Eccrine poromas, 303–304
Eccrine spiroadenomas, 304
Ectropion
    following blepharoplasty, 1935, *1935*
    blepharoplasty for, 1972, *1974–1976*, 1975
    following eyelid operations in Oriental patients, 2075
Edema
    following blepharoplasty, 1937
    conjunctival, following eyelid operations in Oriental patients, 2075
    control of, leg ulcers and, 1834
    in hands
        control of, 1748, *1748*
        evaluation of, 1746, *1747*
Elbow
    amputations proximal to, replantation and, 1633–1634, *1637–1639*
    burn wounds of, 434
Electrical burns, 441–448
    clinical evaluation of, 442, 444–446, *445*
    complications of, 448
    hand reconstruction and, 1672, *1674*, 1675
    management of, 226–228
        nonsurgical, 446
        surgical, 446–448, *446–448*
    of mount, 426
    pathophysiology of, 441–442, *442, 443*
Electrical charges, wound healing and, 10
Electrical modalities, in hand rehabilitation, 1750–1751, *1751*
Electrodesiccation, in basal cell carcinoma, of skin, 316
Emphysema, soft tissue, maxillofacial, roentgenographic interpretation and, 1072–1073
Encephaloceles, 817, *819*
Enchondromas, of hands, 1463–1464, *1464, 1465*
Endocrine system, thermal burns and, 406
Endoscopy, in oropharyngeal carcinoma, *926*, 926–927, *927*
Enophthalmos, following blepharoplasty, 1937
Entropion
    following blepharoplasty, 1937
    blepharoplasty for, 1975–1976, *1977*
Epidermal cysts, 301
Epidermal growth factor, wound healing and, 4t, 9
Epidermal nevus syndrome, 296, 298
Epidermal tumors, 295–298

Epidermodysplasia verruciformis, 295, 312
Epidermoid cysts, of hands, 1454–1455
Epiglottic cartilage, 1008, *1010*
Epinephrine, pretreatment with, before lipectomy, 232–233, 233t
Epiphora, following blepharoplasty, 1935–1936
Epispadias, 1393–1395
    surgical technique for, 1393, *1394*, 1396
    complications of treatment for, 1395
    postoperative care and, 1395, *1396–1397*
Epithelialization, in wound healing, 5
Epithelial-mesenchymal interactions, craniofacial development and, 468
Epithelial tunnels, following blepharoplasty, 1938
Epithelioid sarcomas, of hands, 1462
Epulis, giant cell, 200
Eruptive vellus hair cysts, 301
Erythroplakia, oropharyngeal carcinoma and, 923, *924*
Esophagus
    cervical, lesions of, oropharyngeal reconstruction and, 968
    intrathoracic transposition of soft tissue for repair of, 1270
Estlander lip transfer, 909
Ethmoid bone, evaluation of, in maxillofacial trauma, 1064–1065
Excimer lasers, 256
Exercises, in hand rehabilitation, 1748
Exfoliative cytology, in oropharyngeal carcinoma, 927
Exophthalmos, blepharoplasty for, 1940
Expectations. *See* Patient satisfaction
Extended facelift, 1966
Extensor carpi radialis brevis tendon transfer, 1596, *1597*
    Brand, *1594*, 1594–1595
Extensor carpi radialis longus tendon transfer, Brand, *1594*, 1594–1595
Extensor digitorum longus tendon grafts, 124
Extensor indicis proprius (Burkhalter) tendon transfer, 1587, *1588*
External ear, 772–792
    anatomy of, 772–773, *773, 774*
        muscles, 772, *774*
        sensory nerve supply of auricle, 773, *775*
    cutaneous malignant tumors of, *331*, 331–332
    deformities of. *See specific deformities*
    embryology of, 773–774
    prominent, 774–777
        skin excision and mattress suture for, *776*, 776, *777*
        skin excision with or without excision of cartilage and, *775*, 775–776, *776*
        widening of cartilage by rasping and, *777*, 777, *778*
External levator resection procedure, for ptosis of eyelid, 800–801, *802–803*, 804
Extremities. *See also* Lower extremities; Upper extremities
    burn wound reconstruction and. *See* Burn wounds, of extremities and trunk, reconstruction of
Extrusion, following rhinoplasty in Oriental patients, 2086, *2086*
Eye(s). *See also* Blepharoplasty; *headings beginning with terms* Lacrimal *and* Orbital
    amblyopia and
        anisometropic, hemangiomas and, 355
        deprivation, hemangiomas and, 355, *356*

Eye(s)—*Continued*
    evaluation of, in maxillofacial trauma, 1063–1064, *1065*
    irritation of, eyelid operations in Oriental patients and, 2075
Eyebrows, burns of, 422–423
Eyelashes, loss of, following blepharoplasty, 1937
Eyelid(s)
    blepharoplasty and. *See* Blepharoplasty
    burns of, 423–424
    cutaneous malignant tumors of, 324, *329, 330*, 330–331
    injuries of, 1090–1092. *See also* Ptosis, of eyelid, traumatic
    lower
        atonic, blepharoplasty for, 1939
        elevation of, 530, *530*
        ptosis of. *See* Ptosis, of eyelid
Eyelid injuries
    anatomy and, 1090, *1090–1091*
    management of, 1090–1092, *1091–1094*
Eyelid operations, in Oriental patients, 2059–2075, *2060*
    complications and suboptimal results with, 2072–2075, *2072–2075*
    postoperative assessment of, 2070–2071, *2071*
    postoperative care and, 2070
    preoperative assessment for, 2063
    surgical anatomy and, 2059, 2061–2062, *2061–2063*
    transconjunctival method for, 2063–2065, *2064–2067*
    transcutaneous method for, 2065, 2068–2070, *2068–2071*
Eyelid reconstruction, 864–881
    anatomy and, *864*, 864–866, *865*
    complications of, 880–881
    full-thickness defects and, 869
    partial-thickness defects and, 869
    preoperative preparation for, 867–868
    surgical principles for, 866–867, *866–868*
    surgical technique for, 869–878
        lateral canthal reconstruction, 875
        lower eyelid reconstruction, *871, 873–874, 876–877*
        medial canthal reconstruction, 874–875, *875–877*
        multiple-zone reconstruction, 876, 878, *878–881*
        upper eyelid reconstruction, *869*, 869–871, *870*

Face. *See also* Forehead
    aesthetic units of, 416, *417*
    burn reconstruction and. *See* Burn wounds, of head and neck, reconstruction of
    lipectomy and. *See* Suction-assisted lipectomy
    midline lesions of, 816–821
    photographic documentation of, lipectomy and, 226, *226*
    reconstruction using soft tissue expansion, 207–208, *208*
Facelift. *See* Facial rejuvenation
Facial aesthetics, 1863–1865, *1864*
    facial rejuvenation and. *See* Facial rejuvenation, aesthetic considerations in
Facial asymmetry, 1873

Facial clefts, 486–498. *See also* Cleft lip; Cleft palate; Nasal clefts
    classification of, 487, *487*
    identification of, 486–487, *487*
        chronologic basis for, 486
        topographic basis for, 486
    internasal dysplasia and, *489*, 489–490
        surgical treatment of, 489–490, *490–492*
    maxillary dysplasia and, 494–498, *495*
        surgical treatment of, 494, *496*, 496–498, *497*
    nasomaxillary dysplasia and, 494, *495*
    nasoschizis and, 492, *493*, 494
        surgical treatment of, 492–494, *493–495*
    surgical treatment of
        anchoring occupational therapy tissues and, 489
        planning of incision for, 488–489
        principles of, 487–488, *488*
        timing of, 488
Facial fractures, 171–179
    in children and adolescents, 1188–1198, *1189*
        of alveolar process, 1198
        of lower third of face, 1195–1198, *1197*
        of middle third of face. *See* Midface fractures, in children and adolescents
        of upper third of face, 1188–1189
    mandibular, 171, *172–176*, 174
    mandibular reconstruction and, *183*, 183–187
        alloplastic, 183, *184–185*
        with bone grafts, 183, 185, *186–187*, 187
    midfacial, 177–179, *177–182*
Facial gunshot wounds, 1181–1187, *1182–1185*
    mandibular fractures and, 1186
    repair of midface and, 1181, 1183, 1185–1186
    soft tissue reconstruction and, 1186–1187
    3-D computed tomography in, 277–278, *278*
Facial nerve
    injuries of, 1084–1085
        anatomy and, 1084–1085, *1085*
        management of, 1085, *1086*
        with subperiosteal facelift, 1916
    surgical management of salivary gland tumors and, 1043–1044
Facial prostheses, 1028, *1029*
Facial reanimation, 822–829, 823t, 1045–1055
    clinical experience with, 1052, 1055, 1055t, *1056–1058*
    cross-face nerve grafting for, 823–824, *824*
    indications and timing for, 823
    microsurgical approach for, *1046*, 1046–1047, *1047*
    muscle transplantation for, *824*, 824–825, *826*, *827*, 827
    preoperative planning for, 823
    results of, *828*, 828–829, *829*
    surgical technique for, 1047–1052
        ancillary procedures and, 1052
        preoperative planning and, 1048, *1048*
        stage 1, 1048–1049, *1049*, *1050*
        stage 2, 1049–1052, *1051–1054*
Facial reconstruction, 842–863
    clinical diagnosis and, 843–844, *844*, *845*
    goal setting for, 844–846, *845*
    local control and, 843
    planning of operation for, 846–863
        corollaries of subunit principle and, 851, 854–855, *855–862*, *857–858*, 863

Facial reconstruction, planning of operation for—*Continued*
        subunit principle and, 846–848, *846–854*, 851
    skin cancer and, 842–843
    wound margins and, 843
Facial rejuvenation, 1871–1872, *1872*, 1873–1901, 1979–1989. *See also* Blepharoplasty; Brow-lift; Forehead-lift
    aesthetic considerations in, 1873
        facial asymmetry and, 1873
        in men, 1903–1904, *1904*, *1905*
        panfacial rejuvenation and, 1873
        recognizing aging in face and neck and, 1873, *1874*
    anesthesia for, 1885–1886
    augmentation of skeletal features and, 1979–1981, *1981*, *1982*
    chemical peel and, 1987–1989, *1988*, 1988t
    complications of, 1901
    dermabrasion and, 1989, *1989*
    direct excision for, 1982–1983, *1982–1985*
    filler injections in, 1983, *1986*, 1987, *1987*
    lip modifications in, 1983, *1985*, *1986*
    in men, 1903–1908
        aesthetic considerations and, 1903–1904, *1904*, *1905*
        anesthesia for, 1904
        dissection for, 1906–1908, *1907*
        incisions for, 1905–1906
        physiologic differences from women and, 1903
        postoperative care and, 1908
        preoperative assessment for, 1904
        surgical technique for, 1905–1908, *1907*
    perioral. *See* Perioral rejuvenation
    postoperative care and, 1901
    preoperative planning for, 1873–1883
        of crow's feet correction, 1882–1883
        of earlobe incision, 1876
        of modification of submental region, 1881–1882
        of modification of superficial musculoaponeurotic system, *1879–1885*, 1880–1881
        of occipital incision, 1877, *1878*
        of postauricular incision, 1876–1877, *1877*
        of preauricular incision, 1874–1875, *1876*
        of submental incision, 1878, *1879*
        of temporal incision, 1874, *1875*, *1876*
    preoperative preparation for, 1883–1885
    retinoids for, 1987
    skin care and hygiene and, 1987
    subperiosteal facelift, 1910–1919, *1916–1919*
        ancillary procedures and, 1915–1916
        clinical applications of, 1916
        complications of, 1916
        evaluation and planning for, 1911
        historical review of, 1910
        rationale and indications for, 1910–1911
        surgical technique for, 1911–1913, 1912–*1914*, 1915
    suction lipectomy for, 1979, *1980*
    surgical technique for, 1886–1895
        cheek and neck dissection, *1887*, 1887–1888, *1888*
        crow's-feet dissection, 1891, *1892*
        dressings and, 1895
        flap repositioning and placement of suspension sutures, 1891, *1892*, 1893, *1893*
        flap trimming and closure, 1893–1895, *1894*
        incisions and, 1886

Facial rejuvenation, surgical technique for—*Continued*
        modification of superficial musculoaponeurotic system and platysma, 1888–1890, *1889*
        submental dissection, *1890*, 1890–1891, *1891*
        temporal dissection, *1886*, 1886–1887, *1887*
Facial soft tissue injuries, 1083–1099
    ear injuries, 1098–1099
        anatomy and, 1098
        management of, 1098–1099, *1099*
    eyelid injuries, 1090–1092
        anatomy and, 1090, *1090–1091*
        management of, 1090–1092, *1091–1094*
    facial nerve injuries, 1084–1085
        anatomy and, 1084–1085, *1085*
        management of, 1085, *1086*
    general principles of, 1083–1084, *1084*
    lip and cheek injuries, 1092–1098, *1097*
        anatomy and, 1092–1093, *1094*
        management of, 1093, *1095*, *1096*
    nasal injuries, 1098
        anatomy and, 1098
        management of, 1098
    parotid duct injuries, 1086
        anatomy and, 1086, *1086*
        management of, 1086, *1087*
    scalp injuries, 1086, 1088
        anatomy and, 1086, 1088, *1088*
        management of, 1088, *1089*
Facial surgery, 1865–1872
    aesthetic. *See* Aesthetic facial surgery; Blepharoplasty; Brow-lift; Facial rejuvenation; Forehead-lift; Rhinoplasty
    of aging face. *See* Facial rejuvenation
    of forehead, 1865
    infraorbital rim augmentation and, 1868–1869
    of malar-midface area, 1866–1868, *1869*
    of mandible
        anterior, 1870–1871, *1871*
        posterior, *1869*, 1869–1870
    of supraorbital ridges, 1865, *1866*
    of temporal areas, 1865
        temporal fossa, 1865, *1867*
    of zygomatic arch-malar area, 1865–1866, *1868*
Familial dysplastic nevus syndrome, 350
Fascia
    subcutaneous, 217, *218*
    superficial, trunk- and thigh-lifts and, 2201–2202, *2202*
Fascia lata frontalis sling, for ptosis of eyelid. *See* Ptosis, of eyelid, autogenous fascia lata frontalis sling for
Fascial grafts, 88t, *93*, 93–94
    uses of, 93–94
Fascicles, identification for nerve grafting, 130–131, *131*
Fasciitis, necrotizing, of hands, 1473–1474, *1477*
Fasciocutaneous flaps, 61, 63, *63–66*, 66, 73, 75, 77–80, 78t
    in foot reconstruction, 1796–1797, *1797*, *1798*
    of lower extremity, 77–80
        anatomy of, 78–79, *79*
        surgical technique for, 79–80
    in lower extremity reconstruction, 1774–1775, *1775*

Fasciocutaneous flaps—*Continued*
 medial plantar flap, 75, 77
  anatomy of, 75, 77
  surgical technique for, 77, *79*
 neurovascular pudendal-thigh flaps, 80
  anatomy of, 80, *81*
  surgical technique for, 81
 for oropharyngeal reconstruction, 968
Fasciotomy, intrinsic, incisions for, 1419, *1421*
Fat
 assessment of, for blepharoplasty, *1923*,
  1924
 excision of, in blepharoplasty, 1934, *1934*
 lipectomy and. *See* Suction-assisted
  lipectomy
 liposuction and. *See* Breast reduction, by
  liposuction and vertical mammaplasty;
  Liposuction
 preantral, 220
 tumors of, of skin, 300, *301*
Fat deposits, in Oriental upper lid, 2062,
 2062, 2063
Fat emboli, following suction-assisted
 lipectomy, 2199
Fat grafts, 88t, 88–90
 uses of, 89–90
Fat injection, 239, *239, 240*
Fat necrosis, following reduction
 mammaplasty, avoidance of, 2142
Fatty acids, wound healing and, 9
Fear, lipectomy and, 227
Females. *See also specific female genital organs*
 harmony and proportion in female figure
  and, 220
Festoons, blepharoplasty for, 1939, *1940*
Fetus, wound healing in, 13
Fibroblast growth factor, wound healing and,
 4t, 9
Fibroblast proliferation, in wound healing,
 4–5
Fibromas
 of hands, 1457
 soft, 299
Fibronectin, matrix formation and, 5
Fibrosarcomas
 facial, 3-D computed tomography in,
  280–281, *282*
 of hands, 1463
Fibrous dysplasia, of maxilla, monostotic, 3-D
 computed tomography in, 283, *283,
 284*
Fibrous tissue tumors, of skin, 299, *299, 300*
Fibula free vascularized flaps, 986t, *992,
 992–993, 993*
Fibular grafts, 105t, 111–112
 in lower extremity reconstruction. *See*
  Lower extremity reconstruction
Filler injections, in facial rejuvenation, 1983,
 1986, 1987, 1987
Fine-needle aspiration, in oropharyngeal
 carcinoma, 928–929
 processing of specimens and, 929
 reporting results of, 929
 technique for, *928*, 928t, 928–929
Finger(s). *See also* Hand(s); Thumb(s)
 clawing of, tendon transfers for, 1592–1593
 duplications of rays of, 1432–1433
 incisions for exposure of distal
  interphalangeal joint and, 1422, *1422*
 incisions for exposure of proximal
  interphalangeal joint and, 1419, *1421*
 incisions on, on volar aspect, 1416, *1416*
 index, tendon transfers to provide
  adduction of, 1596

Finger(s), index—*Continued*
 accessory abductor pollicis longus and
  free tendon graft, *1596*
 infections in, incisions for treatment of,
  1417, 1417–1418
 mallet, treatment of, 1573–1574, *1574*
 myxomas of, 1462
 replantation of, 1491–1492, *1492*,
  1627–1628, 1628, 1629
  hand rehabilitation following, *1760*,
   1760–1761, *1761*
  multiple amputations and, 1630–1631,
   1632–1634
  results of, 1641
 toe-to-hand transplantation and. *See* Toe-
  to-hand transplantation
 trigger, incisions for release of, 1416–1417
Finger injuries
 to fingertips. *See* Fingertip injuries
 to ligaments
  of carpometacarpal joints, 1542
  chronic tears of ulnar collateral ligament,
   1540, *1541*
  dorsal metacarpophalangeal joint
   dislocations, 1540, 1542
  of interphalangeal joints, 1534–1536,
   1535, 1537, 1538
  of metacarpophalangeal joints, 1536,
   1538
 nail-bed. *See* Nail-bed injuries
Fingertip injuries, 1493, 1495–1505
 with exposed bone, 1496–1505
  advancement flaps and, 1496–1498,
   1498–1501, 1500–1501, 1504, 1505
  cross-finger flaps and, 1498, *1502, 1503*
  distant flaps and, 1505, *1507*
  local neurovascular island flaps and,
   1502, 1505, *1506*
  thenar flaps and, 1498, 1500, *1503, 1504*
 with loss of pulp only, 1496
  closure by skin grafting, 1496, *1496, 1497*
  healing by secondary intention and, 1496
First and second branchial arch syndrome,
  See Hemifacial microsomia (craniofacial
  microsomia; first and second branchial
  arch syndrome)
First branchial cleft anomalies, 810–811, *811*
Fischer technique, 216
Fistulas
 branchial cleft, 810, *810*
 bronchopleural, closure of, intrathoracic
  transposition of soft tissue for, 1273
 oronasal. *See* Oronasal fistulas
 salivary, free tissue techniques and, 979,
  981
Fixation. *See also under specific fractures*
 intermaxillary
  for mandibular fractures, 1168, *1169*,
   1170
  during surgery, 171
 for mandibular reconstruction, 997, *997*
 maxillomandibular, 1158
  release of, 1162
 plate. *See* Plate fixation
 rigid
  for maxillary deformities, 721, *721–722,
   722*
  in orthognathic surgery. *See*
   Orthognathic surgery
 screw. *See* Screw fixation
Flanks, male, lipectomy and, 237, *238*

Flap(s), 56–70, 71–85. *See also* Flap surgery
 advancement. *See* Advancement flaps
 choice of, 69
 for coverage of bone grafts for alveolar
  clefts, 672, *672, 673*
 delay phenomenon and, 69
 design of, 57
  refinements of, 59
 donor site for, 72
 failure of, hand reconstruction and, 1680
 fasciocutaneous. *See* Fasciocutaneous flaps
 free radicals and, 69
 history of, 56
 island, 57, *58*
 microcirculation of, 67–69
  physiologic organization of, 68
  structural organization of, 67–68
  viscosity and, 68–69
 morbidity of, 70
 muscle. *See* Muscle flaps; *specific flaps*
 musculocutaneous. *See* Musculocutaneous
  flaps
 musculotendinous, tensor fasciae latae, in
  thigh reconstruction, 1779
 necrosis of, free tissue techniques and, 979
 omental. *See* Omental flaps
 osseous. *See* Osseous flaps
 osteocutaneous, scapular
  free, 971, *973–975*
  for oropharyngeal reconstruction, 968
 osteomusculocutaneous. *See*
  Osteomusculocutaneous flaps
 pedicled, 57
  distant, 57, *59*
  local, 57, *58*
  for mandibular reconstruction, 983
  microvascular free flaps, 57
 pharmacologic manipulation of, 69
 radial forearm
  free, 970, *970–971*
  for oropharyngeal reconstruction, 968
 rhombic, 28–30, *29*, 57, *58*
 rotation, 57
 for scar revision, 42, *42*
 sensation in, 72
 skin. *See* Skin flaps
 transposition, 57
 triangular, converging. *See* Z-plasty
 vascular basis of, 59–66
  fasciocutaneous flaps and, 61, 63, *63–66,
   66*
  macrocirculation and, 59–60, *60*
  musculocutaneous flaps and, 61, *61, 62*,
   63t
  skin flaps and, *60*, 60–61
 venous drainage of, 66–67
 visceral
  free, 971, *976, 977*
  for oropharyngeal reconstruction,
   968–969
Flap surgery. *See also* Free tissue transfer
 for abdominal wall and groin
  reconstruction, 1357
 for breast reconstruction, 1317–1322
 for chest wall reconstruction. *See* Chest
  wall reconstruction, flaps for
 choice of flaps for, 71–72
 for hips, 1361–1364
 for lower extremity coverage. *See* Lower
  extremities, fasciocutaneous flaps
 for nasal reconstruction
  axial paramedian forehead flaps and,
   887, *888, 889, 889*
  local nasal flaps and, 886, *886*
  nasolabial flaps and, 889, *890, 891, 892*

Flap surgery—*Continued*
  oropharyngeal reconstruction using. *See*
      Oropharyngeal reconstruction, with
      transposition flaps
  for pelvis 1364–1369
  for pressure sores, 1376–1384
  size and arc of rotation for, 72
  for soft tissue coverage of hand and upper
      extremity, 1646–1651
    axial pattern distant flaps and, 1648,
        1650, *1650, 1651*
    local flaps and, 1647, *1647, 1648*
    random pattern distant flaps and,
        1647–1648, *1649*
    reverse radial artery forearm flap and,
        1650–1651, *1652*
  vascular supply and, 72
  wound preparation for, 71
Flashlamp pumped dye lasers, 264–266, *265*
Flexor carpi radialis tendon transfer, 1581,
    1583, 1584, 1585
Flexor carpi ulnaris tendon transfer, 1581,
    1582
Flexor digitorum sublimis tendon transfer, to
    ring finger, 1587, *1589,* 1595–1596
Flexor digitorum superficialis tendon grafts,
    124
Flexor pollicis longus tendon, lacerations of,
    1554
Flexor pulley reconstruction
  for hand injuries, 1569
    surgical technique for, 1569, *1570*
  tendon grafting and, 124, *124*
Flexor tendon grafting, 120–126, *122*
  anatomy and, 120–121
    adjacent structures, 121
    cellular components, 120, *120*
    extracellular components and, 121
    tendon sheath, 121, *121*
  blood supply and, 121–122
  complications of, 126
  donor sites and harvest technique for, *123,*
      123–124
  graft revascularization and, 122
  nutrition and, 122
  physiology of tendon healing and, 122
  postoperative care and, 125–126
  pulley reconstruction and, 124, *124*
  single-stage, 124–125
    indications for, 122–123
    technique for, 124–125, *125*
  stages, 123
    indications for, 123
  two-stage, 126, *126*
Flexor tenolysis, for hand injuries, 1564–1569
  complications of, 1569
  indications for, 1564–1565
  postoperative care and, 1567–1569, *1568*
  surgical technique for, 1565–1566,
      1566–1567
Floating forehead, 500
Floating thumb (pouce flotant), 1448
Fluid(s), following lipectomy, 240
Fluid resuscitation
  for lipectomy, 230t, 230–231, *231*
  in thermal burns. *See* Thermal burns, fluid
      resuscitation and
Fluoroscopy, in wrist pain, 1729
5-Fluorouracil, in oropharyngeal carcinoma,
    940, 940t, 941, 942, 943t
Foam coated implants, for augmentation
    mammaplasty, 2100

Follicular occlusion tetrad, 392–395
  acne conglobata and, 394–395
  beard sicosis and, 394, *394*
  dissecting cellulitis of scalp and, 392, *393*
Foot, diabetic. *See* Diabetic foot
Foot reconstruction, 1790–1797, *1792, 1793t,*
    1820–1827
  adjunctive techniques for, 1857–1859
    bone techniques, 1857–1858
    tarsal tunnel release, *1858,* 1858–1859
  amputations and, 1824, *1826,* 1827
  of diabetic foot, 1843–1857
    amputation and, 1856–1857, *1857*
    dorsal wounds and, 1845, *1845, 1846*
    plantar forefoot wounds and, 1845–1846,
        1847–1850
    plantar hindfoot wounds and,
        1847–1848, 1851–1852, *1853–1856,*
        1854, 1856
    plantar midfoot wounds and, 1847, *1851,*
        1852
  fasciocutaneous flaps in, 1796–1797, *1797,*
      1798
  neurovascular injury and, 1821
  soft tissue, 1821, *1823*
  of sole, 1821, 1824, *1825*
  strategies for primary treatment and,
      1820–1821, *1822*
  of weight-bearing heel, 1790–1791,
      1793–1796, 1794–1796
Fordyce condition, 302, 302–303
Forearm. *See also* Upper extremities
  amputations at level of, replantation and,
      1631–1633, *1636, 1637,* 1641
  injuries of extensor tendons of, 1576
Forehead
  burns of, 418, *420*
  floating, 500
Forehead flaps, paramedian, axial, for nasal
    reconstruction, 887, *888,* 889, *889*
Forehead-lift, 1948–1955. *See also* Brow-lift
  arterial network and, 1949
  background of, 1948
  closure in, 1955
  consultation for, 1949
  coronal
    complications of, 1962
    surgical technique for, 1961–1962,
        1961–1964
  drainage and, 1955
  frontalis muscle and, *1954,* 1954–1955
  planes of dissection and, 1949–1950, *1950,*
      1951
  results with, 1955, *1955–1957*
  scalp incisions and treatment of galea and,
      1950, *1952*
  subcutaneous dissection of forehead and,
      1952
  subgaleal dissection of forehead and,
      1952–1953, *1953*
  surgical planning for, 1949–1955
  treatment of glabellar lines and, 1953, *1953*
Forehead surgery, 1865. *See also* Brow-lift;
    Forehead-lift
Foreign bodies
  hand injuries and, 1489, *1490*
  wrist pain and, 1730t–1731t
Forked flap columellar reconstruction, 615,
    616
Forked flap method, for bilateral cleft nasal
    deformity repair, 578, *578*
Fourth branchial cleft anomalies, 813, *813*
Fractionation, altered. *See* Radiation therapy,
    altered fractionation and

Fractures. *See also specific anatomic sites; specific
    anatomic sites and types of fractures*
  accompanying nail-bed injuries, treatment
      of, 1495
  comminuted, facial, 3-D computed
      tomography in, 278–280, *278–280*
  of hands, 1490, *1491*
  healing of, 103. *See* Bone, healing of
  of lower extremities. *See specific fractures*
Franceschetti-Zwahlen-Klein syndrome. *See*
    Mandibular dysostosis (Franceschetti-
    Zwahlen-Klein syndrome; Treacher
    Collins syndrome)
Free muscle flaps, for hip reconstruction,
    1364
Free radicals, skin flaps and, 69
Free tendon grafting, for flexor tendon
    injuries of hand, 1557–1561
  accessory abductor pollicis longus tendon
      transfer and, 1596
  complications of, 1561
  indications for, 1557
  postoperative care and, 1561
  surgical technique for, 1557, *1558–1559,*
      1559–1561
Free tissue transfer, 969–979
  breast reconstruction with. *See* Breast
      reconstruction, with free tissue
      transfer; Buttock flap breast
      reconstruction; Transverse rectus
      abdominis (TRAM) flap breast
      reconstruction, using free TRAM flaps
  complications of, 979, 981
    early, 979
    late, 979, 981
  donor site selection for, 968–969
  flap elevation techniques for, 970–971
    free jejunal transfer, 971, *976, 977*
    radial forearm free flaps and, *970,*
        970–971
    scapular osteocutaneous free flaps and,
        971, *973–975*
  flap transfer and, 971, 973–974, 978
    final inset and closure and, 978
    microvascular monitoring and, 978
    partial insert and, 973–974, *977*
    recipient vessels and, 973
    revascularization and, 978
  hand reconstruction and, 1668
  hand rehabilitation following, 1763
  for leg ulcers, 1836–1838, *1837*
  in lower extremity reconstructions, 1775,
      1777
  operating room setup and plan for, *969,*
      969–970
  patient preparation for, 969
    informed consent and, 969
    preoperative assessment and, 969
    preoperative preparation and, 969
  postoperative care and, 978–979, *980–981*
  for repair of lumbar spine defects, 1369
  for sacral reconstruction, *1368,* 1369
  for soft tissue coverage of hand and upper
      extremity, 1651–1656, *1653,* 1654t
    latissimus dorsi muscle flaps and, 1652,
        1654, *1656, 1657*
    rectus abdominis muscle flaps and, 1654
    scapular fasciocutaneous flaps and, 1654,
        1656
    temporoparietal fascial flaps and, 1652,
        1655
Frey syndrome, surgical management of
    salivary gland tumors and, 1044

Frontal advancement, in craniofacial
dysostosis, 512
Frontal nerve block, 16, *16*
Frontal sinus
exploration and obliteration of, 1112–1114,
1113, 1114
fractures of, 1109–1114, *1110*
Frontal sinus fractures
anterior wall, 1112, *1113*
classification of, *1110–1112,* 1111
cranialization and, 1114, *1114–1118*
evaluation of, 1109
exploration and obliteration of frontal sinus
and, 1112–1114, *1113, 1114*
principles of treatment for, 1110–1111
surgical exposure and, 1112, *1112*
Frontoethmoidal meningoencephalocele,
516–525
classification of, 516
clinical features of, 520, *520*
diagnostic testing in, 520
etiology of, 516
pathology of, 517, *518, 519*
surgical treatment of, 520–525, *521–523*
complications of, *524,* 524–525, *525*
Frontomaxillary advancement, single-stage,
in cranifacial dysostoses, 163, *163,* 163,
163
Frontonasal dysplasia, 3-D computed
tomography in, 273, *274*
Frontozygomatic fractures, 1211, *1211*
Functional appliances, preoperative, in
hemifacial microsomia, 538
Functional measurements, cephalometric,
478, *478*
Functional sensibility test, for hands, 1746
Functional testing, in wrist pain, 1732
Furlow double-reversing Z-plasty, 596–603
postoperative care and, 603
repair of cleft palate from incisive foramen
to uvula with, 596–601
incision design for, 596, *597*
surgical technique for, *586, 598–601,* 599,
601
repair of complete bilateral cleft palate
using, 601–602, *603, 604*
repair of complete unilateral cleft palate
using, 601, *602, 603*
Fusiform scar revision, 37

Galeal frontalis musculofascial flaps, in
craniomaxillofacial surgery, 142, *144*
Ganglia, 1733–1734
anatomy and, 1733, *1733, 1734*
complications of, 1734
diagnosis of, 1734
etiology of, 1733
of hands, 1458–1460, *1459*
presentation of, 1733
treatment of, 1734
wrist pain and, 1730t–1731t
Gasoline, burns caused by, 450–451
Gastrocnemius flaps, in knee and leg
reconstruction, 1778–1779, *1780–1782*
Gastrointestinal system, thermal burns and,
406
GBLC (geometric broken line closure), for
scar revision, *40,* 40–41
Gel-filled implants, for augmentation
mammaplasty, 2100
Genetics, scar formation and, 34, *35*

Genioplasty, 193, *193, 194*
advancement, technique and results of, 743
complementary, 743
harmonizing, 743
reduction, technique and results of, 743,
745–747
simple, 743
Genitalia
ambiguous, 1399
developmental anomalies of. *See also specific
anomalies*
history of, 1388
reconstruction of. *See specific disorders and
organs*
Geometric broken line closure (GBLC), for
scar revision, *40,* 40–41
Giant cell epulis, 200
Giant cell tumors, of tendon sheath, 299, *300*
of hands, *1460,* 1461
Glaucoma, disturbances, 1938
Glenoid fossa, reconstruction of, in
hemifacial microsomia, 540–541
Gliomas, of face, 817, *820*
Glomus tumors
of hands, 1461, *1461*
of skin, 300, *300*
Glossectomy, tongue prostheses following,
1025, *1025–1027*
Glottic carcinoma, 1011
Gluteal flaps, inferior, for breast
reconstruction, 1336–1337
Gracilis flaps
free, in knee and leg reconstruction,
1788–1790, *1789–1791*
in thigh reconstruction, 1779
Granular cell tumors, 305
Granuloma(s), pyogenic (lobulated capillary
hemangiomas), 353, 355, *356*
Granuloma pyogenicum, 300
of hands, 1457
Great vessels, reinforcement of suture lines
of, intrathoracic transposition of soft
tissue for, 1270, *1271–1272*
Groin reconstruction, 1357
Ground substance, matrix formation and, 5
Growth factors
craniofacial development and, 467–468
for leg ulcers, 1836
scarring and, 11
wound healing and, 4t, 7, 9
Growth hormone, wound healing and, 10
Gunshot wounds, to face. *See* Facial gunshot
wounds
Gynecomastia, lipectomy and, 237–238,
238–239

Hair
aesthetic facial surgery in African-
Americans and, 2050–2051, *2051*
damage to roots of, following eyelid
operations in Oriental patients, 2075
Hair follicles, 47
Hair restoration, 2088–2098, *2092–2097*
adjunctive procedures and, 2092–2093,
2097, 2098
classification of baldness and, 2088–2089,
2089
complications of, 2092
Dardour flap for, 2091, *2091*
Juri flap for, 2089–2091, *2090*
Halo nevi, 306–307, *307*

Hand(s)
congenital anomalies of, 1424–1449, *1425*
acrosyndactyly, 1434, 1441, 1444, *1444*
classification of, 1424, *1426*
clinodactyly, 1439, *1439,* 1440, 1441
constriction ring syndrome, 1441, 1442t,
1443, 1443–1444
duplications, 1429–1433, *1429–1433*
evaluation of, *1427,* 1427–1428, *1428*
flexion deformities, 1449, *1452, 1453,*
1453t
macrodactyly, 1441, 1441t, *1442*
radial dysplasia. *See* Radial dysplasia
syndactyly. *See* Syndactyly
timing of surgical treatment of,
1428–1429, 1429t
Dupuytren contracture of. *See* Dupuytren
contracture
function of, evaluation of, 1747, *1747*
rehabilitation of. *See* Hand rehabilitation
replantation of, 1631, *1635, 1636, 1672*
hand rehabilitation following, 1762
rheumatoid arthritis in, 1713–1719
arthroplasty for, 1715–1716
boutonnière deformities and, 1717–1718
flexor tendon rupture in, 1554–1555
incisions for treatment of, 1422–1423,
1423
of interphalangeal joints, 1716–1718,
1717
of metacarpophalangeal joints,
1713–1716, *1714, 1715*
staging of, 1713–1715, *1714, 1715*
swan-neck deformities and, 1716–1771,
1717
of thumb, 1718–1719, *1719*
soft tissue coverage of. *See* Soft tissue
coverage, of hand and upper extremity
Hand fractures, 1508–1521
closed reduction and functional bracing
and, 1508, *1509*
closed reduction and internal fixation of,
1508–1509, *1509–1511*
excision, arthroplasty, and arthrodesis for,
1520, *1529*
limited open reduction and internal
fixation of, 1511–1512, *1511–1513*
open, treatment of, 1519–1520, *1528, 1529*
open reduction and internal fixation of,
1512–1514, *1514, 1515*
plates for, 1517–1519
buttress, 1519, *1527*
neutralization, 1518, *1523*
tension-band, 1518–1519, *1524–1526*
rehabilitation following. *See* Hand
rehabilitation, fractures and
screw fixation of, 1514, 1517, *1517–1522*
wiring techniques for, 1514, *1516*
Hand infections, 1467–1479
antibiotics and general surgical principles
for, 1467, 1468t, 1469
contaminated injuries with tissue loss and,
1478, 1479
diagnosis of, 1467
felon, 1469, *1470*
necrotizing fasciitis, 1473–1474, *1474*
osteomyelitis, 1479
paronychia, 1469, *1469*
pyogenic arthritis, 1473, *1477*
synergistic, 1474
tenosynovitis
acute flexor, 1469–1470, *1470,* 1472–1473,
1473–1476
chronic, *1478,* 1479

Hand injuries, 1480–1492. *See also* Hand fractures
  care of amputated parts and, 1481–1482, *1483*
  determining if injury is partial or complete and, 1488
  determining if injury is to tendon or nerve and, 1487–1488
  dorsal, hand reconstruction and, 1668, *1669–1670*
  of extensor tendons, 1572–1577
    anatomy and, 1572, *1573*
    general considerations for repair of, 1573, *1574*
    in zone I, 1573–1574, *1574*
    in zone II, 1574
    in zone III, 1574–1575. *1575, 1576*
    in zone IV, 1575
    in zone V, 1575–1576, *1577*
    in zone VI, 1576–1577, *1578*
  of flexor tendons, 1550–1556, 1557–1571
    active tendon prosthesis and, 1564
    anatomy and, 1550–1551, *1551*
    complications of, 1556
    conventional free tendon grafting and, 1557–1561, *1558–1559*
    diagnosis and emergency care for, 1551
    flexor pulley reconstruction and, 1569, *1570*
    flexor tenolysis and, 1564–1569, *1566–1568*
    general considerations for repair of, 1551–1553, *1552, 1553*
    lacerations of flexor pollicis longus tendon, 1554
    partial lacerations, 1554
    postoperative care and, *1555*, 1555–1556
    rupture in rheumatoid arthritis, 1554–1555
    staged reconstruction and, 1561–1564, *1562, 1564*
    technical considerations for repair of, *1553*, 1553–1555
    in zone I, 1553, *1553*
    in zone II, 1553–1554
    in zone III, 1554
    in zone IV, 1554
    in zone V, 1554
  history taking and, 1480–1481, *1481*
  initial evaluation of, 1482–1488, *1483*
    bones and joints in, 1485
    nerves in, 1486–1487, *1487*
    tendons in, *1485*, 1485–1486, *1486*
    vasculature in, 1482, *1483, 1484*, 1484–1485
  initial management in emergency room, 1488–1492
    debridement and closure in, 1488–1489
    of foreign body injuries, 1489, *1490*
    of fractures, 1490, *1491*
    of human bites, 1490
    replantation in, 1491–1492, *1492*
    splints in, 1491
    of tendon injuries, 1491
    tetanus and antibiotic prophylaxis in, 1488
  mutilating, salvage of hand and. *See* Hand reconstruction
  rehabilitation of. *See* Hand rehabilitation
  tendon transfers for, 1579–1596
    accessory abductor pollicis longus and free tendon graft, 1596
    Brand transfers, *1594*, 1594–1595

Hand injuries, tendon transfers for—*Continued*
  clawing of fingers and, 1592–1593
  extensor carpi radialis brevis, 1596, *1597*
  flexor digitorum sublimis tendon to ring finger, 1595–1596
  general principles for, 1579–1580
  in median nerve palsy. *See* Median nerve palsy, tendon transfers for
  modified Stiles-Bunnet transfer, 1593–1594
  to provide index finger adduction, 1596
  to provide metacarpophalangeal joint flexion alone, 1593, *1593*
  to provide simultaneous metacarpophalangeal and interphalangeal extension, 1593–1595, *1594*
  to provide thumb adduction, 1595–1596, *1597*
  in radial nerve palsy. *See* Radial nerve palsy, tendon transfers for
  selection and timing of, 1580
  surgical technique for, 1580
  in ulnar nerve palsy, 1592, 1596
Hand reconstruction, 1658–1680. *See also* Thumb reconstruction
  assessment of injury and, 1658–1659
  complex, 1668–1675
    devascularization and, 1672, *1673*
    dorsal injuries and, 1668, *1669–1670*
    electrical burns and, 1672, *1674*, 1675
    hand replantation and, 1672
    transmetacarpal replantation and, 1668, *1670, 1671, 1672*
  complications of, 1680
  joint preservation and, 1660
    making best use of available parts and, 1660, *1661–1662*
  postoperative care and, 1675
  postoperative monitoring and, 1675
  preparation for, 1659
    debridement and, 1659
    preoperative care and, 1659
  primary, 1659–1660, 1660–1661, 1665–1668
    bone and, 1660–1661, *1663, 1664*, 1665
    free tissue transfer and, 1668
    nerves and, 1665–1667, *1667*
    skin and, 1667–1668
    tendons and, 1665
    vessels and, 1665, *1666, 1667*
  secondary, 1675–1680
    combined procedures involving thumb, 1675, *1676*, 1677
    revision amputation, 1677, 1680
    tenodesis and thumb joint fusion, 1677, *1678*
    toe-to-hand transfer, 1677, *1679*
  toe-to-hand transplantation and. *See* Toe-to-hand transplantation
Hand rehabilitation, 1745–1763
  edema control and, 1748, *1748*
  evaluation techniques and, 1745–1747
    for edema, 1746, *1747*
    for hand function, 1747, *1747*
    for range of motion, 1745
    for sensibility, 1746
    strength, for 1745–1746
  exercises and therapeutic activities in, 1748
  fractures and, 1521, 1758–1759, *1759*
    articular, 1759
    of distal phalanx, 1758
    of distal radius, 1759

Hand rehabilitation, fractures and—*Continued*
  metacarpal, 1759
  of middle phalanx, 1758–1759
  of proximal phalanx, 1759
  of thumb, 1759
  following free tissue transfer, 1763
  modalities used in, 1749–1751
    biofeedback, 1751
    continuous passive motion, 1751, *1752*
    electrical, 1750–1751, *1751*
    thermal, 1749–1750, *1751*
  following nerve injuries, 1756–1758
    nerve compression syndromes, 1757–1758, *1758*
    postoperative treatment of peripheral nerve injuries and, *1756*, 1756–1757, *1757*
    therapy after nerve repair and, 1756
  following proximal interphalangeal joint arthroplasty, 1759–1760
  following replantation, 1760–1763
    of arm, *1762*, 1762–1763
    digital, *1760*, 1760–1761, *1761*
    of thumb or toe, 1761–1762
  scar management and, 1747, *1748*
  sensibility training in, 1748–1749, *1749*
  splinting in, 1749, *1749*, *1750*
  following tendon repairs, 1751–1756
    of extensor tendons, 1753–1755, *1754*
    of flexor tendons, 1751–1753, *1752–1753*
    staged tendon grafts, 1755, *1755*
    tendon transfers, 1755–1756
    tenolysis, 1755
  toe-to-hand transplantation and, 1705
Hand surgery. *See also* Hand reconstruction
  burn wounds of, 431, *431–435, 433–434*
  incisions for, 1415–1423
    adequacy of exposure and, 1415
    on base of thumb, *1418*, 1418–1419
    for Dupuytren contracture, 1419, *1420*
    for exposure of distal interphalangeal joint, 1422, *1422*
    for exposure of proximal interphalangeal joint, 1419, *1421*
    for infections, *1417*, 1417–1418
    for intrinsic fasciotomy, 1419, *1421*
    minimization of scarring and, 1415, *1416*
    misplaced, 1415
    for release of trigger finger, 1416–1417
    for replantation, 1422, *1422*
    for treatment of rheumatoid arthritis, 1422–1423, *1423*
    for treatment of syndactyly, 1423, *1423*
    on volar aspect of finger, 1416, *1416*
Hand tumors, 1454–1466, 1455t
  arising from connective tissue, 1457–1462
    fibromas, 1457
    ganglia, 1458–1460, *1459*
    giant cell tumors of tendon sheath, *1460*, 1461
    glomus tumors, 1461, *1461*
    lipomas, 1457–1458, *1459*
    mucous pseudocysts, 1460–1461
    myxomas, 1462
  arising from epithelium, 1454–1457
    basal cell carcinomas, 1456
    Bowen disease, 1456
    epidermoid cysts, 1454–1455
    granuloma pyogenicum, 1457
    keratoacanthomas, 1455, *1456*
    melanomas, 1456–1457, *1457*
    squamous cell carcinomas, 1457, *1458*
    verruca vulgaris, 1454

Hand tumors—*Continued*
  of bone and cartilage, 1463–1466
    enchondromas, 1463–1464, *1464, 1465*
    osteochondromas, 1464, *1465*
    osteoid osteomas, 1466
    solitary bone cysts, 1466
  of nerve tissue, 1462
    neurilemmomas, 1462, *4468*
    neurofibromas, 1462
  sarcomas, 1462–1463
    Boeck sarcoids, 1463
    epithelioid, 1462
    fibrosarcomas, 1463
    liposarcomas, 1463
    malignant fibrous histiocytomas,
      1462–1463
    rhabdomyosarcomas, 1462
    synovial, 1463
  of tendon sheath, 1463
    synovial cysts, 1463
    xanthomas, 1463
Hanging (hooded) ala, secondary rhinoplasty
    for, 2040, *2045, 2046*
Haversian canal, 103
Head and neck. *See also* Neck; Neck
    dissection
  burn reconstruction and. *See* Burn wounds,
    of head and neck, reconstruction of
  regional blocks of, 16–18, *16–19*
Head and neck cancer team, 1008
Healing
  of bone. *See* Bone grafts, bone healing and
  of tendons, physiology of, 122
  of wounds. *See* Wound healing
Heart, reinforcement of suture lines of,
    intrathoracic transposition of soft
    tissue for, 1270, *1271–1272*
Heel reconstruction, of weight-bearing heel,
    1790–1791, *1793–1796, 1794–1796*
Hemangiolymphangiomas, 365, *366*
Hemangiomas, 352–359
  capillary, lobulated (pyogenic granulomas),
    353, 355, *356*
  capillary (strawberry; superficial dermis
    vascular channels), 352–353, *353, 354*
  capillary-cavernous, 353, *355*
  cavernous (deep dermal and subcutaneous
    vascular channels), 353, *354*
  indications for early treatment of, 355–356
    deprivation and anisometric amblyopia
      as, 355, *356*
    Kasabach-Merritt syndrome as, 355
    microshunting limb lesions as, 355, *357*
    obstructing lesions as, 356, *357, 358*
  keratotic (verrucous malformations), 363,
    364
  residual problems with, 356, 358–359
    overgrowth, 359, *359*
    partial regression, 356, *358, 359*
    rebound cortisone injection, 359, *360*
  senile (cherry hemangiomas), 300
  strawberry, argon laser therapy for,
    259–262, *261–263*
Hematologic system, thermal burns and, 406
Hematomas
  augmentation mammaplasty and, 2112
  following blepharoplasty, 1937
  periorbital, following blepharoplasty, 1937
  following prophylactic subcutaneous
    mastectomy, 1282
  retrobulbar, following blepharoplasty, 1937
  septal, nasal fractures and, 1133–1134, *1134*
  subscleral, following blepharoplasty, 1937
  subungual, treatment of, 1494

Hemifacial microsomia (craniofacial
    microsomia; first and second branchial
    arch syndrome), 536–547, *537, 538*
  nonsurgical treatment of, 538–539
    correction of maxillary deficiencies and
      distortions and, 538–539
    orthodontic, 539
    postoperative, 538
    preoperative functional appliance and,
      538
    preparation for mandibular
      reconstruction and, 538
  postoperative care and, 541–542
    of chin, 542
    of nose, 542
  surgical treatment of, 539–541, 542t
    complications of, 542
    with condyle absent, 540, *541*
    with condyle present, *539,* 539–540
    glenoid fossa reconstruction and,
      540–541
    maxillary surgery and, 541
    results with, 542, *543–546*
Hemilaryngectomy, 1014
Hemorrhage
  control of, burn wound excision and
    grafting and, 411
  intrasurgical, eyelid operations in Oriental
    patients and, 2075
  following prophylactic subcutaneous
    mastectomy, 1282
  following rhinoplasty, 2019–2020
Hermaphroditism, 1399
Hidradenitis suppurativa, 384–395
  clinical manifestations of, 385
  eccrine and apocrine glands and, 384
  epidemiology of, 384–385
  etiopathogenesis of, 385
  follicular occlusion tetrad and. *See*
    Follicular occlusion tetrad
  treatment of, 385–392
    in axillary hidradenitis, 385–386, *386,
      388, 389*
    in hidradenitis involving perineal region,
      groin, and genitalia, 389–391, *390, 391*
    immunotherapy in, 391–392
Hidradenoma papilliferum, 303
Hidrocystomas
  apocrine (apocrine cystadenomas), 303, *303*
  eccrine, 303
High median nerve palsy, tendon transfers
    for, 1590, *1591,* 1592
Hip reconstruction, 1360–1364, *1361,*
    1369–1370
  general principles of, 1361, *1362*
  muscle flaps for, 1361–1364
    free muscle flaps, 1364
    rectus abdominis, 1362, 1364
    rectus femoris, 1361–1362, *1362, 1363*
    vastus lateralis, 1362
  results of, 1364
Histochemical staining, nerve grafting and,
    1616
Homeobox-containing genes, craniofacial
    development and, 468
Hooded (hanging) ala, secondary rhinoplasty
    for, 2040, *2045, 2046*
Hormones, scarring and, 11
Hospitals, organization of, laser use and, 267
Human bites, of hand, 1490
Huntington fibular transfer, 1803, 1805
  follow-up and, 1805
  technique for, 1803, *1803,* 1805

Hydrocephalus, with craniosynostosis, 512
Hydrofluoric acid, burns caused by, 449–450,
    450
Hydroxyapatite, 113–118
  biologic and mechanical properties of, 116,
    117–119, 118
  clinical considerations with, 113–116,
    114–116
Hydroxyurea, in oropharyngeal carcinoma,
    942
Hygiene, facial rejuvenation and, 1987
Hyperbaric oxygen therapy
  for leg ulcers, 1835, *1835*
  in mandibular reconstruction, 983–984
Hyperfractionation, 949
  accelerated, 951
Hypertelorism, 151, 154
  extracranial approach in, 151, *156*
  intracranial approach in, 151, 154, *156–158*
Hyperthermia, with brachytherapy, 954
Hypertrophic scars. *See* Scar(s); Scar revision;
    Scarring
Hypofractionation, 951
Hypoplastic thumb, 1696, 1698
Hypospadias, 1388–1393
  complications of procedures for, 1393
  postoperative care and, 1393
  surgical technique for, *1389–1392,* 1391,
    1393
Hypotensive anesthesia, for breast reduction,
    2118
Hypovolemia, lipectomy and, 231

Ichthyosis hystrix, 297–298
Iliac crest, lipectomy and, 235
Iliac crest free vascularized flaps, 986t, 987,
    987–991, 989
Ilium grafts, 105t, 105–107
  nonvascularized, 105–106, *106, 107*
  vascularized, 106–107
Ilizarov's technique, 1812, *1813–1819,*
    1814–1815
Imaging studies, 945. *See also specific modalities*
  in oropharyngeal carcinoma, 926, *926*
  in wrist pain, 1732, 1732–1733
Immune system, thermal burns and, 404
Immunologic factors, scarring and, 11
Immunosuppression, wound healing and, 8
Immunotherapy
  in hidradenitis suppurativa, 391–392
  for malignant melanomas, 348–349
Implants. *See* Prostheses
Incisions. *See under specific procedures*
Inclusion cysts (milia), 301, *301*
  following blepharoplasty, 1938
Induration, following blepharoplasty, 1937
Infants
  craniofacial dysostosis in, 512–513, *513*
  orthodontic treatment for clefts in, 648, *651*
Infection(s), 32–33. *See also* Sepsis
  following blepharoplasty, 1936
  craniomaxillofacial surgery and, 166, 168
  hand reconstruction and, 1680
  in hands, incisions for treatment of, *1417,*
    1417–1418
  of hands. *See* Hand infections
  of mandibular fractures, 1174–1175
  mandibular fractures and, 1177
  following median sternotomy. *See* Median
    sternotomy, infected
  following rhinoplasty, 2020
Infection control, leg ulcers and, 1833
Infectious arthritis, wrist pain and,
    1730t–1731t

Inferior alveolar nerve block, 17–18
Inferior gluteal flaps, for breast
    reconstruction, 1336–1337
Inflammatory stage
    of bone healing, 1809
    of wound healing, 3–4, 4, 4t
Inflatable implants, for augmentation
    mammaplasty, 2100
Informed consent
    for augmentation mammaplasty,
        2101–2102, 2102, 2103
    for free tissue techniques, 969
    for lipectomy, 230
Infraorbital nerve block, 17, 17
Infraorbital rim augmentation, 1868–1869
Inhalation injury, thermal, 398–399
    diagnosis of, 398, 398–399
    treatment of, 399, 399t
Inner thigh-plasty, with liposuction or
    dermatocrurolipectomy, 2240–2243
    complications of, 2243
    indications for, 2240
    technique for, 2240–2243, 2243
Innervation, of skin grafts, 47–48
Interalar reduction, in African-Americans,
    2055–2056, 2056
Interdental wiring, for mandibular fractures,
    1168, 1168
Intermaxillary fixation, for mandibular
    fractures, 1168, 1169, 1170
Internal brow pexy, 1965, 1966, 1967
Internasal dysplasia, 489, 489–490
    surgical treatment of, 489–490, 490–492
    nose and, 489–490, 490–492
Interorbital space, anatomy of, 1138
Interphalangeal joints
    anatomy of, 1531, 1532
    distal
        hand rehabilitation following fracture of,
            1758
        incisions for exposure of, 1422, 1422
        of fingers, ligament injuries of, 1534–1536,
            1535, 1537, 1538
    middle, hand rehabilitation following
        fracture of, 1758–1759
    proximal. See Proximal interphalangeal
        joint
    rheumatoid arthritis in, 1716–1718
        boutonnière deformities and, 1717–1718
        swan-neck deformities and, 1716–1717,
            1717
Intersex, 1399
Interstitial brachytherapy, 951–952, 952
Intracavitary brachytherapy, 952
Intraoral examination, in velopharyngeal
    insufficiency, 621
Intraoral prostheses, 1018–1019, 1019–1021
Intraorbital space, isolated fractures of,
    1142–1143
Irradiation. See also Radiation therapy
    wound healing and, 8
Irrigation, for lipectomy, 235
Ischemia
    scarring and, 11
    wound healing and, 9
Island flaps, 57, 58
Isotopes, for brachytherapy, 952–953, 953t

Jaw(s). See also Mandible; Maxilla;
    Temporomandibular joint deformities;
    Temporomandibular joint
    reconstruction; headings beginning with
    terms Mandibular and maxillary
    positioning, in mandibular dysostosis, 532,
        533–534

Jejunal flaps, free, 971, 976, 977
Johanson step-plasty, 913, 913, 914
Joint(s). See also specific joints
    of hand
        evaluation of, 1485
        preservation of, 1660
Juri flap, 2089–2091, 2090

Karapandzic maneuver, 909–910, 911, 912
Kasabach-Merritt syndrome, hemangiomas
    and, 355
Keinböck disease, 1743–1744
    background of, 1743
    diagnosis of, 1743
    pathophysiology of, 1743
    presentation of, 1743
    treatment of, 1743–1744
    wrist pain and, 1730t–1731t
Keloids, 10–11
    aesthetic facial surgery in African-
        Americans and, 2051–2052
    factors influencing formation of, 30
    features of, 11
    revision of, 43–44, 44
    treatment of, 11
Keratoacanthomas, 298, 299
    of hands, 1455, 1456
Keratoconjunctivitis sicca, following
    blepharoplasty, 1934–1935
Keratosis
    actinic, 309–310, 310
    seborrheic, 295, 297
Keratotic hemangiomas (verrucous
    malformations), 363, 364
Kesselring technique, 216
Kleeblattschädel, 151
Klippel-Trenaunay syndrome, 363, 364, 365,
    365
Knee(s)
    lipectomy and, 236
    suction-assisted lipectomy of, 2243–2247
        indications for, 2244, 2244–2245
        technique for, 2245–2247, 2245–2247
Knee reconstruction. See Lower extremity
    reconstruction, of knee and leg
Knots, eyelid operations in Oriental patients
    and, 2074, 2075

Labial sulcus, absence of, cleft lip and, 606t,
    607
Labiomental groove, construction of, 530, 531
Lacerations
    intranasal, nasal fractures and, 1134, 1135
    of nail bed, treatment of, 1494–1495
    of tendons of hand, 1554
        flexor pollicis longus tendon, 1554
        partial, 1554
Lacrimal gland, prolapse of, following eyelid
    operations in Oriental patients, 2075
Lacrimal system injuries, 1105–1107
    evaluation of, 1105–1106
    reconstruction and, 1106–1107, 1106–1108
Lactation, following reduction mammaplasty,
    2142
Lagophthalmos, following blepharoplasty,
    1938
Lag screws, for mandibular fractures, 1170,
    1170
Lambdoid craniosynostosis, isolated, 151
Lambdoid suture, synostosis of, 512
Laryngeal cancer, 1008–1017
    anatomy and, 1008–1009, 1009, 1010
    chemotherapy in, 1016–1017
    glottic, 1011
    head and neck cancer team and, 1008

Laryngeal cancer—Continued
    laryngoscopy in, 1010–1011
        direct, 1011, 1012t
        indirect, 1010–1011
    mediastinal tracheostomy in, 1016
    patient evaluation in, 1010
    subglottic, 1012
    supraglottic, 1011–1012
    total laryngectomy in, 1012–1013, 1013
    tracheoesophageal puncture for, 1017
    voice rehabilitation and, 1017
    voice-sparing operations for, 1013–1016
        hemilaryngectomy, 1014
        supraglottic laryngectomy, 1014–1016
Laryngectomy
    necessity for, when removing base of
        tongue, 938
    supraglottic, 1014–1016
        postoperative management and,
            1015–1016
        technique for, 1014–1015
    total, 1012–1013, 1013
    voice rehabilitation following, 1017
Laryngoscopy, 1010–1011
    direct, 1011, 1012t
    indirect, 1010–1011
Laser(s), 252–267
    argon, 256–257
    carbon dioxide, 253–255, 254, 255
    excimer, 256
    history of, 252
    hospital organization and establishing
        credentials for, 267
    interaction with tissue, 253
    neodymium: yttrium-aluminum-garnet,
        255–256
    photocoagulation, 256–266
        argon, 256–262
        continuous-wave, argon-pumped,
            tunable dye laser, 264
        copper vapor, 263–264
        flashlamp pumped dye laser, 264–266,
            265
        yellow-light, 262–263, 263
    physics of, 252–253
    pigmented lesion, 266
    ruby, Q-switched, 266
    safety with, 266–267
Laser suction, for breast reduction, 2119
Laser therapy, for scarring, 11–12
Lateral thigh flaps, for breast reconstruction,
    1339, 1339, 1340, 1341
    flap dissection and, 1341
Latissimus dorsi flaps
    breast reconstruction using, 1317–1322
        complications of, 1321–1322
        preoperative planning for, 1318,
            1319–1321
        surgical technique for, 1318–1319, 1321,
            1322, 1323
    for chest wall reconstruction, 1250–1251
    free, in knee and leg reconstruction,
        1782–1783, 1785–1787, 1787
    for immediate breast reconstruction
        following mastectomy, 1292
    intrathoracic transposition of, 1269–1270,
        1270
    for soft tissue coverage of hand and upper
        extremity, 1652, 1654, 1656, 1657
Le Fort I osteotomies, for maxillary
    deformities, 726, 728–739, 730, 731
    with downward movement, 736, 737, 738,
        739
    with forward movement, 729, 732
    with posterior movement, 732, 733
    with superior repositioning, 732, 734,
        734–736

Le Fort III osteotomies
  in Crouzon and Apert syndromes, 160,
    161–162, 162
  for mandibular deformities, 742–758
    timing of, 742–743
  for maxillary deformities, 739, *740, 741*
Legs. *See* lower extremities; Lower extremity
    reconstruction, of knee and leg; *specific
    regions of leg*
Leg ulcers, 1828–1838
  diagnosis of, 1828–1832
    of arterial ulcers, 1830–1831, *1831*, 1831t
    patient evaluation and, 1828–1829, 1829t
    of sickle cell ulcers, 1831
    ulcer evaluation and, 1829, 1829t
    of uncommon ulcerations, 1832, *1833*
    of vasculitic ulcers, 1832, *1832*
    of venous ulcers, 1829–1830, *1830*
  prevention of recurrence of, 1838
  treatment of, 1832–1838, *1834*
    local wound management in, 1833–1835,
      1835
    new developments in wound care and,
      1836–1838, *1837*
    surgical, 1836
Lentigos, 305, *305*
  maligna, 344
Leser-Trélat sign, 295
Lesional hypertrophy, port-wine stains and,
    257
Leucovorin, in oropharyngeal carcinoma, 940
Leukoplakia, oropharyngeal carcinoma and,
    923, *924*
Levator palpebrae superioris muscle,
    anatomy of, 2061, *2061, 2062*
Lichen planus, oropharyngeal carcinoma
    and, 923
Ligaments
  injuries of
    of fingers and thumbs. *See* Finger
      injuries; Thumb(s), injuries to
      ligaments of
    of upper extremity ligaments, 1531
  laryngeal, 1009
  rupture of, wrist pain and, 1730t–1731t
  strain or tear of, wrist pain and,
    1730t–1731t
  wrist pain and. *See* Wrist pain, ligaments
    and
Limb(s). *See also* Lower extremities; Upper
    extremities
  photographic documentation of, lipectomy
    and, 223, 226, *226*
Limb perfusion, isolated, for malignant
    melanomas, 349–350
Lip(s)
  adherence to maxilla, cleft lip and, 606t,
    607
  asymmetry of, cleft lip and, 606t, 607
  burns of, 426
    of lower lip, 426
    of upper lip, 426, *427*
  cheiloplasty and, in African-Americans,
    2058, *2058*
  cleft. *See* Cleft lip; Facial clefts
  closure of, for bilateral cleft lip repair, 574
  cutaneous malignant tumors of, 324, *329*
  excessively long, cleft lip and, 606t, 607
  function of, 906
  injuries of, 1092–1095, *1097*
    anatomy and, 1092–1093, *1094*
    management of, 1093, *1095, 1096*
    lateral, bilateral cleft lip repair and, 568,
      571
    lower, advancement of, 1995, *1995*

Lip(s)—*Continued*
  modifications of, 1983, *1985, 1986*
  shortening of, for bilateral cleft lip repair,
    574
  structure of, 906, *907*
  symmetry of, bilateral cleft lip repair and,
    574
  tight, cleft lip and, 606t, 607
  upper
    advancement of, 1996, *1996*
    augmentation of, 1995
  vermilion deficiency and, cleft lip and,
    606t, 607
  vermilionectomy and, 907, *907*
  vermilion excess and, cleft lip and, 606t,
    606–607
Lip adhesion, for unilateral cleft lip, 551
Lipectomy, suction-assisted, abdominal
    contouring with. *See* Abdominal
    contour operations; Suction-assisted
    lipectomy
Lipexeresis, 216
Lip-lift, 1990–1992, *1991*
  results with, 1991–1992
  technique for, 1990–1991
Lipomas
  of hands, 1457–1458, *1459*
  of skin, 300
Liposarcomas, of hands, 1463
Liposuction
  breast reduction by. *See* Breast reduction,
    by liposuction and vertical
    mammaplasty
  inner thigh-plasty with. *See* Inner thigh-
    plasty, with liposuction or
    dermatocrurolipectomy
  for lymphedema, 380
Lip reconstruction, 906–919
  for full-thickness lip loss, 907, 909–919
    Abbe lip-switch for, 909, *909, 910*
    Estlander lip transfer for, 909
    Freeman modification of Barnard
      procedure for, 917, *917, 918*
    Johanson step-plasty for, 913, *913, 914*
    Karapandzic maneuver for, 909–910, *911,
      912*
    May modification of Dieffenbach
      cheiloplasty for, 915, *915, 916*
    microvascular transfers for, 919
    multistage transfers for, 919
    Stranc-Robertson steeple flap repair for,
      919, *919, 920*
  lip function and, 906
  lip structure and, 906, *907*
  for superficial defects, 907, *907, 908*
Lip revision, total, 614, *614*
Local flaps, 57, *58*
  in lower extremity reconstruction,
    1774–1775
    fasciocutaneous, 1774–1775, *1775*
Local injury, microcirculation and, 68
Lower body lift, complete, 2214, *2216–2218*
Lower extremities. *See also specific regions of
    lower extremities*
  burn wounds of, *439*, 439–440, *440*
  contouring of. *See* Body contouring, of
    trunk and limbs; Calf implantation;
    Suction-assisted lipectomy; Thigh-lifts
  fasciocutaneous flaps of, 77–80
    anatomy of, 78–79, *79*
    surgical technique for, 79–80
  reconstruction using soft tissue expansion,
    213, *214*
  underdevelopment of leg caused by
    poliomyelitis or clubfoot, calf
    implantation and, 2255–2256, *2258*

Lower extremity injuries
  fractures, 1769t, 1769–1772
    external fixation of, 1770–1771
    fixator placement and, *1770–1772*, 1771
    immediate amputation for, 1770
    open, initial care of, 1769
    vascular injury and, 1771–1772
    wound care and, 1769–1770
  initial evaluation of, 1767–1768
    history in, 1767
    physical examination in, 1767t,
      1767–1768, *1768*, 1768t
    roentgenography in, 1768
Lower extremity reconstruction, 1773–1799,
    1800–1806
  bone allografts in, 1802–1803
    follow-up and, 1803
    indications for, 1802
    technique for, *1802*, 1803
  cancellous bone grafting in, 1800–1802
    indications for, 1800
    Papineau procedure for, 1800–1801, *1801*
  distant tissue transfer in, 1775, 1777
  distraction osteogenesis in, 1805–1806
    follow-up and, 1806
    technique and fixation and, 1805–1806,
      1806, 1807
  evaluation of requirements for, 1773–1774,
    1774
  of foot. *See* Foot reconstruction
  free vascularized fibular grafts in, 1805
    follow-up and, 1805
    technique for, *1804*, 1805
  of knee and leg, 1778–1790, *1779*
    gastrocnemius flaps in, 1778–1779,
      1780–1782
    gracilis free flaps in, 1788–1790,
      1789–1791
    latissimus dorsi free flaps in, 1782–1783,
      1785–1787, 1787
    serratus anterior flaps in, 1787, *1788*
    soleus flaps in, 1779–1782, *1783, 1784*
  local flaps in, 1774–1775
    fasciocutaneous, 1774–1775, *1775*
  muscle flaps in, 1775, *1776*
  primary and delayed closure in, 1774
  skin-graft closure in, 1774
  techniques of muscle flap coverage for,
    1797–1799
  of thigh. *See* Thigh reconstruction
  vascularized bone segment transfer in,
    1803–1805
    Huntington fibular transfer, 1803, *1803*,
      1805
    indications for, 1803
Lumbar spine defects, 1369–1370
  free tissue transfer for treatment of, 1369
  muscle flaps for treatment of, 1369
Lunate fractures, 1743
Lunotriquetral instability, 1543, *1546*
Lymphangiohemangiomas, 365, *367*
Lymphangiomas
  cavernous, 368, *379*
  hygroma (cystoides), 368, *379*
  simplex and circumscriptum, 368, *368*
Lymphatic bridging procedures, 376
Lymphatic drainage, of oropharynx, 932, *933*
Lymphatic malformations, 368
Lymphaticolymphatic grafts, 377, 379–380
Lymphatic supply, skin grafting and, 47
Lymphedema, 374–381
  anatomy and, 375
  diagnostic tests in, 375–376

Lymphedema—*Continued*
  etiology of, 374–375
    of primary lymphedema, 374
    of secondary lymphedema, 374t, 374–375
  pathophysiology of, 375
  treatment of, 376–381
    aims of, 376
    conservative, 376
    pharmacologic, 376
    surgical, 376–381
Lymph node-venous anastomosis, 376

Macrocirculation, of skin flaps, 59–60, *60*
Macrodactyly, 1441, 1441t, *1442*
Macromastia, unilateral, breast reduction for, 2119–2122, *2121–2123*
Macules, café au lait, 306
Mafenide acetate cream, in burn wound sepsis, 402t, 403
Magnetic resonance imaging
  in oropharyngeal carcinoma, 926
  in temporomandibular joint deformities, 1224
  in wrist pain, 1729, *1729*
Malar fractures, treatment of, *1210*, 1211–1212
  frontozygomatic component and, 1211, *1211*
  zygomaticomaxillary component at inferior orbital rim and, 1211–1212, *1211–1215*
  zygomaticomaxillary component below malar buttress and, 1212, *1215–1216*
  zygomaticotemporal component and, 1212
Malar surgery, 1865–1868, *1868*, *1869*
Males. *See also specific male genital organs*
  abdominal contour operations in, 2172
  breasts of, lipectomy and, 237–238, *238–239*
  contouring trunk in, suction-assisted lipectomy for, 2198
  facial rejuvenation in. *See* Facial rejuvenation, in men
  flanks of, lipectomy and, 237, *238*
Malignant fibrous histiocytomas, of hands, 1462–1463
Malignant melanomas, 341–351
  acral lentiginous melanoma, 344
  adjuvant therapy for, 348–350
    chemotherapy, 349
    immunotherapy, 348–349
    isolated limb perfusion, 349–350
    radiation therapy, 348
  compound nevus and, 350
  diagnosis of, 342, *342*, 346
  epidemiology of, 341–342
  familial dysplastic nevus syndrome and, 350
  follow-up care for, 350–351
  histology of, 342, *343*, 344
    acral lentiginous melanoma, 344
    lentigo maligna, 344
    nodular melanoma, 344
    superficial spreading melanoma, 344
  lentigo maligna, 344
  locally recurrent, 350
  lymphatic metastases with unknown primary site and, 350
  microscopic classification of, 344–346, *345*, *346*
  nodular, 344
  staging of, 345t, 346, 346t
  superficial spreading, 344
  surgical treatment of, 346–348
    reconstruction and, 347, *347*
    regional lymph nodes and, 347–348, *348*

Malignant mixed tumor, of salivary glands, 1038, *1039*
Mallet finger, treatment of, 1573–1574, *1574*
Malnutrition, wound healing and, 8–9
Malocclusion, mandibular fractures and, 1177
Malposition, of nose, following rhinoplasty in Oriental patients, 2083, *2085*
Mammaplasty
  augmentation. *See* Augmentation mammaplasty
  reduction. *See* Reduction mammaplasty
  vertical
    breast reduction by liposuction and. *See* Breast reduction, by liposuction and vertical mammaplasty
    correction of breast ptosis by, 2157, *2158–2164*
Mandible
  advancement of, cephalometrics and, 481, *482*, 483
  evaluation of, in maxillofacial trauma, 1065–1067, *1067*
  marginal resection of, in oropharyngeal resection, 937–938, *938*
  splitting of, in oropharyngeal resection, 936–937, *937*
Mandibular body and ramus osteotomy, for mandibular deformities, 745, 749–756
  indications for, 645
  techniques and results of, 749–756, *750–756*
Mandibular compression screw (MCS) plate, 169, *170*
Mandibular deformities, orthognathic surgery for. *See* Orthognathic surgery, for mandibular deformities
Mandibular dysostosis (Franceschetti-Zwahlen-Klein syndrome; Treacher Collins syndrome), 527–535
  anesthesiologic considerations in, 535
  principles of treatment of, 527–528
  surgical procedure for, 529–535
    augmentation of chin with lyocartilage and construction of labiomental groove, 530, *531*
    correction of coloboma, 535
    elevation of lower eyelid and lateral canthus, 530, *530*
    nasal reconstruction, 535
    reconstruction of auricular deformities, 535
    removal of elongated coronoid process, 532, *532*
    with zygomatic-orbital defects, *528*, 529, *529*
  timing of treatment of, 528–529
    in children 6 to 10 years of age, 529
    in children 12 years or older, 529
    without cleft palate, 528–529
    with isolated cleft palate, 528
Mandibular dysplasia
  bilateral cleft lip and palate and, 687
  isolated cleft palate and, 698
  unilateral cleft lip and palate and, 683
Mandibular fractures, 171, *172–176*, 174, 1165–1178
  of alveolar bone, 1172, *1173*
  anatomy and, 1165, *1166*
  of body of mandible, 1172–1174
    close to mental foramen, 1173
    in molar region and area of angle of mandible, 1173–1174
    parasymphyseal area fractures, 1173, *1174*

Mandibular fractures—*Continued*
  classification of, 1165, *1166*, 1167
  diagnosis of, 1167
  gunshot wounds causing, 1186
  multiple, 1177
    of both jaws, 1177
    of mandible, 1177, *1180*
  surgical techniques for, 1172–1177
    alveolar bone fractures and, 1172, *1173*
    ascending ramus fractures and, 1176–1177, *1178*, *1179*
    in children, 1176
    comminuted fractures and, *1174*, *1175*, 1175–1176
    compound fractures and, 1174
    infected fractures and, 1174–1175
    multiple fractures and, 1177, *1180*
    severely atrophic mandibles and, 1176
    simple fractures of body of mandible and, 1172–1174, *1174*
  symptoms of, 1167
  treatment of, 1167–1172
    bone plates and, 1170–1172, *1171–1173*
    bone wiring and, 1170, *1170*
    circumdental wiring and, 1168, *1168*
    interdental wiring and, 1168, *1168*
    intermaxillary fixation and, 1168, *1169*, 1170
    lag screws and, 1170, *1170*
    results and complications of, 1177–1178
Mandibular nerve block, 17, *17*
Mandibular osteotomies, 187–188, *188–191*
Mandibular prostheses, 1022–1024, *1022–1025*
Mandibular reconstruction, 183, 183–187, 982–997
  alloplastic, 183, *184–185*
  with bone grafts, 183, 185, *186–187*, 187
  dental rehabilitation following, 998, *999*
  fixation for, 997, *997*
  free vascularized osseous flaps for, 985–996, 986t
    combined, 996, *996*
    fibula, 992, *992–993*, *993*
    iliac crest, 987, *987–991*, 989
    metatarsal or dorsalis pedis, 994
    radial forearm, 989, *991*, 992
    rib, 985, 987
    scapula, 994, *994–996*, 996
  goals and principles of, 983, *984*, 984t
  immediate versus delayed, 983
  indications for, 982
  pedicled osteomusculocutaneous flaps for, 984–985
    pectoralis major, 984
    sternocleidomastoid, 985
    trapezius, 984–985
  preparation for, in hemifacial microsomia, 538
  vascular considerations in, 996–997
Mandibular setback, cephalometrics and, 481, 483
Mandibular surgery, to posterior mandible, *1869*, 1869–1870
  to anterior mandible, 1870–1871, *1871*
Marking
  for bilateral cleft lip repair, 568, *569–570*, *572*
    evaluation of measurements and, 568
    lateral lip and, 568
    prolabial markings and, 568
  for blepharoplasty, of upper lid, 1924
  for brachioplasty and brachial suction-assisted lipectomy, 2222, *2223*, 2224, *2227*, *2228*

Marking—*Continued*
　for breast reduction, *2115*, 2115–2116, *2116*,
　　2119–2120, *2121*, *2147*, *2148–2151*
　for eyelid operations in Oriental patients,
　　2064, *2066–2067*
　for lipectomy, *231*, 231–232, 242–243, *243*
　for reduction mammaplasty, *2130–2131*,
　　2131–2132
　for suction-assisted lipectomy
　　of calf and ankle, *2248*, 2249, *2249*
　　of thigh, *2237*, *2238*, *2239*
　for TRAM flap breast reconstruction, 1310,
　　1313
　of TRAM flaps, for breast reconstruction,
　　1326, 1327–1328, *1328*
Mast cells, scarring and, 11
Mastectomy
　breast reconstruction following. *See* Breast
　　reconstruction
　subcutaneous, prophylactic. *See*
　　Prophylactic subcutaneous mastectomy
Matrix formation, in wound healing, 5
Maxilla
　advancement of, cephalometrics and, 483
　deformities of
　　correction of, in hemifacial microsomia,
　　　538
　　orthognathic surgery for. *See*
　　　Orthognathic surgery, for maxillary
　　　deformities
　lesions of, oropharyngeal reconstruction
　　and, 968
　leveling of, 739, *739*
Maxillary dysplasia, 494–498, *495*
　bilateral cleft lip and palate and, 687
　isolated cleft palate and, 697
　surgical treatment of, 494, 496–498
　　skeleton and, 498
　　soft tissues and, *496*, 496–497, *497*
Maxillary expansion, 722, *723–725*, 724
Maxillary fractures, 1156–1163
　anatomy and, 1156, *1157*
　in children and adolescents, 1194–1195,
　　1196
　diagnosis of, 1158
　patterns of, 1156, *1158*
　repair of
　　exposure for, 1158, *1158*
　　fracture reduction and, 1158
　　Le Fort fractures without mobility,
　　　1162–1163
　　maxillomandibular fixation and, 1158
　　plate and screw stabilization and, 1158,
　　　1159–1161, 1162
　　primary bone grafting and, 1162, *1162*
　　release of maxillomandibular fixation
　　　and, 1162
　　sagittal fractures, 1163, *1163*
　　soft tissue resuspension and, 1162–1163,
　　　1163
　roentgenographic appearance of,
　　1074–1075, 1078–1080
　　Le Fort I fractures, 1078, *1079*
　　Le Fort II fractures, 1078, *1079*
　　Le Fort III fractures, 1078, 1080, *1080*
　　simple fractures, 1075
　treatment goals for, 1156
Maxillary hypoplasia, unilateral cleft lip and
　palate and, 683
Maxillary osteotomies, 190–191, *192*
Maxillary surgery, in hemifacial microsomia,
　541

Maxillofacial fractures
　blow-out, 1080–1082, *1081*
　maxillary, 1074–1075, 1078–1080
　roentgenographic appearance and
　　classification of, 1074–1082, *1075–1081*
　roentgenographic interpretation and,
　　1071–1072, *1072*
　tripod, 1074, *1077–1078*
　of zygoma, 1074, *1075*, *1076*
Maxillofacial growth, influence of cleft lip
　repair on, 564
Maxillofacial trauma
　initial management of, 1060–1068
　primary survey and, 1060–1063
　　evaluation in, 1060–1062, *1061*
　　management of bleeding and, 1062–1063,
　　　1063
　radiologic evaluation of, 1069–1082
　　in acute trauma setting, 1069–1074
　　appearance and classification of fractures
　　　and, 1074–1082, *1075–1081*
　secondary survey and, 1063–1068
　　of eyes, 1063–1064, *1065*
　　of mandible, 1065–1067, *1067*
　　of midface, 1065, *1066*
　　of nervous system, 1063, *1064*
　　of nose, 1067
　　of nose and ethmoid bone, 1064–1065
　　of soft tissue, 1067–1068
Maxillomandibular fixation, 1158
　release of, 1162
Maxon (polyglyconate) sutures, 8
Meatal advancement glansplasty incision,
　1388
Mechanical forces, scarring and, 11
Mechanical ptosis, traumatic, 1105
Medial plantar flaps, 75, 77
　anatomy of, 75, 77
　surgical technique for, 77, *79*
Medial thigh-lifts. *See* Thigh-lifts, medial
Median nerve palsy, tendon transfers for,
　1585, 1587–1589
　extensor indicis proprius (Burkhalter)
　　transfer, 1587, *1588*
　flexor digitorum sublimis tendon to ring
　　finger (Bunnell transfer), 1587, *1589*
　in high median nerve palsy, 1590, *1591*,
　　1592
　palmaris longus (Camitz) transfer, 1587,
　　1590
Median sternotomy, infected, *1252*,
　1252–1259
　chronic wounds and, 1257, *1260–1261*
　surgical technique for, 1254, *1254–1256*,
　　1257, *1258*, *1259*
　symptoms and signs of, 1253
　treatment of, *1244*, 1253–1254, *1254*
Mediastinal tracheostomy, 1016
Medical evaluation, for lipectomy, 227
Melanocytic nevi, acquired, 306, *306*
Melanocytosis, dermal, 307
Melanomas
　of hands, 1456–1457, *1457*
　malignant. *See* Malignant melanomas
Melanosis, Becker, 305
Meningiomas
　cutaneous, 305
　frontal, 3-D computed tomography in,
　　284–286, *285–289*
Meningoencephalocele, frontoethmoidal. *See*
　Frontoethmoidal
　meningoencephalocele

Meningomyelocele, 1240–1247
　clinical management of, 1242–1248
　　definitive repair and, 1244, *1244–1247*,
　　　1246
　　split-thickness grafts in, 1242–1243, *1243*
　　ventriculoperitoneal shunt in, 1243–1244
　development and, 1241
　evaluation of, 1241–1242
　pathology of, 1241, *1241*
Mental foramen, mandibular fractures close
　to, 1173, *1174*
Mental nerve block, 18, *19*
Mentosternal adhesion, burn wounds of neck
　and, 427
Mesh undermining, in lipectomy, 235
Mesodermal tumors, of skin, 299–300
　of fat, 300, *301*
　of fibrous tissue, 299, *299*, 300
　vascular, 300, *300*
Metabolism, thermal burns and, 403–404, 406
Metacarpals
　fractures of, hand rehabilitation following,
　　1759
　of thumb, acquired deformities of base of,
　　1689, *1690*, *1692*
Metacarpophalangeal joints
　anatomy of, 1531, *1533*
　extensor tendon injuries of, treatment of,
　　1575–1576, *1577*
　of fingers
　　dorsal, dislocations of, 1540, 1542
　　ligament injuries of, 1536, *1538*
　　rheumatoid arthritis in, 1713–1716, *1714*
　　　arthroplasty for, 1715–1716
　　　staging of, 1713–1715, *1714*, *1715*
　　tendon transfers to provide flexion of,
　　　1593, *1593*
　　tendon transfers to provide simultaneous
　　　flexion of interphalangeal joints and,
　　　1593–1595
　　　Brand transfers, *1594*, 1594–1595
　　　modified Stiles-Bunnet transfer,
　　　　1593–1594
　of thumb
　　acquired deformities of, 1687, *1688*, 1689
　　ligament injuries of, 1536, 1538, *1539*,
　　　1539–1540, *1540*
Metals, burns caused by, 451, *451*
Metal suction cannula, for breast reduction,
　2119
Metastases
　of malignant melanoma, lymphatic, with
　　unknown origin, 350
　of oropharyngeal carcinoma, chemotherapy
　　for, 939
Metatarsal free vascularized flaps, 986t, 994
Methotrexate, in oropharyngeal carcinoma,
　939–940, 940t, 942, 943t
Metopic craniosynostosis, 151, *154–155*
Microcephaly, 151, *154–155*
Microcirculation, of skin flaps, 67–69
Micrographic surgery. *See* Mohs micrographic
　surgery
Microlymphaticovenous anastomosis, 377
Microneurovascular anastomoses, for facial
　reanimation, 1051–1052, *1052–1054*
Micropenis, 1397–1398
Microshunting limb lesions, hemangiomas
　and, 355, *357*
Microsomia
　craniofacial, *See* Hemifacial microsomia
　　(craniofacial microsomia, first and
　　second branchial arch syndrome)

Microsomia, craniofacial—*Continued*
preoperative functional appliance and, 538
hemifacial, *See* Hemifacial microsomia (craniofacial microsomia, first and second branchial arch syndrome)
Microstomia, burn wounds and, 426
Microsurgery
for facial reanimation, *1046*, 1046–1047, *1047*
for oropharyngeal reconstruction, 968
Microtia, 789–795
etiology of, 790
features of, 789, 791
treatment of, 790–795
general principles of, 790
two-stage method of, 790–793, *783–789*, 789, 791
Microvascular free flaps, 57
Midcarpal instability, 1543, 1546, *1546*
Midface
evaluation of, in maxillofacial trauma, 1065, *1066*
gunshot wounds of, repair of, 1181, 1183, 1185–1186
Midface fractures, 177–179, *177–182*. *See also specific anatomic sites*
in children and adolescents, 1189–1195, *1190*
maxillary, 1194–1195, *1196*
nasal, 1189–1191, *1190*, *1191*
naso-orbital, 1191–1192, *1192*
of orbital floor, 1194, *1195*
zygomatic, *1193*, 1193–1194, *1194*
Midface surgery, 1866–1868, *1869*
Midline pocket, for rhinoplasty in Oriental patients, preparation of, 2079, 2081
Milia (inclusion cysts), 301, *301*
following blepharoplasty, 1938
Minerals, wound healing and, 9, 10–11
Miniabdominoplasty, surgical instrumentation and procedure for, 2172–2174, *2175*, *2176*
Mitomycin C, in oropharyngeal carcinoma, 942, 943t
Mixed tumor, malignant, of salivary glands, 1038, *1039*
Mohs micrographic surgery, 333–339
indications for, 333–334, 334t, *335*
histologic characteristics and, 333–334
reconstruction, healing by secondary intention, or prosthesis and, *338*, 338–339, *339*
technique for, 334, *336*, 336–338, *337*
Molar region, mandibular fractures in, 1173–1174
Molecular genetics, craniofacial development and, 468–469
Monobloc advancement, in craniofacial dysostoses, 163, *163*, 512
Monofascicular orientation, for nerve grafting, 130
Monofilament sutures, 22, 22t
Mortality, burns and, early excision and, 408
Motor end plates, regeneration of, 1602
Mouth
burns of, 426
classification of, 426
electrical, 426
microstomia and, 426
floor of, reconstruction of. *See* Mandibular reconstruction
Mucocutaneous ridge malalignment, cleft lip and, 606, 606t

Mucoepidermoid carcinoma, of salivary glands, 1037, *1038*
Mucosal excess, cleft lip and, 606t, 606–607
Mucous membranes, topical anesthesia of, 18–19
Mucous pseudocysts, of hands, 1460–1461
Multiview videofluoroscopy, in velopharyngeal insufficiency, 623, 624, *624*, *625*
Muscle(s)
assessment of, for blepharoplasty, *1923*, 1923–1924
bulging of imbalance of, cleft lip and, 606t, 607
of external ear, 772
extrinsic, 772, *774*
intrinsic, 772
laryngeal, 1008–1009
reconstruction of, for bilateral cleft lip repair, 574
transplantation if, for facial reanimation, *824*, 824–825, *826*, *827*, *827*
Muscle flaps, 73. *See also specific muscle flaps*
for hip reconstruction, 1361–1364
in lower extremity reconstruction, 1775, *1776*
for pelvic reconstruction, 1364, *1365*
for pressure sores, 1384
for repair of lumbar spine defects, 1369
for sacral reconstruction, 1366, *1367*, 1369
Muscle grafts, 88t, 91
autografts, 134
uses of, 91
Muscle inset, for facial reanimation, 1051–1052, *1052–1054*
Musculocutaneous flaps, 61, *61*, *62*, 63t, 73, 80, 82t, 82–84
transverse rectus abdominis, 83–84, *86*
trapezius, 80, 81–83
anatomy of, 80, 81–83, *83–85*
Musculofascial flaps, galeal frontalis, in craniomaxillofacial surgery, 142, *144*
Musculoskeletal system, thermal burns and, 406
Musculotendinous flaps, tensor fasciae latae, in thigh reconstruction, 1779
Myofascial pain dysfunction syndrome, 1224
Myogenic ptosis, traumatic, 1105
Myxomas, of palm or finger, 1462

Nail bed
basal cell carcinoma of, 1456
squamous cell carcinoma of, 1457, *1458*
Nail-bed injuries, 1493–1495
anatomy and, 1493, *1494*
mechanism of injury and, 1493–1494, *1494*
treatment of, 1494–1495
avulsion injuries, 1495, *1495*
fractures accompanying nail-bed injuries, 1495
simple lacerations, 1494–1495
subungual hematomas, 1494
Nasal clefts, 581–594. *See also* Facial clefts
bilateral, 574–575, 578–579, 585–593, *588*
composite earlobe graft technique for, 578, *579*
elongation of columella in, 575, *577*
forked flap method for, 578, *578*
open-tip method for, 578–579, *580*
postoperative care and follow-up care for, 579
preoperative orthopedic treatment of, 588–589
primary reconstruction of, 589, *590*, *591*

Nasal clefts, bilateral—*Continued*
stage-2 reconstruction of, 589, *592–594*, 593
secondary correction of, 702–715
airway obstruction and, 706–707, *707*
deformities associated with bilateral cleft lip and, *708*, 708–709
deformities associated with unilateral cleft lip and, 703–706, *704*
preoperative evaluation and planning for, 703, *703*
results of, 709, *709–717*, 718t–719t
surgical technique for, 703–709, *704*, *707*, *708*
timing of procedure for, 702
unilateral, 581–585, *582*, *584*
difficulties associated with, 585, *587*
preoperative orthopedic treatment of, 583
surgical technique for, 583, 585, *586*
Nasal displacement, following rhinoplasty in Oriental patients, 2086
Nasal extrusion, following rhinoplasty in Oriental patients, 2086, *2086*
Nasal floor reconstruction, for bilateral cleft lip repair, 574
Nasal fractures, 1126–1135
anatomic classification of, 1127, *1128*
anatomy and pathophysiology of, *1126*, 1126–1127, *1127*
in children and adolescents, 1189–1191, *1190*, *1191*
complications of, 1133–1134, *1134*, *1135*
diagnosis of, 1127–1128
etiology of, 1126
physical examination in, 1128, *1128*, *1129*
treatment of, 1128–1133, *1129*
anesthesia for, 1129–1130
casting techniques for, 1133, *1134*
comminuted fractures, 1133, *1133*, 1134
goals of, *1130*, 1130–1131
nasal septal fractures, 1131, 1133
surgical techniques for, 1131, *1131–1133*, 1133
timing of, 1129
Nasal injuries, 1098. *See also* Nasal fractures
anatomy and, 1098
management of, 1098
Nasalis
pars alaris, anatomy of, 2077
pars transversa, anatomy of, 2078
Nasal malposition, following rhinoplasty in Oriental patients, 2083, *2085*
Nasal reconstruction, 883–905, *884*. *See also* Rhinoplasty
for central nasal defects, 895, *898–901*
for deep defects, 887–895
axial paramedian forehead flaps and, 887, *888*, 889, *889*
heminasal reconstruction and, 893, *893–897*, 895
nasolabial flaps and, 889, *890*, *891*, 892
restoration of nasal lining and, 892–893, *893*
nasal support and, 903–905, *905*
replacement of nasal cover, 885
for superficial defects, 885–886
full-thickness skin grafts and, *885*, 885–886
local nasal flaps and, 886, *886*
total, *902–904*, 903
Nasal spine, rhinoplasty and, 2011–2012
Nasal stenoses, secondary rhinoplasty for, 2043, *2048*, *2049*

Nasoethmoidal fractures, 1142, *1143*
Nasoethmoidal-orbital fractures, reduction and stabilization of, 1149–1151, *1150–1151*
Nasolabial flaps, for nasal reconstruction, 889, *890, 891,* 892
Nasolabial furrows, excision of, *1993,* 1993–1994
  results with, 1994
  technique for, 1993–1994
Nasomaxillary dysplasia, 494, *495*
Nasometry, multiview, 630, *630*
Naso-orbital fractures, in children and adolescents, 1191–1192, *1192*
Nasopharyngoscopy
  in oropharyngeal carcinoma, 925, *925*
  in velopharyngeal insufficiency, *623,* 623–624
Nasoschizis, 492, *493,* 494
  surgical treatment of, 492–494, *493–495*
   nose and, 492, *493–495*
   skeleton and, 494
Neck
  burns of, 426–428
   classification of, 426–427
   treatment of, 427–428, *428*
  lateral masses of, 810–814, *814, 815.* See *also* Branchial cleft anomalies
  lipectomy and. See Suction-assisted lipectomy
  midline masses and sinuses of, 814–815, *816*
  photographic documentation of, lipectomy and, 226, *226*
  reconstruction using soft tissue expansion, 210
  regional blocks of, 16–18, *16–19*
  surgical management of salivary gland tumors and, 1044
Neck dissection
  in facial rejuvenation, *1887,* 1887–1888
  in oropharyngeal resection, 935–936
  timing of, 936
Necrotizing fasciitis, of hands, 1473–1474, *1477*
Neodymium: yttrium-aluminum-garnet lasers, 255–256
Nerve(s)
  of hand
   determining if injury is to nerve and, 1487–1488
   evaluation of, 1486–1487, *1487*
  hand reconstruction and, 1665–1667, *1667*
Nerve blocks, sympathetic, in wrist pain, 1729
Nerve compression
  carpal tunnel syndrome and. See Carpal tunnel syndrome
  chronic, 1605, *1609*
  wrist pain and, 1730t–1731t, 1734–1735
Nerve conduits, 134
Nerve ends, preparation for nerve grafting, 130
Nerve function, surgical management of salivary gland tumors and, 1044
Nerve grafting, 127–134
  allografts and, 133–134
  grading of nerve injury and, 127–128
  indications for, 128–129
  muscle autografts and, 134
  nerve conduits and, 134

Nerve grafting—*Continued*
  for peripheral nerve injuries of upper extremities, 1611, 1615–1619
   awake stimulation and, 1616, 1618, *1618*
   donor nerve grafts and, 1619, *1622–1624*
   histochemical staining and, 1616
   neuroma in continuity and, 1619, *1620, 1621*
   technique for, 1611, 1615–1616, *1615–1617*
  physiologic events following nerve injury and, 128
  postoperative care and, 132–133
  surgical technique for, 130–132
  timing of, 129–130
  vascularized, 134
Nerve injuries
  grading, 127–128
  peripheral. See Peripheral nerve injuries of upper extremities, nerve grafting for. See Nerve grafting, for peripheral nerve injuries of upper extremities
  physiologic events following, 128
Nerve supply, skin grafting and, 47
Nerve tissue, normal, identification of, 131
Nervous system, evaluation of, in maxillofacial trauma, 1063, *1064*
Neural tumors, of skin, 304, *304*–305
Neurapraxia, 1603
Neurilemmomas (schwannomas), of hands, 1462, *1462*
Neurofibromas, 304, *304*
  of hands, 1462
Neurogenic ptosis, traumatic, *1104,* 1105
Neurologic studies, of diabetic foot, *1842,* 1842–1843, *1843*
Neuromas, 304, 304–305
  amputation, 304–305
  in continuity, 1605, *1607, 1608,* 1619, *1620, 1621*
Neuropathy, diabetic, *1842,* 1842–1843, *1843*
Neurotmesis, 1605
Neurotropism, peripheral nerve injuries and, 1599–1601, *1600–1602*
Neurovascular injury, of foot, foot reconstruction and, 1821
Neurovascular island flaps, local, for fingertip injuries with exposed bone, 1502, *1505, 1506*
Neutralization plates, for hand and wrist fractures, 1518, *1523*
Nevi
  araneus (spider nevi), 362
  basal cell nevus syndrome and, 312, *313,* 315
  blue, 307
  comediconus, 297, *298*
  comedonicus, 296
  compound, 350
  congenital, 306, *307*
  of connective tissue, 299
  epidermal nevus syndrome and, 296, 298
  familial dysplastic nevus syndrome and, 350
  flammeus (port-wine stain), 360–362, *362*
   argon laser therapy for, 257, *257, 258,* 259
   neonatorum, 363
  halo, 306–307, *307*
  lipomatosus superficialis, 300, *301*
  melanocytic, acquired, 306, *306*
  nuchal (salmon patch; stork bite), 363
  sebaceus, 296
   of Jadassohn, 297, 311, *311*
  Spitz, 307, *307*
  unius lateris, 297–298

Nipple-areolar complex
  delivery of, in reduction mammaplasty, 2139–2140, *2139–2140*
  lactation and, following reduction mammaplasty, 2142
  sensitivity of, following reduction mammaplasty, 2142
  viability of, following reduction mammaplasty, 2142
Nipple reconstruction, 1342–1343, 1344–1348
  with tattooing, 1344–1348
   secondary reconstruction and, 1348
   skate technique for, 1344, *1345,* 1346
   tattooing and, 1346–1348, *1348*
  TRAM flap breast reconstruction and, 1335, *1336–1338*
Nitrofurazone ointment, in burn wound sepsis, 402t, 403
Nodular melanomas, 344
Norepinephrine, depletion of, skin flaps and, 69
Nose. See also *headings beginning with term Nasal*
  burns of, 424–425
   classification of, 424
   treatment of, 434–435, *435*
  cutaneous malignant tumors of, 324, *324–328*
  deformities of, rhinoplasty for. See Rhinoplasty
  evaluation of, in maxillofacial trauma, 1064–1065, *1067*
  fibrous papules of, 299, *299*
  postoperative care of, in hemifacial microsomia, 542
  reconstruction of, in mandibular dysostosis, 535
  reconstruction using soft tissue expansion, 208, *209–210,* 210
  twisted, rhinoplasty for, 2029–2030, *2031*
Nostril sidewall, drooping, in Oriental patients, 2083, *2084*
Nuchal nevus, (salmon patch; stork bite), 363
Numbness, following blepharoplasty, 1936, *1936*
Nutrition
  following lipectomy, 240
  of tendons, 122
Nutritional repletion, pressure sores and, 1375
Nylon sutures, 22, 22t

Obesity, as indication for breast reduction, 2143
Occipital incision, for facial rejuvenation, 1877, *1878*
Oculoplastic surgery. See Blepharoplasty
Oligofascicular orientation, for nerve grafting, 130
Omental flaps, 95–101
  anatomy and embryology and, 95, *96, 97*
  applications of, 98, *99–101*
  for chest wall reconstruction, 1252
  contraindications to, 95
  disadvantages of, 100–101
  surgical technique for, 96, 98
Onlay bone grafts, 104–105
Open fractures, of hands and wrist, 1519–1520, *1528, 1529*
Open rhinoplasty, for correction of cleft nasal deformity, 2002
Open-tip method, for bilateral cleft nasal deformity repair, 578–579, *580*
Operating room setup, for free tissue techniques, *969,* 969–970

Optic nerve injuries, orbital fractures and, 1144
Orbicularis oculi muscle, anatomy of, 2059
Orbital bone contouring, in blepharoplasty, 1934
Orbital carcinomas, 1000–1007, 1006t
  anatomy and, 1000, 1001
  diagnosis of, 1000–1001, 1001t, 1002, 1003
  surgical technique for, 1001–1003, 1003–1005
Orbital defects, with mandibular dysostosis, treatment of, 528, 529, 529
Orbital fractures, 1136–1155, 1137
  blow-out, roentgenographic appearance of, 1080–1082, 1081
  clinical anatomy and, 1136, 1136–1138
    of anterior orbit, 1136–1138
    of interorbital space, 1138
    of middle orbit, 1138
    of posterior orbit, 1138
  coronal approach to, 1212–1214, 1216, 1216–1218
  diagnosis of, 1138–1144, 1139, 1140
    anterior orbital fractures, 1140–1142, 1141, 1143
    middle orbital fractures, 1142–1143, 1144
    posterior orbital fractures, 1143–1144
  fronto-orbital, 1141–1142, 1142
    reduction and stabilization of, 1151, 1152
  intraorbital, isolated, 1142–1143
  malar. See Malar fractures, treatment of
  maxillo-orbital, 1141, 1440–1141
    reduction and stabilization of, 1149, 1149
  of medial orbital wall, 1143, 1144
  nasoethmoidal-orbital, 1142, 1143
    reduction and stabilization of, 1149–1151, 1150–1151
  naso-orbital, in children and adolescents, 1191–1192, 1192
  optic nerve injury and, 1144
  of orbital floor, 1143
    in children and adolescents, 1194, 1195
  of orbital roof, 1143
  postoperative care and, 1155
  secondary reconstruction of soft tissue deformity associated with, 1199–1216, 1200–1204
    fracture osteosynthesis and graft fixation and, 1207, 1208, 1209
    malar fractures and, 1210–1216, 1211–1212
    surgical approaches to orbit and, 1210–1218, 1211–1216
    use of foreign materials in, 1199–1200, 1205–1206, 1205–1207
  superior orbital fissure syndrome and, 1143–1144
  treatment of, 1144–1155
    coronal incision and, 1144, 1145
    exposure and, 1144–1145, 1145, 1147
    internal orbital reconstruction and, 1153, 1154, 1154–1155
    lateral extension of upper blepharoplasty incision and, 1145, 1147
    maxillary gingivobuccal sulcus incision and, 1145, 1147
    reduction and stabilization and, 1145–1146, 1148–1152, 1149–1151
    soft tissue closure and, 1155
    subciliary incision and, 1144–1145, 1146
    transconjunctival incision and, 1145, 1147
  zygomatico-orbital, 1140, 1141
    reduction and stabilization of, 1145–1146, 1148, 1149

Organoid nevi, 295–298, 298
Organ preservation, in oropharyngeal carcinoma, chemotherapy and, 942
Oriental patients, aesthetic facial surgery in. See Aesthetic facial surgery, in Oriental patients; Eyelid operations, in Oriental patients; Rhinoplasty, in Oriental patients
Oronasal fistulas
  bilateral cleft lip and palate and, 687
  unilateral cleft lip and palate and, 683
Oropharyngeal carcinomas, 921–930
  anatomy and physiology and, 921–922
  classification and staging of, 929t, 929–930, 930t
  glottic, 1011
  pathophysiology and risk factors for, 922–923
  presentation and examination in, 923–929
    exfoliative cytology, 927
    fine-needle aspiration, 928–929
    imaging studies, 926, 926
    inspection and palpation, 925, 925
    physical examination, 923, 925, 925
    precancerous lesions and, 923, 924
    using anesthesia, endoscopy, and biopsy, 926, 926–927, 927
  radiation therapy in, 945–954
  recurrent, salvage therapy for, 953–954
  squamous cell, 935
    chemotherapy for. See Chemotherapy, for oropharyngeal carcinoma
  subglottic, 1012
  supraglottic, 1011–1012
Oropharyngeal reconstruction, 966–969, 967
  of cervical esophageal lesions, 968
  with free tissue transfer, 966–981. See also Free tissue transfer
  microsurgical techniques for, 968
  of palatal and maxillary lesions, 968
  requirements for, 966–968, 967, 967t
  of soft tissue lesions, 968
  timing of, 968
  with transposition flaps, 956–961
    deltopectoral flap, 961, 964–965
    general principles of, 956–958, 957t
    pectoralis major flap, 958, 960, 961
    platysma flap, 958, 959
    surgical principles for, 958
    trapezius flap, 961, 962–963
Oropharyngeal resection, 931–938
  anatomy and, 931, 931–932, 932
  approaches to base of tongue and pharyngeal walls and, 938
  clinicopathologic considerations and, 933–934
  incision for, 935, 935, 936
  lymphatic drainage and, 932, 933
  marginal resection of mandible and, 937–938, 938
  necessity of laryngectomy when removing base of tongue and, 938
  neck dissection and, 935–936
    timing of, 936
  pathology and patterns of spread of tumors and, 932–933, 933, 934
  splitting of mandible and, 936–937, 937
  tracheostomy and, 935
Orthodontic treatment
  in cleft lip and palate, 648–666, 649, 650, 650t
    orthodontic and orthognathic surgery, 662–663, 663–668, 664t, 665–666

Orthodontic treatment, in cleft lip and palate—Continued
    orthopedic treatment in infancy, 648, 651
    in permanent dentition, 658–659, 661, 661, 662
    in primary dentition, 650–652, 651–654
    in transitional dentition, 652–658, 654–660
  in hemifacial microsomia, 539
  preoperative, for maxillary deformities, 721
Orthognathic surgery
  for clefts, 662–663, 663–668, 664t, 665–666
  correction of secondary skeletal deformities in adolescent patients with clefts and, 682–698
    integrated team approach for, 682
    results of, 686–687, 688–691, 691, 694–697, 697, 698, 699–701
    surgical technique for, 683, 684–685, 686, 687, 689, 692–693, 698
    timing of surgery for, 682–683
    in unilateral cleft lip and palate, 683–687
  for mandibular deformities
    anterior segmental osteotomy, 743, 745, 749, 750
    chin correction and, 743, 744–748
    mandibular body and ramus osteotomy, 749–756, 750–756
    sagittal split osteotomy and chin repositioning, 754
    sagittal split osteotomy and mobilization of lower anterior segment, 754–756
    sagittal split osteotomy and osteotomy of upper jaw, 756–757, 757
  for maxillary deformities, 720–740
    complications of, 740
    leveling of maxilla and, 739, 739
    maxillary expansion and, 722, 723–724, 724
    osteotomies and. See Le Fort I osteotomies, for maxillary deformities; Osteotomies
    preoperative orthodontic treatment and, 721
    preoperative planning for, 720–721
    rigid fixation and, 721, 721–722, 722
  rigid fixation in, 187–193
    genioplasty techniques, 193, 193, 194
    mandibular osteotomies, 187–188, 188–191
    maxillary osteotomies, 190–191, 192
Orthopedic treatment, preoperative
  of bilateral cleft nose, 588–589
  for unilateral cleft lip, 551
  for unilateral cleft nose, 583
Osseointegration, of prostheses, 1028–1029, 1030–1033, 1031
Osseous flaps, free vascularized, 985–996, 986t
  combined, 996, 996
  fibula, 986t, 992, 992–993, 993
  iliac crest, 986t, 987, 987–991, 989
  metatarsal or dorsalis pedis, 986t, 994
  radial forearm, 986t, 989, 991, 992
  rib, 985, 986t, 987
  scapula, 986t, 994, 994–996, 996
Osteoarthritis, wrist pain and, 1730t–1731t
Osteoblasts, 103
Osteochondromas, of hands, 1464, 1465
Osteoclasts, 103
Osteoconduction, 104
Osteocutaneous flaps, scapular free, 971, 973–975
  for oropharyngeal reconstruction, 968

Osteocytes, 103
Osteoid osteomas, of hands, 1466
Osteoinduction, 104
Osteomusculocutaneous flaps, pedicled,
    984–985
  pectoralis major, 984, 984t
  sternocleidomastoid, 984t, 985
  trapezius, 984–985, 984t
Osteomyelitis, 1809–1815
  bacteriologic factors in, 1810
  bone healing and, 1809–1810
  classification of, 1810
  diagnosis of, 1810
  etiology and pathogenesis of, 1810
  of hands, 1479
  treatment of, 1810–1815, 1811, 1812
    Ilizarov's technique in, 1814, 1813–1819,
      1814–1815
Osteoradionecrosis
  as indication for mandibular
    reconstruction, 982
  prostheses for, 1028
Osteosynthesis, of orbital fractures, 1207,
    1208
Osteotomies
  anterior segmental. See Anterior segmental
    osteotomies
  Le Fort I. See Le Fort I osteotomies, for
    maxillary deformities
  Le Fort III, in Crouzon and Apert
    syndromes, 160, 161–162, 162
  mandibular, 187–188, 188–191, 745,
    750–756, 750–756
  maxillary, 190–191, 192, 724, 726, 727
  in rhinoplasty, 2016–2017, 2017, 2040
  sagittal split. See Sagittal split osteotomies
  of upper jaw, sagittal split osteotomy
    combined with, 756–757, 757
Overgrowth (soft tissue gigantism),
    hemangiomas and, 359, 359
Oxidizing agents, burns caused by, 449
Oxycephaly, 151, 152–153, 511–512

Packing, rhinoplasty and, 2019, 2019
Palatal augmentation prostheses, 1025, 1027
Palatal lift, in cleft lip and palate, 766, 767,
    768
Palatal obturators, 1018–1019, 1019, 1020
  in cleft lip and palate, 762–765, 763, 765
Palatal processes, embryology of, 465,
    465–466, 466
Palate
  cleft. See Cleft palate; Facial clefts
  lesions of, oropharyngeal reconstruction
    and, 968
  repair of, with pharyngeal flap operation,
    640, 641, 642
  soft, brachytherapy of, 953
  splitting of, for pharyngeal flap operation,
    634, 635
Palatopharyngeal obturators, 1019, 1021
  in cleft lip and palate, 766, 766, 767
Palatopharyngeus muscle, 931
Palm, myxomas of, 1462
Palmaris longus tendon grafts, 123
Palmaris longus (Camitz) tendon transfer,
    1587, 1590
Panfacial rejuvenation, 1873
Pansuture craniosynostosis, 151
Papillary cystadenoma lymphomatosum
    (Warthin tumor), 1035, 1036t, 1037,
    1037

Papineau procedure, 1800–1801
  follow-up and, 1801
  technique for, 1800–1801
Papular angiokeratomas, 300
Papules, fibrous, of nose, 299, 299
Paranasal sinuses, carcinoma of, 1000–1007,
    1006t
  anatomy and, 1000, 1001
  diagnosis of, 1000–1001, 1001t, 1002, 1003
  surgical technique for, 1001–1003,
    1003–1005
Paranoia, lipectomy and, 227
Parascapular flaps, 74t
Parasymphyseal area fractures, 1173, 1174
Parenchymal pedicle reduction
    mammaplasty. See Reduction
    mammaplasty, parenchymal pedicle
    reduction mammaplasty
Parkes Weber syndrome, 365
Paronychia, 1469, 1469
Parotid duct injuries, 1086
  anatomy and, 1086, 1086
  management of, 1086, 1087
Parotidectomy, 1038–1042
  flap elevation and, 1040
  incision for, 1039–1040
  nerve dissection and, 1040, 1040–1042,
    1041
  patient preparation for, 1039, 1039
Patient counseling, soft tissue expansion
    and, 202, 204
Patient position, for pharyngeal flap
    operation, 634
Patient satisfaction
  with blepharoplasty results, 1934
  with lipectomy, unrealistic expectations
    and, 227
  with perioral rejuvenation. See Perioral
    rejuvenation, patient satisfaction
    with
Pectoral(s), fat pad, lipectomy and, 238
Pectoralis major flaps
  for chest wall reconstruction, 1250
  intrathoracic transposition of, 1269, 1269
  for oropharyngeal reconstruction, 958, 960,
    961
  osteomusculocutaneous, 984, 984t
Pectus deformities
  pectus carinatum, 1238
  pectus excavatum, 1237–1238
  preoperative evaluation of, 1237
  results of surgical treatment of, 1237–1238,
    1239
  surgical technique for, 1237, 1238
Pelvic reconstruction, 1360, 1364, 1369–1370
  general principles of, 1364
  muscle flaps for, 1364, 1365
Penile construction and reconstruction,
    1400–1410, 1401
  complications of, 1410
  for epispadias. See Epispadias
  for hypospadias. See Hypospadias
  postoperative care and, 1409–1410
  surgical technique for, 1400–1409, 1401
    flap design and, 1401, 1402
    flap elevation and, 1402–1403, 1402–1405
    preparation of recipient site and,
      1403–1404, 1406, 1406, 1407
    prosthesis placement and, 1406,
      1408–1409, 1408–1410
Penis
  curvatures of, 1397
  epispadias and. See Epispadias

Penis—Continued
  hypospadias and. See Hypospadias
  micropenis and, 1397–1398
Pentoxifylline, for leg ulcers, 1835
Perceptual evaluation, of velopharyngeal
    insufficiency, 620–621
Perilunate dislocations, 1546–1547, 1547, 1548
Periodontitis, mandibular fractures and, 1177
Perioral rejuvenation, 1990, 1990–1998
  augmentation of upper lip for, 1995
  collagen injections for, 1996
  corner-lift for, 1992, 1992–1993
  dermabrasion for, 1994, 1994–1995
  lip-lift for, 1990–1992, 1991
  lower lip advancement for, 1995, 1995
  nasolabial furrow excision and, 1993,
    1993–1994
  patient satisfaction with, 1996–1998
    life-altering results and, 1997, 1997
    patient upset and, 1997–1998
    technical results and, 1997
  principles of surgery of, 1998
  psychological importance of perioral area
    and, 1997–1998
  silicone injections for, 1996
  upper lip advancement for, 1996, 1996
Periorbital hematomas, following
    blepharoplasty, 1937
Peripheral nerve injuries
  axoplasmic transport and, 1598
  chronic nerve compression, 1605, 1609
  fifth-degree (neurotmesis), 1605
  first-degree (neurapraxia), 1603
  fourth-degree, 1603
  of hand, hand rehabilitation and. See Hand
    rehabilitation, following nerve injuries
  mixed (neuroma in continuity; sixth-degree
    injury), 1067, 1605, 1608
  nerve grafting and. See nerve grafting
  nerve repair and, 1608–1609, 1610–1613
    techniques of, 1610–1611, 1613, 1614
    timing of, 1610
  neurotropism and contact guidance and,
    1599–1601, 1600–1602
  regeneration and, 1601–1602
    of distal segment, 1602, 1604, 1605
    of motor end plates, 1602
    of proximal segment, 1602, 1603
    of sensory receptors, 1602
  second-degree (axonotmesis), 1603
  third-degree, 1603
  of upper extremities, nerve grafting for. See
    Nerve grafting, for peripheral nerve
    injuries of upper extremities
Permanent dentition, orthodontic treatment
    for clefts in, 658–659, 661, 661, 662
Phalangization, 1685
Phallic construction and reconstruction. See
    Penile construction and reconstruction
Pharmacologic agents. See also Drug(s); Drug
    therapy; specific drugs and drug types
  toe-to-hand transplantation and, 1705
Pharyngeal arches, embryology of, 462–463,
    462–466, 465–466
Pharyngeal flap operation, 632–642
  anesthesia for, 634
  indications for, 633
  patient position for, 634
  postoperative care and follow-up
    evaluation for, 640
  preoperative care for, 634
  procedures associated with, 634
  results with, 640

Pharyngeal flap operation—*Continued*
  sphincter pharyngoplasty compared with,
      645–647, *646*, *647*
  technique for, 634–640
    dissection of pharyngeal flap, 636, *637*
    flap suture, 638–639, *639*
    levator muscle reconstruction, 639
    outline of pharyngeal flap, 634
    palatal repair, 640, *641*, *642*
    palatal splitting, 634, *635*
    posterior pharyngeal wall repair, 638,
        638
    preparation of turn-back flaps and
        muscle dissection, 634, 636, *636*
    suture of turn-back flaps, 639, *640*
  timing of, 633
Pharyngeal walls
  approaches to, 938
  brachytherapy of, 953
Pharyngoplasty, sphincter. *See* Sphincter
      pharyngoplasty
Phenols, burns caused by, 451
Photocoagulation lasers. *See* Laser(s),
      photocoagulation; *specific types of*
      photocoagulation lasers
Photography, lipectomy and, 223, 226
  face and neck and, 226, *226*
  trunk and limbs and, 223, 226, *226*
Physical evaluation, for lipectomy, 227
Physical therapy, following lipectomy, 240
Pigmentation
  of skin, blepharoplasty and, 1921
  of skin grafts, 48
Pigment cell tumors, benign, 305–307,
      305–307
Pigmented lesion lasers, 266
Pig snout nose, secondary rhinoplasty for,
      2036, 2038, *2038–2039*
Pilar (tricholemmal) cysts, 301
Pilomatrichomas, 301
Pinch and roll test, termination of lipectomy
      and, 235
Pinch test, for lipectomy, 228–229, *229*
Plagiocephaly, 148, *150*, 151, 500, 504,
      506–508, 508
Plain-film roentgenography, in maxillofacial
      trauma, 1069–1073
  anterior or posteroanterior view, 1070, *1070*
  basic principles of, 1069
  bony fracture and, 1071–1072, *1072*
  Caldwell view, 1070, *1070*
  equipment for, 1070
  interpretation of, 1071–1073
  lateral view, 1071, *1072*
  soft tissue emphysema and, 1072–1073
  submentovertical view, 1070, *1071*
  symmetry and, 1073
  technique for, 1070–1071
  Waters view, 1070, *1071*
Plantaris tendon grafts, 123, *123*
Plasmatic imbibition, 47
Plate(s), for hand and wrist fractures. *See*
      Hand fractures; Wrist fractures
Plate and screw stabilization, of maxillary
      fractures, 1158, *1159–1161*, 1162
Plate fixation, 169, 170–171
  continuous cooling and, 170
  of craniofacial skeleton, 169, *170*
  in craniomaxillofacial surgery, 141–142, *143*
  intermaxillary fixation during operation,
      171
  low-speed drilling and, 170
  plate contouring and, 171
Platelet-derived growth factor (PDGF),
      wound healing and, 4t, 9

Platysma, modification of, 1888–1890, *1889*
Platysma flap, for oropharyngeal
      reconstruction, 958, *959*
Platysmoplasty, anterior, 247
Pleomorphic adenoma (benign mixed tumor),
      of salivary glands, 1035, 1036t, *1037*
Plesiotherapy, 952, *952*
Poland anomaly, 1233, *1234–1236*, 1235–1237
Poliomyelitis, underdevelopment of leg
      caused by, calf implantation and,
      2255–2256, *2258*
Polly beak, secondary rhinoplasty for, *2034*,
      2034–2035, *2035*
Polydactyly, hidden, 1434
Polydioxane sutures, 21–22, 22t
Polydioxanone sutures, 8
Polyester sutures, 22, 22t
Polyfascicular orientation, for nerve grafting,
      130
Polyglactin (Vicryl) sutures, 8
Polyglactin 910 sutures, 21, 22t
Polyglycolic acid (Dexon) sutures, 7, 21, 22t
Polyglyconate (Maxon) sutures, 8
Polypropylene sutures, 8, 22, 22t
Polytetrafluoroethylene (PTFE-graphite), for
      facial augmentation, 1865
Polythelia (supernumerary nipples), 303
Porokeratosis, 312, *313*
  actinic, disseminated superficial, 312, *313*
Poromas, eccrine, 303–304
Port-wine stains (nevus flammeus), 360–362,
      362
  argon laser therapy for, 257, *257*, *258*, 259
Positioning, for lipectomy, 232, *232*, 233
Postauricular incision, for facial rejuvenation,
      1876–1877, *1877*
Postcapillary venules, of skin flaps, 67
Post-traumatic arthritis, wrist pain and,
      1730t–1731t
Post-traumatic cysts, wrist pain and,
      1730t–1731t
Pouce flotant (floating thumb), 1448
Preantral fat, 220
Preauricular incision, for facial rejuvenation,
      1874–1875, *1876*
Preauricular sinuses, 810, *810*
Precapillary sphincter, of skin flaps, 67
Preiser's disease, wrist pain and, 1730t–1731t
Premaxilla, management of, in bilateral cleft
      lip, 566, *567*
Premaxillary positioning appliance, in cleft
      lip and palate, 759–761, *760*, *761*
Pressure, for scarring, 12
Pressure-flow evaluation, multiview,
      624–630, *625–629*, 628t–630t
Pressure sores, 1371–1386
  etiology of, 1371, *1372*, 1373
  incidence of, 1371
  prevention and management of, *1373*,
      1373–1375, 1374t
    contractures and, 1375
    nutritional repletion and, 1375
    skin care and, 1374–1375
    wound care and, 1375, 1375t
  surgical reconstruction and, 1376t,
      1376–1386, *1383*, *1384*
    of ischial sores, 1377, *1378–1381*,
        1379–1380
    of multiple and extensive sores,
        1383–1384, *1385*
    postoperative management and
        rehabilitation and, 1384–1386, *1386*
    of sacral sores, 1376–1377, *1377*, *1378*
    of trochanteric sores, 1380, *1382*, *1383*

Pretunneling, before lipectomy, 233–234, *234*
Primary dentition, orthodontic treatment for
      clefts in, 650–652
  anterior crossbite and, 652, *654*
  posterior crossbite and, 650, *651–653*
Prolabium
  dissection of, for bilateral cleft lip repair,
      571
  management of, in bilateral cleft lip, 566,
      567
  marking, for bilateral cleft lip repair, 568
Prophylactic subcutaneous mastectomy,
      1276–1282
  complications of, 1282
  implants and, 1281–1282
  indications for, 1277
  patient selection for, 1276–1277
  postoperative care and, 1282
  surgical technique for, 1277–1281
    ablative technique and, 1278–1279
    anesthesia and, 1277
    incisions and, 1277–1278, *1278–1280*
    preoperative preparation and, 1277
    submuscular reconstruction and,
        1279–1281, *1281*
Prostheses
  for abdominal wall reconstruction,
      1352–1353
  active tendon implants, 1564
  for augmentation mammaplasty. *See*
      Augmentation mammaplasty
  breast
    following prophylactic subcutaneous
        mastectomy, 1281–1282
    replacement of expander with permanent
        implant and, 1302, *1303–1305*
  calf. *See* Calf implantation
  cheek implants, 1915
  facial, 1028, *1029*
  head and neck. *See also specific prostheses*
    for patients treated by chemotherapy or
        radiation therapy, 1028
  intraoral, 1018–1019, *1019–1021*
  mandibular, 1022–1024, *1022–1025*
  nasal
    introduction of, 2081–2082
    preparation of, 2079
    visible, 2086
  osseointegration and rehabilitation and,
      1028–1029, *1030–1033*, 1031
  penile, placement of, 1406, 1408–1409,
      1408–1410
  tongue, 1025, *1025–1027*
Prosthodontics, in cleft lip and palate,
      759–774
  articulation development prosthesis, *761*,
      761–762, *762*
  general dental care and, 762–763
  palatal lift, 766, *767*, 767, 768
  palatal obturator, 762–765, *763*, 765
  palatopharyngeal obturator, 766, *766*, *767*
  premaxillary positioning appliance,
      759–761, *760*, *761*
  tooth replacement and, 768–769, *768–773*
Protein deficiency, wound healing and, 8
Protein kinase C, craniofacial development
      and, 467
Protoplasmic poisons, burns caused by, 449
Proximal interphalangeal joint
  arthroplasty of, hand rehabilitation
      following, 1759–1760
  fractures of, hand rehabilitation following,
      1759
  incisions for exposure of, 1419, *1421*

Pseudocysts, mucous, of hands, 1460–1461
Psychological evaluation
  for blepharoplasty, 1920
  for lipectomy, 227
PTFE-graphite (polytetrafluoroethylene), for facial augmentation, 1865
Ptosis, of breast, correction by vertical mammaplasty, 2157, *2158–2164*
Ptosis, of eyelid, 800–808
  autogenous fascia lata frontalis sling for, 804–808
    obtaining fascia lata for, 804, *806–807*
    placement of fascia lata within eyelids and, 804–805, 808
  blepharoplasty for, 1921–1922, *1922*, 1968–1972, *1970–1973*
  external levator resection procedure for, 800–801, *802–803*, 804
  following blepharoplasty, 1936
  following eyelid operations in Oriental patients, 2075
  senile, 1968–1969
  traumatic, 1101–1105
    aponeurotic, 1101–1102, *1102–1104*
    mechanical, 1105
    myogenic, 1105
    neurogenic, *1104*, 1105
Pudendal-thigh flaps, 80
  anatomy of, 80, *81*
  surgical technique for, 80
Pulley reconstruction, flexor. *See* Flexor pulley reconstruction
Pulmonary embolism, following suction-assisted lipectomy, 2199
Pyogenic arthritis, of hands, 1473, 1477
Pyogenic granulomas (lobulated capillary hemangiomas), 353, 355, *356*

Q-switched ruby lasers, 266
Quadrilateral vermilion flap reconstruction, of cupid's bow, 614–615, *615*

Race. *See also* Aesthetic facial surgery, in African-Americans; Aesthetic facial surgery, in Oriental patients
  wound healing and, 30–31
Radial dysplasia, 1444–1449, *1445*
  clubhand, *1445*, 1446, 1447, *1447*
  hypoplastic thumb, 1447t, 1447–1449, *1448, 1450–1451*
Radial forearm flaps
  free, *970*, 970–971
  free vascularized, 986t, 989, *991, 992*
  for oropharyngeal reconstruction, 968
Radial fractures, distal, hand rehabilitation following, 1759
Radial grafts, 105t, 112
Radial nerve palsy, tendon transfers for, 1580–1585
  Boyes sublimis transfer, *1584*, 1585, *1586*
  flexor carpi radialis transfer, 1581, *1583, 1584*, 1585
  standard flexor carpi ulnaris transfer, 1581, *1582*
Radiation injuries, 452–456
  clinical findings in, 452–453, *453*
  definitive surgical treatment of, 453–456
    excision and, 456
    postoperative care and, 456
    reconstruction and, 454, *455*, 456
  preoperative management of, 453

Radiation therapy
  altered fractionation and, 949–951
    accelerated fractionation, 949, *950*, 951
    accelerated hyperfractionation, 951
    hyperfractionation, 949
    hypofractionation, 951
  in basal cell carcinoma, of skin, 316
  brachytherapy, 951–954
    isotopes and source placement for, 951–953, *952*, 953t
    site-specific application of, 953–954
  fundamentals of, 945–946, *946–948*
  head and neck prostheses for patients treated by, 1028
  for malignant melanomas, 348
  in oropharyngeal carcinoma, 945–954
    chemotherapy and, 942–943, 943t
    prognostic factors for local control and, 954
    radiobiologic principles and, 946, 948–949
  for salivary gland tumors, 1044
  for scarring, 12
Radiography. *See* Imaging studies; *specific modalities*
Radioisotopes, for brachytherapy, 952–953, 953t
Radioulnar joint, distal, disorders of, 1547
Ramus, ascending, fractures of, 1176–1177
  condylar process fractures, 1176–1177, *1178, 1179*
  coronoid process fractures, 1176
Random pattern flaps, for soft tissue coverage of hand and upper extremity, 1647–1648, *1649*
Range of motion, of hand, evaluation of, 1745
Rectus abdominis flaps
  for breast reconstruction (TRAM), 1310–1317
  for chest wall reconstruction, 1251–1252
  for hip reconstruction, 1362, 1364
  intrathoracic transposition of, 1270
  for soft tissue coverage of hand and upper extremity, 1654
Rectus femoris flaps, for hip reconstruction, 1361–1362, *1362, 1363*
Redistribution, radiation therapy and, 948
Reducing agents, burns caused by, 449
Reduction mammaplasty, 2126–2142
  anatomic considerations and, 2126–2128, *2127–2129*
  avoidance of complications of, 2141–2142
    delayed wound healing, 2141–2142
    fat necrosis, 2142
    scarring, 2142
  indications for, 2126
  parenchymal pedicle reduction mammaplasty, 2133, 2136–2140
    delivery of nipple-areolar complex and, 2139–2140, *2139–2140*
    elevation of skin flaps and, 2133
    excision of parenchymal tissue and, 2133, *2136*
    reassembly of reduced breast and, 2133, 2136, *2137–2138*
    skin incisions for, 2133, *2134–2135*
  postoperative care and, 2140–2141, *2141*
  preoperative preparation for, 2128, 2131–2133
    evaluation and, 2128, 2131
    marking and, *2130–2131*, 2131–2132
    patient preparation and, 2133

Reduction mammaplasty—*Continued*
  viability of nipple-areolar complex and, 2142
    lactation and, 2142
    nipple-areolar sensibility and, 2142
Reduction procedures, for lymphedema, 380
Reflex sympathetic dystrophy
  hand rehabilitation and, 1758
  wrist pain and, 1730t–1731t
Regeneration, peripheral nerve injuries and. *See* Peripheral nerve injuries, regeneration and
Rehabilitation
  dental, following mandibular reconstruction, 998, *999*
  fractures of hand and wrist and, 1521
  head and neck prostheses and, 1028–1029, *1030–1033*, 1031
  following treatment for pressure sores, 1384–1386, *1386*
  of voice, following laryngectomy, 1017
Relaxed skin tension lines, scar revision and, 36–37, *37*
Remodeling phase, of bone healing, 1809
Renal system, thermal burns and, 405
Reoxygenation, of central necrotic tumor regions, 948
Reparative phase, of bone healing, 1809
Replantation
  of arm, hand rehabilitation following, *1762*, 1762–1763
  of fingers, 1491–1492, *1492*
    hand rehabilitation following, *1760*, 1760–1761, *1761*
  of hand, 1672
    hand rehabilitation following, 1762
  of thumb, hand rehabilitation following, 1761–1762, *1762*
  of toes, hand rehabilitation following, 1761–1762, *1762*
  of upper extremities, 1625–1643
    hand rehabilitation following, *1762*, 1762–1763
    history of, 1626
    indications for, 1627–1628, *1628–1639*, 1630–1634
    initial evaluation for, 1626–1627
    postoperative care and, 1640
    results with, 1640–1643, *1640–1644*
    surgical technique for, 1639–1640
Repopulation, of tumor and normal cell populations, 948
Respiratory system, thermal burns and, 405
Retinacula cutis, 217, *218*
Retinoids
  in facial rejuvenation, 1987
  retinoic acid, for scarring, 12
Retrobulbar hematomas, following blepharoplasty, 1937
Revascularization
  free tissue techniques and, 978
  of skin grafts, 47
  of tendon grafts, 122
Reverse radial artery forearm flaps, for soft tissue coverage of hand and upper extremity, 1650–1651, *1652*
Rhabdomyosarcomas, of hands, 1462
Rheumatoid arthritis
  in hands. *See* Hand(s), rheumatoid arthritis in
  in wrist. *See* Wrist, rheumatoid arthritis in
Rhinitis, following rhinoplasty, 2020

Rhinoplasty, 1999–2020, *2000*
  in African-Americans, 2054–2057, 2055t
    surgical technique for, 2055t, 2055–2057, *2055–2057*
  alar cartilage resection and, 2012–2013, *2013*
  alar wedge in, 2017, *2017*
  for bulbous tip deformities, 2024–2029
    with thick skin and adequate projection, 2025, *2028*
    with thick skin and overprojection, 2025, *2027*
    with thick skin and poor projection, 2025, *2025*, *2026*
    with thin skin and adequate projection, 2029
    with thin skin and overprojection, 2029, *2029*, *2030*
    with thin skin and poor projection, 2029
  cartilage grafts in, 2009
  for difficult nasal deformities, 2021–2032
    bulbous tip deformities. *See* Rhinoplasty, for bulbous tip deformities
    consultation for, *2022*, 2022–2023
    diagnosis and, 2021–2022
    lobule and, 2021–2022
    septum and, 2022
    skin sleeve and, 2021
    soufflé effect and, 2024, *2024*
    surgical exposure for, 2023, *2023*, *2024*
    surgical plan for, 2023–2024
    thin skin and, 2030, 2032
    twisted nose, 2029–2030, *2031*
    vault and, 2022
  dorsal resection for, 2010–2011, *2012*
  functional nasal anatomy and, 2003–2004
    bony and upper cartilaginous vaults, *2003*, 2003–2004
    dorsum and tip, 2004, *2004*
    middle and lower cartilaginous vaults, 2004
    nasal layers, *2002*, 2003
  grafts for, 2018
    dorsal, 2018, *2018*
    lateral wall, 2018, *2018*
    placement of, 2016, *2016*
    tip, 2018, *2019*
  nasal spine-caudal septum and, 2011–2012
  open, 2002
  in Oriental patients, *2076*, 2077–2083
    ancillary procedures and, 2082–2083, *2082–2084*
    preoperative assessment for, 2079
    surgical anatomy and, 2077–2078, *2078*
    surgical technique for, 2078–2083, *2080–2081*
  osteotomy in, 2016–2017, *2017*
  patient preparation for, 2009–2010
  postoperative course and, 2019–2020
    follow up and revision and, 2020
    hemorrhage and, 2019–2020
    infection and, 2020
    packing and splints and, 2019, *2019*
    rhinitis and, 2020
    septal perforation and, 2020
  preoperative diagnosis and, 2004–2009
    discussion of potential complications and, 2009
    external examination and, 2005
    interview and, 2004–2005
    intranasal examination and, 2005

Rhinoplasty, preoperative diagnosis and—*Continued*
    setting strategy with patient and, 2007–2009, *2008*
    surgical plan and, 2005–2007, *2006*, *2007*
  secondary, 2033–2043
    crooked nose and, 2040, *2041*
    extramucosal technique for, 2033–2034
    hanging ala and, 2040, *2045*, *2046*
    incisions for tip remodeling and, 2035–2036
    insufficient removal of hump and, 2034
    order of surgical steps for, 2033
    osteotomies for, 2040
    pinched nose and, 2036, *2036*, *2037*
    pointed narrow tip and, 2036
    retraction of alar border and, 2040, 2043, *2047*
    septal perforations and, 2040, *2042–2044*
    short nose and pig snout nose and, 2036, 2038, *2038–2039*
    stenoses and, 2043, *2048–2049*
    supratip deformity and, *2034*, 2034–2035, *2035*
    septal resection and spreader graft tunnels in, *2014–2015*, 2014–2016
    shortening of upper lateral cartilages in, 2014
    skeletonization for, 2010, *2010*, *2011*
    with subperiosteal facelift, 1915–1916
    wound closure in, 2016, *2016*
Rhomboid flaps, 28–30, *29*, 57, *58*
Rib free vascularized flaps, 985, 986t, 987
Rib grafts, 105t, 107–108
  nonvascularized, 107–108, *109*
  vascularized, 108
Rigid fixation, for maxillary deformities, *721*, 721–722, *722*
Road tattooing, 34, *35*
Roentgenography
  cephalometric. *See* Cephalometrics
  of diabetic foot, 1839–1840, *1840*, *1841*
  in lower extremity injuries, 1768
  in oropharyngeal carcinoma, 926
  plain-film. *See* Plain-film roentgenography
  in temporomandibular joint deformities, 1223
Rotation-advancement technique, for unilateral cleft lip, 551–552, *553–554*
Rotation flaps, 57
Ruby lasers, Q-switched, 266
Rudimentary supernumerary digits, 305

Sacral reconstruction, 1364–1369, 1369–1370
  free tissue transfer for, *1368*, 1369
  general principles of, 1365, *1365*, *1366*
  muscle flaps for, 1366, *1367*, 1369
Saddlenose deformities, nasal fractures and, 1134
Safety, of lasers, 266–267
Sagittal craniosynostosis, 148, *149*
Sagittal plane, for computed tomography imaging, in maxillofacial trauma, 1073
Sagittal split osteotomies
  chin repositioning combined with, in mandibular deformities, 754
  mobilization of lower anterior segment combined with, 754–756
  osteotomy of upper jaw combined with, 756–757, *757*
Sagittal split-ramus osteotomy, 187–188, *188–191*
Salivary fistulas, free tissue techniques and, 979, 981

Salivary gland tumors, 1034–1044
  benign, 1035, 1036t, 1038, *1038*
  epidemiology of, 1034
  malignant, 1037–1038, *1038*, *1039*
  medical oncologic therapy for, 1044
  radiation therapy for, 1044
  signs and symptoms of, 1034–1035
  staging of, 1035
  surgical management of, 1038–1044
    complications of, 1044
    facial nerve and, 1043–1044
    neck and, 1044
    parotidectomy, 1038–1042
    submandibulectomy, 1042, *1042*, *1043*
Salmon patch (nuchal nevus; stork bite), 363
Sarcomas, of hands. *See* Hand tumors
Sartorius flaps, in thigh reconstruction, 1778
Scalp injuries, 1086, 1088
  anatomy and, 1086, 1088, *1088*
  burns, 418
    classification of, 418
    treatment of, 418, *419*
  management of, 1088, *1089*
Scalp reconstruction, 830–841
  anatomy and, 830–832, *831*
  management of acute scalp wounds, 832, *833*, 834, *835–837*
  replantation and, 841
  secondary, 834, *838–840*, 841
  selection of method for, 832
Scaphocephaly, 148, *149*, 500, 503–504, *505*
Scaphoid bone
  fractures of, 1741
    diagnosis of, 1741
    treatment of, 1741, *1741*, 1741t, *1742*
  rotary subluxation of, *1542*, 1542–1543, *1544–1545*
Scapholunate instability, wrist pain and, 1739, 1740t
Scapular flaps
  fasciocutaneous, for soft tissue coverage of hand and upper extremity, 1654, 1656
  free vascularized, 986t, 994, *994–996*, 996
  osteocutaneous
    free, 971, *973–975*
    for oropharyngeal reconstruction, 968
  skin, 74t
Scar(s)
  hypertrophic, following blepharoplasty, 1938
  web, following blepharoplasty, 1938
Scar revision, 34–44
  age of scar and, 35
  algorithm for, 37, *38*
  causes of scar and, 34–35, *35*
  cleft lip and, 606, 606t
  contraindications to, 36, 37
  excision and, for facial burns, 417
  healing of scar and, 35
  keloids and hypertrophic scars and, 43–44, *44*
  location of scar and, 36
  maturation of scar and, 36
  mechanism of injury causing scar and, 35
  methods of, 37–43
    dermabrasion, 41, *41*
    fusiform, 37
    geometric broken line closure, 40, 40–41
    skin grafting, flaps, and soft tissue expansion, 41–43, *42*, *43*
    W-plasty, 39–40, *40*
    Z-plasty, 37, *38*, 39, *39*
  physical characteristics of scar and, 36

Scar revision—*Continued*
    prior revision and, 35–36
    reasons for, 34
    relation of scar to anatomic landmarks and, 36
    relation of scar to relaxed skin tension lines and, 36–37, *37*
    relation of scar to wrinkle lines and, 37
Scarring, 10–13. *See also* Scar revision
    aesthetic facial surgery in African-Americans and, 2051–2052
    in children, scar revision and, 36
    etiology of, 11
    following eyelid operations in Oriental patients, 2075, *2075*
    factors influencing, 30–31
    features of keloids and hypertrophic scars, 11
    of hands, scar management and, 1747, *1748*
    minimization of, hand-skin incisions and, 1415, *1416*
    following reduction mammaplasty, avoidance of, 2142
    scar maturation and, scar revision and, 36
    treatment of, 11–13
Schrudde technique, 216
Schwannomas (neurilemmomas), of hands, 1462, *1462*
Screw fixation, 169, 170–171
    continuous cooling and, 170
    in craniomaxillofacial surgery, 141–142, *143*
    of hand and wrist fractures, 1514, 1517, *1517–1522*
    intermaxillary fixation during operation, 171
    low-speed drilling and, 170
    self-tapping screws and, 170–171, *171*
Scrotum, angiokeratoma of, 300
Sebaceous glands, 47
    hyperplasia of, 302
    skin grafting and, 48
Seborrheic keratosis, 295, *297*
Second branchial cleft anomalies, 811–812, *812, 813*
Self-esteem, lipectomy and, 227
Senile hemangiomas (cherry hemangiomas), 300
Sensibility
    of hand, evaluation of, 1746, *1746*
    of nipple-areolar complex, following reduction mammaplasty, 2142
Sensibility training, in hand rehabilitation, 1748–1749
Sensory receptors, regeneration of, 1602
Sepsis, burn wound, 401–403, 406
    nature of, 401–402
    treatment of, 402t, 402–403
Septal perforations
    following rhinoplasty, 2020
    secondary rhinoplasty for, 2040, *2042–2044*
Septal resection, shortening, in rhinoplasty, *2014–2015*, 2014–2016
Serratus anterior flaps
    for chest wall reconstruction, 1249–1250
    free, in knee and leg reconstruction, 1787, *1788*
    intrathoracic transposition of, 1269, *1270*
Serratus anterior muscle, anatomy of, facial reanimation and, 1049–1051, *1051*
Sialoceles, surgical management of salivary gland tumors and, 1044

Sickle cell ulcers, of leg, 1831
Silicone, cystic changes induced by, wrist pain and, 1730t–1731t
Silicone gel, for scarring, 12, *12, 13*
Silicone implants, textured, for augmentation mammaplasty, 2100–2101
Silver nitrate soaks, in burn wound sepsis, 402t, 403
Silver sulfadiazine cream, in burn wound sepsis, 402t, 403
Simultaneous advancement, in craniofacial dysostosis, 512
Sinuses
    branchial cleft, 810, *810*
    midline, of head and neck, 814–815, *816*
    paranasal. *See* Paranasal sinuses, carcinoma of
    preauricular, 810, *810*
Skeletonization, for rhinoplasty, 2010, *2010, 2011*
Skeletonized appearance, following blepharoplasty, 1937
Skin
    disorders of
        following blepharoplasty, 1938
        wound healing and, 31
    evaluation of, for blepharoplasty, 1921–1923, *1921–1923*
    hand reconstruction and, 1667–1668
    laxity of, termination of lipectomy and, 235
    sloughing of, following blepharoplasty, 1936, *1936*
    thick, rhinoplasty and, 2030, 2032. *See also* Rhinoplasty, for bulbous tip deformities
    thin, bulbous nose deformities with. *See* Rhinoplasty, for bulbous tip deformities
    type of, wound healing and, 31
    wrist pain and, 1733
Skin care
    facial rejuvenation and, 1987
    pressure sores and, 1374–1375
Skin envelope, marking for breast reduction and, 2120, *2121*
Skin flaps, 60, 60–61, 73–75, 74t
    abdominal, anatomy of, 74t, 75, *77*
    anatomy of, 73–75, *75*
        abdominal skin flaps, 75, *77*
        technique of flap dissection and, 74–75, *76*
    arterial, 72–73
    indications for, 73
    parascapular, 74t
    scapular, 74t
Skin graft(s). *See also* Skin grafting
    allografts, 53
    composite, 52–53
    cultured epithelial grafts, 54–55
    dermal fat grafts, 53
    harvesting, 49–50, *50, 51*
    pigmentation of, 48
    preparation of, 50
    skin thickness and, 45–46
    source of, 45
    thickness of, 48
    xenografts, 53–54
Skin grafting, 45–55. *See also* Skin graft(s)
    anatomy and, 46, 46–47
    of burn wounds. *See* Burn wounds, grafting of
    donor site and, 48–49, *49*

Skin grafting—*Continued*
    donor site healing and, 55
    for fingertip injuries, with loss of pulp only, 1496, *1496, 1497*
    graft take and healing and, 47–48
        graft contraction and, 48
        graft innervation and, 47–48
        graft pigmentation and, 48
        graft revascularization and, 47
        plasmatic imbibition and, 47
        sweat and sebaceous gland function and, 48
    indications and graft selection for, 48
    in lower extremity reconstruction, 1774
    in meningomyelocele, 1242–1243, *1243*
    in nasal reconstruction, full-thickness skin grafts and, *885*, 885–886
    recipient site complications and, 70
    for scar revision, 41–42
    for soft tissue coverage of hand and upper extremity, 1645–1646, *1646, 1647*
    wound preparation for, 50, 52, *52–55*
Skin-levator-skin method, for eyelid operations in Oriental patients, 2070, *2070*
Skin staples, for breast reduction, 2119
Skin tumors
    benign, 295–307. *See also specific tumors*
        of cutaneous appendages, 301–304
        epidermal, 295–298
        of mesodermal origin, 299–300
        of neural crest origin, 304–307
    malignant
        basal cell carcinoma, 316–319
        carcinoma in situ, *314–315*, 315–316
        of external ear, *331*, 331–332
        of eyelid, *330*, 330–331
        of eyelids, 324, 330–331
        of lip, 324, *329*
        of nose, 324, *325–328*
        rare syndromes associated with, 312–315
        squamous cell carcinoma, 320, *321*
        of upper limb, 320, *322, 323*, 324
    premalignant, 309–312
Skull. *See also* Scalp reconstruction
    base of, tumors of, craniomaxillofacial surgery in, 165–166, *167*
    cloverleaf, 512
Soft palate, brachytherapy of, 953
Soft tissue
    evaluation of, in maxillofacial trauma, 1067–1068
    injuries of, management of, 31t, 31–32
    intrathoracic transposition of. *See* Chest wall reconstruction, intrathoracic transposition of soft tissue in
    resuspension of, maxillary fractures and, 1162–1163
        Le Fort fractures without mobility, 1162–1163
        sagittal fractures, 1163, *1163*
Soft tissue coverage, of hand and upper extremity, 1645–1656
    flaps and. *See* Flap surgery, for soft tissue coverage of hand and upper extremity
    free tissue transfer for. *See* Free tissue transfer, for soft tissue coverage of hand and upper extremity
    skin grafts and, 1645–1646, *1646, 1647*
Soft tissue emphysema, maxillofacial, roentgenographic interpretation and, 1072–1073
Soft tissue expansion. *See* Tissue expansion

Soft tissue gigantism (overgrowth), hemangiomas and, 359, *359*
Soft tissue reconstruction, facial gunshot wounds and, 1186–1187
Sole, of foot, reconstruction of, 1821, 1824, *1825*
Soleus flaps, in knee and leg reconstruction, 1779–1782, *1783, 1784*
Soufflé effect, rhinoplasty and, 2024, *2024*
Sphincter pharyngoplasty, 643–647, *644*
  indications for, 643, *644*
    pharyngeal flap operation compared with, 645–647, *646, 647*
    surgical anatomy and technique for, 643, *644–646, 645*
Spider nevi (nevi araneus), 362
Spiroadenomas, eccrine, 304
Spitz nevi, 307, *307*
Splinting
  in hand rehabilitation, 1749, *1749, 1750*
  following nerve grafting, 132–133
  rhinoplasty and, 2019
Spreader graft tunnels, in rhinoplasty, *2014–2015,* 2014–2016
Squamous cell carcinomas
  of external ear, *331,* 331–332
  facial, 3-D computed tomography in, 289, *289, 290*
  of hand and nail bed, 1457, *1458*
  of lip, 324, *329*
  of nose, 324, *324–328*
  oropharyngeal, 935
    chemotherapy for. *See* Chemotherapy, for oropharyngeal carcinoma
  of skin, 32, *320*
  of upper limb, 320, 324
Staged advancement, in craniofacial dysostosis, 512
Staged excision, for lymphedema, 380
Staged flexor tendon reconstruction, for hand injuries, 1561–1564
  complications of, 1563–1564
  indications for, 1561
  surgical technique for, 1561–1563, *1562, 1564*
Staging
  of malignant melanomas, 345t, 346, 346t
  of oropharyngeal carcinoma, 929t, 929–930, 930t
  of rheumatoid arthritis, in metacarpophalangeal joints, 1713–1715, *1714, 1715*
Stahl ear, 781–783, *782*
  etiology of, 782
  treatment of flat helix with unrolled helix but without third crus deformity, 783, *784, 785*
  treatment of relatively well-shaped helix with third crus, 782–783, *783, 784*
Stanozolol, for leg ulcers, 1835
Staples, 8, 22
  for breast reduction, 2119
Steatocystoma multiplex, *302,* 302–303
Sternocleidomastoid osteomusculocutaneous flaps, 984t, 985
Sternotomy, median. *See* Median sternotomy
Steroids
  for scarring, 12
  wound healing and, 8
Stiles-Bunnet tendon transfer, modified, 1593–1594
Stitch abscess, eyelid operations in Oriental patients and, 2072, *2074,* 2075

Stork bite (nuchal nevus; salmon patch), 363
Stranc-Robertson steeple flap repair, 919, *919, 920*
Strawberry hemangiomas (capillary hemangiomas; superficial dermis vascular channels), 352–353, *353, 354*
  argon laser therapy for, 259–262, *261–263*
Strength, of hand, evaluation of, 1745–1746
Subcutaneous mastectomy, prophylactic. *See* Prophylactic subcutaneous mastectomy
Subcutaneous tissue, wrist pain and, 1733
Subglottic carcinoma, 1012
Sublimis tendon transfer, Boyes, *1584,* 1585, *1586*
Submandibulectomy, 1042, *1042, 1043*
Submental dissection, in facial rejuvenation, *1890,* 1890–1891, *1891*
Submental incision, for facial rejuvenation, 1878, *1879*
Submental region, planning modification of, 1881–1882
Submuscular reconstruction
  for immediate breast reconstruction following mastectomy, 1287–1289, *1287–1289*
  prophylactic subcutaneous mastectomy and, 1279–1281, *1281*
Subperiosteal facelift. *See* Facial rejuvenation, subperiosteal facelift
Subscleral hematomas, following blepharoplasty, 1937
Subungual hematomas, treatment of, 1494
Subunit principle
  corollaries of, facial reconstruction and, 851, 854–855, *855–862, 857–858, 863*
  facial reconstruction and, 846–848, *846–854, 851*
Suction-assisted lipectomy, 216–248, 2186–2199, 2187t
  of abdomen, 236–237
  abdominal contouring with. *See* Abdominal contour operations
  aesthetically unfavorable results with, 241, *241*
  aesthetic complications of, 2199
  anesthesia and fluid resuscitation for, 230–231
  anterior platsmoplasty, 247
  biochemistry and histology of fat and, 217
  brachial. *See* Upper extremities, brachioplasty and brachial suction-assisted lipectomy and
  of calf and ankle, 2247–2250
    indications for, 2247, 2249
    markings for, *2248,* 2249, *2249*
    postoperative care and, 2250
    technique for, 2249–2250, *2250, 2251*
  of calves and ankles, 238
  cannula technique for, 216–217, 217t
  cellulite and, 239
  classification of procedures using, 2186–2187, *2188–2193*
  closed suction and, 247, *248*
  complications and sequelae, 241–242
  complications and sequelae of, 247–248, *251*
  contraindications to, 2190
  curette techniques for, 216
  of face and neck, 242–248
    aesthetic ideal and, 242, *242*
    conceptual viewpoint and, 242
    diagnosis and marking for, 242–243, *243*
    false indications for, 243

Suction-assisted lipectomy, of face and neck—*Continued*
    integration of evaluation data for, 243–244, *244*
  face-lift and suction, 247, 249–250
  for facial rejuvenation, 1979, *1980*
  fat injection and, 239, *239, 240*
  in gynecomastia, 237–238, *238–239*
  harmony and proportion in female figure and, 222–223, *223–225*
  of iliac crest and dorsal rolls, 235
  of knee, 2243–2247
    indications for, *2244,* 2244–2245
    technique for, 2245–2247, *2245–2247*
  of knees, 236
  of male flanks, 237, *238*
  medical complications associated with, 2198–2199
  nomenclature for, 220, *221,* 222
  patient evaluation for, 227–230, 2187, 2189
    aesthetic, *228,* 228–230, *229*
    medical, 227
    physical, 227
    psychological, 227
  patient studies and, 247
  of pectoral fat pads, 238
  photographic considerations and, 223, 226, *226*
    face and neck and, 226, *226*
    trunks and limbs and, 223, 226, *226*
  physics and equipment for, 218–220, *219*
  postoperative care and, 240–242, 2198
  preoperative assessment and planning for, 2191, 2193
  preoperative preparation for, 2194
  subcutaneous fascial system and, 217, *218*
  suction anterior to flap and, 247, *247*
  suction beneath flap and, 246
  surgical technique for, when to stop and, 235
  technique for, 231–235, *236,* 246, 2194–2198
    closure of incision and, 2196, *2196*
    contouring of trunk in men and, 2198
    cross tunneling and, 235
    epinephrine pretreatment and, 232–233, 233t
    extraction and, 234–235
    irrigation and, 235
    marking patient and, *231,* 231–232
    mesh undermining and, 235
    patient positioning and, 232, *232, 233*
    pretunneling and, 233–234, *234*
    skin excision and, 2194–2196, *2195, 2196*
    suction cannula and, 2194, *2195*
    umbilicoplasty and, *2197,* 2197–2198
  of thigh, 2237–2240
    anesthesia for, 2238
    complications of, 2240
    contraindications to, 2237
    indications for, 2237
    marking for, 2237, *2238, 2239*
    technique for, 2238–2240, *2239–2242*
  of thighs
    anterior, 236, *237*
    lateral, 235–236, *236*
    medial, 236, *236*
  topographic anatomy and, 217–218, *218, 219*
  treatment plan for, 244–246
    augmentation and, 246
    incisions and, 244, *245*
    local SMAS advancement and platysmal resection and, 244
    open and closed suction and, 244, *245, 246*
    skin undermining and, 244

Sulfur, burns caused by, 451, *451*
Superficial musculoaponeurotic system, modification of, 1888–1890, *1889*
  in men, 1906, *1907*
  planning, *1879–1885*, 1880–1881
Superficial spreading melanomas, 344
Superior orbital fissure syndrome, 1143–1144
Supernumerary digits, rudimentary, 305
Supernumerary nipples (polythelia), 303
Suprabrow excisions, 1965
Supraglottic carcinoma, 1011–1012
Supraglottic laryngectomy, 1014–1016
  postoperative management and, 1015–1016
  technique for, 1014–1015
Supraorbital nerve block, 16–17
Supraorbital ridge surgery, 1865, *1866*
Supratip deformity, secondary rhinoplasty for, *2034*, 2034–2035, *2035*
Sural nerve, harvesting, 131–132
Surgical drainage, for lymphedema, 376–377
  into deep lymphatics, 376
  lymphatic bridging procedures for, 376
  lymph node-venous anastomosis for, 376
  microlymphaticovenous anastomosis for, 377
  surgical technique for, 377, *378*, *379*, 380t, *381*, *382*
Suture materials, 20–22, *21*, 22t
  wound healing and, 7–8
Suturing
  placement of suspension sutures for facial rejuvenation and, 1891, *1892*, 1893, *1893*
  of skin wounds, 20–24
    elective surgical wounds, 22–23, *23*
    principles of wound closure and, 23–24, *23–25*
    suture materials and, 20–22, *21*, 22t
Swan-neck deformities, rheumatoid arthritis and, 1716–1717, *1717*
Sweat glands, 46–47
  skin grafting and, 48
Symmetry, maxillofacial, roentgenographic interpretation and, 1073
Sympathetic blocks, in wrist pain, 1729
Syndactyly, 1433–1434, 1434t, *1434–1438*
  acrosyndactyly, 1434, 1441, *1444*, 1444
  complex, 1434, *1434*
  complicated, 1434, *1434*
  incisions for treatment of, 1423, *1423*
  simple
    complete, 1434, *1434*
    incomplete, 1434, *1434*
Synostosis, of lambdoid suture, 512
Synovectomy, for rheumatoid arthritis of wrist, 1711, *1711*
Synovial cysts, of hands, 1463
Synovial sarcomas, of hands, 1463
Syringocystadenoma papilliferum, 303, *303*
Syringomas, 303, *304*
  choroid (eccrine mixed tumors), 304

Tar, burns caused by, 451, *451*
Tarsal tunnel release, diabetic foot and, *1858*, 1858–1859
Team
  for breast reconstruction using free tissue transfer, 1325
  craniofacial. *See* Craniofacial team
  head and neck cancer, 1008
Teeth. *See also* Dentition; Orthodontic treatment; Orthognathic surgery; Prosthodontics; *headings beginning with term* Dental
  replacement of, in cleft lip and palate, 768–769, *768–773*

Teimourian technique, 216
Telangiectasia, blepharoplasty and, 1921
Telecanthus, 159–160
  surgical treatment of, 159–160
    extracranial approach to, 159, *159–160*
    intracranial approach to, 159–160
Temperature, microcirculation and, 68
Temporal dissection, in facial rejuvenation, *1886*, 1886–1887, *1887*
Temporal fossa surgery, 1865, *1867*
Temporal galea, in craniomaxillofacial surgery, 144–145, *146–147*
Temporal incision, for facial rejuvenation, 1874, *1875*, *1876*
Temporalis muscle, management of, in craniomaxillofacial surgery, 141, *142*
Temporal-lift, 1966, *1967*
Temporal surgery, 1865
Temporomandibular joint deformities, 1220–1228
  anatomy and, 1220–1221, *1221*
  ankylosis, 1224–1226, *1225*
  diagnosis of, 1222–1224
    history in, *1222*, 1222–1223, *1223*
    imaging in, 1223–1224
    physical examination in, 1223
  embryology of, 1220
  internal derangement, 1224
  mandibular fractures and, 1177
  mechanics of, 1221–1222
  myofascial pain dysfunction syndrome, 1224
  treatment of, 1226–1228
    arthroplasty in, 1227–1228, *1228*
    arthrotomy in, *1226*, 1226–1227
    conservative, 1226
Temporomandibular joint reconstruction, 997–998, *998*, *999*
Temporoparietal fascial flaps, for soft tissue coverage of hand and upper extremity, 1652, *1655*
Tendon(s)
  flexor pulley reconstruction and, 1569. *See* Flexor pulley reconstruction
  flexor tenolysis and. *See* Flexor tenolysis
  of hand
    evaluation of, *1485*, 1485–1486, *1486*
    injuries to, 1491
  hand reconstruction and, 1665
  reconstruction of, of flexor tendons, staged. *See* Staged flexor tendon reconstruction
  strain, rupture, or avulsion of, wrist pain and, 1730t–1731t
Tendon grafting
  of flexor tendons. *See* Flexor tendon grafting
  free. *See* Free tendon grafting
  for hand injuries, hand rehabilitation following, 1755, *1755*
Tendon implants, active, 1564
Tendon injuries, of hand. *See also* Hand injuries, of extensor tendons; Hand injuries, of flexor tendons
  determining if injury is to tendon and, 1487–1488
  hand rehabilitation following. *See* Hand rehabilitation, following tendon repairs
Tendon sheaths
  anatomy of, 121, *121*
  giant cell tumor of, 299, *300*
  of hands
    giant cell tumors of, *1460*, 1461
    synovial cysts of, 1463
    xanthomas of, 1463

Tendon transfers
  in hand. *See* Hand injuries, tendon transfers for; Median nerve palsy, tendon transfers for; Radial nerve palsy, tendon transfers for
  for hand injuries, hand rehabilitation following, 1755–1756
Tenodesis, hand reconstruction and, 1677, *1678*
Tenolysis, hand rehabilitation following, 1755
Tenosynovitis
  chronic, of hands, *1478*, 1479
  extensor, of wrist, 1712–1713
  flexor, acute, of hands, 1469–1470, *1470*, 1472–1473, *1473–1476*
  of wrist, 1730t–1731t, 1735–1736
    background of, 1735
    De Quervain, 1735
    De Quervain stenosing tenosynovitis, 1735
    presentation and diagnosis of, 1735
    treatment of, 1735–1736
Tension-band (compression) plates and wires, for hand and wrist fractures, *1524–1526*, 1528–1529
Tensor fasciae latae musculotendinous flaps, in thigh reconstruction, 1779
Testing, by craniofacial team members, 473
Tetanus prophylaxis, hand injuries and, 1488
TGF-β (transforming growth factor-beta), wound healing and, 4t, 9
Thenar flaps, for fingertip injuries with exposed bone, 1498, 1500, *1503*, *1504*
Thermal burns, 396–406. *See also* Burn wounds
  complications of, 404–406, 405t
    cardiovascular, 405
    endocrine, 406
    gastrointestinal, 406
    hematologic, 406
    metabolic and nutritional, 406
    musculoskeletal, 406
    renal, 405
    respiratory, 405
    septic, 406
  fluid resuscitation and, 399–401
    assessment of wound and, 401
    fluid administration and, 400t, 400–401
    fluid monitoring and, 399–400
  immune consequences of, 404
  inhalation injury and, 398–399
    diagnosis of, *398*, 398–399
    treatment of, 399, 399t
  management at scene, 396–397, *397*, 397t
  metabolism and metabolic support and, 403–404
  wound sepsis and, 401–403
    nature of, 401–402
    treatment of, 402t, 402–403
Thermal modalities, in hand rehabilitation, 1749–1750, *1751*
Thigh(s)
  anterior, lipectomy and, 236, *237*
  contouring of. *See* Inner thigh-plasty; Suction-assisted lipectomy, of thigh
  lateral, lipectomy and, 235–236, *236*
  medial, lipectomy and, 236, *236*
Thigh flaps, lateral, for breast reconstruction, *1339*, 1339, *1340*, 1341
Thigh-lifts, 2205. *See also* Body contouring, of trunk and limbs; Transverse flank-thigh-buttock-lift
  medial, 210–213, *212*
    anatomy and, 2210, *2212*
    indications for, 2211
    technique for, 2211, 2213, *2213–2215*

Vol. I pp. 1–829; Vol. II pp. 830–1411; Vol. III pp. 1413–2258 **[31]**

Thigh reconstruction, *1777, 1777–1778*
  gracilis flaps in, 1779
  sartorius flaps in, 1779
  tensor fasciae latae musculotendinous flaps
      in, 1779
  vastus lateralis flaps, 1779
  vastus medialis flaps, 1779
Third branchial cleft anomalies, 813
3-D computed tomography, 271–291, *272*
  in Apert syndrome, 272–273, *273, 274*
  in facial comminuted fractures, 278–280,
      278–280
  in fibrosarcoma of face, 280–281, *282*
  in frontal meningiomas, 284–286, *285–289*
  in frontonasal dysplasia, *273, 274*
  in gunshot wound of face, 277–278, *278*
  in kleeblattschädel deformity, 275, *275–277*
  in maxillary squamous cell carcinoma, 289,
      289, 290
  in maxillofacial trauma, 1074
  in monostotic fibrous dysplasia of the
      maxilla, 283, *283, 284*
  in Treacher Collins syndrome, 277, *277*
  in von Recklinghausen disease, 280, *281*
Thrombophlebitis, following suction-assisted
      lipectomy, 2199
Thumb(s)
  base of, incisions on, *1418*, 1418–1419
  clasped thumb deformity and, 1449, *1453*,
      1453t
  congenitally absent, 1694, *1694–1695*, 1696,
      1697
  duplication of ray of, 1429, *1431–1433*, 1432
  fractures of, hand rehabilitation following,
      1759
  fusion of joint, hand reconstruction and,
      1677, *1678*
  hand reconstruction and, 1675, *1676*, 1677
  hypoplastic, 1447t, 1447–1449, *1448,
      1450–1451*, 1696, 1698
    dressing for, 1449
    extrinsic tendon shortening for, 1449
    flexor pulley release for, 1448
    floating thumb, 1448
    incisions for, 1448
    intrinsic muscle reattachment for, 1449
    skeletal shortening and repositioning for,
        1448
    skin closure for, 1449
    soft tissue dissection for, 1448
  injuries to ligaments of
    of carpometacarpal joint, 1542, *1542*
    of metacarpophalangeal joint, 1536, *1539*,
        1539–1540, *1540*
  replantation of, 1628, *1629–1631*, 1630
    hand rehabilitation following, 1761–1762,
        1762
  rheumatoid arthritis in, 1718–1719, *1719*
  tendon transfers to provide adduction of,
      1595–1596
    extensor carpi radialis brevis transfer,
        1596, *1597*
    flexor digitorum sublimis transfer to ring
        finger, 1595–1596
  trigger, 1449, *1452*
Thumb reconstruction, 1682–1698, *1683*
  acquired deformities and, 1682–1691
    of entire thumb, 1689, 1691, *1693*
    level I, 1682–1684, *1684, 1685*
    level II, 1684–1685, *1686*, 1687
    level III, 1687, *1688*, 1689
    level IV, 1689, *1690, 1692*

Thumb reconstruction—*Continued*
  congenital deformities and, 1691,
      1693–1698
    congenitally absent thumb, 1694,
        1694–1695, 1696, *1697*
    hypoplastic thumb, 1696, 1698
    great-toe transplantation for, 1699–1701
      indications for, 1699–1700
      preoperative evaluation for, 1700
      surgical sequence for, 1700–1701,
          1702–1705
    second-toe transplantation for, 1701
      surgical technique for, 1701, *1706–1709*
Thyroid cartilage, 1008, *1009, 1010*
Tibial grafts, 105t, 111
Tip defatting, in African-Americans,
      2056–2057, *2057*
Tip remodeling, incisions for, 2035–2036
Tissue expansion, 201–215
  for abdominal wall reconstruction,
      1350–1351, *1351*
  breast reconstruction with. *See* Breast
      reconstruction, with tissue expansion
  clinical uses of, 214
  complications of, 206–207, *207*
  expansion for, 207
  final advancement for, 207
  for head and neck burns, 417, *417*
  for immediate breast reconstruction
      following mastectomy, 1289, 1291
  natural history and anatomy and, 201–202
  postoperative care for, 207
  regional reconstruction using, 207–213
    of breast, 210–211, *211*
    of ear, 210
    of face, 207–208, *208*
    of lower limbs, 213, *214*
    of neck, 210
    of nose, 208, *209–210*, 210
    of trunk, 212, *212*
    of upper limbs, 212–213, *213*
  for scar revision, 43, *43*
  surgical procedure for, 202–206, *203, 204*
    choice of expander and, 204–205
    patient counseling and, 202, 204
    placement of expander and, 205–206
Tissue loss, scaring and, 34
Tobacco use, as risk factor for oropharyngeal
      carcinoma, 922
Toe(s), replantation of, hand rehabilitation
      following, 1761–1762, *1762*
Toe pressures, diabetic foot and, 1841–1842
Toe-to-hand transplantation, 1699–1709
  donor site morbidity and, 1709
  hand reconstruction and, 1677, *1679*
  hand therapy and, 1705
  pharmacologic agents and, 1705
  postoperative care and, 1701
  postoperative function and, 1709
  for thumb reconstruction. *See* Thumb
      reconstruction
Tomography. *See also* Computed tomography
  in maxillofacial trauma, 1073
    basic principles of, 1073
    equipment and technique for, 1073
    indications for, 1073
  in wrist pain, 1729
Tongue, base of
  approaches to, 938
  brachytherapy of, 953
  necessity for laryngectomy when
      removing, 938
Tongue prostheses, 1025, *1025–1027*
Tonsils, brachytherapy of, 953
Touch pressure sensibility, of hand,
      evaluation of, 1746, *1746*

Touch-ups, following lipectomy, 240
Toxicity, of anesthetic agents, 19–20
Tracheoesophageal puncture, 1017
Tracheostomy
  mediastinal, 1016
  in oropharyngeal resection, 935
Transconjunctival skin flap technique. *See*
      Blepharoplasty, transconjunctival
Transforming growth factor-beta (TGF-β),
      wound healing and, 4t, 9
Transitional dentition, orthodontic treatment
      for clefts in, 652–658, *657–660*
  developmental considerations and, 652,
      654–656, 655
Transposition flaps, 57
Transverse flank-thigh-buttock-lift, *2204*,
      2205–2209
  incision design for, *2204, 2205*, 2205
  indications for, 2205
  technique for, 2206–2209, *2206–2212*
Transverse rectus abdominis (TRAM) flap(s),
      83–84, *86*
Transverse rectus abdominis (TRAM) flap
      breast reconstruction, 1310–1317
  anatomy of TRAM flap and, 1311, *1311*
  complications of, 1315
  preoperative markings for, 1312, *1313*
  preoperative preparation for, 1312
  secondary revisions and, 1315, 1317,
      1317–1319
  single versus double pedicle flaps and,
      1311, *1311*, 1312
  surgical technique for, 1312–1315,
      1314–1316
  using free TRAM flaps, 1327–1335
    abdominal closure and, *1334*, 1334–1335
    flap dissection and, 1329–1331, *1330,
        1331*
    flap transfer and, *1332, 1333*, 1333
    marking flaps for, *1326*, 1327–1328, *1328*
    postoperative care and, 1335
    preoperative considerations for,
        1328–1329, *1329*
    preparation of recipient vessels and,
        1331–1333, *1332*
    secondary revision and nipple-areolar
        reconstruction and, 1335, *1336–1338*
    shaping of flaps and, 1333–1334, *1334*
    surgical technique for, 1329–1335
Trapdoor scars, 34, *35*
Trapezium fractures, 1743
Trapezius flaps
  for chest wall reconstruction, 1251
  musculocutaneous, 80, 82–83
    anatomy of, 80, 82–83, *83–85*
  for oropharyngeal reconstruction, 961,
      962–963
  osteomusculocutaneous, 984t, 984–985
Trauma. *See* Fractures; *specific anatomic sites*
Treacher Collins syndrome. *See* Mandibular
      dysostosis (Franceschetti-Zwahlen-
      Klein syndrome; Treacher Collins
      syndrome)
  3-D computed tomography in, 277, *277*
Treatment planning, cephalometrics and. *See*
      Cephalometrics, treatment planning
      and
Triamcinolone, for Dupuytren contracture,
      1722
Triangular fibrocartilage complex disorders,
      1547, 1549, *1549*

Triangular flap technique
  surgical technique for, 558–563
    adjustment of vermilion and, 563, *563*
    closure of cleft and, 560, 560–561, *561*
    incisions and, 558, *559*, 560
    positioning nasal ala and, 561, *562*, 563
    summary of, 563–564, *564*, *565*
    verification of preoperative
      measurements and, 560
  for unilateral cleft lip, 552, 554–564
    avoidance of incisions and, 558
    goals of, 552, 554–555
    preoperative measurements for, 555, *556*,
      557, 558
    surgical technique for, 558–563
    treatment of nasal deformity and, 558
Trichoepitheliomas, 302
Trichofolliculomas, 301–302
Tricholemmal (pilar) cysts, 301
Tricholemmomas, 302, *302*
Trigger finger, incisions for release of,
  1416–1417
Trigger thumb, 1449, *1452*
Trigonocephaly, 151, *154–155*, 500, 501,
  502–504, 503
Triple folds, eyelid operations in Oriental
  patients and, 2072, *2073*, *2074*
Tripod fracture, roentgenographic
  appearance of, 1074, *1077–1078*
Triquetrum fractures, 1743
Trunk
  arteries of, 60
  burn wounds of, 434. *See also* Burn
    wounds, of extremities and trunk,
    reconstruction of
  photographic documentation of, lipectomy
    and, 223, 226, *226*
  reconstruction using soft tissue expansion,
    212, *212*
Trunk-lifts, 2205. *See* Body contouring, of
  trunk and limbs
Tumors. *See also specific tumors and anatomic
  sites*
  of base of skull, craniomaxillofacial surgery
    in, 165–166, *167*
  oropharyngeal. *See also* Oropharyngeal
    carcinomas
    pathology and patterns of spread of,
      932–933, *933*, *934*

Ulcers
  decubitus. *See* Pressure sores
  of leg. *See* Leg ulcers
  oral, oropharyngeal carcinoma and, 923
Ulnar collateral ligament, chronic tears of,
  1540, *1541*
Ulnar impingement syndrome, 1738
Ulnar nerve palsy, tendon transfers for, 1592
  in high ulnar nerve palsy, 1596
Ulnar resection, for rheumatoid arthritis of
  wrist, 1712
Umbilicoplasty, 2178, 2181, *2181–2183*, *2197*,
  2197–2198
Upper extremities. *See also* Finger(s);
    Forearm; Hand(s); Thumb(s); Wrist
    injuries
  brachioplasty and brachial suction-assisted
    lipectomy and, 2219–2235
    clinical aspects of, 2219
    marking for, 2222, 2223, 2224, 2227, 2228
    patient selection for, 2219–2222,
      2220–2222

Upper extremities, brachioplasty and brachial
    suction-assisted lipectomy and—
    Continued
    postoperative care and, 2223, *2225–2227*,
      2228
    surgical procedures and, 2222–2228,
      2223, *2225–2236*
  joint and ligament injuries of, 1531–1549
    anatomy and, 1531–1533
    diagnosis of, 1534
    to digits. *See* Finger injuries; Thumb(s),
      injuries to ligaments of
    general principles of management of,
      1534
    of wrist. *See* Wrist injuries
  peripheral nerve injuries of, 1598–1622
    anatomy and physiology of, 1598–1601,
      1599–1602
    classification of, 1603, 1605, 1606t,
      1606–1609
    nerve grafting for. *See* Nerve grafting, for
      peripheral nerve injuries of upper
      extremities
    regeneration and, 1601–1602, *1603–1605*
    repair of, 1608–1609, *1610–1613*
    techniques for repair of, 1610–1611, *1613*,
      1614
    timing of repair of, 1610
  reconstruction using soft tissue expansion,
    212–213, *213*
  replantation and. *See* Replantation, of
    upper extremities
  soft tissue coverage of. *See* Soft tissue
    coverage, of hand and upper extremity
Upper lateral cartilages, shortening, in
  rhinoplasty, 2014
Upper limbs, cutaneous malignant tumors of,
  320, 322, *323*, 324

Vaginal agenesis, *1398*, 1398–1399
Vascular channels
  deep dermal (cavernous hemangiomas),
    353, *354*
  subcutaneous (cavernous hemangiomas),
    353, *354*
  of superficial dermis (capillary
    hemangiomas; strawberry
    hemangiomas); 352–353, *353*, *354*
Vascularized bone grafts, 105, 105t
  fibular, free, in lower extremity
    reconstruction, *1804*, 1805
Vascularized bone segment transfer, in lower
  extremity reconstruction, 1803–1805
  Huntington fibular transfer, 1803, *1803*,
    1805
  indications for, 1803
Vascular lesions
  skin tumors, 300, *300*
  superficial, argon laser therapy for, *257*,
    257–259, *258*, *260–261*
  wrist pain and, 1730t–1731t
Vascular malformations, of skin, 352–372,
    353t, *361*
  arteriovenous, 370–372, *373*
  capillary, 360–363
  capillary-lymphatic and capillary-
    lymphatic-venous, 363, 363–365
  hemangiomas. *See* hemangiomas
  lymphatic, 368
  venous, 368, 370, *370–372*
Vascular studies, of diabetic foot, 1840–1842
Vasculature
  capillaries of skin flaps, 67
  of hand, evaluation of, 1482, *1483*, *1484*,
    1484–1485

Vasculature—*Continued*
  injuries of, lower extremity fractures and,
    1771–1772
  intrathoracic transposition of soft tissue for
    reinforcement of suture lines of great
    vessels, 1270, *1271–1272*
Vasculitic ulcers, of leg, 1832, *1832*
Vastus lateralis flaps
  for hip reconstruction, 1362
  in thigh reconstruction, 1778
Vastus medialis flaps, in thigh
  reconstruction, 1778
Velopharyngeal incompetence, sphincter
  pharyngoplasty for. *See* Sphincter
  pharyngoplasty
Velopharyngeal insufficiency, 619–631
  anatomy and physiology of, 632
  diagnosis of, 620–630, 632–633
    acoustic assessment in, 630, *630*
    aerodynamic assessment in, 624–630,
      625–629, 628t–630t
    anatomic evaluation in, 621, *622*
    multiview videofluoroscopy in, 623, 624,
      624, *625*
    nasopharyngoscopy in, *623*, 623–624
    patient history in, 620
    perceptual evaluation in, 620–621
  management of, 630–631
  pharyngeal flaps in. *See* Pharyngeal flap
    operation
  velopharyngeal function and, 619–620
    abnormal, 619–620
    normal, 619
Venous drainage, of flaps, 66–67
Venous lakes, 300
Venous malformations, of skin, 368, 370,
  370–372
Venous ulcers, of leg, 1829–1830, *1830*
Ventriculoperitoneal shunts, in
  meningomyelocele, 1243–1244
Vermilion
  deficiency of, cleft lip and, 606t, 607
  excess of, cleft lip and, 606t, 606–607
Vermilionectomy, 907, *907*
Verrucae (warts), 295, *296*, 296t, *297*
  vulgaris, 1454
Verrucous malformations (keratotic
  hemangiomas), 363, *364*
Vertical dimension problems, cephalometrics
  and, 483, *484*, 485
Vertical mammaplasty
  breast reduction by liposuction and. *See*
    Breast reduction, by liposuction and
    vertical mammaplasty
  correction of breast ptosis by, 2157,
    2158–2164
Vesicant agents, burns caused by, 449
Vessels, hand reconstruction and, 1665, *1666*,
  1667
Vestibular reconstruction, for bilateral cleft
  lip repair, 571, 574
Vibratory sensation, of hand, evaluation of,
  1746
Vicryl (polyglactin) sutures, 8
Videofluoroscopy
  multiview, in velopharyngeal insufficiency,
    623, 624, *624*, *625*
  in temporomandibular joint deformities,
    1223
Visceral flaps
  free, 971, *976*, *977*
  for oropharyngeal reconstruction, 968–969
Viscosity, of blood, 68–69

Visual disturbances, following blepharoplasty, 1938
Visual examination, termination of lipectomy and, 235
Vitamins, wound healing and, 8–9, 10
Voice rehabilitation, following laryngectomy, 1017
Voice-sparing operations, 1013–1016
    hemilaryngectomy, 1014
    supraglottic laryngectomy, 1014–1016
        postoperative management and, 1015–1016
        technique for, 1014–1015
Volar advancement flaps, for fingertip injuries with exposed bone, 1500–1501, 1504, 1505
von Recklinghausen disease, 3-D computed tomography in, 280, 281
V-Y advancement, 27–28, 28
V-Y vermilion mucosal rolldown, 607–608, 609

Wart(s) (verrucae), 295, 296, 296t, 297
    vulgaris, 1454
Warthin tumor (papillary cystadenoma lymphomatosum), 1035, 1036t, 1037, 1037
Web scars, following blepharoplasty, 1938
Wiring
    bone, for mandibular fractures, 1170, 1170
    circumdental, for mandibular fractures, 1168, 1168
    for hand and wrist fractures, techniques for, 1514, 1516
    interdental, for mandibular fractures, 1168, 1168
    tension-band wires for hand and wrist fractures and, 1524–1526, 1528–1529
Wound(s). See also Burn wounds
    preparation for skin grafting, 50, 52, 52–55
    separation of, following blepharoplasty, 1936
    strength og, 6–7, 7
Wound care
    for leg ulcers, new developments in, 1836–1838
    lower extremity fractures and, 1769–1770
    pressure sores and, 1375, 1375t
Wound contraction, 5–6, 6
Wound healing, 3–13
    age and, 30, 30
    agents augmenting, 9–10
        arginine, 10
        electrical charges, 10
        growth factors, 9
        growth hormone, 10
        hyperbaric oxygen, 10
        vitamin A, 10
        zinc, 10
    basic principles of, 7–8
        blood supply and, 7
        surgical technique and, 7
        sutures and, 7–8
    delayed, following reduction mammaplasty, avoidance of, 2141–2142
    of donor site, 55
    excessive scarring and. See Scarring
    fetal, 13
    impaired, 8–9
        aging and, 9
        immunosuppression and, 8
        irradiation and, 8

Wound healing, impaired—Continued
    ischemia and, 9
    malnutrition and, 8–9
    steroids and, 8
    location of wound and, 31
    normal, biology of, 3–7
        acute inflammatory phase, 3–4, 4, 4t
        cellular proliferation, 4–5
        collagen remodeling, 5
        epithelialization, 5
        growth factors and, 7
        matrix formation, 5
        wound contraction, 5–6, 6
        wound strength and, 6–7, 7
    race and, 30–31
    scar revision and, 35
    skin disorders and, 31
    skin type and, 31
Wounds, gunshot, of face. See Facial gunshot wounds
W-plasty, 27
    for scar revision, 39–40, 40
Wrinkle(s), of skin
    following blepharoplasty, 1938
    blepharoplasty and, 1921
    canthal. See Crow's feet
Wrinkle lines, scar revision and, 37
Wrist
    amputations at, replantation and, 1631, 1635, 1636
    anatomy of, 1532–1533, 1533, 1534
    burn wounds of, 434
    fusion of, for rheumatoid arthritis, 1712
    rheumatoid arthritis in, 1710–1712, 1730t–1731t
        arthroplasty for, 1712
        synovectomy for, 1711, 1711
        ulnar resection for, 1712
        wrist fusion for, 1712
Wrist fractures, 1508–1521
    closed reduction and functional bracing and, 1508, 1509
    closed reduction and internal fixation of, 1508–1509, 1509–1511
    excision, arthroplasty, and arthrodesis for, 1520, 1529
    limited open reduction and internal fixation of, 1511–1512, 1511–1513
    open, treatment of, 1519–1520, 1528, 1529
    open reduction and internal fixation of, 1512–1514, 1514, 1515
    pain and See Wrist pain, bony injuries and
    plates for, 1517–1519
        buttress, 1519, 1527
        neutralization, 1518, 1523
        tension-band, 1518–1519, 1524–1526
    rehabilitation and, 1521
    screw fixation of, 1514, 1517, 1517–1522
    wiring techniques for, 1514, 1516
Wrist injuries. See also Wrist fractures
    of extensor tendons, 1576
    fractures. See Wrist fractures
    to ligaments, 1542–1549
        lunotriquetral instability, 1543, 1546
        midcarpal instability, 1543, 1546, 1546
        perilunate dislocations, 1546–1547, 1547, 1548
        rotary subluxation of scaphoid bone, 1542, 1542–1543, 1544–1545
        triangular fibrocartilage complex and distal radioulnar joint injuries, 1547, 1549, 1549

Wrist pain, 1728–1744
    bony injuries and, 1730t–1731t, 1739–1740
        background of, 1739
        of capitate, 1742–1743
        diagnosis of, 1740–1741
        of lunate, 1743
        presentation of, 1739–1740
        of scaphoid, 1741, 1741, 1742
        of trapezium, 1743
        of triquetrum, 1743
    capsular, 1733–1734
        diagnosis of, 1733
        ganglia and, 1733, 1733–1734, 1734
    carpal bossing and, 1744
    cartilage and, 1738–1739
        diagnosis of, 1739
        pathophysiology of, 1738
        presentation of, 1738
        treatment of, 1739, 1739t, 1740t
    evaluation of, 1728–1733, 1730t–1731t
        arthrography in, 1728
        arthroscopy in, 1732
        bone scans in, 1728–1729
        fluoroscopy and special views in, 1729
        functional testing in, 1732
        instability series in, 1728
        magnetic resonance imaging in, 1729, 1729
        sympathetic blocks in, 1729
        systematic approach to, 1732, 1732–1733
        tomography in, 1729
    Keinböck disease and, 1743–1744
        background of, 1743
        diagnosis of, 1743
        pathophysiology of, 1743
        presentation of, 1743
        treatment of, 1743–1744
    ligaments and, 1736–1738
        background of, 1736
        carpal collapse patterns and, 1737, 1737
        diagnosis of, 1736–1737
        dislocations and, 1737, 1738
        pathophysiology of, 1736
        treatment of, 1737–1738
        ulnar impingement syndrome and, 1738
    nerve compression and, 1734–1735
        carpal tunnel syndrome and, 1734–1735
    scaphoid avascular necrosis and, 1744
    skin and subcutaneous tissue and, 1733
    tenosynovitis and. See Tenosynovitis, of wrist

Xanthelasma, blepharoplasty for, 1939
Xanthomas, of hands, 1463
Xenografts, 53–54
Xeroderma pigmentosum, 312, 312

Yellow-light lasers, 262, 263

Zinc, wound healing and, 9, 10–11
Z-plasty, 25–27, 26–28
    for burn wounds of extremities and trunk, 431
    Furlow double-reversing. See Furlow double-reversing Z-plasty
    for scar revision, 37, 38, 39, 39
        angles and, 39
        limbs and, 39
        variations of, 39, 39, 40

Zygomatic arch surgery, 1865–1866, *1868*
Zygomatic defects, with mandibular
 dysostosis, treatment of, *528*, 529,
 529
Zygomatic fractures, 1119–1125
 anatomy and, 1119–1120, *1120*
 in children and adolescents, *1193,*
  1193–1194, 1194
 diagnosis of, 1120t, 1120–1121, *1121, 1122*

Zygomatic fractures—*Continued*
 pathophysiology of, 1120
 roentgenographic appearance of, 1074,
  1075, 1076
 surgical treatment of, 1122–1124
  for complex fractures, 1124
  complications of, 1125
  for fractures of zygomatic arch,
   1124

Zygomatic fractures, surgical treatment of—
  Continued
  postoperative care and, 1124–1125
  for simple fractures, 1122–1124, *1123*
Zygomaticomaxillary fractures
 below malar buttress, 1212, *1215–1216*
 at inferior orbital rim, 1211–1212,
  1211–1215
Zygomaticotemporal fractures, 1212